D0710279

SAUNDERS
ELSEVIER

11830 Westline Industrial Drive
St. Louis, Missouri 63146

PATHOLOGY AND INTERVENTION IN MUSCULOSKELETAL
REHABILITATION   ISBN: 978-1-4160-0251-2

Copyright © 2009 by Saunders, an imprint of Elsevier Inc.
Photo Copyright © 2009 for Chapter 8 and Chapter 14, will be retained by Diane Lee
Photo Copyright © 2009 for Chapter 8 and Chapter 14, will be retained by Linda-Joy Lee

All rights reserved. No part of this publication may be reproduced or transmitted in any
form or by any means, electronic or mechanical, including photocopying, recording, or any
information storage and retrieval system, without permission in writing from the publisher.
Permissions may be sought directly from Elsevier's Rights Department: phone: (+1) 215
239 3804 (US) or (+44) 1865 843830 (UK); fax: (+44) 1865 853333; e-mail:
healthpermissions@elsevier.com. You may also complete your request on-line via the Elsevier
website at http://www.elsevier.com/permissions.

Notice

Neither the Publisher nor the Authors assume any responsibility for any loss or injury
and/or damage to persons or property arising out of or related to any use of the material
contained in this book. It is the responsibility of the treating practitioner, relying on
independent expertise and knowledge of the patient, to determine the best treatment and
method of application for the patient.

The Publisher

ISBN-13: 978-1-4160-0251-2
ISBN-10: 1-4160-0251-0

Vice President and Publisher: Linda Duncan
Acquisitions Editor: Kathy Falk
Developmental Editor: Sarah Vales
Publishing Services Manager: Julie Eddy
Project Manager: Rich Barber
Designer: Julia Dummitt

Printed in the United States

Last digit is the print number: 9 8 7 6 5 4 3 2 1

**Working together to grow
libraries in developing countries**

www.elsevier.com | www.bookaid.org | www.sabre.org

ELSEVIER   BOOK AID International   Sabre Foundation

Contributors

Omar El Abd, MD
Instructor, Physical Medicine and Rehabilitation
Harvard Medical School
Boston, Massachusetts
Interventional Spine Director
Newton-Wellesley Hospital
Newton, Massachusetts
Attending Physician
Physical Medicine and Rehabilitation, Spaulding
    Rehabilitation Hospital
Physical Medicine and Rehabilitation, Massachusetts
    General Hospital
Boston, Massachusetts

C. Dain Allred, MD
Major, USAF, MC
Department of Orthopedic Surgery
David Grant Medical Center
Travis AFB, California

Susan L. Armijo-Olivo, BPT, BScPT, MScPT
PhD Candidate in Rehabilitation Sciences
Faculty of Rehabilitation Medicine
University of Alberta
Edmonton, Alberta

Peter Asnis, MD
Orthopaedic Surgeon, Massachusetts General Hospital
Instructor in Orthopaedics, Harvard Medical School
Boston, Massachusetts

Steven A. Aviles, MD
Iowa Orthopaedic Centre, PC
Des Moines, Iowa

Jennifer L. Baird, PT, MS
Department of Kinesiology
Motor Control Laboratory
University of Massachusetts
Amherst, Massachusetts

Mary F. Barbe, PhD
Associate Professor
Physical Therapy Department
Temple University
Philadelphia, Pennsylvania

Ann E. Barr, DPT, PhD
Professor and Chair
Department of Physical Therapy
Jefferson College of Health Professions
Thomas Jefferson University
Philadelphia, Pennsylvania

Eric M. Berkson, MD
Clinical Associate in Orthopaedic Surgery
Massachusetts General Hospital
Boston, Massachusetts

Mark D. Bishop, PT, PhD, CSCS
Assistant Professor
Department of Physical Therapy
College of Public Health and Health Professions
University of Florida
Gainesville, Florida

Joanne Borg-Stein, MD
Medical Director
Spaulding-Wellesley Rehabilitation Center
Medical Director, Newton Wellesley Hospital Spine Center
Team Physician, Wellesley College
Assistant Professor of PM&R
Harvard Medical School
Boston, Massachusetts

**Peter D. Brukner, MBBS, DRCOG, FACSP,
    FASMF, FACSM**
Associate Professor
Centre for Health, Exercise and Sports
    Medicine
The University of Melbourne
Director
Olympic Park Sports Medicine Centre
Melbourne, Victoria
Australia

David B. Burr, PhD
Chair and Professor
Department of Anatomy and Cell Biology
Professor
Department of Orthopaedic Surgery
Indiana University School of Medicine

Professor of Biomedical Engineering
Indiana University-Purdue University Indianapolis
Indianapolis, Indiana

Nancy N. Byl, MPH, PhD, PT, FAPTA
Professor and Chair
Department of Physical Therapy and Rehabilitation Science,
UCSF/SFSU Graduate Program in Physical Therapy
UCSF/UCB Graduate Program in Bioengineering
Peter Ostwald Health Program for Performing Artists
University of California
San Francisco, California

Judy C. Chepeha, BScPT, MScPT, PhD Candidate
Assistant Professor
Department of Physical Therapy
Faculty of Rehabilitation Medicine
University of Alberta
Edmonton, Alberta
Consultant Physical Therapist
Glen Sather Sports Medicine Clinic
University of Alberta
Edmonton, Alberta

Pierre A. d'Hemecourt, MD
Division of Sports Medicine
Childrens Hospital Boston
Boston, Massachusetts

Joanne G. Draghetti, MS, OTR, CHT
St. Joseph Hospital
Nashua, New Hampshire

Caroline Drye Taylor, MS, PT, OCS, FAAOMPT
Taylor & Thornburg Physical Therapy, Inc.
Oakland, California

James W. Edmondson, MD
Professor
Department of Medicine, Endocrinology Division
School of Medicine
Indiana University
Indianapolis, Indiana

Timothy L. Fagerson, PT, DPT, MS
Adjunct Faculty
Graduate Programs in Physical Therapy
MGH Institute of Health Professions
Boston, Massachusetts
President, SOSPT, Inc.
Spine-Orthopaedic-Sport Physical Therapy
Wellesley, Massachusetts

Manuela L. Ferreira, BPT, MSc, PhD
Discipline of Physiotherapy
Faculty of Health Sciences
University of Sydney
Sydney, Australia

Paulo H. Ferreira, BPT, MSc, PhD
Discipline of Physiotherapy
Faculty of Health Sciences
University of Sydney
Sydney, Australia

Walter R. Frontera, MD, PhD
Dean and Professor
Physical Medicine and Rehabilitation and Physiology
University of Puerto Rico School of Medicine
San Juan, Puerto Rico
Senior Lecturer
Department of Physical Medicine and Rehabilitation
Harvard Medical School
Boston, Massachusetts

Freddie H. Fu, MD
David Silver Professor of Orthopaedic Surgery
Chairman, Department of Orthopaedic Surgery
Head Team Physician, Department of Athletics
Adjunct Professor, School of Health and Rehabilitation
  Science
University of Pittsburgh
Pittsburgh, Pennsylvania

John P. Fulkerson, MD
Orthopedic Associates of Hartford, PC
Clinical Professor and Sports Medicine Fellowship Director
University of Connecticut
School of Medicine
Farmington, Connecticut

Inae C. Gadotti, BScPT, MScPT
PhD Candidate in Rehabilitation Sciences
Faculty of Rehabilitation Medicine
University of Alberta
Edmonton, Alberta

Steven Z. George, PT, PhD
Assistant Professor
Department of Physical Therapy
Center for Pain Research and Behavioral Health
Brooks Center for Rehabilitation Studies
College of Public Health and Health Professions
University of Florida
Gainesville, Florida

Peter G. Gerbino II, MD
Monterey Joint Replacement and Sports Medicine
Monterey, California

Thomas J. Gill, IV, MD
Chief, Sports Medicine Service
Assistant Professor of Orthopedic Surgery
Harvard Medical School
Department of Orthopedic Surgery
Massachusetts General Hospital
Boston, Massachusetts

Jennifer B. Green, MD
Tufts-New England Medical Center
Boston, Massachusetts

Lindsay C. Groat, RPA-C
Syracuse Orthopedic Specialists
Syracuse, New York

Jane Gruber, PT, DPT, MS, OCS
Director of Rehabilitation Services
Department of Rehabilitation Services
Newton Wellesley Hospital
Newton, Massachusetts

Zehra H. Habib, PhD, PT
Staff Therapist
Physical Therapy and Occupational Therapy Services
Children's Hospital Boston
Affiliate Teaching Hospital of the Harvard Medical School
Boston, Massachusetts

Sanaz Hariri, MD
Resident, Orthopedic Surgery
Harvard Combined Orthopedic Surgery Program
Massachusetts General Hospital
Boston, Massachusetts

Diane M. Heislein, PT, DPT, MS, OCS
Clinical Associate Professor
Department of Physical Therapy and Athletic Training
Sargent College of Health and Rehabilitation Sciences
Boston University
Boston, Massachusetts
Physical Therapist
Physical Therapy Services
Massachusetts General Hospital
Boston, Massachusetts

Jay Hertel, PhD, ATC, FACSM
Associate Professor
Department of Human Services

University of Virginia
Charlottesville, Virginia

Paul W. Hodges, PhD, MedDr, BPhty(Hons)
NHMRC Principal Research Fellow/Professional Research Fellow
Director, NHMRC Centre of Clinical Research Excellence in Spinal Pain, Injury and Health
School of Health and Rehabilitation Sciences
The University of Queensland
Brisbane, Queensland
Australia

Christopher D. Ingersoll, PhD, ATC, FACSM
Joe H. Gieck Professor of Sports Medicine
Professor, Department of Human Services
Professor, Department of Physical Medicine and Rehabilitation
University of Virginia
Charlottesville, Virginia

Lorrie Ippensen Vreeman, PT, DPT
Physical Therapist
Indiana First Steps Early Intervention Program
Clarian Health Partners
Indianapolis, Indiana

James J. Irrgang, PhD, PT, ATC
Director of Clinical Research
Department of Orthopaedic Surgery
University of Pittsburgh
Pittsburgh, Pennsylvania

Maura Daly Iversen, PT, DPT, SD, MPH
Professor and Associate Director
MGH Institute of Health Professions
Assistant Professor in Medicine
Harvard Medical School
Behavioral Scientist
Division of Rheumatology, Immunology and Allergy
Brigham & Women's Hospital
Boston, Massachusetts

Diane Lee, BSR, FCAMT, CGIMS
Diane Lee and Associates – Consultants in Physiotherapy
White Rock, British Columbia

Linda-Joy Lee, BSc, BScPT, FCAMT, CGIMS, MCPA
Canadian Institutes of Health Research (CIHR) Fellow
PhD Candidate
Centre for Clinical Research Excellence in Spinal Pain, Injury and Health

University of Queensland
Brisbane, Australia
Synergy Physiotherapy
North Vancouver, British Columbia

Bruce M. Leslie, MD
Newton-Wellesley Orthopedic Associates
Newton, Massachusetts

Toby Long, PhD, PT
Director for Training of the Georgetown
    University Center for Child and Human
    Development
Director, Division of Physical Therapy of the
    Georgetown University Center for Child and Human
    Development
Associate Professor, Department of Pediatrics,
    Georgetown University
Georgetown University
Washington, D.C.
Adjunct Faculty University of Indianapolis, Krannert
    Graduate School of Physical Therapy
Rocky Mountain University of Health Professions, and the
University of Maryland at Baltimore, Department of Physical
Therapy and Rehabilitation Science

David J. Magee, BPT, PhD
Professor
Department of Physical Therapy
Faculty of Rehabilitation Medicine
University of Alberta
Edmonton, Alberta

Ron Mattison, BPE BScPT
Allan McGavin Sports Medicine
Faculty of Medicine
University of British Columbia
Vancouver, British Columbia

David J. Mayman, MD
Instructor in Orthopedic Surgery
Department of Medicine
Weill Cornell Medical School
Assistant Attending Orthopedic Surgeon
Orthopedic Surgery
Hospital for Special Surgery
New York, New York

Jim Meadows, BScPT, DipPT, FCAMT
Lecturer (Adjunct)
Department of Physical Therapy
Massachusetts General Hospital Institute of Health Sciences
Boston, Massachusetts
Lecturer (Adjunct)
Department of Physical Therapy
Nova Southeastern University

Fort Lauderdale, Florida
Owner, Swodeam Institute
Medicine Hat, Alberta

Robert J. Nee, PT, MAppSc, ATC
Assistant Professor
School of Physical Therapy
Pacific University
Hillsboro, Oregon

David P. Newman, PT, DPT, OCS
Assistant Clinical Professor
School of Physical Therapy and Rehabilitation Sciences
College of Medicine
University of South Florida
Tampa, Florida

Stephen J. Nicholas, MD
Director
Nicholas Institute of Sports Medicine and Athletic
    Trauma (NISMAT)
Lenox Hill Hospital
New York, New York

Martin Parfitt, DipPT, MCSP, MCPA
Strathcona Physical Therapy
Edmonton, Alberta
Clinical Associate Professor
Department of Dentistry
Faculty of Medicine
University of Alberta
Edmonton, Alberta

Christopher M. Powers, PhD, PT
Associate Professor
Department of Biokinesiology and Physical Therapy
Department of Radiology, Keck School of Medicine
Co-Director, Musculoskeletal Biomechanics Research
    Laboratory
University of Southern California
Los Angeles, California

Helen E. Ranger, PT, MS, CHT
Newton Wellesley Hospital
Newton, Massachusetts

Glenn R. Rechtine, MD
Professor, Orthopaedic Spine Division
Department of Orthopaedics
University of Rochester
Rochester, New York

**David C. Reid, MD, BPT, MCh(Orth), MCSP,
    MCPA, FRCS(C)**
Professor of Orthopaedic Surgery
Adjunct Professor of Rehabilitation Medicine

Honorary Professor of Physical Education
University of Alberta
Edmonton, Alberta

Michael M. Reinold, PT, DPT, ATC, CSCS
Coordinator of Rehabilitation Research and Education
Department of Orthopedic Surgery,
   Division of Sports Medicine
Massachusetts General Hospital
Boston, Massachusetts
Rehabilitation Coordinator/Assistant Athletic Trainer
Boston Red Sox Baseball Club
Boston, Massachusetts

Neil S. Roth, MD
Attending Physician
Department of Orthopedic Surgery
Lenox Hill Hospital
New York, New York
Attending Physician
Department of Orthopedic Surgery
White Plains Hospital
White Plains, New York

Harry E. Rubash, MD
Chief, Orthopaedic Surgery
Massachusetts General Hospital
Boston, Massachusetts

Marc R. Safran, MD
Professor, Department of Orthopaedic Surgery
Associate Director, Sports Medicine
Stanford University
Stanford, California

Edgar T. Savidge, PT, DPT, OCS
Senior Physical Therapist
Physical Therapy Services
Massachusetts General Hospital
Boston, Massachusetts

Evan D. Schumer, MD
Newton-Wellesley Orthopedic Associates
Member of the American Society for Surgery
   of the Hand (ASSH)
Newton, Massachusetts

Keiba L. Shaw, PT, MPT, MA, EdD
Assistant Professor
School of Physical Therapy and Rehabilitation Sciences
College of Medicine
University of South Florida
Tampa, Florida

Mychelle L. Shegog, MD
Fellow in Sports Medicine
Childrens Hospital Boston
Boston, Massachusetts

Nina Shervin, MD
Department of Orthopaedic Surgery
Harvard Combined Orthopaedic Surgery Program
Massachusetts General Hospital
Boston, Massachusetts

Richard B. Souza, PhD, PT, ATC, CSCS
Musculoskeletal Biomechanics Research Laboratory
Department of Biokinesiology and Physical Therapy
University of Southern California
Los Angeles, California

Linda Steiner, PT DPT, MS, OCS
Clinical Assistant Professor
MGH Institute of Health Professions
Graduate Programs in Physical Therapy
Clinical Associate in Physical Therapy
Department of Physical and Occupational Therapy
Massachusetts General Hospital
Boston, Massachusetts

Ann-Marie Thomas, MD, PT
Instructor
Department of Physical Medicine and Rehabilitation
Harvard Medical School
Spaulding Rehabilitation Hospital
Boston, Massachusetts

Timothy F. Tyler, MS, PT, ATC
Nicholas Institute of Sports Medicine and Athletic Trauma
   (NISMAT)
Lenox Hill Hospital
New York, New York

Emily Veeneman, MD
School of Medicine
Indiana University
Indianapolis, Indiana

Stuart J. Warden, BPhysio (Hons), PhD, FACSM
Assistant Professor and Director of Research
Department of Physical Therapy
School of Health and Rehabilitation Sciences
Assistant Professor
Department of Anatomy and Cell Biology
School of Medicine
Indiana University
Indianapolis, Indiana

Kevin E. Wilk, DPT, PT
Adjunct Assistant Professor
Programs in Physical Therapy
Marquette University
Milwaukee, Wisconsin
Vice-President Education
Associate Clinical Director
Physiotherapy Associates-Champion Sports Medicine
Birmingham, Alabama
Rehabilitation Consultant
Tampa Bay Rays Baseball Club
Tampa, Florida

James E. Zachazewski, DPT, SCS, ATC
Clinical Director
Physical Therapy
Massachusetts General Hospital
Boston, Massachusetts

"To Teach is to Learn Twice"

To those who invested in us that we might in turn pass on their knowledge and wisdom to future generations of students.

Preface

Musculoskeletal Rehabilitation Series

Musculoskeletal conditions have an enormous impact on society. Today, musculoskeletal conditions have become the most common cause of disability and severe long-term pain in the industrialized world. As we approach the second half of the Bone and Joint Decade, it is apparent that the knowledge and skill required by the community of health care providers involved in managing the impairments and functional limitations resulting from acute or chronic musculoskeletal injury/illness have grown exponentially as the frequency of visits to practitioners' offices for musculoskeletal system complaints has risen.

The art and science of musculoskeletal rehabilitation began as a consequence of the injuries suffered on the battlefields of Europe during World War I. Since that time, numerous textbooks have been published regarding musculoskeletal rehabilitation. These texts have encompassed the areas of basic science, evaluation, and treatment. However, these books have most often been developed and written in professional "isolation" (i.e., from a single discipline's perspective). As a consequence, topics have either been covered in great depth but with a very narrow focus, or with great breath with very little depth. Our goal in the development and production of this series was to develop a series of textbooks that complement and build on one another, providing the reader with the needed depth and breath of information for this critical area of health care.

Volume I of the series is the 5th edition of David Magee's *Orthopedic Physical Assessment*. This now classic text provides the clinician with the most comprehensive text available on this topic. First published in 1987, it has withstood the test of time and is the most widely used text in this area. In 1996, we developed and published *Athletic Injuries and Rehabilitation*. Based upon feedback from both students and clinicians, we have expanded and broadened the scope of *Athletic Injuries and Rehabilitation* into two new volumes. *Volume II, Scientific Foundations and Principles of Practice,* provides clinicians with currently available science regarding musculoskeletal issues and principles of practice that should guide clinicians regarding therapeutic intervention. In *Volume III, Pathology and Intervention,* we have attempted to provide readers with a comprehensive text containing information on the most common musculoskeletal pathologies seen and the best evidence behind contemporary interventions directed towards the treatment of impairments and limitations associated with acute, chronic, and congenital musculoskeletal conditions, which occur across the lifespan.

International contributors have provided their unique perspectives on current diagnostic methodologies, clinical techniques, and rehabilitative concerns. We hope that our continued use of interdisciplinary author teams has firmly broken down the professional "territorial turf" barriers that have existed in past decades of health care. Health care professionals involved in the contemporary care of musculoskeletal conditions must continue to share and learn from one another to advance the provision of the most time- and cost-efficient care possible in twenty-first century society.

Each volume in our series is liberally illustrated. Key concepts in each chapter are highlighted in text boxes, which serve to reinforce those concepts for the reader, and numerous tables summarize chapter information for easy reference. Readers will find that references are not contained on printed pages at the end of chapters, but rather, as part of a comprehensive electronic resource on CD-ROM (provided with each volume), which allows the reader to link to MEDLINE abstracts where possible. Because of the comprehensive nature of this multi-volume series, each text, although complete in itself, has been edited to build and integrate with related chapter materials from the other volumes in the series. It is the editors' hope that this series will find its way into use by faculty as a basis for formal coursework as well as a friendly companion and frequently consulted reference by students and those on the front lines of clinical care.

As with our previous collaborations, we look forward to the feedback that only you, our colleagues, can provide, so that we may continue the development and improvement of the *Musculoskeletal Rehabilitation Series.*

David J. Magee
James E. Zachazewski
William S. Quillen

Preface

Pathology and Intervention

Pathology and Intervention is our third book in the *Musculoskeletal Rehabilitation Series* dedicated to providing students and practicing clinicians with a comprehensive integrated musculoskeletal resource to consult regarding the most common area of practice for most clinicians involved in rehabilitation. In this text, we have assembled an exceptional multidisciplinary group of clinicians to present the best evidence behind contemporary interventions directed toward the treatment of the impairments and functional limitations associated with acute, chronic, and congenital musculoskeletal conditions occurring across the lifespan.

In an effort to maximize the volume of information presented on specific pathologies and methods of interventions, and to minimize the duplication of information, we have asked the authors, and edited the text, to refer readers to *Volume I, Orthopedic Physical Assessment for Musculoskeletal Assessment*, and to *Volume II, Scientific Foundations and Principles of Practice*, for basic science information regarding inflammation, healing, tissue deformation, and the development of muscular strength and endurance.

This has allowed the authors to provide the reader with as much information as possible on the specific pathologies most often seen in the clinic and the best methods of intervention.

We have again asked the authors to concentrate on answering the key questions of who, what, when, where, why, and how. **Who** usually suffers from the types of injuries and conditions described? **What** are the best methods of intervention for these conditions? **When** should intervention be initiated? **Where** does the practicing clinician find the information on which the authors base their recommended methods of intervention? **Why** should the reader utilize the author's recommendations? **How** should the clinician progress the patient toward full recovery? We believe that the authors have effectively answered these questions, giving the reader a textbook that will prove valuable for years to come.

David J. Magee
James E. Zachazewski
William S. Quillen

Acknowledgments

We would like to gratefully acknowledge the ongoing professional assistance of the following individuals who have steadfastly supported this series from its inception.

Kathy Falk – Senior Editor, Health Professions, Elsevier
Rich Barber – Project Manager, Elsevier
Bev Evjen – Editorial Assistant
Ted Huff – Artist

Contents

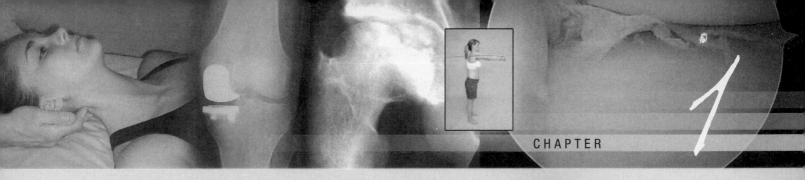

CHAPTER

PATIENT EDUCATION, MOTIVATION, COMPLIANCE, AND ADHERENCE TO PHYSICAL ACTIVITY, EXERCISE, AND REHABILITATION

Keiba L. Shaw

Introduction

The Surgeon General's report on physical activity and health in 1996 brought forth the importance of engaging in an active lifestyle to prevent the insidious onset of chronic disease and illness.[1] Healthy People 2010 established goals for promoting a healthy lifestyle for individuals in the United States.[2] Most recently, a study by the Robert Wood Johnson Foundation in 2001 reported that, despite evidence that physical activity is beneficial to individuals in midlife and those 50 years and older, these individuals continue to remain sedentary.[3] By definition, **physical activity** encompasses any movement of the body in which the muscles actively contract, the metabolism increases, and calories are burned. **Exercise** is considered a subcategory of physical activity; it refers specifically to a structured program of activity geared toward achieving or maintaining physical fitness.[4] This chapter focuses on compliance with and adherence to physical activity, and its subcategory of exercise, as they relate to rehabilitation. Although distinct differences have been noted in the literature between the meaning of **adherence** (choosing to engage in behaviors of one's own volition) and **compliance** (engaging in behavior as instructed or prescribed by a health care professional),[5] the two terms are used interchangeably throughout this chapter.

The Professional's Role in the Promotion of Exercise Adherence

The health care professional plays an essential role in motivating individuals to participate in physical activity and exercise. The importance of this role is particularly significant in the older adult population. A study by Schutzer and Graves[6] showed that individuals who are older or chronically ill see their physician at least once a year and prefer to receive advice about exercise from their physician or personal health care provider. Among older individuals on Medicare, 40% of those surveyed said that they participated in an exercise program as a result of their physician's advice.[7] A study that assessed long-term exercise adherence after rehabilitation for chronic low back pain revealed that the physician's and physical therapist's assurance that the patient was capable of performing the recommended exercises in spite of pain symptoms went a long way in reinforcing self-efficacy in the patient's ability to complete the exercises.[8]

In assessing barriers to the promotion of physical activity by general practitioners and nurses, McKenna et al.[9] found that general practitioners in the action or maintenance stage of changing their own physical activity level were three times more likely to regularly promote the same behavior in

1

their patients. Thus professionals who exercise on a regular basis and "practice what they preach" can transfer these same beliefs, attitudes, behaviors, and action to their patients.

In a study that examined socioenvironmental exercise preferences among older adults,[10] the results suggested that the perception of the exercise instructor as qualified, the advice of the medical doctor to begin exercising, and evaluation by a health professional to monitor the physical effects of exercise were rated as most important in 320 adults 74 to 85 years of age who lived independently in the community. In addition, the health professional's ability to evaluate and demonstrate appropriate exercises and to evaluate and monitor the physical effects of exercise were rated as very important. The latter finding is especially relevant to clinicians who treat older adults and want to encourage them to be active participants in their rehabilitation programs.

Sluijs et al.[11] found a relationship between positive feedback given to patients by their physical therapists and the degree of noncompliance. The study indicated that if physical therapists did not provide their patients with positive feedback, compliance with the rehabilitation program was decreased. However, the question remains whether the positive feedback facilitated compliance, or compliance prompted the physical therapist to give positive feedback. The presumption is that giving positive feedback was beneficial for increasing the likelihood that adherence to the rehabilitation program would be obtained.

Exercise professionals have the most influence over program factors when designing a plan for increasing client retention. Remembering to keep clients involved in designing their exercise programs is necessary, because this increases the client's feelings of self-efficacy and greatly affects the choice of exercise.

Definition of Motivation

Motivation is considered highly important and relevant to maintaining behavior. It is a term often used, and a concept cited as necessary, among health care providers and rehabilitation specialists in discussing a patient's or client's commitment to a rehabilitation and/or exercise program. So what does this term really mean? Why do rehabilitation and exercise experts consider it so important? To begin to answer this question, a brief but thorough explanation and a definition of motivation are warranted, along with a glimpse into the various theories about motivation.

Motivation has a multitude of definitions. The *American Heritage Dictionary* defines motivation as "the act or process of motivating; the state of being motivated; something that motivates; an inducement or incentive."[12] The *Word-Net Dictionary* defines motivation as "the psychological feature that arouses an organism to action toward a desired goal; the reason for the action; that which gives purpose

and direction to behavior"; and "a concept used to describe the factors within an individual which arouse, maintain and channel behavior towards a goal."[13]

Regardless of the definition used, most motivation theorists believe that behavior will not occur unless activated by some internal and/or external force. The underlying question then becomes: Does motivation influence behavior as a result of conditioning or as a result of influences such as environment, explanatory style, personality, perception, memory, or cognitive development?[14]

Motivational Theories

In both the psychology and sport psychology literature, motivation has been classified as either intrinsic (internal) or extrinsic (external). In addition, individuals will act to satisfy or meet basic needs.[15,16] These needs can be classified as behavioral or external, social, biological, cognitive, affective, conative, or spiritual.[14]

Obtaining a desired reward, experiencing pleasant sensations, or escaping unpleasant consequences often is the impetus for engaging or not engaging in a behavior. Behavioral needs often inspire individuals to act so as to avoid unwanted consequences or to pursue desired responses. Socially, individuals strive to be valued members of a group, which makes them able to imitate the positive (or negative) behaviors of others within the group. As biological beings, individuals strive to increase or decrease stimulation or arousal while seeking to maximize pleasurable sensations that affect the five senses. In addition, individuals strive to minimize unpleasant sensations, such as thirst, hunger, and anything that makes one uncomfortable, in order to maintain homeostasis and balance as a system in the long term. At the cognitive level, an individual is inspired to maintain attention to things that the person deems interesting or threatening, while seeking to develop a meaning for and understanding of those things with which the individual is unfamiliar. Again, the person strives to increase equilibrium while eliminating anything that may be seen as a danger to survival.

In the affective domain, motivation plays a large role in efforts to reduce emotional dissonance. Individuals have a drive to feel good and a need to increase their sense of well-being and self-esteem. The individual seeks security in his surroundings and within himself and will strive to maintain adequate levels of optimism and enthusiasm to obtain it. Research has shown that individuals who are pessimistic do not fare as well at participation in exercise as those who are more optimistic.[17]

Research has shown that pessimistic individuals do not fare as well with exercise participation as those who are more optimistic.

Taking control, developing and maintaining self-efficacy, and meeting individually developed goals are other aspects of motivation. Individuals have personal dreams and needs related to fulfilling those dreams. As a result, the person attempts to reduce obstacles, thereby opening the way to achieving her dreams.

> Taking control, developing and maintaining self-efficacy, and meeting individually developed goals are additional aspects of motivation. Individuals have personal dreams and needs related to fulfilling those dreams.

Individuals who are more spiritual in nature strive to connect themselves to the unknown; or, in another sense, attempt to make sense of and find meaning in their lives.

All of these concepts or needs contribute significantly to the existing literature on motivational theories. The framework of the most popular theories on motivation is based on three major aspects: the social cognition aspect, the humanistic aspect, and the multidimensional aspect.

Social Cognitive Theory

Social cognitive theory, as developed by Albert Bandura,[18] proposes reciprocal determinism as a leading factor in motivation. Individuals act as contributors to their own motivation, behavior, and development. In addition, environment interacts with the individual's behavior and characteristics to produce engagement or disengagement in an activity. Simply stated, human development is a back-and-forth interaction between the individual (the person's interpretation and retention of specific information), the individual's behaviors, and the environment (Figure 1-1).

Bandura also suggests that **self-efficacy**, or the belief that a particular action is possible and can be accomplished,

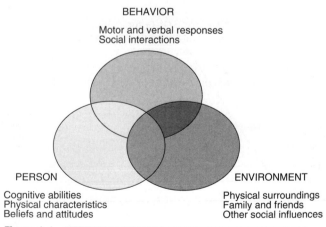

BEHAVIOR
Motor and verbal responses
Social interactions

PERSON
Cognitive abilities
Physical characteristics
Beliefs and attitudes

ENVIRONMENT
Physical surroundings
Family and friends
Other social influences

Figure 1-1

Social Cognitive Theory. (Modified from Shaffer DR: *Developmental psychology: childhood and adolescence,* ed 4, Pacific Grove, California, 1996, Brooks/Cole.)

and the ability to self-regulate are the primary mediators in producing a change in behavior. He states that self-efficacy is a good predictor of intention. Self-efficacy, along with the mediating effect of cognition, is seen as a circular process by which an increase in self-efficacy in turn produces success, thereby contributing to an increase in self-efficacy and the thought that one can indeed be triumphant in one's actions.

Failure undermines self-efficacy, especially if failure occurs before the individual has developed a strong sense of self-efficacy. For example, people who have successfully completed rehabilitation from an injury in the past will have the belief that, if injured again, they will be able to recover successfully from the injury and return to accustomed activities. The more experience people have in successfully overcoming obstacles (i.e., multiple successes within the same area, such as injury recovery), the more they will believe that they have the "tools" for coping with challenges to come. Bandura theorized that the best way to create a strong sense of efficacy is through *mastery,* in which successes serve as a base for developing an individual's personal efficacy. Continued mastery promotes repeat performances and improves adherence to physical activity, exercise, and rehabilitation.[14,19]

Self-Determination Theory

The self-determination theory (SDT) is defined as "a macro-theory of human motivation concerned with the development and functioning of personality within social contexts."[20] In other words, we as humans make choices based on our experiences, thoughts, and contemplations, as well as through our interactions with others in a variety of social settings.

The theory of human behaviors focuses on the degree to which human behaviors are volitional and investigates the inherent growth tendencies and natural psychological needs that are the basis of the incorporation of personality and self-motivation.[21] The psychological needs identified by the proponents of the SDT include needs for competence, relatedness, and autonomy. These needs, according to this theory, are essential for initiating the individual's ability to function at maximum potential and to develop the ability to enhance personal well-being and thrive socially.[21]

A subtheory of the SDT is the cognitive evaluation theory (CET); simply put, this theory states that people engage in activities to satisfy certain inherent needs and to gain intrinsic rewards and satisfaction. The CET also proposes that if an individual who is intrinsically motivated to meet certain psychological needs is given extrinsic rewards for his behavior, by the very nature of the process (through cognitive rethinking), the person would lose his *locus of causality* and move toward becoming more extrinsically motivated.[22,23] Events or actions that occur because of or are affected by feedback, communication, and rewards, and that elicit a sense of competence during the action, enhance intrinsic motivation for those events or actions.[23] In this way, external sources may serve either to increase or decrease intrinsic motivation for action.

Health Belief and Health Promotion Models

The health belief model encompasses the motivational, attitudinal, and self-efficacy components of various theories. The theory of reasoned action (TRA) and theory of planned behavior (TPB), as developed by Ajzen and Fishbein[24] and by Ajzen,[25] propose the individual's attitude, social norms, and the individual's perceived control as accurate predictors of behavioral intentions.

The TRA is most successful when applied to behaviors under an individual's voluntary control. If behaviors are not fully under voluntary control, even though individuals may be highly motivated by their own attitudes and subjective norm, they may not actually perform the behavior because of intervening environmental conditions.

The TPB was developed to predict behaviors in which individuals have incomplete voluntary control. Taking self-esteem and self-efficacy into consideration, the TPB expands on the concept of perceived behavioral control. Perceived behavioral control indicates that an individual's motivation is influenced by the perception of how difficult the behaviors are and the perception of how successfully the individual can or cannot perform the activity. It is easy to see how this theory may relate to the concept of motivation and adherence to physical activity and/or exercise, especially in the rehabilitative setting. If patients' perceived control, self-efficacy, or self-esteem are low, the perception and belief that they can influence their behaviors in a positive manner is undermined.

In a study that assessed risk behavior after a diagnosis of coronary heart disease, planned behavior was found to be the main factor predicting self-reported exercise and observed fitness levels.[26] When exercise intention and behavior were assessed in a sample of 225 older women (65 years of age or older), significant predictors of exercise intention were behavioral beliefs, normative beliefs, and perceived control beliefs. In other words, these women were more likely to exercise if (1) they perceived more positives than negatives in performing the behavior (behavior beliefs); (2) they believed that people close or important to them approved rather than disapproved of the behavior (normative beliefs); and (3) they believed that the difficulty of the task was manageable by them (perceived control belief).[27]

Humanistic Theory

The humanistic theory, as proposed by Abraham Maslow,[15] is one of the most popular theories of motivation. According to this theory, humans are driven to achieve their maximum potential and will always do so unless obstacles are placed in their way. This theory states that specific needs (Figure 1-2) must be met in order to achieve one's potential,[28] which Maslow termed *self-actualization,* or a complete understanding of oneself and those around us. In essence, self-actualization includes focusing on problems, incorporating a continuous appreciation for life, concern about personal growth, and the ability to have peak and meaningful experiences. Needless to say, few if any individuals reach this level.

According to Maslow, the obstacles put in our paths reflect basic needs such as hunger, thirst, financial problems, safety, and time constraints; that is, essentially anything that detracts from our pursuit of maximum growth. According to this theory, the individual cannot focus on the higher levels without first achieving some degree of mastery of the lower levels. Indeed, how can a person concentrate on transcendence and actualization if basic needs for food, comfort, sleep, and safety are unmet? In the same vein, the question could be asked: How can an individual focus on maintaining or improving his health through physical activity and exercise if basic needs go unfulfilled?

Multidimensional Models

The transtheoretical model (TTM) was first introduced by Prochaska and DiClemente as a theoretical model of behavior change related to smoking cessation (Figure 1-3).[29] This model has since been used to develop effective interventions to promote health behavior change is a variety of settings and individuals of varying ages. The transtheoretical model is an integrative model of behavior change that

---

Women Were More Likely to Exercise if:

- They perceived more positives than negatives in performing the behavior (behavior beliefs)
- They believed that people close or important to them approved rather than disapproved of the behavior (normative beliefs)
- They believed the difficulty of the task was manageable by them (perceived control belief)

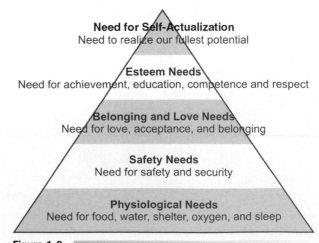

Figure 1-2

Maslow's Hierarchy of Needs. (Data from Maslow A: *Motivation and personality,* ed 2, New York, 1970, Harper.)

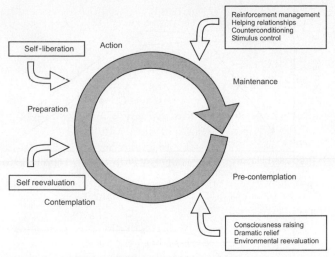

Figure 1-3

Transtheoretical Model. (From Adams J, White M: Are activity promotion interventions based on the transtheoretical model effective? a critical review, *Br J Sports Med* 37:106-114, 2003.)

incorporates a decisional balance, temptation, and self-efficacy scales.[29-32] The model describes five stages of change: precontemplation, contemplation, preparation, action, and maintenance (Table 1-1; also Figure 1-3).

Precontemplation. The hallmark of the precontemplation stage is a lack of intention to take action. Individuals have a variety of reasons for not engaging in an activity; for example, they may be uninformed or underinformed about the benefits of participation, or they may have attempted the behavior previously and were not successful. Failed attempts often are demoralizing for the individual attempting the behavior change. For example, an obese patient may have tried unsuccessfully to engage in an exercise program to lose weight and therefore has no thoughts or intentions of trying again.

Contemplation. The contemplation stage is typical of the person who is thinking about engaging in a behavior or activity within the next 6 months. These people usually are

open to receiving new knowledge and interested in listening to the benefits that engaging in the behavior may accomplish. For some individuals, this is as far as they will progress. In this stage, the person is aware of the pros of changing behavior as well as the cons of not changing. This awareness may cause the person to become ambivalent, leading to inaction, and the danger exists that the person will stagnate in the information gathering mode. Patients in this stage say things such as, "I know I should be doing these exercises, but I don't have the...[time, money, equipment, and so forth]."

Preparation. Individuals in the preparation stage intend to take action in the immediate future (within 30 days) and are typified by both intentional and behavioral components. These individuals have taken some concrete action toward the behavior change; in essence, they have a plan of action that they have begun to implement. For example, they may have made an appointment with the clinician, or they have bought appropriate workout shoes.

Action. Individuals in the action stage are actively engaged in the behaviors and/or lifestyle changes that will promote improved health. Individuals in this stage are encouraged and taught relapse prevention strategies, because the changes they have made are considered new and therefore tenuous. Relapse prevention is critical in the action stage, and criteria have been established to determine whether the change in behavior is sufficient to reduce the risk of disease. Strategies include making sure the individual is aware of occasional "slips" in her commitment to the routine. The person needs to be made aware that missing an occasional workout session or rehabilitation appointment does not doom her to failure, or that "cheating" on her diet does not mean that she cannot get back on task. Shifting the focus from failure to successes ("You did it for 6 days; what made that work?") promotes problem solving and provides encouragement.

Maintenance. Individuals in the maintenance stage have engaged in a behavioral change for longer than 6 months. Preventing boredom and a change in focus is

Table 1-1

Transtheoretical Model: Stages of Change

Stage	Characteristics
Precontemplation	Identified with individuals who do not intend to take action regarding the specific behavior (e.g., "I don't exercise, and I don't intend to start.")
Contemplation	Identified with individuals who intend to change their behavior within the next 6 months (e.g., "I don't exercise, but I'm thinking about starting.")
Preparation	Identified with individuals who intend to take action in the immediate future (e.g., "I exercise once in a while but not regularly.")
Action	Identified with individuals who have made specific and explicit changes in their behaviors and lifestyle within the past 6 months (e.g., "I exercise regularly and have done so for the last than 6 months.")
Maintenance	Identified with individuals who are actively working to prevent relapse into previous behaviors and habits (e.g., "I exercise regularly and have done so for longer than 6 months.")

essential during this stage. The person can accomplish this by establishing creative new supportive behaviors. These behaviors can include continued addressing of barriers as they arise, reformulating the rules of one's life as they relate to the behavior change, and acquisition of new skills (problem-solving and coping mechanisms) to deal with life and avoid relapse. Anticipating situations in which a relapse could occur and preparing coping strategies in advance should be emphasized to individuals in this stage. They should be encouraged to be patient with themselves and to recognize that letting go of old behavior patterns takes time and practicing new ones must be reinforced. Individuals in this stage have recurring thoughts of returning to their old habits (e.g., not exercising, making poor dietary choices, skipping rehabilitation appointments), but they usually resist the temptation and stay on track if they have noted progress.

As mentioned previously, the TTM encompasses an integrative schema for behavior change, including an examination of cost and benefits inherent in the decisional balance model. Using this model, individuals weigh the relative importance of the cons against the importance of the pros of engaging in a particular behavior change. In examining the stages of change in relation to healthy (exercise) and unhealthy (smoking) behaviors, Velicer et al.[33] found a predictable pattern in the pros and cons in relation to stages of change (Figure 1-4).[34] In the precontemplation stage, the pros of smoking far outweigh the cons of smoking. In the contemplation stage, these two scales are more equal. In the action and maintenance stages, the cons outweigh the pros. With healthy behavior (exercise), the patterns are analogous across the first three stages, with the pros of the healthy behavior remaining high.

Advocates of this stage of change model have cited its advantages as a model to predict and promote healthy behavior. One advantage of this model is that it is able to match the stage each individual is in with the proper intervention. For instance, if a person has purchased a pair of gym shoes and has joined the local gym, that person, according to the stages of change model, is in the preparation stage. Interventions can then be focused on providing positive support and encouragement to help the individual move into the action stage. Another advantage of this model is that it helps the health and exercise professional identify individuals who are in fact ready to change their behavior, thereby saving time and resources that could be better used elsewhere.

As mentioned, a study that examined barriers to physical activity by general practitioners and practice nurses found that general practitioners in the action or maintenance stage of behavior change were three times more likely to regularly promote the same behavior in their patients than general practitioners in other stages.[9] A 2003 critical review of the literature examined activity promotion interventions in a variety of populations based on the TTM; the study

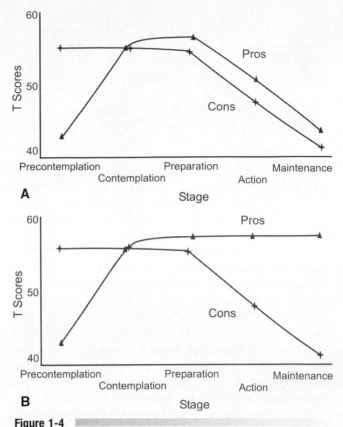

Figure 1-4

A, Stages of change and smoking. **B,** Stages of change and exercise. (From Cancer Prevention Research Center: *Detailed overview of the transtheoretical model.* Available at http://www.uri.edu/research/cprc/TTM/detailedoverview.htm.)

involved 26 studies that used written material, counseling, or both.[32] The authors found some evidence of short-term benefit from the TTM in terms of activity levels or stage of activity change. Longer term effects were harder to achieve and maintain. In 73% of the short-term studies, a positive effect of TTM-based interventions over control conditions was seen. This is in contrast to longer term studies, which showed only a 29% increase or positive effect of TTM-based interventions over the control. The numbers are encouraging, however, because the review seems to suggest that even brief intervention using the transtheoretical model will have an effect on behavior change and should be encouraged in other settings and studies.

In a study by Marcus et al.[35] that assessed motivational readiness to change, aerobic capacity and reported participation in leisure activities were higher for men and women in the stages of contemplation, preparation, action, and maintenance. In addition, men in the contemplation stage had a higher body mass index (BMI) and a higher percentage of body fat than men in the maintenance and action stages. Likewise, men who were randomized to an exercise intervention group and who initially were in the contemplation and preparation stages had a 14% and 15% increase, respectively, in aerobic capacity at follow-up, whereas men in the action and maintenance stage had a 5% increase in aerobic capacity. For women, those in the contemplation, preparation, action, and maintenance stages had a 16%, 14%, and 10% increase in aerobic capacity, respectively. This study also examined the baseline stage of motivational readiness for exercise and found that over a 9-month intervention, no differences were seen in the baseline stage of motivational readiness for exercise for the subjects reporting an increase in activity. Of the men in this study who participated in the exercise intervention and met their exercise goals, 54% were in the contemplation stage, 69% were in the preparation stage, and 68% were in the action and maintenance stages. For women, 35% initially in the contemplation stage met their intervention goals, whereas 67% and 24% met their goals who initially were classified in the preparation, action, and maintenance stages. This surprising finding revealed that adherence did not differ by baseline exercise motivational readiness stage, as was so often found in other studies.[35]

In a study that assessed factors that influenced exercise behavior in adults with physical disabilities, the most reliably predicted stages of change for exercise were maintenance (90.2%), precontemplation (73.8%), and contemplation (70.8%).[36]

As previously mentioned, the primary role of clinicians in the maintenance stage is to help prevent relapse in their clients. This can be done by helping clients to re-engage in their efforts in the change process by focusing on successes and promoting realistic goal setting so as to prevent discouragement

and to help them continue to uphold their positive steps toward a change in behavior. Clinicians attempting to help clients in the precontemplation stage should be empathetic while trying to engage their clients in questions that require thoughtful insight into the behavior that needs to be changed. Instilling hope and identifying incongruities between goals and statements can play a large part in inducing change in individuals in this stage. For individuals in the contemplation stage, clinicians should try to develop and maintain a positive relationship with their clients. This can come in the form of helping the individual personalize risk factors while posing questions that provoke thoughts about these risk factors and about the possible negative outcomes if the person does not change the behavior.

Factors Associated with Motivation and Adherence to Physical Activity, Exercise, and Rehabilitation

Having examined a few of the major theories associated with the complex concept of motivation and how it relates to adherence, the discussion now moves to focus on the factors associated with increased or decreased motivation and adherence to physical activity, exercise, and rehabilitation. The psychological and rehabilitation literatures have identified several factors that influence motivation and adherence; these factors may be personal, situational, environmental, cognitive, or behavioral in nature (Table 1-2).

Table 1-2

Characteristics Associated with Motivation and Adherence to Physical Activity, Exercise, and Rehabilitation

Factors	Description
Personal factors	Considered inherent to the individual's personality; stable and representative of the individual's persona
Self-motivation	The ability to persist in behaviors despite situational or environmental deterrents
Biomedical status	Poorer health tends to lead to decreased adherence
Socioeconomic status	The person's income bracket tends to influence the ability to access medical care, as well as exercise equipment and venues
Age	In various studies, older individuals tended to adhere to exercise programs more than younger individuals
Ethnicity	Caucasians tend to participate in more physical activities than other racial or ethnic groups
Gender	Males tend to adhere to cardiac rehabilitation programs more than females; also, men report greater levels of total and vigorous activity than women
Marital status	Singles tend to have lower rates of adherence to physical activity/exercise than married couples
Education	Individuals with higher levels of education adhere to exercise programs more than those who are uneducated
Smoking status	Cigarette smokers tend to show less adherence to exercise programs
Situational/ environmental factors	Social and physical environment in which the individual interacts will influence the positive or negative perception of the individual
Cognitive factors	What a person thinks about a situation or action influences the individual's emotional and behavioral responses
Behavioral factors	These factors are influenced by cognitive appraisal and by the person's belief that he can or cannot change his behavior

Personal Factors

Characteristics considered inherent to the individual's personality fall into the category of personal factors that influence motivation and adherence. These characteristics are considered to be stable and representative dispositions of an individual's persona. They include concepts such as self-motivation, biomedical status, socioeconomic status (SES), age, ethnicity, gender, and education, to name a few. Various studies have examined these concepts and the ways they relate to adherence and compliance in a variety of populations, as well as how they relate to adherence to physical activity, exercise, and rehabilitation programs. The sport psychology literature has examined other personal concepts, such as pain tolerance, task and ego involvement, and trait anxiety, as they influence rehabilitation adherence in the athletic population.

Personal Factors that Influence Motivation and Adherence Include:

- Self-motivation
- Biomedical status
- Education
- Socioeconomic status
- Age
- Ethnicity
- Gender

Self-Motivation

Self-motivation is the ability to persist in behaviors in spite of situational or environmental deterrents;[37] it has been found to be most consistently correlated with adherence to rehabilitation in athletes who sustained a sports injury.[38,39] It stands to reason that individuals who are highly self-motivated will be more inclined to adhere to self-monitored exercise programs, and to adhere to them longer, than individuals who are not as highly motivated. Therefore increasing self-motivation is advantageous for promoting adherence to various rehabilitation programs.

Clinicians can help improve a person's ability to be self-motivated by helping the person build a history of success. For example, starting an individual with a task or an exercise that the person can easily accomplish, and then gradually increasing the level of difficulty, will promote confidence and inspire continued motivation to reach a particular goal. The individual should be encouraged to focus on successes, rather than on failures that may prevent the person from trying again.

Biomedical Status

When a panel of geriatric exercise experts was asked to assess personal characteristics with regard to exercise behavior in older adults, biomedical status was rated the most important factor in determining whether an older adult will initiate and adhere to exercise.[40] In other words, exercise participation depends on whether a person perceives himself or herself to be in good health. This is an important factor, because health care providers can offer physical screening programs, which can reassure clients that it is indeed safe and beneficial for them to exercise. This same panel also found that in older adults, a person's past exercise history and socioeconomic level were important factors in exercise adherence. Exploring the individual's past exercise history helps identify strategies that can optimize future exercise behavior. This assessment includes asking about activities the individual liked or disliked and soliciting information about perceived and real barriers and rewards.[40]

Questions to Ask to Determine the Likelihood of Compliance with Exercise or Rehabilitation Programs

- Have you exercised or participated in a rehabilitation program in the past?
- What are some barriers that might prevent you from engaging in exercise/rehabilitation?
- What are some things that might help you to stick with the program?
- When you exercise, do you exercise alone or with others?
- Do you prefer to exercise alone or with others?
- What kind of activities/exercise do you like to do?
- What are your goals for participating in an exercise/rehabilitation program?

Exploring a person's past exercise history can help identify strategies for optimizing future exercise behavior. This assessment includes asking about activities the person liked or disliked and soliciting information about perceived and real barriers and rewards.

Socioeconomic Status

Interestingly, socioeconomic status (SES) was found to be extremely relevant in the older population in promoting exercise adherence. As a person's income level declines or becomes fixed, the ability to pay for exercise advice, equipment, and exercise facilities becomes limited. For individuals who can no longer afford these expenses, adherence tends to decrease. Therefore it is essential that health care providers obtain information about the client's income so that they can best meet the client's needs and increase the probability of adherence to an exercise and/or rehabilitation program.

Age

Age is another personal factor that has been found to correlate with adherence to exercise and rehabilitation. In a study involving a group of church-going African Americans participating in an exercise intervention, older individuals tended to adhere to an exercise program more than younger individuals.[41] The researchers noted that the exercise intervention was timed and coordinated to accommodate the schedules and needs of the older subjects, which may have biased the results. A study that assessed training levels and adherence in patients with coronary heart disease between the ages of 30 and 67 found that older patients were more likely to sustain an exercise attendance schedule necessary to recoup therapeutic benefits.[42] In yet another study, participation in and adherence to a physical activity program decreased among older individuals.[43] This decrease in participation may be attributed to an assortment of reasons, including poor health, lack of time, fear, and an unsafe environment.

Ethnicity

Caucasians appear to participate in more physical activities than other racial or ethnic groups, regardless of age.[44] In a sample of African Americans, a 27% attendance rate for a church-based exercise program was noted, providing some support for the notion that minorities tend to adhere less to physical activity and exercise programs. A recent study by Hawkins et al.[43] found no significant differences in the prevalence of achieving sufficient duration of moderate levels of physical activity by race or ethnicity in California adults. In fact, California-born Latinos were 21% more likely to participate in vigorous physical activity than other ethnic groups. The researchers noted that significant differences may have been found if recent ethnic immigrants to the United States were included in the sample. Martin et al.[45] also found no relation between ethnicity and participation in moderate to vigorous levels of physical activity.

Gender

Men have been found to be more engaged in and adherent to physical activity, exercise, and cardiac phase II rehabilitation programs than women.[46] In assessing the effect of tailored interventions on exercise adherence, Keele-Smith and Leon[44] found that women were more inactive than men, and more men than women were reported to have engaged in vigorous physical activity. In a study that examined demographic and other variables in an assessment of participation in exercise guidelines, established by the American College of Sports Medicine and the Centers for Disease Control and Prevention, in a cohort of adults 18 years and older, women were found to be less likely to meet the guidelines. In addition, men reported greater levels of total and vigorous activity, and women reported engagement in low energy to moderately vigorous activities.[45] In a sample of college students, 92% of males versus 63% of females reported engaging in regular exercise.[47]

Marital Status

Another personal factor that may play an important part in determining a person's level of motivation for physical activity, exercise, and rehabilitation participation is marital status. In one study,[44] those who were unmarried tended to have lower adherence, which may be directly related to social support (which is discussed later).

Education

Studies have found that individuals with less education are less adherent to health-related programs.[40,44] Smoking status is also a factor; cigarette smokers tend to be less committed to making healthy lifestyle changes[42] and are less able to maintain a consistent exercise program.[44]

Situational/Environmental Factors

Situational factors represent the social and physical environment in which the individual interacts. Therefore the presence of other people, including the health care or exercise specialist and other patients or clients, influences whether the individual has a positive or negative perception and experience with physical activity, exercise, or rehabilitation.

Situationally, convenience of the location of exercise facilities and convenience of exercise opportunities (e.g., research solicitations) often facilitate adherence to exercise programs. In addition, the quality of the client-practitioner interaction either enhances or diminishes the quality of the person's participation.

Environmentally, the characteristics of the actual exercise or rehabilitation setting and time of day also are important to individuals and can partly determine adherence. Individuals have a preferred time of day and setting in which they feel most comfortable and are most likely to follow through with established exercise and/or rehabilitation protocols. Therefore, to best ensure adherence, the practitioner must create an environment and a situation best suited to the individual's needs.

Cognitive Factors

What a person thinks about a situation or action mediates emotional and behavioral responses to an event. If people perceive something to be out of their control, they either will not attempt the behavior or will expect to fail in it. This is especially relevant to eliciting changes in health behaviors. If individuals do not believe that they will be successful in the tasks set forth by the exercise and physical activity guidelines, they may be more apt not to engage in the activity. Therefore education can be helpful for facilitating cognitive reappraisals and for promoting the individual's belief that he can engage in behaviors that positively affect his health.

Behavioral Factors

As stated previously, whether individuals engage in behaviors reflects their cognitive appraisal of the situational context. In rehabilitation, a person's cognitive belief that she not only will be able to cope with the injury, but will be able to cope well, determines whether the person will exhibit behaviors conducive to recovery. Changing behaviors, especially health-related behaviors, has proven difficult. Strategies, in the form of behavioral modification (also known as *behavioral interventions*) are practiced in psychology and rehabilitation to encourage the desired change in individuals. For example, encouraging the individual to make a commitment in private by choosing, committing, and later going public by announcing to others the decision to change is a powerful step toward behavior change. The public commitment is more powerful than the private decision. Another way to encourage behavior change is to have an individual sign a written contract. This contract is an agreement made between the person and the clinician to engage in specific steps to reach mutually established goals.

Barriers Associated with Decreased Motivation and Compliance/Adherence to Physical Activity, Exercise, and Rehabilitation

The factors discussed pertaining to motivation, compliance, and adherence to exercise and rehabilitation reflect mainly theoretical manifestations of personality, situation, and cognition. They do not adequately identify the perceived and real issue of individuals who are most at risk for health-related decline as a result of no or inadequate participation (Tables 1-3 to 1-5). It is important to identify barriers, both perceived and real, as well as ways health care providers and exercise specialists can help individuals overcome them.

Table 1-3

Barriers Associated with Decreased Motivation and Compliance or Adherence to Physical Activity, Exercise, and Rehabilitation

Barrier	Overview
Environment	These factors may include physical obstacles; access to and the cost of health clubs and rehabilitation centers; and climate problems
Health	Health barriers include unhealthy behaviors (e.g., smoking); the individual's perception of being in poor health; and chronic illness
Supervision and direction	Lack of supervision and guidance for exercise is a deterrent to initiation of and compliance with an exercise program
Time	Time problems can include lack of time for exercise and exercise programs that take up too much time
Family	Family responsibilities and obligations may take priority over rehabilitation and exercise
Occupation	Work responsibilities and obligations may take priority over rehabilitation and exercise

Table 1-4

Strategies for Increasing Compliance

Strategy	Effect
Solicit social support from family, significant others, children, and friends	Family support is the most important type of social reinforcement. If possible, have the family participate in the exercise or take part in the patient's rehabilitation. Suggest fitness routines that can be done with the children
Make the activity fun and enjoyable	Work with the patient to identify activities the person has enjoyed in the past and incorporate these activities into the current exercise or rehabilitation routine
Increase the individual's knowledge about the activity and/or injury	Teach the patient about the benefits of exercise/rehabilitation and the dangers of not engaging in the suggested activities
Make the physical environment pleasant and appealing	Remove clutter; make sure the décor is bright and cheery
Address perceived and real barriers	Compile a list of potential barriers and help the individual problem-solve by identifying realistic alternatives

Table 1-5
Factors That Increase Motivation

Factor	Effect
Social support	High self-efficacy
Establishment of therapeutic rapport	Individual involvement in planning aspects of the exercise or rehabilitation program
Decreased perception of discomfort	Individual engagement in planning and establishing goals
Positive reinforcement by the clinician	Increased knowledge about the benefits of engaging in a regular exercise or rehabilitation program

Environment

The physical environment can be a deterrent to some individuals trying to decide whether to commit to an exercise and/or rehabilitation program. This is true across the lifespan, from the young to older adults who would be well advised to change their exercise behavior. In a sample of African American women with physical disabilities (ages 18 to 64 years), the cost of joining a fitness center, lack of transportation, and fear of leaving their homes ranked 1 through 3, respectively, as barriers to exercise.[48] In a study that examined ways to overcome exercise barriers in older adults, identified environmental barriers included physician advice (e.g., rest instead of activity), access to and the cost of health clubs and rehabilitation centers, and climate.[49] As mentioned previously, if physicians did not inquire about diet and exercise, patient perception that these factors were not important was high. Also, lack of follow-up to monitor progress or goal achievement and busy schedules on the part of the health care provider and/or exercise specialist often promote nonadherence in individual patients.

With regard to access and cost, many individuals, especially those living in low income areas and the elderly, cannot afford to join an area gym. Although some areas provide free access to fitness and recreational equipment, people may not be able to afford the cost of transportation to these facilities. Similarly, walking may not be an option, because some patients live in dangerous neighborhoods with a high crime rate.[6,50]

Finding a safe environment in which patients and clients can exercise should be a priority for the health care provider and other exercise specialists.[51] It has been shown that older adults who do not live in the vicinity of recreational facilities often do not participate in regular exercise and are more sedentary.[51] For individuals living in the northern climates, weather conditions may not be conducive to regularly engaging in outdoor activities.[6] In the same sense, individuals living in warmer climates may be impeded by high humidity and/or heat. In either case, extremes in the weather can prevent individuals from participating in a regular exercise routine for up to 6 months.[49] In the rehabilitation environment, patients with physical disabilities often mention lack of adaptive space and/or accessible equipment, along with poor equipment maintenance, as barriers.[52] These patients also have said that they perceive fitness and recreational facilities to be unfriendly to individuals with physical disabilities.

Health

Unhealthy behaviors, such as smoking and leading a sedentary lifestyle, contribute to both acute and chronic diseases in the general population. Abolishing or at the very least reducing these practices ideally should promote increased quality of life. The health care provider's efforts to help a client start or adhere to an exercise program often are encumbered by the person's perception that poor health limits the patient's ability to participate in exercise and rehabilitation programs. Older adults in particular often cite poor health as the leading barrier to physical activity and exercise.[53] In a group of cardiac rehabilitation patients, gender and barrier efficacy were related to overcoming health barriers, such as fear of another cardiac event, medication side effects, and angina or chest pain.[46] These investigators also found that men more than women tended to have higher barrier efficacy; for example, they felt more capable of engaging in the cardiac program without experiencing detrimental effects to their health. A study that examined exercise behavior in older adults found that during the initiation and adherence stages, biomedical status was the most important determinant of exercise adherence.[40] A panel of experts agreed that, for older adults, initiation of and adherence to an exercise program depends on the individual's perceived and actual state of health.[40]

With regard to participation in physical activity by adults age 65 or older, the most commonly reported barrier to increasing physical activity was health problems.[54] In their review of the literature, Sluijs et al. reported that characteristics associated with certain illnesses related to compliance: "When the illness causes more disabilities and handicaps and patients perceive the illness as very serious, they appear to be more compliant (with rehabilitation) than patients with less serious illness."[11] They also reported that patients with chronic illnesses seemed to be less compliant than those with acute illnesses, which suggests that recovery from the illness is an incentive in itself to participate in the exercise regimen as dictated by their rehabilitation program. In the Sedentary Women Exercise Adherence Trial (SWEAT), which involved a group of middle-aged and older women, the most common reason stated for withdrawal from an exercise program was illness or injury.[55] When fear of injury or reinjury is added, compliance with rehabilitation and other exercise programs declines.[49]

Supervision and Direction

Individuals have reported that lack of supervision and guidelines for exercise has been a deterrent to initiating and adhering to exercise. Those who have had no training in exercise prescription would not unreasonably want some assistance with the planning and implementation of an exercise program. This is especially true for some older adults and other individuals who may have significant health-related issues. Also, in any exercise program it is essential to monitor participants for excessive effort. If the activity is too intense for their comfort, they are more likely to drop out or sustain an injury.

In examining exercise preferences in older adults, researchers found that those who had higher levels of reported pain were more likely to feel that their exercise should be monitored and evaluated by a qualified professional.[53] This finding is in alignment with other research that has reported a higher degree of noncompliance with exercise and rehabilitation programs in older individuals who have significant health problems and pain.[55] The literature supports the finding that adherence to exercise protocols is best established when the protocols are supervised. Morey et al.[56] investigated whether a supervised exercise program could predict adherence in the same group of individuals when transitioned over to a home-based program. They found that during the supervised portion of the study, adherence to weekend home-based exercise, as a preparation for transitioning to a complete home-based program, was the strongest predictor of adherence to the home-based program. Of interest in this study was the fact that individuals who were assessed and determined to be adherers, compared to those determined to be nonadherers, remained so throughout the study. Adherence to exercise, therefore, can be predicted at an early stage; for example, by using the stages of change model of behavioral change.[56]

Studies have indicated that marital status plays an important part in exercise preference and supervision. Cohen-Mansfield et al.[53] reported that unmarried participants rated supervision by an authority figure (i.e., a person who provided advice, monitoring, and/or evaluation of the exercise program) to be highly important, which suggests that encouragement and direction helped these individuals initiate and adhere to the exercise program.

Time, Family, and Occupation

Time often is perceived as a barrier to engaging in physical activity, exercise, and rehabilitation. Cohen-Mansfield et al.[53] found that older individuals (ages 74 to 85 years) generally preferred to exercise between 9 AM and 12 PM; the oldest group preferred to exercise between 12 and 3 PM. Interestingly, these researchers also found that the group that preferred to exercise earlier (between 9 AM and

12 PM) were healthier than the group that preferred exercise later in the day.[53] College-aged students regularly listed exercise taking too much time as a barrier.[47] Physical therapy patients also indicated that exercise, in the form of rehabilitation, required extra time that they did not have.[11] In a sample of Australian subjects ages 18 to 78 years, lack of time was cited as a barrier. For individuals who have children and who work, child care and work responsibilities may be prohibitive to incorporating exercise and physical activity into the daily or weekly routine. Accomplishing work goals and tasks may take priority over participating in rehabilitation, physical activity, or exercise. For retired individuals, other activities, such as volunteering and spending time with grandchildren, may supercede exercise or rehabilitation participation.[49,51]

As can be inferred from these findings, rehabilitation and exercise specialists need to be flexible in scheduling patient and client appointments to increase the likelihood of these individuals participating in an exercise or rehabilitation program. In addition, physical therapy clinics, gyms, fitness centers, and other recreational environments should vary their hours of operation to accommodate as much as possible clients' preferences and their need to work around conflicting activities.

Overview of Adherence to Rehabilitation in the Clinical Population

Rehabilitation specialists such as physical therapists, occupational therapists, speech language pathologists, and athletic trainers use exercise as one component of their intervention to effectively treat their patients. These professionals are presumed to have a thorough understanding of the pathology of the injury and the physiological demands of the exercise. However, when health care professionals are confronted with the client's unique physical impairments and disabilities, they may overlook the psychological and motivational factors that are important to the success of the exercise program.

In rehabilitation, a successful outcome often is linked to the patient's attendance at clinic appointments and compliance with the exercise programs developed by the clinician.[58-60] However, this is not always the case. Brewer et al.[38] found that outcomes in rehabilitation after anterior cruciate ligament reconstruction were not mediated by adherence to rehabilitation. Nevertheless, encouraging individuals to participate actively in rehabilitation is important for increasing the probability of recovery from injury.

A study by Goodman and Ballou[61] examined perceived barriers and motivators with regard to exercise in patients undergoing hemodialysis. The study found that adherence to exercise among these patients was low; 38% stated that in a typical week, exercise did not reach 15 minutes.

The results also suggested that barriers and lack of motivation, rather than health-related impairments, stopped these individuals from exercising (see Tables 1-3 and 1-5).

In a sample of African American women with physical disabilities (as rated by the Americans with Disabilities Act [ADA]), adherence to regular physical activity was found to be directly related to the number of barriers that existed in the individual's life.[48] These barriers included the cost of the exercise program (84.2%), lack of energy (65.8%), transportation problems (60.5%), and not knowing where to exercise (57.9%). These problems have some implications regarding the strategies rehabilitation and exercise specialists might use to encourage individuals to engage in habitual exercise and/or rehabilitation.

Short-term adherence to a pelvic floor muscle exercise program significantly predicted long-term adherence to the same program (1 year afterward) in a clinical population of women with urinary incontinence.[62] This may be directly related to the severity of symptoms each individual experienced (i.e., the weekly number of incontinence episodes). Individuals with more frequent episodes appeared to be more adherent to the program and to maintain their adherence 1 year afterward.[62] This also may be due to the social stigma and embarrassment that individuals feel with this health problem.

A major health concern today, cardiovascular disease, results in a loss of independence and quality of life for individuals who have suffered a cardiac event. For this reason, cardiac rehabilitation programs have been developed to provide exercise, education, and assistance in a medically supervised environment to help the patient achieve behavioral changes that enhance the quality of life.[63] It is essential that health care professionals facilitate adherence to these programs so as to help bring about the behavioral changes needed to maximize function in these individuals.

A few studies have examined adherence and motivation to participate in cardiac rehabilitation programs.[64,65] In a review of the literature, Beswick et al.[65] identified several factors that improved recruitment, adherence, and compliance in cardiac rehabilitation. These included a formal patient commitment (i.e., a written contract), spouse or familial involvement, strategies to aid self-management, educational intervention, and psychological intervention through group psychotherapy. These factors had varying levels of success in improving adherence to the cardiac program. (Other factors are discussed later in the chapter.) In yet another study, personal factors such as health and work status significantly influenced adherence to the cardiac program.[63] This study found that individuals who were not working and who were in the high risk group for health had the lowest mean physical activity scores (i.e., participation) in the cardiac rehabilitation program at baseline and at the conclusion of the study 1 year later.

Factors Identified as Increasing Patient Adherence to Cardiac Rehabilitation Include:

- A formal patient commitment set down in a written contract
- Spouse or family involvement
- Strategies to aid self-management
- Educational intervention
- Psychological intervention through group psychotherapy

Another study examined motivation in conjunction with a health-promoting lifestyle after a 12-week cardiac rehabilitation exercise program.[66] These researchers found that individuals who participated in the program had higher motivation for a healthy lifestyle than those who did not participate. In addition, perceived benefits of exercise, barriers, and self-efficacy, as well as emotional well-being and health, improved in the exercise group versus the comparison group.[66] A review of the U.S. National Exercise and Heart Disease Project[67] found that participation in a cardiac rehabilitation program had a compliance rate of 79.6% after 2 months of continuous monitored training, but that adherence decreased to 13% at 36 months.[68] In a study by Blanchard et al.,[46] barrier self-efficacy was shown to be associated with compliance in a phase II cardiac rehabilitation program. In essence, individuals who believed that they had sufficient abilities to overcome specific cardiac-related barriers had better adherence to the rehabilitation program.[46] Bray and Cowan[69] found that proxy efficacy had an affect on predicting exercise self-efficacy and post program intentions in cardiac rehabilitation. Simply stated, *proxy efficacy* means the confidence that individuals had in their clinician's communication, teaching, and motivating capabilities was predictive of exercise self-efficacy and post program participation in cardiac rehabilitation. Considering that research correlates increased physical activity and exercise with positive outcomes after a coronary event, the impetus to increase compliance and adherence in this population is great.

Another clinical population that warrants the benefits of an exercise program are individuals with chronic obstructive pulmonary disease (COPD). This disease is the fourth leading cause of death in the United States for people ages 65 to 84 years; it is the fifth leading cause of death for people ages 45 to 64 and those aged 85 and older.[70] COPD also is a primary cause of disability among older adults.[71] Participation in an exercise program has many psychological as well as physical benefits for individuals with COPD. Major benefits detailed in the literature include increased physical capacity, decreased anxiety about dyspnea, greater independence in activities of daily living, reduced fatigued, and improved overall quality of life.[72] Emery et al.[73] examined cognitive and psychological outcomes in patients with COPD after 1 year and found that adherence to a regular exercise program was associated with increased physical and cognitive performance and greater emotional well-being. Those who did not adhere to the program were found to have a decrease in both physical and psychological constructs.[73] The danger of noncompliance in any of these clinical populations, but with COPD most specifically, is that any benefits gained will diminish over time;[74] this makes increasing the likelihood of exercise participation and maintenance over time particularly important.

Increasing Motivation and Adherence to Exercise and Rehabilitation

Theoretical approaches, models, and barriers notwithstanding, increasing motivation and subsequently adherence to exercise and/or rehabilitation is the goal of health care professionals, exercise specialists, patients, and clients in a variety of settings with a variety of health-related issues. The rehabilitation, sports psychology, psychology, and sociology literature has sought to identify ways to increase motivation and adherence to exercise and rehabilitation. Some of these strategies were mentioned previously, such as patient commitment through a written contract, spouse or familial involvement, strategies to aid self-management, educational intervention, and psychological intervention through group psychotherapy. Other factors include self-efficacy, social support, and patient/client–practitioner interaction.

Self-Efficacy

Bandura[18] defines self-efficacy as "people's judgments of their capabilities to organize and execute courses of action required to attain designated types of performances." Human motivation, well-being, and a sense of personal accomplishment are based on self-efficacy beliefs. Unless people believe that their actions can produce the outcomes they desire, they have little incentive to act or to persevere in the face of difficulties. Therefore the development of self-efficacy is presumed to promote action to initiate and complete various tasks. Self-efficacy is developed through mastery of tasks or performance experience, vicarious or observational experience of others successfully completing a task, verbal persuasion from a voice of authority (e.g., physician,

physical therapist), emotional desire to perform the task (motivation), and physiological states (e.g., reduction in physical discomfort, such as pain or fatigue).[6,75]

When individuals master a task, their success contributes to their sense of personal efficacy. In the same sense, failure to master a specific task (e.g., exercise) undermines self-efficacy, especially if the failures outweigh the successes.[76] In the general adult population, self-efficacy often is a strong indicator of engagement in physical activity.[77,78] In populations with an acute or a chronic illness, improved self-efficacy has been predictive of long-term exercise compliance.[8,75]

In the health care setting, clinicians often have used the successful experiences of some patients to engage other patients in increased participation in rehabilitation. The rehabilitation environment may be set up in such a way as to help patients observe and translate the positive experiences of other patients with similar injuries or diagnoses, thereby increasing self-efficacy and facilitating positive outcomes for themselves.

Social Support

Whether in the beginning, middle, or end stage of an exercise or rehabilitation program, individuals have stated that social support from family, friends, significant others, peers, and/or health care providers is desired. Indeed, *not* having the support of important persons in their lives has been cited as a barrier to participation in or adherence to exercise and rehabilitation programs. Studies have found that married individuals tend to adhere longer to physical activity and exercise programs than individuals who are not married, which suggests the importance of spousal support.[79] Also, unmarried individuals are more likely to participate in exercise programs if social opportunities are available.[10]

In a study that examined the role of social support and group cohesion in exercise compliance, Fraser and Spink[80] found that group cohesion and social support contributed to the prediction of attendance at exercise sessions. Social support was identified as a main motivator in a group of Southern women who participated in a walking intervention.[81] These women reported spouses, significant others, friends, coworkers, and neighbors, as well as children, siblings, parents, and extended family members, as sources of exercise support. An interesting finding was the difference in support plans for people in various income groups. Nies et al.[81] found that high income women appeared to incorporate significant others (spouses, boyfriends, partners) and pets into their walking schedule more than women in a low income group. This is in contrast to a study that assessed attendance for a community-based exercise program in an African American church congregation; the study reported increased adherence in individuals who had a high sense of community affiliation.[41]

In an attempt to predict long-term maintenance of physical activity in older adults, McAuley et al.[82] examined

---

Self-efficacy May be Increased Through:

- Mastery of tasks
- Performance experience
- Vicarious or observational experience of successful task completion
- Verbal persuasion from a voice of authority (e.g., physician)
- Emotional desire to perform the task (motivation)
- Physiological states (reduction of discomfort)

the role of social, behavioral, and cognitive factors and found an indirect correlate between increased levels of social support for exercise and pleasant affective mediated by high levels of self-efficacy at the end of the program. Scores on the Social Support subscale of the Exercise Motivation Questionnaire (EMQ), although not statistically significant, differentiated between individuals who exercised regularly and those who did not; regular exercisers tended to have higher than average scores on this subscale.[43] Increased adherence to home-based rehabilitation programs may partly be due to the familiarity of the environment, as well as to the increase likelihood of support from family members, significant others, friends, neighbors, and/or peers.

Recognizing the value of social support should inspire health care providers and other specialists to include people who are important to their patients and clients when planning exercise and rehabilitation programs.

Education

Intuitively, the more knowledge people have about a topic, the more comfortable and confident they will be in making a decision regarding that topic. This is also true for exercise. Therefore education should be an integral part of any exercise or rehabilitation program.[40]

When a panel of experts was asked to examine personal characteristics that may influence exercise behavior in older adults, educational level was rated as the third most important determinant of whether older adults would initiate an exercise regimen.[40] In a sample of women with urinary incontinence, education about sex was a significant predictor of long-term adherence to a pelvic floor muscle exercises provided by a physical therapist.[62] This study found that women who did not have sex education in school and who attended school for fewer years tended not to adhere to their prescribed exercise program. Given the findings of these studies, patients and clients must be taught the benefits of exercise, as well as what constitutes good exercise habits.

Health care professionals and exercise specialists can provide educational information about exercise and rehabilitation through a variety of verbal and nonverbal interactions, such as telephone counseling, written materials, direct conversation with the patient or client, and committee liaisons.

The educational component should include explanations of the benefits that engaging in exercise and physical rehabilitation will have for the individual's health and symptoms. It also should include a general explanation of the major concepts of exercise based on the individual's past and current exercise behavior, health status, and baseline physical functioning. This teaching should include explanations of the target heart rate, perceived exertion, and body composition. Written handouts with pictures appropriate for the individual's educational level should be provided.

Other areas that must be covered, especially for individuals in rehabilitation, include an accurate explanation of the nature of the injury, the treatment approach and rationale, and realistic expectations for recovery.[60,83] Whether given verbally or nonverbally, this information should be provided by a health care or exercise professional whom the patient or client trusts and perceives to have a strong knowledge of exercise.

Patient/Client–Practitioner Interaction

To promote motivation and adherence to a rehabilitation program, the health care professional must develop a rapport with the patient and establish effective communication.[84] Patients who were found to have effective communication with their physical therapists also were found to attend scheduled physical therapy appointments and to comply with established rehabilitation activities during the sessions.[84] Athletes who felt that medical professionals were honest, interested in their well-being, and aware of the psychological symptoms related to their injuries tended to be more likely to adhere to their rehabilitation programs.[85] Establishing open lines of communication and fostering a collaborative atmosphere more often than not has a positive influence on adherence to treatment.[86] In addition, enhanced communication between the client and the health care practitioner helps to bring to light and resolve any issues that may affect adherence. A sound therapeutic relationship plays a major role in adherence, and the clinician and the patient must communicate as partners to build that relationship and trust.[87]

Another essential component of exercise and rehabilitation adherence is feedback. Health care and exercise professionals should provide positive feedback to their patients and clients to improve adherence to any rehabilitation and exercise program. Studies have found that positive reinforcement increases the likelihood of participation in and maintenance of an activity.[88] Monitoring and supervision by a qualified health care professional also have been shown to improve compliance with exercise and rehabilitation programs.[11] In studying correlates of exercise compliance in physical therapy, Sluijs et al.[11] found that compliance was significantly related to the amount of positive feedback patients received. In addition, patients who perceived that their therapist was satisfied with how they were exercising were more compliant than patients who were not aware of their clinician's feelings about their exercise. In the same study, patients who were more compliant with their exercises had therapists who frequently asked them to participate in establishing the exercise regimen and supervised them more often throughout its implementation.[11] The findings from these studies emphasize that developing trust, establishing good communication, and caring are some of the most important factors in building a therapeutic relationship that fosters patient adherence.

Table 1-6

Factors That Must be Addressed to Elicit Healthy Behavior Changes

Characteristics	Barriers
Personal factors	Environment
Self-motivation	Health
Biomedical status	Supervision and
Socioeconomic status	direction
Age	Time
Ethnicity	Family
Gender	Occupation
Marital status	
Education	
Smoking status	
Situational/environmental factors	
Cognitive factors	
Behavioral factors	
Identification of stage of change (i.e., precontemplation, contemplation, preparation, action, maintenance)	

Summary

As the chapter shows, the concepts of motivation, adherence, and compliance, as they relate to physical activity, exercise, and rehabilitation, are complex. No one factor will help individuals want to engage in healthy habits. For behavior to change, a combination of factors needs to be incorporated to assist individuals in making decisions that will positively affect their quality of life (Table 1-6). Health care practitioners and exercise professionals should make use of the many theories and models available in the literature while listening to and addressing the unique situations of each of their patients and clients.

References

To enhance this text and add value for the reader, all references have been incorporated into a CD-ROM that is provided with this text. The reader can view the reference source and access it online whenever possible. There are a total of 88 references for this chapter.

CHAPTER 2

CERVICAL SPINE

Jim Meadows, Susan L. Armijo-Olivo, and David J. Magee

Introduction

The etiology of injury to the cervical spine and the causes of cervical spine pathology are numerous. They can be myogenic, mechanical, neurogenic, or psychosomatic in origin and can be further divided into acute and chronic states. Acute injuries may be due to trauma, unaccustomed activity, or a poor working or sleeping position. Chronic pathology usually is due to poor posture, poor muscle tone, or illness. In a young child, it may be the result of an idiopathic torticollis.

In young people, mechanical and myogenic types of cervical pathology are most commonly due to a ligament sprain or muscle strain, whereas in older adults, they are more commonly due to cervical spondylosis (disc degeneration). Spinal stenosis (narrowing of the spinal canal) also can lead to symptoms, as can facet syndrome (pathology in the zygapophyseal joints). Neurogenic neck pain is primarily due to facet impingement or disc degeneration or herniation, resulting in irritation of the cervical nerve roots and subsequent radicular pain into the shoulder and/or arm. Psychosomatic problems commonly are the result of depression, anxiety, hysteria or, in some cases, malingering.

One reason the cervical spine is vulnerable to injury is its high degree of mobility with a heavy weight, the head, perched on top of it. The cervical spine is the most flexible and mobile part of the spine, and the intervertebral discs make up about 40% of its height.[1] Neck pain, however, tends to be less disabling than back pain.[2]

With regard to injuries, the cervical spine can be divided into two areas, the upper cervical spine and the lower cervical spine. Upper cervical injuries are associated with the vertebral segments CO (occiput) to C2; these injuries are referred to as **cervicoencephalic** injuries.[3,4] The term *cervicoencephalic* portrays the relationship between the cervical spine and the occiput. Cervicoencephalic injuries can be severe enough to involve the brain, brain stem, and spinal cord.[3,4] The symptoms of injury associated with these segments may arise from areas of the brain (cognitive dysfunction), the anatomic nervous system (sympathetic dysfunction), the cranial nerves (cranial nerve dysfunction) or the vertebral and/or internal carotid artery (vascular dysfunction) and tend to be headache, fatigue, vertigo, poor concentration, and irritability to light.[3,4] This is important to understand, because once sympathetic system dysfunction, cognitive dysfunction, cranial nerve dysfunction or vascular dysfunction is evident, the condition takes an inordinate amount of time to resolve, is more difficult to treat, and may have more severe consequences. Cognitive dysfunction includes altered mental functions of comprehension, judgement, memory and reasoning. Sympathetic symptoms are a result of hypertonia of the sympathetic nervous system, affect emotions, and may include tinnitus, postural dizziness, blurred vision, photophobia, rhinorrhea, sweating, lacrimation, and weakness.[3,5] Cranial nerve dysfunction involves one or more of the cranial nerves, and vascular dysfunction involves either the vertebral, basilar, or internal carotid arteries. Patients with severe injuries often may also demonstrate numbness or pain, sharp reversal of the cervical lordosis, and restricted motion, especially at one particular vertebral level.

Sympathetic Symptoms Caused by Cervical Pathology

- Tinnitus (ringing in the ear)
- Postural dizziness
- Blurred vision
- Photophobia (intolerance to light)
- Rhinorrhea (runny nose)
- Abnormal sweating
- Lacrimation (tearing)
- Weakness

Symptoms of Cognitive Dysfunction

- From concussions, head injuries
- Memory dysfunction – retrograde amnesia, post traumatic amnesia
- Concentration difficulties/difficulty remembering things
- Disorientation
- Balance problems/incoordination
- Dizziness
- Increased emotionality
- Feeling "in a fog"

Lower cervical spine injuries are associated with vertebral body segments C3 to C7; these injuries are referred to as **cervicobrachial** injuries. Pathology in this region commonly leads to pain in the upper extremity.[3,4] Neck pain or extremity pain may occur individually, or the two may occur together. One may be greater than the other, or they may be equal. In any case, the clinician's main concern is whether the signs and symptoms are peripheralizing (moving more distally) or centralizing (moving more centrally). If they are peripheralizing, the condition usually is worsening. If they are centralizing, the condition is improving. Common signs of minor injury are neck stiffness and limited range of motion. Unfavorable signs include paresthesia, muscle weakness into the upper extremity, radicular signs, and neurological deficit.[5]

Torticollis

The term *torticollis* (wry neck) means scoliosis or "twisted neck" in the cervical spine. The condition may be acute or chronic. Congenital torticollis, seen in young children, involves the sternocleidomastoid muscle. Congenital or infantile torticollis primarily affects females ages 6 months to 3 years. It results from unilateral contraction of the sternocleidomastoid muscle caused by ischemic changes in the muscle. The resulting deformity is side flexion to the same (affected) side and rotation to the opposite side (Figure 2-1). A lump, or pseudo-tumor, sometimes is felt over the muscle in the first month, but this disappears.[6] The contracture itself is not painful, but it can lead to developmental and cosmetic problems.

The cause of congenital torticollis is unknown, but the condition may be related to abnormal blood supply to the sternocleidomastoid muscle, resulting in a structural abnormality in the muscle. Increased amounts of interstitial fibrous tissue are found in the muscle, and this fibrous tissue tends to contract over time, causing the deformity. If the condition is not corrected early, asymmetry of the face may develop, with the affected side not being as well developed. The asymmetry corrects itself if the condition is corrected early. However, the correction, which commonly involves repeated, painful stretching of the affected muscle, may take years. Torticollis often is associated with

other cervical deformities, such as Klippel-Feil syndrome, which is characterized by shortness of the neck and fusion of two or three of the vertebral bodies.[6]

The treatment for congenital torticollis, from a rehabilitation standpoint, is stretching and overcorrection of the deformity at birth. Most cases of congenital torticollis can be corrected this way, provided the stretching is carried out diligently. The clinician must teach the parents how to do the stretching, because it must be done two to four times a day for at least a year. Needless to say, the child will not like the stretching and will express herself the only way she can—by crying. The clinician should prepare the parents for this so that they are not worried that the child is being injured.

Acute or acquired torticollis usually occurs in people 20 years of age or older. Spasm of one or more muscles (i.e., the sternocleidomastoid, splenius capitis, semispinalis capitus, or scalenus anterior) is commonly seen. The acute type of torticollis primarily is due to trauma or muscle strain; however, in some cases it may be related to an upper respiratory tract infection, a viral infection, poor posture (with symptoms arising after the patient has been in an awkward posture for several hours), hearing problems, injury to the facet joints, dislocation, or even tumors.[6] Patients commonly awaken complaining of a "crick" or pain in the neck, and they may relate the condition to "sleeping in a draft" or a similar circumstance. More commonly, the real cause is poor neck position for several hours. The pain is unilateral; range of motion (ROM) is decreased, especially to one side; and severe pain is noted at end range on active and passive movement testing.[6] In the neutral position, resisted isometric strength is strong but may cause discomfort; however, the discomfort is not as great as that seen at the end of range of motion in active and passive movement.

Acute or acquired torticollis usually resolves on its own within 7 days to 2 weeks.[6] This type of torticollis is treated primarily with rest and heat and/or ice if the patient is seen within the first 24 hours. Muscle and joint mobilization and manipulation techniques may also be helpful, and pain-relieving modalities may be effective. The patient also should be treated with nonsteroidal anti-inflammatory drugs (NSAIDs) or muscle relaxants.

Whiplash (Acceleration Injury)

Whiplash has been recognized as a significant public health problem in industrialized countries, because it is an important cause of chronic pain disability.[7] The term *whiplash* is derived from the "whipping of a lash," indicating a quick change in direction or movement, often with a snap. The head goes through a range of motion involving flexion often combined with rotation, followed very rapidly by extension, or vice versa. Whiplash is also called a *cervical sprain* or a *cervical strain*, or an *acceleration-deceleration injury* of the neck. The extent of injury depends on the

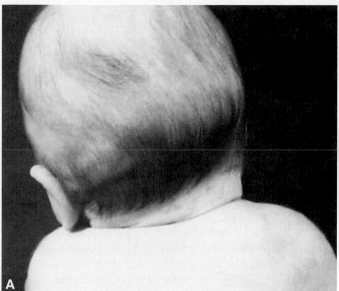
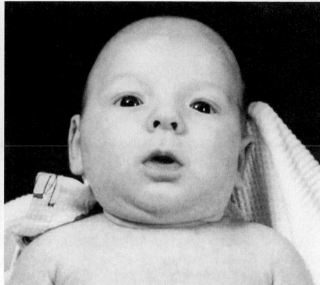
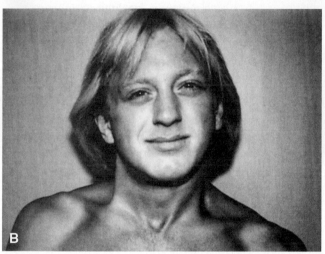

Figure 2-1

A, Congenital muscular torticollis on the left. The head is tilted to the left, and the chin is rotated to the
right. **B,** Untreated right congenital muscular torticollis in a 19-year-old man. Note the asymmetry of the
face. On the affected side, it is shortened from above downward and relatively wide from side to side.
The level of the eyes and the ears is asymmetrical. (From Canale ST: *Campbell's operative orthopaedics,*
St Louis, Mosby, 2003.)

force of impact. If the injury is caused by an automobile
accident, the position of the head at the time of impact,
whether the patient was aware of the impending collision,
and the condition of the neck tissues (e.g., effects of aging)
are all factors that affect the severity of the injury.[8-10] Seventy percent of patients with whiplash report an immediate
occurrence of symptoms, but many also report delayed
symptoms.[5,11-14] Common signs include neck pain and
headaches originating from the occipital area. If the condition is serious enough, the patient may complain of more
severe symptoms (Table 2-1).[5,15]

The Quebec Task Force on Whiplash-Associated Disorders[15] defines whiplash as "an acceleration-deceleration
mechanism of energy transfer to the neck. It may result

from rear end or side impact motor vehicle collision, but
can also occur during other mechanisms. The impact may
result in bony or soft tissue injuries to the cervical spine
(whiplash injury), which in turn may lead to a variety of
clinical manifestations called *whiplash-associated disorders*
(WADs)." Chronic WADs usually are defined as symptoms
or disabilities that persist for longer than 6 months.[15,16]
The Quebec Task Force established a system of five grades
for classifying the severity of these disorders (Table 2-2).[15]

Whiplash-associated disorders include aching or stiffness
in the neck. These symptoms usually appear within a few
hours after the accident. In some cases the patient may have
difficulty swallowing because of injury to the esophagus
and larynx. Headache is common and usually occurs in

Table 2-1
Grading System for Whiplash-Associated Disorders

Grade 1	Grade 2	Grade 3	Grade 4
Muscle strain	Muscle strain/ligament sprain	Possible disc protrusion	Cervical fracture/dislocation
Neck stiffness	Neck and/or back stiffness	Nerve root signs: Objective neurological signs (myotomes/dermatomes)	Nerve root signs: Objective neurological signs (myotomes/dermatomes)
Neck pain	Neck and/or back pain	Neck or back pain	Neck pain
Neck tenderness	Paraspinal tenderness	Restricted ROM	Restricted ROM
No physical signs	Restricted ROM	Abnormal reflexes (reduced), dermatomes, (abnormal), and myotomes (weak)	Abnormal reflexes (reduces), dermatomes (abnormal) and myotomes (weak)
Normal reflexes, dermatomes, and myotomes	Normal reflexes, dermatomes, and myotomes	Possible upper motor neuron signs	Possible upper motor neuron signs (e.g., urinary incontinence, pathological reflexes)
X-ray film: Unnecessary	X-ray film: No fracture/dislocation	X-ray film: No fracture/dislocation	X-ray film: Fracture/dislocation
Accounts for about 43% of cases	Accounts for about 29% to 56% of cases	ST scan/MRI: May show area of nerve involvement	ST scan/MRI: May show area of nerve/fracture/dislocation/spinal cord involvement
		Accounts for about 3% to 12% of cases	Accounts for about 6% of cases

Data from Spitzer WO, Skovron ML, Salmi LR et al: Scientific monograph of the Quebec Task Force on Whiplash-Associated Disorders: redefining "whiplash" and its management, *Spine* 20:1S-73S, 1995.

Table 2-2
Quebec Task Force Classification of the Severity of Whiplash-Associated Disorders

Grade	Clinical Presentation
0	No neck symptoms, no physical signs
1	No physical signs except neck pain, stiffness, or tenderness only
2	Neck symptoms and musculoskeletal signs, such as decreased range of motion and point tenderness
3	Neck symptoms and neurological signs, such as decreased or absent deep tendon reflexes, weakness, and sensory deficits
4	Neck symptoms and fracture or dislocation

From Spitzer WO, Skovron ML, Salmi LR et al: Scientific monograph of the Quebec Task Force on Whiplash-Associated Disorders: redefining "whiplash" and its management, *Spine* 20:8S-58S, 1995.

the occipital area, but it may also radiate to the vertex of the skull or the temples. In some cases the pain may be retro-ocular. The pain may also be referred into the interscapular area, the chest, and the shoulders. The head commonly is held in flexion (with a loss of the lordotic curvature) as a result of muscle spasm, and range of motion, especially side flexion or rotation, is limited. In some cases the person may suffer a concussion during the accident, leading to loss of consciousness, amnesia, nausea, vomiting, and cognitive dysfunction. Older patients because of pre-existing degenerative changes and those who have a psychosocial response to the injury tend to have a poor prognosis. Symptoms associated with any pre-existing degenerative changes seem to come on faster after an accident.[17] Some studies indicate that even minor trauma, such as low-velocity collisions, can lead to prolonged symptoms.[18]

Rear end impact (i.e., acceleration type) injuries tend to cause the greatest disability from the whiplash mechanism, primarily because the victim is unaware of the impending impact. Impact from behind causes the lower portion of the body to move forward abruptly while the head momentarily remains in place. The head then arches backward through a path of extension because it is heavy and suspended on a thin, flexible support (the cervical spine). This quick movement catches the protective muscle reflex unprepared; consequently, the limiting influence of the ligaments is exceeded, resulting in hyperextension, especially if the head is not stopped by a headrest. Backward shearing may also occur in the cervical spine, possibly resulting in spinal cord damage from subluxation or fracture of the vertical body.[19] The hyperextension is followed by a protective flexor muscle contraction that causes a rebound, combined with compression that pulls the head forward from its hyperextended position; the result is compressive hyperflexion, which may stress the intervertebral disc and posterior structures.

The position of the head at the time of impact affects ROM and the severity of injury. Normal extension is about 70°, but extension is decreased when the head is rotated 45°. Therefore head rotation can increase the probability and severity of cervical injury because of the decrease in available range of motion.

In front end impact (i.e., deceleration type) injuries, the body moves forward and then comes to a sudden stop. Actually, the lower body stops, but the head, because of its weight, continues forward as a result of inertia. The impact is abrupt, may be unexpected, or overpowers the extensor mechanism, resulting in hyperflexion. Movement of the head is stopped by the chin hitting the chest wall. A rebound then occurs, causing hyperextension as a result of reflexive contraction of the extensor muscles.

A third type of whiplash mechanism is a rotation injury. For example, people with long hair can cause a rotational sprain of the ligaments or muscles, or possibly damage the facet joint, by whipping the head around to get the hair out of their eyes.

The influence of crash-related factors on outcome is the subject of debate. Some studies have found a relationship between factors,[20] whereas others have reported that crash-related factors were not important predictors of poor outcome.[7] The evidence is not conclusive in this matter. Higher intensity neck pain and headache, as well as radicular symptoms and signs, have been strongly associated with delayed recovery.[21,22] Cassidy et al.[7] reported that patients who consulted a medical physician and a physical therapist or a medical physician and a chiropractor took longer to recover than those who did not seek a health care provider. These findings were corroborated by Gun et al.[17] No explanation was given for the difference, except that people in greater pain and discomfort would be more likely to seek help.

Although efforts have been made to classify and define WADs, the descriptive validity of the WADs classifications has been questioned because the two primary symptoms used to describe these conditions are nonspecific and prevalent in the general population.[2,23-25] Nederhand et al.[26] concluded that cervical muscle dysfunction is not specific to patients with grade 2 WAD and that it appears to be a general sign of chronic pain. These findings do not support the validity of the WADs categories described by the Quebec Task Force.

In some cases the same mechanism of injury that occurs with whiplash, if assisted by contact with the nonyielding surface, can lead to more severe cervical injuries, such as dislocation or fracture of a cervical vertebra, or a combination of these two injuries. The result can be neurological damage and paralysis. This might occur in an individual who falls forward, striking the chin, face, or forehead against an object, causing forceful hyperextension or backward thrust of the neck; or an individual who falls backward, striking the head, causing forceful hyperflexion or forward thrust of the neck. Another example is an individual who dives into shallow water, striking the head, causing forceful hyperflexion and compression of the cervical spine. Similar injury patterns can occur in football with spearing or in hockey when players are checked headfirst into the boards.

According to Stovner[16] and Freeman,[27] the estimated proportion of patients who report pain and disability 6 months after an accident ranges from 19% to 60%, and the percentage of patients who are absent from work after 6 months is 9% to 26%.[15,20] The natural course of whiplash disorders is unknown; however, some prognostic factors have been described to distinguish between patients who are expected to experience either a normal or a delayed recovery. According to Stovner,[16] a causal link between trauma and chronic symptoms is not conclusive. Litigation issues have been related to the chronicity of symptoms. In countries where litigation appears to play a role in recovery, the disability of WADs is prolonged, and in countries where litigation is absent, the prevalence of chronic whiplash syndrome is low or nonexistent.[7]

It has been reported that long-term neck symptoms do not occur in any higher proportion in whiplash patients than in the general population.[24,28] However, 15% to 40% of whiplash patients may report persistent headaches and neck pain.[11]

Clinicians can help patients understand the effect of the injury and reduce the impact of any disability by explaining the prognostic factors associated with these injuries. According to Scholten-Peeters et al.,[29] the physical prognostic factors associated with delayed recovery in WADs are decreased mobility of the cervical spine immediately after injury, pre-existing neck trauma, older age, and female gender. Some psychological factors (e.g., inadequate cognition, fear avoidance beliefs, catastrophizing, maladaptive coping strategies, depression, and anxiety) have been found to be related to delayed recovery in WADs, much as they have been in other pain conditions, such as low back pain.[17] More research is needed to develop a prognostic patient profile consisting of factors that predict outcome in whiplash patients.[29] Gun[17] and others[30] found that patients who consulted a lawyer had a worse Neck Pain Outcome Score (NPOS); also, after 1 year, these patients had a sevenfold greater chance of still receiving treatment and a sevenfold lesser chance of claim settlement. For individuals with a history of a previous motor vehicle accident claim, improvement after 1 year in the NPOS was 10 points lower, and improvement on the Visual Analogue Scale (VAS) was 1 point lower.

Factors Associated with Delayed Recovery in Whiplash-Associated Disorders

- Decrease in cervical spine mobility immediately after injury
- Pre-existing neck trauma
- Older age
- Female gender
- Psychological factors
- Pending litigation

According to a systematic review of prognostic factors in whiplash by Cote et al.,[21] reliable information on whiplash is still scarce, and the methodological quality of studies needs to be improved. Based on the reviewed studies, these researchers concluded that consistent evidence indicated that older age and female gender were associated with delayed recovery from whiplash. No consistent evidence was found for marital status, number of dependents, income, work activities, or education as predictors of recovery. No strong evidence associated a past history of headaches or neck pain with recovery. The studies that have reported these associations lacked control of the confounders.

Cote et al.[21] also found that compensation or litigation issues could have an influence on claimants' behavior and recovery. The differences in the rating of prolonged symptoms between systems with and without compensation raises questions about the real incidence of chronic WADs.[16]

A complete history of the whiplash patient should be taken. This should include details about specific symptoms (especially those related to cognitive, sympathetic, cranial nerve and vascular dysfunction), pre-existing symptoms, disabilities, participation problems, accident-specific information (e.g., velocity of the car, type of collision), recovery time, previous diagnostic tests and procedures, success of treatment (medical or other), attitude, cognition, present severity of symptoms, psychosocial issues, and medications used. This information can indicate the degree of compromise suffered by the patient and how the WADs affect the person's life. Some assessment tools are available for evaluating pain (VAS) and neck disability (Neck Disability Index) (see *Orthopedic Physical Assessment*, volume 1 of this series).

A study by Nederhand[31] demonstrated that patients with grade 2 WADs had higher activity of the upper trapezius than healthy controls and also that they were unable to relax these muscles after a dynamic task. These findings indicated that patients with grade 2 WADs exhibited abnormal muscle activation in situations in which no biomechanical demand for the activation existed. One of the symptoms described in the Quebec Task Force's WADs classification system[14,15] coincides with the description of "musculoskeletal signs." Nederhand et al.[31] considered the criteria used to determine musculoskeletal signs (e.g., the presence of "point tenderness" and "muscle spasm") to be inaccurate, because assessment commonly is done in the sitting or standing position, which results in only small differences in electromyography (EMG) levels between patients and controls. According to these authors, surface EMG may be a useful tool for differentiating patients with grade 2 WADs, because it helps determine the hyperactivity of the cervical muscles.

Cervical Spondylosis

Cervical spondylosis is an age-related, degenerative condition sometimes referred to as *cervical arthritis, segmental instability, hypertrophic arthritis, degenerative spondylosis,* *cervical arthrosis,* or *degenerative disease.*[3] It has both an inflammatory component and a degenerative component, which eventually lead to arthritis of the cervical spine. The term *cervical spondylosis* implies a loss of mechanical integrity of a cervical intervertebral disc, leading to instability of the affected segment and, later on, nerve root or cord compression symptoms caused by stenosis either in the intervertebral foramen or the spinal canal (Table 2-3).[32] Although spondylosis appears most obviously in the cervical spine because of its mobility, it may occur in other areas of the spine, especially the lower lumbar spine. The condition begins with intervertebral disc degeneration, which can occur as a result of damage to the disc or poor nutrition. A state of poor nutrition may result from changes at the cartilaginous end plate between the disc and the vertebral body, resulting in lack of nutritional interchange.

Synonyms for Spondylosis

- (Cervical)* disc disease/degeneration
- Segmental instability
- Hypertrophic arthritis
- Degenerative spondylosis
- (Cervical)* arthrosis

*Also occurs in other areas of the spine

As the disc degenerates and loses bulk, a reduction of the mucopolysaccharides in the nucleus pulposus occurs, leading to an increase in collagen in the nucleus pulposus. These changes result in the loss of turgor in the disc[33,34] and a loss in the disc's ability to resist compressive forces. In time the annulus, because it starts to act like an underinflated tire, begins to protrude beyond the margins of the vertebral body. This results in a loss in the buffer qualities of the nucleus pulposus. Shock absorption is no longer spread or absorbed evenly by the annulus or the cartilaginous end plate. The increased mobility (because of the "underinflated tire" of the disc) leads to greater shearing, rotation, and traction stress on the disc and adjacent vertebra. The result of these actions is approximation of the vertebral bodies and loss of the normal lordotic curvature in the cervical spine. In addition, the pedicles begin to approximate, resulting in an overriding or subluxation of the facet joints, which leads to approximation of the lamina. This, in turn, can lead to possible infolding of the ligamentum flava, especially when the cervical spine is in the neutral position or extension, along with degeneration of the joints of von Luschka. These changes subsequently lead to decreased range of motion, shortening of the cervical spine, and loss of spinal stiffness.[34,35]

As previously stated, as the disc degenerates, the nucleus pulposus begins to lose its turgor, and its gel-like tissue, which normally is under pressure, begins to fibrose and take on an appearance similar to the annulus. The disc also

Table 2-3
Assessment of Aging and Degeneration of the Human Intervertebral Disc

Disc Grade	Nucleus Pulposus	Annulus Fibrosus	End Plate	Vertebral Body
Assessment by Gross Morphology*				
I	Gel-like, bulging; blue-white	Discrete lamellae; white	Hyaline; uniform thickness	Margins rounded
II	Fibrous tissue band extending from the annulus fibrosus	Chondroid or mucinous material between lamellae	Irregular thickness of cartilage	Margins pointed
III	Consolidation of fibrous tissue	Extensive chondroid or mucinous material; loss of annulus-nucleus demarcation	Focal defects in cartilage	Early chondrophytes or osteophytes at margins
IV	Horizontal clefts parallel to end plate	Focal disruptions	Fibrocartilaginous tissue extending from subchondral bone; irregularity and focal sclerosis of subchondral bone	Osteophytes <2 mm
V	Clefts extending throughout	Clefts extending throughout	Diffuse sclerosis	Osteophytes <2 mm
Assessment of Magnetic Resonance Imaging Findings†				
I	Homogeneous; bright; demarcation distinct	Homogeneous; dark gray	Single dark line	Margins rounded
II	Horizontal dark bands extend across the annulus fibrosus centrally	Areas of increased signal intensity	Increase in central concavity	Tapering of margins
III	Signal intensity diminished; gray tone with dark and bright stippling	Indistinguishable from nucleus pulposus	Line less distinct	Small dark projections from margins
IV	Proportion of gray signal reduced; bright and dark regions larger	Indistinguishable from nucleus pulposus; some bright and dark signals contiguous with nucleus pulposus and annulus fibrosis	Focal defects in line	Projections <2 mm with same intensity as marrow
V	Gross loss of disc height; bright and dark signals dominant	Signals contiguous with nucleus pulposus	Defects and areas of thickening	Projections <2 mm with same intensity as marrow

From Frymoyer JW, Gordon SL: *New perspectives on low back pain*, p 193, Park Ridge, IL, 1989, American Academy of Orthopedic Surgeons.
*Based on data from Vernon-Roberts B: The pathology and interrelation of intervertebral disc lesions, osteoarthritis of the apophyseal joints, lumbar spondylosis and low back pain. In Jayson MIV, editor: *The lumbar spine and back pain*, ed 2, pp 83-114, London, 1980, Pitman Medical Publishers.
†Using T2-weighted spin-echo images. TR 2000 msec and TE 90 msec.

begins to lose height, causing slight overriding of the zygapophyseal joint articular surfaces; this in turn leads to translational instability (i.e., loss of arthrokinematic control). Over time, this instability leads to the formation of protective osteophytes and limitation of movement.[34,36] Radiological evidence shows that these changes are found in 60% of patients over age 45 and 85% of those over age 65, even if symptoms are not present.[34,36] In the cervical spine, the areas most commonly and most severely affected are C5-6 and C6-7.[3] If symptoms are going to develop, they tend to appear between 35 and 55 years of age.

Kirkaldy-Willis[35] divided spondylosis into three stages: the dysfunctional stage, the unstable stage, and the stabilization stage. Although he developed these stages for the lumbar spine, they are equally applicable to any area of the spine. Based on Kirkaldy-Willis's description, these stages begin when the patient complains of symptoms. However, the condition begins long before symptoms are evident. Initially spondylosis develops silently and is asymptomatic.[6]

In the **dysfunctional stage,**[35] the patient complains of nonspecific neck pain with localized tenderness (Table 2-4). On radiographical examination, the disc degeneration is

Table 2-4

Signs, Symptoms, and Radiological Changes in the Dysfunctional Stage of Spondylosis

Signs	Symptoms	Radiological Changes

Local tenderness
Muscle contraction
Hypomobility
Pain on extension
Neurological exam
  usually normal
	Low back pain:
	• Often
	  localized
	• Sometimes
	  referred
	Pain with
	  movement
		Abnormal
		  decreased
		  movement
		Malalignment of
		  spinous processes
		Irregular facets
		Early disc changes

From Kirkaldy-Willis WH: *Managing low back pain,* p 79, New York, 1983, Churchill Livingstone.

obvious, as seen in the loss of height and the bulging of the annulus beyond the vertebral margins. Abnormal function of the facet joints (subluxation caused by disc degeneration) and synovitis may occur, along with protective muscle spasm, although this subluxation is seldom seen on x-ray films. Side flexion or rotation commonly is limited or stiff and painful, especially to one side. The same is true for cervical extension. A neurological examination at this stage frequently is negative. In some cases symptoms may be attributed to a recent injury, such as a car accident, when in fact they already were present, even though the patient did not complain of symptoms.

The **unstable stage**[35] is marked by increased zygapophyseal or facet capsular laxity (Table 2-5). An abnormal "spinal rhythm" or "instability jog" (a flickering of the skin over the spine during movements) may become evident. This instability jog is an indication of lack of arthrokinematic motion control (i.e., a motor control deficit exists) as the patient moves the neck and head. The disc continues to

degenerate and in some cases may herniate, and more bulging can occur in unstable stages and lead to hypermobility. This leads to segmental hypermobility (translational instability). Progressive degeneration of the facet joints is seen, which may lead to facet joint syndrome. Radicular pain also may be seen, because the lateral nerve roots can become trapped in the intervertebral foramen.[37] Traction spurs (usually found anteriorly) sometimes are seen on radiological examination.[38] Traction spurs are caused by abnormal stresses on the outermost attachments of the annulus and are thought to be related to the excessive mobility caused by the degenerative disc.[32,36] Traction spurs generally are seen 2-3 mm from the discal edge of the vertical body and project horizontally.

Traction spurs are not true claw, or marginal, osteophytes, which occur at the edge of the vertebral body (Figure 2-2). A claw osteophyte is commonly related to loss of disc height and annular bulging, which lifts the periosteum from the vertebral edge, causing new bone to be laid down. A claw osteophyte or spur may also hook over the disc at the discal margin. Osteophytes are a physiological response to a compression load that reflects the body's attempts to stabilize the spine.[39]

With disc degeneration in the cervical spine, the joints of von Luschka are approximated, leading to a third location of osteophyte formation. Intraforaminal osteophytes encroach on the intervertebral foramen and possibly the vertebral artery, resulting in neurological symptoms and an increased possibility of vertebral artery syndrome. The anterior spinal artery may thicken, leading to vascular insufficiency, or compression of the nutrient vessels may occur. Silberstein[40] contends that the joints of von Luschka are actually formed by this degeneration and rubbing and that they are not true synovial joints. Intraforaminal osteophytes limit movement and eventually stabilize the joint containing the fragmented disc.

Table 2-5

Signs, Symptoms, and Radiological Changes in the Unstable Stage of Spondylosis

Signs	Symptoms	Radiological Changes

Detection of abnormal movement
  (inspection, palpation)
Observation of "catch" in the back
  (on movement)
Pain on coming to standing position
  after flexion
	Symptoms of dysfunction
	Giving way of back (i.e., "catch"
	  in back on movement)
	Pain on coming to standing
	  position after flexion
		Anteroposterior:
		• Lateral shift
		• Rotation
		• Abnormal tilt
		• Malaligned spinous processes
		Oblique:
		• Opening of the facets
		Lateral:
		• Spondylolisthesis (in flexion)
		• Retrospondylolisthesis (in extension)
		• Narrowing of the foramen (in extension)
		• Abnormal opening of the disc
		• Abrupt change in pedicle height
		CT changes

From Kirkaldy-Willis WH: *Managing low back pain*, p 81, New York, Churchill-Livingstone, 1983.

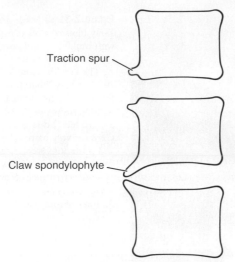

Traction spur

Claw spondylophyte

Figure 2-2

A traction spur projects horizontally from the vertebral body about 1 mm from the discal border. Traction spurs are indicators of segmental instability. The common claw spondylophyte, on the other hand, extends from the rim of the vertebral body and curves as it grows around the bulging intervertebral disc. Claw spondylophyte are associated with disc degeneration; they are *not* radiological manifestations of osteoarthritis. (Redrawn from Macnab I: *Backache*, p 4, Baltimore, 1977, Williams & Wilkins.)

In the unstable stage, patients complain primarily of neck dysfunction (see Table 2-5). They also commonly complain of a "catch" or sudden pain in the neck in part of the range of motion during movement.[35] Greater restriction of movement is seen in this stage than in the dysfunctional stage, as well as uncoordinated movement (abnormal movement patterns) caused by dysfunction of the functional spinal unit (i.e., the disc and two apophyseal joints). Circumferential tears of the annulus fibrosus and radial tears extending from the annulus fibrosus to the nucleus pulposus may also be seen in this stage.

In the final stage, or **stabilization stage,**[35] fibrosis of the facet joints occurs, along with even greater disc degeneration and osteophyte formation (Table 2-6). Osteophytes form along the edges of the facet joints, leading to enlarged facets. Lateral nerve root entrapment becomes more common in this stage, leading to radicular signs and lateral stenosis in the intervertebral foramen. At the same time, osteoarthritis of the facet joints becomes more obvious.

Narrowing of the degenerating disc through the different stages of spondylosis can lead to anterior impingement by the uncovertebral spurs, anterior impingement by the annular bulging, and posterior impingement by the osteophytes of the facet joints and fibrosis of the epidural nerve sleeves.[36,37] Facet joint degeneration leads to erosion of the joint cartilage and lipping around the joint edge, with formation of facet osteophytes. The synovial membrane thickens, and this, combined with the formation of facet osteophytes, leads to a decrease in the size of the intervertebral foramen and a greater possibility of radicular signs and

Table 2-6

Signs, Symptoms, and Radiological Changes in the Stabilization Stage of Spondylosis

Signs	Symptoms	Radiological Changes
Muscle tenderness	Low back pain	Enlarged facets
Stiffness	of decreasing	Loss of disc height
Reduced movement	severity	Osteophytes
Scoliosis		Small foramina
		Reduced movement
		Scoliosis

From Kirkaldy-Willis WH: *Managing low back pain*, p 86, New York, 1983, Churchill Livingstone.

symptoms. Nerve root fibrosis may also result from disc degeneration, leading to inflammatory changes, rubbing of the nerve root and sheath against the rough pedicles during movement, or injury to the nerve root. The cartilaginous end plate of the vertebral body degenerates throughout the development of spondylosis, showing thinning, fibrillation, and fissuring. The fissuring may extend the whole thickness of the end plate, and granulation tissue may grow through into the disc, adding to the fibrosis of the disc.[35]

The signs and symptoms of cervical spondylosis are mainly pain, restriction of motion and, in later stages, radicular signs. In some cases the spinal cord or anterior spinal vessels may be compressed, leading to myelopathic symptoms.[41] The pain may be vague or ill defined, or it may be a dull, aching pain that increases over time and then tends to be referred to the shoulder or arm rather than the neck. Pain tends to be accentuated by movement and more often is evident toward end range. Radicular pain is referred into the appropriate dermatome initially, and the myotomes are affected later. Radiographical examination shows narrowing of one or more of the intervertebral discs and osteophyte spurring and irregularity, along with sclerosis of the vertebral body.[35,42]

Cervical Osteoarthritis

Osteoarthritis (OA) in the cervical spine is, in effect, the later stage of spondylosis, marked by progressive degeneration of the intervertebral disc and especially the zygapophyseal joints (trijoint complex). Although the condition commonly is silent and asymptomatic, osteoarthritic changes can include osteophyte formation, hypertrophy of the synovial membrane and, in some cases, a chronic inflammatory response (Figure 2-3). OA involves the zygapophyseal joints, which show degeneration of the articular surfaces and increased stiffness of the subchondral bone.[6] These changes lead to a decrease in the intervertebral disc space, osteophyte encroachment into the intervertebral foramen, hypertrophy

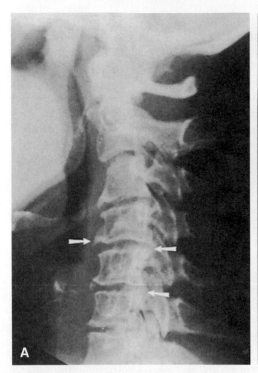
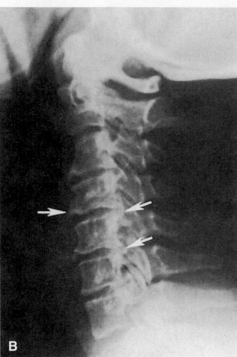

Figure 2-3

X-ray films of a 68-year-old man with multiple radiological signs of cervical osteoarthritis *(arrows).* **A,** The cervical spine in flexion, which is very limited. Note that the atlas tips up, compared with the one shown in **B.** All intervertebral disc spaces below C2-3 are very narrow, and anterior and posterior osteophytes are apparent *(arrows).* The spine extends very little in **B** and is quite straight in **A** (i.e., no significant flexion). (From Bland JH: *Disorders of the cervical spine,* p 213, Philadelphia, 1994, WB Saunders.)

of soft tissue (e.g., the ligamentum flava) and, in some cases, encroachment on the spinal cord or vertebral artery.

Because of the structures involved and their proximity to the spinal cord, nerve roots, peripheral nerves (especially the sinu vertebral nerve) and, in some cases, components of the autonomic system, symptoms can vary widely. They can range from relatively benign effects (e.g., limited range of motion with minimal pain) to more severe symptoms involving the spinal cord (myelopathy), nerve roots (painful radiculopathy, sometimes without a predictable pattern), severe pain and muscle spasms and, in some cases, autonomic and brain stem responses.[6] Symptoms commonly are aggravated by movement.

Cervical Spine Instability

According to Olson and Joder,[43] Hesinger,[44] Aspinall,[45] and Derrick and Chesworth,[46] loss of cervical spine stability may be a significant factor in neck pain in many cases. Cervical instability has not been fully defined, and many of the concepts used to describe it are extrapolated from work done on the lumbar region.[47] Panjabi defined clinical stability as "the ability of the spine, under physiological loads, to limit patterns of displacement so as not to damage or irritate the spinal cord or nerve roots, and, in addition, to prevent incapacitating deformity or pain due to structural changes."[48] When the cervical spine demonstrates instability, failure to maintain correct vertebral alignment

has occurred,[49] a result either of bony changes or of neuromuscular pathology.

According to Norris, the essential feature of stability is "the ability of the body to control the whole range of motion of a joint."[50] Therefore the limits of the stability should provide sufficient support yet allow for the flexibility of normal activities.[51-55]

Clinical instability of the spine occurs when the neutral zone increases relative to the total range of motion (Figure 2-4). The neutral zone has been shown to increase with intersegmental injury and intervertebral disc degeneration (see Cervical Spondylosis)[53,56-58] and to be decreased by the activation of the stabilizing muscle forces across the motion segment. Degeneration and mechanical injury of the cervical stabilization components (e.g., discs, ligaments, and muscles) are the primary causes of increases in the neutral zone.[59]

Cervical instability can occur secondary to trauma, surgery, systemic disease, or tumors. However, most patients diagnosed with cervical instability suffer from degenerative changes to the motion segment. Niere and Torney defined minor cervical instability as "an increase in the neutral zone associated with one or more segments within the cervical spine. This condition may be associated with a number of signs and symptoms but does not include severe incapacitating pain nor symptoms indicative of spinal cord compression or vertebral artery disruption."[60] It has been proposed that cervical instability may exist where pain and

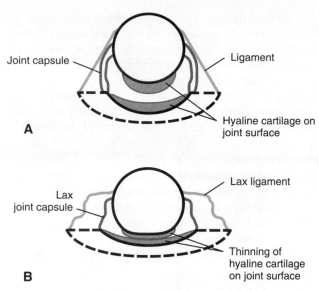

A

Joint capsule

Ligament

Hyaline cartilage on joint surface

Lax joint capsule

Lax ligament

Thinning of hyaline cartilage on joint surface

B

Figure 2-4

Articular instability. **A,** Normal joint with normal stability. Glides and nonphysiological mobility are limited by the joint surfaces and tension in the ligaments and joint capsules. **B,** Degenerative joint with articular instability. Note that the degeneration permits the bone ends to move closer to each other and thereby slacken off the capsule and ligaments. This allows increased nonphysiological motion on stability testing with a normal end feel. Glides and nonphysiological mobility are less limited by the flattened joint surfaces and slackened ligaments and joint capsules. (From Magee DJ, Zachazewski JE, Quillen WS: *Scientific foundations and principles of practice in musculoskeletal rehabilitation,* p 516, St Louis, 2007, Mosby.)

disability occur as a result of lack of control of the neutral zone motion, without compromise of the vascular or neural structures.[60] Minor cervical instability can be demonstrated only through clinical features that make the diagnosis more difficult (Table 2-7).[60]

Unfortunately, there is no gold standard for diagnosing minor cervical instability, nor even an accepted set of associated clinical signs and symptoms.[60] As signs of minor

cervical instability, clinicians have described radiological evidence of traction spurs and hypermobility, anterolisthesis, and clinical signs similar to those seen in Kirkaldy-Willis's unstable phase of cervical spondylosis.[60] Poor motor control has been recognized as a major component of clinical instability.[60] Studies on the lumbar spine have demonstrated that this alteration in motor control can be a factor in the development of lumbar instability.[61-65] Some have hypothesized that aberrant motion (i.e., an instability jog), which is seen with sudden acceleration or deceleration that occurs outside the intended plane of movement in the midranges of active cervical movement, is a cardinal sign of instability.[66]

Other signs of clinical instability are reported to be general tenderness in the cervical region, referred pain to the shoulder and parascapular area, cervical radiculopathy, cervical myelopathy, occipital and frontal or retro-orbital headaches, paraspinal muscle spasm, decreased cervical lordosis, and pain with sustained postures.[43,67] According to Niere and Torney[60] and Swinkels et al.,[68] clinical findings associated with cervical instability include neck pain; complaints of catching or locking in the neck; weakness; altered range of motion; a history of major trauma or repetitive microtrauma; neck pain and headaches that are provoked by a sustained weight-bearing posture (e.g., sitting) and relieved by non-weight-bearing postures (e.g., lying supine); hypermobility with a soft end feel during passive intervertebral motion testing; and poor cervical muscle strength (e.g., the multifidus, longus colli, and longus capitis).[60] Shaking and poorly controlled (aberrant) motion during active cervical range of motion also have been mentioned.[43] According to Paris,[69] instability exists only when an aberrant motion, such as a visible slip, catch, or shaking, occurs (i.e., an instability jog) or when a palpable difference in bony position can be noted between standing and lying down. Poor motor control and an inability to initiate co-contraction of the local muscle system in the neutral zone have been observed in many patients.[64]

Table 2-7
Signs and Symptoms of Minor Clinical Cervical Instability

Main Signs and Symptoms	Secondary Signs and Symptoms	Other Signs and Symptoms
History of major trauma	History of repeated microtrauma	Apprehension when moving into neck extension
Catching/locking/giving way	Neck weakness (subjective)	Feeling of "heavy head"
Poor muscular control	Traction spurs	Feeling as if the head is dropping off
Excessively free end feel on palpation	Altered range of motion	Episodes with no precipitating cause
Signs of hypomobility on x-ray film	Neck pain	Crepitus
	Muscle spasms	Feeling of a lump in the throat
Unpredictability of symptoms	Muscular atrophy	Difficulty returning from extension
Spondylolisthesis	Headaches	Poor response to previous treatment
		Good response to stabilizing treatment
		Shoulder girdle weakness and atrophy

Modified from Niere KR, Torney SK: Clinicians' perceptions of minor cervical instability, *Man Ther* 9:144-150, 2004; and Cook C, Brismée JM, Fleming R, Sizer PS: Identifiers suggestive of clinical cervical spine instability: a Delphi study of physical therapists, *Phys Ther* 85(9):895-906, 2005.

Generally, patients with cervical instability develop compensatory movements to stabilize the motion segment. Because the patient does not have good control of deep spinal muscles (e.g., the multifidus, intertransversarii, and longissimus), the body tries to recruit global muscles to maintain segmental stability. This action also has been seen in patients with neck pain and whiplash.[67,70-72] Tables 2-8 and 2-9 present summaries of the variables and factors related to minor cervical instability as described by Niere and Torney.

The lack of specific or sensitive diagnostic tools complicates the diagnosis of cervical instability. O'Sullivan[64] maintains that radiological evidence of intersegmental motion of a single motion segment is significant only if this finding is supported by clinical evidence of segmental instability at the corresponding segmental level. The diagnosis still relies on clinical findings: history, subjective complaints, visual analysis of the active motion quality, and manual examination.[43]

Upper cervical instability is a controversial topic, and the literature lacks consensus on its clinical aspects.[68] However, instability in the upper cervical spine is a major concern for clinicians, because inappropriate treatment in this area can have severe consequences (i.e., paralysis or death).[73,74] According to Swinkels and Oostendorp,[75] upper cervical instability should be considered a special subcategory of general cervical instability because it is doubtful whether upper cervical instability occurs in patients without an inflammatory process (e.g., rheumatoid arthritis) or congenital problems (e.g., Down's syndrome). In fact, atlantoaxial instability and hypermobility occur more frequently and most clearly in patients with rheumatoid arthritis, and in most cases without neurological signs.[75] Muscle action compensation could be argued to be a response of upper cervical instability without symptoms.

Table 2-8
Frequency of Response of Clinicians in Each Category for Cervical Clinical Stability

Finding	No Importance		Minor Importance		Somewhat Important		Very Important		Vitally Important		% Responses of Very or Vitally Important
	N	%	N	%	N	%	N	%	N	%	%
History of major trauma	0	0	5	4	36	25	70	48	33	23	71
Catching/locking/giving way	1	1	13	9	29	20	66	46	34	24	70
Poor motor control	0	0	16	11	34	24	69	48	24	17	65
Excessively free end feel on palpation	4	3	8	6	40	28	63	44	27	19	63
Signs of hypomobility on x-ray film	3	2	16	11	34	24	56	39	34	24	63
Unpredictability of symptoms	1	1	16	11	46	32	63	44	16	11	56
Spondylolisthesis	7	5	21	15	43	30	50	35	21	15	50
History of repeated trauma	4	3	22	15	46	32	58	40	13	9	49
Neck weakness (subjective)	3	2	20	14	63	44	46	32	11	8	40
Traction spurs	11	8	26	18	59	41	36	25	11	8	33
Altered range of motion	8	6	48	33	45	31	36	25	7	5	30
Neck pain	10	7	36	25	56	39	34	24	7	5	29
Muscle spasm	4	3	46	32	61	42	27	19	5	4	23
Muscular atrophy	14	10	56	39	50	35	17	12	7	5	17
Headaches	16	11	62	43	45	31	19	13	1	1	14

From Niere KR, Torney SK: Clinicians' perceptions of minor cervical instability, *Man Ther* 9(3):144-150, 2004.

Table 2-9
Factors Related to Cervical Instability

Passive Dysfunction	Active Dysfunction	Cervical Pattern	Movement Abnormality
Traction spurs Signs of hypomobility on x-ray films Spondylolisthesis History of repeated microtrauma History of major trauma	Poor motor control Neck weakness (subjective) Unpredictability of symptoms Catching/locking/giving way, as well as muscular atrophy	Headaches Neck pain Muscle spasm Muscular atrophy	Excessively free end feel on palpation Altered range of motion History of major trauma

From Niere KR, Torney SK: Clinicians' perceptions of minor cervical instability, *Man Ther* 9(3):144-150, 2004.

Table 2-10
Signs and Symptoms of Upper Cervical Instability

Neurological Signs	Clinical Symptoms	Radiological Signs
Hyperreflexia Paraesthesia Coordination problems in walking Spasticity or pareses Hypoesthesia in the area of the occipitalis major nerve (less frequent)	Pain in the upper cervical or suboccipital areas (70%) Variable radiation to mastoid, occipital, temporal, or frontal regions Limitation of neck movement Torticollis	Atlas-Dens Interval (ADI): Adult limit: 2.5-3 mm Child limit: 4.5-5 mm

Modified from Swinkles R, Beeton K, Alltree J: Pathogenesis of upper cervical instability, *Man Ther* 1:127-132, 1996; and Swinkles RA, Oostendorp RA: Upper cervical instability: fact or fiction? *J Manip Physiol Ther* 19:185-194, 1996.

Atlantoaxial subluxation is the most common type of cervical spine instability in patients with rheumatoid arthritis, with a quoted incidence of 50% to 70%.[76] Inflammation and pannus formation in and around the transverse and alar ligaments cause the instability seen in rheumatoid arthritis. Other conditions associated with upper cervical instability are ankylosing spondylitis, psoriatic arthritis, and Reiter's syndrome.[76]

Suspicion of upper cervical instability is based on clinical signs, such as neck pain, the most common symptom (Table 2-10). Seventy percent of patients have pain in the upper cervical or suboccipital area, with variable radiation to the mastoid, occipital, temporal, or frontal region. Other signs that may be present include limitation of neck movements, torticollis (a cardinal sign in the early phase), and neurological signs (e.g., hyperreflexia, paresthesia, coordination problems when walking, and spasticity or pareses). Hypoesthesia is seen less frequently.

Upper cervical instability is commonly diagnosed using a radiological criterion known as the *Atlas-Dens Interval* (ADI).[77] A consensus meeting of the American Roentgen Ray Society[77] set the upper limit for the ADI at 2.5-3 mm for adults and 4.5-5 mm for children. X-ray examinations have some restrictions, and other concerns include standardization of techniques, faults in measurements, and problems with standards of normalization. Thus a conventional x-ray study can fail to provide adequate information about atlantoaxial stability. According to some radiographical studies, no correlation exists between the amount of atlantoaxial dislocation and the presence of neurological symptoms.[77,78] Most patients with rheumatoid arthritis tolerate atlantoaxial instability without neurological symptoms, because the spinal cord tolerates gradually applied pressure surprisingly well.[75]

Clinical tests to detect upper cervical instability, such as the lateral shift test of C1, the upper cervical flexion test, the Sharp-Purser test, the rotation test of C2 coupled with side flexion of the head, and anterior shift of the atlas compared with the dens axis,[79] are disputable, and according to Swinkels and Oostendorp,[75] no information is available about the reliability and validity of these tests. Surgical treatment for cervical instability is reserved for patients with severe neurological involvement. The objective of conservative treatment of clinical cervical instability is to increase the function of the muscular and neural systems so as to decrease the stress on the spinal segments.[49,54]

The objective of the stabilization exercises commonly incorporated into rehabilitation programs is to restore (i.e., reduce) the size of the neutral zone in order to restore the normal arthrokinematic motion that occurs when minimal forces are imposed on the spine.[76] The methods of restoring the neutral zone in rehabilitation are evident, include re-education of the neurofeedback loop system, which includes muscles, tendons, and receptors.[76]

Facet (Apophyseal or Zygapophyseal) Joint Syndrome

The posterior joints of the vertebrae have a surface area that is approximately two thirds the size of the surface area of the intervertebral disc; they also have relatively lax and richly innervated capsules, and they are covered with hyaline cartilage.[6] The joints aid stability but are not primarily weight bearing.[6] As a result of disc degeneration or trauma, the mechanical load on the facet joints can be increased. This increased load may cause a synovial reaction, cartilage fibrillation, erosion of the joint surface and, in rare cases, loose bodies. In most cases facet joint syndrome is believed to be the result of a synovial reaction that manifests itself symptomatically as muscle spasm and pain. These symptoms (pain and spasm) may be referred into specific areas, depending on the facet joint involved (Figure 2-5). This pattern of symptom referral is different from normal dermatome patterns.[80,81] Similarly, range of motion may be decreased. In some patients the condition is thought to be an early case of osteoarthritis of the facet joints.

Disc Herniation

Disc herniation can occur in the cervical spine, although it is much less common than in the lumbar spine. The

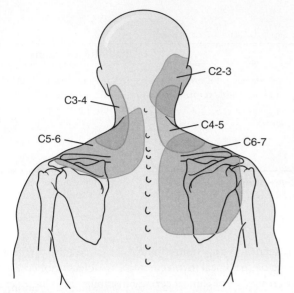

Figure 2-5
Referred pain patterns that can occur with pathology of the zygapophyseal joints. (Redrawn from Porterfield JA, DeRosa C: *Mechanical neck pain: perspective in functional anatomy,* p 104, Philadelphia, 1995, WB Saunders; modified from Dwyer A, Aprill C, Bogduk N: Cervical zygapophyseal joint pain patterns, *Spine* 15:453-457, 1990.)

Disc herniations may occur in any direction, but posterior and posterolateral herniations produce the greatest number of clinical signs and symptoms. Central posterior herniations lead to pain that radiates into the limbs bilaterally and myelopathic symptoms (Table 2-11).[3] However, because of the strength of the posterior longitudinal ligament, patients more commonly present with posterolateral protrusions that cause unilateral symptoms (radicular pain) in the upper extremity.[3] In most cases cervical disc herniations are acute, and the patient complains of pain or aching and has limited functional ROM of the cervical spine.[85] Although the pain may be referred, it does not always follow a normal dermatomal pattern because more than one nerve root tends to be involved.[85] If the upper nerve roots are involved, the patient may also complain of headaches.[85]

Spinal Stenosis

Spinal stenosis generally is an uncommon problem in the cervical spine except as a secondary (acquired) result of degeneration or trauma. However, with a developmental stenosis (present at birth) of the spinal canal, degenerative symptoms may appear sooner, because congenital spinal stenosis has been combined with the acquired spinal stenosis from spondylosis or trauma (Table 2-12).[86,87] With activities that put stress on the head, resulting in spinal compression, unilateral or bilateral neurological signs may result.[88] Spinal stenosis is diagnosed if the sagittal diameter of the spinal canal is less than 13 mm.[6] Acquired spinal stenosis may be due to disc herniation (all four types), hypertrophy of the ligamentum flava, osteophytes, an inflammatory response, or hypertrophy of the lamina or facet joints. Differential diagnosis of spinal stenosis must include elimination of other conditions (see the following sections).

condition seems particularly to affect males in their 30s, and the discs most commonly affected are those between C5-6 and C6-7.[82] Disc herniations can range from protrusion and bulging of the disc without rupture of the annulus fibrosus to sequestration of the disc, which results in discal fragments from the annulus fibrosus and nucleus pulposus outside the disc proper (Figure 2-6).[83,84] Between these two extremes are disc prolapse, in which the outermost fibers of the annulus fibrosus contain the nucleus, and disc extrusion, in which the annulus fibrosus is perforated and discal material moves into the epidural space.

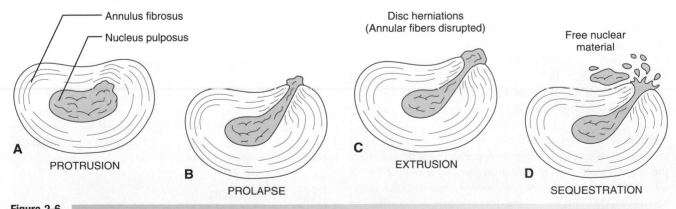

Figure 2-6
Types of disc herniations. **A,** Protrusion. **B,** Prolapse. **C,** Extrusion. **D,** Sequestration. (From Magee DJ: *Orthopedic physical assessment,* ed 4, p 471, Philadelphia, 2002. WB Saunders.)

Table 2-11

Signs and Symptoms of Motor and Sensory Changes in Cervical Myelopathy

Initial Symptoms (Predominantly Lower Limbs)	Later Symptoms (In Order of Occurrence)
Spastic paraparesis	Various combinations of upper and lower limb involvement
Stiffness and heaviness, scuffing of the toe, difficulty climbing stairs	Mixed picture of upper and lower motoneuron dysfunction
Weakness, spasms, cramps, easy fatigability	Atrophy, weakness, hypotonia, hyperreflexia to hyporeflexia, and absent deep tendon reflexes
Decreased power, especially of flexors (dorsiflexors of ankles and toes; flexors of hips)	Headache and head pain
	Neck, eye, ear, throat, or sinus pain
	Sensory symptoms in the pharynx and larynx
Hyperreflexia of knee and ankle jerks, with clonus	Paroxysmal hoarseness and aphonia
	Rotary vertigo
Positive Babinski's sign, extensor hypertonia	Tinnitus synchronous with pulse or continuous whistling noises
Decreased or absent superficial abdominal and cremasteric reflexes	Deafness
	Oculovisual changes: Blurring, photophobia, scintillating scotomata, diplopia, homonymous hemianopsia, and nystagmus
Drop foot crural monoplegia	Autonomic disturbance: Sweating, flushing, rhinorrhea, salivation, lacrimation, nausea, and vomiting
	Weakness in one or both legs, drop attacks with or without loss of consciousness
	Numbness on one or both sides of the body
	Dysphagia or dysarthria
	Myoclonic jerks
	Hiccups
	Respiratory changes: Cheyne-Stokes respiration, Biot's respiration, or ataxic respiration

Data from Bland J: *Disorders of the cervical spine: diagnosis and medical management,* Philadelphia, 1994, WB Saunders.

Differential Diagnosis of Central Spinal Stenosis

- Vascular claudication
- Diabetic neuropathy
- Other peripheral neuropathies
- Motor neuron disease
- Multiple sclerosis
- Other central nervous system lesions
- Spinal infections (acute, subacute, and chronic)
- Neoplasms (involving the cauda equina, spinal nerves, or vertebrae)

From Kirkaldy-Willis WH: *Managing low back pain,* p 103, New York, 1983, Churchill-Livingstone.

Table 2-12

Classification of Spinal Stenosis

Congenital/developmental

Acquired
  Degenerative (central, lateral, or both)
  Combined (with disc herniation, with developmental stenosis, or with both)
  After laminectomy (scarring)
  After fusion (above the fusion, beneath the fusion)
  Trauma (early and late changes)
  Paget's disease
  Fluorosis

From Kirkaldy-Willis WH: *Managing low back pain,* p 103, New York, 1983, Churchill Livingstone.

Cervical Myelopathy

In cervical myelopathy the spinal cord is compromised as a result of compressive, tensile, or torsional forces, which are caused by stenosis, spondylosis, disc herniation, or trauma.[89,90] These forces lead to compression and ischemia of the anterior and sometimes the posterior aspect of the spinal cord.[6,36] Cervical myelopathy is most commonly seen as a spinal cord "disease" after middle age.[6] The condition usually has an insidious onset, and the signs and symptoms can be quite variable.[6] These signs and symptoms may be progressive and unrelenting or intermittent and steplike. They may also be associated with multiple remissions.[89] Cervical pain and signs related to cervical movement are not common.[89] This variability of symptoms often results in confusing diagnoses; consequently, the interval between the development of initial symptoms and final diagnosis can be as long as 1.5 to 4 years.[6]

Signs and Symptoms of Sensory Changes in Cervical Myelopathy

- Headache and head pain
- Neck, eye, ear, throat, or sinus pain
- Sensory symptoms in the pharynx and larynx
- Paroxysmal hoarseness and aphonia

(Continued)

Signs and Symptoms of Sensory Changes in Cervical Myelopathy—cont'd

- Rotary vertigo
- Tinnitus synchronous with pulse or continuous whistling noises
- Deafness
- Oculovisual changes (blurring, photophobia, scintillating scotomata, diplopia, homonymous hemianopsia, and nystagmus)
- Autonomic disturbance (sweating, flushing, rhinorrhea, salivation, lacrimation, nausea, and vomiting)
- Weakness in one or both legs, drop attacks with or without loss of consciousness
- Numbness on one or both sides of the body
- Dysphagia or dysarthria
- Myoclonic jerks
- Hiccups
- Respiratory changes (Cheyne-Stokes respiration, Biot's respiration, or ataxic respiration)

From Bland J: *Disorders of the cervical spine: diagnosis and medical management,* p 216, Philadelphia, 1994, WB Saunders.

Vascular Risk Factors

- Hypertension
- Hypercholesterolemia (high cholesterol)
- Hyperlipidemia (high fat)
- Hyperhomocysteinemia (hardening of the arteries)
- Diabetes mellitus
- General clotting disorders
- Infection
- Smoking
- Direct vessel trauma
- Iatrogenic causes (surgery, medical interventions)

Data from Kerry R, Taylor AJ: Cervical arterial dysfunction assessment and manual therapy, *Man Ther* 11:243-253, 2006.

Assessing for Vascular Problems

- Risk factors
- Position testing (especially rotation and extension) for symptoms
- Cranial nerve examination
- Eye examination
- Blood pressure examination
- "Headache like no other"
- Autonomic nervous system examination

Data from Kerry R, Taylor AJ: Cervical arterial dysfunction assessment and manual therapy, *Man Ther* 11:243-253, 2006.

Vertebrobasilar Artery Insufficiency

Vertebrobasilar artery insufficiency is not a common condition. However, both it and internal carotid artery insufficiency can lead to significant problems.[6] Injury to the lining of the vessels can lead to thrombotic occlusion, artery dissection, pseudo-aneurysm, or subintimal hematoma from manipulation of the spine, overhead work, or traction.[91] Normally the vertebral artery, which supplies about 20% of the blood to the brain (the internal carotid supplies about 80%), courses cephalically through openings in the transverse processes of the cervical spine. Once past the transverse processes of C2, the course the arteries must take to enter the skull en route to the brain causes them to "kink." As a consequence of this route and because the artery is tethered at the atlanto-occipital membrane, at the C1 transverse foramin and at the C2 transverse process along with the kinking, these arteries are at risk from forces that cause excessive stress on the vessels. Excessive force or motion in rotation and extension can reduce the circulation and potentially injure the vessel lining of these arteries.[6,91,92] If this reduction in circulation with movement, which is normal, especially in rotation or extension, is combined with degenerative or other changes in the area, the circulation to the brain stem may be further compromised; this can lead to signs and symptoms of vertebrobasilar artery insufficiency (Tables 2-13 and 2-14) or internal carotid artery insufficiency (Table 2-15), resulting from ischemia of the brain stem, cerebellum, cerebrum visual cortex, and vestibular apparatus.[6,92] Injury to the vessels can lead to quadriplegia or death.[91] Although injury to the vertebral artery and internal carotid artery are rare, clinicians treating the cervical spine should always have an understanding of possible accompanying risk factors as well as what factors should be assessed when looking for vascular problems.

Barré-Liéou syndrome, also known as *posterior cervical sympathetic syndrome,* involves both the sympathetic nervous system and the vertebral artery. It causes a widespread and diverse combination of signs and symptoms.[6] Basically the symptoms are the result of compression on the posterior cervical sympathetic system and its innervation of the vertebral artery, which lies close by.

Cervical Anomalies

Although relatively rare, congenital anomalies can be found in the cervical spine. They are not usually found in isolation but are associated with other developmental skeletal defects, such as dysplasia.[6,74] Many anomalies cause no signs or symptoms and are discovered on a cervical x-ray film taken for other reasons. Some patients present with signs and symptoms later in life as degeneration contributes to the effect of the anomaly; other anomalies, although rare, may be incompatible with life.[6]

Cervical anomalies may combine bone and nerve defects.[93] Bony anomalies are of concern primarily in terms of their effect on cervical stability, especially in the upper cervical spine, as well as the narrowing (stenosis) of the spinal canal and the effect this narrowing may have on the neural structures.[74,94,95]

Table 2-13

Classic Signs and Symptoms of Vertebrobasilar Insufficiency (VBI) with Associated Neuroanatomy

Sign or Symptom	Associated Neuroanatomy
Dizziness (vertigo, giddiness, lightheadedness)	Lower vestibular nuclei (vestibular ganglion = nuclei of CN VIII vestibular branch)
Drop attacks (loss of consciousness)	Reticular formation of midbrain Rostral pons
Diplopia (amaurosis fugax; corneal reflux)	Descending spinal tract, descending sympathetic tracts (Horner's syndrome); CN V nucleus (trigeminal ganglion)
Dysarthria (speech difficulties)	CN XII nucleus (Medulla, trigeminal ganglion)
Dysphagia (+ hoarseness/hiccups)	Nucleus ambiguous of CN IX and X, Medulla
Ataxia	Inferior cerebellar peduncle
Nausea	Lower vestibular nuclei
Numbness (unilateral)	Ipsilateral face: descending spinal tract and CN V Contralateral body: ascending spinothalamic tract
Nystagmus	Lower vestibular nuclei + various other sites depending on type of nystagmus (at least 20 types)

From Kerry R, Taylor AJ: Cervical arterial dysfunction assessment and manual therapy, *Man Ther* 11:245, 2006.

Table 2-14

Presentations of Vertebral Artery Dissection

Non-Ischemic (Local) Signs and Symptoms	Ischemic Signs and Symptoms
Ipsilateral posterior neck pain/occipital headache C5-6 cervical root impairment (rare)	Hindbrain transient ischemic attack (dizziness, diplopia, dysarthria, dysphagia, drop attacks, nausea, nystagmus, facial numbness, ataxia, vomiting, hoarseness, loss of short-term memory, vagueness, hypotonia/limb weakness [arm or leg], anhidrosis [lack of facial sweating], hearing disturbances, malaise, perioral dysthesia, photophobia, papillary changes, clumsiness and agitation) Hindbrain stroke (e.g., Wallenberg's syndrome, locked-in syndrome) Cranial nerve palsies

From Kerry R, Taylor AJ: Cervical arterial dysfunction assessment and manual therapy, *Man Ther* 11:245, 2006.
Non-ischemic symptoms may precede ischemic events by a few days to several weeks.

Table 2-15

Clinical Features of Internal Carotid Artery Dissection

Non-Ischemic (Local) Signs and Symptoms	Ischemic (Cerebral or Retinal) Signs and Symptoms
Head/neck pain Horner's syndrome Pulsatile tinnitus Cranial nerve palsies (most commonly CN IX to XII) Less common local signs and symptoms include: • Ipsilateral carotid bruit • Scalp tenderness • Neck swelling • CN VI palsy • Orbital pain • Anhidrosis (facial dryness)	Transient ischemic attack (TIA) Ischemic stroke (usually middle cerebral artery territory) Retinal infarction Amaurosis fugax

Non-ischemic signs and symptoms may precede cerebral/retinal ischemia by anything from a few days to over a month.
From Kerry R, Taylor AJ: Cervical arterial dysfunction assessment and manual therapy, *Man Ther* 11:248, 2006.

As mentioned previously, Klippel-Feil syndrome (Figure 2-7) is a condition in which two or more vertebral bodies are fused, which occurs during embryological development.[96] About 50% of patients with Klippel-Feil syndrome have a low posterior hairline, limited range of motion, and an apparent short neck,[96] although some may appear normal.

Cervical ribs (Figure 2-8) are another anomaly that may be related to the cervical spine, and this condition is often grouped with a number of conditions under thoracic outlet syndrome. These anomalous ribs, which may be bony or cartilaginous, arise from the costal processes of the vertebral bodies. They usually are asymptomatic but may cause brachial plexus symptoms, especially of the lower nerve roots (C7, C8, and T1), as well as evidence of nervous or arterial compression.[6]

Cervicogenic Headache

The term *cervicogenic headache* (CEH) is used to describe a group of headaches that are thought to arise from disorders in the neck. According to Andersen et al.,[97] cervicogenic headache is a complex syndrome and its pathophysiology is far from simple. The involvement of musculoskeletal structures (nociceptive pain), sensory nerves and roots (neuropathic pain), and referred pain can be implicated. Even if no definitive damage can be found in patients with CEH, the presence of some axonal dysfunction cannot be excluded. Also, central sensitization of the central nervous system (CNS) may explain the chronicity of this syndrome.

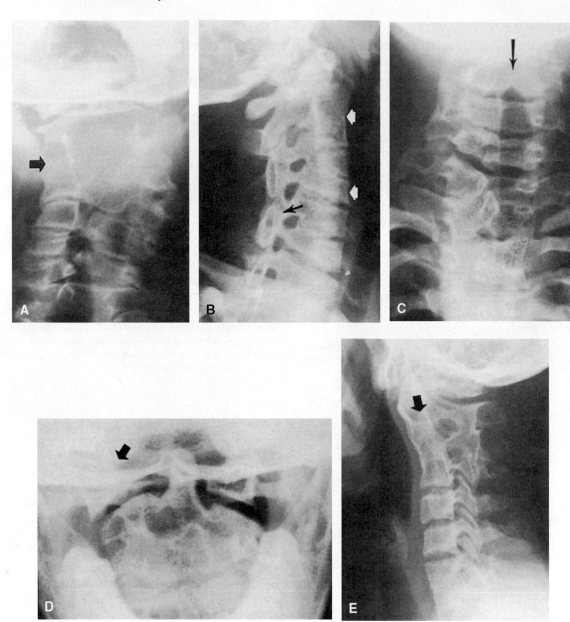

Figure 2-7

A, Anteroposterior view of the cervical spine of a 31-year-old man with Klippel-Feil syndrome shows fused C2 and C3 vertebrae *(arrow)*, a hemivertebra at C5, spina bifida, and scoliosis of the cervical spine. The patient was asymptomatic and had an incidental radiologic study for an injury. **B,** Lateral view of the cervical spine of a 12-year-old boy with Klippel-Feil syndrome shows fusion of the C2 and C3 vertebrae *(upper white arrow)* and only partial fusion with poorly developed disc spaces at C3-4, C4 to C6, and C6-7. A hemivertebra is seen at C5 *(lower white arrow)*. The zygapophyseal joint is fused at C3-4 and C5-6 *(black arrow)*. **C,** Anteroposterior view of **B** shows a butterfly vertebra (C3 and C4, *arrow*), and hemivertebrae (C7 to T1). T2 and spina bifida are seen just above the level of the first rib. In other views, a surprising amount of remodeling and osteophytosis is seen. **D,** Open-mouth view of **B** shows deviation of the odontoid process to the right, the result of having two sets of posterior elements on the left *(arrow)* and only one on the right. **E,** Lateral view of the cervical spine of a 15-year-old girl with Klippel-Feil syndrome shows fusion of the C2-3-4 vertebrae *(arrow)* and a kyphotic deformity of the cervical spine. Fusion also occurred at C7 through T3, and a hemivertebra is seen at C7. The neck was not short, and no evidence of basilar impression or occipitalization of the atlas was noted. The patient was asymptomatic. (From Bland JH: *Disorders of the cervical spine,* p 425, Philadelphia, 1994, WB Saunders.)

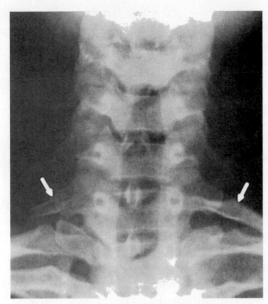

Figure 2-8
Anteroposterior view of the cervical spine of a 21-year-old man whose incidentally discovered cervical ribs became typically symptomatic after an automobile accident resulted in a neck injury *(arrows)*. (From Bland JH: *Disorders of the cervical spine,* p 427, Philadelphia, WB Saunders, 1994.)

The pathophysiological mechanisms underlying cervicogenic headache have not been clearly demonstrated, but some evidence indicates that the fundamental mechanism must be convergence.[98-100] The neuroanatomic relationship between the cervical spine and craniofacial pain is provided by the interconnection between the trigeminal nerve and the first cervical nerve roots. Studies in animals have supported this connection.[80,81,101-103] The communication

between the trigeminal nerve and the first three levels of the cervical spine is so close that they merge into a single column of gray matter, and they consequently are not differentiated anatomically, functionally, or pathologically.[104] This convergence is the foundation of referred pain in the head and upper neck. Nevertheless, the reference pattern is more common in the region innervated by the ophthalmic branch of the trigeminal nerve than in the maxillary or mandibular branches, because the maxillary and mandibular afferents in the spinal tract of the trigeminal nerve do not extend as far caudally into cervical segments as do the ophthalmic afferents.[105,106]

Another source of referred pain from the cervical spine to the head is provided by the innervation coming from the upper cervical nerves roots (Table 2-16).[105,107-109] The atlanto-occipital joint is innervated by the C1 ventral ramus and the lateral atlantoaxial joint by the C2 ventral ramus; the C2-3 zygapophyseal joints are innervated by the C3 dorsal ramus. All three nerves of the upper cervical spine intermingle at multiple segments and converge with the trigeminal afferents on cells in the dorsal grey column of the C1 to C3 segments. Because of this convergence, pain from any of the upper three cervical synovial joints could be perceived in the same region and referred to the occiput and to regions innervated by the trigeminal nerve.[109-116]

Another origin of CEH may be the dura mater; headache can occur as a result of tension and/or pressure on the dura mater. The cranial dura mater is innervated by the trigeminal, vagus, and hypoglossal nerves and the upper cervical nerves. Hack et al.[117] found that an anatomic connection existed between the rectus posterior minor muscle and the dura mater, and as a result, contraction of the rectus posterior muscle might cause tension on the dura mater,

Table 2-16
Innervation Provided by Upper Cervical Nerves (C1, C2, and C3) to Different Structures

Structures	C1	C2	C3
Tissues	Sensory information to deep suboccipital tissues Vertebral internal carotid Paramedian dura of the posterior cranial fossa	Skin of the occiput, transverse ligament of Atlas, and membrane tectoria Vertebral internal carotid Paramedium dura (through its sinuvertebral nerve itinerates)	Atlantoaxial ligaments and the dura matter of the spinal cord and clivus Vertebral internal carotid
Muscles	Sensory of cervical prevertebral muscles (longus capitis, longus cervicis, rectus capitis anterior, lateralis, ECM, and trapezius)	Major part of the upper neck muscles, splenius capitis, semispinalis capitis, and longissimus capitis	Splenius capitis, splenius cervicis, and longissimus capitis Deeper branch supplies semispinalis cervicis and multifidus Superficial branch innervates semispinalis capitis
Joints	Atlanto-occipital joint Median atlantoaxial joint	Atlantoaxial joint; through its sinuvertebral nerve innervates the median atlantoaxial joint	C2-C3 zygapophyseal joint C2-C3 disc

From Bogduk N: Cervicogenic headache: anatomic basis and pathophysiologic mechanisms, *Curr Pain Headache Rep* 5:382-386, 2001.

leading to a headache. Several cervical structures, such as the skin, the cervical muscles and their attachments, the capsules of the cervical joints, and discs, ligaments, nerves, and nerve roots, are thought to be possible origins of CEH.[109,118]

According to Pereira Monteiro,[119] the clinical limits of CEH have not yet been well defined. Cervicogenic headache is estimated to account for 15% to 20% of all chronic and recurrent headaches,[120,121] and CEH is the most common persistent symptom after neck trauma.[122,123] According to Sjaastad et al.,[123] CEH is characterized by predominantly unilateral symptoms, always on the same side, that are precipitated by neck movement or sustained neck postures or by pressure on certain tender spots in the neck. Pain, stiffness, and decreased range of motion of the neck are symptoms, and ipsilateral shoulder or arm pain may or may not be present.

From a classification standpoint, the implication of unilateral signs and symptoms in CEH is fundamental.[124-126] However, Watson and Trott[126] have reported that CEH can be bilateral with one side predominant. Side consistency is evident with CEH; this means that the side on which the signs and symptoms appear should not change with different attacks, as occurs with migraine headaches.

CEH headache typically is associated with pain in the neck or suboccipital region.[127] By definition, the pain can be mechanically provoked or intensified, and it radiates in an atypical distribution from the occipital to the frontotemporal and orbital regions. In some cases the face and ipsilateral shoulder and arm, without any definitive radicular pattern, are also affected. Nausea, vomiting, phonophobia and photophobia, and ipsilateral visual blurring may occur, as well as dizziness and difficulty swallowing.[128]

CEH can be mild, moderate, or severe in intensity, but it most commonly is moderate. It can fluctuate in intensity between headache periods and even within a single period. Lying down and resting may help, as does simple analgesia for some patients. Table 2-17 presents Sjaastad's diagnostic criteria[129,130] for cervicogenic headache. Alteration of the neck range of motion generally is seen with CEH, and it has been defined as a distinctive feature in the diagnosis of these patients.[118,129] Impaired neck mobility in the cardinal plane is a diagnostic criterion in cervicogenic headache,[129,131] but several studies have found that active cervical mobility is unreliable in differential diagnosis.[118,132-136]

The onset of CEH may be related to a traumatic incident. Whiplash is among the first diagnostic criteria for CEH,[130]

Table 2-17
Major and Minor Criteria for Cervicogenic Headache

Major Criteria	Symptoms and signs of neck involvement. One or more of the following three phenomena must be present:
	• Precipitation of head pain similar to that which usually occurs by:
	  ○ Neck movement and/or a sustained, awkward head position, and/or
	  ○ External pressure over the upper cervical or occipital region on the symptomatic side
	• Restriction of range of motion (ROM) in the neck
	• Ipsilateral neck, shoulder, or arm pain of a rather vague, nonradicular nature or occasionally arm pain of a radicular nature
	Confirmatory evidence by diagnostic anesthetic blockages
	Unilateral head pain without side shift
	Head pain characteristics:
	• Moderate to severe, nonthrobbing pain that usually starts in the neck
	• Episodes of varying duration or fluctuating, continuous pain

Minor Criteria	Other characteristics of some importance:
	• Only marginal effect or lack of effect of indomethacin
	• Only marginal effect or lack of effect of ergotamine and sumatriptan
	• Female gender
	• Not infrequent head or indirect neck trauma by history, usually of more than moderate severity
	Other features of lesser importance:
	• Various attack-related phenomena that are only occasionally present and/or moderately expressed when present:
	  ○ Nausea
	  ○ Phonophobia
	  ○ Photophobia
	  ○ Dizziness
	  ○ Ipsilateral blurred vision
	  ○ Difficulty swallowing
	  ○ Ipsilateral edema, mostly in the periocular area

Modified from Sjaastad O, Fredriksen T, Bono G, Nappi G: *Cervicogenic headache: basic concepts,* European Headache Federation, p 43, London, 2003, Smith-Gordon; and Pikus H, Philips J: Characteristics of patients successfully treated for cervicogenic headache by surgical decompression of the second cervical root, *Headache* 35:621-629, 1995.

but cervicogenic headache can be present in individuals without a history of trauma.[101,122,126,137] As with most forms of headache, the incidence of cervicogenic headache is higher in females.[138] The onset of CEH is not age specific, and the condition can be associated with degenerative joint disease or a sedentary lifestyle. The history often is prolonged.[138]

Despite efforts to clarify the clinical diagnosis of CEH, diagnosis is still a problem because of the overlap of symptoms with other types of headaches, such as migraine and tension-type headache (Table 2-18). Therefore relying on the patient's history and symptoms may be not the best way to reach an accurate diagnosis. Also, patients can suffer a "mixed" headache form or two types of headaches concurrently.[139] The differences between the available classifications for headaches of cervical origin make the study of CEH confusing and the diagnosis of this condition more difficult.[140]

According to Jull,[138] evaluation of physical impairments of the cervical spine can help in the diagnosis of CEH. Also, treatment of the musculoskeletal impairments associated with CEH has been proposed as an essential part of the condition's overall treatment.[138,141] This means that the physical examination is crucial. Deep flexor muscles, including the longus capitis and longus colli, are important for cervical segmental and postural control. Alteration of the strength and endurance of the deep flexor muscles has been found in patients with neck pain and those with cervical dysfunction.[138] Dumas et al.[101] and Watson et al.[126]

investigated the relationship between strength of the upper neck flexor muscles and endurance of the same group of muscles in patients with cervicogenic headache. Both studies concluded that strength of the upper neck flexors was significantly different between patients with nontraumatic CEH compared with controls. In both studies patients with nontraumatic CEH had smaller values of endurance compared with normal subjects.

The treatment of CEH involves many specialists, including physicians, neurologists, orthopedic surgeons, rheumatologists, neurosurgeons, physical therapists, chiropractors, and osteopaths. Conservative therapies are recommended as the first choice. According to Jull,[138] the physical therapy approach to CEH should include treating the patient's physical impairments not only to reduce symptoms but also to provide preventive maintenance. In addition, education of the patient in the predisposing and precipitating factors that aggravate the crisis is essential for the overall management of these patients. Some evidence from randomized controlled trials (RCTs) supports the use of both manipulative therapy and specific exercise to reduce the frequency and intensity of the headaches and neck pain in a 1-year follow-up period. However, the combined therapy was not superior to either therapy alone.[142] Exercise therapy consisted of exercises directed toward improving motor control of the deep and superficial cervical muscles and training of

Table 2-18
Diagnosing Different Headaches

Cervicogenic Headache	Migraine	Tension Type Headache
Unilateral pain; never changes sides	Unilateral pain but may be bilateral and can change sides with different attacks	Usually bilateral pain
Throbbing pain	Throbbing pain	Pressing, tightening pain
Moderate to severe intensity	Moderate to severe intensity	Mild to moderate intensity
Autonomic symptoms	Autonomic symptoms	Not accompanied by autonomic symptoms
Pain starting in the neck and pain triggered by neck movement and/or sustained awkward position	Pain is not triggered by neck movement	Pain usually is not triggered by neck movement
Affecting mainly females	Affecting mainly females	Affecting mainly females
Requires individual to lie down to feel better	Aggravation by routine physical activity	Does not worsen with routine physical activity
Reduced range of motion in the cervical spine	No reduced range of motion in the cervical spine	No remarkable unilateral restriction of neck motion
No precipitant mechanism	Precipitant mechanism (i.e., food, light, stress)	Not attributed to some other disorder
No response to medications	Response to ergot/sumatriptan treatment	Presence of trigger points; tenderness extending to shoulders and cervical muscles and also present in pericranial muscles
Good response to blockage of cervical joints or nerves	No response to blockage of cervical joints or nerves	Blockage of greater occipital nerve reduces pain only in area of blockage; does not abolish headache

Modified from Bono G, Antonaci F, Ghirmai S et al: Unilateral headaches and their relationship with cervicogenic headache, *Clin Exp Rheumatol* 18(suppl 19):S11-S15, 2000; and Vincent MB, Luna RA: Cervicogenic headache: A comparison with migraine and tension-type headache, *Cephalalgia* 19:11-16, 1999.

the scapular muscles. Stretching and postural exercises are also recommended to improve body mechanics.[143]

Two systematic reviews of the effectiveness of manipulative therapy in CEH found some evidence supporting its effectiveness.[144-146] Nilsson et al.[145] found that manipulative therapy reduced the frequency and intensity of headaches; however, it did not change the subjects' use of analgesics compared with subjects who had massage plus laser placebo therapy in the upper cervical region. Manipulative therapy had a nonsignificant but better effect than azapropazone (an NSAID) in a short term, and against mobilization and waiting list after 3 weeks of treatment was also found.[146]

In the early stages, conservative treatment through medication, change of lifestyle, physical therapy modalities, and acupuncture also can be used. If the symptoms persist, blocks or radiofrequency treatment of the facet joints may be useful. More aggressive procedures, such as surgical cervical stabilization (e.g., foraminectomy, laminectomy, and unectomy), are reserved for patients with severe symptoms.

Assessment of the Cervical Spine

The assessment of the cervical spine follows the method presented in *Orthopedic Physical Assessment* (volume 1 of this series). However, if the examiner is assessing primarily for hypomobility, then an understanding of the biomechanics in the cervical spine becomes important. In this context, *coupling* becomes an important factor in the assessment of the cervical spine. In effect, coupling is the conjunct rotation of a spinal segment. Side flexion and rotation have very small amounts of pure movement, and for all practical purposes, the two movements are combined. If side flexion initiates coupled movement, a small amount of rotation is combined with it. Similarly, if rotation initiates a movement, a small amount of side flexion accompanies it. In this context, rotation implies rotation and side flexion occurring together, not separately. Experts have many opinions about how a spinal segment couples, whether ipsilaterally (right rotation with left side flexion) or contralaterally (right rotation with right side flexion). For the most part, no one really knows the exact coupling action. Fortunately, with regard to the cervical spine (unlike with the lumbar spine), most of the opinions about coupling are convergent, which strengthens their validity. That being said, the reliability and validity of these tests have not been confirmed. The following section is based on the clinical experience of the chapter's first author, Jim Meadows.

Atlanto-occipital Segment

Considerable motion occurs at the atlanto-occipital joint, certainly enough for the movement to be appreciated and not just the end feel. Table 2-19 outlines the movement and range of motion that occur at the left occipital joint.

Table 2-19

Movement and Range of Motion of the Left Atlanto-occipital Joint

Movement	Range (Degrees)
Flexion	3.5
Extension	21.0
Right side flexion	5.4
Left side flexion	5.6
Right rotation	6.6
Left rotation	7.9
Combined flexion-extension	24.5
Combined side flexions	11.0
Combined rotations	14.5

As with most of the cervical spine, the key to understanding the function of the atlanto-occipital joint is to remember that it is primarily capable of flexion and extension. A considerable degree of rotation and side flexion is also available. The second point to keep in mind is that the arthrokinematics are the reverse of those in the other zygapophyseal joints, and they occur in a different plane (horizontal). Although clinicians may know this intellectually, intuitively it "goes against the grain," and practitioners' have a tendency to forget this point.

Mobility Tests

With the patient supine, the head is extended around the axis for the atlanto-occipital joint (an axis approximately common with that of the atlantoaxial joint and running through the external auditory meatus). The head then is side flexed left and right around a common craniovertebral axis running roughly through the nose. As the side flexion is carried out, a gradual translation force is applied in the opposite direction to the side flexion. The translation is economical in that it maintains the axes of motion, reduces the degree of angular displacement necessary to obtain full range of motion, and allows the clinician to detect an end feel. The range of motion of side flexion is assessed from side to side, as is (more important) the end feel of the translation. The end feel allows the barrier to be assessed and can be muscular, capsular/tissue stretch (pericapsular tissue), or pathomechanical (subluxation or "jamming" of the joint). The side flexion procedure is then repeated for flexion.

During extension, the occipital condyles glide anteriorly to the limit of their symmetrical extension range. During side flexion and right translation, the coupled right rotation is produced. As rotation causes the right occipital condyles to retreat toward a neutral position, the left condyle must advance into the extension barrier. If side flexion is limited, the limiting factor must be on the left side of the segment (i.e., ipsilateral to the side flexion), preventing the advance of the condyle into its normal position (or, with hypermobility, allowing it to advance too far).

An alternate method is to extend the segment and then rotate it rather than side flex it. This method may be preferable, because it eliminates the need to consider the coupling motion. Right rotation must flex the right joint and extend the left, but in practical terms, this is problematic. Limiting the rotation to the atlantoaxial segment is quite difficult, and the examiner cannot be confident that any range restriction is a result of hypomobility at the atlanto-occipital joint rather than the segment below.

During flexion, the occipital condyles move posteriorly. The right rotation that occurs as a consequence of the left side flexion causes the left condyle to move away from the flexion barrier toward the neutral position while the right condyle is moved posteriorly into the flexion barrier. Therefore the limiting factor must lie on the right side of the segment that is contralateral to the side flexion. Again, rotation of the segment can be used instead of side flexion, but the practical difficulties remain.

It is apparent that the arthrokinematic and osteokinematic movements occur simultaneously. In fact, the arthrokinematic movement in itself does not afford as much information about the type of hypomobility in these craniovertebral segments as it does elsewhere. This is due to the orientation of some of the suboccipital muscles that are oriented parallel to the plane of the joint so that they can restrict the glide of the joint and the bone movement. Consequently, whether the hypomobility is myofascial, pericapsular, or pathomechanical in nature must be determined by other means. End feel would be the obvious answer to this question, but hypertonic muscles sometimes alter the axis of rotation in such a manner as to cause a false pathomechanical end feel. The more useful approach is to try a hold/relax technique and determine how much improvement occurs. If substantial improvement is seen, an extra-articular restriction is playing a major role; if little improvement is noted, an articular restriction is present.

It is important for the clinician to determine the side that is affected. If manipulation is used, the force must be as local as possible. The side of hypomobility is less important if mobilization is used, because the direction of the mobilization is into the hypomobility.

Atlantoaxial Segment

Although rotation is the main movement at the atlantoaxial joints, a surprisingly large amount of flexion, extension, and side flexion also occurs at the segment (Table 2-20).

Mobility Tests

The atlantoaxial joints can be tested using the coupled movements of rotation and side flexion. According to cadaveric and in vivo studies, this segment has considerable range of motion (see Table 2-20).

Rotation. The advantage of using rotation to assess range of motion is that coupling is not an issue. The disadvantage is that many clinicians find this a less sensitive

Table 2-20

Movement and Range of Motion of the Left Atlantoaxial Joints

Movement	Range (Degrees)
Flexion	11.5
Extension	10.9
Right side flexion	9.4
Left side flexion	4.0
Right rotation	39.5
Left rotation	38.3
Combined flexion-extension	22.4
Combined side flexions	13.4
Combined rotations	77.8

means of testing. (*Sensitive* here means being able to feel the movement.)

The patient sits with the clinician standing to one side. C2 is stabilized with a wide pinch grip, and the clinician's other hand reaches around the head to hold the occiput and C1. The patient's head is held against the clinician's chest, and a very light compressive force is applied as the head is rotated toward the clinician. The compressive force allows the descent of the head that normally occurs as the C1 facets descend on those of C2. The range of motion is assessed and the end feel evaluated (Figure 2-9).

Side Flexion. With the patient lying supine, the clinician reaches under the neck so that a finger wraps around the spinous process of C2, compressing the soft tissue against the process. The clinician side flexes the occiput around the craniovertebral axis while palpating the movement of the C2 vertebra via the motion of its spinous

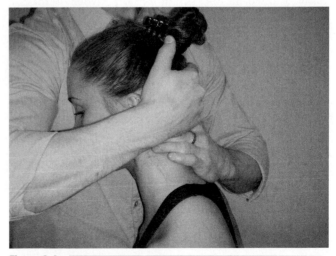

Figure 2-9
Atlantoaxial mobility test in rotation.

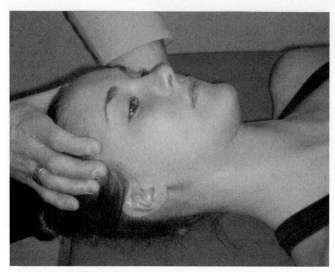

Figure 2-10
Atlantoaxial mobility test in side flexion.

process (Figure 2-10). The movement is in the opposite direction to the side flexion, indicating rotation of the C2 vertebra to the same side with consequential rotation of the segment to the opposite side. For example, if the head is side flexed to the right, the spinous process of C2 moves to the left as the vertebral body rotates to the right. Because by convention segmental movement is named by the movement of the superior vertebra, the C1-2 segment is rotated to the left. As the head is side flexed, the clinician assesses the amount of spinous process displacement to gain an idea of the range of C2 rotation. The clinician stabilizes the head when all movement has ended and then pulls the C2 spinous process further into its passive range to gain the end feel of rotation. When right side flexion is produced, the clinician assesses left rotation and vice versa.

Flexion and Extension. These movements are most easily assessed in the sitting position when a rocking motion is produced and no glide is available. However, given that combined rotation has about four times the range of combined flexion-extension (see Table 2-20), if rotation is restored at the zygapophyseal joint, flexion and extension must also be restored, and this precludes the need to test the motion except in the extremely unlikely event that scarring has occurred in the flexor or extensor muscles. In trauma patients, who may have such scarring, flexion or extension is likely to be much more limited than rotation and side flexion. Also, isometric testing reasonably can be expected to be either weak or painful (in the acute case, painfully weak) and the muscle to be tender to palpation. In such cases stretching techniques must be undertaken for these muscles.

There also is no forward or backward translation, because the dens and the transverse ligament severely restrict this motion, therefore no deductive determination

of the side of the hypomobility can be made. Complex and very careful testing by a skilled practitioner may elicit this information, but in reality it is not necessary for treatment.

Cervical Segments (C2 to C7)

The cervical spine proper is more complicated to assess than the craniovertebral articulations, because it has not only muscles and zygapophyseal joints but also discs and uncovertebral joints (joints of von Luschka). Consequently, this examination needs to be somewhat more detailed and complex to obtain information on these additional structures.

Segmental Screening Test

As with any other screening tests, the purpose of the segmental screening test is to demonstrate quickly the need for more exhaustive testing and to focus the clinician's attention on a specific level or levels and specific movement or movements. However, it also can be used to determine the direction of treatment without concern about which structure is limiting the movement. This is particularly true for mobilization, but the information gained from the screening test may also be used with certain types of manipulation.

The segmental screening test is performed in a fashion similar to mobility testing of the atlanto-occipital joint. The segment is extended, which lifts the superior vertebra forward (eliminating the need to extend the entire cervical spine). While the extended position is maintained, the segment is side flexed left and right around its axis of motion and simultaneously translated contralaterally (Figure 2-11). During left side flexion, the left side of the segment is maximally extended while the right side is moving toward its neutral position. The range of motion of the side flexion and the end feel of the translation are evaluated for normal,

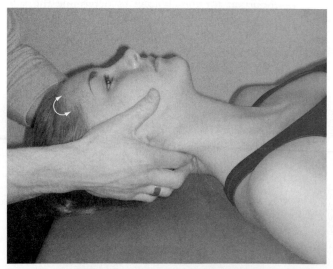

Figure 2-11
Segmental screening test for cervical segments C5 to C7.

excessive, or reduced motion. If left side flexion is restricted, extension of the flexor muscles or one of the joints on the left likely is the problem. If the end feel of the translation is normal but side flexion is restricted, the hypomobility is extra-articular (i.e., myofascial). If left side flexion is restricted in flexion, then the right side of the segment is not flexing normally.

Occasionally side flexion appears to be normal but translation is restricted in all three positions. The likeliest cause of this restriction is uncovertebral joint dysfunction, because these "joints" are involved in (or are the result of) side flexion and rotation and thus are largely unaffected by flexion or extension.

Deduction within the limits of theoretical knowledge can be used to determine the dysfunction, but direct testing, of course, is better. To this end, the arthrokinematics of the zygapophyseal and uncovertebral joints are evaluated.

Zygapophyseal Arthrokinematic Tests: Posteroanterior Intervertebral Movements (PAIVMs)

The orientation of the zygapophyseal joints is craniocaudal, mainly in the coronal plane. The patient lies supine. If extension is to be tested, the clinician lifts the superior vertebra of the segment by using the hand to gain extension, and the fingers are placed over the inferior processes of the superior vertebra (the superior facet). The two facets of the hypomobile side are compressed against each other by lifting upward while the superior facet is pushed caudally (Figure 2-12). The end feel is assessed by comparing it with the other side and/or the joints above and below.

For flexion, the segment is flexed and the superior facet of the suspected hypomobile joint is pulled cranially, again to assess the end feel. To do this, the clinician must move the bone and not the overlying soft tissue; therefore it is useful for the clinician to attempt to put the fingertips between the two facets (Figure 2-13).

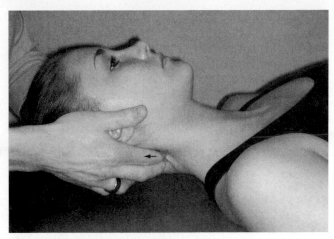

Figure 2-13
Posterior intervertebral movement in flexion.

Uncovertebral Arthrokinematic Tests: PAIVMs

The uncovertebral joints are oriented inferomedially and superolaterally in a mainly sagittal plane. Hypomobility of the joint restricts translation with or without perceptible limitation of side flexion itself. The restriction is felt in flexion, extension, and neutral; flexion generally is the least affected. The patient lies supine. If left translation is restricted, the right joint's inferomedial glide is tested by pushing inferomedially on the right superior transverse process while the inferior bone is stabilized by holding the left inferior transverse process (Figure 2-14). Superolateral glide of the left joint is tested by pushing the left inferior transverse process inferomedially while the superior bone is stabilized via the right superior transverse process.

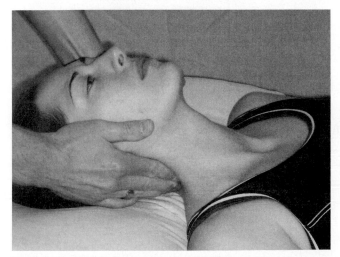

Figure 2-12
Posteroanterior intervertebral movement in extension.

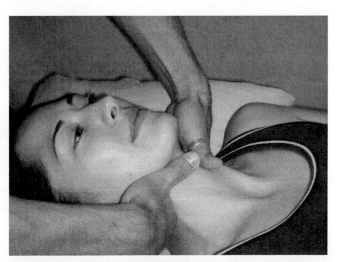

Figure 2-14
Uncovertebral arthrokinematic testing.

Analysis of the Assessment Results

The assessment can yield information about the severity of the pain, the onset of the pain relative to the onset of tissue resistance (i.e., simultaneously, before, or after), and the type of tissue resistance (e.g., normal or abnormal, muscle spasm, capsular, pathomechanical). Knowing these results and correlating them with the history findings enables the clinician to determine the degree of inflammation, if any, and the direction and type of hypomobility (flexion or extension, pathomechanical, pericapsular, extra-articular, or subacute inflammatory) and thus establish a viable treatment plan. Table 2-21 outlines the vertebral segments and the hypomobility diagnoses based on hypomobility findings.

Table 2-21
Cervical Segment, Hypomobility Findings, and Subsequent Hypomobility Diagnosis

Segment	Hypomobile Findings	Hypomobility Diagnosis
Atlanto-occipital	Flexion/right side flexion/left translation Hold/relax substantially improves Hold/relax no improvement	Left extensor hypertonicity Left joint hypomobility
	Flexion/left side flexion/left translation Hold/relax substantially improves Hold/relax no improvement	Right extensor hypertonicity Right joint hypomobility
	Extension/left extensor hypertonicity Hold/relax substantially improves Hold/relax no improvement	Left flexor hypertonicity Right joint hypomobility
	Extension/left extensor hypertonicity Hold/relax substantially improves Hold/relax no improvement	Right flexor hypertonicity Left joint hypomobility
Atlantoaxial	Right rotation Hold/relax substantially improves Hold/relax no improvement	Left rotator hypertonicity Right rotation articular
	Left rotation Hold/relax substantially improves Hold/relax no improvement	Left rotator hypertonicity Right rotation articular hypomobility
	Flexion loss leading to rotation loss Hold/relax substantially improves Hold/relax no improvement	Extensor hypertonicity Bilateral articular
	Extension loss leading to rotation loss Hold/relax substantially improves Hold/relax no improvement	Extensor hypertonicity Bilateral articular
C2 to C7	Flexion/right side flexion/left translation Z- and U-joint PAIVM: − Left Z-joint PAIVM: + Right U-joint PAIVM: + Left U-joint PAIVM: + Flexion/left side flexion/right translation Z- and U-joint PAIVM: − Left Z-joint PAIVM: + Right U-joint PAIVM: + Left U-joint PAIVM: ⏐ Extension/right side flexion/left translation Z- and U-joint PAIVM: − Left Z-joint PAIVM: + Right U-joint PAIVM: + Left U-joint PAIVM: + Extension/left side flexion/left translation Z- and U-joint PAIVM: − Left Z-joint PAIVM: + Right U-joint PAIVM: + Left U-joint PAIVM: +	Left side flexion hypomobility Left extensor hypertonicity Left Z-joint superior glide (flexion) Right U-joint inferomedial glide Left U-joint superolateral glide Left side flexion hypomobility Right extensor hypertonicity Left Z-joint superior glide (flexion) Right U-joint inferomedial glide Left U-joint superolateral glide Right side extension hypomobility Left extensor hypertonicity Right Z-joint inferior glide (extension) Right U-joint inferomedial glide Left U-joint superolateral glide Left side flexion hypertonicity Right flexor hypertonicity Left Z-joint inferior glide (extension) Right U-joint superolateral glide Left U-joint inferomedial glide

PAIVM, Posteroanterior intervertebral movement; *Z-joint,* zygapophyseal joint; *U-joint,* uncovertebral joint.

Table 2-22
Pain-Resistance Relationship, Acuteness, and Possible Treatment in the Cervical Spine

Pain-Resistance Relationship	Acuteness	Treatment
Severe pain with no resistance	Empty feel (severe pathology)*	None
True constant pain†	Visceral	None
Severe continuous pain‡	Hyperacute	Rest, ice, compression, and elevation (RICE)
Pain before resistance	Acute	Grade 1 mobilization
Pain with resistance	Subacute	Grade 2 mobilization
Pain after resistance	Nonacute	Grade 3 or 4 mobilization
Resistance without pain	Stiff or pathomechanical	Grade 4++ mobilization
		Minithrusts or manipulation

*This is true empty end feel, not the feeling caused by torn ligaments, which usually is a soft capsular end feel.
†No physical stress or rest changes the intensity of the pain.
‡High intensity rest pain that worsens with mechanical stress.

Cervical Spine Hypomobility Considerations

- Limited motion with a spasm end feel plus a history of relatively severe pain and a proportional amount of irritability is strongly indicative of arthritis (systemic or traumatic), the treatment of which needs to be rest from adverse stress. This may mean mobilizing a nearby hypomobile segment that is putting undue stress on the painful joint.
- Limited motion with a hard capsular end feel requires rhythmical oscillations that stretch the capsular tissues. The joint may or may not be painful but is almost certainly contributing to the patient's neck pain by stressing a painful joint.
- Limited motion with a pathomechanical end feel (abrupt and lightly springy) requires nonrhythmical techniques such as high velocity, low amplitude thrusts (manipulation) or minithrusts (oscillations).
- Minor pain or discomfort, which usually occurs when the barrier is stretched (pain after resistance), requires true grade 3 or grade 4 techniques; that is, near–end range oscillatory mobilizations that do not reproduce the pain but that also do not retreat to the beginning of the range.
- Acute and subacute pain states (pain before or with the onset of resistance) require grade 1 or grade 2 oscillations for neurophysiological pain modulation.
- Any technique that provokes spasms should be avoided. If an alternative cannot be found, manual treatment should be abandoned until the pathology subsides.

Inflammation of the joint is characterized by relatively intense, continuous pain with high levels of irritability. In deeper joints, such as the vertebral articulations, other characteristics of inflammation, such as heat and swelling, cannot be observed. However, in the neck swelling may be palpated, and any redness is an indication of a systemic arthritis or infection (Table 2-22).

Treatment

Treatment of the cervical spine revolves primarily around patient complaints of pain, weakness, and restricted range of motion. Therefore the remainder of the chapter discusses treatment methods used in the cervical spine to increase range of motion, improve strength, and provide relief of pain. Before beginning the treatment, however, the clinician must clear any cautions or contraindications to such treatment (Table 2-23).

Exercise Therapy

According to Jordan and Ostergaard,[147,148] the goal of any rehabilitation protocol using exercises is to restore lost functional capacities, such as range of motion and muscular strength and endurance, as well as the ability to manage daily tasks at home and in the workplace.

Table 2-23
Cautions and Contraindications to Joint Play Mobilization of the Cervical Spine

Cautions	Contraindications
Osteoporosis	Vertebral artery symptoms
Bone disease	Spinal cord lesions
Congenital anomalies	Multiple nerve root involvement
Coagulation problems	
Dizziness/vertigo	Active collagen disease
Nonmechanical reason for hypomobility	Active rheumatic disease
	Joint instability
Atypical patterns of restriction	Ankylosed joint
Neurotic patient	Hyperacute pain
Acute inflammation	
Pending litigation	
History of cancer in the area	
History of poor response to manual techniques	

Exercise therapy trials have shown that certain parameters are important for a successful outcome. Richardson and Jull[149] and Bird et al.[150] have reported that appropriate exercises must ensure proper motor control, performance, and endurance of a certain part of the body. Therefore the clinician must decide on the type of muscle contraction (i.e., concentric, eccentric, or isometric), the patient's body position (i.e., supine, prone, or standing), the level of resistance or load (high or low intensity), the number of repetitions, and method of progression.[151]

Type of Muscle Contraction

Based on the biomechanical and physiological characteristics of local cervical muscles, isometric exercises are more beneficial for re-educating the stabilization role of the deep muscles in the spine, because these muscles support low loads for longer periods and work to control fine movement. In later stages, however, isometric exercises can be combined with dynamic and global exercises.

Exercises involving a coordinated contraction between deep anterior and posterior muscles (the multifidus posteriorly and the longus colli and longus capitis anteriorly) are also part of the protocol requirements. In the cervical spine, stability is obtained by the coordinated activity of deep muscles.

Tonic motor units and tonic fibers work best in a stabilization function. Disuse and reflex inhibition are shown to affect the slow twitch and tonic fiber function. A good training program focuses on improving the holding capacity (endurance) of these muscles; therefore prolonged tonic isometric contractions using a percentage of the maximum voluntary contraction (MVC) (about 30%) are most effective in retraining the stability in the affected muscles.[152] Also, specific exercises that isolate the local muscles from the global muscles are preferred, because they have been shown to obtain a better result in posture control and symptomatology.[142] These suggestions are in agreement with those postulated by Bird et al.[150] and Falla.[151] According to Bird et al.,[150] low loads are used for muscular endurance in the range of 20 or more repetition maximum (RM) (the greatest amount of weight lifted with a correct technique for a specific number of repetitions).

Body Position and Level of Resistance

In general, the body positions used depend on the objectives of treatment. Because the required level of resistance is low, to obtain a focused re-education of the muscles, positions such as supine, prone, or kneeling have been suggested to help better obtain motor control in the spinal segments.[149] Therefore reduced loads to the local muscles should be used as much as possible, along with positions and exercises involving minimal external loading to reduce the possibility of pain and reflex inhibition. Thus high intensity exercises are not appropriate in the early stages of rehabilitation or when the objective is re-education of specific muscles.

Low loads also help restore tonic function in the spinal muscles. Muscle contractions below 30% to 40% of the MVC can be used to restore this function.[152] Loads as low as approximately 25% of the MVC have been shown to develop increased muscle stiffness to stabilize the spine.

In summary, low loads used with positions and exercises that involve minimal external loading are the ideal combination for rehabilitating local muscles in any spinal stabilization program.[149]

Number of Repetitions

To rehabilitate motor control and coordination among muscles in the cervical spine, the local muscle must be isolated. To gain maximum benefit, therefore, the exercise must be repeated as many times as possible during the day until the patient acquires the desired control of the muscle. In addition, the patient must be able to hold the determined position before progressing to advanced stages. According to Bird et al.,[150] to improve endurance, a repetition of 4 to 6 sets per exercise, with rest periods of 30 to 60 seconds between sets, is appropriate.

Methods of Progression

According to Richardson and Jull,[149] progression proceeds in the following stages: First, the hold time of a determined action (isometric co-contraction) is increased. This is followed by increasing the number of repetitions of this holding activity (static stabilization). Ideally, patients should be able to stabilize and isolate the correct muscle action in all exercise positions and develop this holding activity. As patients progress, they should be able to reproduce and maintain the contraction during dynamic functional movements. The time taken to achieve this varies from patient to patient and with the severity of the dysfunction. The first treatment sessions commonly focus on teaching the patient the correct contraction procedure, which can take several weeks.

Duration

According to Jordan and Ostergaard,[147,148] supervised instruction should be provided for a minimum of 2 months, with 2 or 3 sessions a week. To ensure compliance with the treatment, sessions should last no longer than 1 hour. Home exercises must be done in addition to these supervised exercises.[153-156]

Cervical Muscle Retraining

It has been shown that motor dysfunction appears early after injury and does not automatically resolve with pain reduction.[157] Therefore therapeutic exercises have an important role to play in improving motor function, because pain reduction alone does not seem to restore motor function fully. Also, early intervention is preferred in patients suffering from pain and cervical dysfunction to prevent chronicity and perpetuation of symptoms and dysfunctional patterns.[151]

According to Falla,[151] two basic approaches can be used to treat neck pain conditions with exercises. One exercise regimen consists of general strengthening and endurance exercises for the neck flexor muscles.[147,158,159] This exercise program involves high load training and recruiting of all synergist muscles (deep and superficial muscles).

The other exercise approach focuses on the muscle control aspects, and its objective is to improve coordination and control of the muscles (during a controlled flexion movement).[153] With this approach, low intensity contractions of the deep cervical flexors are used during the craniocervical flexion movement. After the patient acquires control between the deep and superficial muscles, through training of the craniocervical flexion movement holding capacity and progression, general strengthening exercises can be added.

Both regimens can be used, but they must be applied at different times. Low intensity exercises and control pattern movements must be applied in the initial stages, whereas global exercises involving a greater number of muscles must be used after re-education of and coordination between the deep and postural neck muscles have been established.[151,153]

Jull et al.[153] proposed a treatment protocol for training dysfunctional cervical muscles. This protocol has been used successfully to treat both patients with cervicogenic headache and those with painful neck conditions.[142,160] The protocol emphasizes motor control rather than muscle strength. The same principles have been stated by O'Grady and Tollan.[161] Both groups of researchers divided the treatment into two phases: retraining the cervical muscles and retraining the scapular muscles. The following sections describe retraining of the cervical muscles.

Re-education of the Craniocervical Flexion Movement. According to Jull et al.,[153] the re-education of the correct craniocervical flexion (CCF) movement is the first indispensable component for an exercise program. The clinician must teach the patient to perform the movement correctly and to control and eliminate any compensation strategy, such as neck retraction, excessive cervical flexion, and/or jaw clenching. For the treatment to progress, the craniocervical flexion movement must be performed correctly. Emphasis on the precision of the movement, rather than the number of repetitions, is essential.[151,153,160]

Training of the Holding Capacity of the Deep Neck Flexors. Once the patient can correctly perform the CCF movement, training to improve the holding capacity of the deep flexors is begun. A preinflated, air-filled pressure sensor is used to guide and control the training of deep neck flexor muscles (Figure 2-15). This sensor, which has a visual feedback device, is essential to guide the patient in controlling the level of pressure and the desired level of muscle contraction. Also, the feedback device helps motivate the patient and provides quantification of the degree of improvement.[151,153,160]

The starting point for holding capacity training (HCT) usually is the pressure level the patient has reached and can hold without compensation for at least 10 seconds.[149,153] Patients commonly start at 22 or 24 mmHg. The training consists of teaching the patient to achieve

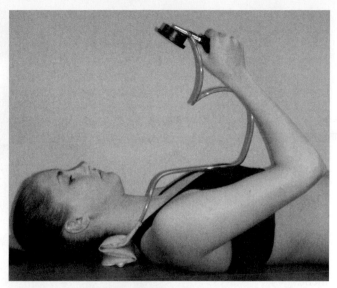

Figure 2-15

Craniocervical flexion test and craniocervical flexion training. Patients are instructed to perform a gentle nodding movement (craniocervical flexion) and practice progressive targeting using the air-filled pressure sensor at five incremental levels with the aid of a visual feedback device.

the determined pressure level and then to hold it for a time without evidence of compensation or poor motor patterns. Ideally, the patient is asked to practice the exercise at least twice a day, without interfering with daily activities. For each pressure level, the patient holds the position for 10 seconds and repeats this 10 times. Reaching an ideal pressure level between 28 and 30 mmHg may be somewhat difficult for patients.[153] The duration of training needed to acquire holding capacity for the deep flexors varies from patient to patient; however, according to Jull et al.,[153] an average of 4 to 6 weeks is necessary to obtain a good performance (i.e., holding 28 to 30 mmHg for 10 seconds, 10 times), but some patients with major muscular dysfunctions could take up to 12 weeks. The patient can use the feedback device at home to practice the training, and once the correct performance is achieved, the individual can be weaned from the visual feedback.

Retraining of Cervical Spine Extension in the Upright Position. Once the patient is able to perform the craniocervical flexion movement in the supine position without compensations, the movement is progressed to the sitting and upright positions. The first part of this next stage consists of moving the head and cervical spine into an extension movement in the sitting or upright position. The patient is instructed to first lift the chin and then look up to the ceiling and to continue this movement, trying to look farther along the ceiling, until the end of the comfortable range of extension is reached. The patient then returns to the neutral position (natural head position). The first part of this exercise trains the cervical flexor muscles to contract eccentrically. Any compensation, such as chin retraction or cervical retraction, should be discouraged.

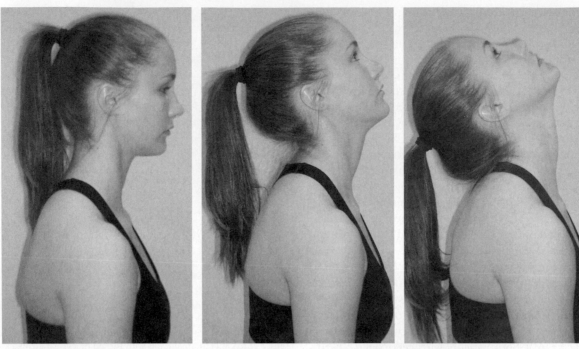

Figure 2-16
Retraining of cervical spine extension in the upright posture.

The second part of the exercise is the return to the upright position by concentric contraction of the cervical flexors muscles. The movement must be started with craniocervical flexion. It is important that the movement be performed mainly at the level of the craniocervical region rather than having dominant action of the sternocleidomastoid (Figure 2-16).

These exercises can be progressed in two ways: first, by increasing the range of the head extension movement as control improves; and second, by adding isometric hold exercises in different parts of the range of cervical returning movement (concentric flexion) to improve the cervical flexion synergy through functional ranges of extension. The exercises consist of performing neck extension in a comfortable (i.e., pain-free) range and then initiating the craniocervical flexion movement toward the upright position, without reaching the full upright position completely, and holding it for 5 seconds. These exercises should be repeated and progressed according to the patient's tolerance, because they are potentially high load exercises.

Retraining of the Extensors of the Craniocervical Spine. To retrain the extensors of the cervical spine along with the training of the deep flexor muscles, exercises are started with the patient in the sitting and upright positions, with progression to the prone and four-point kneeling positions. In the sitting position, for example, the patient is instructed to perform slow head flexion, controlling the speed against gravity and working the extensors eccentrically, and then to return to the neutral position without

any compensation. Chin poking, for example, is one of the most common compensations seen with this movement, and it indicates excessive craniocervical extension, which usually is caused by dominance of the superficial muscles (e.g., semispinalis capitis). This exercise can be progressed by asking the patient to alternate small ranges of craniocervical extension and flexion while maintaining the cervical spine in neutral position in the prone on elbows position or the four-point kneeling position (Figure 2-17). In addition, isometric holds during this movement in the intermediate ranges can be encouraged. The objective of these exercises is to train the coordinated movement among the deep cervical extensor muscles (such as the semispinalis cervicis and the multifidus), the deep craniocervical extensors (such as rectus capitis and the suboccipital muscles in the upper cervical levels), and the deep flexor muscles (such as longus colli and longus capitis). In this exercise, semispinalis and multifidus help to control the cervical spine in the neutral position while the deep small craniocervical extensor muscles perform controlled eccentric, concentric, or isometric contractions,[151,153,160] and the deep flexor muscles (especially longus colli), given their postural role, help to stabilize the neck.[162]

Co-contraction of the Neck Flexors and Extensors. This exercise is started once the patient has achieved control of the correct pattern of contraction for the cervical flexor and extensor muscles. The exercise consists of a self-resisted isometric rotation in the supine, correct sitting, or upright position. The resistance must be gentle (about 10% to 30% of the MVC) (Figure 2-18).

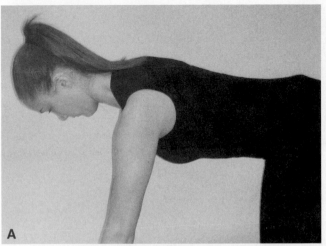

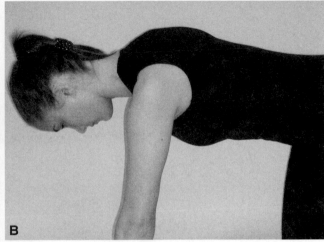

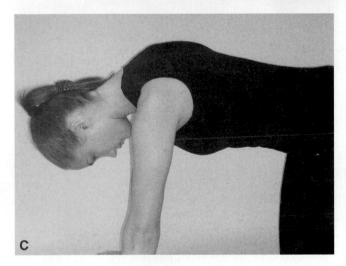

Figure 2-17

Retraining of the extensors of the cervical spine. **A,** Neutral position. **B,** Nod. **C,** Flexion.

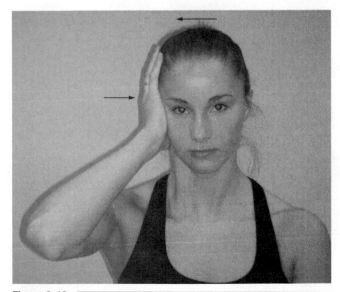

Figure 2-18

Co-contraction of the neck flexors and extensors using self-resisted isometric rotation contraction in a correct upright position.

The patient alternates the resistance as an alternating rhythmic stabilization exercise. The exercise must be done smoothly and slowly, with the focus on control rather than speed. This exercise is easy to perform and can be done throughout the day.[151,153,160]

Murphy[154-156] has proposed a progression for retraining of the cervical muscles through retraining of the cervical flexors and extensors in the four-point ("all fours" or "bird dog") kneeling position. This method is designed to help the dynamic stability system of the cervical spine to work functionally and optimally. The first step is a maneuver called *cervical bracing,* which consists of training the co-contraction of the deep cervical flexors and lower cervical and upper thoracic extensors. While in the four-point kneeling position (Figure 2-19, *A*), the patient first protracts the head and then performs upper cervical flexion while keeping the lower cervical spine in a neutral position. This configuration is maintained by the patient, who is encouraged to keep the spine and the rest of the body stabilized.[155] When this movement can be performed correctly and held for at least 10 seconds, the patient progresses to the next stage. In this stage, the patient combines the head and neck control movement with arm and leg movements (Figure 2-19, *B* and 2-19, *C*). The patient raises an arm and maintains the stability of the body, as well as the stability of the cervicothoracic system. The patient then raises a leg. These movements are alternated (right arm, left leg; then right leg, left arm) until the patient can maintain and perform the correct movement pattern. In addition, the patient can balance a light weight (e.g., a book) on the head to increase the difficulty of the exercise and to retrain stability in the same sequence (Figure 2-19, *D*).[154-156]

O'Grady and Tollan[161] have proposed a further progression of these exercises using a foam rolls or gym ball. The exercises done with these tools are advanced-stage exercises of increased difficulty, because they are two- and three-dimensional, unstable exercises. The patient co-contracts the deep cervical flexors and extensors while balancing on the foam rolls or gym ball (Figure 2-20). These exercises can be made more challenging by having the patient contract the neck (co-contraction) in different positions.

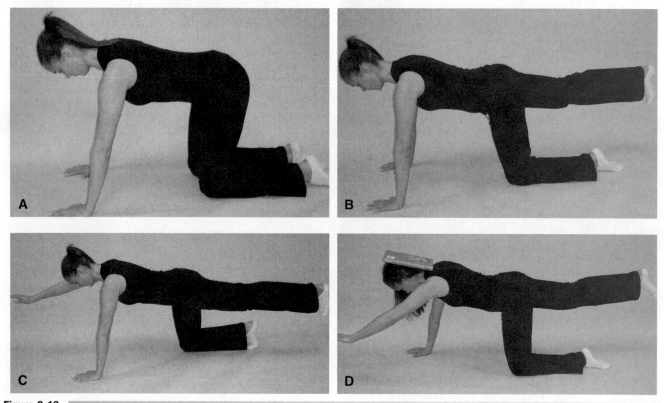

Figure 2-19

Sensorimotor training and cervical stabilization. **A,** Four-point kneeling position. **B,** The patient lifts one leg. **C,** The patient lifts one leg and the opposite arm. **D,** The patient lifts a leg and the opposite arm while maintaining head posture holding a book.

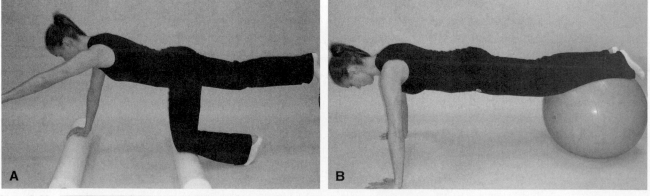

Figure 2-20

Advanced cervical stabilization exercises. **A,** Two-dimensional exercises. **B,** Three-dimensional exercises.

Retraining of Scapular Orientation and Position. The position of the scapula commonly is altered in patients with cervical pain. Retraining of the scapular position is a very complex and difficult task, because patients have difficulty understanding the position of the scapula and cannot correct it through visual cues; they must be taught to feel the correct position and movement.[151,153,160]

The scapula generally is seen to be protracted and downwardly rotated in patients with cervical problems. Exercises are done to correct this position and to try to bring the coracoid upward and the acromion backward. This action results in a slight retraction and lateral rotation of the scapula. The objective is to activate all of the muscles that control the scapular position (i.e., the trapezius, serratus anterior, levator scapulae, rhomboids). However, before retraining can begin, lengthening and relaxation of the hyperactive and tight muscles, such as the upper trapezius (Figure 2-21) and the levator scapulae, pectoralis minor, pectoralis major and sternocleidomastoid (Figure 2-22), must be promoted.[153,160] The altered muscular patterns contribute to increased vertical compressive loads on the joints of the cervical spine.[163] (More information on scapular stabilization may be found in Chapter 5.)

Training of the Endurance Capacity of the Scapular Stabilizers. The training of scapular muscle endurance is the next step. It consists of maintaining the correct position of the scapula for at least 10 seconds and then progressing to holding longer based on the patient's tolerance. These exercises can be progressed from the side lying position to the prone position. The patient can use gravity resistance to train the endurance of the scapular muscles. The exercise is similar to the retraction/depression test. The clinician usually needs to facilitate this

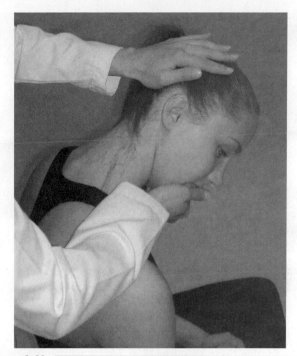

Figure 2-22
Stretching of the cervical and shoulder girdle muscles (here, the sternocleidomastoid).

training until the patient is able to perform the movement and hold it for the required time.[151,153,160]

Retraining of Scapular Control with Arm Movement and Load. The objective of this stage is to maintain the position of the scapula while performing movements of the arm. The patient accomplishes this by doing exercises within a small range of motion (60° or less) while holding the correct position of the scapula. Closed chain exercise can be used to progress the difficulty of these exercises. For example, in the four-point kneeling, "prone on elbows" position, the patient can perform concentric and eccentric control exercises of the scapula while maintaining the cervical spine in neutral position. The objective is to retrain the holding capacity of serratus anterior by holding the position in the intermediate ranges for 10 seconds; this is repeated 10 times (Figure 2-23).

Postural Re-education. Postural retraining should be one of the main objectives of treatment of patients with neck pain. Correcting the patient's posture ensures a regular reduction of harmful loads on the cervical joints induced by the poor postural pattern of the head, cervical spine, and scapula. In addition, postural correction helps retrain the deep and postural stabilizing muscles during functional postures. Postural training should be performed repeatedly during the day so that it becomes a habit for the patient and also to give constant positive feedback to the activated muscles. Postural training is performed first in the sitting position and then in the upright and functional positions (Figures 2-24 and 2-25). This retraining cannot just

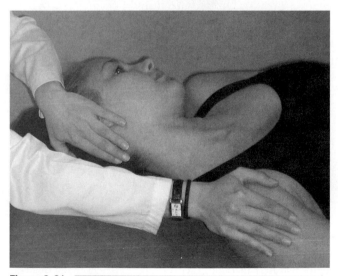

Figure 2-21
In addition to having the patient perform active exercises, the clinician stretches the cervical and shoulder girdle muscles (here, the upper trapezius) to maintain the biomechanical environment and to allow re-education of muscular function.

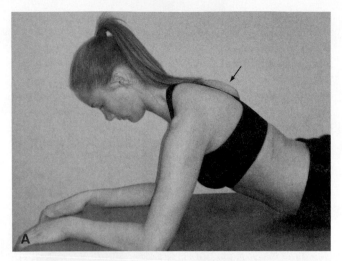

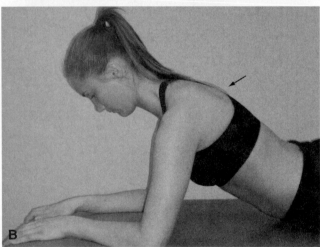

Figure 2-23
Training of the scapular stabilizing muscles. The patient is positioned with the elbows supported in the bed. She then trains the scapulae in both eccentric and concentric control and in holding capacity. The head and neck must maintain a neutral position to retrain the capacity of the cervical extensors. **A,** Scapular winging. **B,** Scapula engaged.

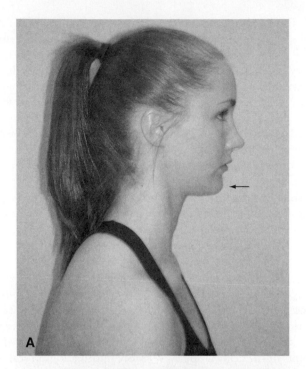

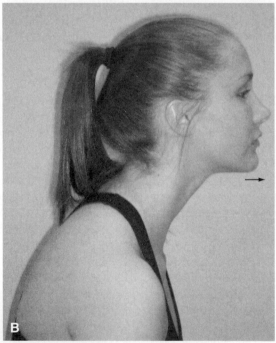

Figure 2-24
Postural control is essential to maintain the functionality of the muscles and the stability of the craniocervical system. **A,** Retraction. **B,** Protraction.

concentrate on the cervical spine and head and their relation to the trunk and pelvis. It must involve training of the thoracic spine, scapula, and pelvic core. The complete kinetic chain must be trained. An interesting postural exercise, the action of lifting the occiput from the atlas, has been shown to activate the longus colli, an important postural muscle.[164]

Treatment of Postural Control Disturbances

In some patients, especially those with chronic WADs, dizziness and unsteadiness are common symptoms. Patients with idiopathic chronic neck pain and those with acute and persistent WADs also have been found to have greater cervical joint position errors.[165-168] Also, patients with whiplash who complain of dizziness have a greater joint position deficit than those who do not have these

symptoms.[153] Deficits in standing balance have been demonstrated in people with persistent neck pain of both idiopathic and traumatic origin.[153] According to Humphreys and Irgens, "There is a dissociation or dysfunction in the integrated visual, vestibular and proprioceptive systems of the neck due to trauma and/or continuing

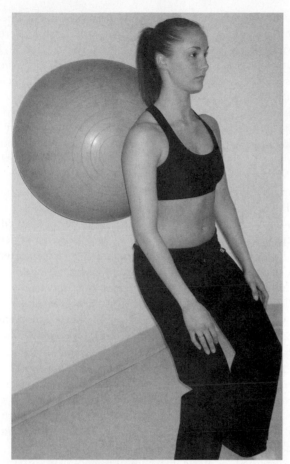

Figure 2-25
Postural training in the upright position using a gym ball. The patient is encouraged to lift the occiput from the atlas and to maintain the shoulder girdle in neutral position. Scapula position also is encouraged.

down) and then progress to the sitting and standing positions.

Oculomotor Exercises. Ocular exercises are progressed in several stages. They start with the head stationary and continue with movements of the head but with the eyes fixed on a target.[167,168] These exercises cannot be performed if the patient is in pain, and they should be stopped if symptoms such as dizziness and unsteadiness appear. According to Fitz-Ritson,[169] the exercises must begin slowly, and the patient must focus on different components of the exercises. Some exercises for eye and head coordination are also used; for these, the patient must combine eye movements and head movement in a synchronized fashion. For example, the patient first rotates the head and the eyes at the same time in the same direction; then, progressively, the patient moves the eyes first to the target and then rotates or moves the head toward that point. Movement in opposite directions (the eyes look in one direction and the head moves in the opposite direction) is trained at the end of the progression (Figure 2-26). All these exercises can be progressed using different surfaces and positions (e.g., the patient sits on a therapy ball, wobble board, or foam roll or walks while doing the exercises).[167]

Fitz-Ritson[169] used these types of exercises in a randomized controlled trial to evaluate the effect of "phasic exercises" plus chiropractic treatment, compared with standard exercise treatment plus chiropractic treatment, in patients with chronic WADs. The Neck Pain Disability Index as

mechanical problems in chronic neck patients."[167] Most of the time these symptoms (dizziness and unsteadiness) are related to altered joint position error or disruptions of balance or eye movement control.[167-169] The treatment should include exercises to address these conditions (although research into the effectiveness of these exercises is needed). The following section focuses on the retraining of these impairments.

Retraining Exercises for Repositioning the Head in Natural Head Posture. These exercises are applied only if the patient has an impairment of the joint position of the head. The patient practices relocating the head to the natural head posture and to specific positions through the range of motion. The patient trains first with the eyes open and then with the eyes closed. All movements (flexion, extension, rotation, and side flexion) are used to retrain the head position.[153,167]

Retraining Balance. Training of balance is important and depends on the level of impairment. The positions and exercises commonly use unstable positions or surfaces to train body balance first in "low" positions (e.g., lying

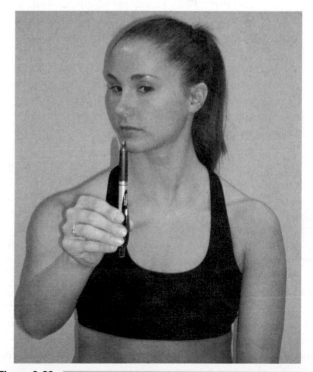

Figure 2-26
Oculomotor training. The patient trains the coordination between head and eye movements.

used as an evaluation tool. The study found that patients treated with phasic exercises plus chiropractic treatment improved 48.3% compared to the baseline evaluation. The author recognized that, in the past, these phasic exercises were applied to patients with acute and chronic neck pain or WADs, which led to poor results. Therefore the author suggested that tonic exercises be performed first, before the patient is progressed to the phasic exercises.[169]

Humphreys and Irgen[167] obtained the same results using oculomotor exercises. They found that these exercises reduced pain intensity and improved the accuracy of repositioning of the head after 4 weeks of treatment in patients with chronic neck pain, compared with patients who did not receive treatment. However, even with these good results, the authors recognized that a link still had to be established connecting cervicocephalic kinesthesia, head reposition accuracy (HRA), and neck pain.

Traction

Traction is used in the cervical spine to distract the zygapophyseal joints, to increase the space between the vertebrae, and to enlarge the intervertebral foramina. Traction may also be used to stretch joint capsules and ligaments that are hypomobile; to reduce muscle spasm and pain by reducing α-neuron excitability; and to improve blood supply through use of intermittent traction.[139,140] Although traction is commonly used in the treatment of the cervical spine, some have questioned its effectiveness.[170-173]

Manual traction usually is the first form applied. It is used to relax the patient, to test the tissues' reaction to traction, and to test the reaction of the patient's signs and symptoms to traction.

Specific manual traction involves applying longitudinal traction to a segment while stabilizing the segments above and below to safeguard them from the effects of the treatment. This technique generally is used to reduce pain and muscle spasm and thereby indirectly increase the range of motion. The technique also is used to reduce the mechanical effects of traction when pain relief is not the primary response required. For example, in certain patients with multiple levels that are unstable or painful, or in a patient who is unable to tolerate lying down, mechanical traction may be difficult or even contraindicated.

Manual traction may be used with the patient in either the sitting or the supine lying position (the sitting position is described). The patient is seated comfortably at a height suitable for the clinician (the top of the patient's head should be approximately level with the clinician's humerus when the arm is held at 90° of elevation). To achieve this, the patient may have to slump in the seat if the chair is not adjustable. The clinician stands just behind the patient's shoulder on either side, depending on which is more comfortable for the clinician. The clinician cradles the patient's forehead with the arm that is anterior with

respect to the patient, reaching around the patient's head to hold the occiput. The clinician's other hand holds across a posterior aspect of the inferior bone of the segment to be treated in a lumbrical grip. The segments above are now locked by a sequence of movements that, all else being equal, are at the discretion of the clinician (Figure 2-27). This sequence includes flexion, rotation and side flexion or extension, and rotation and side flexion to the left or right, depending on whether instability is present above the target segment.

Mechanical traction usually is applied to the cervical spine with the patient in the supine position on a traction table (Figure 2-28), although seated traction may be used in some cases, especially if the patient has respiratory difficulties.[174] This is often an effective technique for patients with cervical spondylosis or those showing radicular signs. The patient is placed in a relaxed position with pillows under the head, shoulders, and knees.

The amount of traction applied to the cervical spine will vary; the minimum is 1.8 to 4.5 kg (4 to 10 lbs). Gentle sustained traction of 4.5 to 7 kg (10 to 15 lbs) for 3-5 minutes is appropriate for relieving muscle spasm; intermittent traction of 7 to 14 kg (15 to 30 lbs) is appropriate for causing a pumping action to aid circulation and to relieve pressure on the nerve and nerve roots by separating the joint structures. Traction increases the pressure in a normal disc, and machine traction has a greater effect than manual traction.[175]

Sustained, or **static**, mechanical traction is traction that is applied continuously for a number of minutes. Sustained traction is indicated for patients with high joint and/or

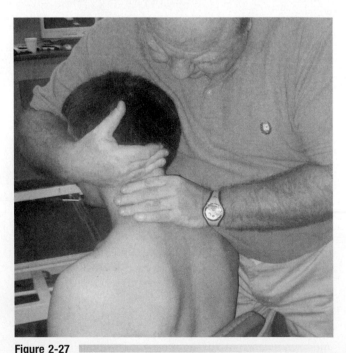

Figure 2-27
Specific manual traction.

Figure 2-28
Mechanical traction using the Saunders device with the patient in the supine position.

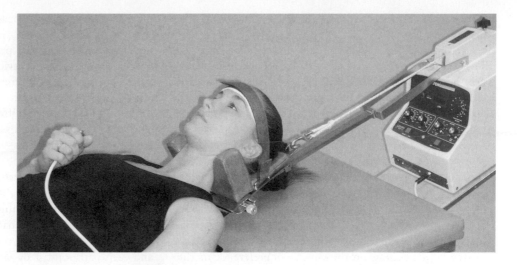

nerve root irritability; those with recent or developing neurological signs that have been associated with irritability; and patients with severe arm pain combined with reduced neck movement toward the painful site.

Intermittent, or **rhythmic**, mechanical traction is probably the most common form of cervical traction used by clinicians, because it enables patients to tolerate greater traction forces.[176] This type of traction is applied for short periods (seconds or minutes) with rest periods (seconds or minutes) in between. Intermittent traction is indicated for patients with an acute joint derangement (less than 6 weeks), unless joint or root irritability is high, and for those with generalized joint mobilization (facet osteoarthritis), spondylosis, cervical problems that do respond to mobilization, nonirritable neurological (radicular) signs, headaches coming from the neck, muscle spasm, or pain. Intermittent traction is reported to produce twice as much separation as sustained traction.[176]

Studies have shown that 24° to 35° of cervical flexion allows maximum separation of the zygapophyseal joints, providing maximum enlargement of the intervertebral foramina.[176-180] In the supine lying position, the most effective angle of pull for treating the cervical spine is about 60° from horizontal. Researchers also have found that about 11.3 kg (25 lbs) is necessary to separate the cervical vertebrae, with maximum separation occurring with 20.4 kg (45 lbs); at these weights, separation occurred within 7 seconds.[181] Ten to 4.5 to 6.8 kg (15 lbs) may be necessary to overcome the weight of the head and the force of gravity if the head is upright. In the lying position, the force is reduced. However, the clinician must keep in mind that the head accounts for about 7% of the total body weight.

Studies also have shown that 9.1 to 11.3 kg (20 to 25 lbs) is necessary to straighten the lordotic curvature of the cervical spine.[182] Table 2-24 provides a traction guide that is based on signs and symptoms as an indication of when the duration (time) or weight should be altered. Normally, the clinician starts with a weight approximately equivalent to the weight of the head (i.e., 3.6 to 4.5 kg [8 to 10 lbs] or less) and increases or decreases either the duration or the load, depending on the reaction of the signs and symptoms.[176] Treatment usually is given for 20-30 minutes daily or every second day for 2-3 weeks.[177]

Table 2-24
Traction Guide

	Symptoms	Signs	Duration	Weight	Comment
Case 1	↓	↓	↗	↗	Work slowly if joint is irritable
Case 2	No change	No change	↑	= or ↑	
Case 3	↓	No change	↑	=	
Case 4	↓	↑	=	=	
Case 5	↑	↓	=	=	
Case 6	↑	No change	=	½ ↓	
Case 7	↑	↑	½ ↓	½ ↓	

From Grieve GP, editor: *Modern manual therapy of the vertebral column*, New York, 1986, Churchill Livingstone.
↑, Increase; ↓, decrease; ↗, slight increase; =, leave the same
NOTE: 1. Do *not* increase weight and duration at the same time; 2. Increase in units of 3-5 each time.

Cervical traction must be applied with caution in patients whose history indicates osteoporosis, hypertension, cardiovascular disease, congenital anomalies, evidence of instability, vertigo, "drop attacks," possible arteriosclerosis of the vertebral or carotid arteries, or claustrophobia, as well as in patients with respiratory problems or coughing. The immediate disappearance of nerve root pain on the first application of traction may indicate a high probability of severe pain occurring when the traction is removed. According to some reports, intermittent cervical traction may lead to lumbar radicular discomfort in some cases.[183]

Manual Traction with a Locking Technique

To apply manual traction with locking, the clinician flexes or extends (depending on the clinician's preference or the patient's requirement) the segments from the occiput down to the superior bone of the segment of interest while palpating a superior vertebra for movement. As soon as any movement is felt, the flexion or extension is backed off to ensure that the target segment remains in neutral. The superior segments then are side flexed away from the clinician, who ensures by palpation of the superior vertebra that the side flexion is not carried into the target segment. At this point, the levels above the target segment are locked into flexion, side flexion, and rotation, whereas the levels below it are stabilized by the clinician's lumbrical grip (see Figure 2-27). Traction is produced by slight straightening of the clinician's legs at the knees, to the degree required. When only neurophysiological effects are required, very little lifting is necessary. If a mechanical effect is required, the clinician provides more knee extension.

Cervical Orthosis

Cervical collars are used primarily to treat muscle spasm, to provide stabilization, and to limit range of motion. The physiological effectiveness of these devices has been questioned, but they can limit movement, depending on the collar chosen.[6,184-187] No studies have been performed to determine the clinical effectiveness of these devices or the outcomes when they are used. The clinician must also be aware that the patient may become dependent on the device, which is visible and may contribute to a sympathy factor. In most cases, except when bony or ligamentous instability has been diagnosed, the patient should be weaned off the collar as soon as possible.

Mobilization of the Cervical Spine

The results of the segmental examination, leading to treatment and the assessment described previously, can be used as the basis for treatment of both acute pain states in which a neurophysiological but nonmechanical effect is desired and for nonacute conditions in which primarily a

mechanical effect is needed. The advantage of using the assessment technique for mobilization is that it requires no "levering" through a proximal segment and therefore no need to lock the cervical spine segments above and below the segment of interest. This means that minimal risk is incurred of stressing either the other segments or the vertebral arteries at levels different from that being treated. The assessment approach is also a simpler technique and consequently easier to master.

Treatment of the Non–acutely Painful Segment

When the cervical spine is treated with manual techniques for nonacute or nonpainful hypermobilities for which a mechanical effect on the barriers is required, multiple barriers are likely to be encountered during the treatment, and each barrier must be dealt with as it becomes evident. Muscle resistance usually is the first barrier the clinician meets, and this resistance can be reduced or eliminated by using very light hold/relax (10% to 30% MVC contraction) techniques or muscle energy techniques.[188-190] The patient is asked to produce resistance that matches the clinician's light push into the direction to be mobilized, holds the contraction for about 10 seconds to allow inhibition of the muscle spindle, and then relaxes. The clinician then takes up the slack, and the sequence is repeated until a new barrier is met or until no new range is achieved with each contraction. If full range and normal end feels are found after this, the barrier was entirely increased muscle tone (e.g., muscle spasm). If motion is still restricted and the end feel changes from a muscular end feel, different techniques may be required. For example, the next barrier may be mild pain or discomfort, for which grade 4 Maitland oscillatory techniques may be used until the discomfort is abolished.[191] If the grade 4 techniques provoke pain, the clinician should perform grade 3 techniques. If an early collagen end feel is detected, a technique specific to that barrier is used, such as grade 4+ oscillatory techniques for pericapsular extensibility or minithrust/manipulation for pathomechanical problems. Treating each barrier as it appears with the appropriate technique makes the entire treatment more effective and economical.

Mobilization Sequence of Progression

1. Hold/relax or muscle energy techniques for muscle spasm
2. Maitland's grades 2-4 mobilization techniques for pain modulation (depending on acuteness); grades 3-4 techniques for mobilization
3. Maitland's grade 4+ mobilizations/minithrusts for end range mobilization
4. Isometric contractions for re-education

The duration of mobilization treatment varies and depends on the effect required, the irritability of the patient's tissues, and the patient's response during treatment. If the patient's tissues or joints are all irritable, the additional treatment should be relatively short, especially if it is done at the same session as the extensive assessment. Once the clinician knows that the treatment responses are good or at least neutral, the dose (i.e., the duration) can be increased. If the clinician hears a click or other noise or feels the vertebra shift, the treatment should be stopped and the segment and regional movements should be reassessed. Before the segment is taken out of its end range position, four or five isometric contractions should be performed by the agonist. This tends to reduce the amount of relapse between treatment sessions.

Neurophysiological Techniques for Pain

Midrange Techniques. For the purposes of this chapter, midrange is the biomechanical neutral or resting position of the joint. It is the point where the joint capsule has maximum laxity, the volume of the joint is at its greatest, and as a result, the joint is in its least irritable position.[83] As a starting point, therefore, this position is ideal for techniques that are not intended to stress the barrier and that are intended to avoid causing pain and increasing inflammation.

Using the starting point, a **grade 1** Maitland technique can be defined as a small amplitude technique (about 25%) at the beginning of the available range; a **grade 2** Maitland technique is a large amplitude movement in the middle of the range of motion (i.e., the middle 50%); a **grade 3** Maitland technique is a large amplitude movement at the end of the range of motion (i.e., the last 50%); and a **grade 4** Maitland mobilization is a small amplitude movement at the end of the range of motion (the last 25%).[191] Although grades 3 and 4 are not primarily intended to stress the barrier, but just to reach it, in practice most clinicians do stress the barrier with these techniques; therefore properly speaking, they should be described as grade 3+ and grade 4+ mobilizations. A **grade 5** mobilization generally is referred to as exceeding the barrier and is, in fact, a manipulation; however, for most models of biomechanical dysfunction, this definition is lacking in accuracy; therefore in this chapter, it is defined as a grade 4+ mobilization.

With the exception of traction or distraction, techniques that work at the beginning of joint play are intended to reduce pain by achieving a neurophysiological modulation of the pain rather than by exerting a mechanical effect on the abnormal movement barrier.

Neutral Side Glide Techniques. Neutral side glide techniques may be general or specific. For the general techniques, the patient lies supine, and the clinician stands at the head of the bed. The clinician lifts the patient's head slightly off the pillow and then side glides the head, keeping it parallel with the shoulders (Figure 2-29). This causes a side translation in the whole cervical spine. With regard to specific techniques, those described in the following sections can be used for pain modulation. When they are used for this purpose, no flexion or extension is added to the technique for the atlanto-occipital joint and the C2 to C7 segments,

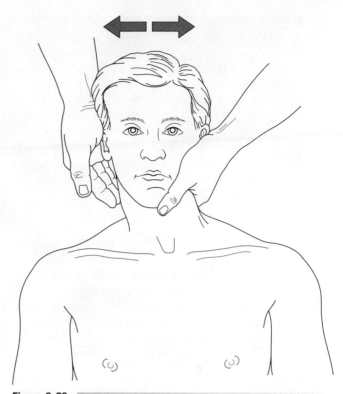

Figure 2-29
Side glide of the cervical spine: Glide to the right. (From Magee DJ: *Orthopedic physical assessment,* ed 4, p 165, Philadelphia, 2002, WB Saunders.)

and very low amplitude translation oscillations are used. For the atlantoaxial segments, the supine techniques work well when grade 1 or grade 2 techniques are required.

Common Requirements for a Safe, Effective, and Economical Mobilization Treatment

- Most importantly, all cautions and contraindications must be recognized and respected.
- A precise and accurate diagnosis is essential.
- The mobilizing force must be focused at the affected segment.
- Each barrier must be recognized as it is encountered and treated appropriately.
- The mobilization technique must be appropriate for the direction, grade, and type of mobilization; this will depend on the barrier met.
- All other segments must be safeguarded from the force of the mobilization as much as possible.
- Definitive therapeutic exercise and patient instruction must follow up manual therapy for both hypomobility and instability (hypermobility) if long-term results are to be accomplished.

Treatment of the Atlanto-occipital Joint. The first technique simply takes the assessment and, using grades, converts it into a treatment method. The techniques

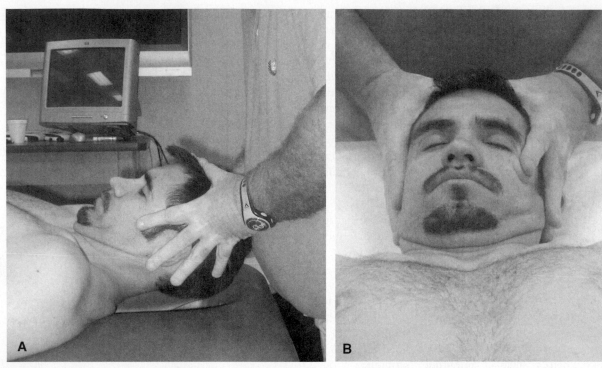

Figure 2-30
A, Axially specific mobilization of extension of right flexion atlanto-occipital joint. **B,** Supine side flex of the right atlanto-occipital joint.

described are for the right side of the segments; therefore, when the joints on the left are treated, the patient's and clinician's positions, the hand positions, and the directions of forces must be reversed.

Treatment of Right Flexion Hypomobility in the Supine Position. The patient lies supine, and the clinician sits or stands at the head of the bed. Both of the clinician's hands are placed on top of the patient's head, slightly forward of midline (Figure 2-30, *A*). The clinician flexes the patient's head by pushing down on the head so that the chin tucks in. Hold/relax or muscle energy techniques then are used to relax the muscles, and any discomfort that may be present is dealt with using grade 4 oscillations. Then, mobilization is performed using either grade 4+ techniques or minithrusts to the barrier. The clinician then side flexes the head to the left, trying to take the left ear onto the neck and simultaneously translating the head to the right until the barrier is felt (Figure 2-30, *B*). Mobilization is performed using either grade 4+ techniques or minithrusts to the barrier. After mobilization, the patient is asked to contract the agonists and antagonists isometrically for short-term re-education.

Treatment of Right Flexion Hypomobility in the Sitting Position. The patient is seated, and the clinician stands slightly behind the patient's right shoulder. The clinician stabilizes the atlas by applying a wide lumbrical grip with the left hand. The clinician's other hand reaches around the patient and lightly grasps the occiput. The clinician flexes the occiput around its own sagittal axis (through

the ear) and then side flexes it to the left around its coronal axis (through the nose) and simultaneously translates it to the right, being careful to minimize movement in the adjacent segment (Figure 2-31). When the abnormal end feel is

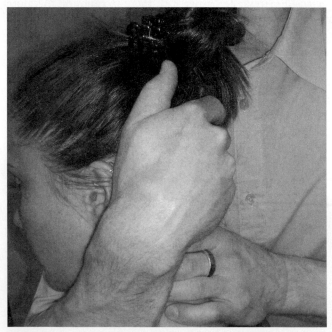

Figure 2-31
Treatment of right flexion hypomobility in the sitting position.

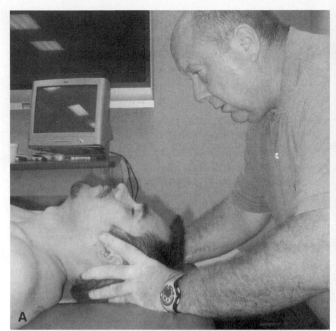
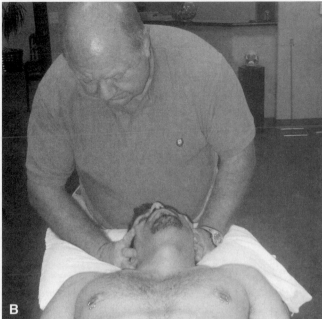

Figure 2-32

A, Axially specific mobilization of extension of right flexion atlanto-occipital joint. **B,** Extension of the right atlanto-occipital joint.

appreciated, the clinician performs the sequence for muscle relaxation (hold/relax or muscle energy techniques) or pain modulation (grades 2-4 mobilizations); when the definitive barrier of translation is encountered, the clinician applies either grade 4+ mobilizations or minithrusts. Afterward, the patient performs isometric contractions using the antagonists and agonists to move the joint actively through the available range of motion.

Treatment of Right Extension Hypomobility in the Supine Lying Position. The patient lies supine, and the clinician sits or stands at the head of the bed. The patient's head is extended. Both of the clinician's hands are placed on top of the patient's head, slightly behind the midline. The clinician extends the patient's head by pushing it down so that the chin is lifted up and back. The clinician then side flexes the head to the right, trying to tuck the right ear onto the neck and simultaneously translating the head to the left until a barrier is felt (Figure 2-32). The muscles are first relaxed with hold/relax or muscle energy techniques, and any discomfort that may be present has been dealt with using grades 2-4 oscillations. Mobilization is performed with either grade 4+ techniques or minithrusts to the barrier. After mobilization, the patient is asked to contract the agonists and antagonists isometrically for short-term re-education.

Treatment of Right Extension Hypomobility in the Sitting Position. The patient is seated, and the clinician stands slightly behind the patient's left shoulder. The clinician stabilizes the inferior vertebra of the segment to be treated by applying a wide lumbrical grip with the right hand. The clinician's left hand reaches around the patient's head and lightly grasps the segments above the target segment,

making sure that the hypothenar eminence contacts the neural arch and the tip of the transverse process of the segment to be treated. The clinician extends the target segment around its sagittal axis and then flexes the right side around its coronal axis while simultaneously pulling the vertebra toward the left, causing left translation (Figure 2-33). Once an abnormal end feel or restriction is felt, the clinician carries

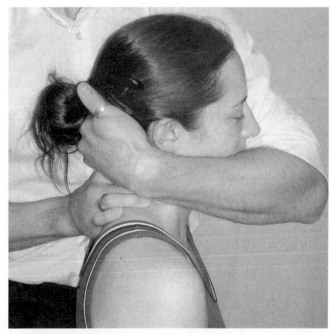

Figure 2-33

Treatment of right extension hypomobility in the sitting position.

out the sequence of muscle relaxation (hold/relax or muscle energy techniques) until no further relaxation is produced (usually 4-5 contractions). If necessary, pain modulation can be achieved using oscillatory mobilization graded according to the degree of pain (grades 1-4) until the pain is relieved, at which point the definitive restricted end feel (capsular or pathomechanical) is encountered. This definitive barrier or abnormal end feel can then be treated with grade 4+ mobilizations, minithrusts, or a manipulation technique. The mobilizations are continued as long as the clinician feels necessary or prudent. Afterward, the patient performs agonist and antagonist isometric contractions at the end of the newly gained range.

Note: In the preceding descriptions, side flexion is always away from the clinician, and translation is always toward the clinician. The clinician can stand on the other side of the patient and side flex toward and translate away, but the method described is the easiest one.

Treatment of Bilateral or Symmetrical Hypermobilities. Bilateral hypermobilities can be treated with unilateral techniques performed to each side, and this approach is preferable when only the last part of the range of movement is absent. However, a bilateral technique for symmetrical dysfunction can also be used and may save time and effort. Such symmetrical restrictions can be due to scarring or adhesions resulting from trauma or to adaptive shortening; that is, structural shortening that results when the tissue does not go through its full range of motion frequently enough.

Treatment of Bilateral Flexion Hypomobility. The treatment for bilateral flexion hypomobility can be performed with the patient either seated or lying down. If the patient is seated, the clinician stands to one side of the patient (in this case description, the clinician stands on the right). The clinician's left hand stabilizes the atlas with a wide lumbrical pinch grip around the neural arch; the right hand reaches around the patient's head and the fingers wrap around the lower occiput, so that the fingers of both hands touch each other. The occiput is flexed around the craniovertebral sagittal axis and simultaneously glided posteriorly (Figure 2-34). Hold/relax or muscle energy techniques are used to reduce muscle tone or spasm, and grades 2-4 oscillations are performed to reduce any discomfort that may be present. Then, grade 4+ techniques are used to stretch the abnormal barrier to posterior gliding.

If the lying position is preferred, the patient is placed in the supine lying position with the head on a pillow, and the clinician stands at the head of the bed. The clinician uses both hands to hold the patient's head slightly forward of midline. The chin is tucked into the throat until the clinician detects the end feel. Muscle spasm and pain are dealt with first as noted previously (Figure 2-35). Using 4+ mobilizations, the glide is mobilized by applying further pressure into the end feel.

If a locking technique is desired (some clinicians feel that it is more specific), only one hand is placed on the head,

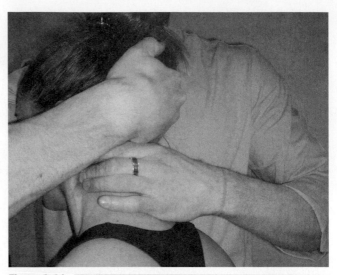

Figure 2-34
Treatment of bilateral flexion hypomobility in the sitting position.

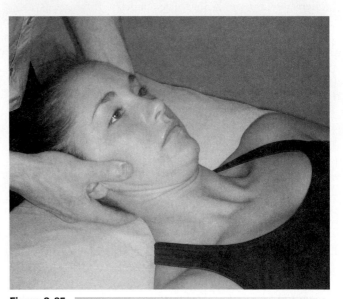

Figure 2-35
Treatment of bilateral flexion hypomobility in the supine lying position.

and the other hand stabilizes the atlas in the same wide lumbrical grip described for the sitting technique.

Treatment of Bilateral Extension Hypomobility. The treatment for bilateral extension hypomobility can be performed with the patient either seated or lying down. If the patient is seated, the clinician stands to one side of the patient (in this case description, the clinician stands on the right). The clinician's left hand stabilizes the atlas with a wide lumbrical pinch grip around the neural arch, if possible coming a little anterior around the transverse process; the right hand reaches around the patient's head and the fingers wrap around the lower occiput, so that the fingers of both hands touch each other. The occiput is extended around the craniovertebral sagittal axis and simultaneously glided

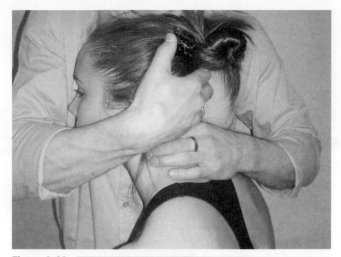

Figure 2-36
Treatment of bilateral extension hypomobility in the sitting position.

anteriorly (Figure 2-36). The clinician then applies the appropriate mobilization technique, which depends on the barrier encountered. The technique using grade 4+ mobilizations to stretch the abnormal barrier to posterior gliding is a little more difficult, because the atlas must be prevented from moving forward during the mobilization.

If the lying position is preferred, the patient is placed in the supine lying position with the head on a pillow, and the clinician stands at the head of the bed. The clinician uses one hand to reach under the patient's head to stabilize the atlas, using the usual wide lumbrical grip, by holding the head back; the other hand reaches around the chin so that the head rests in the crook of the clinician's arm. The head is extended and glided anteriorly on the stabilized atlas until an end feel is appreciated (Figure 2-37). Grade 4+ mobilizations are applied in the manner described previously.

Treatment of the Atlantoaxial Segment. As with the treatment techniques for the atlanto-occipital segment,

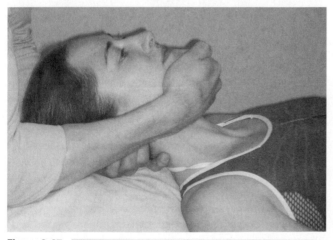

Figure 2-37
Treatment of bilateral extension hypomobility in the supine lying position.

the techniques for the atlantoaxial segment are simply modifications of the assessment techniques. Right hypomobility restriction is described. Similar techniques can be used for left hypomobility restriction, but in the opposite direction.

Treatment of Right Rotation Hypomobility Using Side Flexion. With the patient lying supine with a pillow supporting the head, the clinician stands or sits at the head of the bed. The clinician reaches under the patient's neck with the right hand so that his or her finger wraps around the spinous process of C2, compressing the soft tissue against the spinous process; the other hand holds the top of the patient's head. The clinician left side flexes the occiput around the craniovertebral coronal axis (through the nose) while pulling on the spinous process of the C2 vertebra until an end feel is appreciated. At this point, C2 is rotated to the left, but the segment is rotated to the right as C1 is relatively right rotated (Figure 2-38, *A*). As mentioned previously, convention dictates that the segmental movement be named by the relative or absolute movement of the superior vertebra.

The clinician stabilizes the head when all movement has occurred and the end feel has been reached, and then starts to mobilize into right rotation (Figure 2-38, *B*). Muscle relaxation consists of hold/relax or muscle energy techniques to the right side flexors; left side flexion slack is taken up in the relaxation phase. If soreness intervenes, grades 2-4 mobilizations are performed by oscillations to the spinous processes, and the barrier then is mobilized by grade 4+ mobilizations or minithrusts. Isometric exercises of the right and left side flexors produce some short-term re-education.

Treatment of Right Rotation Hypomobility Using Rotation. The patient is seated, and the clinician stands on the right side, slightly behind the patient. The clinician's left hand holds C2 in a wide lumbrical grip around its neural arches so that the thumb stabilizes the posterior aspect of the right transverse process. The clinician's right hand wraps around the occiput, with the little finger lying over the left neural arch of C1. Care must be taken that the clinician's arm does not compress the patient's nose or face. One of two things now must be done to take the slack off the alar ligament and allow rotation to occur; either the occiput must be side flexed to the left, or a light compressive force must be imparted so that when rotation starts, C1 can descend onto C2. The clinician achieves compression by allowing a small amount of his or her weight to fall onto the patient's head, so that the head is not being inadvertently held up by the clinician (Figure 2-39). The appropriate mobilization technique is used for the type of barrier encountered, followed by the appropriate isometric contractions.

Treatment of Flexion Hypomobility. On the rare occasion that the posterior muscles are structurally shortened and require stretching, the following technique may

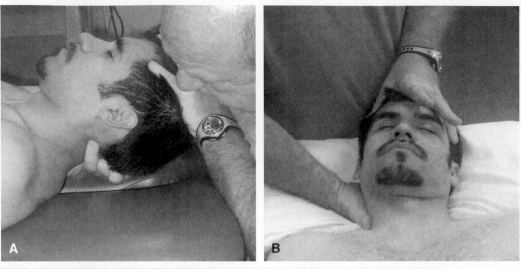

Figure 2-38
Right rotation assessment and mobilization of the atlantoaxial joints.

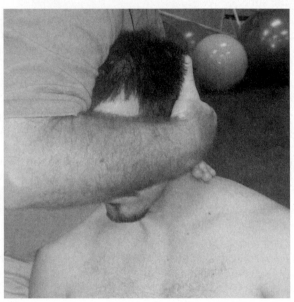

Figure 2-39
Assessment and mobilization for right rotation of the atlantoaxial joint in the sitting position.

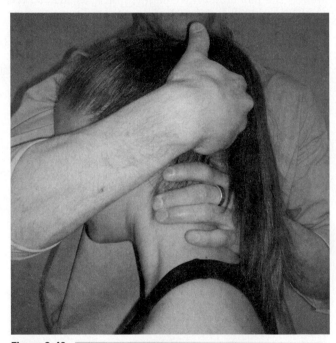

Figure 2-40
Treatment of flexion hypomobility of the atlantoaxial joint.

be useful. The patient is seated, and the clinician stands on either side of the patient (for the purpose of this description, the clinician is on the right side). The clinician's left hand stabilizes the axis (i.e., C2); the right hand reaches around the occiput and atlas (i.e., C1), as low as possible, so that both hands are touching. Care must be taken that the clinician's forearm does not compress the patient's face. The clinician flexes the occiput and atlas around the craniovertebral sagittal axis until the end feel is appreciated (Figure 2-40). The appropriate mobilization technique is then performed. These mobilizations are *osteokinematic* (i.e., they follow a

normal range of motion), rather than arthrokinematic, and they consist of a rollover movement, because the dens/transverse ligament complex prevents anterior and posterior gliding at this segment.

Treatment of Extension Hypomobility. The patient and clinician positions, as well as the positions of the clinician's hands, as described in the previous section, are adapted for the flexion technique, except that the occiput and atlas are extended around the craniovertebral sagittal axis, and extension osteokinematic mobilizations are applied at the appropriate barrier (Figure 2-41).

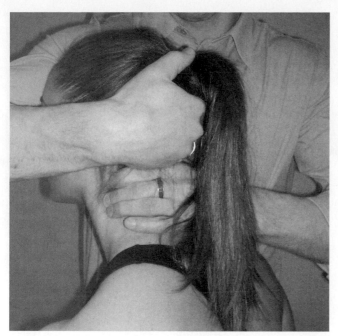

Figure 2-41
Treatment of extension hypomobility of the atlantoaxial joint.

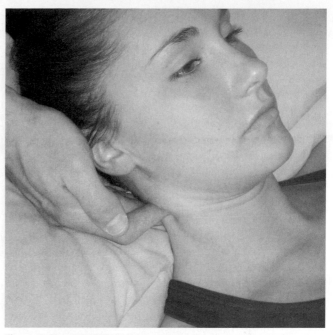

Figure 2-42
Treatment of right side flexion hypomobility of C2 to C7 in the supine lying position.

Minithrusts are not indicated for either flexion or extension hypomobility, because neither type of hypomobility is a pathomechanical dysfunction.

Treatment of C2 to C7

Treatment of Right Side Flexion/Flexion Hypomobility in the Supine Lying Position. The patient lies supine, and the clinician sits or stands at the head of the bed. The patient's head and neck are fully flexed and resting on a pillow or the clinician's abdomen. The clinician uses the middle fingers of both hands to told the superior vertebra of the target segment under the neural arches; the pads of the index fingers are pressed gently against the transverse process tips (Figure 2-42). As an alternative, especially for those with smaller hands or when a lower segment is treated, the index fingers reach around the neural arches and the first metacarpal head is pressed against the transverse process tip. The first technique is likely to be more sensitive for most clinicians.

With either grip, a small amount of left side flexion is applied to fix the axis and then combined with rotation to the right until an end feel is appreciated. The barrier to the translation is then addressed with the appropriate mobilization technique, as determined by the end feel. As more range becomes available as a result of the treatment, the slack is taken up. The maximum duration of the treatment has been reached when no further improvement in movement is noted or when the technique can no longer be controlled because of clinician limitations (e.g., fatigue).

Treatment of Right Flexion/Flexion Hypomobility in the Sitting Position. The patient is seated, and the clinician stands slightly behind the patient's right shoulder.

The clinician uses the left hand to stabilize the lower vertebra of the target segment, using a wide lumbrical grip around its neural arches. The clinician's right hand reaches around the patient to lightly grasp the segment above the level to be treated, making sure that the little finger wraps around the right neural arch of the superior vertebra of the target segment and that the hypothenar eminences are over the left transverse process tip. The clinician flexes the segment around its own sagittal axis and then side flexes it to the left around its coronal axis while simultaneously translating it to the right, taking care to minimize movement in the adjacent segments (Figure 2-43). When the abnormal end feel is appreciated, the clinician applies the appropriate mobilization technique, followed by the appropriate isometric contractions.

Treatment of Right Extension Hypomobility in the Supine Position. The patient lies supine with the head supported on a low pillow, and the clinician sits or stands at the head of the bed. The clinician uses the middle fingers to hold the superior vertebra of the target segment under the neural arches; the pads of the index fingers are pressed gently against the transverse process tips (Figure 2-44). As an alternative, especially for those with smaller hands or when a lower segment is treated, the index fingers reach around the neural arches and the metacarpal head of the second finger is pressed against the transverse process tip. Using either grip, the clinician lifts the vertebra so that the segment extends. A small amount of right side flexion is applied to fix the axis and then combined with left translation until an end feel is appreciated. The barrier to the translation is then

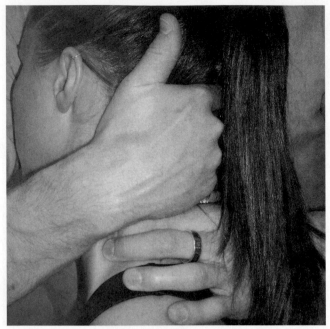

Figure 2-43
Treatment of right side flexion hypomobility of C2 to C7 in the sitting position.

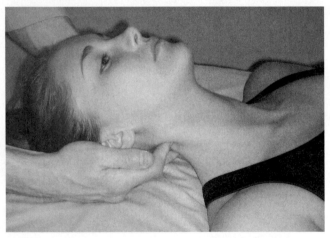

Figure 2-44
Treatment of right side extension hypomobility of C2 to C7 in the supine position.

addressed with the appropriate mobilization technique, as determined by the end feel. As more range becomes available as a result of the technique, the slack is taken up.

Treatment of Right Extension Hypomobility in the Sitting Position. The patient is seated, and the clinician stands slightly behind the patient's left shoulder. The clinician stabilizes the lower vertebra of the target segment with the right hand, using a wide lumbrical grip around the neural arches. The clinician's left hand reaches around the patient to lightly grasp the segments above the level to be treated, making sure that the little finger wraps around the right neural arch of the superior vertebra of the target segment and that the hypothenar eminence is over the right

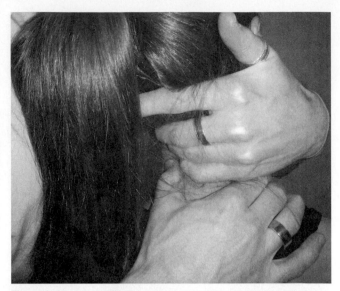

Figure 2-45
Treatment of right side extension hypomobility of C2 to C7 in the sitting position.

transverse process tip (Figure 2-45). The clinician extends the segment around its own sagittal axis and then side flexes it to the right around its coronal axis while simultaneously translating it to the left, taking care to minimize movement in the adjacent segment. The barrier to the translation is then addressed with the appropriate mobilization technique, as determined by the end feel. This is followed by the appropriate isometric techniques.

In the preceding descriptions, side flexion is always away from the clinician, and translation is always toward the clinician. To treat hypomobility to the left, the same techniques are used, but in the opposite direction.

Treatment with a Flexion, Extension, or Rotation Locking Technique. The segments from the occiput down to the superior bone of the segment of interest are flexed or extended (depending on the clinician's preference or the patient's requirement) while a superior vertebra is palpated for movement. As soon as any movement is felt, the clinician backs off the flexion or extension to ensure that the target segment remains in neutral. The superior segments then are side flexed (the clinician palpates the superior vertebra to ensure that the side flexion is not carried into the target segment) (Figure 2-46). At this point, the levels above the target segment are locked into flexion, side flexion, and rotation; the levels below are stabilized by the clinician's lumbrical grip. If flexion is mobilized, the spine must be locked into extension, and if extension is mobilized, the spine must be locked into flexion; otherwise, the mobilizing force will extend to unlock the superior segments. The clinician provides flexion by flexing the head and spine while holding the locked position. Extension is performed in a similar fashion. The clinician provides rotation by rotating the head and spine while holding the locked position.

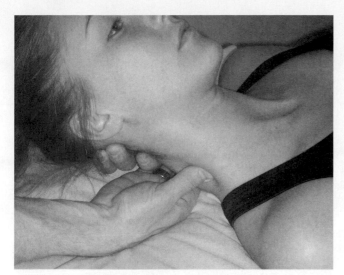

Figure 2-46
Locking techniques for C2 to C7 in supine lying flexion, side flexion, and rotation.

Summary of Mobilization Techniques

Specific manual mobilization techniques are many and varied. They may include complex locking techniques that allow the clinician to lever through unaffected segments, or they may be simple techniques with no preparatory locking if direct force to the affected vertebra is intended. Passive mobilization is an effective and satisfying method of treating mechanical segment dysfunction, but it is only part of the treatment, and it opens a window of opportunity for rehabilitation. Passive mobilization is not a definitive treatment in and of itself. Nonetheless, it is perhaps the most effective way to control the sequencing of other interventions, because it results in rapid improvement in pain intensity, range of motion, willingness to move, and patient compliance, and it allows the clinician to dictate when rehabilitation of movement begins.

References

To enhance this text and add value for the reader, all references have been incorporated into a CD-ROM that is provided with this text. The reader can view the reference source and access it online whenever possible. There are a total of 190 references for this chapter.

TEMPOROMANDIBULAR DISORDERS

Martin Parfitt, Inae C. Gadotti, and Susan L. Armijo-Olivo

Introduction

Temporomandibular disorders (TMDs) consist of a group of pathologies that affect the masticatory muscles and the temporomandibular joint and related structures. TMDs interfere greatly with daily activities and can significantly affect the patient's lifestyle, diminishing the individual's ability to work and interact in a social environment. In the United States alone, approximately $2 billion is spent each year on direct care for TMDs.[1]

Chronic pain caused by TMDs has been shown to produce the same individual impact and burden as back pain and severe headache. TMDs are commonly associated with other conditions of the head and neck region, such as headache, neck pain, and neck muscular dysfunction. To date, studies have shown a clinical association between cervical spine dysfunction and TMD.[2]

Research supports the use of conservative and reversible treatments to treat most patients with TMDs.[3,4] TMD is recognized as a complex disorder, and the treatment of these patients involves many health care professionals, such as dentists, speech pathologists, physicians, psychologists, and physical therapists. Occlusal splint therapy, medications, psychotherapy, behavioral therapy, acupuncture, and physical therapy have been used to try to improve patients' symptomatology. The effectiveness of the treatment also depends on the patient. Most treatments have not been researched, and their use depends on the experience of the clinicians.

Physical therapy does not escape the rigor of scientific evaluation. The procedures of physical therapy intervention are not well described in the literature in this area. Basically, physical therapy treatment is used to relieve pain, improve range of motion, and improve the function of the masticatory system through physical modalities, exercises, and manual techniques. Physical therapy also addresses the craniocervical system as a whole, improving the balance between the various muscles to maintain equilibrium of the craniomandibular system (CMS) (i.e., postural equilibrium) and to prevent additional problems sometimes seen in patients with TMDs, such as spasm of the cervical muscles, cervical pain, and referred pain from the cervical spine to the masticatory system.

From a physical therapy perspective, clinicians work with patients who require treatment of the temporomandibular joint (TMJ) and its surrounding structures. Treatment goals are the same as for any other musculoskeletal structure. However, the clinician must always keep in mind that this is a special joint: bilateral in nature and having structural and anatomical features that are different from the other joints in the body.[5] Pain is the most common symptom and the one that usually causes the patient to seek help in the first place. For this reason, any clinician treating patients with TMDs must address pain management in addition to possible causes or factors associated with pain.

If the TMJ is hypomobile, normal mobility should be restored through mobilization and exercise and then should be maintained through exercise and function. If the TMJ is hypermobile, the hypermobility must be restricted through patient education, modification of use, and exercise to restore normal function. If muscle spasm is present, the spasm has to be reduced through mobilization, exercise, or perhaps with the assistance of physical agents. If inflammation is a factor, the effects of the inflammation must be controlled with rest, change of function, an increase in the blood supply to the area, and adjunctive pharmaceutical therapy.

This chapter provides a general overview of the etiology, epidemiology, classification, and treatment of TMDs. It deals only with disorders that are commonly presented or referred for rehabilitation (usually to a physical therapy department). The reader interested in more in-depth knowledge about TMDs is encouraged to refer to more specific references.[6,7]

Temporomandibular Disorders

Definition

Temporomandibular disorders is a broad, nonspecific term that encompasses several clinical problems involving the stomatognathic system, which is responsible for speech, swallowing, breathing, and mastication functions; the TMJ; the masticatory muscles; and the craniocervical system.[8] Use of the term **temporomandibular joint dysfunction** as an overall descriptor of TMDs has been discontinued, because it is considered misleading and inaccurate, implying structural conditions when, in fact, most of the time, these conditions are not the cause of the dysfunction.[9] TMDs usually are manifested by one or more of the following signs or symptoms: pain, joint sounds, limitation of jaw movement, muscle tenderness, and joint tenderness.[10] In addition, TMDs are commonly associated with other symptoms affecting the head and neck region, such as headache, ear-related symptoms (e.g., tinnitus [ringing in the ear] and otalgia [pain in the ear]), and cervical spine disorders (e.g., fatigue of the masticatory, cervical, and scapular muscles).[11-14] TMDs are considered musculoskeletal disorders of the masticatory system, and they affect more than 25% of the general population.[11] According to Goldstein, "chronic TMD is considered as a psychophysiologic disorder of the central nervous system that modulates emotional, physiologic, and neuroendocrine responses to emotional and physical stressors."[9]

Epidemiology

According to a study by Drangsholt and LeResche,[1] TMDs affected about 20 million adults in the United States and 450 million adults worldwide in 1998. One in three adults will develop TMD pain.[15] TMDs, therefore, are very common conditions. However, only 1% to 3% of the population seek care for their TMDs, and 3.6% to 7% of the general population is in need of treatment.[15] Various studies demonstrate that 50% to 75% of adults have at least one sign and/or symptom related to TMD.[16] According to Auvenshine,[17] approximately 10% of the population has pain in the temporomandibular region. Some signs seem to be more common in the healthy population than others; for example, joint sounds or mandibular deviation occurs in 50% of the population.[11,18,19] Limitation of mouth opening is thought to be rare (seen only in 5%).[11]

Some studies have found that signs and symptoms of TMD in the general population occur twice as often in females as in males (2:1).[20-23] However, other studies have found the ratio of females to males to be approximately the same[24] or 3:1.[25] A recent study found that more than 70% of patients with TMD were women, and the ratio of affected females to males was 2.4:1 for arthralgia, 2.5:1 for osteoarthritis, 3.4:1 for myofascial pain, and 5.1:1 for disc displacement.[26] The literature supports the fact that women are more sensitive to pain conditions and that they report pain that is more severe, more frequent, and of longer duration than that reported by men.[27-34] In addition, women are more likely to seek help than men.[1]

According to data presented by LeResche,[35] only 25% of the community cases met the criteria for a diagnosis of myalgia or myofascial pain; 3.3% met the criteria for a diagnosis of internal derangement; and 4.2% met the criteria for a diagnosis of an arthrogenic condition. Most subjects presented with a mixed diagnosis and were classified into more than one group. Muscle and disc diagnoses were made in 8.3%; myogenic and arthrogenic diagnoses were made in 21.7%; and myogenic, arthrogenic, and disc displacement diagnoses were made in 7.5%.

Etiology

The etiology of TMDs has been hypothesized to be multifactorial. As stated by Goldstein,[9] the medical cause of most TMDs has not yet been established or is unknown (idiopathic). Some factors, such as bad posture, bruxism, anatomical factors (related to dental occlusion alterations that can cause internal derangement of the TMJ), occlusal disharmony, malposition or malformation of the condyle or fossa, trauma, orthodontic treatment, and psychological factors (e.g., stress),[36] have been hypothesized to initiate or precipitate TMD or to increase a person's predisposition to develop these disorders.[37] However, most of these factors are not based on solid scientific grounds. According to Drangsholt and LeResche,[1] factors associated with female gender, the number of pre-existing pain conditions, and depression appear to be strongly associated with TMD. The remaining factors mentioned previously have failed to demonstrate a strong relationship with TMD, and more research is needed to clarify their role in causing or perpetuating TMD pain.

It is unknown why people develop TMD and why they progress to chronicity. A variety of physical and psychological factors could be implicated in chronic TMD, such as oral habits, secondary gain, and higher levels of pain and disability. Such factors are also seen in other chronic pain conditions, such as low back pain, headache, and neck pain. Thus the most recent accepted theory related to the etiology, assessment, and management of TMD is supported by the biopsychosocial model.[38] TMD therefore is recognized as a multidimensional disorder that is a result of biological, psychological, and social alterations.

Classification of Temporomandibular Disorders

Various professional organizations have classified TMDs in various ways. The American Academy of Orofacial Pain has established a set of diagnostic criteria that has been presented as an addendum to the classification of and diagnostic criteria for headache disorders, cranial neuralgias, and facial pain.[39] A number of classification schemes used in epidemiological studies of TMDs include clinical signs. The differential diagnosis of TMD is based on the patient's chief complaint, clinical evaluation of the patient's signs and symptoms, and TMJ imaging when necessary. Most of the tools have been based on clinical experience and patients' reports.

Several classification systems have been used in epidemiological studies to define TMD. However, not all of them have been validated or tested for reliability and responsiveness. The currently accepted criteria for diagnosing TMD are the *Research Diagnostic Criteria for Temporomandibular Disorders* (RDC/TMD) developed by the Department of Oral Surgery, University of Washington. The RDC/TMD is a guide that provides clinical researchers with a standardized system for examining, diagnosing, and classifying the most common subtypes of TMD with clear face and criterion validity.[1] It was introduced in 1992 and has been widely used in clinical research settings around the world where TMD and facial pain are managed. Some recent studies have demonstrated the good reliability of the RDC/TMD in different settings, not only for determining signs and symptoms,[40] but also for making reliable diagnoses.[41] Wahlund et al.[42] found good to excellent reliability ($\kappa > 0.78$) for each of the RDC/TMD major groups. This guide has been recommended as a model system for standardizing the investigation into the diagnosis and classification of any chronic pain condition. The guide is divided into two sections: Axis I: Clinical TMD conditions, and Axis II: Pain-related disability and psychological status.[43] In this chapter, the authors focus on the Axis I classification.

TMDs can also be broadly divided into (1) disorders of the masticatory muscles, (2) TMJ disc displacements, and (3) degenerative disorders of the TMJ. Each of these categories has several subcategories. For example, disorders of the masticatory muscles include myofascial pain, myositis, myospasm, local myalgia, myofibrotic contracture, neoplasia, and chronic muscle pain (i.e., fibromyalgia). TMJ disc displacements include disc displacement with reduction and disc displacement without reduction. TMJ degenerative disorders include arthralgia, osteoarthrosis, and arthritis (Table 3-1 and Figure 3-1).[43,44]

Some authors classify temporomandibular disorders as **arthrogenic TMDs**, which involve an alteration in the TMJ (e.g., congenital disorders, disc displacement, fracture, dislocation, inflammation, hypermobility, ankylosis, and osteoarthritis) and **myogenic TMDs**, which involve the masticatory muscles (e.g., myalgia [local muscle soreness], myofascial pain, myositis, myospasm [protective co-contraction], myofibrotic contracture, and centrally mediated myalgia).[3,17,45] Only common TMD alterations are described in detail in this chapter.

Muscular Disorders
Myofascial Pain
The most common type of masticatory muscle disorder among the TMDs is myofascial pain. Myofascial pain is characterized by spontaneous pain and localized tenderness on palpation of the masticatory muscles, muscle stiffness, muscle pain that increases with function, and the possible presence of trigger points.[43,44] According to the RDC/TMD, pain during palpation should be present in at least three masticatory muscles. Because jaw function may be altered, the RMC/TMD subclassifies the condition as myofascial pain with or without limited mouth opening. Headache, earache, and toothache are other symptoms associated with this disorder. The recommended treatments include manual therapy (e.g., therapeutic massage, acupressure, and acupuncture) and osteopathic manipulation. Some of these treatments are discussed in detailed later in the chapter.

Table 3-1
Classification of Temporomandibular Disorders

RDC/TMD			Okeson	
Disorders of the Masticatory Muscles	TMJ Disc Displacement	Degenerative Disorders	Myogenic Disorders	Arthrogenic Disorders
Myofascial pain Myofascial pain with limited opening	Disc displacement with reduction Disc displacement without reduction	Arthralgia Osteoarthrosis Arthritis	Myofascial pain Myositis Myospasm (tonic contraction myalgia) Local muscle soreness (local myalgia) Centrally mediated myalgia	Congenital disorders Disc displacement Fracture Dislocation Inflammation Hypermobility Ankylosis Osteoarthritis

Data from Kraus S: Temporomandibular disorders, head and orofacial pain: cervical spine considerations, *Dent Clin North Am* 51:161-193, 2007; Auvenshine RC: Temporomandibular disorders: associated features, *Dent Clin North Am* 51:105-127, 2007; Dworkin SF, LeResche L: Research diagnostic criteria for temporomandibular disorders: review, criteria, examinations and specifications, critique, J Craniomandib Disord 6:301-355, 1992; and Okeson JP: *American Academy of Orofacial Pain: orofacial pain—guidelines for assessment, diagnosis and management,* Chicago, 1996, Quintessence.

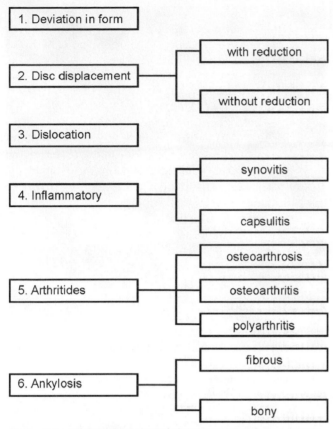

1. Deviation in form

2. Disc displacement
- with reduction
- without reduction

3. Dislocation

4. Inflammatory
- synovitis
- capsulitis

5. Arthritides
- osteoarthrosis
- osteoarthritis
- polyarthritis

6. Ankylosis
- fibrous
- bony

Figure 3-1
Classifications of TMDs. (Reprinted with permission from Dr. L. Kamelchuk, Calgary, AB, 2005.)

Chronic Centrally Mediated Myalgia

According to Okeson,[46] muscle pain can be highly influenced by central mechanisms in chronic conditions. Chronic centrally mediated myalgia is a result of prolonged myofascial pain. Therefore the longer a patient complains of myogenous masticatory pain, the greater the likelihood the person will develop chronic centrally mediated myalgia. Chronic centrally mediated myalgia mainly originates from the central nervous system (CNS), and signs and symptoms are felt peripherally in the muscle tissue.[46] A clinical characteristic of chronic centrally mediated myalgia is constant, aching, myogenous pain, pain at rest that increases with function, and increased tenderness to palpation, along with a prolonged history of pain.[46] Because this condition is a complex one, treatment strategies must address it as a chronic disorder.

Myospasm

Myospasm is a rare, acute condition of the masticatory muscles. It is an involuntary and continuous muscle contraction characterized by localized pain and limited range of motion (ROM) of the jaw.[44] It usually is of short duration.[46]

Local Nonspecific Myalgia

Myalgia is acute, local, noninflammatory pain in the masticatory muscles as a result of protective muscle splinting, post-exercise muscle soreness, muscle fatigue, trauma, and/or pain from ischemia. Its causes and pathology are not clearly defined.[44] It is also called local muscle soreness.[46] According to Okeson,[46] it is characterized by changes in the local environment of the muscle tissues, mainly through release of algogenic substances that produce pain.

Myofibrotic Contracture

Myofibrotic contracture is a painless shortening of a masticatory muscle as a result of fibrosis in muscles and surrounding tissues.[44]

Temporomandibular Joint Disc Displacements

Internal derangement of the TMJ is defined as an abnormal relationship between the mandibular condyle and the disc. This abnormal relationship may involve disc displacement with reduction or disc displacement without reduction. Patients with disc derangement can present with a clinical sign, such as clicking, that is characteristic, but not necessarily confirmation, of a reducing disc derangement.[47]

Disc Displacement with Reduction

Disc displacement can occur anteriorly, medially, anteromedially, or (the most rarely seen) posteriorly. The etiology of disc displacement can be either direct trauma to the mandible (e.g., a blow during a motor vehicle accident or contact sports) or indirect trauma. Some researchers postulate that small, repeated episodes of trauma to the joint eventually can cause enough internal tissue damage to produce displacement.[48] It is thought that microtrauma occurs to the structure of the disc itself and/or in some cases to the posterior ligament attached to the disc. This damage causes histological changes within the cell structures of the disc and reduces the disc's load bearing or compression capacity.

Repeated microtrauma eventually leads to macrotrauma and a further breakdown in tissue and in the disc's ability to function properly. Eventually the disc begins to sublux off the head of the condyle; clinically, this produces a click, which can be heard by the patient (and sometimes by others) or can be felt by the clinician during palpation over the poles of the joint during mandibular movement. The patient may present with a reducing disc (i.e., a disc that is displaced and reduces back to its proper position on the condyle), which the patient and clinician may or may not be able to feel. A correct diagnosis of subluxed or dislocated disc can be made only with the backup of an appropriate radiological examination.

In the initial stage of disc displacement, the click during displacement is present early in the opening phase. As the disc and posterior ligament become further traumatized and further displaced, the click is noted later in the opening phase. Therefore a patient who has a click after opening the mandible at least 5 mm of intraincisal distance is likely to have a fairly recent dysfunction, whereas a patient who does not have a click until 45 mm of opening is likely to have had a dysfunction for a longer time (Figures 3-2 to 3-4). In the dental profession, a click that is felt during both the opening and closing phases is called a **reciprocal click;** in other cases, a click at the joint may be felt either during opening or during closing. When the disc displacement with reduction is unilateral, the mandible can deviate to the affected side during mouth opening.[49]

Patients with disc displacement with reduction can have symptoms of joint tenderness on palpation, joint pain that

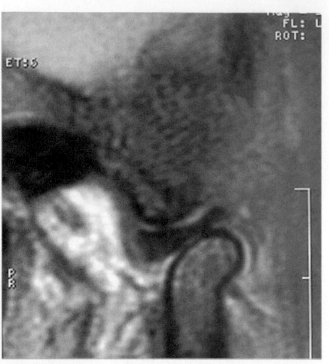

Figure 3-4
MRI of disc displacement with reduction showing reduced disc opening. (Courtesy Dr. D. Hatcher, Sacramento, CA.)

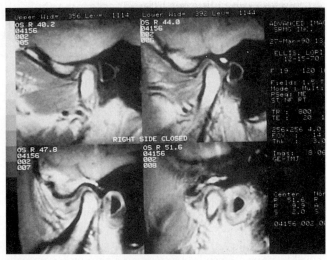

Figure 3-2
MRI of disc displacement with reduction. (Courtesy Dr. L. Kamelchuk, Calgary, AB.)

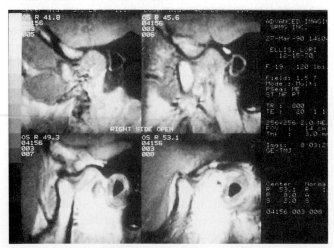

Figure 3-3
MRI of disc displacement with reduction. (Courtesy Dr. L. Kamelchuk, Calgary, AB.)

is increased with function, and aberrant mandibular movement with opening.[49]

From a clinical standpoint, it is important to make the patient aware of the likely biomechanical dysfunction occurring in the joint and to emphasize the fact that no form of treatment is likely to reduce the displaced disc. Patients tend to focus on the click, and it is vital to explain, as an educational part of the treatment, that it is possible to have a clicking joint that is pain free and functional. Indeed, because the disc is crucial to lubrication and nutrition of the structures within the joint,[5] a joint with a clicking disc is preferable to one that is silent and displaced.

Treatment should focus on attempting to produce a symmetrical opening so that the heads of the mandibular condyles translate equally during opening. Making sure that muscle activity is symmetrical also is necessary. As part of the education process, the clinician must teach the patient to avoid any activities that might cause additional trauma to the involved joint or even to the opposite joint. As a result of the dysfunction or the pain caused by the dysfunction, patients not uncommonly isolate any mastication to the side away from the dysfunction. Patients must be coached to chew equally on both sides. They also must be taught to avoid any habit that might increase trauma to the joint, such as nail biting, chewing on toothpicks, bruxing, or chewing gum; these activities can adversely affect the temporomandibular joint.

Disc Displacement Without Reduction

In some cases disc displacement with reduction causes enough trauma to the disc and its attached ligaments that the disc does not slide back into its normal position over the pole of the condyle. This can happen asymptomatically, although classically, patients present with a history of a clicking functional joint that suddenly changes to a non-clicking, reduced opening joint (e.g., "My jaw clicked for 5 years, and then all of a sudden I woke up [or bit down on some popcorn or yawned], there was a big crack, and my jaw didn't click any more, but I couldn't open my mouth as far."). In a study by Stegenga and De Bont,[47] 9% of patients with reducing disc displacement progressed to nonreducing disc displacement within 3 years. The main complaint of these patients is inability to open the mouth wide. In the case of a unilateral problem, the mandible is deviated to the affected side during attempted opening without returning to the midline.[49]

Disc displacement without reduction is also called a **clinical closed lock** (Figures 3-5 and 3-6). As previously noted, the closed lock can be present with or without symptoms; however, a person with a clinical closed lock is more likely to have accompanying symptoms such as pain, muscle spasm, and reduced function. If the pain is from the TMJ itself, the patient probably will point to the joint and indicate that it hurts there. Sometimes pain can be referred from the TMJ to other areas. It often manifests as a parietal headache on the same side or as pain under the angle of the jaw, or both. Pain also can be referred to the temporomandibular area from other structures; for example, a trigger point in the midbelly of the sternocleidomastoid muscle refers pain directly over the TMJ. Therefore it is very important that the clinician perform a complete musculoskeletal assessment, which includes not only the masticatory system but also other structures that could be involved, especially the cervical spine.

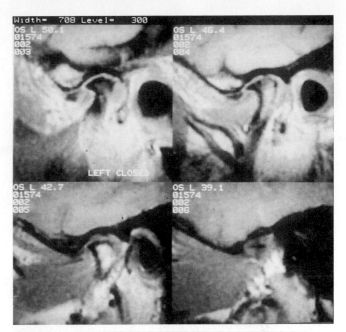

Figure 3-6

MRI of disc displacement without reduction. (Courtesy Dr. L. Kamelchuk, Calgary, AB.)

Treatment of a clinical closed lock is aimed at restoring more normal function. Because of the kinematics of the joint, a degree of opening can be achieved with the disc in a displaced position. Opening produces condylar translation and rotation. In the first movement, which takes place in the superior part of the joint, the mandibular condyle articulates with the disc; in the second movement, which takes place in the inferior part of the joint, the disc and condyle articulate with the temporal fossa. With the disc displaced, translation is reduced; this can be seen during the examination, and it differentiates the clinical closed lock from a straightforward capsulitis. Unless a large amount of muscle spasm disrupts the normal condylar movement, when capsulitis is present without disc displacement, the head of the condyle is still able to translate forward during mandibular opening. In both disorders the condyle can still rotate, and an opening of up to 30 mm of intraincisal distance can be achieved using only condylar rotation.

In most cases, if the joint is left untreated, the structures in the joint gradually are stretched so that eventually a more functional opening is achieved. However, secondary adaptive changes can occur in the masticatory structures and can cause other dysfunctions. For example, a joint with a clinical closed lock (a hypomobile joint) stresses the contralateral mandibular joint and causes hypermobility of that joint, which may become symptomatic. For this reason, one of the aims of treatment should be to speed up the stretching that normally occurs in the dysfunctional

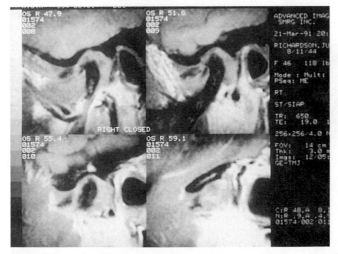

Figure 3-5

MRI of disc displacement without reduction. (Courtesy Dr. L. Kamelchuk, Calgary, AB.)

joint to alleviate the stress on the opposite joint. Thus mobilization of the hypomobile joint becomes vital to restoration of a more symmetrical opening. The patient should be informed that the clinician is not actually trying to relocate the disc, but rather to speed up what the body eventually would achieve anyway; that is, a stretching out of tight structures to obtain a more normal function.

Estimates are that 9% to 13% of asymptomatic joints have some type of TMD-related problem. However, not all patients with pain over the TMJ region have an internal derangement; likewise, the absence of pain in the TMJ region does not necessarily mean that no internal derangement is present. It has been shown that in so-called normal, symptom-free populations, a certain percentage of joints actually have internal derangements. This fact emphasizes the importance of the history, musculoskeletal assessment, and radiological survey in determining the condition present. The clinician cannot determine the type of pathology taking place in the joint by using just one type of diagnostic imaging. In the past, some practitioners thought that a lateral x-ray film of the temporomandibular joint was enough to allow determination of the pathologic condition at the TMJ and even the position of the condylar head in the temporal fossa. However, it has since been shown that a full set of diagnostic images is needed to ascertain properly what is going on in the joint. Many practitioners now require a Panorex (a radiograph that gives an overall impression of the maxilla-mandible structure) (Figure 3-7); tomograms that show both the opening and resting positions of the condyle; and cephalograms, which orthodontists use to define growth patterns, particularly the skull structure (Figure 3-8). Magnetic resonance imaging (MRI) of the joint demonstrates the state and position of the disc and surrounding soft tissues in much greater detail (Figure 3-9) than an x-ray film.

Degenerative Disorders

As mentioned previously, the disc is an important structure in the lubrication and nutrition of the joint. When the disc stops functioning properly (e.g., immobile, disc in the anterior position), changes occur in the joint structures that can

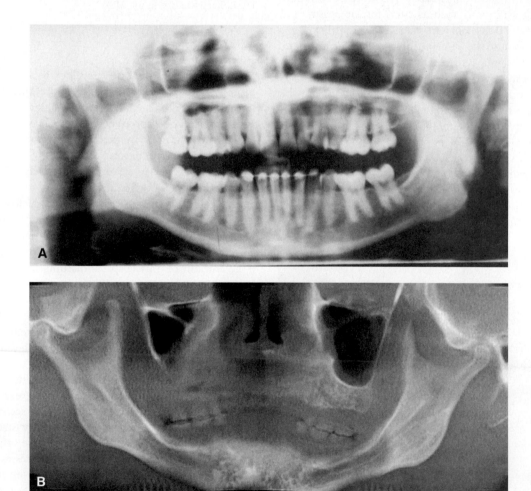

Figure 3-7

A, Panorex image of the maxilla and mandible. **B,** Panorex image of an edentulous patient.

Continued

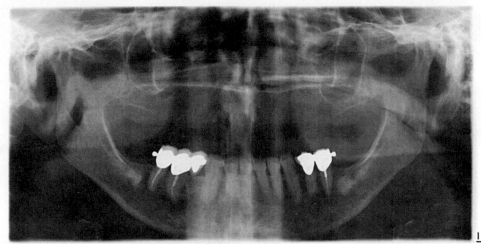

Calcification stylohyoid

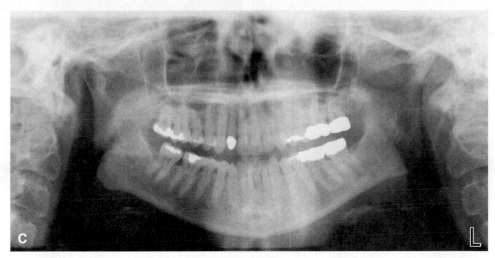

Elongated left stylohyoid

Figure 3-7 cont'd
C, Panorex image of a patient with eagle syndrome. (**A** courtesy Dr. L. Kamelchuk, Calgary, AB; **B** and **C** courtesy Dr. D. Hatcher, Sacramento, CA.)

be seen with diagnostic imaging. The hypomobility affects the pumping action that delivers nutrients from the synovial fluid to the articular cartilage. The deficiency in lubrication and nutrients may induce or aggravate degeneration.[47] Changes that occur in the joint structures include erosion, cavitation, osteophyte formation, and a reduction in the normal joint line (Figure 3-10).

TMDs that arise from degenerative joint changes most often are seen after age 40.[50] Some small x-ray changes usually can be seen in a joint that has disc displacement with reduction, such as flattening of the condylar head, subchondral sclerosis, and slight remodeling; however, the major degenerative changes do not occur until the disc is displaced and is not reducing. All these changes can occur without symptoms. When symptoms do occur, they usually include pain, muscle spasm, headaches, and a change in

function of the masticatory system. For example, the patient is unable to chew hard foods, or crepitus is experienced at the TMJ with function. The main aim of treatment for degenerative joint disease of the TMJ is to restore the area to normal function. In addition, it bears repeating: As part of the educational process, the clinician must emphasize to the patient that the treatment is not about restoring the disc or disc function, but more about speeding along what the body would normally do anyway.

According to the RDC/TMD, the degenerative disorders include TMJ arthralgia, capsulitis, and TMJ osteoarthritis/osteoarthrosis.

TMJ Arthralgia
TMJ arthralgia is characterized by pain and tenderness in the TMJ capsule and/or the synovial lining. Pain is present

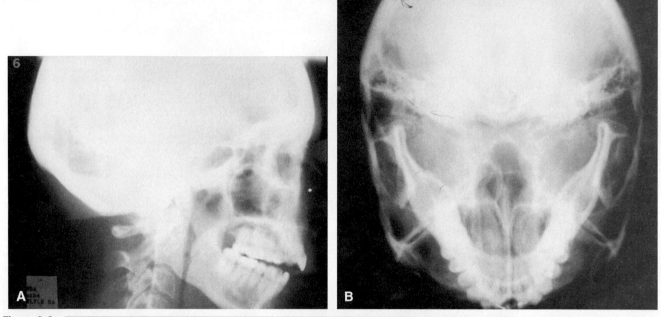

Figure 3-8
Cephalograms of the skull. **A,** Lateral view. **B,** Basilar view. (Courtesy Dr. L. Kamelchuk, Calgary, AB.)

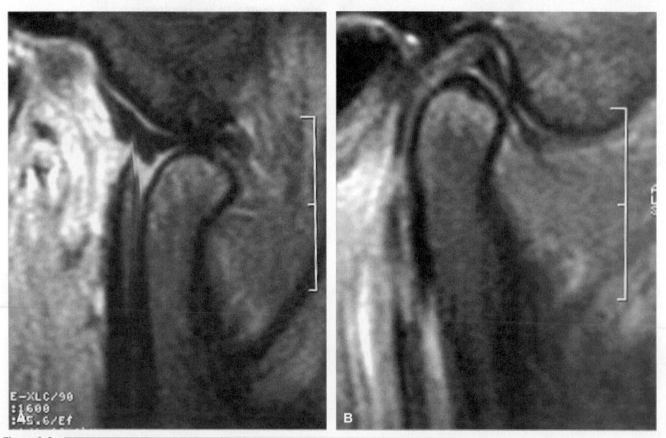

Figure 3-9
MRI studies of a normal temporomandibular joint. **A,** Open. **B,** Closed. (Courtesy Dr. D. Hatcher, Sacramento, CA.)

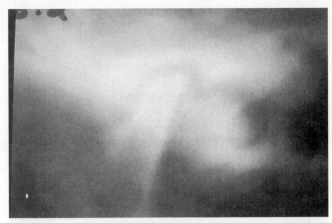
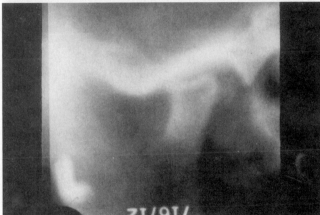

Figure 3-10

CT scans of degenerative joint disease. (Courtesy Dr. L. Kamelchuk, Calgary, AB.)

in one or both joints during palpation, and the patient has at least one of the following symptoms: pain in the joint region, pain during maximum unassisted opening, pain during assisted opening, or pain during lateral movements. Crepitus should not be present with a diagnosis of simple arthralgia.[43] Capsulitis commonly is present in patients with TMJ arthralgia.

Capsulitis

Pain on palpation over the superior pole and/or posterior part of the TMJ is thought to indicate a capsulitis of the joint. This can be present in an acute stage (e.g., after trauma, such as a blow to the jaw) or in a chronic stage, after repeated minor trauma or insults to the joint itself (e.g., with bruxism in the presence of a Class II malocclusion).* The clinician should keep in mind that capsulitis also may be present in the first stages of some general

---

*Details on malocclusion, internal derangement, clinician observation, and the patient history can be found in volume 1 of this series, *Orthopedic Physical Assessment*, Chapter 4.

systemic diseases (e.g., rheumatoid arthritis, ankylosing spondylitis) and with local or systemic infection, although cases involving infection are rarely seen in the private practice setting.

Along with pain on palpation, the patient may have some swelling within the joint (although this is rarely seen except in cases of direct acute trauma). Patients often complain of swelling or a sense of fullness over the temporomandibular region. However, this is not often seen clinically unless the area has suffered a severe degree of trauma. Patients are likely to have pain on occlusion and to complain of discomfort with mastication (which, of course, causes compression within the joint and distention of the joint capsule). The capsular pattern of the temporomandibular joint is thought to be reduction of mandibular opening. Sometimes the patient also reports having pain with activities such as yawning or opening wide to bite, which involve stretching of the joint capsule. Capsulitis can be accompanied by spasm of the muscles of mastication, particularly the masseter and the medial and lateral pterygoid muscles. Muscle spasm is present on the ipsilateral side, and during the assessment, the examiner will note deviation of the mandible to that side on opening. Condylar translation (i.e., the movement of the condyle forward within the joint) is likely to be present, and this clinical finding is one of the differential diagnostic indicators that distinguish an isolated capsulitis from other internal derangements of the TMJ.

In the acute stage, treatment is aimed at reducing the inflammation and resultant swelling, resting the involved structures, and reducing any muscle spasm; pain reduction should follow as a result of these measures.

Three of the four basic principles represented by the acronym RICE (rest, ice, and compression; elevation is not really possible with the TMJ) can be used in the treatment of acute capsulitis. The patient should be instructed to eat only soft foods to avoid compressing the joint and aggravating the muscle spasm. The use of an occlusal splint to rest the joint sometimes is effective; however, if the surrounding muscle spasm is severe, a splint can actually increase it, because it increases the vertical dimension, thus stretching the contracted muscles. Ice can be applied to the side of the face over the TMJ region to reduce any heat caused by an acute inflammation, as well as the effects of the inflammation and swelling. The authors' experience has been that, apart from cases involving an acute traumatic inflammatory problem, patients usually find moist heat more comfortable and efficacious. As mentioned, elevation is not possible for cases involving the TMJ; however, symptoms can be controlled through use of the usual principles for treating an acutely traumatized musculoskeletal joint. Nonsteroidal anti-inflammatory drugs (NSAIDs) may be prescribed to reduce pain and/or inflammation.

TMJ Osteoarthritis/Osteoarthrosis

Arthritis is an inflammatory condition in the joint, and it can manifest in different forms, such as osteoarthritis and rheumatoid arthritis. Osteoarthritis results in erosion and fibrillation of the cartilage and degeneration of subchondral bone. Symptoms of osteoarthritis include pain, restricted jaw movement, and joint sounds (crepitus). Rheumatoid arthritis (RA) is a chronic systemic inflammatory disease that involves the synovial joints, including the TMJ. RA produces symptoms such as fatigue, fever, anemia, and neuropathy.[51]

According to the RDC/TMD, a diagnosis of osteoarthritis requires the presence of arthralgia plus either crepitus in the joint or imaging evidence of at least one degenerative characteristic, specifically erosion of normal cortical delineation, sclerosis of part or all of the condyle and articular eminence, flattening of joint surfaces, or osteophyte formation.

TMJ osteoarthrosis is a degenerative disorder in a joint with an abnormal joint structure. For this diagnosis, the same characteristics must be present as for the osteoarthritis diagnosis, but the arthralgia symptoms must be absent.[43] Osteoarthrosis presents degenerative changes similar to those seen with osteoarthritis, but it is a noninflammatory condition.

Other TMJ Problems

Hypermobility

Hypermobility can be viewed in two ways: as a joint dysfunction entity in itself, or as an end process in the natural history of joint dysfunction, which progresses from capsulitis to disc displacement with reduction to disc displacement without reduction to degenerative joint disease and eventually to hypermobility.

For a joint to be labeled hypermobile, radiological hypermobility must be present. Normally the head of the condyle can be seen to translate to the tip of the articular eminence; however, with radiographic hypermobility, the condylar head translates beyond the articular eminence (Figure 3-11). This often is accompanied by a change in the normal biomechanics of the joint, which means the examiner would see an increase in condylar translation and a reduction in condylar rotation. As mentioned previously, rotation normally takes place at the beginning of mandibular opening; midopening requires a degree of rotation and some translation; and the final phase of opening involves mainly translation of the condyle. In a hypermobile joint, posterior disc structures usually are stretched and the posterior ligament frequently is perforated. Because of the soft tissue laxity, a great deal of translation can occur at the beginning of opening, and very little rotation is felt at all. This is almost a reversal of the normal articular mechanics of the joint.

If the hypermobility is the result of stiffness in the opposite joint, treatment obviously includes mobilization of the hypomobile joint. If the hypermobility is the end result of degenerative changes within the joint, treatment focuses more on restricting the extra mobility within the joint. If the biomechanics of the joint have been changed, part of the treatment should include exercise to try to return joint movement to a more normal form. For example, some hypermobility can cause increased translation and reduced rotation. One way to restrict translation is to coach the patient in using the tongue to control movement. The tip of the tongue is placed behind the top teeth, the lips are placed together, and the teeth are left in their resting position in slight dysocclusion (the upper

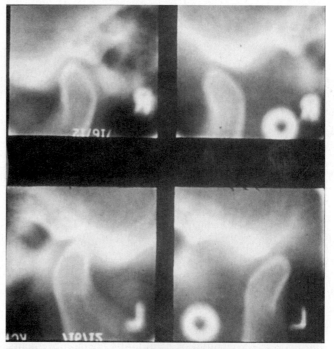
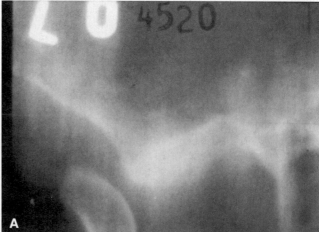

Figure 3-11

A, Tomograms showing hypermobility of the TMJ.

Continued

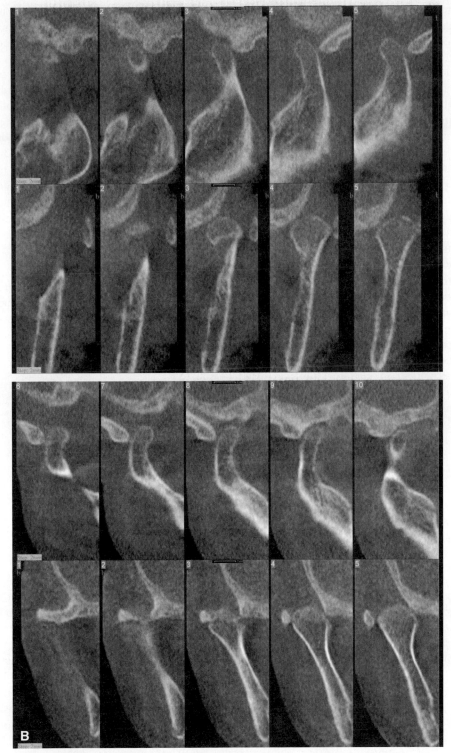

Figure 3-11 cont'd
B, Tomograms of a hypermobile TMJ showing dislocation of the condyle. (**A** courtesy Dr. L. Kamelchuk, Calgary, AB; **B** courtesy Dr. D. Hatcher, Sacramento, CA.)

and lower teeth have a slight distance between them [1-3 mm at rest]; this is called the *free way space*). Then the patient is instructed to keep the lips together and drop the jaw. By placing an index finger over the head of the condyle, the examiner can feel a reduction in the condylar translation and a return to some rotation. The patient is instructed to repeat this exercise once an hour so that the different movement patterns produced by the motor units are reprogrammed as a new engram into the motor cortex.

The tongue can also be used to restrict hypermobility. If the patient is instructed to keep the tip of the tongue behind the top teeth and to open the mouth as far as possible with the tongue in place, in most cases the joint will not be stretched into its hypermobile range. In some cases a patient with a long tongue will not be able to restrict the opening sufficiently; the individual should then be instructed to place the tip of the tongue in the roof of the palate. If this still does not restrict the opening movement sufficiently, the patient can be coached to fold the upper one third of the tongue into the roof of the mouth. Normal opening should be assessed as 40-50 mm interincisal distance. Opening past 50 mm frequently can be present with normal joint biomechanics, indicating laxity. Increased translation also can occur at the cost of lost condylar rotation (less than 50 mm), which often is seen in individuals with Asian features.

Patient Education to Limit Hypermobility

- Control opening wide (hypermobility)
- Put the tip of your tongue against the back of your upper teeth. Keeping your tongue in this position, open your mouth as far as the tongue will allow. This is as far as you should allow yourself to open, so that the soft tissue around the jaw is not overstretched and is allowed to rest
- Cut your food into bite-sized (i.e., small) pieces. Do not take big bites out of hamburgers or other foods
- When you feel a yawn coming on, make sure to control the amount of mouth opening using the tongue positioning technique described in the second point

---

TMJ Ankylosis

Ankylosis of the TMJ is a complete fusion of the condyle to the temporal fossa (true ankylosis). Ankylosis is classified as congenital, traumatic, inflammatory (i.e., rheumatoid arthritis), systemic (e.g., ankylosing spondylitis), or neoplastic (e.g., osteochondroma).[49]

Ankylosis causes restriction of opening and stress on the opposite joint; in fact, patients often present with symptoms arising from the joint opposite the ankylosed

joint. In children, TMJ ankylosis impairs mandibular growth and can result in mandibular micrognathia (underdevelopment). This condition has functional and esthetic implications. It also causes difficulties related to nutrition and oral hygiene. Treatment (i.e., surgical correction) should be initiated as soon as the condition is recognized. The main objective is to re-establish joint and jaw functions.[52]

During mobilization, as part of the physical therapy treatment, no distraction of the condyle on the ankylosed side occurs, and radiographic restriction also is noted. Apart from treating the opposite joint symptomatically, therapy is not effective in improving movement (Figure 3-12).

TMD-Related Factors

Any discussion of temporomandibular disorders must include factors and dysfunctions associated with TMDs. As mentioned previously, bruxism, forward head posture, alterations in occlusion, and psychosocial stress have been hypothesized to initiate or precipitate a TMD or to increase a person's predisposition to developing a TMD.

Bruxism

Parafunctional habits, such as bruxism, teeth clenching, jaw thrusting, gum chewing, and jaw testing (repeatedly moving the jaw to cause a click, or moving the jaw into a painful position to see if the click or pain is still present) can add repetitive strain to the masticatory muscles and cause tenderness and pain (Figure 3-13).

According to Lobbezoo and Naeije,[53] the etiology of bruxism is related to morphological, pathophysiological, and psychological factors. Pathophysiological factors in the etiology of bruxism are increasingly related to sleep disturbances, chemical alterations in the brain, use of medication, and use of cigarettes and alcohol. Bruxism can cause muscle pain, TMJ noise, limited jaw movements, and headache.

One of the most common characteristics seen in patients with myogenic TMD is the hyperactivity of the masticatory muscles that can be caused by bruxism. This hyperactivity is caused by the dynamic imbalance of the masticatory system,[54] and it can contribute to internal derangement.[50]

In 1997 Kampe et al.[55] investigated subjects between 23 and 68 years of age with more than 5 years of bruxism. The authors suggested a causal relationship between the bruxism and TMD signs and symptoms, including headache and pain in the neck and shoulder. People with TMDs commonly have parafunctional habits (e.g., bruxism, clenching the teeth, and nail biting [neuromuscular

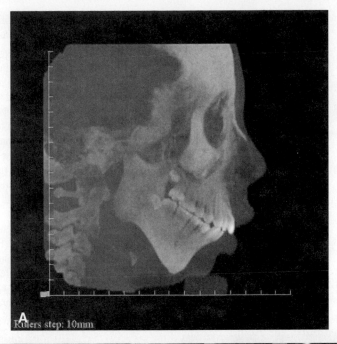

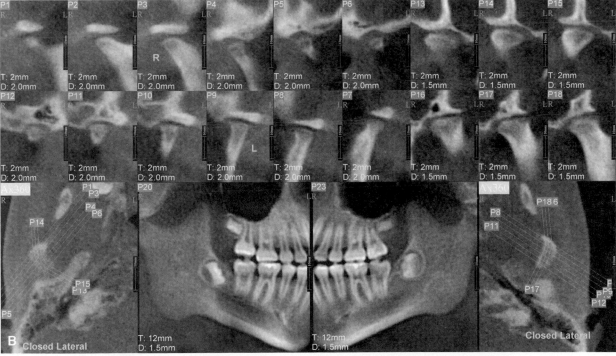

Figure 3-12

Tomogram of **(A)** ankylosis and **(B)** juvenile rheumatoid arthritis (right closed). (Courtesy Dr. D. Hatcher, Sacramento, CA.)

factors]). However, the relationship between bruxism, stress, and TMD is unclear. Some studies have found that bruxism is not always present in people with TMD; therefore a causal relationship cannot be claimed.[56]

Bruxism or clenching the teeth often can be done unconsciously and may be the body's response to an aggravating stimulus (e.g., a high restoration on a tooth, malocclusion, stress, habit, or a combination of factors). Some authors believe that bruxing can trigger problems within the TMJ apparatus, whereas others deny such a claim.[9,57] Either way, bruxing definitely can aggravate TMDs and hinder treatment and recovery.

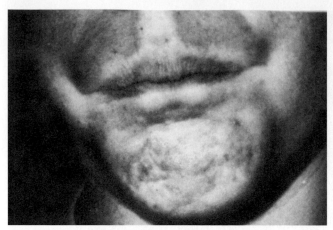

Figure 3-13

Facial features of a patient with bruxism.

Signs and Symptoms of a "Bruxer"

- The patient regularly and consistently clenches and relaxes the masseters
- A masseter "bump" is present. (The clinician lightly palpates the masseters as the patient opens and closes the mouth. Normally, on closing, the teeth lightly come together before resting. A "bruxer" shows a definite and obvious overcontraction as the teeth occlude)
- Hypertrophy of the masseters is obvious (this may give the patient a heavyset jaw)
- The patient regularly and consistently purses the lips or squeezes them together
- The teeth show facet wearing
- The tongue shows scalloping (this occurs as a result of the teeth constantly biting on the edges of the tongue)

Because bruxism often is an unconscious habit, it can be very difficult to control. Sometimes just pointing out the habit to patients can be enough to make them aware of the problem and prompt them to take steps to control it themselves. In other cases, some form of relaxation technique, biofeedback, or stress management might be necessary to help control the problem. Exercise that promotes the contraction of muscles antagonistic to the masseters and temporalis can help (e.g., a resisted mandibular opening). If the bruxing is aggravated by gum chewing or holding a toothpick between the teeth, removal of the offending object often is enough to control the symptoms.

Patient Management Program: Controlling Bruxism

- One of the most important steps in breaking the habit of clenching and grinding the teeth (bruxism) is to become conscious of when it occurs and then to stop doing it. Many people are unaware they have the habit until it is pointed out to them. This awareness must occur before you can control the habit. An excellent way to avoid clenching the teeth is to learn to keep your lips together and your teeth apart. This simple step makes clenching the teeth impossible; even more important, it relaxes the very muscles that become tense and taut. As an extra dividend, this relaxation technique improves your facial expression and appearance. It also promotes a more normal resting position of the temporomandibular joints.
- The more conscious you become about this basic procedure of relaxing the jaw muscle, the greater control you will have in overcoming this harmful habit. First, you need to identify when you are most likely to clench or grind your teeth during waking hours, such as while driving on the freeway, during physical exertion or sports, or when you are under emotional tension or stress. At these times you should repeat to yourself, "lips together, teeth apart."
- By sealing your lips and gently blowing or puffing air, you will automatically separate your teeth and simultaneously relax your jaw and facial muscles.
- Remember, you probably have had this habit for a long time, and it won't vanish overnight. You must persevere and practice this exercise each time you find your teeth clenched.

Forward Head Posture

According to some researchers, the forward head posture can cause TMDs.[58-60] Head posture and its relation to occlusion, to the development and function of the dentofacial structures, and to TMDs have been studied. Head posture alterations have been associated with changes in the stomatognathic system, influencing the biomechanical behavior of the TMJ and associated structures. Some have suggested that the position of the head affects the resting position of the mandible,[60,61] produces greater muscular activity in the temporal and masseter muscles,[58,60-67] and alters the TMJ internal relationships.[68] This can be explained by the relationship between the masticatory system and the cervical spine, as a result of neurophysiological, anatomical, and biomechanical interactions.[54]

A systematic review done in 2006 studied the association between the head and the cervical posture and TMD.[69] Of the 12 papers included in the study, nine concluded that postural alteration could be associated with TMD. However, the studies included in the review were of poor methodological quality. According to the authors, it was not clear that head and cervical posture were associated with TMD because of the level of evidence in the studies. Further studies are needed to determine the relationship between postural alterations and TMD.

In addition, a systematic review that focused on the effectiveness of physical therapy interventions for TMD found that postural training was one of the interventions recommended to restore or optimize the alignment of the craniomandibular system and to reduce pain in patients who have TMDs with muscular involvement (i.e., myogenic TMD).[70]

The cervical spine and related structures can be seen as an integral part of the physical therapy approach to patients with TMDs, because many studies have demonstrated a clinical association between alterations in cervical spine with masticatory systems disorders.[2]

Occlusal Alterations

Dental occlusion is very important for masticatory function. It has been suggested that a significant relationship exists between alterations in the masticatory system and dental occlusion. Occlusion relationships should be routinely considered as an important part of the diagnosis in patients with TMD.[71]

Occlusion alterations influence the TMJ and the functions of the masticatory muscles. According to Okeson,[45] occlusion alterations can be associated with parafunctional habits such as squeezing, bruxism and clenching the teeth, which lead to muscle spasm and hyperactivity. Celic et al.[72] investigated the prevalence of TMD and the relationship between dental occlusion and parafunctional habits using clinical assessment and patient histories. They found a significant correlation between occlusion alterations, parafunctional habits, and TMD. Another study[73] found that the electromyographic (EMG) responses of the temporal and masseter muscles were modified in subjects with a Class II occlusion alteration (Angle classification). Subjects with a Class II occlusion showed hyperactivity of the temporal muscles, which altered the normal EMG pattern between the temporal and masseter muscles and also led to a higher occurrence of forward head posture. Conversely, many clinical studies have failed to demonstrate any significant differences between patients with TMD and controls in terms of occlusal variables.[74-76] For example, a recent study that evaluated 4310 subjects did not find any association between any occlusal variable and subjective TMD symptoms.[75] Neither convincing nor powerful evidence supports the theory of occlusal alterations as an important factor in TMD.[9]

Stress

Stress can play a significant role in TMDs; it can either initiate problems or aggravate an existing dysfunction. The clinician should include an explanation of the effects of stress in the initial history and interview process, because if stress appears to be a major concern, it may be necessary to involve a health professional (e.g., a clinical psychologist) who is experienced in stress management techniques, relaxation techniques, biofeedback, and counseling. The authors have found that a patient is much more willing to accept a referral to a clinical psychologist if this is brought up as a possibility before any therapy is initiated. If the whole

concept of stress as a factor in the pathology and treatment of the condition is left until after therapy has been initiated, the patient is more inclined to believe that the clinician thinks the problem is all in the patient's head; patients can be very averse to referral to a clinical psychologist after therapy has been unsuccessful or only partially successful.

The body does not appear to differentiate between good stress and bad stress. Winning the lottery can have just as detrimental an effect on the body as losing a job or losing a loved one. Various systems for rating life events have been published, and the clinician can use them to quantify the degree of stress a patient may be experiencing (Table 3-2).

In the life event rating scale presented in Table 3-2, the numbers in the column on the right represent the amount, duration, and severity of change required to cope with each item, averaged from the responses of hundreds of people. Marriage was arbitrarily assigned a magnitude of 50 points, and the subjects then rated the other items by number according to how much more or less change each required in comparison to marriage. For instance, the scale implies that losing a spouse by death (100) requires, in the long run, twice as much readjustment as getting married (50), four times as much as a change in living conditions (25), and nearly 10 times as much as minor violations of the law (11).

The more changes a person experiences in a given period, the more points accumulate. The higher the score, the more likely the person is to have a change in health. All kinds of health changes (e.g., serious illness, injuries, surgery, psychiatric disorders, even pregnancy) have been found to follow high life change scores. The higher the score, the more serious the health change is likely be.

Discussions with clinical psychologists have revealed that people commonly are able to cope with a severe life stress at the time of the event and that symptoms become apparent approximately 6 months after the stressful period. Therefore, when taking the history, the clinician should ask about previous life stressors to determine whether they are coincident with the latest exacerbation of symptoms. Clinically, some patients have been found not to be *psychologically aware;* that is, they are unable (or unwilling) to comprehend the effects of the psyche on the body and on an individual's well-being. Involvement in the psychological side of therapy might not be practical. Similarly, the clinician may have encountered people who are not *body aware;* that is, they seem to have no awareness of the physical functioning of the body or its specific control. This can make treatment for certain individuals challenging.

To help a patient understand the problem and identify some of the initiating factors, the clinician may find it worthwhile to get the patient to keep a daily diary of the symptoms or pain. A pain rating scale that is fairly simple to understand can be used (e.g., 0 is no pain and 10 is the worst pain the patient can imagine) (Table 3-3). With this approach, the clinician can obtain an idea of the degree of pain the patient feels and how the symptoms behave

Table 3-2
Life Event Rating Scale

Life Event	Mean Value
1. Death of spouse	100
2. Divorce	73
3. Marital separation	65
4. Jail term	63
5. Death of close family member	63
6. Personal injury or illness	53
7. Marriage	50
8. Fired at work	47
9. Marital reconciliation	45
10. Retirement	45
11. Change in health of family member	44
12. Pregnancy	40
13. Sex difficulties	39
14. Gain of new family member	39
15. Business readjustment	39
16. Change in financial state	38
17. Death of close friend	37
18. Change to different line of work	36
19. Change in number of arguments with spouse	35
20. High value mortgage	31
21. Foreclosure of mortgage or loan	30
22. Change in responsibilities at work	29
23. Son or daughter leaving home	29
24. Trouble with in-laws	29
25. Outstanding personal achievement	28
26. Wife begins or stops work	26
27. Begin or end school	26
28. Change in living conditions	25
29. Revision of personal habits	24
30. Trouble with boss	23
31. Change in work hours or conditions	20
32. Change in residence	20
33. Change in schools	20
34. Change in recreation	19
35. Change in church activities	19
36. Change in social activities	18
37. Lower value mortgage or loan	17
38. Change in sleeping habits	16
39. Change in number of family get-togethers	15
40. Change in eating habits	15
41. Vacation	13
42. Christmas	12
43. Minor violations of the law	11

Modified from Holmes TH, Rahe RH: The social readjustment rating scale, *J Psychosomat Res* 1:213-218, 1967.

throughout the day. Table 3-4 shows a diary that some clinical psychologists use to have patients rate their headache symptoms throughout the day.

The myofascial pain caused by stress and fatigue can occur not only in the region of the masticatory muscles, but also in the neck and shoulder region. This symptom is commonly present in patients with TMD. The sternocleidomastoid and trapezius muscles often are affected. Stress also can cause the patient to develop parafunctional habits, such as bruxism and clenching the teeth, which contribute to the hyperactivity of the masticatory muscles and consequently cause pain in this region.

Physical Therapy Treatment

The American Academy of Craniomandibular Disorders (AACD) and the Minnesota Dental Association (MDA) have cited physical therapy as an important treatment for TMD.[77] Physical therapy is prescribed with the intent to relieve musculoskeletal pain, reduce inflammation, and restore oral and neck motor function.

Numerous therapeutic interventions may prove effective in the treatment of TMD, including electrophysical modalities, acupuncture, exercises, and manual therapy techniques. Electrophysical modalities include ultrasound, microwave, laser, and electroanalgesic techniques (e.g., transcutaneous electrical nerve stimulation [TENS]), interferential current, and biofeedback. Interventions often include therapeutic exercises for the masticatory and/or cervical spine muscles to improve strength, coordination, resistance, and mobility in the region.[78] Manual therapy techniques are commonly used to reduce pain, restore mobility, or both. Interventions may also include or focus on associated impairments of the craniocervical system, such as poor posture, cervical muscle spasm, cervical pain, and referred pain from the cervical spine,[78] because a connection between cervical spine dysfunction and temporomandibular disorders has been seen clinically.[2,69]

In a recent systematic review, McNeely et al.[70] analyzed 12 randomized controlled trials that addressed the use of therapeutic exercise, acupuncture, and electrophysical modalities in the treatment of TMD. They found that the quality of the current evidence supporting the effectiveness of physical therapy in TMD is poor. Because of the dearth of published research on the efficacy of physical therapy in the treatment of TMD, only limited evidence is available upon which to base practice guidelines. Consequently, clinical decision making must still be based on empirical evidence. For this reason, the information about treatment interventions that follows is based on evidence and on the authors' clinical experience. For practical reasons, the information is divided into three general categories:

1. *Exercise,* including isotonic and isometric exercises to re-establish the correct working postures of the masticatory, cranial, and cervical systems, along with exercises to improve strength, resistance, and motor control of the masticatory and cervical muscles.
2. *Electrophysiological modalities,* including heat sources (e.g., hot packs and infrared and shortwave diathermy), ultrasound, TENS, and acupuncture.
3. *Manual therapy,* including various mobilization techniques to improve range of motion, reduce muscle spasm, and diminish pain.[79]

Clinicians practicing in this area can use any combination of these treatments that they feel suits their needs. However, after a stringent search of the literature, the authors must emphasize that the methods and combinations chosen are

Table 3-3
Pain Disability Index

The rating scales below are designed to measure the degree to which several aspects of your life are presently disrupted by chronic pain. In other words, we would like to know how much your pain is preventing you from doing what you normally do or from doing it as well as you normally would. Respond to each category by indicating the overall impact of pain in your life, not just when the pain is at its worst.

For each of the seven categories of life activity listed, please circle the number on the scale that describes the level of disability you typically experience. A score of 0 means no disability at all, and a score of 10 signifies that all the activities in which you would normally be involved have been totally disrupted or prevented by your pain.

1. **FAMILY/HOME RESPONSIBILITIES.** This category refers to activities related to the home or family. It includes chores and duties performed around the house (e.g., yard work, errands) and favors for other family members (e.g., driving the children to school).

0   1   2   3   4   5   6   7   8   9   10

2. **RECREATION.** This category includes hobbies, sports, and other similar leisure time activities.

0   1   2   3   4   5   6   7   8   9   10

3. **SOCIAL ACTIVITY.** This category refers to activities that involve participation with friends and acquaintances other than family members. It includes parties, theater, concerts, dining out, and other social functions.

0   1   2   3   4   5   6   7   8   9   10

4. **OCCUPATION.** This category refers to activities that are part of or directly related to your job. This includes nonpaying jobs as well (e.g., housewife) and volunteer work.

0   1   2   3   4   5   6   7   8   9   10

5. **SEXUAL BEHAVIOUR.** This category refers to the frequency and quality of your sex life.

0   1   2   3   4   5   6   7   8   9   10

6. **SELF CARE.** This category includes activities that involve personal maintenance and independent daily living (e.g., taking a shower, driving, getting dressed).

0   1   2   3   4   5   6   7   8   9   10

7. **LIFE-SUPPORT ACTIVITY.** This category refers to basic life-supporting behaviors, such as eating, sleeping, and breathing.

0   1   2   3   4   5   6   7   8   9   10

Modified from Tait RC, Pollard CA, Margolis RB et al: The Pain Disability Index: psychometric and validity data, *Arch Phys Med Rehabil* 68:441, 1987.

purely a matter of preference; there is no "gold standard" physical therapy treatment for any particular TMJ condition.

Exercise

Therapeutic exercises are prescribed to address specific TMJ impairments and to improve the function of the TMJ.[80] The most useful techniques for re-education and rehabilitation of the masticatory muscles have been reported to be muscle stretching and strengthening exercises.[81] Passive and active stretching of muscles and/or ROM are performed to increase oral opening and reduce pain.[81] Postural exercises also are recommended to restore or optimize the alignment of the craniomandibular system.[78]

Two recent systematic reviews provide evidence supporting the use of postural exercises and active and passive oral exercises to reduce symptoms of TMD.[70,82] A systematic review by McNeely et al.[70] found two studies that examined the effect of postural training (in combination with other therapies) on myogenic TMD. They reported significant improvements in pain and oral opening,[83,84] which supports the addition of postural exercise training. Komiyama et al.[83] found that after 1 month, mouth opening had increased significantly in patients who received postural training

Table 3-4
Headache Diary

Progress Chart

It is important to monitor the intensity of
your pain for at least two reasons:

1. Research has shown that this will help to
   reduce the psychological side effects that
   often accompany pain.
2. This information is useful in helping to
   determine the effects of your treatment
   program.

The following five-point scale is useful in
helping people monitor the severity of
their pain.

0. No headache.

1. Low level, only enters awareness when
   you think about it.

2. Aware of pain most of the time, but it
   can be ignored at times.

3. Painful but still able to continue job.

4. Severe pain, difficult to concentrate with
   undemanding tasks.

5. Intense incapacitating pain.

To monitor your pain level, mark the
appropriate number on the graph at each
hour and join the points together. Placing
the colored dot on your watch will help
you remember to do this.

Name: _____

Modified from Andrasik F: Assessment of patients with headache. In Turk D, Melzack R, editors: *Handbook of pain assessment*, p 465, New York, 2001, Guilford Press.

compared to patients who received only cognitive intervention or to a control group. Wright et al.[84] found a statistically significant improvement in maximum pain-free opening, pain threshold, and the modified Symptom Severity Index in patients who received postural treatment compared to those who received self-management instructions alone.

In summary, the evidence shows that physical therapy interventions, including exercises to correct head and neck posture, can be effective for relieving musculoskeletal pain and improving oral motor function in patients with muscular TMD.[83,84] However, more information is required to determine the optimal exercise prescription. In particular, details on frequency, intensity, duration, and the specific type of exercise used in treatment protocols are essential to allow replication in the clinical setting. Also, a more precise protocol description of postural exercises will allow a clear conclusion about the effectiveness of this type of intervention for relieving the symptoms of muscular TMD.

A study by Carmeli et al.[85] examined the effect of a combination of manual therapy and active exercise, compared with occlusal splint therapy, in the treatment of an anteriorly displaced temporomandibular disc in patients with arthrogenic TMD. The authors reported significant improvement in pain and oral opening in the manual therapy/exercise group. The only study that reported a nonsignificant finding with exercise examined the benefit of an oral exercise device on oral opening, pain, and wellness in patients with mixed TMD.[86] In this study, Grace et al.[86] found no significant benefit either from addition of the oral exercise device to traditional therapies or from use of the oral exercise device as part of a home program. However, the use of multiple uncontrolled treatments in the study masks any conclusions about the relative effectiveness of the oral exercise device.

Despite the methodological limitations of the studies analyzed by this review, evidence exists that supports the use of manual therapy and oral and postural exercises to reduce pain and improve ROM in people with TMD. This can guide clinicians in making the best choice for treating patients with TMD.[83,84]

As mentioned previously, exercises can be used to address impairments at the level of the craniomandibular system. Exercises can help reduce muscle spasm, restore muscle function, improve muscle strength and resistance, diminish pain, and aid motor control of the muscles. Different types of exercises are performed in the jaw and cervical region. (Information on cervical exercises was presented in Chapter 2 and can be reviewed there; evidence supports the use of cervical and postural exercises to improve TMD symptoms.) The following exercises focus on the TMJ and masticatory muscles.

Isotonic, isometric, and resistive exercises can be used, depending on the patient's condition. For example, the patient can actively perform exercises to improve range of motion by moving the jaw in all directions (open-close and lateral movements) to the end of ROM. These types of exercises stimulate lubrication of the TMJ, improve the proprioceptive information to the joint receptors, and help control pain.[87-89] In addition, these active exercises can be assisted by the clinician or self-assisted by the patient at the end of opening ROM. Mandibular opening can also be achieved by placing the thumbs and forefingers between the teeth and causing a passive stretch against the mandible and maxilla (Figure 3-14). The stretch should be held for at least 30 seconds to cause changes in the soft tissues.[90]

Active exercises also have been used to improve coordination and retraining of the jaw muscles. As mentioned previously, patients with TMD usually present with impaired masticatory muscle contraction patterns. These impaired patterns can cause abnormal distribution of loads to the

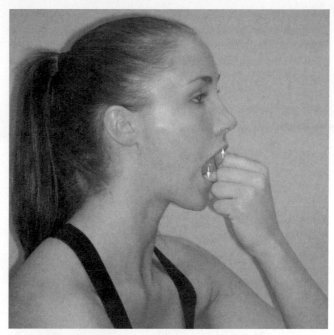

Figure 3-14
Passive stretch of the mouth opening.

TMJ and reinforce abnormal equilibrium between muscular groups. The objective of active exercises for coordination is to train the patient to open and close the mouth and perform lateral movements smoothly, trying to avoid abnormal patterns of contraction. This often can best be done if the patient works in front of a mirror. The patient opens and closes the mouth and performs lateral movements using the visual feedback on the position of the jaw (Figure 3-15).

As mentioned earlier, in patients with hypermobility, the active exercises can be controlled with the tongue

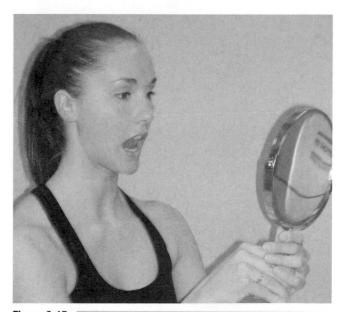

Figure 3-15
Visual feedback on jaw movement using a mirror.

positioned in the roof of the palate (Figure 3-16). If strengthening is the aim, gentle resistance can be provided in all directions (Figures 3-17 and 3-18). Input also can be achieved. The clinician places the fingers lightly beneath or on the side of the mandible and has the patient push into the slight resistance to get the muscles to contract and achieve the required movement; as an alternative,

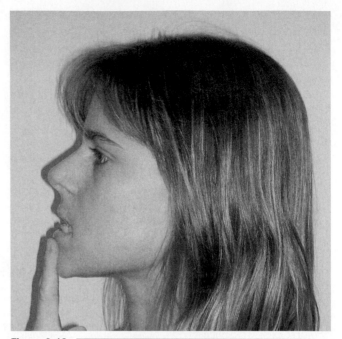

Figure 3-18
Resistive exercise for protrusion.

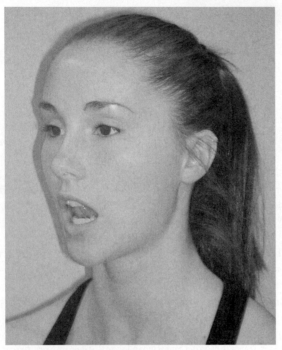

Figure 3-16
Tongue positioned in the roof of the palate.

the clinician can have the patient use his own fingers to supply the necessary light resistance. Jaw strengthening is performed with low loads (low resistance). Also, the clinician must always keep in mind the patient's symptoms. If the patient is in an acute phase or if pain is intense, strengthening exercises should be delayed, and treatment should begin with only gentle active or passive exercises.

Proprioceptive neuromuscular facilitation (PNF) techniques are another type of active-assisted exercises that physical therapists commonly use to reduce muscular activity in the jaw (e.g., the masseter and pterygoid muscles).[91] The patient is asked to open the mouth within a comfortable range; this takes pressure off the inflamed or painful posterior structures and prevents condylar loading when resistance is applied. The clinician then places the hands under the mandible and, using light, gradually increasing pressure, attempts to close the mandible while the patient resists the closure (Figure 3-19). This causes contraction of the hyoid muscles and produces a reciprocal inhibition of the masseter, temporalis, and pterygoid muscles. Resistance is applied for a number of seconds and then slowly withdrawn, and the sequence is repeated a number of times as required. Pain and fatigue are limiting factors and should guide the clinician in the number of repetitions to be performed. By placing one hand on the side of the mandible and producing a pressure to the opposite side, the clinician can encourage lateral glide and exercise of the muscles. Again, using the PNF technique of reciprocal inhibition, the muscles on the side of the resistance contract and the muscles on the opposite side relax. Even though these exercises are effective at improving ROM of the jaw and

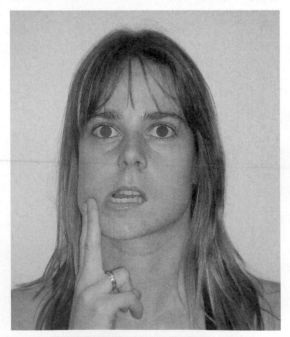

Figure 3-17
Resistive exercise for lateral excursion.

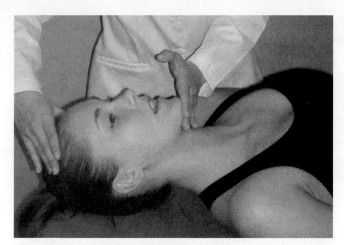

Figure 3-19
Proprioceptive neuromuscular facilitation (PNF) technique for inhibition of closing of the masticatory muscles.

probably improve the flexibility of the relaxed muscles, the mechanisms of that improvement are still under study.[91,92]

Clinicians must keep in mind that exercise and/or mobilization can easily be overdone in the treatment of the temporomandibular region. This is a sensitive area, which is made more sensitive by any dysfunction within it. Instead of exercising once or twice a day for 5 minutes at a time, a far more effective approach is to exercise a little bit and often. Some clinicians, such as Rocabado,[93] have instituted a 6 × 6 × 6 exercise routine: six exercises performed six times a day, with six repetitions of each exercise. This is easy for the patient to remember and to follow. Other clinicians prefer to have the patient perform one or two exercises each hour, using a few repetitions of each exercise. Either way, the patient must be continually reminded to perform the exercises, not only to maintain any restored function, but also as a reminder to avoid performing any movements or habituations that might aggravate the condition. A home exercise program is described Box 3-1.

Electrophysical Modalities

Electrophysical modalities, such as shortwave diathermy, ultrasound techniques, laser treatments, and TENS (Figure 3-20), are commonly used in the clinical setting.[94] The purpose of these modalities is to reduce inflammation and increase blood flow by altering capillary permeability.[94] The literature suggests that electrophysical treatments, when performed early in the course of TMD, are beneficial for reducing symptoms.[94] McNeely et al.[70] found that the studies included in their systematic review had major methodological flaws, and the findings are limited. The systematic review done by Medlicott and Harris[82] produced similar results. Consequently, no clear conclusions can be drawn. Because electrophysical modalities may be less labor intensive than other treatments (e.g., occlusal splint therapy and manual therapy), further study is needed to warrant their use.

Manual Therapy

According to Kalamir et al.,[79] "The biopsychosocial health paradigm emphasizes a reversible and conservative approach to chronic pain management. Manual therapy for TMD claims to fulfill these criteria." Mobilization of the mandible aims to restore the normal range of motion, reduce local ischemia, stimulate proprioception, break fibrous adhesions, stimulate synovial fluid production, and reduce pain.[79] Manual therapy has been used for many years as an adjunct treatment, along with exercises, physical modalities, and splint therapy. Recent evidence suggests that manual therapy is a legitimate treatment for TMD, superior to splint therapy and even more effective when combined with exercises.[85]

Before the TMJ can be mobilized, any inflammation and local muscle spasm in the area must be reduced, because both of these conditions can be aggravated by attempts to stretch the affected joint. Unless the dysfunction is fairly recent (less than 6 weeks), the clinician should not look to mobilization to restore the disc-condyle relationship to normal. Rather, mobilization should be used to achieve what the body would do on its own over an extended period; that is, stretch out the tight structures to restore a more functional movement. The clinician must be sure to explain this, so that the patient does not get the idea that mobilization will cure the clicking or tight joint by "getting everything back to normal." In addition to restoring function, mobilization (Figure 3-21) attempts to prevent the development of adaptive problems elsewhere. For example, stiffness in the affected joint causes torsion of the unaffected joint on the opposite side, which eventually could cause hypermobility of that joint.

To mobilize the joint, the clinician asks the patient to open the mouth and then places the thumb along the superior surface of the lower teeth on the side of the joint to be mobilized (Figure 3-22). The index finger is curled under the angle of the mandible so that the bone is cupped by the finger. The index finger of the opposite hand can be used to palpate the joint line. Mobilization is brought about by exerting pressure on the teeth with the thumb; this causes a distraction of the head of the condyle meeting the head of the mandibular joint. If some condylar translation is lost, this can be restored by performing an anterior glide of the condyle after some distraction of the joint.

Jaw mobilization can also be performed in the lateral and medial directions to provide joint stretching in all structures. For lateral mobilization, the clinician positions the thumb in the lateral aspect of the last molar and pushes the condyle in a lateral direction. The patient can also be taught self-mobilization of the TMJ (Figure 3-23). For medial mobilization (i.e., internal mobilization of the condyle), the clinician positions the second and third fingers outside the mouth and pushes the condyle in a medial direction. Sometimes the clinician can guide the

Box 3-1 Home Exercise Program for the Temporomandibular Structures

Do all of the exercises (or those assigned) hourly or as instructed, with a repetition of 5 times each. The 5 repetitions of each exercise should take 1 minute or less. Doing these exercises throughout the day will take only a few minutes of your time. Do the exercises for 1 month or longer if so instructed. Do them at home, at work, in the car, and so on. However, if any exercise causes you pain, discontinue it immediately and consult your therapist.

Exercise 1: Place the top of your tongue against the roof of your mouth and make a clucklike sound Your lower jaw will drop downward to a comfortable position, and your upper and lower teeth will be apart. Return the top of your tongue to the position it was in immediately before you made the sound, exerting slight upward pressure with the tongue; your teeth are still apart. Place the palm of your left hand just below your navel and breathe in and out through your nose 5 times using only your stomach muscles to breathe. Feel your stomach rise and fall the 5 times. Do not use the muscles of your chest or shoulders to breathe.

Exercise 2: Return the top of your tongue to the position against the roof of your mouth as in exercise 1, exerting slight upward pressure Continue to breathe through your nose using your stomach muscles. Now, open and close your mouth farther 5 times without moving your tongue. At the end of the second week, chew all your food this way.

NOTE: Do all repetitions of the following exercises with your tongue elevated against the roof of your mouth; breathe through your nose using your stomach muscles.

Exercise 3: Grasp the back of your neck with both hands with your elbows pointing forward. Holding your neck rigid, nod your head, trying to touch your chin to your Adam's apple. If you do this correctly, your head will be able to move only about 2.5 to 3.8 cm (1 to 1½ inches). Do not flex your neck forward. Your head should just rotate forward at the very top of your neck. Hold this position for a few seconds. Feel the muscles stretch at the top of the back of your neck, just beneath your skull. Repeat 5 times. Continue breathing through your nose using your stomach muscles and with your tongue against the roof of your mouth.

Exercise 4: Move your face straight backward keeping your chin down and your face perpendicular to the floor (i.e., as if you were bracing at attention). Do not raise your head while doing this exercise. Continue to breathe through your nose. Pause for a few seconds when your head is in the backward position, as far back as you can get it, and then relax. To help maintain the head in the correct position, you can focus your eyes on a point directly in front of you while performing the exercise. Repeat 5 times. Continue correct breathing.

Exercise 5: Repeat the position in exercise 4. With your head braced back, rotate your head forward and try to touch your chin to your Adam's apple. You do not need to immobilize your neck with your hands, but do not bend your neck forward. Hold for a few seconds. Repeat 5 times.

Exercise 6: Grasp your hands behind your waist. Roll your shoulders backward as far as they will go. Mentally picture your left and right shoulder blades touching each other. Hold for a few seconds and then relax. Repeat 5 times. Continue correct breathing.

Exercise 7: Simultaneously elevate your left and right shoulders upward, attempting to touch your ears. Hold for a few seconds and then relax. Repeat 5 times.

Exercise 8: Without elevating your left shoulder, bend your head to the left and attempt to touch your left ear to your left shoulder. Hold for a few seconds and then relax. Repeat 5 times.

Exercise 9: Without elevating your right shoulder, bend your head to the right and attempt to touch your right ear to your right shoulder. Hold for a few seconds and then relax. Repeat 5 times.

Exercise 10: With your head in a neutral position, place the heel of your right hand against your right temple and gently press to your left so that your head bends an additional 1.3 cm (½ inch) toward your shoulder. Repeat 5 times.

Exercise 11: With your head in a neutral position, place the heel of your left hand against your left temple and gently press to your right so that your head bends an additional 1.3 cm (½ inch) toward your shoulder. Repeat 5 times.

Exercise 12: With your head braced back and your chin rotated toward your Adam's apple, intertwine the fingers of your hands and place them so that they cup the back of your head Gently press forward to rotate your chin an additional 1.3 cm (½ inch) toward your Adam's apple. Feel this additional stretching pressure at the top of your neck just beneath your skull. Hold for a few seconds and then relax. Repeat 5 times.

Exercise 13: This is an *isometric* exercise; that is, the muscles contract, but you won't see or feel any appreciable movement of the head. Throughout this exercise, *do not* let the position of your head change.
   a. With your head bent forward 30°, place the heel of either your left or right hand against your forehead and press upward with 0.45 kg (2 lbs) of pressure. Resist this upward pressure with your neck muscles so that your head does not move. Hold for a few seconds and then relax. Repeat 5 times.
   b. With your head upright, place the palm of your left or right hand against the back of your head and press forward with 0.45 kg (2 lbs) of pressure. Resist this pressure for a few seconds and then relax. Repeat 5 times.
   c. With your head upright, place the heel of your left hand against your left temple and press to your right with 0.45 kg (2 lbs) of pressure. Resist this pressure for a few seconds and then relax. Repeat 5 times.
   d. With your head upright, place the heel of your right hand against your right temple and press to your left with 0.45 kg (2 lbs) of pressure. Resist this pressure for a few seconds and then relax. Repeat 5 times.

Box 3-1   Home Exercise Program for the Temporomandibular Structures—cont'd

Exercise 14: Place the top of your tongue in the same position against the roof of your mouth as in exercise 1, exerting slight upward pressure. Continue to breathe through your nose using your stomach muscles. The upper and lower teeth are still apart. Throughout this exercise, *do not* let the position of your jaw move.

    a. This is an isometric exercise. Place your thumbs beneath your chin and push upward with 170 gm (6 oz) of pressure to close your mouth. Resist this closing force with an equal opening force so that your jaw does not move from its original position. Hold for a few seconds. Repeat 5 times.

    b. Resume the tongue and jaw positions described in exercise 1. Place the ends of the index and middle fingers of your right hand against the right side of your lower jaw and push to your left with 170 gm (6 oz) of pressure. Resist this by holding your jaw steady with an equal force so that your jaw does not move. Hold for a few seconds. Repeat 5 times.

    c. Repeat exercise 14b using the index and middle fingers of the *left* hand against the *left* side of your lower jaw and pushing to the *right* with 170 gm (6 oz) of pressure. Do not let your jaw move. Hold for a few seconds. Repeat 5 times.

Exercise 15: Throughout this exercise, *do not* let the position of your tongue change.

    a. Place the index finger of your right or left hand on top of your tongue with your finger pointing toward your throat. Press downward with approximately 170 gm (6 oz) of pressure and simultaneously lift your tongue with an equal force so that the index finger does not press the tongue down. Hold for a few seconds and then relax. Repeat 5 times.

    b. Place your index finger under your tongue with your fingernail upward. Press upward against the undersurface of your tongue with 170 gm (6 oz) of pressure and simultaneously press down with your tongue with an equal force so that the index finger does not push the tongue up. Hold for a few seconds and then relax. Repeat 5 times.

    c. Place your left index finger against the left side of your tongue. Press to your right with 170 gm (6 oz) of pressure and simultaneously resist this pressure with an equal force so that your tongue does not move. Hold for a few seconds and then relax. Repeat 5 times.

    d. Place your right index finger against the right side of your tongue. Press to your left with 170 gm (6 oz) of pressure and simultaneously resist this pressure with an equal force so that your tongue does not move. Hold for a few seconds and then relax. Repeat 5 times.

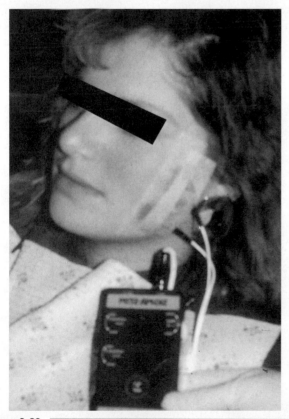

Figure 3-20
Use of transcutaneous electrical nerve stimulation (TENS) to treat a painful temporomandibular joint.

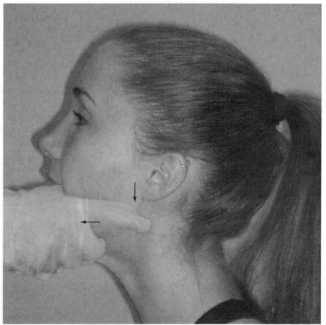

Figure 3-21
Acute disc reduction mobilization.

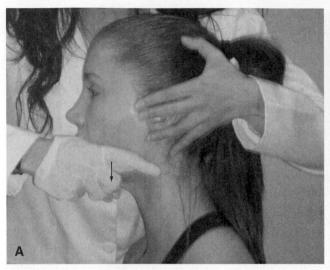
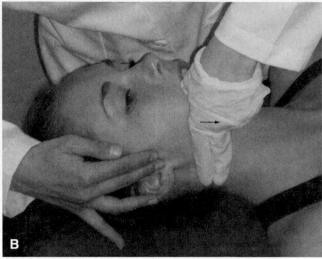

Figure 3-22
A, Axial intraoral mobilization in the sitting position. **B,** Axial intraoral mobilization in the supine position.

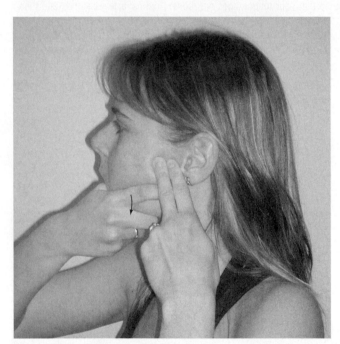

Figure 3-23
Patient self-mobilization of the TMJ.

lateral or medial movements using intraoral mobilization (Figure 3-24).

Patients can be taught to perform self-mobilization of the joint according to the techniques just described. It is important to teach the patient to perform these mobilizations appropriately and to hold the positions for the amount of time required to achieve a positive effect on the TMJ.

Patients with a hypomobile joint on one side and a symptomatic hypermobile joint on the other side frequently complain that mobilization on the hypomobile side causes pain on the hypermobile side because of stretching of symptomatic tissue. This is a problem, which requires graduated mobilization to lessen the effects of any torsion of the opposite mandible. In these cases, Maitland-type graduated mobilization can be used. The regimen starts with grade 1 techniques and progresses through grades 2 and 3 to a strong grade 4. Oscillation at the end of the available range can be added to reduce spasm and to add more proprioceptive input, thereby reducing pain.[95] Although mobilization is used primarily to restore movement, the clinician should keep in mind that the lighter grades (1 and 2) can be used

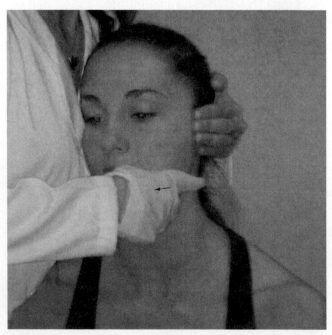

Figure 3-24
Guided jaw mobilization.

on a hypermobile joint to reduce muscle spasm and for proprioceptive effect. The stronger grades of mobilization should not be used on a hypermobile joint, because they would stretch tissue that already is in a lax state.

Once a joint has been mobilized, the patient should be instructed to perform some regular exercises to maintain the regained mobility. Opening the mouth to the end of the newly acquired range, repeated a few times every hour, is one such exercise. The patient might need the visual feedback afforded by performing the exercise in front of a mirror to ensure that the mandibular motion can be produced symmetrically in the midline. Unless the patient is coached properly, maintenance exercises will not return the mandible to its normal function. For example, an anteromedially displaced disc on one side will stop condylar movement during opening and also during lateral glide. If mobilization has succeeded in stretching out the tight tissue, more opening should be available, together with more lateral glide. However, if the patient has not been able to achieve a lateral glide because of the joint dysfunction, she will need visual feedback (i.e., doing the exercise in front of a mirror) to see what happens to the mandible when she performs the movement.

Other TMJ Treatments
Orthodontics and Other Dental Treatments

Some authors, including Mew,[18] have postulated that orthodontic treatment can cause TMD. Some studies refute this.[9,75,76] Even more, the orthodontic treatment used in patients with TMD to improve symptomatology has been debated in the literature.[9] Because no clear link has been shown between malocclusion and the development of TMD, orthodontics and other dental treatments that alter the bite or teeth (e.g., occlusal adjustment,[96] dental restorations, and TMJ surgery) are inappropriate as initial management methods for TMD. However, sometimes a patient starts to show signs and symptoms of TMD during orthodontic treatment; these patients may need to be taught ways to reduce any stress through the joints during the period of orthodontic care. During orthodontic treatment, a patient who is banded and fitted with elastics to control mandibular motion may develop muscle spasm and reduced mobility. In these cases, treatment of the condition and mobilization must be coordinated with the orthodontist so that the elastics can be removed and joint mobilization provided.

Cognitive Behavioral Therapy

It is important that clinicians understand TMD as a complex disorder and that they keep in mind the biopsychosocial model as a basis for the etiology, assessment, and management of TMD. In this context, cognitive behavioral therapy has emerged as an important option for treating patients with TMD, because it addresses the mind and body as a whole. Counseling, stress management, biofeedback, relaxation therapy, cognition, psychoeducation, and even primary therapeutic exercises are recognized components of a cognitive behavioral program.[38,97]

Acupuncture

Acupuncture increasingly is being used in the treatment of musculoskeletal conditions in North America.[98] Currently the mechanisms underlying the action of acupuncture are unclear.[99] Acupuncture may relieve pain according to the principles of the gate control theory or by acting as a noxious stimulus. Some evidence indicates that acupuncture may stimulate the production of endorphins, serotonin, and acetylcholine within the central nervous system.[99] In the systematic review by McNeely et al.,[70] three studies[100-102] examined the use of acupuncture in the treatment of myogenic TMD. Patients treated with acupuncture showed significantly better results for pain threshold, pain intensity, and clinical dysfunction score than the control group. However, no significant differences were found between the acupuncture group and the group treated with occlusal splint therapy (weak studies).[101,102] In addition, Goddard et al.[100] found no significant difference in pain threshold response between patients treated with acupuncture and those given sham acupuncture. The three studies included in this systematic review were clinically heterogeneous, and both studies were rated as weak. Also, the study findings were conflicting in terms of efficacy. Therefore no conclusions currently can be drawn regarding the efficacy of acupuncture in the treatment of TMD.

Surgery

Surgery on the TMJ itself has become rare; only about 5% of patients who undergo treatment for TMD require surgery.[103] There are no generally recognized surgical protocols for TMD, although some guidelines have been proposed as requirements for TMJ surgery.[9] Surgery should be reserved for cases in which surgical treatment can warrant success.

Guidelines for TMJ Surgery

- The TMJ is the source of pain and/or dysfunction that results in significant impairment.
- Appropriate nonsurgical management was unsuccessful.
- The pain is localized in the TMJ (when loading and with movement).
- Interferences with proper TMJ function are the mechanical type.
- The patient requests the surgical approach.
- The patient has no medical or psychological contraindications to surgery.

When surgery is performed, the procedure most often is an arthroscopic technique and includes lavage to free up any joint restrictions and to flush the joint to allow for better function. An ankylosed joint or a joint with a clinical closed lock that has not responded to conservative treatment fits the category of conditions requiring surgery. After surgery, therapy focuses on improving joint function as quickly as possible. The initial treatment is based on the same criteria used for acute capsulitis.

Postradiation Therapy for Hypomobility of the Temporomandibular Joint

Patients who have had surgery and radiation therapy for treatment of cancer of the neck and oropharyngeal structures can present with severe restriction of range of motion of the mandible. Extensive therapy, including mobilization, in an attempt to improve function has not been successful. Radiation therapy appears to cause severe fibrosis of the masticatory and neck musculature that does not respond to therapy. Surgical intervention can cause postoperative muscle spasm that makes swift mobilization difficult. The authors believe that, if these unfortunate individuals are to be helped effectively, therapy must be instituted almost immediately after treatment, which entails the use of resources at the hospital where the treatment is given. If physical therapy is not introduced until after the patient has been discharged from hospital, it often is too late to effect any improvement.

Patient Education

As mentioned previously, it is vital that patients know the intent of the treatment so that they do not harbor any incorrect expectations for the treatment outcome. Patients also must be made aware of the likely biomechanical changes caused by the dysfunction, so that they become fully involved in the rehabilitation process and understand why certain activities must be avoided. A useful educational tool is a simple diagram of the anatomy of the temporomandibular joint; it need not be anatomically specific nor drawn with an excruciating degree of detail.

The education process can be split into several parts. The first part should provide an explanation of the basic anatomy, joint position, and normal disc-condyle relationship. The second part should include some description of the patient's probable pathological condition. The third part should be a description of possible aggravating factors and various activities to be avoided. The fourth part should include a description of some things patients can do for themselves at home, including a list of required exercises. The fifth part should provide some indication of the extent of recovery expected, the likelihood of recurrence of problems, and the need to bring other health care professionals into the rehabilitation process.

Patient Management Program: Everyday Activities

Successful treatment and management of temporomandibular joint/muscle dysfunction depends in large part on the way these injured areas are treated. The following instructions can greatly enhance the correction and healing of this area.

- For the next few months, be sure to cut all your food into bite-sized (i.e., small) pieces. Try not to open your mouth any wider than the thickness of your thumb.
- Do not eat hard crusts of bread, tough meat, raw vegetables, or any other food that requires prolonged chewing.
- Do not chew gum during this period of treatment.
- Be sure not to protrude your jaw, as you must do in biting off a piece of meat.
- Do not bite any food with your front teeth.
- When you chew, make sure you chew equally on each side of your mouth. Do not get in the habit of doing all your chewing on one side only.
- If you wear lipstick, do not bring your jaw forward when applying it.
- Avoid protruding your jaw during any other activities (e.g., smoking, conversation, and so on).
- Make every effort not to strain your joint ligaments unnecessarily. For example, do not stretch your mouth open when yawning.
- If you find yourself clenching your teeth, try to remember, "lips together, teeth apart."
- Try to sleep on your back or side. Avoid sleeping on your jaw or in the prone position.

Patient Management Program: Diaphragmatic Breathing

- If you breathe through your mouth, you are breathing abnormally. Consequently, your jaw will be dropped and can never be in a normal resting position unless you change your breathing habits. Your symptoms will never entirely go away, and you will not receive maximum benefit from your treatment.
- When breathing and at rest, hold the tip of your tongue against the back of your top teeth. Keep your lips lightly together; the upper and lower teeth should be slightly separated. This technique will prevent mouth breathing. All breathing should be done through your nose, with your tongue elevated, for the rest of your life. Your teeth should be slightly apart (0.32 to 0.63 cm [1/8 to 1/4 inch]).
- Do not suck in air through your mouth.
- Concentrate your breathing on your stomach. Your stomach should expand and contract, *not* your chest. Put your hand on your stomach and feel it go in and out; this is called *abdominal,* or *diaphragmatic, breathing.* This is the way you should breathe from now on. Simultaneously, keep your tongue against the roof of your mouth.
- Do 5 breaths every hour (i.e., at 1-hour intervals, consciously inhale and exhale from your stomach five times; hopefully, you will also be breathing this way subconsciously in between).
- Never use nasal inhalants or sprays.
- Never put your tongue between the biting surfaces of your teeth.

In summary, patient education involves explaining the nature of the pain and ways to avoid painful conditions. Information about the biopsychosocial model of TMD, chronic pain, and self-management needs to be included in the education program.[104] In addition, the patient needs to be advised about posture and ergonomic conditions (e.g., work-related postures or loads) and the adverse effects of certain positions and oral behaviors, such as biting, chewing, and grinding, that create constant microtrauma in the tissues. Patient education has been found to be crucial to the success of treatment.[99]

TMJ Education Process

The following points are covered at the first visit:
- Explanation of anatomy, joint position, and the normal disc-condyle relationship
- Description of the probable pathology
- Description of the aggravating factors and activities to avoid
- Guidelines the patient can follow at home, including exercises
- Likely extent of recovery
- Likelihood of problem recurrence
- Inclusion of other health care professionals in the treatment process (if needed)

Summary

Treatment of temporomandibular disorders and related dysfunctions follows the same principles as treatment of any other musculoskeletal problem. After a comprehensive history has been taken and an assessment performed, a hierarchy of signs and symptoms is formulated, together with a hierarchy of treatments aimed at helping to alleviate the signs and symptoms and restore normal functioning of the craniomandibular system. The object is to return the patient to maximum possible function. To do this, the clinician must have the patient's cooperation and participation; to give these, the patient must understand the condition, what will be required for recovery, and the goals set by the clinician.

Frequently treatment not only is multifaceted, but also requires the participation and skills of practitioners from different specialties, such as physical therapists, dentists, clinical psychologists, speech pathologists, and physicians. Concentrating on one area alone does not provide successful outcomes or ensure a happy patient. TMD is recognized as a multidimensional disorder, the result of biological, psychological, and social alterations. Therefore assessment and management of TMD must address the biological, psychological, and sociological aspects of the individual as a whole.[38]

References

To enhance this text and add value for the reader, all references have been incorporated into a CD-ROM that is provided with this text. The reader can view the reference source and access it online whenever possible. There are a total of 104 references for this chapter.

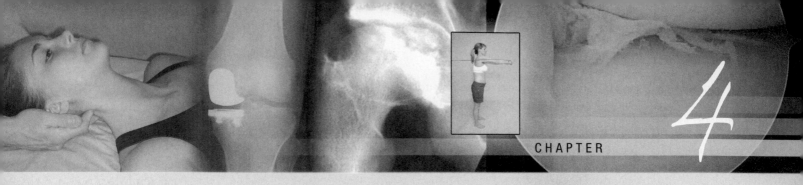

CHAPTER 4

Shoulder Trauma and Hypomobility

Judy C. Chepeha

Introduction

Optimal functioning of the shoulder and arm can take place only if the delicate balance of healthy anatomy, proper biomechanics, and normal physiology is maintained. Disruption of any one of these three factors may lead to overload and injury, resulting in pain and dysfunction. The past decade has yielded a vast amount of new information about the pathoanatomy and biomechanics of the shoulder.[1-8] This increased knowledge has contributed to the clinician's ability to understand and manage the patient with shoulder complaints more accurately and effectively. Surgical techniques, grounded in basic scientific principles related to the restoration of normal anatomy, biomechanics, and the physiology of injured or compromised structures, have changed to allow for earlier introduction of rehabilitation. Keeping pace with changes in surgical intervention, rehabilitation programs now, more than ever, are grounded in principles derived from physiology, anatomy, and restoration of the entire kinetic chain, from the lower extremity through the trunk, shoulder girdle, and arm.

Proper rehabilitation of the injured shoulder must be based on a sound knowledge of the normal anatomy and function of the entire shoulder girdle complex and the inherent demands and possible mechanisms that may contribute to or cause injury to this region. Simply setting the goals of increasing range of motion and improving strength at the glenohumeral joint is no longer acceptable. Clinicians must be mindful of how the entire glenohumeral and scapulothoracic complex relates to the entire kinetic chain, and they must understand the subtle relationships among all these interrelated components. Rehabilitation programs prescribed for the treatment of shoulder conditions should be based on **principles of treatment** rather than specific condition exercise protocols, and these principles should be well grounded in the clinician's knowledge of the shoulder, particularly how it functions under both normal and abnormal circumstances. Hopefully, these advances in management of the injured shoulder will be reflected in improved and earlier return to functional status for patients.

One advantage of managing the injured shoulder according to treatment principles rather than specific protocols is the adaptability of these principles to many different situations. In other words, patients with vastly different shoulder pathologies all can benefit from the application of some or all of these treatment principles, because they are based on common concepts of "normalizing" shoulder anatomy, biomechanics, and physiology. This chapter presents treatments for a variety of shoulder pathologies.

Principles of Shoulder Treatment

- Proper and thorough assessment
- Early protected motion after a period of immobilization
- Proper evaluation and treatment of local and distant deficits
- Scapular control
- Pain management
- Sensorimotor control
- Progressions
- Closed chain axial loading exercise
- Functional exercises

Common Principles of Treatment

Proper and Thorough Assessment

As with any musculoskeletal pathology, treatment of the patient with a shoulder complaint must begin with a thorough assessment. The assessment should include evaluation of the associated cervical and thoracic spine regions and all the joints that encompass the shoulder girdle. Patients should be examined statically and dynamically and while they are performing functional activities.

Early Protected Motion After a Period of Immobilization

The shoulder complex, particularly the glenohumeral joint, is prone to stiffness after trauma or immobilization.[9,10] Early intervention with mobility exercises and joint mobilization techniques may prevent this restriction of range of motion, reduce the associated pain, and allow the shoulder to move into positions that can best address normalization of muscle activity and function. Special consideration must always be given to the adaptive tightening of the glenohumeral posterior capsule, which presents clinically as a medial rotation deficit (i.e., glenohumeral internal rotation deficit [GIRD]), and to the anterior shoulder muscles (e.g., pectoralis minor), which also tend to shorten.

Proper Evaluation and Treatment of Local and Distant Deficits

Many shoulder injuries are associated with local and/or distant deficits in flexibility, strength, muscle balance, and proper mechanics that affect the whole kinetic chain. For example, hip and lumbar spine inflexibility, altered scapulohumeral rhythm, and reduced medial rotation motion may be part of the cause of the shoulder injury or may occur as a result of the injury. Regardless of the onset, all deficits of the kinetic chain must be noted on assessment and incorporated into a proper treatment plan.

Scapular Control

Scapular dyskinesis, or an alteration in the position or motion of the scapula, is caused by weakness or inhibition of the periscapular muscles, especially the lower trapezius and serratus anterior.[11] The resultant loss of scapular control, coupled with an often overactive upper trapezius, can contribute to shoulder impingement and instability syndromes, acromioclavicular dysfunction, and rotator cuff weakness.[11-14] Proper shoulder rehabilitation must always include a thorough examination of the scapula and correction of any deficits.

Pain Management

Pain is a powerful inhibitor of muscle activation throughout the body. This is especially so at the shoulder because of the degree of muscle activity required to coordinate joint motion, stability, and function. Clinicians must closely monitor pain and make sure that it is not causing inhibition of the weaker, targeted muscles and encouraging perpetuation of an improper muscle recruitment pattern.

Sensorimotor Control

Sensorimotor control is the neuromuscular control basis of sensory input, often known as *proprioception*. With the increased knowledge about the effect of changes in proprioception and neuromuscular control of joint stabilization in the shoulder, exercises that address retraining of this important factor have been integrated into treatment approaches.[13,15]

Progressions

The indications for progressing a patient to more difficult exercises are grounded in the physiological principles of tissue healing and tissue response to injury. They also are based on the acquisition of key functions at the shoulder girdle and the entire kinetic chain; these include adequate hip and trunk extension; normal pelvic control; proper scapular control, especially into retraction and depression; normal scapulohumeral rhythm; and glenohumeral joint range of motion.

Closed Chain Axial Loading Exercises

Closed chain rehabilitation exercises link the trunk to the scapula and the scapula to the arm; this allows strengthening of the scapular and arm musculature as a functional unit. These exercises should be done along with early postoperative range of motion techniques, because they minimize the shear effect and reduce the open kinetic chain loading applied to the glenohumeral joint.[16-19]

Functional Exercises

Rehabilitation of the injured shoulder should always include exercises that are considered functional. However, clinicians must keep in mind that, for an exercise to be considered functional, it must reflect the individual patient's functional activities and goals for work, daily life, and recreation.

The nine elements just discussed provide a brief overview of some of the key principles of shoulder rehabilitation. Greater detail on specific treatments and exercise guidelines are presented later in this chapter and in Chapter 5.

Shoulder Anatomy

In considering the shoulder, the clinician must include the entire shoulder girdle, which consists of three bones—the scapula, the clavicle, and the humerus. These bones are linked to each other and to the body by four joints—the glenohumeral joint, the acromioclavicular joint, the sternoclavicular joint, and the scapulothoracic articulation. The combined effect of these four articulations is a high degree of mobility, which allows the arm and hand great functional capacity but also makes the shoulder particularly vulnerable to injury, because stability is sacrificed for mobility. The glenohumeral joint has an almost global range of motion because the glenoid cavity is a shallow socket approximately one third to one fourth the size of the humeral head. To compensate, the glenoid labrum, which attaches tightly to the bottom half of the glenoid and loosely to the top half, increases the glenoid depth approximately two times, adding to glenohumeral stability.[3,4] Normally, when the humeral head is moved through its large ranges of motion, only a small amount of translation or excursion occurs between the humeral head and the glenoid. If the dynamic structures controlling this translation (primarily the rotator

Table 4-1

Restraints about the Glenohumeral Joint

Passive (Static)	Active (Dynamic)	
Capsule Labrum Coracohumeral ligament Superior glenohumeral ligament	Suprapinatus Infraspinatus Subscapularis Teres minor	Humeral stablizers
Middle glenohumeral ligament Inferior glanohumeral ligament Geometry of humeral articular surface Geometry of glenoid articular surface Coracoacromial ligament Articular cartilage compliance	Pectoralis major Latissimus dorsi Long head of the biceps Triceps Deltoid Teres major	Movers of glenohumeral joint
Joint cohesion	Serratus anterior Latissimus dorsi Trapezius Rhomboids Levator scapule Pectoralis minor	Scapular stabilizers

Modified from Zachazewski JE, Magee DJ,Quillen WS, editors: *Athletic injuries and rehabilitation*, p 510, Philadelphia, 1996, WB Saunders.

cuff) are injured, translation may increase, leading to increased wear on the glenoid labrum, failure of the static restraints, and eccentric overload of the dynamic restraints, resulting in instability, impingement, or both.[2,4,6,7,20]

The restraints of the glenohumeral joint typically are classified as either active (dynamic) or passive (static). Table 4-1 presents a list of the two groups. It is worth noting that even though the stabilizing components are divided into two groups, the actual mechanism of stability is not achieved through distinctive, separate processes, but rather by means of one that is very interconnected.

Shoulder Function

The shoulder is the most proximal link of the upper extremity kinetic chain. It has evolved to allow humans great mobility, so that they can position the most distal segment, the hand, for function. This seemingly simple task is achieved through a highly coordinated pattern of movement that begins in the lower extremities and moves sequentially to the trunk, scapulothoracic joint, glenohumeral joint, and elbow and eventually to the wrist and hand, where the function is performed.

Specific shoulder girdle function relies on the combined motion of the sternoclavicular, acromioclavicular, glenohumeral, and scapulothoracic joints. This collective motion is achieved through the interaction of the muscles that influence the movement of the scapula, clavicle, and humerus relative to the axial skeleton. Considerable in vivo and in vitro research has been done to try to elucidate the complex mechanism by which the shoulder moves and muscles act to facilitate these movements.[21,22] Early radiographic studies of arm elevation identified a 2:1 ratio of glenohumeral motion to scapulothoracic motion when the humerus is elevated in the coronal plane (Figure 4-1).[23] A similar analysis of elevation in the scapular plane found a ratio of 5:4 after the first 30° of elevation.[24,25] Similar studies carried out by other researchers found slight variations of these earlier observations.[26]

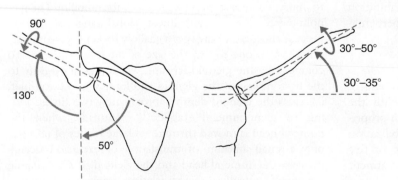

Figure 4-1

Movements of the scapula, humerus, and clavicle during scapulohumeral rhythm. (From Magee DJ: *Orthopedic physical assessment*, ed 4, p 225, Philadelphia, 2002, WB Saunders.)

Elevation in a 30° to 40° anterior to the coronal plane customarily is referred to as *scapular plane elevation* or *scaption*. However, the scapula is a highly mobile reference point that not only moves with arm elevation, but also inclines forward early in motion, obviously in a different direction from that of the intended elevation. Relative motion between the scapulothoracic joint and the glenohumeral joint has been referred to as the *scapulohumeral* or *glenohumeral rhythm*. The ratios of 2:1 and 5:4 are commonly accepted as representing the ratio of glenohumeral motion to scapulothoracic motion, but these values are only a limited reflection of the scapulothoracic and scapulohumeral combinations possible to achieve a given arm position. These ratios are based on two-dimensional radiographic projections of angular rotations taken at discrete positions of elevation; however, the arm moves in three dimensions, and for positions other than elevation, much of this motion is under voluntary control. These findings and others are not intended to dismiss completely all of our earlier understanding of scapulohumeral motion, but rather to broaden awareness of the dynamic, multiplane model of the shoulder.

Muscle function at the shoulder is considered one of the highly intricate systems in the body. The function of a muscle with respect to any joint depends on the position of the skeletal components, the distance of the muscle from the joint's center of rotation, and the external and internal forces acting at the time of muscle contraction. Given the three-dimensional, highly mobile nature of the shoulder joint, it is easy to understand why proper functioning of its muscles is essential for a normal, healthy shoulder.

The prime movers of the shoulder are the deltoid, pectoralis major, latissimus dorsi, and teres major muscles. Electromyographic studies[21,27-29] have shown that these muscles function predictably along their line of pull and that they form a drapelike effect over the shoulder, creating the potential for infinite lines of pull that may allow an almost 360° arc of motion.

The rotator cuff contributes to shoulder motion through a variety of means. The muscles of the rotator cuff can function as important movers of the upper extremity if the muscles' line of action is consistent with the intended direction of motion. This group of muscles also serves as a key set of stabilizing muscles for the glenohumeral joint by creating a compressive force that maintains the humeral head on the glenoid surface, and it can function to produce axial rotation of the humerus. (The role of the rotator cuff is discussed in greater detail later in this chapter.)

Finally, muscles that attach to the scapula and therefore control scapulothoracic joint motion have been decisively reported as playing a fundamental role in how the shoulder functions; or, more appropriately, how *well* the shoulder functions. The work of researchers such as Kibler[12] and Kibler and Livingstone[18] has taught clinicians to be mindful of the trapezius, rhomboids, levator scapulae, teres minor, serratus anterior, and latissimus dorsi muscles, because their attachment to the scapula allows them to control the motion at the scapulothoracic articulation. Dysfunction or inhibition of any of these muscles has been shown to alter the position of the glenoid significantly, which in turn may result in abnormal centering of the humeral head within the glenohumeral joint.[6,12,30] The importance of proper scapulothoracic positioning cannot be overemphasized. Clinicians' new appreciation of the importance of the role of scapulothoracic position is the most significant change in how patients with shoulder pathology are assessed and treated.

Sternoclavicular and Acromioclavicular Joint Injuries

Sternoclavicular Joint

The sternoclavicular joint is unique in the shoulder girdle, because it is the only true articulation between the clavicle of the upper extremity and the axial skeleton. It is a diarthrodial type of joint, with the enlarged medial end of the clavicle creating a saddle-type articulation with the clavicular notch of the sternum. This joint has the distinction of having the least amount of bony stability, therefore it relies heavily on support from the surrounding capsule and ligaments; these ligaments include the intra-articular disc ligament, the extra-articular costoclavicular (rhomboid) ligament, the interclavicular ligament, and the capsular ligament.

The intra-articular disc ligament is a very dense, fibrous tissue that originates from the synchondral junction of the first rib to the sternum and travels through the sternoclavicular joint, dividing it into two distinct joint spaces (Figure 4-2). Anteriorly and posteriorly, the disc blends with the fibers of the capsular ligament. The intra-articular disc ligament functions as a checkrein for medial displacement of the proximal clavicle.

The costoclavicular, or rhomboid, ligament is short and strong and is made up of an anterior fasciculus and a posterior fasciculus. These two different parts give the ligament a slightly twisted appearance. Below, the costoclavicular ligament attaches to the upper surface of the first rib and at the adjacent part of the synchondral junction with the sternum; above, it attaches to the margins of the impression on the inferior surface of the medial end of the clavicle, sometimes called the *rhomboid fossa*.[31,32] Bearn[33] has shown that the anterior fibers resist excessive upward rotation of the clavicle and the posterior fibers resist excessive downward rotation. Specifically, the anterior fibers resist lateral displacement, and the posterior fibers resist medial displacement.

The interclavicular ligament connects the superomedial aspects of each clavicle with the capsular ligaments and the upper aspect of the sternum (see Figure 4-2). Along with the capsular ligaments, the interclavicular ligament

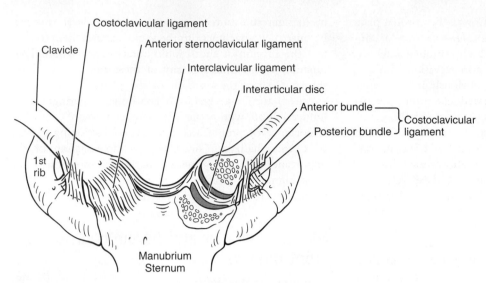

Costoclavicular ligament
Clavicle
Anterior sternoclavicular ligament
Interclavicular ligament
Interarticular disc
Anterior bundle
Posterior bundle
Costoclavicular ligament
1st rib
Manubrium
Sternum

Figure 4-2
Sternoclavicular joint.

helps to hold up the shoulder. To demonstrate this, the clinician can place a finger in the superior sternal notch; the ligament is lax with elevation of the arm but becomes taut when both arms are left to hang at the sides.

The capsular ligament of the sternoclavicular joint, which extends over the anterosuperior and posterior aspects of the joint, represents thickenings of the joint capsule. The anterior portion of the capsular ligament is heavier and stronger. Bearn[33] has demonstrated that the capsular ligament is the most important and strongest ligament of the sternoclavicular joint and that is the structure most responsible for preventing upward displacement of the medial clavicle in the presence of a downward force on the distal end of the shoulder.

Function of the Sternoclavicular Joint

The sternoclavicular joint acts similar to a ball and socket joint, allowing for motion in almost all planes, including rotation. In normal shoulder motion, the joint can allow

for 30° to 35° of upward elevation, 35° of combined forward and backward movement, and 45° to 50° of rotation about the long axis of the clavicle and therefore the sternoclavicular joint.[23,34,35] It is important that the clinician appreciate that almost all motions of the upper extremity affect the sternoclavicular joint and are transferred proximally back to this joint.

Sternoclavicular Joint Dislocations

Dislocations of the sternoclavicular joint are quite rare, accounting for only about 3% of all fractures and dislocations around the shoulder girdle.[36,37] Most of these dislocations are the anterior type (with an anterior to posterior ratio approaching 20:1) (Figure 4-3).[38] However, posterior dislocations have a high complication rate, therefore it is important for practitioners to recognize the injury and its potential life-threatening nature. A posterior dislocation may put pressure on the many vital structures lying between the sternum and the cervical spine, such as the

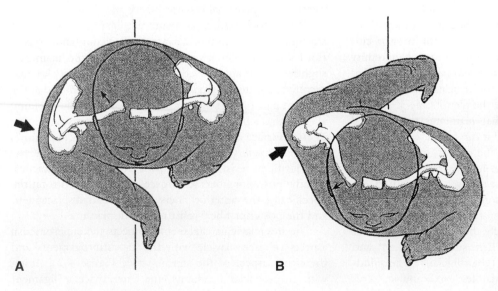

A   B

Figure 4-3
Mechanism of injury to the sternoclavicular joint. **A**, Posterior. **B**, Anterior. (From Emery R: Acromioclavicular and sternoclavicular joints. In Copland SA, editor: *Shoulder surgery,* Philadelphia, 1997, WB Saunders. Redrawn from Rockwood CA, Green DP, editors: *Fractures,* vol 1, ed 2, Philadelphia, 1984, JB Lippincott.)

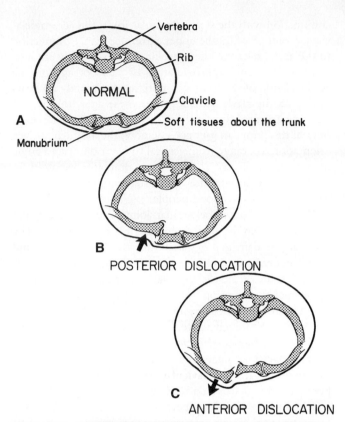

Figure 4-4

Sternoclavicular joint disorders. **A,** Normal anatomical relationships. **B,** Posterior dislocation of the sternoclavicular joint. **C,** Anterior dislocation of the sternoclavicular joint. (From Rockwood CA, Green DP, editors: *Fractures,* vol 1, ed 2, Philadelphia, 1984, JB Lippincott.)

trachea, esophagus, and major vessels (Figure 4-4). Motor vehicle accidents are reported to be the most common cause of dislocation of the sternoclavicular joint, followed by sports activities, in which the dislocation occurs primarily as a result of direct or indirect trauma. An example of direct trauma in a sports activity might be a hockey player hitting the medial side of the clavicle on the goalpost or on another player's knee. With an indirect injury, the athlete may be lying on his side, and the uppermost shoulder is compressed and rolled backward, resulting in an anterior sternoclavicular dislocation on that side. If the shoulder rolls forward and is compressed, a posterior dislocation is more likely.[38,39]

Sternoclavicular dislocations are classified as first, second, or third degree, and the classification is based more on injury to the ligaments supporting the joint than on injury to the joint itself. A first-degree sternoclavicular dislocation results in minor tearing (first- or second-degree sprain) of the sternoclavicular and costoclavicular ligaments, with no true displacement of the joint. A complete tear (third-degree sprain) in the sternoclavicular ligaments and a second-degree sprain of the costoclavicular ligament

constitute a second-degree sternoclavicular dislocation and actually result in subluxation of the joint. A third-degree sternoclavicular dislocation is a true dislocation of the joint, caused by third-degree sprains in the sternoclavicular and costoclavicular ligaments.[40]

Clinical Presentation. Sternoclavicular dislocations are characterized by deformity; local pain or tenderness, especially with arm movements in which the shoulders are rolled forward; and subsequent ecchymosis. With a posterior dislocation or subluxation, some shortness of breath or even venous congestion in the neck may be seen, with decreased circulation sometimes evident in the arm. Reduction of a posterior sternoclavicular dislocation usually is accomplished by extending the shoulders while using some form of roll or sandbag as a fulcrum along the spine. Reduction most often occurs easily, although in some cases supplemental anesthesia may be required. The practitioner also may need to grasp the clavicle with the fingers or, if the anatomy is less defined, with some type of surgical instrument, such as a towel clip.

Treatment of Sternoclavicular Joint Dislocations

If the sternoclavicular joint has incurred only a first- or second-degree sprain and the joint is deemed stable, treatment follows a course similar to that for any other injured joint. The patient's shoulder should be immobilized for 3-4 days, as pain dictates, and then should make a gradual return to normal use of the shoulder and arm. Local electrical modalities and the use of ice and heat may be helpful for reducing pain and inflammation at the sternoclavicular joint. The clinician should be aware of the impact of a sternoclavicular injury on the entire shoulder complex, because the effects of the initial injury may be far-reaching and can lead to compensatory patterns of movement.

In second- or third-degree sprains of the sternoclavicular joint, if the main complaint after reduction is instability, treatment frequently requires sling support for an anterior dislocation or a figure-of-eight bandage for posterior dislocation. The sling is worn for at least 2-3 weeks. Chronic instability may require surgical stabilization of the sternoclavicular joint, which is by no means uniformly successful. Chronic subluxation or damage to the intra-articular disc can produce long-term discomfort with repetitive strong movements of the upper limb.

Complications of anterior sternoclavicular dislocation include cosmetic deformity, recurrent instability, and late osteoarthrosis; complications of posterior dislocation include all of these plus pressure on or rupture of the trachea, pneumothorax, rupture of the esophagus, pressure on the subclavian artery or brachial plexus, voice change, and dysphagia. Although the incidence of one of these complications can be as high as 25%, only about three deaths have been reported in the literature from the more serious complications associated with this injury.[38,40]

Complications of Sternoclavicular Posterior Dislocation

- Cosmetic deformity
- Recurrent instability
- Late osteoarthritis
- Pressure on or rupture of the trachea
- Pneumothorax
- Rupture of the esophagus
- Pressure on the subclavian artery
- Pressure on the brachial plexus
- Voice change
- Dysphagia

The patient with a sternoclavicular joint that spontaneously subluxes or dislocates should be managed with "nonoperative skillful neglect," according to Wirth and Rockwood.[41] They report that in patients with this condition, the medial end of the clavicle typically subluxes or dislocates anteriorly when the person raises the arms over the head (Figure 4-5). This occurs spontaneously and without any significant trauma. In fact, some patients seeking advice for a different shoulder problem are completely unaware that it is happening. Wirth and Rockwood[41] believe that patients should be taught about the anatomical events involved and advised that in time, either the symptoms will disappear or the patient will forget about the condition and no longer consider it a problem.

Acromioclavicular Joint

The acromioclavicular (AC) joint is a diarthrodial joint made up of the lateral aspect of the clavicle and the medial margin of the acromion process of the scapula. In conjunction with the sternoclavicular joint, the acromioclavicular joint provides the upper extremity with a connection to the axial skeleton. The articular surfaces initially are hyaline cartilage until approximately 17 years of age on the acromial side of the joint and until approximately 24 years of age on the clavicular side. After these ages, the hyaline cartilage acquires the structure of fibrocartilage. The anatomy of this joint can vary considerably; the articular surface orientation can range from vertical to overriding at an angle of approximately 50°.[38,42-44] The dramatic variation in anatomy may account for the differences in vulnerability to separation seen among people.

Within the acromioclavicular joint is an intra-articular disc, which may be partial (meniscoid) or complete. The disc can be damaged by an injury to the AC joint and may degenerate further with time; such discs may be implicated in some of the clicking that is heard and some painful syndromes that develop in the joint after trauma.

The acromioclavicular joint is surrounded by a thin capsule that is reinforced above, below, anteriorly, and posteriorly by the superior, inferior, anterior, and posterior acromioclavicular ligaments (Figure 4-6). The fibers of the superior acromioclavicular ligament blend with the fibers of the deltoid and trapezius muscles, which are attached to the superior aspect of the clavicle and the acromion process. These muscle attachments are important because they strengthen the acromioclavicular ligaments and add stability to the acromioclavicular joint.

The coracoclavicular ligament is a very strong, heavy ligament with fibers running from the outer, inferior surface of the clavicle to the base of the coracoid process of the scapula. The ligament consists of two individual ligaments, the conoid ligament and the trapezoid ligament, which sometimes have a bursa between them. As the name

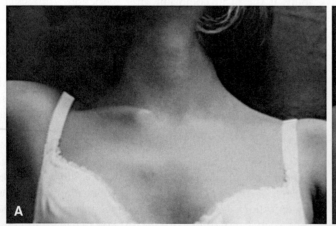 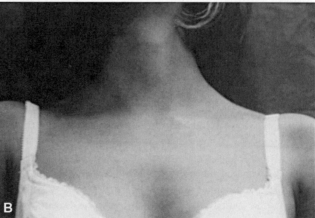

Figure 4-5

Spontaneous subluxation of the sternoclavicular joint. **A,** With the arms in the overhead position, the medial end of the right clavicle spontaneously subluxes out anteriorly without any trauma. **B,** When the arm is brought back down to the side, the medial end of the clavicle spontaneously reduces. This usually is associated with no significant discomfort. (From Rockwood CA, Matsen FA, editors: *The shoulder,* p 564, Philadelphia, 1998, WB Saunders.)

Figure 4-6
Acromioclavicular joint.

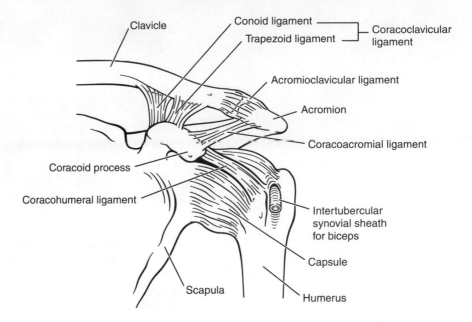

suggests, the conoid ligament is cone shaped, with the apex of the cone attaching on the posteromedial aspect of the base of the coracoid process and the base attaching to the conoid tubercle on the posterior undersurface of the clavicle. The trapezoid ligament arises from the coracoid process, anterior and lateral to the attachment of the conoid ligament just posterior to the attachment of the pectoralis minor tendon. The ligament travels superiorly to a rough line on the undersurface of the clavicle. The coracoclavicular ligament plays an important role not only in strengthening the acromioclavicular joint, but also in assisting the glenohumeral joint with scapulohumeral motion. As the clavicle rotates upward, it dictates scapulothoracic rotation by virtue of its attachment to the scapula; that is, the conoid and trapezoid ligaments.[43,45]

Function of the Acromioclavicular Joint

Codman[46] described the motion at the acromioclavicular joint as "swinging a little, rocking a little, twisting a little, sliding a little and acting like a hinge." Rockwood[47] and Rockwood et al.[48] discovered rather little relative motion between the clavicle and the acromion during studies involving percutaneous implanted pins in subjects. They described a synchronous, three-dimensional linkage between clavicular rotation and scapular rotation, such that when the clavicle rotates, the scapula also rotates. These researchers therefore concluded that most scapulothoracic motion occurs through the sternoclavicular joint, not the acromioclavicular joint.

In a classic article published in 1944, Inman[34] suggested that the total range of motion of the acromioclavicular joint is 20°. He noted that the motion occurs in the first 30° of abduction and then again after 135° of elevation of the arm. He also showed that with full elevation, the clavicle rotates upward 40° to 50°. Inman[34] concluded that the clavicular rotation was a fundamental feature of shoulder motion. Since these original observations, several authors have offered differing opinions about the amount of motion that occurs at the acromioclavicular joint relative to the glenohumeral joint. Despite the differences, researchers agree on the important relationship between the two joints and recognize that scapulohumeral rhythm is a delicate balance achieved through a combination of elevation and rotation of the clavicle and proper scapulothoracic and glenohumeral joint motion.

Acromioclavicular Joint Injuries

The acromioclavicular joint is one of the most frequently injured joints in the body, particularly in sports and activities that require overhead involvement of the shoulder and arm and/or that have a high risk of collision and impact. Injuries to the acromioclavicular joint result in what is often called a "separated" shoulder, and they account for approximately 12% of the dislocations of the shoulder girdle.[49,50] The mechanism of injury is either a fall on the outstretched hand (FOOSH injury), a direct blow to the shoulder, a fall on the elbow, or falling on to the point of the shoulder (Figure 4-7).

As with the sternoclavicular joint, acromioclavicular joint injuries are classified according to ligamentous injury rather than injury to the joint itself. Table 4-2 describes the features and management of the six classifications of acromioclavicular joint injury (Figures 4-8 and 4-9). Some have suggested that third-degree (type III) disruptions can be further divided according to the magnitude of displacement and the potential accompanying muscle and soft tissue stripping and tearing, as well as the direction of displacement of the distal clavicle.[38,50] For instance, displacement of the clavicle of more than 100% often is classified as a fourth-degree (type IV) injury. Type V injuries

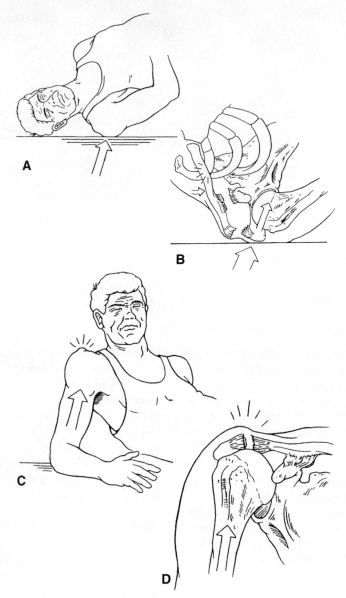

Figure 4-7

Mechanisms of injury to the acromioclavicular joint. **A** and **B,** Direct mechanism of injury. **C** and **D,**
Indirect mechanism of injury. (From Field LD, Warren RF: Acromioclavicular joint separations. In
Hawkins RJ, Misamore GW, editors: *Shoulder injuries in the athlete: surgical repair and rehabilitation,*
p 206, New York, 1996, Churchill Livingstone.)

involve very severe deformity, because the distal end of the
clavicle is displaced upward a significant degree toward the
base of the neck (Figure 4-10). In addition, displacements
may occur posteriorly through the trapezius or, in rare
cases, inferiorly below the coracoid (type VI). Fourth-
degree injuries are associated with considerable disruption
of the deltoid and trapezius muscles. A third-degree separation may be treated without surgery, but surgery does have
a role in the treatment of fourth-, fifth-, and sixth-degree
injuries because of the associated ligamentous disruption
and because of cosmetic considerations in leaner individuals
(see Figure 4-8).[51-54]

Clinical Presentation. Patients who have suffered an
injury to the acromioclavicular joint typically present with
a history of either a distinctive, traumatic mechanism of
injury or a more insidious type of onset that began with
pain and dysfunction. The diagnosis is made by assessing
the site of local tenderness, the degree of deformity, and
whether instability is present. As with the sternoclavicular
joint, injury to the AC joint tends to cause localized pain
with minimal referral. Stressing the joint with horizontal
adduction elicits pain in the injured AC joint, as does loading the joint by applying leverage at the distal arm. A palpable gap (step deformity) may be present with the higher

Table 4-2
Classification of Acromioclavicular Joint Trauma

Classification	Salient Features	Management
First degree (type I)	Minimal structural damage First-degree sprain of the acromioclavicular ligament Local tenderness on palpation Full range of motion (may have pain at extreme) No loss of structural strength Normal stress x-ray film	Re-establish full range of motion and strength
Second degree (type II)	Subluxation of the acromioclavicular joint Tearing of the acromioclavicular capsule Second- or third-degree sprain of the acromioclavicular ligament First- or second-degree sprain of the coracoclavicular ligament May affect the deltoid and trapezius muscles No significant increase in the costoclavicular space on stress x-ray film Slight widening of the acromioclavicular joint on stress x-ray film Definite structural weakness Detectable instability on stress Palpable gap or step deformity possible Obvious swelling initially with later ecchymosis	Requires 6 weeks to heal, although ligaments have good structural strength after approximately 3 weeks Limb support (sling) Treatments for pain relief (e.g., ice, transcutaneous electrical nerve stimulation [TENS], interferential therapy) Ultrasound therapy for collagen enhancement Functional exercises (activities at functional speed control)
Third degree (type III)	Dislocation of the acromioclavicular joint Complete disruption of the acromioclavicular joint Third-degree sprain of the acromioclavicular ligament Third-degree sprain of the coracoclavicular ligament Tearing of the deltoid and trapezius muscles from the distal end of the clavicle Obvious step deformity, often without stress Increased costoclavicular space on stress x-ray film Widening of the acromioclavicular joint on stress x-ray film	May be treated surgically or conservatively If treated conservatively, deformity remains but athlete will function remarkably well with only slight discomfort/instability at high loads Conservative treatment as above
Fourth degree (type IV) Fifth degree (type V) Sixth degree (type VI)	Modifications of type III trauma (rare injuries)	Require surgical repair

Modified from Zachazewski JE, Magee DJ, Quillen WS, editors: *Athletic injuries and rehabilitation*, p 519, Philadelphia, 1996, WB Saunders.

degrees of separation (Figure 4-11). With trauma to the AC joint, the clinician must take care to assess for secondary injury to the surrounding soft tissues (e.g., the rotator cuff) and to the other three articulations of the shoulder complex. Long term, most people function well without surgery, although degenerative changes, including clavicular osteolysis, may be seen in some individuals.

Treatment of the Acromioclavicular Joint

The ultimate function of the AC joint depends not so much on the amount of separation as on the amount of pain that

persists in the joint. Some first-degree dislocations and some of the more severe second-degree injuries are much more problematic because they produce a great deal of pain in long-term follow-up. Therefore early conservative treatment for first- and second-degree separations focuses on pain relief. Initially, the patient's arm may be put in a sling, often accompanied by a swath, to remove the stress of the weight of the limb on the joint and to protect the joint from further damage. As the pain decreases (within 5 to 7 days), range of motion and strengthening exercises, especially to the deltoid and trapezius muscles, are initiated,

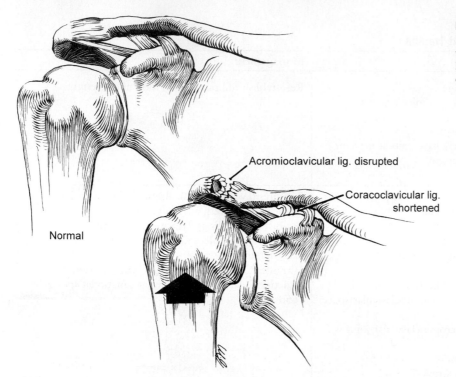

Figure 4-8
Disruption of the acromioclavicular ligament with preservation of the coracoclavicular ligaments. (From Rockwood CA, Green DP, editors: *Fractures,* vol 1, ed 2, Philadelphia, 1984, JB Lippincott.)

Acromioclavicular lig. disrupted

Coracoclavicular lig. shortened

Normal

and the patient usually returns to general activity 2-6 weeks after injury. Soft tissue trauma in second-degree injuries typically is more extensive, therefore the time frame is likely to be prolonged for all the suggested treatments.

In third-degree acromioclavicular joint injuries, complete reduction is not necessary for satisfactory function; in fact, in terms of strength, endurance, and function, non-surgical and surgical treatments have been reported to be equally effective.[53-57] Depending on the preference of the surgeon, third-degree injuries may be treated surgically, but the results are seldom better than with conservative treatment, the recovery period is longer, and the complications of surgery must be considered. For these reasons, the most common treatment for third-degree AC injuries is a sling and swath with treatment as pain allows, again stressing the deltoid and trapezius muscles.

Complications of an AC joint injury include a step deformity produced by the elevated distal end of the clavicle, early skin necrosis if the clavicle is widely displaced in a thin individual, osteoarthrosis, osteolysis, and continuing pain in the long term. For surgical procedures, complications include infection, wound dehiscence, pin migration, and recurrence of the instability, as well as the normal risks of general anesthesia.

Glenohumeral Joint Hypomobility Conditions (Frozen Shoulder)

Conditions that arise as a result of glenohumeral joint hypomobility typically are categorized as "frozen shoulder." Duplay and Putnam provided the first reported descriptions of frozen shoulder in the late 1800s.[58] They used the label *scapulohumeral periarthritis* to describe a broad spectrum of pathologies of the shoulder that resulted

in pain, stiffness, and dysfunction. This label often served as an umbrella term that encompassed disorders such as rotator cuff tendonitis and tears, biceps tendonitis and tears, calcific deposits, acromioclavicular arthritis, and other painful shoulder syndromes. The term *frozen shoulder* was coined in 1934 by Codman,[59] who characterized the condition as involving a slow onset, pain near the deltoid insertion, inability to sleep on the affected side, painful and restricted elevation and external rotation, and a normal radiological appearance. He stated that the condition was "difficult to define, difficult to treat and difficult to explain from the point of view of pathology," He also believed that the symptoms were related to tendonitis of the rotator cuff. To this day, authors and clinicians are still perplexed by frozen shoulder. Little has been discovered that has led to a better understanding of the cause of frozen shoulder and, more important, how best to manage it.

Most agree that the Codman's definition is far too general and that the diagnosis very likely is being applied to patients with other shoulder pathologies, such as rotator cuff tears or subtle instability syndromes. The risk in this error, of course, is in the resultant choice of treatment. A patient with a true frozen shoulder typically undergoes a rehabilitation program consisting of manual mobilization techniques and stretching and strengthening exercises, specifically in the upper ranges of motion. In contrast, a patient with a subtle instability syndrome, who may appear to have a stiff shoulder but in fact has an underlying weakness of the deep shoulder stabilizing musculature, is not best managed with stretching techniques; rather, rehabilitation for this patient should emphasize strengthening of the weakened stabilizing muscles.

Subsequent to Codman's introduction of the frozen shoulder, Neviaser[60] in 1945 recorded his operative and

Figure 4-9
Acromiclavicular joint injuries (see Table 4-2). (From
Rockwood CA, Matsen FA, editors: *The shoulder,*
p 495, Philadelphia, 1998, WB Saunders.)

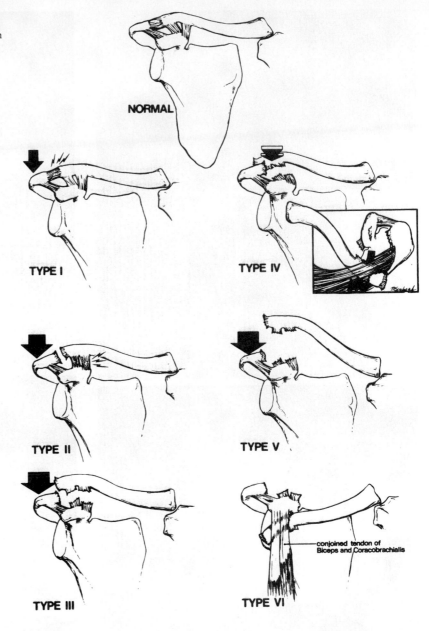

Clinical Presentation of Frozen Shoulder

histological observations in 10 affected patients and 63
cadaveric shoulders. He noted that it was not the bursa that
was affected, but rather the capsule that was thickened and
that had adhered to the humeral head. He therefore suggested *adhesive capsulitis* as a more descriptive term for
shoulders that appeared frozen. Reeves[61] divided the condition into three phases: the painful phase, the frozen
phase, and the thawing phase. Over these three phases
motion and pain gradually improved, but the time frame
for improvement could range from 12 to 42 months. More
recently, Zuckerman and Cuomo[62] defined *frozen shoulder,*
or *idiopathic adhesive capsulitis,* as a condition of uncertain
etiology, characterized by substantial restriction of both
active and passive shoulder motion, that occurs in the
absence of a known intrinsic shoulder disorder.

The two defining factors in patients with a frozen shoulder
are pain and restricted range of motion (ROM) of the glenohumeral joint (Figure 4-12). Most often the pain is
noted first and then the decrease in motion. Patients
describe either a slow, progressive loss of shoulder mobility
or a loss of shoulder motion almost overnight. The
decreased mobility follows a *capsular pattern of restriction,*
a characteristic of all synovial joints in which the pathology
is related to dysfunction of the joint capsule. In the glenohumeral joint, the capsular pattern of restriction presents as
a greater loss first of lateral rotation, followed by abduction,
and then medial rotation.

It is important to note that the restricted range of
motion seen in patients with a frozen shoulder occurs *both*

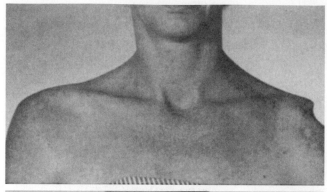

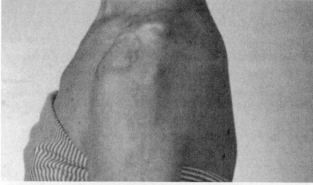

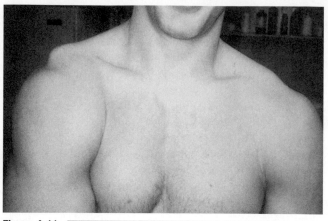

Figure 4-11

Step deformity resulting from acromioclavicular joint trauma. (From Magee DJ: *Orthopedic physical assessment,* ed 4, p 218, Philadelphia, 2002, WB Saunders.)

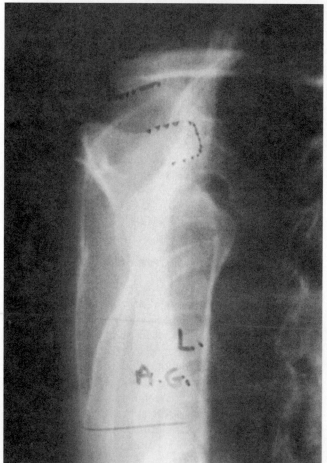

Figure 4-10

Type IV and type V chronic dislocation of the acromioclavicular joint. The scapulolateral x-ray film shows severe displacement of the acromioclavicular joint. (From Rockwood CA, Matsen FA, editors: *The shoulder,* p 497, Philadelphia, 1998, WB Saunders.)

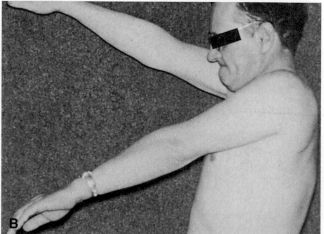

Figure 4-12

A and **B,** A 45-year-old man whose right shoulder is in the painful freezing phase. Note the distress and discouragement in the patient's face. (From Rodwe CR, Leffet RD: Frozen shoulder. In Rowe CR, editor: *The shoulder,* p 158, New York, 1988, Churchill Livingstone.)

actively and passively. This is in contrast to a number of other shoulder conditions in which a loss of active ROM of the glenohumeral joint occurs, but reasonably good if not full passive ROM is maintained. Patients with these other types of shoulder conditions do not have stiffness of the glenohumeral joint as a result of the inert tissue being affected (i.e., the joint capsule); rather, they have a "weakened" shoulder in which the contractile tissue is affected.

In addition to pain and loss of mobility, patients diagnosed with a frozen shoulder at some point in the injury process develop secondary weakness as a result of disuse and poor use. This usually occurs in the deep stabilizers of the glenohumeral joint (e.g., the rotator cuff) and in the more superficial movers, such as the three parts of the deltoid muscle. The upper trapezius tends to become overutilized as the patient incorrectly recruits this muscle in an attempt to elevate the arm; this leads to a reversal of normal scapulohumeral rhythm and further muscle imbalance about the scapula. Therefore, even though frozen shoulder is not generally considered a cause of shoulder weakness, it most certainly can lead to changes in muscle functioning as a result of the altered function that inevitably develops in these patients.

Treatment of Frozen Shoulder

Given the uncertainty about the etiology of frozen shoulder syndrome, it is not surprising that the theories of treatment for this condition are equally inconsistent. The basic agreed-upon principles in managing patients with frozen shoulder syndromes are (1) to relieve pain and (2) to restore motion.

Authors and clinicians have tried to achieve these objectives through cautious neglect, anti-inflammatory medications, injection therapy, physical therapy, and surgery.[60-65] Rowe[32] reported that physical therapy resulted in no change in the course of the pathology in patients with a frozen shoulder and therefore concluded that patients simply needed to be guided through the three self-limiting stages of the disease (Table 4-3). Neviaser[60] felt quite differently, advocating aggressive rehabilitation and, if necessary, surgical manipulation under anesthesia. Farrell et al.[64] recently studied the long-term results of management by manipulation under anesthesia and reported that it was a safe and reasonably effective form of intervention. Patients studied in this particular project were followed an average of 15 years and reportedly were successful in maintaining shoulder motion and function.

Traditional rehabilitation programs have focused on exercises that improve range of motion at the glenohumeral joint.[62,63] Joint mobilization techniques, stretching, and passive ROM exercises often are done initially, because pain usually discourages patients from doing these exercises independently. Exercises should be performed within the limitations of pain, because techniques that aggravate the affected tissue, especially during the painful, freezing phase, have been shown to be ineffective. Griggs et al.[63] evaluated

Table 4-3
Three Phases of Frozen Shoulder

Phase	Clinical Presentation
Freezing phase (painful)	Duration: 10-36 weeks Pain and stiffness around the shoulder No history of injury Nagging, constant pain that is worse at night Little or no response to NSAIDs
Adhesive/restrictive phase	Duration: 4-12 weeks Pain gradually subsides but stiffness remains Pain apparent only at extremes of movement Gross reduction of glenohumeral movements with near total loss of external rotation
Resolution phase	Duration: 12-42 weeks Spontaneous improvement in ROM Mean duration from onset of frozen shoulder to greatest resolution exceeds 30 weeks

From Dias R, Cutts S, Massoud S: Frozen shoulder, *Br Med J* 331:1453-1456, 2005.
NSAIDs, Nonsteroidal anti-inflammatory drugs; *ROM*, range of motion.

the outcome of patients with idiopathic adhesive capsulitis who had been treated with a stretching and exercise program. These researchers concluded that most patients in the adhesive/restrictive phase of the condition can be treated successfully with a four-direction shoulder stretching exercise program.

Clearly, no preponderance of evidence points to the best treatment for patients with frozen shoulder syndromes. However, it seems plausible that some, if not all, of the basic principles of shoulder rehabilitation could be applied in dealing with this condition. Patient education about the condition and its expected phases and outcome; postural awareness and treatment, especially of the adjacent cervical and thoracic spine levels; and exercises for the remaining shoulder girdle musculature are all important considerations. Also, significant care should always be given to re-educating these patients to control movements of the glenohumeral and scapulothoracic joints, because these muscles tend to become "detrained" as a result of the disease and the consequent loss of movement.

Shoulder Fractures

Fractures of the shoulder complex are relatively uncommon.[38] They range from relatively minor, nondisplaced, hairline fractures to major, comminuted, displaced fractures that in some cases are accompanied by life-threatening injuries. Fractures commonly require some type of immobilization and/or a period of protected motion; these measures, although essential for bone healing, can result in secondary shoulder stiffness, muscle weakness, and altered scapulothoracic mechanics. Therefore it is important that the objectives of rehabilitation after a shoulder fracture include normalization of the entire shoulder girdle and trunk, not just the joint adjacent to the local fracture site.

Scapular Fractures

Fractures of the scapula account for only 1% of all fractures, 3% of all shoulder injuries, and 5% of fractures involving the entire shoulder.[66,67] They typically occur as a result of a high energy situation involving a fall or direct blow. With less severe fractures, the muscles effectively stabilize the fracture, and the patient typically can expect a good functional outcome. However, patients may present with associated injuries to the involved arm, shoulder girdle, and thoracic cage; ipsilateral rib fractures are the most common associated injury, occurring in approximately 27% to 50% of patients.[66] Pulmonary trauma (e.g., pneumothorax, hemothorax, or both) is reported in 16% to 40% of patients, and clavicular fractures and injuries to the brachial plexus and subclavian artery reportedly occur in 26% and 12% of patients, respectively.[66-68]

Scapular fractures are classified according to the location of the fracture, specifically the body, neck, glenoid fossa, acromion, spine, or coracoid. The distribution of the different fracture sites has been reported as 35% to 43% at the scapular body, 26% at the neck, 10% at the glenoid fossa, 8% to 12% at the acromion, 6% to 11% at the spine, and 5% to 7% at the coracoid.[66-69]

Clinical Evaluation

Most patients with a scapular fracture have experienced a traumatic, well-defined mechanism of injury, therefore clinical evaluation usually is precluded by a thorough radiographic and neurological examination. Local physical findings, such as swelling, ecchymosis, and crepitus with range of motion, are common, as are subjective complaints of pain in the scapular region. In most cases a detailed assessment of the entire shoulder girdle and the cervical and thoracic spine should be performed (see volume 1 of this series, *Orthopedic Physical Assessment*).

Treatment of Scapular Fractures

Most scapular fractures can be treated successfully without surgical intervention. However, certain fracture sites and classifications of scapular fractures reportedly are best managed by surgical reduction and stabilization.[70,71] These include (1) acromion or scapular spine fractures with downward tilting of the lateral fragment and resultant subacromial narrowing (Figure 4-13); (2) coracoid fractures that extend into the glenoid fossa (Figure 4-14); and (3)

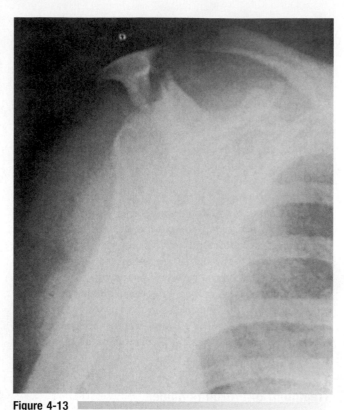

Figure 4-13

Fracture of the base of the acromion. (From Rockwood CA, Matsen FA, editors: *The shoulder,* p 397, Philadelphia, 1998, WB Saunders.)

glenoid rim and intra-articular glenoid fractures associated with persistent or recurrent glenohumeral instability (Figures 4-15 and 4-16).

Nonsurgical treatment of scapular fractures consists of approximately 7 to 10 days of sling immobilization, followed by a progressing regimen of pendular and gentle passive range of motion exercises as comfort and control allow. Once follow-up radiographic findings indicate sufficient healing, the patient is encouraged to discontinue immobilization and proceed with active-assisted and active ROM exercises. Consideration must always be given to restrengthening the muscles that attach to the scapula and those that arise from the scapula (i.e., the rotator cuff and biceps brachii), which may have been affected by disuse and painful inhibition. In a number of cases, patients with a scapular fracture develop stiffness in the adjacent spine, specifically the lower cervical spine to the midthoracic spine. Clinicians must take care to assess these regions and treat accordingly. Failure to address this important part of the kinetic chain may lead to further problems in the shoulder region and most certainly will result in a less than optimal outcome. Most scapular fractures are sufficiently healed by 6 weeks to be able to withstand the progressive load delivered through the ROM and strengthening exercises. However, clinicians and patients must keep in mind that maximum functional recovery, which encompasses more than just bone healing, may take as long as 6 to 12 months.[72,73]

Figure 4-14

Fracture of the base of the coracoid. (From Rockwood CA, Matsen FA, editors: *The shoulder,* p 397, Philadelphia, 1998, WB Saunders.)

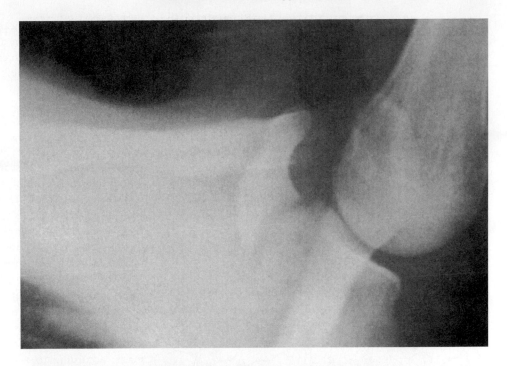

Figure 4-15

Anteroinferior glenoid fracture. (From Rockwood CA, Matsen FA, editors: *The shoulder,* p 396, Philadelphia, 1998, WB Saunders.)

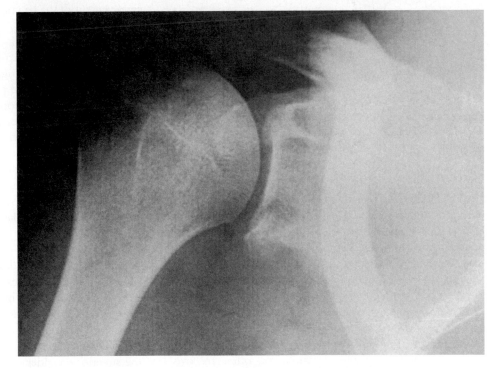

"Floating Shoulder"

The term *floating shoulder* was introduced by Herscovici[74] in 1992 to describe an ipsilateral fracture of the clavicular shaft and the scapular neck (Figure 4-17). It was suggested that the combination of these two types of fractures would result in a loss of the stabilizing effect of the clavicle. Goss[75] has provided the most recent definition of floating shoulder, which is "a double disruption of the superior suspensory shoulder complex (SSSC)." He described three struts of this complex: (1) the acromioclavicular joint–acromial strut, (2) the clavicular–coracoclavicular ligament–coracoid linkage, and (3) the three process–scapular body junction. Goss suggested that a potentially unstable anatomical condition exists when the complex is disrupted in at least two places with significant displacement at either or both sites (Figure 4-18). He also believed that this condition posed considerable risk of poor bone healing, such as delayed union or malunion of the clavicle, the scapular neck, or both.

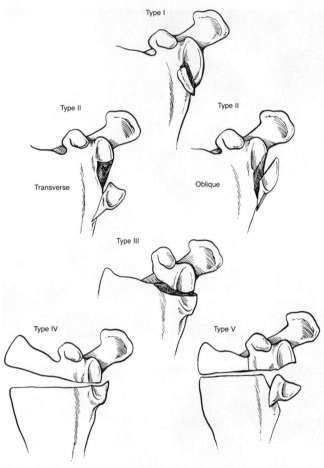

Figure 4-16
Ideberg's classification of glenoid fractures. (From Rockwood CA, Matsen FA, editors: *The shoulder,* p 406, Philadelphia, 1998, WB Saunders.)

A combined clavicular and ipsilateral scapular neck fracture most often is caused by a high energy mechanism of injury. One study showed that 80% to 100% of these cases result from traffic accidents;[76] however, various other causes also have been cited, such as a direct blow, a fall onto the tip of the shoulder, or a fall onto the outstretched hand.[74,75] As with most scapular fractures, combined clavicular and ipsilateral scapular neck fractures have a high incidence of associated traumatic lesions, and when severe accompanying injuries are present, the clinical signs and symptoms of this specific fracture type often are overlooked. The definitive diagnosis therefore is made on the basis of radiographic findings.

Very little research to date has addressed the most effective way to treat a floating shoulder. Literature related to this fracture type is limited to case reports and retrospective studies of small patient series.[74-76] The treatment options mentioned range from conservative management with or without early mobilization to operative treatment through open reduction and internal fixation of the clavicle only or of the clavicle and the scapular neck fracture sites together. Clearly, further research and clinical study are necessary to elucidate this interesting pathology. Any rehabilitation plan should be derived from a careful analysis of the anatomy involved and a thorough examination of the entire shoulder girdle and adjacent spine.

Clavicular Fractures

The most commonly reported fracture of the shoulder girdle is the clavicular fracture (Figure 4-19). The incidence of this type of fracture is highest among children and adolescents, in whom the mechanism of injury typically is a fall onto the lateral aspect of the affected shoulder or, less often, a direct blow to the clavicle. As the shoulder is driven downward, the clavicle forcefully impinges on the underlying first rib, causing a fracture (Figure 4-20). Although a fracture can occur anywhere along the clavicle, the most common site (80% of cases) is reported to be between the medial two thirds and the lateral one third of the bone.[38,77] Fractures are classified according to their anatomical location, specifically the proximal, middle, and distal thirds of the bone. Subclassifications for each of these anatomical thirds are now made, according to the specific fracture pattern and the involvement of the ligament and joint complexes.

Clinical Evaluation

Because of their superficial location, clavicular fractures are easily recognizable through inspection and direct palpation. Patients report localized pain and swelling, and ecchymosis and crepitus often are noted at the fracture site. The degree of deformity depends on the location of the fracture and the amount of displacement (see Figure 4-19, *A*). Associated injuries, although not common, may occur, including scapular fractures, scapulothoracic dissociation, rib fractures, pneumothorax, and neurovascular compromise (Figures 4-21 and 4-22). The brachial plexus is of particular concern because of its proximity to the clavicle, which makes it susceptible to injury.[38,78]

Treatment of Clavicular Fractures

Most clavicular fractures do not require surgery. Reports strongly indicate that nondisplaced fractures have excellent healing capabilities and relatively few adverse outcomes.[79,80] Surgical indications include open fractures, concomitant displaced scapular neck fractures that disrupt the superior shoulder suspensory complex, the presence of neurovascular or skin compromise, and a patient with multiple trauma who needs assistance with early mobilization. Surgical treatment may be considered in some cases for certain high demand patients, such as heavy laborers or athletes, who are exposed to large, repetitive, potentially deforming forces, and individuals who have had a previous nonunion at the same site. However, careful patient selection and preoperative counseling are recommended because of the potential risks (e.g., implant infection, migration of intramedullary wires, neurovascular injuries) and sometimes less than optimal outcomes of the procedure.

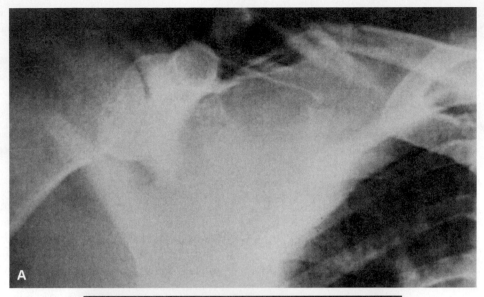

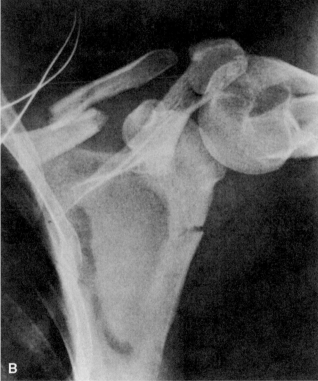

Figure 4-17

Floating shoulder. **A,** Scapular neck fracture with an associated body and clavicular fracture. **B,** Fracture involving the scapula, clavicle, and upper humerus, resulting in a floating shoulder. (From Rockwood CA, Matsen FA, editors: *The shoulder,* p 402, Philadelphia, 1998, WB Saunders.)

Nonsurgical treatment involves symptomatic support in a figure-of-eight bandage or a sling and swath immobilizer for 3 to 6 weeks as dictated by the patient's comfort and control of the arm. Once bone healing is well established (clinical union occurs in 2 to 3 weeks), the patient can be guided through active-assisted and then active ROM exercises. Because most clavicular fractures do not involve the adjacent articulations, this range of motion is quite easily regained. Care must always be taken not to overload the healing fracture site with activities that produce too great a leverage point on this important fulcrum. Restrengthening exercises are prescribed for any muscles that were weakened as a result of painful inhibition and/or the immobilization period. As with any type of shoulder injury, the patient should be checked to ensure that the scapulohumeral rhythm is normal and symmetrical and that the essential stabilizing musculature of the glenohumeral joint is intact. Normal healing times for

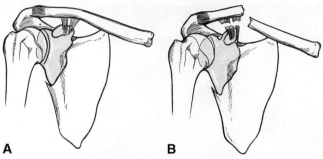

Figure 4-18

Stable (**A**) and unstable (**B**) scapular neck fracture. (From Rockwood CA, Matsen FA, editors: *The shoulder*, p 404, Philadelphia, 1998, WB Saunders.)

a clavicular fracture are 6 weeks in young children and 8 weeks in adults.[45,50]

Proximal Humeral Fractures

The proximal humerus is a common site of injury in the young and the elderly. In a skeletally immature athlete, the fracture frequently presents as an epiphyseal fracture at the proximal humeral growth plate (little leaguer's shoulder); this type of injury most often is associated with youngsters involved in throwing sports.[81,82] The injury is caused by a powerful medial rotation and adduction traction force on the proximal humeral epiphysis. Such an injury occurs during the deceleration and follow-through phases of throwing or pitching, and the rotational forces that occur during the arm-cocking and arm-acceleration phases can add to the problem. The result is a stress fracture, usually a Salter-Harris type I or type II. Radiologic signs, which may take up to 4 to 6 weeks to become evident, include widening of the epiphyseal plate, demineralization and rarefaction on the metaphyseal side of the physis, and metaphyseal bone separation.[81,82]

Radiographic Signs of Little Leaguer's Shoulder

- Widening of the epiphyseal plate
- Demineralization and rarefaction of the metaphyseal side of the physis
- Metaphyseal bone separation

The athlete complains of acute shoulder pain when attempting to throw hard; if ignored, this may result in acute displacement of the weakened physis. Rest is the initial and primary treatment, and the bone may require up to 8 to 12 months to reossify and remodel. The patient must fully understand the problem and why absolute rest, at least initially, is essential.

Rehabilitation may include activities to improve strength, coordination, proprioception, endurance, and range of motion. The exact timing for beginning active exercises, as well as when and how much to progress these exercises, varies, depending on the stage of bone healing evident, the patient's tolerance of pain, and the condition of the surrounding soft tissue and adjacent joints. The most prudent decisions related to exercise prescription for these patients is guided by the radiological evidence and a thorough assessment and monitoring of the patient's clinical signs and symptoms. Clinicians must proceed cautiously, applying gentle stress to the area to encourage healing but never exceeding what the tissue can sustain.

In the elderly these fractures usually occur through osteopenic bone. They may be caused by minimal trauma, such as a fall onto the outstretched hand from a standing height or lower, and occasionally they occur in association

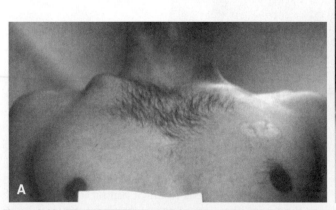
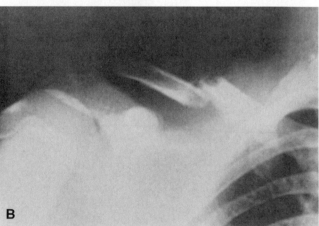

Figure 4-19

A, Fractured clavicle tenting the skin. **B,** Anteroposterior view of a fracture of the right clavicle showing the typical deformity with a proximal fragment displaced superiorly. (**A** from Rockwood CA, Matsen FA, editors: *The shoulder*, p 462, Philadelphia, 2004, WB Saunders; **B** from Rockwood CA, Matsen FA, editors: *The shoulder*, p 444, Philadelphia, 1998, WB Saunders.)

Shoulder Trauma and Hypomobility • CHAPTER 4   111

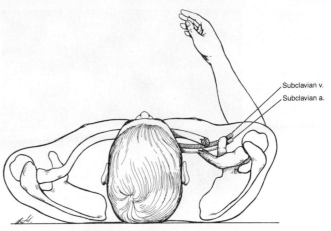

Figure 4-22
Potential injury to the subclavian vessels resulting from a fractured clavicle. (From Rockwood CA, Matsen FA, editors: *The shoulder*, p 444, Philadelphia, 1998, WB Saunders.)

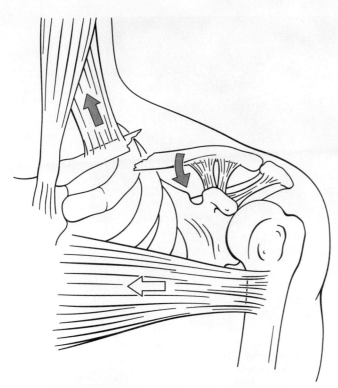

Figure 4-20
Clavicular fracture. With displacement, the proximal fragment is pulled superiorly and the distal segment drops forward.

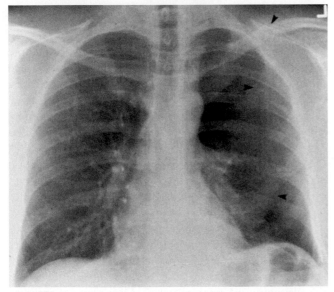

Figure 4-21
Fracture of the left clavicle associated with a left pneumothorax. (From Rockwood CA, Matsen FA, editors: *The shoulder*, p 443, Philadelphia, 1998, WB Saunders.)

with a dislocation. Another possible mechanism of injury, first described by Codman,[46] is excessive rotation of the arm, especially while in the abducted position. In this case the humerus locks against the acromion in a pivotal position, and a fracture can occur, especially in an older patient with osteoporotic bone. Proximal humeral

fractures may also result when a direct blow to the lateral aspect of the shoulder causes a greater tuberosity fracture (Figure 4-23).

Most proximal humeral fractures are nondisplaced or minimally displaced; these should be differentiated from the more serious displaced fractures, which are managed quite differently. The most commonly used classification system is the four-part fracture classification developed by Neer in 1970, in which he initially divided fractures into displaced and nondisplaced (Figure 4-24).[83,84] Displaced fractures, according to this classification, have more than 1 cm of displacement or more than 45° of angulation. Nondisplaced fractures may be called *one-part fractures*, regardless of how many fracture lines are seen. A *two-part fracture* involves displacement of the anatomical neck, surgical neck, lesser tuberosity, or greater tuberosity in relation to the remaining intact proximal humerus. Similarly, *three-* and *four-part fractures* involve displacement of two or three fragments in relation to the main humeral fragment.

According to Neer's classification, the most commonly reported fracture of the proximal humerus is a displaced or nondisplaced (one-part or two-part) fracture involving the surgical neck (Figure 4-25). More recently, researchers have been investigating the clinical impact of greater tuberosity displacements of less than 1 cm. Most authors agree that the shoulder has very little tolerance for greater tuberosity displacement, and some suggest that displacements of 5 mm to 1 cm can result in substantial dysfunction either from impingement or rotator cuff tearing.[83-85] These findings may explain the variability seen among patients with these types of fractures, and why some patients have more difficulty progressing through rehabilitation than others.

Clinical Presentation

Because most proximal humeral fractures present acutely, common symptoms are pain, swelling, and tenderness

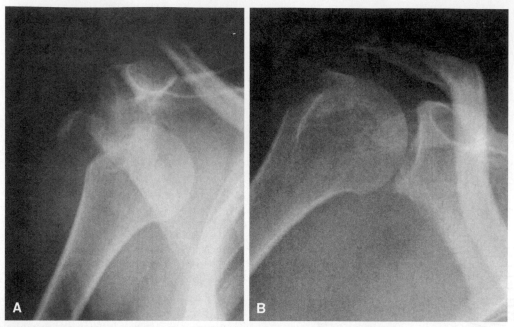

Figure 4-23

A, Anteroposterior x-ray film of a two-part anterior fracture-dislocation with a displaced greater tuberosity fracture. **B,** After a closed reduction, the greater tuberosity fracture reduced and healed without further displacement. (From Rockwood CA, Green DP, Bucholz RW, Heckman JD: *Fractures in adults,* ed 4, p 1069, Philadelphia, 1996, Lippincott-Raven.)

about the shoulder, particularly in the region of the greater tuberosity. Crepitus may be evident with movement of the shoulder, but in most cases the patient is reluctant to initiate any active movement and holds the arm closely against the chest wall. The definitive diagnosis is made through radiographic evaluation.

A thorough assessment should be performed, including evaluation of the integrity of the bony tissue and careful examination of the neurovascular and musculotendinous structures intimately situated in this region, which thus are susceptible to injury. Of particular concern is the rotator cuff, which attaches to the different tuberosities of the humerus and consequently may have a deforming effect, depending on where the fracture occurs. For example, with a fracture of the greater tuberosity, the fragment is pulled superiorly and posteriorly because of the supraspinatus, infraspinatus, and teres minor muscles. Conversely, in a fracture of the lesser tuberosity, the fragment is pulled anteriorly and medially by the subscapularis muscle (Figure 4-26).[45,85]

The deltoid and pectoralis major muscles should also be evaluated in patients with a proximal humeral fracture. Because the deltoid muscle attaches to the lateral shaft of the humerus, it can cause displacement of fractures of the proximal humeral shaft. The pectoralis major muscle, because of its insertion onto the lower portion of the bicipital groove, can displace the proximal shaft of the humerus medially, as is typically seen in surgical neck fractures.

Treatment of Proximal Humeral Fractures

Most proximal humeral fractures are minimally displaced and are successfully treated without surgery. If the fracture is classified as nondisplaced and is impacted or stable, an initial period of immobilization is indicated, using either a conventional sling or a collar and cuff sling that allows the weight of the arm to apply slight traction to the fracture; early range of motion exercises follow, at around 2 weeks after injury. If the fracture is classified as nondisplaced but is considered unstable, the immobilization period is more strictly adhered to with range of motion exercises not being performed until about 4 weeks after injury when clinical union has occurred.

Diminished pain and an easing of the patient's apprehension are reasonable indicators for beginning gentle exercises (e.g., pendular range of motion, active-assisted exercises, and isometric strength exercises of the scapular muscles and the glenohumeral joint muscles). Obtaining intermittent x-ray films before rehabilitation begins is important to establish that the fracture is clinically stable and the bone moves as a unit. Bertoft et al.[86] reported that the greatest amount of improvement in range of motion occurs between 3 and 8 weeks after injury. Therefore it is very important that the clinician ensure proper patient education and monitor any comprehensive exercise program.

The primary concern with patients who have sustained a proximal humeral fracture is shoulder stiffness; however, the clinician must also be very diligent in evaluating for and

Displaced Fractures

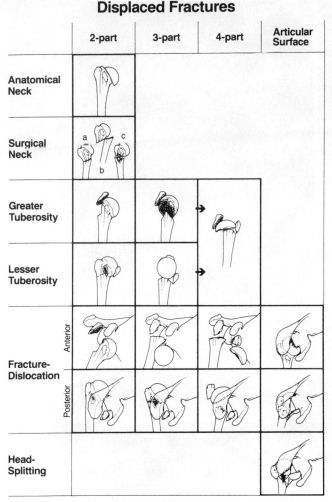

Figure 4-24

Neer's classification. (From Rockwood CA, Matsen FA, editors: *The shoulder*, p 342, Philadelphia, 1998, WB Saunders.)

treating any associated injuries to the glenohumeral joint and the other joints of the shoulder girdle. A thorough examination of the muscles about the region also is important, because they may have been injured, along with the humerus, in the original trauma, or at the very least, they may have been strained or traumatized as a result of the fracture.

Poor results after nonsurgical treatment most commonly are related to shoulder stiffness and limited motion or to the consequences of displacement of the greater tuberosity. Capsular contracture can also be an adverse effect of proximal humeral fractures, further complicating the situation. These problems are best prevented by initiation of passive motion and active-assisted and active range of motion exercises early in the rehabilitation process.

Surgical indications for a fracture of the proximal humerus are not clear-cut. Surgery is reserved primarily for fractures that are significantly displaced; it involves mainly closed reduction with or without percutaneous pinning, or open reduction and internal fixation.[87] Treatment of proximal humeral fractures with surgery is considered

difficult, not only because of the complex anatomy of the shoulder girdle, but also because of the difficulty achieving and maintaining anatomical reduction and stable fixation. Rehabilitation after this type of operation is rigorous and involved, and practitioners should make sure before surgery that the patient is well educated about the condition and suited to handle the important postoperative period. In some cases, because of the co-morbid status and the patient's age, nonsurgical treatment is the most appropriate choice despite substantial fracture displacement.

Rotator Cuff Injuries

The rotator cuff is one of the most commonly injured structures of the shoulder. This is partly because of its anatomical location within the glenohumeral joint, but also because of the extensive activity that occurs in the cuff with virtually every function the arm performs. These factors, coupled with the increasing problems patients develop as a result of poor postural patterns, make the rotator cuff one of the most susceptible tissues in the body to overload and injury.

Considerable research has been done over the past several years on the rotator cuff's morphology, function, and response to aging and injury.[88-92] Practitioners' understanding of how the rotator cuff functions—that is, not as four individual muscles but as a unit—has forced them to examine how best to retrain and strengthen these muscles. The principles of rehabilitation, such as co-contraction, scapular stabilization, and functional exercise prescription, all have contributed to the crafting of treatment strategies that hopefully are more appropriate and effective for the injured rotator cuff.

Anatomy

The four muscles that constitute the rotator cuff (the supraspinatus, the infraspinatus, the teres minor, and the subscapular muscle) arise from the scapula and converge with the capsule of the glenohumeral joint to attach on the tuberosities of the humerus.

The supraspinatus muscle arises from the supraspinatus fossa on the upper one third of the posterior scapula, passes beneath the acromion and the acromioclavicular joint, and attaches to the superior aspect of the greater tuberosity. The infraspinatus muscle arises from the infraspinatus fossa on the lower two thirds of the posterior scapula and attaches to the posterolateral aspect of the greater tuberosity. The teres minor muscle arises from the lower lateral aspect of the scapula and attaches to the lower aspect of the greater tuberosity. The subscapular muscle arises from the anterior aspect of the scapula and attaches over much of the lesser tuberosity.

The four tendons insert as a continuous cuff around the humeral head and permit the cuff muscles to provide an

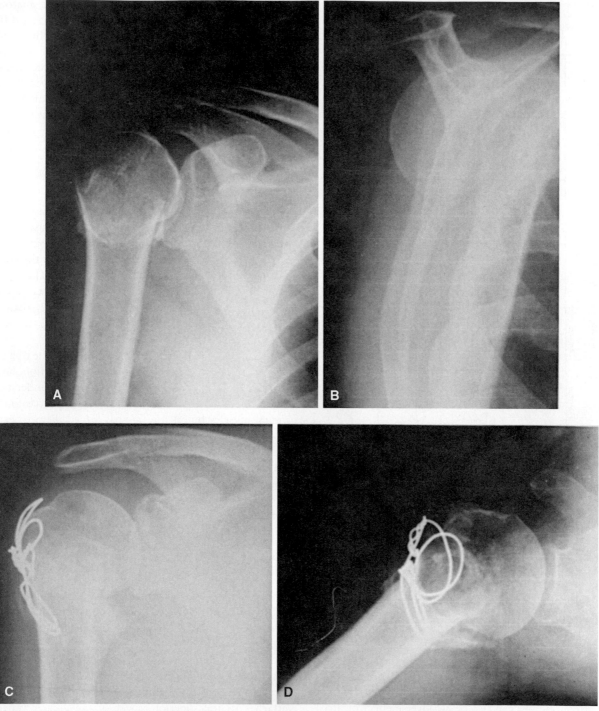

Figure 4-25

Displaced fracture of the surgical neck. **A** and **B,** Anteroposterior and lateral x-ray films of a displaced surgical neck fracture. The fracture was treated for 3 weeks as an undisplaced fracture on the basis of an anteroposterior x-ray film only (**A**). The follow-up lateral x-ray film (**B**) in the scapular plane revealed a significant anterior shaft displacement. **C** and **D,** Anteroposterior and lateral x-ray films after open reduction and internal fixation with two figure-of-eight wires. (From Rockwood CA, Matsen FA, editors: *The shoulder,* p 353, Philadelphia, 1998, WB Saunders.)

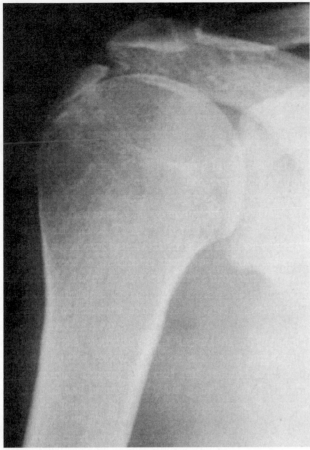

Figure 4-26
Greater tuberosity malunion resulting from unopposed pull of the supraspinatus and infraspinatus muscles. (From Rockwood CA, Matsen FA, editors: *The shoulder,* p 350, Philadelphia, 1998, WB Saunders.)

infinite variety of moments to rotate the humerus and to oppose unwanted components of the deltoid and pectoralis muscle forces. The long head of the biceps tendon may be considered a functional part of the rotator cuff because it attaches to the supraglenoid tubercle of the scapula, travels between the subscapularis and supraspinatus, and exits the shoulder through the bicipital groove under the transverse humeral ligament, attaching to its muscle in the proximal arm. Tension in the long head of the biceps tendon assists in the compression of the humeral head into the glenoid and guides the head of the humerus as it is elevated.[93-95]

Function

Compared to a joint, such as the knee, that has a single axis upon which torques are generated, the shoulder is very different, because it has no fixed axis. In a specific joint position, activation of a muscle creates a unique set of rotational moments, and the timing and magnitude of balancing the muscle effects must be precisely coordinated to prevent humeral motion in unwanted directions. This degree of coordination requires a programmed strategy of

muscle activation that must be established before a motion is carried out. The rotator cuff muscles function to help ensure this shoulder muscle balance.

Functions of the Rotator Cuff

- Rotation of the humerus relative to the scapula
- Compression of the humeral head into the glenoid fossa, providing a critical stabilizing mechanism known as *concavity compression*
- Acts with the deltoid muscle and the long head of the biceps to maintain stability of the glenohumeral joint

The term *rotator cuff* may be a misnomer, because joint compression (concavity compression) may be its most important function, not rotation. In the past the rotator cuff has been referred to as a humeral head depressor; however, more recent evidence shows that the inferiorly directed component of the cuff muscle force actually is small; instead, the primary stabilizing function of the cuff muscles is through head compression into the glenoid (Figure 4-27).[85,91] The cuff functions by compressing the joint to improve stability, resisting sliding or translation (in an anteroposterior and inferosuperior direction), and providing some rotation about any or all of the three major axes (anteroposterior, mediolateral, and the humeral

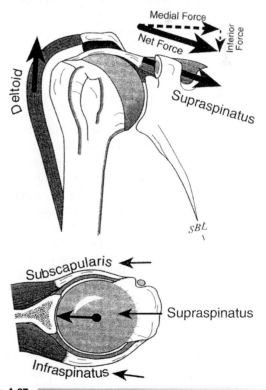

Figure 4-27
Concavity compression of the rotator cuff. (From Rockwood CA, Matsen FA, editors: *The shoulder,* p 778, Philadelphia, 1998, WB Saunders.)

shaft).[90,91] Joint stability is achieved almost entirely by the rotator cuff in the shoulder's midrange positions, because all the passive restraints are lax in these positions. The humeral head maintains a relatively constant position in relation to the glenoid during shoulder rotation. The rotator cuff muscles are closer than any other muscles to the axes of rotation and therefore have shorter lever arms to affect rotation. Recent work has demonstrated that this compressive effect functions relatively independently of shoulder position.[85,91,92] In a normally functioning shoulder, fatigue of the rotator cuff muscles has been shown to cause an increase in the translation of the humeral head anterosuperiorly, a position associated with the development of impingement.[88,96]

Although the muscles of the rotator cuff function primarily as a unit, research has shown that some variability in function occurs among the individual muscles in different arm positions. The infraspinatus is a very effective head depressor with the arm at 90° of abduction and neutral rotation. The subscapularis, however, is a more effective head depressor in lateral rotation and produces almost no anteroposterior translation in abduction and lateral rotation. This may help explain why the subscapularis has been shown to contract very strongly in athletes at the initiation of the acceleration phase of overhead throwing. Several powerful muscles contribute to medial rotation, but tears of the subscapularis may be shown by testing function at the extreme of medial rotation, which indicates the importance of this muscle at this end range of motion. Patients with subscapularis tears may feel the loss of joint compression and stabilization provided by that part of the rotator cuff. The infraspinatus and teres minor are the only two muscles that produce lateral rotation, and large tears in this region of the cuff have profound effects on a patient's motion and strength.

The rotator cuff functions optimally if (1) all the muscles are healthy, intact, and well conditioned; (2) a normal amount of capsular laxity is present at the glenohumeral joint; (3) the undersurface of the coracoacromial arch has a smooth contour; (4) a thin, lubricating bursa is present; and (5) there is concentricity of the glenohumeral joint and cuff/coracoacromial spheres of rotation.

The dynamic interplay of the rotator cuff and the deltoid muscle has been well established and is essential for proper glenohumeral function.[7,21,22,90,92] With the arm in adduction at the initiation of elevation, the pull of the deltoid muscle is nearly parallel to the glenoid surface, producing a well-documented upward shear component. The stability of the humeral head in the glenoid created by the cuff opposes this upward pull of the deltoid and allows the deltoid muscle to function optimally. The long head of the biceps tendon is another very important component of the rotator cuff/deltoid complex (this is explained in detail later in the chapter). It is important to remember that all these muscles work as force-couple units, rather than individually, to maintain glenohumeral stability, and the clinician must give thought to all of them when assessing and rehabilitating an injured shoulder.

Mechanism of Injury/Pathology

Injury to the rotator cuff can occur as a result of many different mechanisms and can lead to a spectrum of injuries ranging from minor paratenonitis and strains to partial and full thickness tears. To understand the many types of rotator cuff conditions, the clinician must have a thorough knowledge of the anatomy and function of this unique muscle group and must appreciate the inherent demands and the stresses, both normal and abnormal, placed on it.

Rotator Cuff Tears

In normal activities, the force transmitted through the rotator cuff tendon is in the range of 140-200 newtons (N).[10,88,97] The ultimate tensile load of the supraspinatus tendon in the sixth or seventh decade of life has been measured as 600-800 N. Research has shown that the primary cause of degeneration of the rotator cuff tendon is aging, which occurs at a much faster rate in this tissue than in other regions of the body. The tendon fibers become weaker with disuse and age, and as they become weaker, less force is required to disrupt them.[98-100] (For more information on tendon injury and repair, see volume 2 of this series, *Scientific Foundations and Principles of Practice in Musculoskeletal Rehabilitation,* Chapter 3.)

Rotator cuff tears are among the most common conditions affecting the shoulder. They may be classified as partial thickness tears, full thickness tears, acute, chronic, traumatic, and/or degenerative, and they can range from mild microtearing (typically referred to as a *strain*) to total absence of the cuff tendons. In a young, active patient, partial thickness tears may include an avulsion of a small chip of bone from the greater tuberosity. In degenerative cuff failure, the process typically starts with a partial thickness defect on the deep (under) surface near the attachment of the supraspinatus to the greater tuberosity. A common misdiagnosis of shoulder pain (e.g., tendonitis, bursitis, impingement syndrome) may actually represent failure of the deep surface fibers of the rotator cuff. The degree to which the intact fibers may hypertrophy, strengthen, or adapt to stabilize the tear and take up the function of the damaged fibers is unknown. Pettersson[101] used the term *creeping tendon ruptures* to describe a condition in which major cuff defects may occur without symptoms or a recognized injury. He suggested that previous minor, often subclinical fiber failure could leave the shoulder weaker and the cuff tendons progressively less able to withstand the loads encountered in daily living.

Incidence of Rotator Cuff Tears

The incidence of rotator cuff tears, measured from cadaver dissections, ranges from 5% to 26.5%.[102-106] One group of authors, recognizing the importance of age in the prevalence of cuff lesions, noted that in cadavers younger than 60 years of age, the incidence of rotator cuff tears was 6%, and in those older than 60 years it was 30%.[107] Partial thickness tears appear approximately twice as often as full thickness defects and can occur on the bursal side, on the joint side, and in the intratendinous region of the rotator cuff. Bursal side tears are reported to produce the most severe symptoms.[108-110] This is due partly to the large number of pain receptors in bursal tissue and partly to the location of the tear (i.e., within the subacromial space).

Some of the most significant research on rotator cuff lesions has been generated from asymptomatic patients. Authors have discovered that approximately 50% of asymptomatic, untraumatized shoulders in patients in their sixth, seventh, or eighth decade of life had arthrographically proven partial or full thickness rotator cuff defects.[101,111-114] As a result of studies such as these, researchers have concluded that rotator cuff lesions are a natural correlate of aging and often are present without any clinical symptoms. It also is worth noting that the increased use of diagnostic imaging, such as magnetic resonance imaging (MRI), over the past decade has identified a seemingly "normal" indicator of aging tissue. Very significant to these findings is the fact that these rotator cuff defects were found to be compatible with normal, painless, functional activity. Yamanaka and Matsumato[115] used arthrography to study the progression of 40 untreated partial rotator cuff tears in asymptomatic patients with a mean age of 61. Over a period of approximately 1 year, their results revealed overall improved subjective shoulder scores. However, the arthrography results revealed a slightly different outcome. Four patients had resolution of the tear, four patients had a reduction of the tear, 21 patients had an enlargement of the tear, and 11 patients progressed to a full thickness tear after the year. The authors concluded that partial thickness tears are likely to progress with advancing age, often in the absence of a history or trauma.

Overall, rotator cuff defects become increasingly common after the age of 40, and many occur without substantial clinical manifestations. Often the determining factors for partial cuff tears that become problematic are the patient's occupation and lifestyle.

Clinical Presentation of Rotator Cuff Tears

The clinical presentation of partial rotator cuff tears can vary and can include shoulder stiffness, weakness, pain, instability and a sense of roughness or grinding. Shoulder stiffness may present as limited passive and active range of motion with pain present at the end point of the motion. This is most commonly seen in partial thickness tears because more of the sensory components are left intact, but it may also be associated with full thickness tears. Another very common complaint, which stems in part from the reduced range of motion, is discomfort at night and difficulty lying on the shoulder on the affected side.

Weakness and pain are primary causes of shoulder functional limitation with rotator cuff defects. The degenerative tendon fibers may be weakened and fail without a specific clinical manifestation. Patients with partial thickness lesions have substantially more pain on resisted muscle action than those with full thickness tears, again because of the often intact nervous tissue, and bursal side tears seem to be more symptomatic than deeper tears because of the resultant problems with roughness of the articulation between the upper surface of the cuff and the undersurface of the coracoacromial arch.[100,109] Some authors and clinicians believe that a subacromial injection of local anesthetic can be used to differentiate weakness caused by painful inhibition from weakness caused by a tendon defect.[116]

Rotator cuff tears may cause shoulder instability as a result of a loss of efficient centering of the humeral head in the glenoid (see Chapter 5). Acute tears of the subscapularis, although not common, may contribute to recurrent anterior instability. Chronic loss of the normal compressive effect of the cuff mechanism and of the stabilizing effect of the superior cuff tendon interposed between the humeral head and the coracoacromial arch may contribute to superior glenohumeral instability.

Patients with cuff tears frequently complain of a symptomatic crepitus during passive glenohumeral range of motion. This roughness often is caused by bursal hypertrophy, secondary changes in the undersurface of the coracoacromial arch, loss of integrity of the upper aspect of the cuff tendons, or degenerative changes in the tuberosities of the humerus.[88,98,100,117] These factors culminate in a condition known as *subacromial abrasion*. Neer et al.[118] used the term *rotator cuff tear arthropathy* to describe a similar phenomenom, which they believed was a cause of this roughness associated with rotator cuff defects.

Treatment of Rotator Cuff Tears

The management of rotator cuff tears is the subject of substantial debate among clinicians and researchers. In a number of studies, the clinical results of cuff repairs in symptomatic patients, who were followed for as long as 10 years, were good to excellent in a high percentage of cases, even though rerupture of the cuff is known to occur in 20% to 65% of cases.[115,119-121] Interestingly, a massive, irreparable rotator cuff tear is not incompatible with good overhead function. Observations such as these have made clinical decision making in the treatment of symptomatic rotator cuff tears challenging. Historically, treatments have consisted of rehabilitation, surgical repair, subacromial decompression without repair, tendon transfers, and tendon substitution techniques. The most commonly reported prognosticative factors for cuff repairs are the patient's age, the chronicity of the tear, and the size of the tear.[88,98,109,120] Rerupture of a tear is clearly a major concern in these patient populations and has been correlated with tear size, tear chronicity, and patient satisfaction.

Some current controversies in the management of rotator cuff tears include the role of rehabilitation, the indications for and timing of surgical repair, the method of surgical repair (arthroscopic, open, or miniopen techniques), and the management of irreparable defects. Important factors that must be considered in the decision between surgical and conservative management of a patient with a symptomatic, full thickness rotator cuff tear are the patient's age and expected activity level and whether muscle/tissue retraction and rotator cuff muscle atrophy and fatty replacement are present.[10,88,121] Surgery is almost always suggested for patients in the fourth or fifth decade of life who have suffered a traumatic injury that resulted in a rotator cuff tear. Patients in the sixth, seventh, or eighth decade of life may or may not be well suited for surgical repair, depending on the chronicity of the tear and the quality of the remaining tendon and muscle tissue, as well as other health issues. If the tissue is less than optimal, failure to heal is a significant possibility. Most patients in the older age groups are more interested in eliminating shoulder pain and achieving a functional range of motion, than in having powerful overhead use of the arm. However, the average age of the general population is increasing, and a significant percentage of these individuals remain much more active; therefore the clinician is likely to be faced with very challenging questions about the best way to manage cuff tears and at the same time maximize a patient's functional goals and requirements.

Partial Thickness Tears. As previously noted, partial thickness cuff tears present with pain and/or weakness on resisted isometric contraction of the involved musculature. Frequently, more pain is seen with partial tears because the defects give rise to stiffness and increased tension on the remaining fibers. Stiffness of the glenohumeral joint motions during passive range of motion in the direction that stretches the tendon produces tendon signs, and an associated posterior capsule tightness commonly is seen.

The goal of nonsurgical treatment of partial thickness tears is to ensure that the scar collagen that forms in the defect becomes as supple as a normal tendon. If this does not happen, scar contracture tends to concentrate the load of the rotator cuff on the scar, leading to recurrence and further propagation of the injury. The emphasis of treatment is on patient education, including how to avoid repeated injury; restoration of normal flexibility, especially of the posterior capsule; restoration of normal strength; adding or encouraging a component of aerobic exercise to the overall treatment; and patient education on modifying work and recreational activities that may interfere with achievement of the optimum outcome. Range of motion goals are met through a combination of gentle stretching and mobilization techniques to ensure normal glenohumeral joint motion and proper capsular extensibility, especially in the posterior capsule region.

A sensible retraining and restrengthening program directed at the rotator cuff musculature is indicated, but care must be taken to avoid overloading the deficient tissue too quickly. This poses three main requirements:

1. First and foremost, clinicians should adjust the *amount of resistance* placed on the cuff, the *repetitiveness of the load* applied, and the *specific glenohumeral joint range of motion* in which the exercises are performed to ensure that the patient is targeting the rotator cuff muscles but not to a degree that exacerbates symptoms or causes more cuff damage. The patient's signs and symptoms, as well as the individual's ability to perform the given exercise properly, are always the best guide for progressing to more challenging levels.

2. The patient should not have any pain after completing the exercises.

3. The stabilizing muscles of the scapula should be included in a strengthening program for the rotator cuff, because their role as supporting muscles and their ability to provide a dynamic stable scapula for efficient functioning of the rotator cuff have been well documented.[11,12] The effects of the trauma to the rotator cuff often have far-reaching associated adverse effects in these scapular muscles, not only as a result of painful inhibition, but also because altered use may lead to improper patterning of scapulohumeral rhythm and resultant alterations in proper muscle recruitment.

A patient who has undergone surgery for a partial rotator cuff tear is managed initially with a period of sling and swath immobilization, followed by a progressive regimen of passive, active-assisted, and active range of motion exercises. The length of time patients are immobilized varies somewhat, but for most, it is 3 to 6 weeks. Although the primary goal after surgery is to encourage optimum healing of the repaired rotator cuff, clinicians must be mindful of the equally important goal of restoring full shoulder girdle mobility to prevent stiffness and adhesions.[10,119,120] Frequently a lack of full shoulder mobility is the cause of patient dissatisfaction after surgery. Neer emphasized that patients with partial tears seemed more susceptible to increased shoulder stiffness and that surgery was inadvisable until stiffness had resolved.[104,118]

Full Thickness Tears. Full thickness tears present with weakness and sometimes pain on resisted isometric testing of the affected rotator cuff muscle or muscles. The appropriate treatment is difficult to determine in some cases, as has been previously noted, and some defects cannot be repaired with surgery. Also, it is important to remember that some full thickness cuff tears may actually exist without clinical symptoms, therefore cuff defects need not be repaired simply because they are there. The goals of rehabilitation for a patient with a symptomatic, full thickness cuff tear are a combination of education about activity modification, pain management, and range of motion and strengthening exercises that focus on the remaining muscles of the cuff and the supporting musculature.

Rotator Cuff Disease

The term *rotator cuff disease* refers to a collection of signs and symptoms (and altered anatomy) that arises from more than one cause. It relates not only to the coracoacromial arch

Figure 4-28

Rotator cuff degeneration. **A,** Normal relationships of the cuff and the coracoacromial arch. **B,** Upward displacement of the head, which squeezes the cuff against the acromion and the coracoacromial ligament. **C,** Greater contact and abrasion give rise to a traction spur in the coracoacromial ligament. **D,** Still greater upward displacement, resulting in abrasion of the humeral articular cartilage and cuff tear arthropathy. (From Rockwood CA, Matsen FA, editors: *The shoulder,* p 767, Philadelphia, 1998, WB Saunders.)

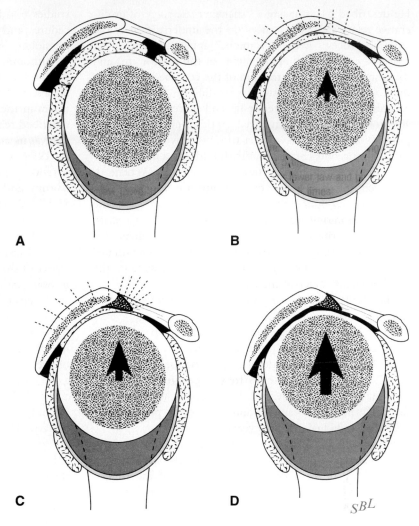

region, but also to other structures and causal factors, such as dislocations and altered biomechanics.[92] It is important to note that subacromial impingement is *not* the sole cause of rotator cuff disease; in fact, it is more accurately described as the phenomenon that occurs as a result of the more probable causes of aging and physical loading of the shoulder and arm (Figure 4-28). The process of aging causes degeneration in the cuff, particularly at its insertion points, which leads to fiber thickening and the formation of granulation tissue. The damaged cuff then malfunctions, leading to further disorders in the subacromial area. Excessive loading of the rotator cuff may occur either through a static or "structural" (e.g., hooked acromion) mechanism, or dynamically as a result of the humeral head and cuff moving against an unyielding structure. Current evidence indicates that both static and dynamic factors act upon the rotator cuff, leading to eventual rotator cuff disease.[110,122]

Other Rotator Cuff Disorders

In addition to partial and full thickness tears, the rotator cuff may incur injuries that result in tendonitis and muscle strain. The clinical presentation of these types of injuries varies, depending on (1) which of the four cuff muscles is involved; (2) where along the muscle and/or tendon the insult has occurred (muscle belly, musculotendinous junction, or tenoperiosteal attachment); (3) the etiology of the injury (trauma, overuse, or secondary to a primary injury); and (4) the severity of the pathology (first, second, or third degree). Treatment of rotator cuff pathologies should be based on information pertinent to these four points, as well as a thorough subjective and objective assessment of the entire shoulder girdle.

Impingement Syndromes

A major clinical advance with regard to shoulder problems is the realization that most conditions involve a spectrum of both injury and pathology. Impingement syndromes are a good example of this, because the diagnosis is derived from a collection of symptoms, signs, and pathologies that may arise from a variety of causes. The term *impingement syndromes* was popularized by Neer in 1972 as a result of an evaluation he performed on 100 dissected scapulas.[123]

He described 11 as having a "characteristic ridge of proliferative spurs and excrescences on the undersurface of the anterior process of the acromion," apparently caused by repeated contact, or impingement, of the rotator cuff and the humeral head, with traction of the coracoacromial ligament. Of special interest was his finding that, without exception, it was the anterior lip and undersurface of the anterior third that were involved. In this region, the supraspinatus inserts onto the greater tuberosity, lying anterior to the coracoacromial arch with the shoulder in a neutral position. With forward flexion the structures must pass beneath the arch, providing the opportunity for impingement. This early description of shoulder impingement syndrome is now commonly referred to as *primary impingement,* because the primary cause of the resultant impingement is the actual abutting of soft tissue structures (e.g., the rotator cuff and glenoid labrum) and bony prominences (e.g., the acromion and coracoid process).

Neer's classification of primary impingement syndrome described three stages:[123]

Stage I: Reversible edema and hemorrhage are present; this stage typically is seen in patients under 25 years of age.

Stage II: Fibrosis and tendonitis affect the rotator cuff, typically in patients in the 25 to 40 age group, and pain often recurs after activity.

Stage III: Bone spurs and tendon ruptures are present, usually in individuals over 40 years of age.

Static factors believed to cause impingement include abnormalities of the coracoacromial arch that may lead to areas of higher than normal compression of the rotator cuff. With dynamic causes, the coracoacromial arch and other subacromial structures initially may be normal; however, abnormal motion of the humeral head and the cuff relative to the scapula is the primary cause of the impingement, leading to sometimes permanent structural changes.[124,125] Two types of abnormal anterior rotator cuff contact occur: external impingement, which exists when the bursal side of the cuff is in contact with the coracoacromial arch, and internal impingement, which occurs when the inner fibers of the cuff contact the upper labrum and its adjacent structures. (More information on impingement syndromes can be found in Chapter 5.)

Biceps Tendon Lesions

Although researchers and clinicians agree that the biceps tendon is a tissue susceptible to trauma and injury, some debate still exists about the etiology of biceps injuries, namely, whether they have a primary cause directly associated with the biceps tendon complex, or whether they are secondary phenomena that occur as a result of dysfunction elsewhere in the shoulder. According to some authors,[129] 95% to 98% of patients with a diagnosis of biceps tendonitis actually have a primary diagnosis of impingement syndrome or scapular instability that is causing secondary involvement of the biceps tendon. More recently, researchers have produced

studies based on the results of MRI and arthroscopic procedures, and these studies have shed new light on the pathophysiology of the long head of the biceps tendon.[129-131]

Although the pendulum has swung away from primary tendonitis and isolated tendon instability diagnoses of the biceps, several authors have published results on these topics in the past two decades. In 1985 Andrews et al.[130] described tears in the superior labrum of the glenohumeral joint at its attachment to the biceps tendon (Figure 4-29). In 1990 Snyder et al.[131] first described the superolabral anterior to posterior (SLAP) lesion, a lesion of the superior labrum and adjoining biceps anchor. They categorized SLAP lesions into four types. Type I lesions show degenerative fraying with no detachment of the biceps insertion; type II lesions show detachment of the biceps insertion; type III lesions show a bucket handle tear of the superior aspect of the labrum with an intact biceps tendon insertion to bone; and type IV lesions show an intrasubstance tear of the biceps tendon with a bucket handle tear of the superior aspect of the labrum.

Morgan et al.[132] further divided type II SLAP lesions into three subtypes, depending on whether the detachment of the labrum involved the anterior aspect of the labrum alone, the posterior aspect, or both.

In their three-part series, "The Disabled Throwing Shoulder," Burkhart et al.[5,11,133] state that they believe the type II SLAP lesion is the most common pathological entity associated with a "dead arm" syndrome, which they define as any pathological shoulder condition in which a thrower is unable to throw because of a combination of pain and subjective unease in the shoulder. In an arthroscopic study done earlier, these same authors observed what they called a dynamic "peel-back phenomenon" in throwers with posterior and combined anteroposterior SLAP lesions. They found that, with the arm in the cocked position of abduction and lateral rotation, the peel-back occurred as a result of the effect of the biceps tendon as its vector shifted to a more posterior position in late cocking. The change in angle and the twist of the biceps tendon produced a torsional force to the posterosuperior labrum, causing detachment if the superior labrum was not well-anchored to the glenoid. These findings suggested a mechanism of injury for SLAP lesions in throwers that was different from the mechanism postulated earlier by Andrews et al.[130] Those researchers had described a *deceleration* mechanism of labral injuries in throwers, which occurred as the biceps contracted to slow the rapidly extending elbow in the follow-through phase. They believed that this created a high tensile load in the biceps that acted to pull the biceps and superior labrum complex from the bone. Burkhart et al.[5,11,133] essentially described the opposite, an *acceleration* mechanism of injury; specifically, in late cocking, as the arm began to accelerate forward from an abducted and laterally rotated position, the long head of the biceps and the superior labrum were peeled back, rather than pulled, from the bone.

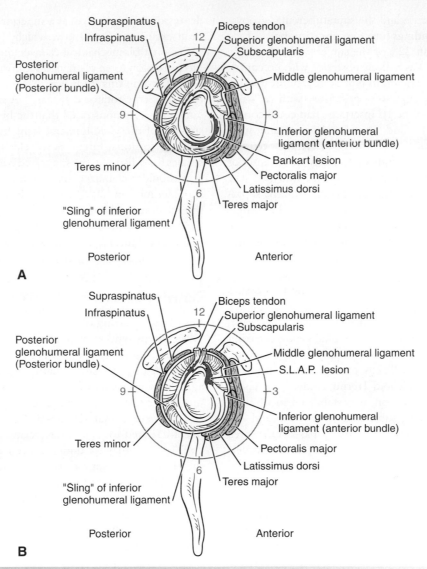

Figure 4-29
Labral lesions of the right shoulder. **A,** Bankart lesion. **B,** SLAP lesion. (From Magee DJ: *Orthopedic physical assessment,* ed 4, p 266, Philadelphia, 2002, WB Saunders.)

Also of interest in the studies investigating type II SLAP lesions are the associated factors in the primary pathology. Burkhart et al.[5,11,133] summarized their findings by stating that the "ultimate culprits" in dead arm syndrome are (1) a tight posteroinferior capsule, which causes a glenohumeral internal rotation deficit (GIRD) and a shift in the glenohumeral rotation point; (2) the peel-back mechanism produced by the biceps tendon, which leads to a SLAP lesion; (3) hyperexternal rotation of the humerus; and (4) scapular protraction. Of the throwers with SLAP lesions whom they examined, 31% were also found to have rotator cuff tears (38% were full thickness tears, and 62% were partial thickness tears).

As can be seen, the biceps tendon plays an important role in the overall anatomy and function of the shoulder joint. However, probably most important for clinicians to appreciate is the incredible relationship the biceps has with the other tissues about the shoulder, namely the glenoid, glenoid labrum, and rotator cuff. Injury to any one of these structures undoubtedly affects the integrity of the biceps tendon and the well-being of the entire shoulder girdle.

Relevant Anatomy

The long head of the biceps tendon originates from the superior glenoid labrum and the supraglenoid tubercle and travels obliquely within the shoulder joint, turning sharply inferiorly to exit the joint underneath the transverse humeral ligament within the bicipital groove. Researchers have noted that the origin of the biceps tendon varies, not only in the type of insertion (single, bifurcated, or trifurcated), but also in the specific anatomical location where it inserts.[129,134-136] Vangsness et al.[134] dissected 105 cadaveric shoulders to study the biceps tendon origin and its relationship to the labrum and the supratubercular groove. They classified their findings into four insertion types. Type I insertions occurred in 22% of the subjects and showed a labral attachment that was entirely posterior with no contribution to the anterior labrum. In type II insertions, the labral contribution was primarily posterior with a small anterior band present. Type III insertions had equal contributions to the anterior and posterior labrum and were found in 37% of the cadavers. Type IV insertions occurred in 8% of the cadavers and consisted mainly of an anterior labral attachment. In another cadaveric study,[129] the researchers noted that the biceps originated from the supraglenoid tubercle 20% to 30% of the time; from the posterosuperior portion of the glenoid labrum 48% to 70% of the time; and from both the supraglenoid tubercle and the glenoid labrum 25% to 28% of the time. This study supports the intimate relationship between the biceps tendon and the labrum and may help explain why the two tissues are commonly injured together.

The biceps tendon is surrounded by a synovial sheath, which ends at the distal end of the bicipital groove, making the tendon an intra-articular but extrasynovial structure. As the long head of the biceps tendon moves from its origin on the superior glenoid labrum and supraglenoid tubercle to its muscle insertion, it is stabilized in position by the supraspinatus and subscapularis tendons and the capsuloligamentous tissues. The triangular-shaped area between the supraspinatus and the subscapularis tendons is referred to as the *rotator interval*. It contains the coracohumeral and the superior glenohumeral ligaments and has on its medial side the coracoid process. Histoanatomical studies have found that both the superior glenohumeral ligament and the coracohumeral ligament are important structures in the stabilization of the biceps tendon in its groove, and lesions associated with any of the components of the rotator interval leave the biceps tendon and the rotator cuff vulnerable to injury.[20,95,136]

Function of the Biceps

Basmajian and Latif[137] characterized the action of the biceps brachii muscle as flexion of the elbow joint when the forearm is in the neutral or supinated position. The muscle is also described as having an important role in decelerating the rapidly moving arm during activities such as forceful overhand throwing. Debate is ongoing regarding the exact function of the biceps at the shoulder. Most references regard it as a weak flexor of the shoulder.[50,133] A consistent observation is that the biceps tendon does not slide in the groove; rather, the humerus moves on a fixed, passive biceps tendon during shoulder motions. The groove can move along the tendon as much as 4 cm (1½ inches).

A summary of the related literature suggests that with shoulder flexion and abduction, independent of elbow flexion, the biceps tendon does have a weak active head depressor role and serves as a superior checkrein to humeral head excursion. One study, which used simulated muscle forces on a biomechanical cadaver model, showed that the biceps tendon force restrained superior humeral translation. A key factor in this study was that this occurred in the presence of a large rotator cuff tear.[94] A similar study using the same model demonstrated that the biceps assists in anterior stability of the glenohumeral joint by increasing the resistance to torsional forces. Some electromyographic (EMG) studies have disputed the suggested role of the biceps tendon as a shoulder stabilizer, finding only a small input during shoulder motion.[138,139] Despite the continued controversy, the relationship between the long head of the biceps and the function and stability of the glenohumeral joint is an important clinical feature, which must always be considered in the management of patients with a shoulder dysfunction.

Classification of Biceps Lesions

Historically, lesions of the biceps have been described as either biceps tendonitis or instability of the biceps tendon. Tendonitis was further divided into *primary tendonitis*, which occurs as a result of pathology of the tendon sheath, and *secondary tendonitis*, which involves an associated original lesion that led to subsequent biceps tendonitis. Many authors believe that the pathology seen in the biceps is directly related to its intimate relationship with the rotator cuff.[95,129] Both pass under the coracoacromial arch and therefore are susceptible to impingement. "Isolated" ruptures of the long head of the biceps tendon are reportedly uncommon. Neer believed that most ruptures of the long head of the biceps tendon were associated with supraspinatus tears.[126,127] One study documented isolated biceps tendon ruptures in as many as 25% of patients,[140] but more recent studies that used computed tomography (CT) arthrograms and arthroscopy for patients with suspected ruptures have found the incidence of isolated ruptures to be 6% and 2.2%, respectively.[136,140]

Slatis and Aalto[141] developed a three-part classification for biceps lesions. A type A lesion is referred to as *impingement tendonitis*, because it occurs secondary to an impingement syndrome and rotator cuff disease. The defective cuff exposes the biceps to a rigid coracoacromial arch, resulting in tendonitis. This is the most common cause of biceps tendonitis. A type B lesion is a *subluxation of the biceps tendon*. All pathologies of the biceps, including subluxation and dislocation, are included in this category. Lesions of the coracohumeral ligament allow the biceps tendon gradually to displace medially. The slipping of the tendon into and out of its groove leads to inflammation and fraying. A type C lesion is called *attrition tendonitis*. These are primary lesions of the biceps tendon that occur inside the canal, resulting in inflammation and eventual degeneration of the biceps tendon. Often spurring and fraying are evident with this type of tendonitis.

Other authors have classified biceps lesions according to their anatomical location, specifically, at their origin, in the rotator interval, or in association with rotator cuff tears.[129] As noted earlier, the third category has spurred considerable study regarding the intimate relationship between the rotator cuff and the biceps tendon complex.

Etiology of Biceps Lesions

DePalma,[142,143] DePalma and Callery,[144] and Michele,[145] among others, have studied the etiology of biceps tendonitis and have proposed two main categories according to age. One category includes younger patients with anomalies of the bicipital groove and those in whom repetitive trauma is the most important causal factor; the other category includes patients in an older age group, in whom associated degenerative changes in the tendon tend to be the predominant causal factor.

In most cases the cause of biceps pathology probably is multifactorial. The most common etiologies, however, are the result of the anatomical location of the tendon. As has been mentioned previously, the potential for impingement of the biceps tendon under the coracoacromial arch is great, especially if an additional dysfunction of the rotator cuff and/or scapular misalignment is a factor. The blood supply of the biceps has been well studied and has been shown to be diminished in the long tendon region, with a "critical zone" similar to that seen in the supraspinatus tendon.[146] In abduction, a zone of avascularity exists in the intracapsular portion of the tendon, which is felt to be caused by pressure from the head of the humerus, a phenomenon referred to as *wringing-out*. Considering these positions, it is easy to see why patients involved in overhead lifting and throwing are more susceptible to ruptures, elongations, and dislocations of the biceps tendon.

The past 15 years have produced a proliferation of information about the superior labrum and its relationship to the biceps tendon.* As was noted previously, Andrews et al.[130] and Snyder et al.[131] originally defined these lesions of the biceps and superior labrum, commonly referred to today as *SLAP lesions*. Two cited causes of SLAP lesions are (1) a fall onto an outstretched hand, which drives the humeral head up onto the labrum and the biceps tendon, and (2) excessive and forceful contraction of the biceps in throwing athletes (e.g., baseball and football players), in which the deceleration phase of the throw can provide traction that results in avulsion of the biceps and superior labral complex. Earlier in this section, the work of Burkhart et al.[5,11,133] was presented; as described, they found an acceleration mechanism of injury for the type II (thrower's) SLAP lesion caused by a peel-back mechanism of the biceps tendon in the late cocking phase of the throw. (More detailed information about the SLAP lesion of the shoulder and its management can be found in Chapter 5.)

---

*References 5, 20, 93, 96, 130, 131, and 147.

Clinical Presentation of Biceps Lesions

Patients with biceps tendon injuries typically present with chronic pain in the proximal anterior area of the shoulder over the biceps tendon, with pain occasionally radiating down into the muscle belly. Similar to impingement syndromes, the pain can also radiate to the deltoid insertion. It is unusual for the pain to radiate into the neck region or distally beyond the biceps. The history usually shows an atraumatic, repetitive onset, although acute trauma may be part of the original injury that predisposed the biceps tendon to subsequent rupture or dislocation.

Night pain is reported as sometimes being associated with biceps lesions. However, this likely can be explained by the overall problems associated with trying to sleep with a painful shoulder. Most shoulder conditions are worse at night, for a number of reasons. A compressive load may be present (e.g., lying on the affected shoulder) or, in some instances, traction may be applied to the shoulder (e.g., arm hanging over the bed); either of these results in pain. Positioning to avoid pain is difficult; however, most patients find that, with the use of many pillows, lying on the contralateral side with the affected arm in neutral, resting on the pillows, is among the most comfortable positions of rest. Many patients with a painful shoulder report that their best rest is achieved in a semireclined position, such as in a recliner, with the arm resting on a pillow in the shoulder resting position.

Patients with bicipital tendonitis tend to be young or middle aged, and the pattern of pain is less at rest and more intense with activity. This is especially so with overhead activities in daily living, work, and/or sports. Rotation of the humerus at or above the horizontal level brings the tuberosities, bicipital groove, biceps tendon, and rotator cuff in direct contact with the anterior acromion and the coracoacromial ligament. Biceps instability is most commonly associated with the throwing athlete, in whom in a certain position of rotation, the motion is accompanied by a palpable snap or pop. The patient often describes pain in the front of the shoulder, which is aggravated by lifting the arm up to around 90°. If the biceps tendon ruptures, this usually is accompanied by acute pain and sometimes an audible pop in the shoulder. Over the following several days, a notable change occurs in the contour of the arm, with ecchymosis that often tracks down to the distal muscle belly.

Numerous tests have been described that can assist in the diagnosis of biceps conditions (these are well documented in volume 1 of this series, *Orthopedic Physical Assessment*, Chapter 5).[133] Most biceps lesions present with tenderness on palpation in the bicipital groove, which often disappears as the lesser tuberosity and groove rotate medially under the short head of the biceps and coracoid process. This is different from the tenderness noted with subdeltoid bursitis and impingement syndromes, which has a more diffuse pattern that does not change with arm rotation. According to Burkhead et al.,[148] this "tenderness in motion" sign is among the most specific for differentiating biceps lesions. Range of motion is perhaps slightly restricted into full abduction and medial rotation, usually as a result of pain rather than capsular constriction. However, pain is felt while performing abduction and medial rotation and abduction and lateral rotation movements. Resisted isometric testing reveals a painful weakness with forward flexion of the shoulder.

Treatment of Biceps Injuries

As is almost universally true of all injuries, the most effective form of treatment of a biceps injury is prevention. As noted, the biceps often is part of the domino effect that occurs as a result of other primary shoulder pathologies. Therefore prevention of injury and overuse in these regions of the shoulder conceivably could prevent injuries to the biceps tendon. Individuals involved in manual labor with either repetitive overhead work or heavy lifting, as well as individuals participating in sports that demand overhand motions, are particularly at risk for biceps injury. Developing a balanced shoulder musculature that includes a strong, healthy rotator cuff and scapular muscle region can help prevent the vicious cycle of impingement tendonitis, irritation, and muscle weakness that leads to altered kinematics, instability, and further impingement of tissue, such as the long head of the biceps.

Once the biceps tendon has been injured, the first step in proper management is a thorough examination of the anterior shoulder, all the structures of the shoulder girdle and, if appropriate, the kinetic chain. Failure either to identify associated lesions (e.g., those affecting the glenoid labrum and rotator cuff) or to note contributing factors (e.g., a poorly stabilized scapula, a hypomobile cervical and/or thoracic spine, or altered muscle recruitment patterning) may lead the clinician to direct the sole treatment to the affected biceps tendon, rather than addressing the true cause of the shoulder injury. Depending on the specific nature and severity of the biceps injury, treatment can range from managing an early, acute inflammatory situation locally at the tendon to treating the biceps tendon by retraining the scapular stabilizing muscles and rotator cuff to properly position the glenohumeral joint and therefore reduce impingement on the long head of the biceps anteriorly. Whichever is the case, the message is always the same: the clinician must make sure that treatment encompasses not only the affected tissue, but also the causal tissue.

Nerve Injuries of the Shoulder

In any discussion of nerve injuries of the shoulder, it is important to note that a fair number of neurologic-like symptoms that patients experience may originate from sites well beyond the actual shoulder. These could include the spinal cord, cervical disc, cervical or thoracic nerve roots, nerve branches, and peripheral nerves, as well as unsuspected sites (e.g., the pleural or abdominal cavity) that can refer pain to the shoulder. Patients with nerve injuries often describe inconsistent, vague symptoms that may involve some combination of pain, paresthesia, or motor weakness in the limb; however, this is highly variable and depends on the patient's individual injury and the component of the nerve affected. Therefore it is very important that clinicians perform a thorough examination of the patient presenting with any neurological symptoms and that they routinely include a check of the cervical and thoracic spine regions as well.

Nerve injuries of the shoulder represent a relatively small percentage of overall problems reported.[36,50,149-151] They are most commonly caused by direct trauma but may also occur as a result of repetitive microtrauma. In some instances, shoulder nerve injuries occur secondary to the predominant injury (e.g., axillary nerve damage from an anterior glenohumeral dislocation) or are part of the effect of the underlying cause of the shoulder condition (e.g., poor posture and scapular instability that lead to thoracic outlet syndrome).

Nerve injuries of the shoulder are being recognized with increasing frequency, especially in sports such as football and rugby, which involve a greater risk of injury from direct contact.[36,149-151] Another condition that has been noted is nerve injury caused by compression and/or stretching arising from muscle hypertrophy or other soft tissue changes; this type of injury often is seen in weight lifters, body builders, and volleyball players, in whom rapid shoulder movements can lead to suprascapular nerve palsies. However, these injuries are not found only in athletes; in fact, nerve entrapment injuries commonly occur in individuals who perform repetitive motions in their occupations, such as those who work extensively at computers and assembly line workers. A more detailed description of nervous tissue and the pathology of nerve injuries about the shoulder can be found in Chapter 20 of this text and in volume 2 of this series, *Scientific Foundations and Principles of Practice in Musculoskeletal Rehabilitation*, Chapter 8.

References

To enhance this text and add value for the reader, all references have been incorporated into a CD-ROM that is provided with this text. The reader can view the reference source and access it online whenever possible. There are a total of 151 references for this chapter.

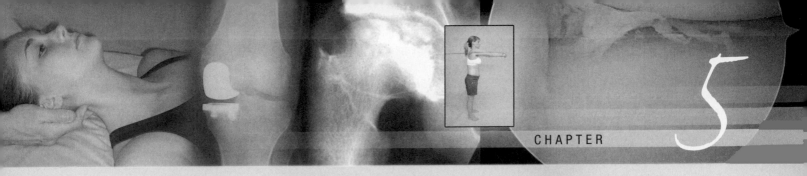

CHAPTER 5

SHOULDER INSTABILITY AND IMPINGEMENT SYNDROME

David J. Magee, Ron Mattison, and David C. Reid

Introduction

The impression gained from a cursory glance at the shoulder belies its complexity. This proximal part of the upper kinetic chain starts at the trunk, includes the scapula, glenohumeral joint, acromioclavicular joint, and sternoclavicular joint.[1] As part of the kinetic chain, the shoulder acts as a funnel, transferring the forces generated by the lower extremity and trunk to the arm.[2-5] The human shoulder has evolved to allow an incredible range of motion for reaching and placing the human hand through a large functional arc, largely at the expense of bony stability. Elevation, depression, protraction, retraction, and rotation of the scapula, along with elevation and rotation of the clavicle, enhance or facilitate the motions of forward flexion, extension, abduction, adduction, medial and lateral rotation, and circumduction of the glenohumeral joint, which allow the arm and hand to be placed in many positions.[6] Unfortunately, every anatomical adaptation toward mobility creates the potential for problems, which can be compounded by the large ranges of motion needed, frequent repetitions, and high stress loads seen in sports and occupations involving the upper limbs.

It is imperative that clinicians consider the shoulder girdle as a whole, rather than any one articulation, when assessing for shoulder instability and impingement. The minimal bony support of the shoulder girdle must be supplemented by strong ligaments and careful arrangement of muscle groups to ensure stability.[7,8] With such a large range of motion available at the shoulder, glenohumeral stabilization comes from compression and precise sequencing of all the muscle groups involved, the labrum, and intricate placement of the ligaments.[9-12]

Functional Anatomy

Although bony containment is lacking in the scapulohumeral articulation, the articular surfaces are positioned to contribute to stability. For example, the scapula faces 30° anteriorly to the chest wall and is tilted upward 3° to augment functional reaching motions above shoulder height.[13,14] The glenoid is tilted upward 5° to help control inferior instability and to further augment movements above shoulder height.[13]

At the glenohumeral joint, a large humeral head articulates with the shallow glenoid cavity, which is deepened by the glenoid labrum. The surface area of the humeral head is significantly larger than the glenoid.[13,15,16] However, the articular surfaces of the humeral head and glenoid are functionally congruent, having radii within 3 mm. The area in contact between the two surfaces constantly changes, with the greatest contact in midelevation rather than at the extremes of glenohumeral motion, where the potential for instability is greatest.[17] Only about 25% to 30% of the large, spherical humeral head is in contact with the glenoid surface at any one time.[13,18] Stability in the glenohumeral joint is achieved through several factors: the glenoid labrum, the negative pressure within the joint capsule, the coefficient of friction of the synovial fluid, and the screw home mechanism of the inferior glenohumeral ligament that occurs with internal and external rotation and elevation, augmented by the compressive effects of the rotator cuff.

With 180° of elevation of the arm, there is 120° of glenohumeral motion, along with 60° of scapulothoracic motion. This large range of activity (i.e., scapulohumeral rhythm) is brought about by precise muscle sequencing, and the resultant force couples generate rotary torques on the scapula and humerus, creating complex arm movement patterns. The term *force couple* refers to muscles working together; some act concentrically to initiate and provide movement or control movement, and others act isometrically, concentrically, or eccentrically to control or decelerate movement.[19]

Any structural injury, scapular dyskinesia (abnormal positions or patterns of movement of the scapula), or dysplasia of the humerus or the glenoid or its labrum can affect the stabilization of the glenohumeral joint.[20] Translation of the humeral head on the glenoid is limited to a few millimeters in every direction during movement.[19,21-23] If the dynamic structures controlling this translation (primarily the rotator cuff) or the passive structures (e.g., the labrum or ligaments) are injured, translation increases. The increased translation leads to increased wearing of the glenoid labrum, failure of the static restraints (see Table 4-1), and eccentric overload of the dynamic restraints, which work individually and in unison to provide stability in the joints of the shoulder, where mobility is paramount. The result is instability, impingement, or both.[24,25]

Any alteration in biomechanics or trauma may lead to a tear in the glenoid labrum. A **Bankart lesion** is a traumatic labral tear that usually occurs with an anterior dislocation. A condition that occurs in the superior labrum anterior and posterior to the biceps (SLAP) lesion is a lesion around the long head of the biceps where it crosses over the glenohumeral joint, where single or repetitive trauma causes the labrum to fray, tear, or peel back from the bone.[2-4] The glenoid labrum increases the glenoid depth approximately twofold, which contributes to glenohumeral stability.[13,15,16,18]

The surrounding soft tissue envelope (i.e., the capsule) is the primary contributor to stability in the normal glenohumeral joint, with a lax inferior capsule allowing movement into full elevation. The capsule is reinforced by the coracohumeral and glenohumeral ligaments, which act as checkreins at the extreme range of motion, assisting the compression caused by the dynamic rotator cuff.[20] These two components augment normal scapulohumeral rhythm to create functional stability. The concavity formed by the glenoid labrum, along with the muscles that provide compression and the unique tightening mechanism of the inferior glenohumeral ligament, provide a concavity-compression mechanism that stabilizes the glenohumeral joint.[13,20]

The glenohumeral ligaments, which are thickenings in the capsule, show a high degree of variability, especially the superior and middle glenohumeral ligaments. Of the three, the inferior glenohumeral ligament is the most important and shows the least variability. It acts like a hammock for the humeral head, preventing some inferior translation, with the anterior and posterior bands tightening on rotation (torsion), which in turn limits anterior and posterior translation.[23] This ligament takes on even greater importance with glenohumeral elevation. At 0° abduction, the subscapularis muscle, the labrum, and the superior glenohumeral ligament are the primary restraints to anterior

translation. At 45° abduction, the subscapularis muscle and the middle and inferior glenohumeral ligaments, along with the labrum, prevent anterior translation. When the arm is abducted more than 90°, which is the usual position of anterior dislocation, the anterior fibers of the inferior glenohumeral ligament are the primary restraints to anterior movement.[13,15,16,18,26] The long head of the biceps tendon acts as a secondary dynamic support to reduce stress anteriorly in the abducted and laterally rotated position.[27] Similarly, the posterior band of the inferior glenohumeral ligament prevents posterior translation above 90°.[15] If the ligaments are hypomobile, they can restrict translation of the humeral head in the glenoid,[28] and restricted translation can affect shoulder motion, especially when the shoulder is under load. If the labrum, capsule, or ligaments are injured or stretched, the resulting hypermobility can lead to functional instability even without major trauma.

The tendon of the rotator cuff and the long head of the biceps have important dynamic roles, but they can perform these roles only when acting from a stable scapular base. They serve in a complementary function to adjust the tension in the capsuloligamentous system.[29] It is possible that stretch receptors within the capsular ligaments are activated by tension to induce selective contraction of the surrounding musculature, protecting these structures at the extremes of motion.[30] As stated previously, contraction of these muscles compresses the humeral head into the glenoid cavity and increases the force needed to translate the humeral head.[15,31,32] Cadaveric studies have shown that simulated maximal contraction of the posterior rotator cuff muscles reduces anterior ligamentous strain, and posterior cuff contraction reduces anterior ligamentous strain.[33]

A second and equally important group of muscles that affects glenohumeral stability is the scapular control muscles (see Table 4-1). These muscles control the scapula, which is the dynamic base (i.e., the origin) for the rotator cuff, biceps, and triceps (long head) muscles. Through their action on the scapula, these muscles position the glenoid beneath the humeral head, adjusting for the changing position of the arm. With scapular dyskinesia, failure to maintain the stable glenoid platform (i.e., the scapula) may occur, causing an alteration in scapulohumeral rhythm and mild to severe winging of the scapula.

These concepts form the basis for rehabilitation of the unstable shoulder. Four key components must be addressed in rehabilitation: (1) normal scapulohumeral rhythm, (2) normal arthrokinematics, (3) balancing of the ligamentous structures, and (4) normal function of the rotator cuff muscles.[1]

Principles of Shoulder Assessment

The essential ingredients for assessing the spectrum of shoulder injuries are a detailed history, identification of the precipitating or perpetuating factors (i.e., the mechanism of injury), and a careful physical examination, including special tests for differential diagnosis. Palpation of the specific structures generating the pain or dysfunction concludes the physical examination. This process should lead the examiner to choose the specific investigations (e.g., diagnostic imaging) needed to confirm the diagnosis, and it also provides a framework that is essential to successful treatment.

Key Elements for a Clinical Diagnosis

- Recognition of the salient points in the history
- Identification of precipitating or perplexing factors
- Careful examination
- Palpation of pain-generating structures

In the shoulder, dysfunction and pain may arise from a variety of sources, including the scapulohumeral complex, the acromioclavicular or sternoclavicular articulations, the rotator cuff and other shoulder muscles, the associated subacromial (subdeltoid) bursa, the biceps tendon, or the labrum; pain may even be referred from the cervical and thoracic spine and ribs. Shoulder pathology shows a common pattern of pain along the anterior glenohumeral joint line and biceps, at the origin of the levator scapulae, and at the teres minor on the posterior joint line. Pain also may be present in the deltoid insertion and upper trapezius, along the medial border of the scapula and, in some cases, over the whole scapula.

When evaluating pain, clinicians should keep in mind the patient's age, occupation, recreational goals, and side dominance. The examiner must make sure that the patient is not confusing pain with weakness, instability, or apprehension. The mode of onset is important; this may present a spectrum of injury mechanisms, from a single traumatic episode to repetitive microtrauma.

Detailed examination of the shoulder can be found elsewhere (see volume 1 of this series, *Orthopedic Physical Assessment,* Chapter 5). When assessing the shoulder, the examiner must keep in mind several important concepts:

1. *Shoulder pain must always be distinguished from referred pain arising from the cervical spine* (Table 5-1). The embryological derivation of the shoulder girdle from the cervical myotomes results in a close relationship for specific innervation, as well as for the referred pain. With any complaint of shoulder girdle discomfort, cervical pathology must be ruled out. Neck pain and dysesthesia (i.e., numbness, tingling, burning) that radiates past the elbow normally implicate cervical disc disease, although nerve entrapment at the elbow or wrist or a local pathological lesion in the hand must be considered.[1] True shoulder pain rarely extends below the elbow. In any patient over age 50, a coexisting cervical degenerative abnormality must be considered.[34]

Table 5-1

Factors Suggesting the Site of Origin of Shoulder Pain

Neck Pathology	Shoulder Pathology
Pain at rest	Pain with use
Pain with neck motion	Pain when working overhead
Pain with overpressure on the neck	Feeling of instability
	Local palpable tenderness
Pain aggravated by postural positions	Painful arc of motion
	Pain into the deltoid area
Pain past the shoulder	Pain mainly on the dominant side
Reflex changes	
Altered peripheral sensation	Pain relief with local injections
Guarded cervical spine motion	

From Zachazewski JE, Magee DJ, Quillen WS, editors: *Athletic injuries and rehabilitation*, p 511, Philadelphia, 1996, WB Saunders.

2. *Generally, shoulder pathology is characterized by pain on use, weakness, stiffness, and guarded apprehension.* (In many cases the patient reports that the shoulder "just doesn't feel right.") These findings help distinguish shoulder pathology from cervical pain, which often is present even at rest and generally is aggravated by chronic compensatory postures such as sitting, reading, or studying at a desk. Neck and shoulder pain cannot be totally isolated. The clinical points that are most suggestive of pain of spinal origin include absence of shoulder tenderness, guarded cervical spine motion, decreased biceps strength and reflex, and a positive cervical compression test (see volume I of this series, *Orthopedic Physical Assessment,* Chapter 3).[1] The most common pattern of cervical disc disease (i.e., spondylosis) refers into the C5-C6 dermatome with pain and/or paresthesia over the shoulder, the lateral arm, and even the forearm.

3. *The patient's ability to maintain a static and dynamic stable core is important in shoulder rehabilitation.* A stable core (i.e., the ability to maintain control of the pelvis and spine) is the transfer zone between the lower extremity and the upper extremity, and as such it plays a significant role in shoulder rehabilitation. If the practitioner tries to correct shoulder and/or cervical posture without addressing the unstable or incorrectly positioned core, treatment will be unsuccessful.

4. *Impingement may occur against the anterior edge of the acromion, the coracoacromial ligament, or the inferior acromioclavicular joint.*[35] Structural narrowing of the subacromial space may occur secondary to inferior acromial tilting (antetilt), the so-called hooked acromion (type III), an unfused acromial ossification center, or subacromial spurring. In addition, acromioclavicular joint hypertrophy and marginal osteophytes may irritate the rotator cuff.[9] Postural changes, particularly slouching with rounded shoulders and a protruding, chin-forward head, contribute to impingement. Magnetic resonance imaging (MRI) has demonstrated

narrowing of the subacromial space as the shoulder girdle moves from a retracted to a protracted position.[36]

5. *Stability of the shoulder complex depends on an intimate relationship between the muscles controlling the scapula and those controlling the humerus.* The examiner must ensure correct functioning of the periscapular stabilizers and the rotator cuff (inner cone muscles). Commonly, the power (outer cone) muscles (i.e., the pectoralis major, deltoid, and latissimus dorsi) are not the problem, although they may contribute to the problem by being tight or substituting for the inner core muscles. Weakness or injury in any of the inner cone muscles leads to an imbalance of the synergistic inner cone (stabilizer) and outer cone (mobilizer) muscles and the prime mover muscles, resulting in abnormal shear forces, which in turn can lead to instability (functional subluxation), labral injury, impingement, muscle imbalance, abnormal joint mechanics, and/or rotator cuff tears.[6,7,37] A thorough, detailed assessment of the strength and flexibility of each individual muscle of the shoulder complex is essential to identify weak and tight links in the kinetic chain and to ensure proper return to correct function. (For muscle testing, the reader is referred to the appropriate muscle testing books.[38-40])

6. *The examiner should watch for scapular dyskinesia, especially if the patient is under 35 and has anterior shoulder pain.*[2-4,41-43] If the scapula cannot be controlled by its stabilizer muscles, extra load is transferred to the humeral control muscles and they become overused, which leads to tendon and labral problems. Scapular instability is a common cause of rotator cuff and bicipital tendonitis/tendinosis and secondary impingement. A functional scapular base is essential for correct shoulder movement, especially in sports.[44]

7. *Hypomobility can be a major issue in shoulder instability and impingement.* The clinician must determine the mobility of the glenohumeral joint capsule (especially posteroinferiorly), the ribs, the scapula, and the acromioclavicular and sternoclavicular joints, as well as assessing for tight muscles (e.g., pectoralis major and minor). Addressing tight structures helps ensure normal shoulder arthrokinematics and function.[2-4] For example, glenohumeral arthrokinematics are markedly altered by a glenohumeral internal rotation deficit (GIRD) or by a tight posterior capsule when internal (medial) rotation is limited and lateral rotation is excessive (also called *glenohumeral external rotation gain* [GERG]).

8. *Immobility of the thoracic spine and ribs can significantly influence the movement patterns of the shoulder complex and can affect the dimensions of the subacromial space.* A careful assessment of the cervical and thoracic spine and ribs is an important part of any shoulder assessment.[45]

9. *Any shoulder rehabilitation program must involve assessment of the whole kinetic chain.*[3] The clinician cannot assess the upper quadrant in isolation. Power movements and accelerating motions begin in the lower limb and trunk

musculature. In patients with shoulder problems, the clinician should look for inflexibility in the hips, especially on the nondominant side, and in trunk rotation and the anterior shoulder muscles, along with weakness of the hip abductors and the pelvic core.[2]

10. *Exertional left shoulder pain in individuals over age 45 with coronary risk factors should be considered as cardiac pain until proven otherwise.* Coronary risk factors include smoking, obesity, hypertension, and a family history of cardiac disease.

11. *Pain from the lungs and abdominal organs can be referred to the shoulder, and injury to these structures should be considered in conditions involving trauma.*

12. *The initial observation should include the thoracic spine and shoulder girdle and requires adequate exposure of the patient.* Viewing the disrobed patient from behind allows the clinician to note any wasting of the shoulder girdle muscles, especially the supraspinatus, infraspinatus, serratus anterior, and posterior deltoid; such wasting may indicate a nerve injury (e.g., suprascapular, long thoracic, or auxiliary nerve)[46] or apparent hypertrophy of the upper trapezius as a result of superior migration of the scapula (i.e., type III dyskinesia).[2-4,41-43] The presence and size of stretch marks or scars often reflect poor quality collagen and may be a clue to the possibility of generalized ligamentous laxity or steroid abuse in athletes. Excessive lordotic curvature, a kyphotic thoracic spine, and/or associated poking chin with rounded shoulders should be noted. The clinician must assess for lack of pelvic or core control with these postural problems, which often contributes to shoulder problems. In addition, these anterior and posterior postural imbalances can lead to a tight pectoralis major and minor, resulting in increased stress on the anterior capsule, tightness of the posterior capsule, and overuse of scapular control muscles.[46]

13. *The examiner must always be aware of the possibility of referred pain.* The response to palpation must be put in the context of the patient's presentation and the implications of this presentation (e.g., secondary gain, pain threshold) must be judged correctly.

14. *Clinicians must know their patients.* The patient may have other issues and agendas that affect the clinical presentation.

Shoulder Impingement

Shoulder impingement is associated with various degrees of inflammation or cuff degeneration. It frequently occurs as a result of microtrauma, macrotrauma, or functional instability. The suspicion of impingement is raised by the presence of a painful arc during attempted active abduction or forward flexion, or in patients with a complaint of anterior or posterior shoulder pain with no history of trauma.

The subacromial space can be identified as a source of impingement by taking the arm passively into full forward elevation with gentle overpressure (Neer impingement test).[46] This test can be supplemented with the Hawkins-Kennedy impingement test, which involves taking the patient's arm to 90° of abduction and then moving it into horizontal adduction, followed by forced medial rotation.[46] The Hawkins-Kennedy impingement test can be enhanced by having the patient resist a force applied downward to the dorsum of the hand. A positive Hawkins-Kennedy test result implies impingement of the rotator cuff under the acromion. A positive Neer impingement test result is thought to represent impingement of the rotator cuff on the anterosuperior glenoid rim or coracoacromial ligament.[47]

Shoulder pain caused by impingement would seem to be easily distinguishable from that caused by posttraumatic instability. However, over time clinicians have come to recognize that these conditions comprise a spectrum of both injury and pathology. At one end of the spectrum is a primary mechanical impingement, and at the other end is frank dislocation. Primary mechanical impingement reflects a gradual attrition and irritation of the tendons that is associated with pain and dysfunction and that often is the result of repetitive overuse. Frank dislocation frequently goes on to become a recurrent dislocating joint (Figure 5-1). Similarly, the spectrum of natural collagenous laxity ranges from extreme tightness to abnormal looseness; therefore the degree of trauma or overuse required to generate a dislocation or subluxation varies.

Between these extremes lies the mildly unstable shoulder that predisposes the patient to impingement and pain; this condition is often seen in athletes such as swimmers and in assembly line workers. The throwing shoulder in which the pitcher alters the mechanics to increase range of lateral rotation to get into the "slot" is another example.[2]

The aging process also fits into this spectrum, and its effects are manifested more in the soft tissue rotator cuff and in the joint surface itself.[47] Furthermore, internal derangements in the form of labral tears, attrition of the rotator cuff muscles, and degeneration of or partial tears in the biceps tendon have begun to be diagnosed with more prevalent use of the arthroscope and the increasing availability of MRI and computed tomography (CT) scanning. As a result, the previously simple, distinct diagnostic categories have become blurred into a spectrum of injuries.

Primary subacromial or anterior impingement is a condition that usually implies rotator cuff abnormality and actual mechanical irritation of the rotator cuff, anterior labrum, and subacromial bursa against the coracoacromial ligament and acromion, resulting in rotator cuff and/or biceps tendonitis/tendinosis, with or without associated bursitis. This condition often is the result of cyclical repetitive abduction, forward flexion, and medial rotation motion at the glenohumeral joint.[48,49] Such movement is seen in swimmers who commonly swim about 10,000 to 14,000 m (6.2 to 8.7 miles) or more per day.[47] Impingement may also occur when the arm is forward flexed, medially rotated, and abducted within the coracohumeral space. This **coracoid impingement syndrome** occurs when the lesser tuberosity of the humerus encroaches on the coracoid process. The condition has been reported in swimmers, tennis players, and weight lifters. With force overload, the humeral and scapular control muscles become fatigued, resulting in muscle weakness and muscle imbalance in the scapulohumeral force couples (Figure 5-2).[48,49] The resultant abnormal shear stresses can lead to impingement.

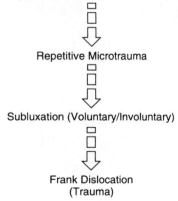

Vague Sense of Shoulder Dysfunction

(**A**traumatic **M**ultidirectional Instability in **B**oth shoulders that responds to Intensive **R**ehabilitation. If Surgery Necessary, **I**nferior Capsular Shift Used [**AMBRI**])

Repetitive Microtrauma

Subluxation (Voluntary/Involuntary)

Frank Dislocation
(Trauma)

(**T**raumatic, **U**nidirectional Instability with **B**ankart Lesion Requiring **S**urgery [**TUBS**])

Figure 5-1

Shoulder instability spectrum. (From Zachazewski JE, Magee DJ, Quillen WS, editors: *Athletic injuries and rehabilitation,* p 520, Philadelphia, 1996, WB Saunders.)

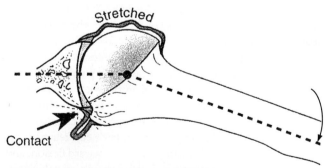

Figure 5-2

Posterior internal impingement. Posterior contact between the glenoid lip and the insertion of the cuff to the tuberosity occurs in the apprehension, or fulcrum, position, especially if the anteroinferior capsule has been stretched, allowing the humerus to extend to an unusually posterior scapular plane. This contact can challenge the integrity of the posterior cuff insertion and the tuberosity. (From Matsen FA: Stability. In Matsen FA, Lippett SB, Sidles JA, Harryman DT: *Practical evaluation and management of the shoulder,* p 98, Philadelphia, 1994, WB Saunders.)

Another type of impingement occurs in individuals over age 40, usually as a result of mechanical impingement arising from alterations in the soft tissues (e.g., rotator cuff, labrum) and/or bony changes (e.g., acromion and coracoid process). This is called **primary anterior (external) impingement**. The patient seldom has instability.[5,50,51] In younger patients (ages 15-35), muscle dynamics is the primary problem (i.e., weakness of the scapular and humeral stabilizers). This is called **secondary anterior (external) impingement,** which primarily is due to scapular dyskinesia and posterior rotator cuff fatigue.[5,50,51]

The fourth type of impingement is **posterior internal impingement** (see Figure 5-2), which involves contact of the undersurface of the rotator cuff with the posterior superior glenoid labrum.[52-54] Burkhart et al.[3] reported that internal impingement is a normal phenomenon that sometimes can result in pathology of the rotator cuff and labrum.

Because of the complexity and interlinking nature of shoulder pathologies, *there has been a movement away from labeling specific structures when making a diagnosis.* Most of the anterior painful shoulder abnormalities, including tendonitis/tendinosis and bursitis, are given the functional term **anterior impingement syndrome** to signify their close relationship.[10,47]

If significant inflammation is present, impingement tests are less specific, because all testing positions tend to be uncomfortable. Very inflamed tissues are uncomfortable even on passive stretching or when put under tension by contraction of the associated muscle. By testing for pain in the nonimpingement position for each specific structure, the clinician can distinguish and isolate the inflammatory response of the tendon from a simple impingement area. For example, a partial rupture of the biceps tendon within the joint may give positive impingement signs and may also be maximally painful with resisted forward flexion. The clinician can further confirm the diagnosis by injecting approximately 3 mL of 0.25% to 1% lidocaine (Xylocaine) directly around the most painful areas (or 5 mL into the subacromial space) and then waiting a suitable interval (usually a few minutes) before repeating the impingement test.[52] Relief of at least 50% of the patient's pain through the painful arc or the impingement positions helps confirm the source of the pain. In addition, when a rotator cuff tear is suspected, elimination of most of the pain allows a more specific examination of strength. The classic findings with a rotator cuff tear are pain even at rest, difficulty abducting in slight forward flexion, and loss of lateral rotation strength. Small tears or partial thickness tears may generate impingement signs without significant loss of rotator cuff strength. Diagnostic tests such as MRI or CT arthrograms can help identify the true problem.

Treatment of Impingement

In the early clinical stages, the patient may complain of aching only after activity, and range of motion is preserved.

The clinician seldom sees the patient at this point, which is unfortunate, because education at this stage could play a significant role. If the patient detects the early onset of symptoms, preventive measures can be instituted, such as modification of an activity. For example, during their workouts, swimmers could use a different stroke (e.g., the breaststroke), do only the leg portion of the stroke, use speed fins, use a center snorkel, or alter their stroke (e.g., different hand entry, altered body roll). The use of resistance devices should be kept to a minimum. For example, the use of hand paddles or swimming against elastic cords can increase the stress on a swimmer's shoulder. Also, using a flutter board held in front of the head while doing kicking strokes may position the arm in a vulnerable impingement posture.

The patient should be instructed to apply ice, especially after a workout, and to take the shoulders slowly through a full range of motion in a controlled fashion while ensuring a dynamically stabilized scapula. The patient should avoid the impingement position in activities of daily living and dry land training programs. Ideally, muscle strength should be tested regularly for weakness of the scapular or humeral control muscles, loss of range of motion and pain, and postural compensatory postures. Correct posture is an important concept that clinicians must keep in mind when asking patients to do shoulder exercises. The practitioner should not allow poor posture with protracted scapulae, which leads to *scapular dumping,* or the position in which the glenoid fossa is no longer superiorly tilted, which allows the humeral head to "fall" out of the glenoid (Figure 5-3); neither should the patient do abduction and medial rotation ("empty can") exercises.

As the impingement pathology progresses to the next stage, the patient experiences discomfort and even pain

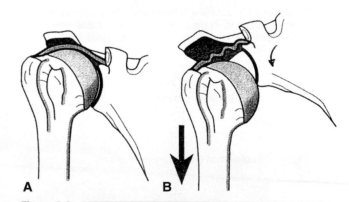

Figure 5-3

Scapular dumping. With the scapula in a normal position (**A**), the superior capsular mechanism is tight, supporting the head in the glenoid concavity. Drooping of the lateral scapula (**B**) relaxes the superior capsular structures and rotates the glenoid concavity so that it does not support the head of the humerus. Conversely, stability is enhanced by elevating the lateral aspect of the scapula. (From Matsen FA: Stability. In Matsen FA, Lippett SB, Sidles JA, Harryman DT: *Practical evaluation and management of the shoulder,* p 81, Philadelphia, 1994, WB Saunders.)

during and after the activity. A positive impingement sign is elicited on examination, and palpation may demonstrate acromioclavicular or anterior glenohumeral joint line tenderness. These patients also present with tenderness over the teres minor and the medial border of the scapula, particularly at the origin of the levator scapulae. Pathological changes may consist of thickening and fibrosis of the tendon, involvement of the subacromial bursa, residual adhesions, and possibly fraying of the labrum.

In the final stages, the patient complains of continuous pain over the supraspinatus and biceps tendons and tenderness over the coracoacromial ligament. A painful arc, especially in the empty can position, is commonly demonstrated, and range of motion is restricted. Medial and lateral rotation motions are not equal bilaterally, and impingement signs are grossly positive. X-ray films may demonstrate infra-acromial and infraclavicular spurs, bony sclerosis near the supraspinatus insertion, and subacromial erosion.

Surgical Treatment of Impingement Syndromes

Surgery is considered a treatment of last resort for impingement syndromes. The indications for surgery include unremitting pain and failure to respond to nonoperative conservative treatment. The timing of surgery depends on the functional disability and pain.

The surgical procedures used are performed arthroscopically and are designed to increase, or decompress, the subacromial space. This is achieved by some combination of shaving or excising the undersurface of the anterior edge of the acromion process with release or resection of the distal part of the coracoacromial ligament, thus decompressing the acromioclavicular space. The decision to remove inferior osteophytes or resect the acromioclavicular joint, combining the procedure with diagnostic arthroscopy of the glenohumeral joint and varying degrees of correction of SLAP lesions, bicipital tendon pathology, or glenohumeral stabilization, usually is a preoperative determination refined by intraoperative findings.

As might be expected with the array of surgical decisions to be made, the progress of postoperative rehabilitation varies. The clinician should have accurate and detailed information before starting the planning of the treatment regimen. In the simplest scenario of arthroscopic subacromial decompression, gentle range of motion can be commenced within the tolerance of discomfort. The initial emphasis is on isometric muscle work, with progression to range of motion exercises and strengthening. This progression is dictated by the ability to restore appropriate scapulohumeral rhythm and functional scapular control. Impingement positions must be avoided, and the exercises should focus on medial and lateral rotation in neutral, along with forward flexion motions, before abduction motions are initiated. It is better to go slowly early, until most of the discomfort has subsided. The clinician should

follow the principles of rehabilitation outlined later in this chapter, including those for nonoperative treatment of impingement.

Shoulder Instability, Subluxation, and Dislocation

Shoulder instability, due either to significant trauma or to inherent ligamentous laxity and overuse with associated functional instability, is a common problem, especially in those under 35 years of age and in individuals who engage in a lot of overhead activity. The condition may be compounded by pseudo-laxity, which is an apparent increase in anterior laxity that results from a decreased cam effect, along with a tear of the superior labrum (SLAP lesion), congenital joint laxity (hypermobility), congenital muscle weakness, congenital anomalies, and muscle weakness or atrophy after injury.[2]

The glenohumeral joint is the most frequently dislocated major joint in the body. In some case series, glenohumeral dislocations are more common than all other joint dislocations combined.[53] Anterior dislocations of the shoulder account for 80% to 95% of all initial shoulder girdle dislocations, and recurrence is common.[54-56]

Classification of these injuries is necessary to develop a logical treatment plan. As previously mentioned, instabilities can range from subtle subluxation to a frank dislocation in which the articular surfaces are no longer in contact (i.e., true dislocation). Recurrent transient subluxation results in a feeling of instability or loss of control due to positioning of the arm. An example of this is forced hyperextension of the arm in elevation and/or lateral rotation, which may result in the "dead arm" syndrome seen in throwing athletes or in tennis players during the serve; in these cases, altered mechanics or traction or pressure on the nerves generates the symptoms.[2,57,58]

Instabilities are basically classified as traumatic or atraumatic instabilities; Neer added a third type, acquired instabilities.[59] A traumatic dislocation is caused by a single force that applies excessive overload to the joint; this often damages the glenoid labrum and may disrupt the capsule. This type of dislocation is seen in patients who present with a condition known as a *TUBS lesion* (*t*raumatic *u*nidirectional instability with a *B*ankart lesion that responds well to *s*urgery), as described by Matsen et al.[28] An atraumatic dislocation usually occurs in patients with multiple joint laxities who frequently have experienced episodes of subluxation before a relatively minor injury results in a dislocation. These individuals often show functional instability (i.e., lack of muscular control) as a result of congenital hypermobility or congenital muscle weakness. This classification includes patients who present with an *AMBRI lesion* (*a*traumatic *m*ultidirectional instability that is *b*ilateral and the primary treatment is *r*ehabilitation, not surgery;[28] if surgery is required, an *i*nferior capsular shift is often recommended). Capsular laxity is common in these patients, and Bankart lesions are not seen, although the labrum may be frayed.[43]

The clinician must keep in mind, however, that overlapping gradations of instability cover the entire spectrum, from TUBS lesions to AMBRI lesions (see Figure 5-1).[24] Individuals with acquired instability who become symptomatic usually are engaged in overhead occupational or recreational activities, such as plastering ceilings, installing ceiling lighting, swimming, gymnastics, and baseball (i.e., pitching), in which the repetitive microtrauma of ill-conceived stretching or rapid, large range motion gradually contributes to capsular stretching. Although the shoulder becomes hypermobile, other joints may test within the normal range. A traumatic episode may push the joint over the edge and produce the first dislocation, but this major episode is only a small component of the problem.[53]

Many clinicians recognize functional instability as a pathological entity, particularly when the joint is put under high stress loads. Scapular control is lacking in these patients, and this is one of the clinician's primary concerns.[3] This instability manifests itself from muscle fatigue or scapular dyskinesia after excessive load or repetitions. The mechanical etiology of functional instability is uncontrolled translation (i.e., loss of the arthrokinematic control) of the humeral head within the glenoid cavity.[18,48,60-64] Strong, coordinated muscle activity and proper neuromuscular balance contribute significantly to a reduction in functional instability and the often accompanying impingement, and these elements form the basis of treatment.

The glenohumeral instability, which is commonly due to asynchronous firing and fatigue of the scapular and humeral control muscles, can lead to subluxation, rotator cuff strains, and tendonitis/tendinosis injuries. Therefore movement control becomes the primary focus of the clinician.[3,20,65-68] Movement control focuses on maximizing coordinated and correct contraction of muscles through strength, endurance, proprioception, and coordination. Burkhead and Rockwood[8] reported that 80% of patients with atraumatic subluxations had good or excellent results with conservative treatment when appropriate rehabilitation was used. Other researchers are more conservative regarding the efficacy of the outcomes.[69-71] An accurate diagnosis and an appropriate, conservative treatment program can lead to a successful outcome in most patients and are essential for successful rehabilitation.[69]

Functional instabilities occur primarily in one direction. However, they can present with global laxity, commonly referred to as *multidirectional instability*.[72]

Voluntary instability, another classification of instability, usually is due to congenital hypermobility or laxity combined with the patient using the shoulder muscles to purposely and spontaneously subluxate the joint.[53,73] For example, patients commonly say, "Look what happens when I do this," as they voluntarily sublux the shoulder.

This condition may provide an element of secondary gain for these individuals, and treatment is difficult. *Involuntary instability* is a recurrent dislocation in a person whose shoulder is so unstable that it dislocates spontanaeously.[9]

A dislocation may be acute or chronic. An acute frank dislocation usually is reducible with a variety of manipulation techniques described elsewhere.[74,75] Reduction of a traumatic dislocation by manipulation should be attempted only by an experienced clinician. Occasionally the dislocation is irreducible, and open reduction may be required to extricate the structures preventing reduction; this condition is called a *complex dislocation,* in which interpositioning soft tissue blocks reduction.

With a chronic dislocation, the humeral head has been out of contact with the glenoid cavity for a protracted period (i.e., days to years). Unreduced posterior dislocations are the most common chronic dislocations because of the incidence of missed diagnosis. If the chronic nature of the dislocation is not recognized, attempts at closed reduction will be unsuccessful or may even result in a fracture.[56] Chronic dislocations invariably require open reduction. In studies of posterior instability, damage occurs to both the anterior and posterior aspects of the capsule.[75,76]

The principles of diagnosis of a dislocated or unstable shoulder were outlined earlier in the chapter. Usually the diagnosis is self-evident from the history, signs, and symptoms. The two most common mechanisms of injury are the arm being forced into 90° or more abduction and 90° lateral rotation, and falling backward with the arm in extension.

The signs and symptoms of any dislocation or instability vary, depending on the severity. Patient complaints range from a vague sense of shoulder dysfunction to marked apprehension and pain, especially if the injury has been traumatic and the dislocation is unreduced. Reduction of the dislocation or subluxation usually provides immediate relief of pain, which is followed by a residual dull ache. Muscle spasm may make reduction difficult without the use of muscle relaxants, especially for the glenohumeral joint. A step deformity and loss of range of motion are evident with a dislocation. Several days later, bruising and ecchymosis may be seen. If the patient complains of paresthesia, numbness, or muscle weakness, the clinician must be alert to the possibility of nerve injury, especially to the axillary nerve.

For dislocations, at least two radiographic views of the shoulder from two different angles are desirable to prevent a missed diagnosis, particularly with a posterior dislocation. X-ray films for an anterior dislocation should include a true anteroposterior (AP) view of the shoulder and a true lateral view of the scapula (Table 5-2). A transcapular view is difficult to obtain in an acutely injured shoulder. A full medial rotation view is commonly obtained to determine whether a Hill-Sachs lesion is present on the articular surface of the humeral head.

Table 5-2
Radiographic Imaging for Different Shoulder Pathologies

Pathology	Radiographic Imaging
Impingement	Anteroposterior (AP) x-ray film in the plane of the scapula Supraspinatus outlet view Axillary AP x-ray film, 30° caudal view (anterior acromial view)
Instability	AP x-ray film in the plane of the scapula Stryker Notch view West Point axillary view Axillary
Arthritis	AP x-ray film in the plane of the scapula Full humerus AP x-ray film in the plane of the scapula with laterally rotated 30° Axillary
Trauma	AP x-ray film in the plane of the scapula Axillary True scapular lateral view (Y view)

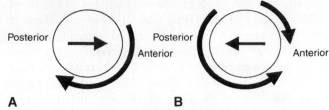

Figure 5-4
Circle concept of instability. Capsuloligamentous structures act together as a circular cuff. **A,** For anterior dislocation to occur, the capsular structures must be disrupted as far as the 7 o'clock position posteriorly. **B,** For posterior dislocation to occur, a significant amount of anterior damage is necessary. (From Zachazewski JE, Magee DJ, Quillen WS, editors: *Athletic injuries and rehabilitation*, p 522, Philadelphia, 1996, WB Saunders.)

Anterior Dislocations

Anterior dislocations account for about 95% of acute traumatic glenohumeral injuries.[76] They occur most frequently in young adults. With an anterior glenohumeral dislocation, the head of the humerus is driven or levered anteriorly and often sits under the coracoid process; this is called a *subcoracoid dislocation*. The anterior capsule may be torn, or the glenoid labrum may be stripped from the anteroinferior aspect of the glenoid cavity (i.e., Bankart lesion). If no Bankart lesion is found, the anterior or lateral capsule may be disrupted.[75] If the capsule alone is injured, the potential for healing is good. With greater damage and stripping of the glenoid labrum, the chances for recurrent dislocation are greater because the potential for healing and spontaneous reattachment of the fibrocartilaginous labrum is poorer. The labral edge becomes atrophic and rounded, forming an inadequate anterior buttress to humeral head translation. The intact labrum is important for maintaining a suctionlike vacuum effect; although it is most important as a static stabilizer, it also enhances dynamic support of the joint.[15,16] The glenohumeral joint usually is bathed in less than 1 mL of synovial fluid,[77] which helps hold the articular surfaces together and enhances the normal negative intra-articular pressure.[17,29] Excessive fluid (usually blood) negates this effect. It should be pointed out, however, that although the damage is primarily anterior, structures in the posterior aspect of the joint may also be injured; this is referred to as the *circle concept of instability,* and the clinician must be alert to the possibility of injury on the opposite side of the joint (Figure 5-4).

On examination, a deformity (i.e., step deformity) or space usually is detected under the tip of the acromion, resulting in prominence of the acromion, flattening of the deltoid muscle, pain, and loss of motion; the patient tends to support the arm in 30° of abduction with the other arm while listing to the affected side. Attempts at movement in any direction are painful, and the humeral head may be palpable in the axilla.

Anterior glenohumeral dislocations have several associated complications (of which recurrence is the most common). These may include injury to the axillary, musculocutaneous, or median nerves or, more rarely, the brachial plexus.[19] Only about 20% of these dislocations show minimal clinical signs, and 5% show significant evidence of neurological involvement; however, Rockwood demonstrated that up to 80% of individuals show electromyographic evidence of nerve injury.[53] This damage initially may be subclinical, with the patient showing no detectable weakness. Consequently, it is essential that the clinician repeatedly check and monitor for paresthesia and changes in the strength of the deltoid muscle. Other complications include rotator cuff tears (the likelihood of these tears increases with advancing age), tears of the glenoid labrum, damage to the articular surface of the humeral head (i.e., Hill-Sachs lesion), damage to the biceps tendon and, on occasion, fractures of the greater tuberosity or the neck of the humerus. Vascular injury must also be considered and can be potentially limb threatening.[78]

Recurrent dislocations, sometimes referred to as "trick shoulders," tend to be anterior dislocations that are intracapsular.[76] They are due either to repeated traumatic dislocation, with each dislocation occurring more easily, or to a congenital defect, such as a lax capsule or shallow glenoid. In active patients under age 20, the recurrence rate can be as high as 90% after a traumatic dislocation, whereas in nonathletes in the same age group, the recurrence rate is 30%. In the 20 to 30 age group, the recurrence rate can be as high as 60%. The recurrence rate declines with age, with fewer recurrent dislocations occurring after age 40.[21,23,78,79] Most of these dislocations (75%) occur within 2 years of the initial traumatic event.[79] Many of these dislocations eventually are treated surgically, because the anatomy of the labrocapsular complex has been disrupted. Nonoperative treatment is successful in some established recurrent dislocations, but it is ineffective for most individuals with recurrent episodes, partly because the dynamic stabilizers (i.e., muscles) are in a poor position to control the humeral head with the arm abducted and laterally rotated. Furthermore, the power muscles (e.g., pectoralis major, anterior deltoid) are thought to contribute to pulling the humeral head out of the joint if sufficient laxity is present. Surgical stabilization, therefore, is appropriate for those with significant functional instability, and excellent success rates usually are achieved.[23] The choice of surgical technique and the timing and extent of surgery depend on the degree and direction of instability, the requirements for range of motion, the associated soft tissue damage, and the surgeon's preference and skills.

Posterior Dislocations

Posterior, or subspinous, dislocations result from the arm being forced or thrust backward when it is forward flexed; these injuries account for about 2% of all glenohumeral dislocations. On examination, posterior prominence of the humeral head may not be evident, and rounding of the shoulder or deltoid is maintained, therefore these dislocations sometimes are missed or misdiagnosed, especially in more heavily built individuals. Some flattening of the anterior shoulder may be seen, and the coracoid process may be more prominent than on the uninjured side. The patient has limited lateral rotation (less than 0°) and limited elevation (less than 90°), which are signs requiring further investigation. In addition, medial rotation and cross-flexion (horizontal adduction) cause pain and apprehension. Posterior dislocations are recognized by the "empty glenoid" sign on the x-ray film (Figure 5-5). The AP view of the normal shoulder shows overlapping of the humeral head and glenoid shadows, which are absent or reduced with a posterior dislocation.

The complex pathophysiology involved in posterior shoulder dislocations has led to the development of numerous surgical techniques to address this problem.[80] Soft tissue techniques range from a simple posterior capsular plication to a posteroinferior capsular shift.[81] Labral repairs may be added to these techniques. Additional bony techniques include wedge osteotomies with or without a bone block and humeral rotation osteotomies.[82] More recently, with improved understanding of the circumstances of posterior instability and more advanced arthroscopic techniques, surgeons have been able to attempt stabilization through arthroscopic surgery with fairly good functional outcomes.[83] Postoperative care varies widely, but if the

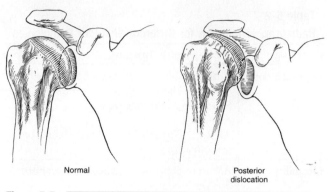

Figure 5-5

"Empty glenoid" sign of posterior dislocation on an anteroposterior x-ray film. Note that the head of the humerus fills the glenoid in the normal x-ray film *(left)*. With a posterior dislocation, the glenoid is "empty," especially in its anterior portion *(right)*. (From Zachazewski JE, Magee DJ, Quillen WS, editors: *Athletic injuries and rehabilitation,* p 523, Philadelphia, 1996, WB Saunders.)

practitioner has an appreciation of the techniques used and follows the treatment principles outlined in this chapter, a customized treatment program can be developed to suit each specific situation.

Treatment of a Dislocated Shoulder

In the management of acute dislocations of the shoulder, an attempt must be made to characterize the injury. A major difficulty in developing a treatment plan from the older literature is the failure of the literature to separate groups adequately according to the underlying degree of injury and the direction of laxity.[84] A glenohumeral dislocation usually is reduced using closed techniques and adequate anesthesia. It is important to recheck the patient's neural and vascular status both before and after reduction and to obtain a second x-ray film to ensure proper positioning.

With dislocations, subluxations, or instability, a concerted, focused effort at nonoperative treatment with a well-planned, well-coordinated therapy program must be attempted. This principle is more important in cases in which the shoulder is more lax, the collagen hyperelasticity is greater, and less trauma is involved in the initial dislocation. If a Bankart lesion or other structural deficiencies are found, they usually are dealt with surgically as soon as possible.

For acute anterior dislocations, treatment begins with adequate early controlled immobilization. After closed reduction, the shoulder is immobilized with a swath and sling for 6 weeks (in young adults) to prevent extension, abduction, and lateral rotation, which promotes good capsular healing. Some researchers have reported that the period or position of immobilization bears little relation to the recurrence of dislocation,[80] and some authors advocate a shorter period of immobilization (1 to 3 weeks).[32,79] The duration of immobilization depends on the philosophy of the physician or surgeon and the type of reconstruction if surgical repair is performed.

In the first 2 weeks after reduction, a program of strong isometric deltoid, shoulder abductor, adductor, and biceps work is instituted within the limits of pain tolerance. Scapular control exercises can be initiated right away within pain-free range of motion. This minimizes muscle wasting as the edema and hemorrhage resolve and the shoulder becomes more comfortable. Two to 6 weeks after injury, the swath is removed for exercises several times a day. Small range, gentle, closed kinetic chain exercises can be initiated provided the movement is pain free. The emphasis is still on isometric activities, with neutral shoulder medial and lateral rotator isometric exercises taking precedence. In addition, concentric exercises through a limited range are permitted, with the clinician bearing in mind that capsular healing is well under way at 3 weeks. The limits of range are determined by pain and whether the patient can comfortably control the movement.

Controlled movements are essential for rehabilitation to occur. Movement commonly can be allowed within a "cone" of 30° abduction, 30° to 60° forward flexion, and lateral rotation to neutral with the elbow never extending through the frontal plane of the body. The controlled active movement applies small amounts of stress to the joint structures to reduce the adverse effects of immobilization on the glenohumeral joint.[32,37,85,86] At no point during this time should abduction and forward flexion go beyond 90°, nor should lateral rotation go past neutral. In older individuals, in whom the danger of stiffness leading to adhesive capsulitis and frozen shoulder is greater than the risks of redislocation, the movement program is initiated at the beginning. Once immobilization has ended, the treatment protocol follows the same principles as for treatment of patients with impingement or instability (see later discussion).

Surgical Treatment of Shoulder Impingement and Instability

Indications for surgery and open reduction include inability to reduce by closed reduction; presence of a large flake of avulsed bone on the inferior glenoid margin, which may contribute to future instability; a significantly displaced glenoid fracture involving a third or more of the articular surface; vascular impairment; and an associated displaced tuberosity fracture or a fracture of the neck of the humerus. On occasion, very athletic individuals may want a guarantee of stability in the shoulder by having early surgery. Postoperative care depends on the type and degree of associated problems that led to open reduction and repair.

Symptomatic recurrent anterior shoulder instability may be treated effectively with capsular plication techniques performed arthroscopically. In the past these arthroscopic approaches have been associated with worrisome redislocation rates.[87,88] With strict technical criteria, including restoration of the proper resting length of the glenohumeral ligament and recreation of the labral "bumper" effect, current arthroscopic techniques offer success rates comparable to open techniques. Strict clinical guidelines for suitable patient selection also are important.

The arthroscopic approach offers several advantages, such as less invasive techniques, good cosmesis, and an excellent return of range of motion with rehabilitation; however, the timeline to full function is not necessarily shortened.[88,89] Similarly, open capsular shift has been the treatment of choice for multidirectional instability over the past 20 years and is successful in 80% to 95% of individuals, but arthroscopic suture capsulorrhaphy techniques now approach these success rates.[90] The arthroscopic techniques have the advantage of greatly reducing associated morbidity and must now be considered the treatment of choice.

Surgical procedures may be arthroscopic, arthroscopically assisted with a miniarthrotomy, a combination of arthroscopy and open repair or reconstruction, or an open arthrotomy technique. The spectrum of surgical approaches involves capsular plications of varying complexity (e.g., arthroscopic capsulorrhaphy; inferior, posterior, or anterior capsular shift; and subscapular muscle and capsule tightening in distinct layers or as a single layer). Thermal capsulorrhaphy has a limited application, and its usefulness has been questioned. Its proposed role is in capsular laxity without dislocation, and it has been used to produce tissue shrinkage in nonathletes.[91] Close postoperative monitoring is essential for successful results.[91]

Bony procedures also may be performed, including osteotomy and wedging of the glenoid (for posterior dislocation), humeral rotational procedures, osteotomies, and conjoint tendon transfer using the tip of the coracoid (variations of the Bristow procedure) (Table 5-3).[32,92-107]

Open procedures that address the disrupted labrum and with anterior capsule plication variations of the Putti-Platt repair) are very effective but pose the risk of restricting lateral rotation unduly in some individuals and may not be desirable for athletes.[79] These procedures may be enhanced by restoration of any part of the labral rim that may have become detached (Bankart repair). Magnuson-Stack–type procedures are particularly difficult to adapt to very active individuals, because insufficient single layer plication leads to an unacceptable redislocation rate, and overtightening inappropriately limits lateral rotation. These open techniques have been used less frequently over the past 10 years.

The Bristow procedure works well for most athletes but results in some minor restriction of full abduction and

Table 5-3
Open Surgical Procedures for Anterior Dislocation

Type	Name	Procedure	Redislocation Rate*	Comment
Bone block	Eden-Hybbinette-Lange procedure[93]	Bone block to increase the anterior margin of the glenoid	0 to 18%[92,94,104] Average: 6%	Decreased lateral rotation Late degenerative changes
Coracoid transfer	Bristow-Helfet procedure[95]	Transfer of the tip of the coracoid process, along with the conjoint tendon of the biceps and the coracobrachialis muscle	3% to 6%[92,95] Average: 1.9%[104]	A dynamic component Poor for throwing athletes 10% decrease in biceps power
Capsular repairs	DuToit staple capsulorrhaphy[96]	Reattachment of the anterior capsule to the anterior glenoid margin	5% to 28%[97,105] Average: 88%[92,105]	Unacceptable redislocation and subluxation rates if not combined with other procedures
	Bankart procedure[98]	Reattachment of the glenoid labrum and plicate anterior capsule	0 to 5%[30,99] Average: 3.3%[105]	Low redislocation rate May restrict lateral rotation
	Putti-Platt procedure[100]	Reattachment of the labrum and plicate capsule and the subscapularis muscle separately	2% to 11%[99,101] Average: 2.8%	Good stability Addresses pathological anatomy
	Magnuson-Stack procedure[102]	Staple placation of the entire anterior capsule and the subscapularis muscle	2% to 17%[92,103] Average: 7.5%[104]	Problem with redislocation and biceps tendon involvement

From Zachazewski JE, Magee DJ, Quillen WS, editors: *Athletic injuries and rehabilitation*, p 524, Philadelphia, 1996, WB Saunders.
*Variable, depending on the surgeon, the patient population, the period of follow-up, and the number in the series.

lateral rotation combined with abduction and extension. It has proved to be a good procedure for athletes involved in high contact sports, such as hockey, football, and rugby. However, it is not the best choice for throwing athletes, who need full lateral rotation in abduction, which may be limited by this approach. The Bristow procedure is an option that should be considered when a high degree of stabilization is required.

Arthroscopic stabilization currently is the standard of care. With soft tissue surgical techniques, it is important to allow sufficient time for capsular healing with minimal stress to these tissues. With bony techniques, such as the Bristow procedure, a period of approximately 6 weeks is required to allow for union of the bone block before stress is applied.

For patients who require absolute full range of motion or who have any significant component of multidirectional instability, one of the inferior capsular shift procedures is more appropriate.[108] The principle behind these repairs is to tighten the middle and inferior glenohumeral ligaments, with due regard given to the circle concept of instability (see Figure 5-4).

After operative treatment, the traditional Putti-Platt procedure has a 1% to 5% incidence of recurrent dislocation; the Magnuson-Stack operation, 1% to 9%; and the Bristow repair, 1% to 6%.[105] These results should be compared to the increasingly successful outcomes of arthroscopically assisted techniques, which, as surgeons have become more experienced, have reached and surpassed the open

techniques. Return to a high level of function is the rule with an appropriately selected and executed technique performed with due regard for the pathological lesion and the activity goals of the patient.

Although postoperative therapy is based on tissue healing principles and proper stress to the tissues, each surgeon has certain criteria that he or she wants followed in a rehabilitation program. The clinician must be aware of these criteria, including the reasons for them, along with any restrictions or modifications to treatment, to prevent any misunderstanding with the surgeon and patient's desired outcome.

Postsurgical Treatment of the Shoulder

The basic rehabilitation plan may be modified, depending on the type of surgical procedure performed, precautions to treatment noted by the surgeon, the individual surgeon's preferences, and whether pain, restriction, or both are factors. For the most part, the treatment of patients undergo arthroscopic procedures parallels that for patients who have open techniques, although the former have less tissue disruption and muscle wasting. The patient's willingness to move and the quality of the patient's movements also are of concern to the clinician. Only broad guidelines are given for progression. The treatment principles remain constant: to relieve pain, to observe for complications, to regain muscle control, to strengthen, to regain range of motion safely, to improve endurance, and to retrain proprioceptive control. These guidelines form the foundation of an activity-based protocol. Specificity plays a major role; each program must be individualized to the patient and his activities.

Principles of Specificity Related to Sports and Rehabilitation

Every athletic event makes specific demands in terms of load (stress), rate, repetitions, duration, and neurophysiological adjustment. When a new or modified task with a different demand in intensity, load, rate, repetitions, duration, or neurophysiological adjustment is instituted, an entirely new pattern of adjustment must be acquired. Therefore training and rehabilitation must be specific to the sport or activity in which the athlete hopes to take part. This principle applies to all of the following:

1. Cardiovascular fitness (aerobic and anaerobic activities)
2. Strength training (isometric, isotonic [concentric and eccentric], isokinetic)
3. Open chain and closed chain activities
4. Motor skills and motor learning
5. Flexibility (static, dynamic)
6. Coordination
7. Proprioceptive control
8. Timing, reaction time, and movement time
9. Progression
10. Biomechanical demands
11. Tissue healing and stress

To achieve progression in these areas, the clinician proceeds from:

1. General to specific
2. Simple to complex
3. Easy to difficult
4. Lesser to greater volume
5. Lesser to greater intensity
6. Lesser to greater frequency

From Zachazewski JE, Magee DJ, Quillen WS, editors: *Athletic injuries and rehabilitation*, p 527, Philadelphia, 1996, WB Saunders.

Postsurgical treatment initially concentrates primarily on the scapula. Scapular control exercises focus primarily on the lower and middle trapezius and serratus anterior. These exercises include scapular retraction, depression, protraction, and elevation with the arm at the side. Careful observation should detect compensatory shoulder postures that indicate incorrect firing (contraction) sequences. As the patient improves, the glenohumeral joint can be taken into abduction, scaption (plane of the scapula), forward flexion, and other elevation movements, provided the patient can maintain control of the scapula and can stabilize the humerus in the glenoid. Lateral rotation should be performed only with extreme care and never beyond neutral in the early stages of rehabilitation (i.e., the hand should never go outside the sagittal plane of the body, and the elbow should never go behind the frontal plane of the body). These are important early rules, regardless of the surgical procedure used. Keeping inside this "cone"

reduces the stress on the anterior labrum and the repaired soft tissues to a minimum. During rotation exercises, the clinician should watch for excessive winging, because the scapula may be compensating for tight medial or lateral rotators. If present, this can be treated with joint play techniques or muscle energy/proprioceptive neuromuscular facilitation (PNF) techniques, depending on whether the restriction is caused by inert tissues or the muscles.

Postoperative exercises for the shoulder should not cause sharp or severe pain. It is acceptable for the patient to be slightly uncomfortable when doing exercises, but they must be done with confidence and a sense of control. The discomfort should disappear when the exercise stops. The clinician must ensure that the exercises are done correctly. Correct movement patterns are more important than load or speed. Once proper scapular control is achieved up to 30° of abduction, the clinician can move on to 30° to 90°, and when proper dynamic control has been gained in that range, the patient can be progressed to 180°.[109]

Once control of the scapula is achieved, isometrics to the muscles of the glenohumeral joint are instituted at several positions in the range of motion below shoulder level, with no lateral rotation beyond 0°. The positioning and resistance depend on the patient's response to pain and discomfort. The clinician must make sure that both the scapular control and humeral control muscles receive attention.[31] The patient is instructed to perform proper isometrics into abduction, medial rotation, lateral rotation (to 0°), extension, and a "full can" (neutral) position (below horizontal) for the supraspinatus. Even if the patient is in a sling, rhythmic stabilization exercises and co-contraction at the joint (in the Hawkins position) can be performed to the affected shoulder (Figure 5-6). If the patient complains of pain in the shoulder, cold can be applied to give some relief. In addition, active exercise to the other joints of the arm and the rest of the body may be instituted to ensure involvement of the whole kinetic chain.

As the patient improves (as evidenced by decreased pain and discomfort), isotonic exercises, especially flexion and extension, can be initiated (usually by the third or fourth day), again below shoulder level and with no lateral rotation beyond 0°, within the pain-free and controllable range. By the fourth day, medial and lateral rotation to 0° with the arm in the adducted position may be performed very carefully. For the lateral rotators, only very careful isometrics should be performed, to prevent excessive stress to the tissues. By the fifth day, the patient may begin assisted abduction. To achieve proper scapular and humeral control, exercises are used when appropriate and when strength and pain allow.[109] Once the pain has diminished and as the patient is weaned from the sling, the clinician can follow the treatment concepts for rehabilitation of shoulder instability described later in the chapter.

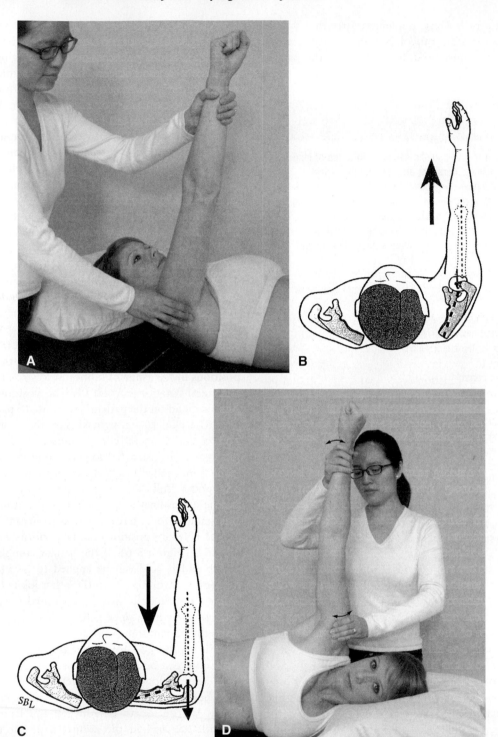

Figure 5-6

Isometric hold (rhythmic stabilization) in the Hawkins position. **A,** In forward flexion; note that the clinician is stabilizing the glenohumeral joint. Resistance of stabilization at the glenohumeral joint can lead to co-contraction of the muscles of the shoulder. **B,** Line drawing shows how the glenohumeral joint is more stable with the glenoid lying under the head of the humerus in the Hawkins position than in **C. D,** In abduction. (**B** and **C** from Matsen FA: Stability. In Matsen FA, Lippett SB, Sidles JA, Harryman DT: *Practical evaluation and management of the shoulder,* p 64, Philadelphia, 1994, WB Saunders.)

Pitfalls of Treatment for Shoulder Instability and Impingement Management

As with any treatment, the clinician must be aware of common pitfalls. If the following mistakes are kept in mind, the rehabilitation program will have every chance of success.

1. *Failure to perform a complete and thorough assessment.* The assessment must involve the shoulder complex, the trunk, and the core, as well as the lower kinetic extremity, to determine which structures are weak and which are tight and to check for incorrect movement patterns.[66,110]

2. *Failure to assess and address scapulohumeral dysfunction.* The clinician must remember that scapular motion is dynamic for the most part and that the scapula constantly moves, even as it functions as a stable base from which most of the glenohumeral muscles originate. Proximal stability (i.e., scapular control) must be achieved early in the rehabilitation process, before distal mobility (i.e., glenohumeral movement) is encouraged.[42,66] Coordinated scapulohumeral movement is affected by muscle length, muscle strength (especially eccentric muscle strength), capsular tightness, the type of muscle contraction (e.g., isometric, concentric, eccentric, econcentric), timing, and pain. Scapular movement itself is affected by gravity, altered posture, tight muscles, whether the activity is an open or closed kinetic chain, the amount of load the arm lifts, and the speed of arm movement. The clinician must keep all these issues in mind when progressing activity.

3. *Failure to understand the mechanics and demands of the activities to which the patient is returning.* The clinician must have a clear picture of these activities, whether they involve sports or are part of the individual's everyday life, such as work or recreational activites.[66] Driving, obviously, is not the same as throwing. Although patients may present with similar types of painful movement, the clinician must be able to assess the problem with a clear understanding of the demands of the activities the patient wants to accomplish. The practitioner must understand that an injury in one part of the body may cause an alteration in another part (i.e., alteration in shoulder mechanics, movement patterns, and how they are accomplished). The shoulder is a link in a kinetic chain of movement.[2-4,66] This kinetic chain allows the generation, summation, transfer, and regulation of forces from the foot to the hand during everyday activity.[2-4,42,62,66] Although individual muscles are the early emphasis in rehabilitation, eventually, as the patient progresses, the whole body must be integrated with shoulder movement patterns (i.e., so that the lower extremity and core drive the shoulder).

4. *Failure to deal with any hypomobility early in the treatment to ensure that the joint can regain normal arthrokinematics.*[66] Particular attention should be paid to tightness of the posterior glenohumeral capsule; restricted glenohumeral medial rotation (GIRD) or imbalance between the medial and lateral rotation range of motion;[3] tightness of the pectoralis minor and pectoralis major; tightness of the inferior glenohumeral ligament (caudal glide of the glenohumeral joint); and hypermobility in the thoracic spine and ribs.[3] Treatment of structures must ensure proper movement patterns. The clinician should teach the patient how to do stretches correctly so that normal tissues are not compromised and surgically repaired structures are not abused.[3,66] The sleeper stretch and modified sleeper stretch (Figure 5-7) are two examples of appropriate stretches for a tight posterior glenohumeral joint capsule.

5. *Failure to make sure that stretches are done properly.* Although stretching may be necessary to restore normal arthrokinematics in a joint, it cannot compromise other structures (e.g., scapular stabilizers) or reinforce faulty movement patterns.

6. *Failure to control pain and painful movement.* Exercises must be virtually pain free (pain is less than 4 on a 0 to 10 pain scale [0 being no pain, 10 being the worst pain the patient can imagine]). Otherwise, rehabilitation will be compromised. Ideally, exercises should be performed in a pain-free range of motion. The clinician must design

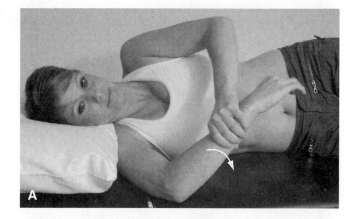

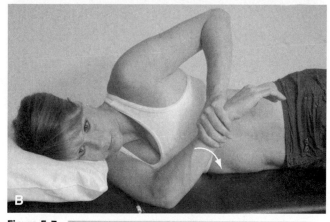

Figure 5-7

A, Sleeper stretch. **B,** Modified sleeper stretch.

exercises that enable the patient to do the activity without pain. It is important to watch for signs of fatigue and to terminate the exercise before excessive fatigue leads to incorrect movement patterns. For example, early activity or overactivity of the upper trapezius is an early sign of fatigue in shoulder exercises.

7. *Failure to correct poor posture.* A normal posture is important for reducing anterior pressure on the anterior labrum and anterior structures of the shoulder. The clinician must make sure the patient can maintain a neutral pelvis position and can hold the neutral pelvis statically and dynamically by ensuring correct alignment of the pelvis and spine. The clinician should also teach the patient to maintain the correct shoulder position by discouraging exercises that cause rounding of the shoulders (e.g., scapular dumping [see Figure 5-3]).

8. *Failure to note habitual exercises done in compensatory postures.* Many clinicians tend to progress exercise routines too quickly, before achieving isolated muscle control, especially of the scapular control muscles. Scapular control implies that the patient is able to control the scapula through contraction of the scapular force couple (lower and upper trapezius, serratus anterior [Figure 5-8]), along with the middle trapezius, rhomboids, and levator scapulae. This is essential, because it enables the patient to establish proper scapular rhythm while moving the arm (i.e., the humerus) in a controlled fashion. Many activities start with

little or no weight, often with gravity eliminated or only very small amounts of weight (0.5 to 0.8 kg [1 to 2 lbs]). Progression in resistance should be small. No advantage is gained from lifting heavy weights.

9. *Failure to select appropriate exercises.* Initially the goal should be to use low risk exercises that use the rotator cuff to compress the head of the humerus into the glenoid; such exercises may include rhythmic stabilization and co-contraction using the Hawkins position (i.e., placing the glenoid under the humerus; see Figure 5-6, *B*).[2-4,66] Low risk exercises that help stabilize the humeral head and keep the shoulder away from compromising impingement postures are preferable. While the patient does the stabilization exercises, the clinician can palpate the humeral head to make sure that it is properly aligned, compressing into the glenoid, and not translating excessively. The clinician also can make sure that the anterior deltoid contracts and is part of the exercise. Shoulder depression against tubing resistance while doing circles or figures-of-eight (Figure 5-9) is another example of a

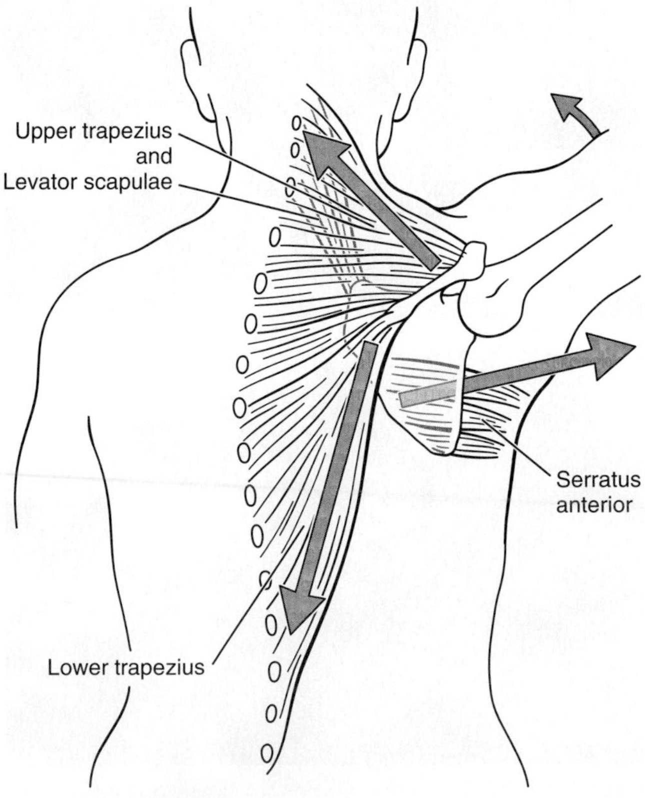

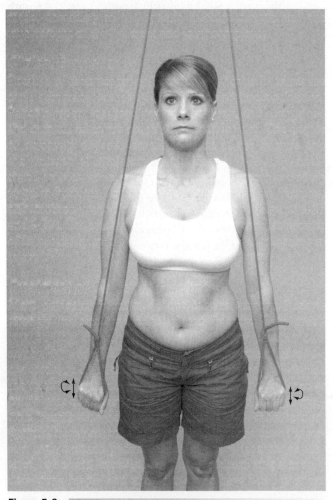

Figure 5-9
Shoulder depression (dynamic caudal glide) using tubing. Example exercises include having a patient do circles or figures-of-eight or write her name. The clinician should always be watching for scapular control.

Upper trapezius and Levator scapulae

Serratus anterior

Lower trapezius

Figure 5-8
Scapular force couple.

low risk exercise. Punch out exercises (Figure 5-10, *A*), dynamic hug (Figure 5-10, *B*), and push-ups with a plus (Figure 5-10, *C*), along with PNF exercises (D2 patterns) (Figure 5-11) work the serratus anterior and help ensure minimal upper trapezius activity. Forward flexion wall exercises with the hands on a ball in a closed kinetic chain (Figure 5-12) also are low risk exercises. The clinician's repertoire of rotator cuff exercises must include more than simple medial and lateral rotation in neutral. The empty can position

puts the glenohumeral joint in a compromising impingement posture and in the anterior tipped (i.e., scapular dump) position. The classic empty can strengthening exercise actually is an impingement posture and is not functional for most activities.[111] This exercise does not help to re-establish scapulohumeral rhythm and often is painful early in the rehabilitation process, leading to counterproductive exercises. The clinician should always be aware that traditional weight room exercises used to strengthen the shoulder musculature and

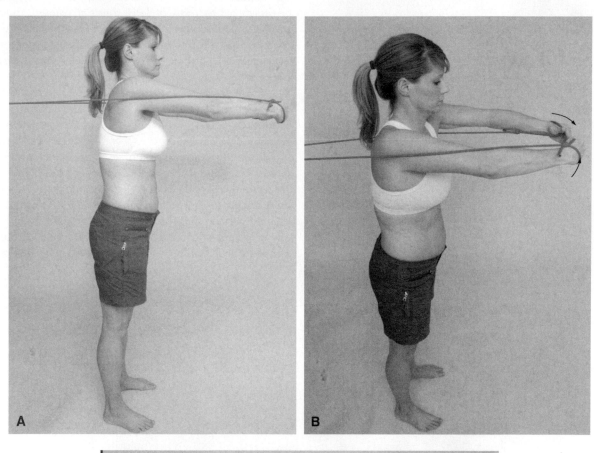

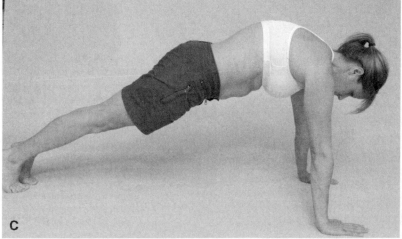

Figure 5-10
Exercises for the serratus anterior. **A,** Punch out. **B,** Dynamic hug. **C,** Push-up with a plus.

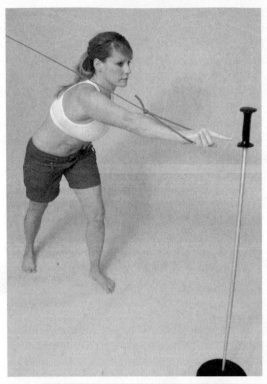

Figure 5-11

Exercise for proprioceptive neuromuscular facilitation using tubing in the lunge position.

surrounding structures often can compound an injury and should be discouraged until the person is in the functional stage of recovery. Traditional gym exercises, such as the bench press and military press, may compound or precipitate shoulder problems. A common mistake of clinicians is to introduce these exercises too early in the rehabilitation program. Early rehabilitation concentrates on training the stabilizers of the scapula and humerus. Once this has been achieved, more complex functional motor patterns can be initiated.

10. *Failure to create an exercise program or to make use of functional patterns in later stages of rehabilitation that integrate lower extremity and trunk movements.* These exercises incorporate the whole kinetic chain and are complementary to traditional rotator cuff and scapulohumeral exercises.[2-4,43,63]

11. *Failure to rehabilitate the deceleration (eccentric) component of shoulder activity.* Controlled eccentric lengthening of muscles, especially the posterior muscles, is essential for proper functional return to activity. The patient needs to control both the concentric and, even more important, the eccentric components (i.e., eccentric braking and shock absorption, especially for the posterior muscles). The patient must be able to control movement regardless of its direction. This is especially important when tubing is used. If the patient has to eccentrically control the shortening of the tubing as well as its lengthening (concentric movement), the exercises

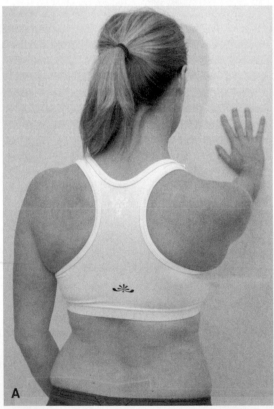

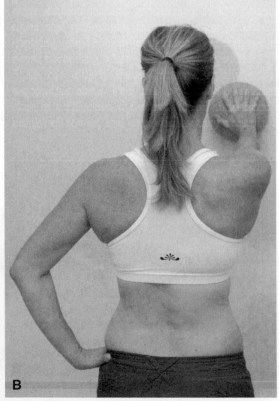

Figure 5-12

Forward flexion closed kinetic chain exercises. **A,** Without a ball. **B,** With a ball. The patient can retract, elevate, depress, and protract the scapula from the position.

become more difficult, the patient will be able to do fewer repetitions, and control will improve more quickly.

12. *Failure to control for fatigue and compensating postures.* The number of repetitions a patient is asked to do should be based on the number the patient can do correctly with control. The clinician should be specific in the instructions regarding the number of repetitions or sets the clinician wants the patient to complete. Normally a specific number of repetitions should not be given; rather, the clinician should watch for and teach the patient to be aware of evidence of fatigue. The patient should recognize fatigue and its compensating postures and stop when they occur. Motor control, muscle memory, the firing (contraction) sequences of muscles (stabilizers, then mobilizers), fatigue patterns, and muscle and cardiovascular endurance all play major roles in the rehabilitation process.

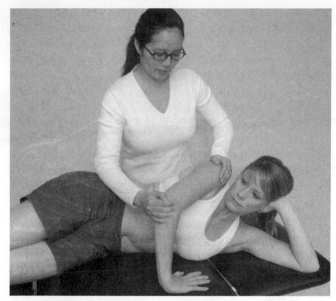

Figure 5-13
Joint stabilization in a closed kinetic chain.

Indicators of Fatigue and Loss of Control

- Erratic movement
- Incorrect movement patterns
- Phasic movements
- Trick movements, loss of control of the scapular base
- Instability jog or catching movement
- Breath holding
- Facial signs of fatigue

13. *Failure to take the time to work one-on-one with the patient.* Clinicians must make sure the patient performs the proper movement patterns and controls posture, and they must assist with the timing and sequencing with compensatory motions. This is done by using individualized, accommodating resistance through all parts of the range of motion.

14. *Failure to address proprioception and kinesthesia.* Proprioception is an important and integral part of the rehabilitation process for shoulder instability. The patient must develop an understanding of the sensation of joint movement as well as joint position. Lephart and Kocker[112] recommended a progression of activities to restore proprioception and neuromuscular control, including starting with joint position sense and kinesthesia, moving on to dynamic joint stabilization, then reactive neuromuscular control, and finally function-specific exercises. For joint position sense, the Hawkins position can be used to position the glenohumeral joint with the patient's eyes open or closed, for rhythmic stabilization and eccentric break exercises (see Figure 5-6). To do these exercises, the clinician positions the patient and then says, "Don't let me move you," while applying co-contraction forces at the joint, along with eccentric breaking forces on the arm. PNF exercises can be used for dynamic joint stabilization and joint loading with closed kinetic chain exercise (Figure 5-13). To train reactive neuromuscular control, plyometrics, throwing and catching, balance drills, and wall falls all play a role later in the rehabilitation process. For functional motor

patterns, PNF (acceleration and deceleration) Body Blade® and Boing® exercises, and actual controlled functional activities can be used.

15. *Failure to use exercise machines with caution.*[43] Generally, machines use long lever arms; this makes controlling the motion difficult and increases the risk of a joint shear. Exercises done on these machines often are not functional and only work isolated parts of the kinetic chain. Also, they often emphasize anterior muscle groups rather than posterior muscle groups, the opposite of the desired effect, especially with anterior instability.

16. *Failure to integrate the patient into the treatment program.* The clinician must convince the patients that their efforts play a crucial role in the rehabilitation process. Treatment for shoulder instability will not succeed unless the patients are actively involved. The patients must feel confident and in control of the rehabilitation exercise program; they also must have a thorough understanding of the exercises they need to do and why they need to do them.

Conservative Treatment of Impingement and Instability

For proper conservative treatment of impingement or instability syndromes, patients must understand the problem and must recognize that the outcome depends on their compliance with the clinician's instructions about what they should and should not do. The physician will prescribe rest, anti-inflammatory medication, pain-relieving medication, and physical therapy in the early stages. In most cases, however, sound rehabilitation is the key to resolution of these problems.

If the problem is one of atraumatic instability, the rehabilitation process follows a course that ensures that the exercises activate the appropriate muscle or muscle groups in the proper sequence and that functional control is achieved (see volume 2 of this series, *Scientific Foundations and Principles of Practice in Musculoskeletal Rehabilitation,* Chapter 19).

Although many modalities may be used to treat instability and impingement, the clinician's primary concern is to restore normal shoulder mechanics and function by restoring the muscles and improving their coordinated action, contraction sequence, strength, endurance, and proprioceptive control.[2-4,42,66]

In the early stages of rehabilitation, the emphasis is on scapular control and humeral head stabilization and restoring the coordinated action of the force couples of the scapulothoracic and glenohumeral joints.[31,66,109,113] This should include integration of the lower limb and trunk as early as possible. Glenohumeral force couples include the subscapularis muscle, a primary stabilizer after anterior dislocation, counterbalanced by the infraspinatus and teres minor muscles, and the deltoid, counterbalanced by the infraspinatus, teres minor, and subscapularis muscles.[26] By establishing strength and neuromuscular control of these force couples, the patient will regain control of humeral head translation during dynamic movement.[60]

The following steps are not necessarily sequential, but the clinician must consider each one to obtain optimum treatment outcomes. For example, with anterior instability, the clinician may treat the anterior glenohumeral joint for pain (step 1.1) while at the same time treating the scapula by ensuring isolated contraction of the lower trapezius (step 2.1)

Proper rehabilitation of instability of the shoulder involves controlled aggressiveness in terms of pushing the patient and pushing the envelope of progression for the patient as much as possible, while make sure the patient can control the movement and do it correctly. Because corrective movement depends on force generation and coordinated action of the muscles, as well as freedom of joint movement, the clinician must ensure that patients work only in the range of motion in which they are able to control the movement and to do the movement correctly (i.e., using correct movement patterns). This is demonstrated by patients working at a speed at which they demonstrate movement control through precise, smooth (nonjerky) movement patterns, although part of the later rehabilitation continuum involves ensuring that patients progress to functional speeds and loads. With instability, the clinician is concerned with dysfunction that is primarily a motor control problem. The stabilization regimen is a multifaceted program that corrects impairment by improving neuromuscular control and coordination of specific muscles and movements of the shoulder. At the same time, the clinician must work to correct the mechanical factors that predispose

or contribute to the abnormal movement patterns. This requires active participation and "buy in" by the patient and an accurate diagnosis by the clinician to determine what restrictions are present; that is, what muscles are at fault and which movements are being done incorrectly. This education and exercise program involves maximum psychological concentration on the part of the patient and very specific movement patterns at minimal speed in a range in which the patient has control. Throughout the process, the principles of specificity apply (see box on p. 137). Stabilization is best achieved by isometric (co-contraction) exercises for static stabilization and concentric-eccentric exercises for dynamic stabilization.

Step 1.1: Reduce Pain

The first step is to relieve pain or at least diminish it, because the aim is to establish pain control.[66] Instability training may be fatiguing, but it should not be painful. Generally, pain should be kept below a 4 on a 0 to 10 VAS scale or at a level that ensures control throughout the exercise (Figure 5-14). This can be accomplished through the use of pain-relieving modalities (e.g., ice, transcutaneous electronic nerve stimulation [TENS], interferential therapy) or by positioning the shoulder in a resting position (Figure 5-15). Other approaches that have a role in pain management include modified traction (e.g., shaking out the arm and "throwing" the arm [Figure 5-16]), glenohumeral compression activities, using a sling, nonsteroidal anti-inflammatory drugs (NSAIDs), and gentle mobilizations.[2-4]

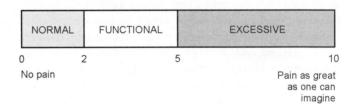

NORMAL	FUNCTIONAL	EXCESSIVE

0   2   5   10

No pain   Pain as great as one can imagine

Figure 5-14

Pain monitoring system.

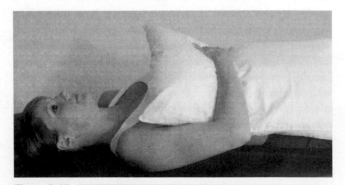

Figure 5-15

Resting position of the shoulder.

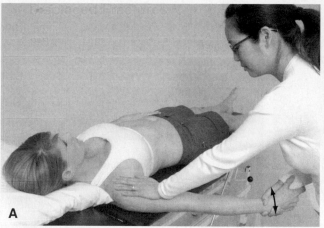
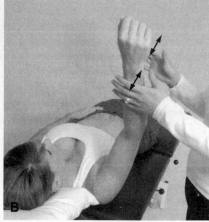

Figure 5-16
A, Shaking out the arm. **B,** Throwing the arm.

Rest from activity is relative and implies decreased length, intensity, and/or frequency of activity. It seldom means total rest. It is important to "take the shoulder for a walk" for 30 minutes each day, which implies moving the shoulder (e.g., swinging the arms while walking).

Step 1.2: Allow Freedom of Movement

The clinician should address any movement restriction in any of the joints of the shoulder complex and in the spine and ribs. This often is necessary to restore normal arthrokinematic movement in the glenohumeral joint (i.e., allowing the humeral head to centralize in the glenoid cavity), the acromioclavicular joint, the sternoclavicular joint, the scapulothoracic "joint," and the thoracic spine and upper ribs.[20,66] The clinician should check for GIRD, restriction of the inferior glenohumeral ligament, and any loss of range in the pectoralis major and pectoralis minor. A tight posteroinferior capsule, which is often seen with impingement syndromes and instability, causes the humeral head to migrate anteriorly and superiorly.[2] All have the potential of being tight.[2-4]

The clinician must always keep in mind the possibility of hypermobility at least in some directions, which tends to be common in individuals with an impingement or instability disorder. Altered glenohumeral arthrokinematics must be assessed and treated as necessary. The clinician must assess carefully to determine which movements are restricted and should treat only these movements, so that the joint play mobilization techniques to stretch the capsule are effective.[113-117] As the circle concept of rehabilitation implies, if the joint is hypermobile in one direction, it may be hypomobile in the opposite direction. With anterior instability, the posteroinferior capsule tends to be tight and therefore requires mobilization, whereas the anterior capsule is hypermobile and requires protection. The clinician

should always check the upper ribs (Figure 5-17) and upper thoracic spine, because these are commonly tight with associated chronic shoulder problems.

Active-assisted exercises using a rigid bar (i.e., a T bar, L bar, wand, or stick) may be used to increase range of motion.[8,74,113] Stretching of the posterior structures can be accomplished using a stick (Figure 5-18), with stretches performed in different ranges of motion of shoulder abduction. In the United States it currently is popular to use a sleeper, modified sleeper, or rollover sleeper stretch or doorway stretch (Figure 5-19). Posterior stretching may also be accomplished by forward flexing the arm and then pushing the humerus posteriorly (Figure 5-20). Humeral head depression (Figure 5-21) is an effective technique for ensuring inferior glide of the humeral head if excursion of the humeral head under the acromion is restricted.[118] It also poses less risk of compromising the medial scapular stabilizers.

After surgery, the clinician should not stretch or stress the anterior capsule in the early stages of recovery. In most postoperative programs, stretching of vulnerable tissues is contraindicated in the first 6 weeks. In these cases, it is important to follow the surgeon's protocols. In nonsurgical cases, stretching should be performed only in hypomobile directions using precise positions and complete control. Restriction may be the result of inert tissue tightness or muscle tightness, and different techniques are used to address these two problems. If the patient has signs of muscle tightness (most commonly the pectoralis minor, subscapularis, infraspinatus, and teres minor),[67] the clinician may use muscle energy techniques, hold/relax, or active release techniques or passive stretching (Figure 5-22). Trigger point therapy, another muscle technique, can be used effectively to increase range with isolated muscle tightness (e.g., the subscapularis) (Figure 5-23). Restriction or loss of abduction or medial or lateral rotation of the shoulder may need to be addressed.[66]

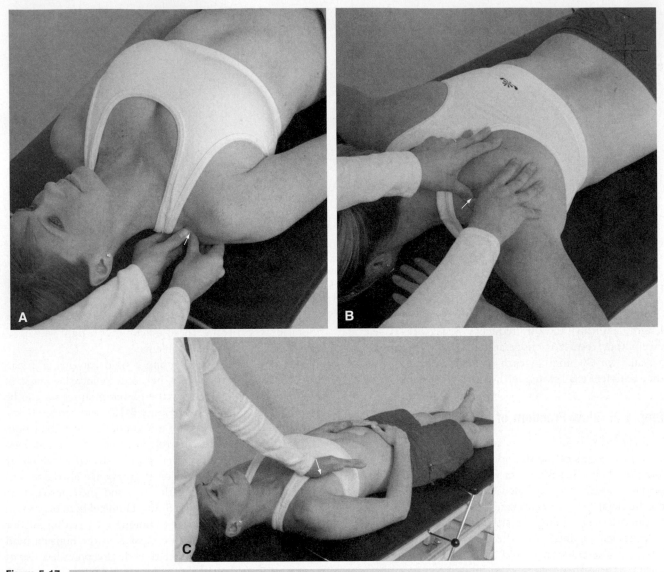

Figure 5-17

Checking the mobility of the ribs. **A,** First rib with patient in the supine position. **B,** First rib with patient in the prone position. **C,** Other ribs.

Because cross syndromes can affect flexibility in the whole kinetic chain, inflexibility in the lower kinetic chain may also have to be addressed.[66] The clinician should assess for and treat any tight lower kinetic chain structures, including the Achilles/calf musculature, hamstrings, hip flexors, abductors, and extensors. Tight trunk flexors and abnormal gait patterns must also be addressed.[66]

Pendular exercises (e.g., the Codman pendular arm swing exercises) may be used initially, provided the exercises are pain free and the patient can control the movement. Caution is required with pendular exercises, especially after arthroscopic surgery, because they apply gravity traction to the repaired vulnerable structures. The clinician may also try modified Codman exercises by having the patient roll a ball on a low chair or table with the elbow extended. This prevents inferior translation and caudal traction on the glenohumeral joint. Anterior translation of the humeral head must be avoided, especially in patients with anterior instability.[119] The clinician must not allow scapular hitching (upward movement) or dumping (downward tilting of the glenoid) with any assisted exercises. The arm may be swung horizontally in a variety of planes. These exercises are useful in the early stages to maintain range of motion, but compensated shoulder postures must be avoided, because some reports have indicated that in pathological shoulder conditions, the upper trapezius and supraspinatus are less likely to relax.[120] Shoulder depression exercises using tubing (dynamic caudal glide) help improve range, enhance scapular control (see Figure 5-9), and promote coordinated scapulohumeral and glenohumeral activity.

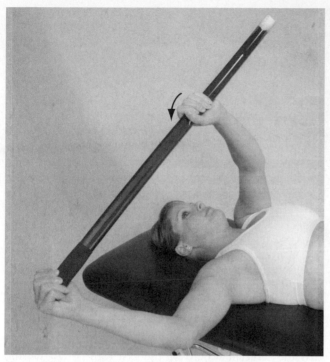

Figure 5-18

A stick can be used to increase the range of motion in the glenohumeral joint.

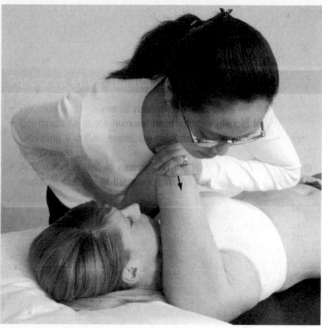

Figure 5-20

Stretching the posterior capsule of the glenohumeral joint. The clinician forward flexes the arm to 90° and then uses the left hand to push the humerus backward. As this happens, the clinician carefully adducts the arm, increasing the tension on the posterior capsule.

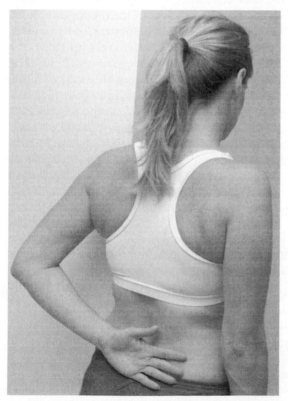

Figure 5-19

Doorway stretch for tight anterior structures.

Step 2.1: Ensure Proper Muscle Function

This stage involves restoring individual muscle function to ensure proper muscle recruitment. Proper contraction of the scapular force couple, including the middle and lower trapezius along with the serratus anterior, requires special attention. If the patient does appropriate exercises and compensatory postures are not allowed, these muscles will not "turn on." The upper trapezius and latissimus dorsi can dominate in compensatory postures, causing an incorrect movement pattern. For example, with a Kibler type III dyskinesia of the scapula, the upper trapezius, levator scapulae, and posterior deltoid do not function in concert most of the time, resulting in the postural deformity.[2-4,67] Biofeedback may be used to teach the patient to contract the desired muscle and to "turn off" the unwanted compensatory muscle contraction.

To encourage isolated muscle contractions (i.e., specificity), the patient is positioned in the "muscle test" position for that muscle.[38-40] The clinician positions the patient so as to isolate the muscle and then asks the patient to hold the position to ensure that the desired isometric contraction is achieved. The patient contracts the muscle only to 10% to 30% of the maximum voluntary contraction (MVC) to ensure an isolated contraction to a concentrate contraction of the muscle.

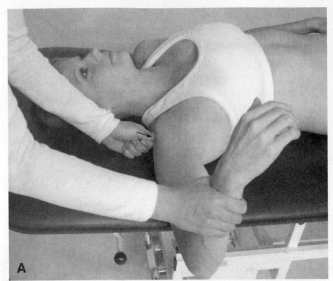
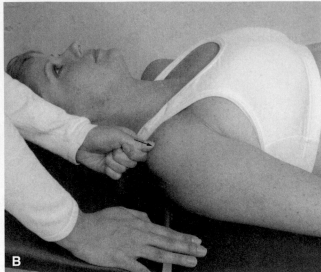

Figure 5-21
Humeral head depression. **A,** Arm by the side. **B,** Arm in 90° abduction.

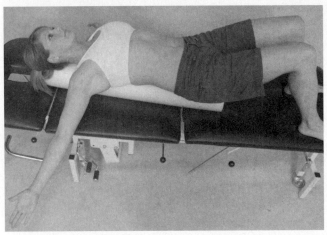

Figure 5-22
Stretching the anterior shoulder structures on a foam roll.

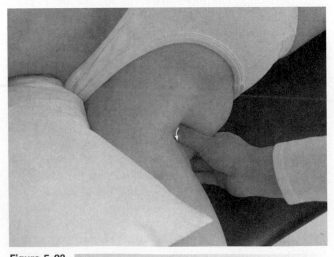

Figure 5-23
Trigger point therapy to the subscapularis.

During these early stages of treatment, it is important that the clinician watch for the first sign of fatigue and stop the patient when it appears. Early on, patients commonly find contracting the isolated muscles difficult, and they frequently show psychological as well as physiological fatigue.

If inferior instability is present, the supraspinatus and deltoid muscles must be given special attention, along with the compression component of the rotator cuff.

Postural correction is an important component of this step. The clinician should determine whether the patient can achieve the neutral pelvis position (i.e., stabilize the core) and hold the position during both static and dynamic activities. As the patient begins to assume and hold the neutral pelvis position, the posture will begin to correct. If the connection is slow or the patient appears to be having problems, the clinician must look for potential restrictive and weak cross syndromes that are limiting the return to normal posture and stretch (e.g., pectoralis minor, hip flexors) and strengthen these components (e.g., abdominal flexors, scapular control muscles).

Step 2.2: Ensure Proper Muscle Recruitment and Motor Patterns

At this stage, treatment is directed primarily at the stabilizer muscles of the scapula, followed by the stabilizers of the glenohumeral joint, because these muscles maintain the normal relationship between the glenohumeral and scapulothoracic joints. The scapular stabilizers provide a stable base for the arm, preserve deltoid fiber length so that acromiohumeral length is maintained, and lessen impingement of the rotator cuff. Proper activation and functioning of the scapular stabilizers is essential[44,66,121] (see Table 4-1).

The clinician must ensure that scapular substitution patterns are not occurring and that the stabilizer muscles contract before the mobilizer muscles.[122] For example, when the patient abducts the arm to 30°, the scapula should stabilize and "lock in" in this phase of scapulohumeral rhythm. Correct scapulohumeral rhythm is paramount. In the first phase of arm abduction (0° to 30°), no or minimal scapular movement should occur. In the second phase (30° to 90°), the scapula should rotate but show minimal protraction or elevation. In the third phase (90° to 180°), lateral rotation to the humerus is necessary. In scaption (i.e., the plane of the scapula), scapulohumeral rhythm is slightly different, with more individual variation in the movement, and more scapular rotation and protraction are common. In scaption less lateral rotation of the humerus occurs and less stress is placed on the tissues of the shoulder. Therefore scaption is a good position for working the patient initially, because there tends to be less pain with movement and scaption is a more common functional movement pattern. If the scapula keeps moving during the first 30° of abduction, the scapular stabilizers are not functioning properly and the mobilizers are dominating, or the exercise is too advanced for the patient.

If the patient is having difficulty determining how to contract individual muscles, electrical stimulation or biofeedback may be used.[123] Useful scapular control exercises include retraction and depression of the scapula, as well as elevation and protraction. This involves individual exercises for the three parts of the trapezius muscle, the serratus anterior, the rhomboids, and the levator scapulae. Exercises for the scapular control muscles include scapular squeezes or pinch, thumb tubes (Figure 5-24, *A*), and power square patterns (Figure 5-24, *B*) for the middle and lower trapezius; dynamic hug and punch outs for the serratus anterior; shoulder depression with tubing and press down exercises (Figure 5-25).[66]

At this step force-couple training also plays a predominant role. Force-couple training involves recruitment of the muscles, along with synchronized action of the muscles using loaded and unloaded activities. Co-contraction with rhythmic stabilizations has a stabilizing and stiffening effect, adds compression for joint position sense, and tends to be done isometrically.[66] Coordinated co-activation results in low peak torque on the shoulder and increased joint control. Co-contraction primarily works the small (inner cone) muscles (i.e., the rotator cuff) of the joint. An example is rhythmic stabilization to the humeral head in the Hawkins punch out position and closed kinetic chain scapular "clock" exercises (the patient moves the scapula through the different hours of a clock while stabilizing the hand against the wall). These exercises also help emphasize the rotator cuff and reduce deltoid activation.[43,66]

Closed kinetic chain activities in the shoulder (e.g., rhythmic stabilization) are more stable, involve less translation, and provide static stability and therefore are used with co-activation.[66] Closed kinetic chain activities provide

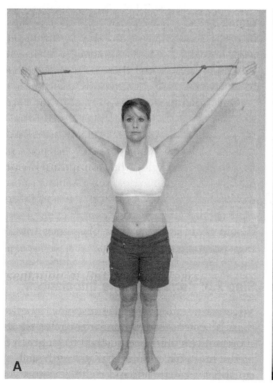 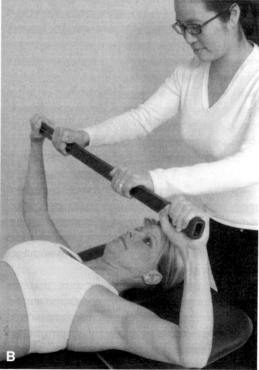

Figure 5-24

A, Thumb tube exercises working the middle and lower trapezius. **B,** Power square position.

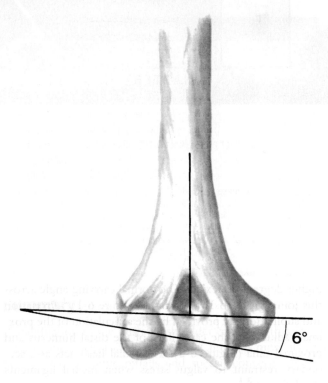

Figure 6-1

Anatomy of the distal humerus, showing how the bony anatomy contributes to the overall valgus alignment of the elbow. There is approximately 6° to 8° of valgus tilt of the distal humeral articulation with respect to the long axis of the humerus. (From Morrey BF: *The elbow and its disorders*, ed 2, p 24, Philadelphia, 1993, WB Saunders.)

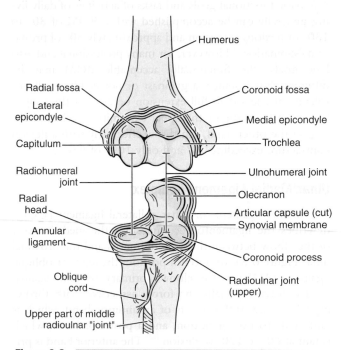

Figure 6-2

Anterior view of the right elbow, disarticulated to expose the ulnohumeral and radiohumeral joints. The margin of the proximal radioulnar joint is shown within the elbow's capsule. (From Magee DJ: *Orthopedic physical assessment*, ed 5, p 362, St. Louis, 2007, WB Saunders.)

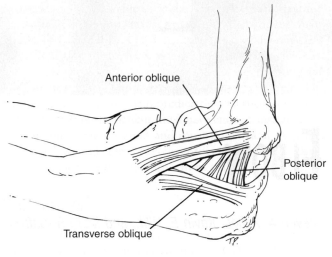

Figure 6-3

The ulnar (medial) collateral ligament complex of the elbow. (From Zairns B, Andrews JA, Larson WG, editors: *Injuries to the throwing arm*, p 196, Philadelphia, 1985, WB Saunders.)

begins as a secondary restraint to valgus stability at 30° and 90° and is a primary restraint to valgus force at 120° of flexion.[7] The posterior oblique ligament forms the floor of the cubital tunnel and plays more of a role in restraint against valgus stress at higher degrees of flexion. The role of the transverse ligament (Cooper's ligament) in elbow stability remains unclear, because this ligament originates from and inserts into the olecranon.

Lateral Ligament Complex

The lateral ligament complex consists primarily of the lateral ulnar collateral ligament (LUCL), the lateral radial collateral ligament (RCL), and the annular ligament (AL) (Figure 6-4). The LUCL, first described by Morrey and

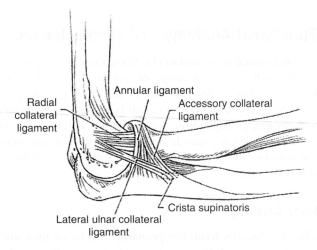

Figure 6-4

The lateral (radial) collateral ligament complex of the elbow. (From Nicholas JA, Hershman EB: *The upper extremity in sports medicine*, p 282, St Louis, 1990, Mosby.)

An,[9] originates from the lateral epicondyle. It passes over the AL and then begins to blend with it distally where it inserts onto the supinator crest of the ulna. O'Driscoll et al.[10,11] have suggested that the LUCL is the essential structure that prevents posterolateral rotatory instability. However, other studies have indicated that many components of the lateral ligament complex contribute to the prevention of posterolateral instability. Isolated sectioning of the LUCL distal to the AL results only in minor laxity. In contrast, significant rotatory instability is observed with more proximal transection of the LUCL and RCL.[12] Most likely all the components of the lateral ligament complex act together to prevent rotatory instability, but the LUCL clearly is the major contributor.

Capsule

The anterior capsule originates from the distal humerus proximal to the radial and coronoid fossae. It then inserts distally onto the rim of the coronoid and the annular ligament. Posteriorly, the capsule incorporates the area proximal to the olecranon process; it attaches distally along the articular margin of the sigmoid notch and the proximal aspect of the olecranon fossa.[13] In terms of elbow stability, most of the literature has focused on the osseous articulation and ligaments. However, at least the anterior capsule apparently does make a significant contribution as well. The anterior capsule has been shown in cadaveric studies to contribute 38% of the resistance to valgus force and 32% of the resistance to varus force in full extension.[14] The posterior capsule's contributions to stability have not been well documented.

Muscles

The muscles about the elbow also provide stability. Because of the conformity of the elbow joint, the muscles about the elbow provide dynamic stability by compressing the joint surfaces through muscular contraction.[13,15-17] The muscles also may passively assist in stability by means of a bulk effect.[13,18]

Pathophysiology and Pathomechanics

The elbow can be subjected to numerous unusual forces when used in activities that place high loads on it, especially sports. Overhead athletes subject their elbows to major valgus forces and as a result are at risk for specific elbow injuries. Sports such as baseball, football, tennis, volleyball, golf, and water polo are most commonly associated with acute and chronic elbow pathology. Overhead throwing athletes are predisposed to overuse syndromes secondary to the repetitive, high velocity stress across the elbow. The highest stress at the elbow occurs during the late cocking and acceleration phases of the throwing cycle.[19] Studies have indicated that the valgus stress at the elbow during the acceleration phase can be as high as 64 N-m, which exceeds the ultimate tensile strength of the UCL.[20] These supraphysiological stresses

result in potential injuries that can be determined based on the pathophysiology of the forces applied: traction or tensile forces of the medial-sided structures, compression of the lateral side of the elbow, and medially directed shear posteriorly (Figure 6-5).[21,22] The athletes commonly have chronic and acute injuries to the UCL with or without medial epicondylitis, as well as ulnar nerve symptoms. Laterally, compression leads to radiocapitellar degeneration and loose bodies, and posterior shear forces may lead to osteophyte formation, loose bodies, and olecranon stress fractures.

Golf and tennis players have a high incidence of medial and lateral epicondylitis. Gymnasts can develop radiocapitellar overload, including osteochondritis dissecans, and posterior impingement secondary to weight bearing on an extended elbow.[23] Weight lifters and shot putters may develop posterior elbow compressive injuries, including chondral damage and loose bodies, in addition to triceps injuries.[24]

Acute injuries, such as fractures and dislocations, can occur as a result of a fall on an outstretched hand (FOOSH injury) or direct trauma. These occur in sports and in everyday activities.

Fractures and Dislocations
Dislocations

The elbow is the second most commonly dislocated major joint, after the shoulder. It is the most frequently dislocated joint in children.[25] Dislocation is often found with high energy mechanisms of injury. It usually results from a fall onto an outstretched hand, which involves a combination of axial compression, supination, and valgus stress.[26]

No single classification system is used consistently for dislocations. They generally are described according to the direction and degree of displacement, whether associated fractures are present, and the acuity or chronicity of the injury.

> **Elbow Dislocations**
> - The elbow is the second most frequently dislocated major joint
> - Elbow dislocations are the most common dislocation in pediatric patients

O'Driscoll et al.[27] described the most common mechanism of acute instability as posterolateral rotatory instability (PLRI). This instability involves a complex pattern of injury: rotational displacement of the ulna on the trochlea occurs, and the radius subluxates or dislocates posteriorly from the capitellum, although the radius and ulna maintain their normal relationship to each other. The spectrum of injury seen with an elbow dislocation can be understood as a disruption of the circle of soft tissue and bone that begins on the lateral side of the elbow and progresses medially.[26] Stage 1 involves partial or complete disruption of the

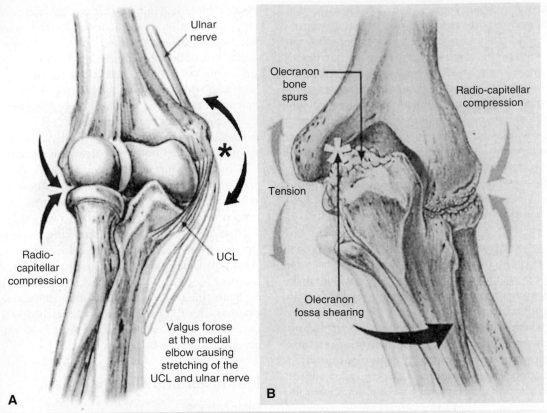

Figure 6-5

Schematic representation of the actions of valgus force on the elbow seen with throwing. **A,** View from the front of the elbow: tensile forces are exerted on the ulnar collateral ligament and ulnar nerve as the radiocapitellar joint receives compressive forces. **B,** Posterior elbow: the olecranon is compressed within the olecranon fossa by elbow extension and increased by valgus forces, leading to posterior impingement with compressive and shear forces to the olecranon and compressive forces to the lateral elbow. (From Safran MR: Injury to the ulnar collateral ligament: diagnosis and treatment, *Sports Med Arthrosc Rev* 11:17, 2003.)

LUCL, resulting in posterolateral rotatory subluxation. In stage 2, additional disruption occurs anteriorly and posteriorly, resulting in an incomplete posterolateral dislocation, or perched dislocation. More severe injury results in stage 3A, in which all soft tissues except the UCL have been disrupted and the elbow is stable only in pronation. In stage 3B, the UCL has been disrupted, and in stage 3C, the entire distal humerus has been stripped of soft tissues, resulting in stability only with flexion greater than 90°.

However, Josefsson[25,28] in his series showed that all simple elbow dislocations (those not associated with fracture) involved injury to the UCL.

In children, elbow dislocations are associated with fractures in up to 50% of cases, especially fractures of the radial head and neck and the medial or lateral epicondyle.[29] Elbow dislocations in children may involve avulsion of the medial epicondyle apophysis instead of direct injury to the ligaments, because the physis is weaker than the ligaments. The avulsed fragment may be nondisplaced or displaced a few millimeters, or it may be even more displaced and become incarcerated in the joint. Avulsions of the medial epicondyle may occur in up to 30% of children with dislocations.[30-32]

In association with elbow dislocations, injury to the musculotendinous origins of the wrist flexors and/or extensors is not uncommon. Other concomitant injuries include radial head and neck fractures, which may occur in 5% to 10% of elbow dislocations, and olecranon fractures.[33] It is important that the examiner identify coronoid fractures, because the prognosis for recurrent elbow instability is directly affected by the amount of coronoid involved (see discussion later in the chapter).

The initial treatment for elbow dislocations is closed reduction after a careful neurovascular examination of the extremity has been performed and appropriate radiographs have been obtained to check for concomitant fractures. Immediately after reduction, the treating physician should examine the elbow for its stable range of motion and smoothness of gliding. These findings should be documented, because they will determine the amount of restriction of motion in the early treatment period. Postreduction radiographs should be obtained to confirm concentric reduction and to rule out fractures. If no fracture is present, the elbow should be splinted in a position of stability (but no more than 90° of flexion) until the initial swelling has subsided. The patient then can be placed in a hinged elbow brace and allowed to begin motion, with extension limited according to the stability of the postreduction examination. Follow-up radiographs are essential to confirm maintenance of reduction. Motion then is gradually progressed, followed by strengthening.[34] (Rehabilitation is detailed at the end of the chapter.)

Postreduction Elbow Assessment

- The postreduction stable range of motion and gliding smoothness determine the amount of motion allowed in early treatment

---

Follow-up is important. Long-term follow-up studies have shown that persistent valgus laxity after elbow dislocation is associated with poorer overall clinical and radiographic results compared with elbows without increased valgus laxity after elbow dislocation.[35] Furthermore, chronic problems related to PLRI may occur; therefore care must be taken to evaluate the patient for this problem.

It is helpful to distinguish simple from complex elbow dislocations. Simple dislocations are not associated with fractures, whereas complex dislocations have associated elbow fractures. Simple dislocations rarely require surgical treatment, and recurrent instability is extremely rare (fewer that 2%).[36] Josefsson et al.[28] compared the operative and nonoperative treatment of simple dislocations. In a prospective trial, they found that elbows treated nonoperatively actually had a slightly improved range of motion and better subjective results than those treated operatively.

Early range of motion is essential to achieve a good outcome. Post-traumatic stiffness is the most common complication. Mehlhoff et al.[37] and Protzman[31] showed that a shorter immobilization time significantly correlated with better outcomes. Regardless, most patients commonly have at least 10° of flexion contracture. For this reason, some surgeons advocate early surgical repair or reconstruction of the injured ligament or ligaments after unstable elbow dislocations to allow for aggressive early range of motion.[38]

The same principle of early motion applies in the treatment of complex dislocations. However, with complex dislocations, fractures often need to be stabilized operatively so that the patient can begin early motion. The appropriate operative treatment depends on exactly which bony and soft tissue injuries are present.

Posterolateral Rotatory Instability

Although case reports on PLRI had existed for years, the condition was brought to the forefront in the early 1990s by O'Driscoll et al.[27,39] This elbow injury pattern is a rotatory instability caused by injury to the lateral UCL. The mechanism of injury is a combination of axial compression, valgus stress, and supination (or external rotation) that exerts a rotational force on the elbow, resulting in a spectrum of soft tissue injuries.[26,27] The initial injury is to the ulnar portion of the lateral collateral ligament complex (LCLC); damage progresses to capsular disruption (anterior and posterior capsule) and eventually may involve the UCL complex if the injury is severe.[10,26,27]

Comprehension of the pathomechanics of PLRI is the key to understanding this condition. Posterolateral rotatory instability of the elbow results from a rotatory subluxation of the radius and ulna (which move together as a unit) relative to the distal humerus. Because the annular ligament is intact in this injury, the radioulnar joint maintains its normal relationship, and the proximal radius and ulna therefore move together in a "coupled" motion. Most give credit to Osbourne and Cotterill[39] as the first investigators to appreciate fully the importance of the lateral ligament complex in recurrent instability and to describe the findings of PLRI. Although much of the initial literature by O'Driscoll and the laboratory at the Mayo Clinic reported the results of biomechanical studies demonstrating that the primary stabilizer in PLRI is the LUCL, much of the recent literature suggests that the injury may not be to the LUCL alone.[10,26,27,40] According to some reports, the RCL and anteroposterior capsule serve as secondary restraints. However, clinically it is known that elbow dislocations and injury to the LCLC occur proximally; PLRI is most commonly seen after this type of injury. Subsequent research by other investigators has suggested that isolated injury to the LUCL alone may not be enough to produce PLRI.[12,13,41] Some suggest that the complex works in a Y configuration and that a proximal injury, near the epicondyle, as seen clinically, can and does produce PLRI.[42]

The diagnosis of PLRI is much more elusive than other ligament injuries, including injuries of the UCL, and requires a careful history and physical examination. The physician must be diligent and must maintain a high degree of suspicion in patients with vague reports of elbow discomfort. Patients with PLRI frequently report that they have painful sensations of clicking, snapping, clunking, locking, dislocating, or giving way. The position of the hand during maneuvers that elicit these symptoms is critical, because the symptoms of PLRI often are produced when the patient extends the elbow with the forearm supinated.[27] Examples include using the hands to get out of a chair with the forearms maximally supinated or doing a push-up in full supination.[43]

The standard preliminary physical examination of the elbow generally is unremarkable with regard to strength, range of motion, and tenderness. The diagnosis requires a provocative test of stability described by O'Driscoll, called the lateral pivot-shift test of the elbow.[27] The pivot-shift test is performed with the patient supine and the examiner standing above the patient's head (Figure 6-6). The affected extremity is brought above the patient's head into forward elevation, and the shoulder is placed in full external

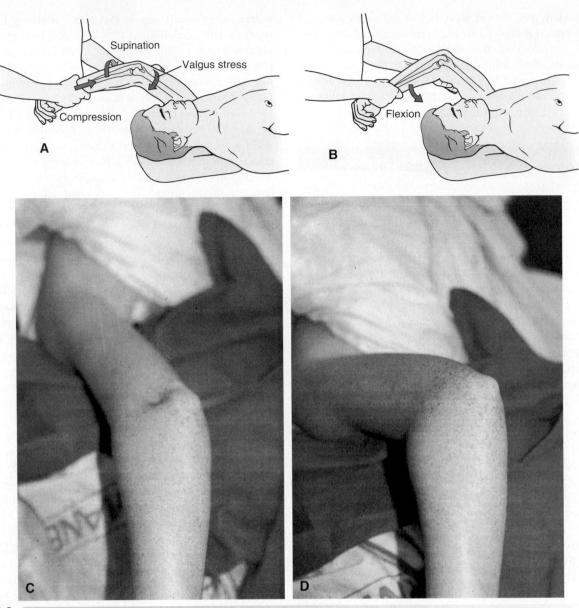

Figure 6-6

Posterolateral rotatory instability. **A,** The patient lies supine with the arm overhead. A mild supination force is applied to the forearm at the wrist. The patient's elbow is then flexed with a valgus stress, and compression is applied to the elbow. **B,** If the examiner continues flexing the elbow at about 40° to 70°, subluxation and a clunk on reduction when the elbow is extended may occur, although usually only in an unconscious patient. **C,** The radial out of anatomical position; this leads to a fullness with dimpling proximal to the radial head. **D,** The same patient as in **C;** as the elbow is brought into flexion, the radial head reduces, eliminating the fullness and dimpling. (**A** and **B** from Magee DJ: *Orthopedic physical assessment,* ed 5, p 378, St Louis, 2007, WB Saunders.)

rotation to stabilize the humerus for the test. The patient's forearm is held in maximal supination, with the examiner using one hand to grasp the wrist distally. A valgus force is applied with the examiner's other hand as the elbow is slowly flexed from a starting position of full extension. The combination of supination and valgus force results in an axial joint compression, which produces a posterolateral rotatory subluxation of the combined radius and ulna relative to the humerus. In an unanesthetized patient, this maneuver reproduces the sensation of instability and often elicits apprehension or guarding. The subluxation usually is maximized as the elbow reaches 40° flexion, and further flexion results in a sudden clunk of joint reduction. Dimpling of the skin proximal to the radial head (posterolateral elbow) can be seen with PLRI in degrees of extension before the reduction. The clunk of reduction in

PLRI generally is felt only by the examiner if the patient is under general anesthesia or occasionally after the patient has had an intra-articular injection of anesthetic. If a patient displays apprehension or guarding during the pivot-shift maneuver, confirmation of the posterolateral instability by examination of the patient under anesthesia usually is recommended. Lateral stress radiographic studies or fluoroscopy during the pivot-shift maneuver demonstrate posterolateral radial head dislocation with widening of the ulnohumeral joint (as a result of the subluxation of the ulna out of the trochlear groove) and may be helpful for confirmation and documentation of the pathomechanics.

Plain radiographs usually are unremarkable unless a bony avulsion off the lateral epicondyle has occurred (Figure 6-7, *A*). Stress radiographs often can show the posterolateral subluxation if the patient is relaxed and allows application of the forces necessary (Figure 6-7, *B*). Lateral stress radiographs show that the ulna is rotated off the distal humerus (slight gapping of the ulnohumeral joint with an otherwise maintained relationship) and the radial head is rotated with the ulna so that the radial head rests posterior to the capitellum. The normal radioulnar relationship differentiates PLRI from radial head subluxation or dislocation in which the radial head is displaced but the ulnohumeral joint is entirely normal. Although arthrography has not been shown to aid in diagnosis, advances in magnetic resonance imaging (MRI) have allowed good visualization of the LCLC and can be helpful in confirming the diagnosis in some cases.[44] Yet, because PLRI is a dynamic problem and the ligament may be stretched but intact, the sensitivity and specificity of MRI for this condition is less than might be preferred; however, studies are still forthcoming.

No nonoperative treatment protocols have been reported to be successful in the management of PLRI.[45] When PLRI markedly interferes with the patient's daily functions, activity modification and a hinged brace with forearm pronation and an extension block may be considered; however, few patients are content with this option, and most require surgical intervention.

Operative intervention often is necessary because no proven conservative management exists for chronic PLRI.[1] Bracing to prevent extension may be attempted, but it usually is poorly tolerated in the long term. Most PLRI injuries are the result of acute rupture secondary to trauma.

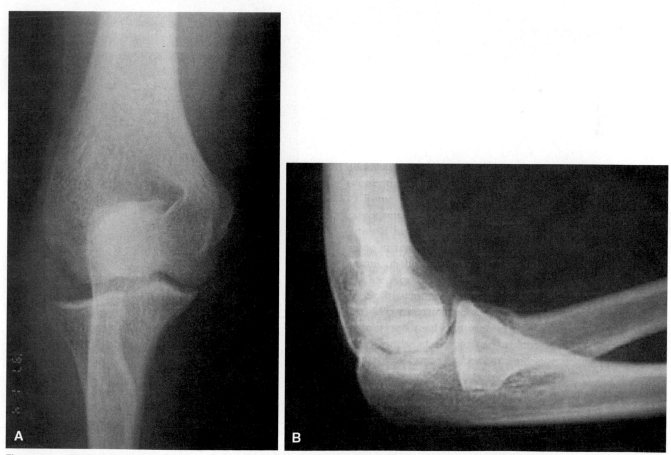

Figure 6-7

Radiographs of patients with posterolateral rotatory instability (PLRI). **A,** Bony avulsion off the lateral epicondyle, leading to PLRI. **B,** Stress radiograph showing the radial head posteriorly subluxated and the ulnohumeral joint slightly widened.

Chronic repetitive injury is rarely the cause of PLRI because few activities require repetitive varus stress, although cubitus varus caused by childhood trauma may present as delayed PLRI.[46] Surgical treatment of PLRI involves repair by means of reattachment of the avulsed LCLC or reconstruction of the LUCL with a free tendon graft to the lateral epicondyle, similar to reconstruction of the medial UCL (Figure 6-8, A).

Repair usually is reserved for acute avulsions from the distal humerus, the most common site of LCL injury in PLRI bone (Figure 6-8, B).[47-49] Because the annular ligament is intact in these patients, radioulnar dislocation does not occur, and surgery on this ligament is not indicated. Ligament reconstruction usually is required in adults, particularly in chronic cases of PLRI. This is done through the same incision as the repair. Ligamentous reconstruction is used to replicate LUCL anatomy using a free tendon graft through bony tunnels in the distal humerus and ulna. Modifications of the technique originally described by O'Driscoll include making the distal connecting tunnels perpendicular to the isometric point to the lateral epicondyle and using the interference screw technique.[46]

Overall, surgical results have been fairly good. Osborne and Cotterill[39] reported excellent results in eight patients with transosseous repair, and Nestor et al.[48] reported excellent results in three patients. Sanchez-Sotelo et al.[49] reported a 90% success rate in restoring stability in the absence of arthritis or radial head fracture at an average 6 years' follow-up; 60% of patients had excellent results, and 40% continued to have pain or some loss of motion. The overall patient satisfaction rate was 86%.[49] Lee and Teo[50] had 80% good to excellent results and 100% stability at follow-up, and all 10 patients were satisfied with the surgical reconstruction. Olsen and Søjbjerg[51] used a triceps graft and had 94% satisfactory results and 78% stability at nearly 4 years' follow-up.

Fractures

As with dislocations, the most common complication after elbow fractures is post-traumatic stiffness. The key to minimizing stiffness is early motion. For this reason, the goal with elbow fracture surgery is rigid fixation. Rigid fixation subsequently allows early motion to be started as part of the

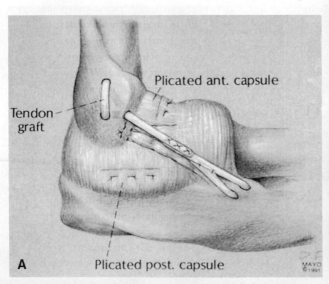
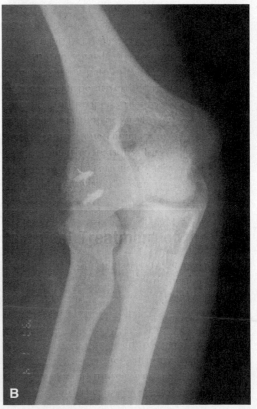

Figure 6-8

PLRI surgical repair and reconstruction. **A,** Schematic representation of PLRI reconstruction using a free graft. The graft is woven through bony tunnels. **B,** Radiograph of the patient in Figure 6-7, A; the bony avulsion of the origin of the lateral collateral ligament (LCL) has been reattached with suture anchors. (**A** from Morrey BF: *The elbow and its disorders,* ed 2, p 579, Philadelphia, 1993, WB Saunders.)

rehabilitation process. Some fractures may be considered stable and do not require surgery; however, early motion still is essential to obtain a good result. One of the most important factors is anatomical restoration of articular surface congruity to reduce the risk of post-traumatic degenerative arthritis.

- In the elbow, the key to minimizing stiffness is early controlled motion.

Despite the best treatment, some elbow injuries still have poor outcomes. This is at least partly related to the severity of the trauma to the articular cartilage at the time of the initial injury. An example is the **terrible triad** of the elbow. The term, coined by Hotchkiss, refers to a high energy injury that results in elbow dislocation, radial head fracture, and coronoid fracture.[52] Triad injuries require treatment of each component to improve the likelihood of success, because failure to address all three leads to an extremely poor outcome. However, even with aggressive operative treatment to provide anatomical reduction and stable internal fixation, the results may still be poor. These patients are prone to early recurrent instability, chronic instability, and post-traumatic arthritis.[53]

Coronoid Fractures

Coronoid fractures are most commonly seen with high energy injuries. The coronoid forms a significant portion of the articular surface of the proximal ulna and acts as an anterior buttress; it also serves as an important attachment site for muscles and ligaments about the elbow. The coronoid is essential for elbow stability; it is the most important part of the ulnohumeral articulation.[54] Coronoid fractures occur in 2% to 15% of acute elbow dislocations.[33,36,55] Coronoid fracture nonunion may result in chronic recurrent elbow dislocation.

Regan and Morrey[56] classified coronoid fractures according to the size of the fragment: type I fractures are tip avulsions; type II fractures involve less than 50% of the height of the coronoid; and type III fractures involve more than 50% of the height of the coronoid and frequently are accompanied by instability of the elbow (Figure 6-9). Type I fractures generally are stable and can be treated as simple dislocations with early motion. Many type II fractures are unstable and require open reduction and internal fixation (ORIF). Type III fractures involve the insertion of the anterior portion of the UCL and are inherently unstable. With these more severe injuries, open reduction with internal fixation or a hinged external fixator may be required to maintain reduction.

Radial Head Fractures

Radial head fractures are very common injuries and are often seen in association with other elbow injuries. These

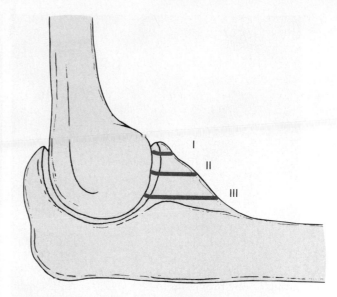

Figure 6-9

Regan-Morrey classification of coronoid fractures. A type I fracture involves the tip of the coronoid. A type II fracture involves less than 50% of the coronoid tip; this usually correlates to a line drawn parallel to the shaft of the ulna from the tip of the olecranon. A type III fracture involves more than 50% of the coronoid. (From Browner BD, Jupiter JB, Levine AM, Trafton PG, editors: *Skeletal trauma*, p 1145, Philadelphia, 1996, WB Saunders.)

injuries usually occur as a result of a fall on an outstretched hand, which transmits force to the elbow, and they can occur in conjunction with elbow dislocations. The radial head plays an important role as a secondary elbow stabilizer for valgus stress, and it also facilitates pronation and supination of the forearm. Mason[57] divided these injuries into nondisplaced fractures involving less than 25% of the radial head (type I); two-part displaced fractures or fractures that are marginally displaced, including angulation, impaction, and depression fractures (type II); and comminuted fractures and fractures that involve the entire radial head (type III).[57] A type IV fracture is usually described as a comminuted fracture in conjunction with elbow dislocation.

Nondisplaced fractures (type I) generally can be treated nonoperatively (Figure 6-10, *A*). Once again, early motion is key to a good outcome with these "stable" fractures. Occasionally clinicians aspirate the hematoma within the joint and even add anesthetic to reduce pain, allowing for earlier range of motion of the elbow. However, even with early range of motion, some loss of elbow motion (averaging 10°) can be expected.[58]

Some type II fractures can also be treated nonoperatively. In the absence of other injuries, a minimally displaced two-part fracture with no block to range of motion is considered a stable fracture and can be treated without surgery.[59] However, displaced type II fractures usually require operative treatment for best results (Figure 6-10, *B*).[60] Excision of a

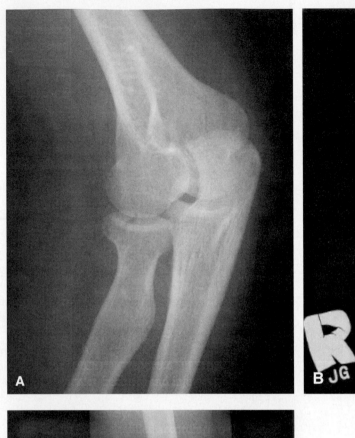

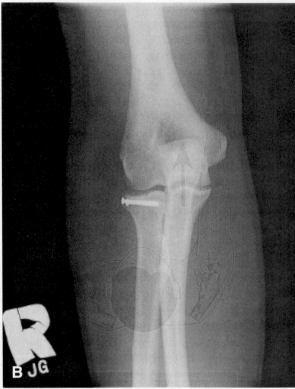

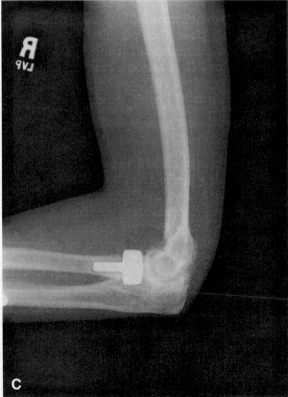

Figure 6-10

Radial head fractures. **A,** Nondisplaced radial head fracture that was treated nonoperatively. **B,** Radial head fracture treated with internal fixation using two screws. **C,** Radiograph of a patient who had a comminuted radial head fracture; treatment required prosthetic replacement of the radial head.

small fragment is acceptable, but larger fragments should be internally fixed.[61] All radial head fractures require careful evaluation of the elbow and the distal radioulnar joint (DRUJ) for associated injuries. If pain or instability is present at the DRUJ, excision of a significant portion of the radial head is contraindicated; such an injury, known as an Essex-Lopresti injury, can result in proximal migration of the radius after excision of the radial head.[62] In the absence of associated injuries, type III fractures can be treated with excision of the radial head. If a DRUJ injury has occurred, the surgeon must either attempt to reduce and fix the fracture fragments to retain the radial head or replace it with a prosthetic radial head (Figure 6-10C).[53] With interosseous ligament injury and/or DRUJ injury, radial head replacement is mandatory if the radial head cannot be fixed. Temporary radial head replacement, such as with a Silastic implant that is removed later, has fallen out of favor, because late displacement after removal of the prosthesis, even after a year, has been reported.[63-65]

Surgery for radial head fractures should be carried out within the first 48 hours or after 3 to 4 weeks, because surgery performed between 2 days and 3 weeks is associated with a higher risk of myositis ossificans.

In skeletally immature patients, most radial head and neck fractures can be treated nonoperatively. In the young throwing athlete, valgus forces at the elbow can result in a physeal fracture at the radial neck. Radiographs generally show an abnormal fat pad sign, which signifies an effusion. With significantly displaced fractures, operative treatment can be considered; however, in younger children, most proximal radial fractures should be treated nonoperatively.

Olecranon Fractures

Because of its subcutaneous location in the posterior elbow, the olecranon is at risk of fracture as a result of falls, direct blows, or dislocations. By definition, the olecranon is the proximal articulating part of the ulna, and this part of the ulna is critical in serving as the final link in the transmission of force from the triceps mechanism to enable elbow extension. Olecranon factures usually are intra-articular. Displaced fractures may result in ulnohumeral instability and incongruity of the articular surface. In addition, the proximal pull of the triceps on the proximal olecranon tends to displace the fracture and prevent healing (Figure 6-11, A). For these reasons, only nondisplaced fractures can be treated nonoperatively, and even these fractures require follow-up radiographic evaluation to ensure that displacement has not occurred since the initial injury. For most olecranon fractures, ORIF is the recommended treatment.[53] Tension band techniques generally are used for transverse fractures (Figure 6-11, B). Comminuted and more proximal fractures may require plate fixation (Figure 6-11, C). Excision of the proximal fragment and triceps reattachment is an option in an elderly patient with poor bone quality, but this technique should be avoided in younger, active patients because

it can lead to elbow instability.[54] Loss of more than 50% of the olecranon articular surface is associated with a 50% loss of stability.[14,66]

Distal Humeral Fractures

Significant energy often is required to cause a distal humeral fracture in young patients. These injuries may be intra-articular or extra-articular. Much of the distal humerus is covered with articular cartilage. The trochlea articulates with the proximal ulna, and the capitellum with the radius. As a result, many distal humeral fractures are intra-articular. The goal of treatment, as with other elbow fractures, is congruent reduction of the articular surfaces and stable fixation to allow early motion. Displaced and intra-articular distal humeral fractures generally require ORIF for optimum results.[67] Some extra-articular, nondisplaced, and avulsion fractures can be treated nonoperatively, but these are less common. Very comminuted fractures in older patients who place lesser demands on the elbow may be treated with noncustom total elbow replacements.[68] Most distal humeral fractures in healthy, active adults are treated optimally with operative fixation and early motion rehabilitation (Figure 6-12). These fractures generally have a high incidence of elbow stiffness, fixation failure, malunion, nonunion, infection, and ulnar nerve injury.

Supracondylar humeral fractures are the second most common fracture in pediatric patients.[69] These injuries usually are the result of a fall onto an outstretched hand or a direct blow to the back of the elbow. They can be treated with closed reduction and casting if the fracture can be maintained in the appropriate position without compromising the neurovasculature. Otherwise, temporary pin fixation, percutaneously or open, may be indicated. These are important injuries, because complications may occur, such as compartment syndrome, brachial artery laceration or thrombosis, loss of motion, cubitus varus, and nerve injury.

Elbow Arthritis

The treatment of elbow arthritis is similar to the treatment of arthritis of other joints. Elbow arthritis generally can be categorized as inflammatory arthritis, post-traumatic arthritis, or osteoarthritis. Primary degenerative arthritis of the elbow is relatively uncommon compared with other joints such as the hip, knee, ankle, and shoulder. Rheumatoid arthritis commonly affects the elbow, and post-traumatic sequelae are a more common cause of arthritis of the elbow. The presenting symptom usually is pain, but it can be accompanied by stiffness or loss of motion, weakness, or instability. Treatment is dictated by the severity of the symptoms, the etiology, and the patient's age. The initial treatment generally is conservative. However, when pathology and symptoms are severe, operative intervention is indicated. Significant advances have been made in recent years in the surgical

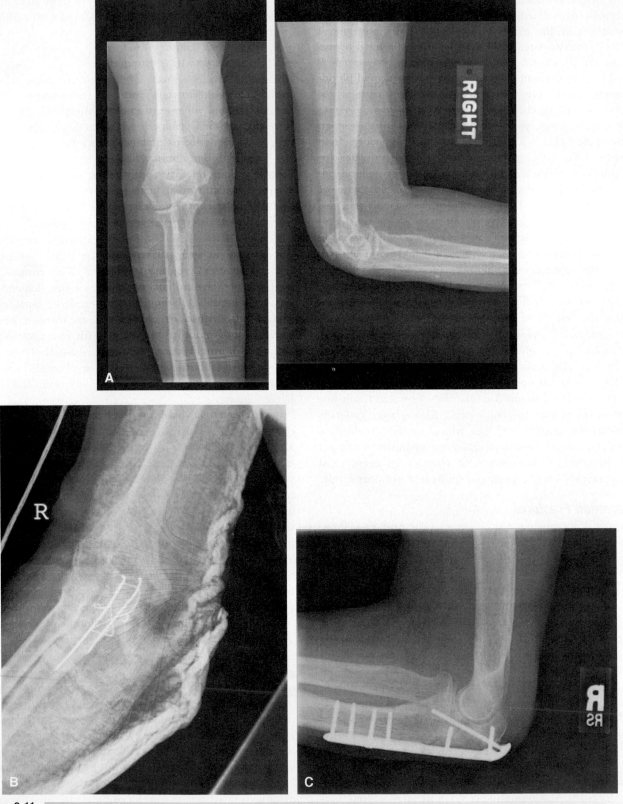

Figure 6-11
Olecranon fracture. **A,** Displaced olecranon fracture. This intra-articular fracture is displaced because of the pull of the triceps. **B,** Radiograph of a patient treated with tension band wiring for a simple olecranon fracture. **C,** Radiograph of a patient with a comminuted olecranon fracture treated with plates and screws.

Figure 6-12
Radiograph of a patient who had open reduction and internal fixation for a comminuted distal humeral fracture.

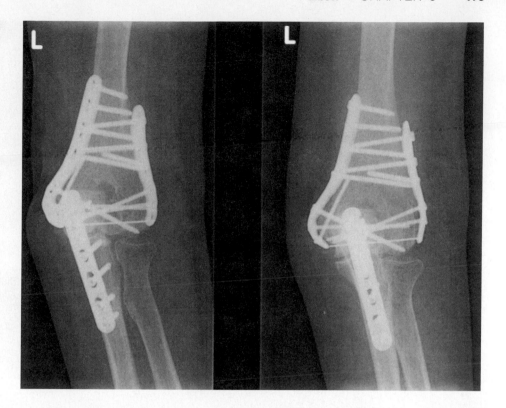

treatment of arthritis of the elbow, most notably in arthroscopic techniques.[70-73]

Rheumatoid arthritis is the most common form of inflammatory arthritis. Although other joints are more commonly affected, rheumatoid arthritis of the elbow often is marked by severe pain and disability. Bone loss and articular destruction cause instability at the ulnohumeral articulation. Surgical treatment, often total elbow arthroplasty (TEA), frequently is necessary and can be quite successful at relieving pain and restoring function.[70,74]

Post-traumatic elbow arthritis can result from any insult to the articular cartilage or bony anatomy but most often is seen after intra-articular distal humeral fractures. Stiffness often is present and may occur secondary to associated heterotopic ossification. Osteoarthritis is found almost exclusively in men who have a history of heavy labor or athletic use of the arm, such as weight lifters and throwing athletes. Limitation of range of motion, especially a flexion contracture, is common.[70]

Nonoperative treatment for elbow arthritis consists of medications, injections, and physical therapy. Operative treatment should be considered for patients with debilitating and persistent symptoms. Arthroscopic techniques include synovectomy, debridement of impinging osteophytes, and contracture release. Many think that arthroscopic synovectomy is more complete and effective than the open technique. However, the procedure is technically demanding, and the neurovascular structures are at risk because of their proximity.[71,72] Open synovectomy, with or without

excision of the radial head, is an established procedure for rheumatoid arthritis of the elbow. Open osteotomy or debridement of impinging osteophytes also can be done to reduce pain and improve range of motion.[70]

Arthrodesis is poorly tolerated because elbow range of motion is essential for use of the hand.[70] It is indicated only for salvage situations when TEA is contraindicated.

Total Elbow Replacement

Total elbow replacement may be performed because of arthritic changes or as a primary treatment for difficult distal humeral fractures in older patients. TEA is an excellent surgical intervention that produces reliable results in a certain subgroup of patients with advanced degenerative changes.[73] Patients with rheumatoid arthritis generally have excellent and reliable pain relief and, because of their relatively low functional demands, tend not to have problems with early loosening or failure of the prosthesis (Figure 6-13).[74] For other elderly patients with low to moderate functional expectations, TEA offers reliable pain relief with medium-term results similar to those for hip and knee arthroplasty.[75] Many now advocate the use of TEA as an acute surgical treatment for elderly patients with comminuted osteoporotic elbow fractures, contending that the results are similar to or better than those obtained with ORIF.[68,76-78]

Unfortunately, in younger, more active patients, early failure, including loosening of the prosthesis, has limited the use of TEA. The treatment of young patients with high

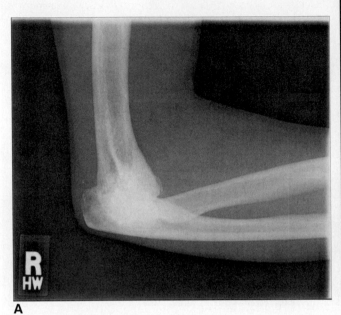

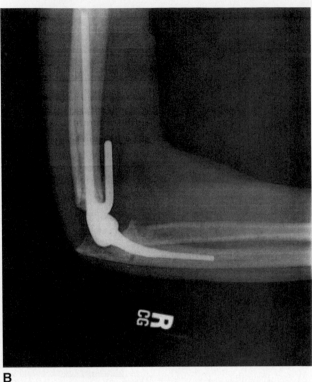

A   **B**

Figure 6-13

Rheumatoid arthritis. **A,** Radiograph of a patient with severe rheumatoid arthritis of the elbow.
B, Postoperative radiograph after a total elbow arthroplasty for the rheumatoid arthritis.

functional expectations and severe elbow arthritis is both difficult and controversial. The results with TEA are inferior to those seen in older, more sedentary patients.[75] However, alternatives such as interposition arthroplasty and resection arthroplasty give less reliable and less sustainable results. In young, active patients who want surgery for painful arthritic changes but who do not want fusion (i.e., arthrodesis) of the elbow, arthroscopy and distraction interposition arthroplasty currently are the only viable alternatives. With either procedure, particularly distraction arthroplasty, limited postoperative goals and expectations should be stressed.[79] With interposition arthroplasty, the arthritic surfaces are conservatively removed and replaced by soft tissue (e.g., fascia lata). Studies show about 70% satisfactory results (pain and function) at 5-year follow-up[79] and 40% at follow-up of more than 20 years.[80] In addition, the role of arthroscopy in the treatment of advanced elbow arthritis needs to be more clearly defined.

Overuse Injuries of the Elbow

Anterior Elbow

Climber's Elbow

The term *climber's elbow* refers to a strain of the brachialis tendon.[81] It usually is seen in association with repetitive pull-ups, hyperextension, or repeated forceful supination or from violent extension against a forceful contraction.[24] Rock climbers are susceptible to this injury as a result of repetitive weight bearing through the upper extremities.[82] Patients typically have pain with extension or resisted flexion and supination. The rule for successful management of this injury is slow and steady improvement with nonoperative treatment. Resolution of the symptoms is obtained with rest and anti-inflammatory treatment. Early rehabilitation should focus on regaining range of motion before strengthening is initiated.

Distal Biceps Tendonitis and Tendon Rupture

Tendonitis at the distal biceps insertion is an uncommon overuse syndrome. It is seen in association with activities similar to those that produce climber's elbow. It also results in pain with resisted flexion and supination, which can be elicited during the physical examination. Rest and conservative care generally result in gradual resolution of symptoms. Surgical treatment generally is not indicated.

Distal biceps tendon rupture also is uncommon but is seen more often than biceps tendinopathy, in which the torn end of the biceps, through an acute event without prodromal (i.e., early) symptoms, usually reveals chronic tendinopathy. Distal biceps tendon rupture represents only 3% of all biceps ruptures; the incidence has been estimated at 1.2 per 100,000 people per year.[83,84] It typically affects the dominant arm of middle-aged men. Smoking may be a risk factor for this injury.[83] The mechanism is a sudden, forceful overload with the elbow in midflexion. Although degenerative changes in the tendon predispose it to rupture, most patients have no history of prior pain or prodromal symptoms. These individuals present with localized pain and tenderness at the bicipital tuberosity, proximal displacement of the biceps tendon with a bulge in the distal arm, inability to palpate the taut tendon within the antecubital fossa, and marked weakness of forearm supination and elbow flexion (often associated with increased pain) (Figure 6-14). The pain and tenderness identified after the acute rupture quickly subside, but a dull ache may persist for weeks. Ecchymosis usually is present in the antecubital fossa, and sometimes above and below the elbow, starting 2 to 3 days after the injury.

The two proposed mechanisms of attritional rupture are due to a relatively poor vascular supply and/or a mechanical impingement against the bicipital tuberosity. Both of these mechanisms appear to play a role in the pathophysiology.[85] Partial ruptures have been documented, although they are less common than complete ruptures.[86-88] Partial tears can be managed conservatively and frequently have good outcomes, particularly if less than 50% of the tendon is damaged.

Muscle-tendon junction injuries are highly uncommon. Their presentation is similar to a distal biceps avulsion (i.e., complete or partial), although the tendon often can still be felt in the cubital fossa. MRI may confuse the picture, suggesting that the tendon is torn. These injuries do well with relative rest initially followed by rehabilitation.[89]

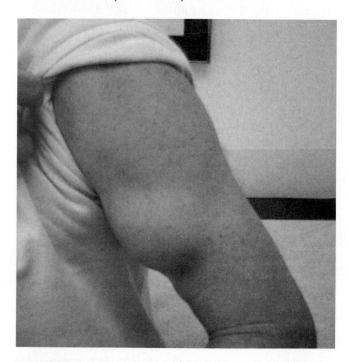

Figure 6-14
Patient with a distal biceps rupture; note the proximal migration and muscle bulge in the arm that are associated with this injury.

MRI is the imaging modality of choice for the diagnosis of partial tears;[90] it is rarely needed for the diagnosis of complete tears of the distal biceps tendon. Complete tears should be managed with surgical repair; inferior results have been documented with nonoperative treatment of these injuries.[91,92] Patients who do not undergo surgical repair have significant limitations in terms of strength and ability to perform certain activities. Nonanatomical tendon reinsertion also gives inferior results compared with anatomical reinsertion. Rantanen and Orava[93] found that for both acute and chronic injuries, nonanatomical reinsertion gave good to excellent results in 60% of patients compared with 90% who had anatomical reinsertion.[93] Only 14% of the patients treated nonoperatively had a good to excellent result, and the main complaint was loss of strength, or endurance strength, with elbow flexion (30% loss of strength) and/or supination (40% loss of strength).[91,93]

Distal Biceps Tendon Repair

Initially, the biceps tendon was repaired with a one-incision technique. However, the exposure required to repair the biceps tendon avulsion to the radial tuberosity with bone tunnels put the radial nerve at risk, and several cases of radial nerve injuries were reported.[94] For this reason, a two-incision technique was devised so that bone tunnels could be made with the arm in full pronation. This forearm rotation pushed the nerve out of the way, reducing the risk of nerve injury. With the advent of new devices, such as suture anchors, the EndoButton, and interference screws, exposure of the proximal radius could be limited, reducing the risk to the nerve with a one-incision technique.[95,96] However, concerns still exist with the use of the one-incision technique with bone anchors; for example, the anchors may back out, and the tendon may heal onto the bone.

Overall, the results of distal biceps tendon repair using either one or two incisions have not been shown to be different, and the technique used generally is based on the surgeon's preference.

The method of anatomical reinsertion is controversial. The two-incision bone tunnel technique produces reliable results but has a relatively higher risk of radioulnar synostosis (fusion).[97,98] However, modification of the Boyd-Anderson technique so that contact with the ulna is avoided has reduced this uncommon complication.[94] Traditionally the one-incision technique was associated with more neurological complications, because it required more extensive dissection, particularly movement of the posterior interosseous nerve. More recently, however, many authors have recommended a one-incision technique that does not require bone tunnels and thus can be performed with less dissection, theoretically reducing the risk of nerve injury. Both suture anchors and EndoButton techniques have been described, with good early results with the one-incision technique.[99-104] Overall, anatomical repair restores strength and function in more than 90% of patients, regardless of the technique used.[93]

The general recommendation is to perform distal biceps reattachment acutely. Chronic biceps tendon ruptures require a more extensive approach.[105,95] A distal biceps rupture is considered chronic if it is not treated within 4 weeks, although excellent results have been obtained after anatomical reinsertion 3 years after injury.[106] The key to success in delayed surgery is the status of the lacertus fibrosus (i.e., the bicipital aponeurosis); if it is intact, the tendon will retract only to the level just proximal to the antecubital fossa. The amount of muscle shortening is not very significant, and delayed repair is easily attainable. However, if the lacertus fibrosus is torn, the tendon may "slingshot" into the arm, significant muscle shortening may occur, along with scarring within the arm, and delayed primary reattachment may be difficult. In such cases allograft reconstruction may be attempted to bridge the gap between the shortened muscle and the bicipital tuberosity; however, this is a salvage procedure, and although the condition often is improved, the patient is unlikely to regain full strength. Reports have identified a range of 13% to 50% deficit in flexion and supination strength.[105]

Pronator Syndrome

Pronator syndrome is proximal entrapment neuropathy of the median nerve. Pronator syndrome must be distinguished clinically from carpal tunnel syndrome (CTS; distal median nerve entrapment), which is by far the most common entrapment neuropathy of the median nerve. An understanding of pronator syndrome is important, because this condition frequently is misdiagnosed, and many patients undergo unsuccessful operations before the correct diagnosis is made.[107]

Four anatomical sites of compression of the median nerve can be found in the elbow region.[108] When a supracondylar process is present at the distal medial humerus (1% of the population), compression can occur under the ligament of Struthers, which originates at the supracondylar process and attaches to the medial epicondyle. At the elbow, the median nerve passes under the bicipital aponeurosis, the second possible location of compression. It then passes between the humeral (superficial) and ulnar (deep) heads of the pronator teres muscle, where compression commonly occurs. Finally, the nerve passes under the fibrous arch of the flexor digitorum superficialis muscle.

Sites of Compression of the Median Nerve at the Elbow

- Under the ligament of Struthers
- Bicipital aponeurosis
- Pronator teres
- Flexor digitorum superficialis

Although conflicting reports have emerged, the most common site of compression in pronator syndrome appears to be between the two heads of the pronator teres.[109] Entrapment at the bicipital aponeurosis and at the arch of the flexor digitorum superficialis also is common.[108,109] Compression caused by the ligament of Struthers is rare.

Clinically, pronator syndrome often is seen in patients who engage in repetitive pronation and supination activities[110] (e.g., pitching, rowing, weight training, archery, and racquet sports).[108] It occurs most commonly in women in their 40s. Patients most often complain of activity-related pain in the anterior aspect of the elbow and forearm. A patient may have a history of a direct blow to the forearm, or repetitive trauma may be the cause; however, in most patients the cause is unknown. In contrast to CTS, patients do not usually experience nocturnal symptoms. The pain with pronator syndrome may be described as a dull pain or an ache in the proximal anterior forearm just distal to the antecubital fossa, and it may radiate distally to the wrist; it rarely radiates proximally. Paresthesias are common in the median nerve distribution, and unlike with CTS, numbness may be present over the thenar eminence in the distribution of the palmar cutaneous branch of the median nerve.[110-114]

Tenderness over the pronator muscle mass often is found on examination.[115] Weakness, if present, usually is subtle. A complete examination should include evaluation for Tinel's sign, Phalen's sign, and the carpal tunnel compression test to assess for CTS. Provocative tests have been described for localizing pathology to a specific anatomical structure: resisted forearm pronation and elbow extension for the pronator teres; active supination against resistance with the elbow flexed for the bicipital aponeurosis; and resisted flexion of the long finger for the arch of the flexor digitorum superficialis.[114-116]

When evaluating a patient with possible pronator syndrome, the clinician must consider all potential sites of nerve compression from the neck to the wrist. Also, median nerve compression at more than one location (the so-called double crush phenomenon) is not uncommon.[107] Electrodiagnostic studies are rarely helpful in the diagnosis of pronator syndrome. However, they can help confirm an alternative or concurrent diagnosis, such as CTS. Nerve conduction studies are most often normal in pronator syndrome.[114]

Treatment initially should be nonoperative. It consists of activity modification, rest, immobilization, anti-inflammatory medications, physical therapy and, in some cases, local cortisone injections. Conservative management usually is successful, but if it fails or if significant abnormalities are noted on nerve conduction studies, the median nerve should be decompressed surgically.[113] Because assessing for sites of significant compression is difficult even intraoperatively, consideration should be given to releasing all the potential sites of compression. The outcomes of surgical treatment generally are good, with reports of a greater than 90% rate of satisfactory outcomes.[115]

Annular Ligament Disruption

Annular ligament disruption is a rare cause of popping or snapping pain in the anterior elbow. It often is associated with injury to the radial head, either subluxation or dislocation, and it often is seen in throwing athletes, who report popping symptoms with pronation and supination. A complete disruption in a symptomatic patient is treated with surgical repair.[24] One report has described arthroscopic and histological findings of loose, degenerative annular ligament tissue in two brothers who were overhead throwing athletes and who had snapping elbow pain.[117]

Heterotopic Ossification

Pathological bone formation in nonosseous tissues, usually referred to as *heterotopic ossification* (HO), is most often seen as a result of elbow trauma,[118] although it also can be seen in association with burns, head trauma, and genetic disorders.[119-121] Although sometimes asymptomatic, HO frequently progresses to disabling pain and stiffness. Despite aggressive therapy, nonoperative treatment generally does not reverse the progression of decreased motion. Fortunately, recent results of surgical excision of HO have shown consistently good outcomes with minimal recurrence and complications.[122]

In susceptible individuals the process likely begins soon after injury. Symptoms of swelling, erythema, and pain may be present in just a few weeks, and elbow stiffness starts 1 to 4 months after the initial injury. Limitation of active and passive range of motion often progresses despite aggressive therapy.[123] The ectopic bone formation usually stabilizes after 3 to 9 months. Morrey et al.[6] have demonstrated that most activities of daily living can be performed with a 100° arc of elbow motion from 30° to 130° of elbow flexion (i.e., normal elbow functional ROM). However, each patient's range of motion goals should be assessed based on the individual's professional and recreational activities.

In most cases the diagnosis, location, and maturity of the HO can be assessed with plain radiographs. Computed tomography (CT) scans can also be helpful in certain cases, especially for preoperative planning. Classification systems for HO are based on location and functional limitation. The most common location about the elbow is posterolateral, but HO can involve almost any part of the elbow.[118]

Initial treatment should involve aggressive therapy to maintain as much motion as possible and minimize progression to ankylosis. Most surgeons recommend both active and passive range of motion exercises, although this is somewhat controversial.[122] When elbow stiffness becomes severe enough to limit recreational or daily activities, surgical excision should be considered. Associated nerve compression, most commonly of the ulnar nerve,

can develop secondary to ectopic bone and generally should be treated with surgery to prevent the development of a permanent nerve lesion. Furthermore, it recently was found that with long-standing loss of elbow motion, ulnar nerve dysfunction may occur once the patient regains elbow motion. For this reason, ulnar nerve transposition should be considered in conjunction with procedures to gain range of motion, even if no ulnar nerve symptoms are present preoperatively, if large gains in elbow motion are expected.[124]

Because of concerns about recurrence, it had long been suggested that HO excision not be undertaken before 1 year after injury. However, multiple reports have demonstrated good results and low recurrence rates with HO excision as early as 3 to 6 months after injury.[125-128] Consideration should be given to prophylaxis after HO excision (e.g., indomethacin or radiation) to prevent recurrence.

Medial Elbow

Medial Epicondylar Physeal Injury

In the adolescent elbow, the medial epicondylar apophysis is the weakest portion of the medial stabilizing structures. As a result, injury to the medial epicondylar apophysis is common. This may be manifested by inflammation of the apophyseal growth plate, or avulsion fractures of the medial epicondyle may occur. Medial epicondylar avulsion fractures are much more common than UCL injuries in the immature elbow, and they are the most common fractures in the immature throwing athlete. This fracture often is seen in association with elbow dislocation, and the displaced fragment of the medial epicondyle occasionally can become incarcerated in the joint, preventing reduction. In throwing athletes, this injury occurs during an especially hard pitch or throw when valgus stress is coupled with flexor/pronator muscle contraction. However, a less stressful throw or a fall onto an outstretched hand also may result in a medial epicondylar avulsion fracture. These patients have acute onset of medial elbow pain and, occasionally, associated ulnar nerve paresthesias.[129,130] Although some may have prodromal symptoms of medial epicondylar apophysitis, this frequently is not the case. Patients with medial apophysis complain of pain on throwing and a decrease in throwing distance, accuracy, and velocity. On examination, these children have tenderness over the medial epicondyle and pain with resisted elbow flexion and pronation. They frequently have a flexion contracture of approximately 15°, based on muscular and capsular tightness.

Radiographs are necessary to confirm the diagnosis, and as is always the case with children, comparison views are important (Figure 6-15). Assessment of apophyseal thickness is important for apophysitis or nondisplaced fractures. This measurement varies by individual and skeletal maturity, which is why the comparison view of the nonaffected

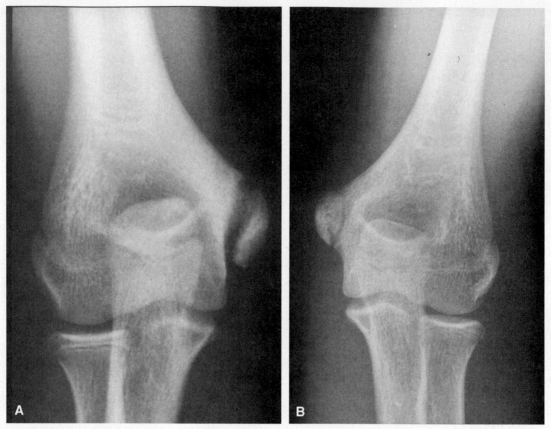

Figure 6-15

Medial epicondylar physeal injury. **A,** AP radiograph of the elbow of a 13-year-old boy who plays baseball in several leagues year round. The medial physis appears slightly widened. **B,** The contralateral elbow; clearly the injured elbow has significant widening compared to the normal elbow.

elbow is important. With apophysitis, the growth plate can be widened and occasionally fragmented.

The treatment of the inflamed apophysis is rest from throwing for 4 to 6 weeks, application of ice (care must be taken to protect the ulnar nerve from thermal injury), and nonsteroidal medication to reduce the pain and acute inflammation. After the symptoms subside, a rehabilitation program is instituted consisting of stretching to eliminate the flexion contracture and strengthening of the muscles that cross the elbow joint, followed by transitioning to functional activities.

Most avulsion injuries can be treated nonoperatively. Certainly in nondisplaced and minimally displaced fractures (the amount of displacement is controversial), when the elbow is stable to valgus stress testing, the condition should be treated conservatively with a short course of immobilization, activity restriction for 2 to 3 weeks, and a gradual return to range of motion exercises, strengthening, and functional activities. Absolute indications for surgery include incarceration of a fragment of the medial epicondyle in the joint and complete ulnar nerve dysfunction. Incomplete ulnar nerve deficits generally resolve with conservative treatment.[130]

The treatment of displaced fractures is more controversial. Surgery may be necessary to reduce and fix some displaced fractures. However, historically surgeons have found that even widely displaced fractures have good results with nonoperative treatment. Josefsson and Danielsson[131] reported good to excellent results at long-term follow-up in 56 patients treated nonoperatively with widely displaced medial epicondyle fractures. Although more than half of these patients had a persistent fibrous nonunion, their outcome was as good as that in patients whose fractures healed. Other authors advocate operative treatment for displaced fractures.[1,132,133] They argue that, especially in high level throwing athletes, no significant displacement should be tolerated (Figure 6-16). However, the benefit of operative over nonoperative treatment for displaced fractures has not been clearly demonstrated. The lead author of this chapter usually surgically treats avulsions that are more than 5 mm (0.2 inch) displaced in the dominant arm of throwing athletes, and those that are 1 cm (½ inch) or more displaced in all other individuals.

Medial Epicondylitis

Medial epicondylitis, or golfer's elbow, is a term for tendinosis at the common medial flexor/pronator origin.

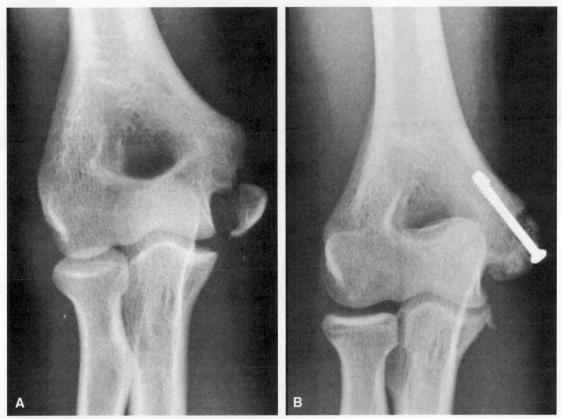

Figure 6-16

Medial epicondylar avulsion fracture. **A,** Radiograph of a 15-year-old baseball player with a medial epicondylar avulsion fracture. **B,** Postoperative radiograph showing a screw in the medial epicondyle to reduce and fix the fracture.

Specifically, the origins of the flexor carpi radialis and the pronator teres are most affected. Medial epicondylitis is much less common than lateral epicondylitis. Young to middle-aged athletes involved in golf, tennis, and overhead throwing are most commonly affected. In fact, medial epicondylitis is more common in professional tennis players than lateral epicondylitis. The repetitive valgus stress of these activities subjects these muscles to injury and chronic inflammation.[19,24]

The peak incidence of medial epicondylitis occurs in the fourth and fifth decades of life.[134] Occasionally, affected patients note medial elbow swelling and medial elbow pain that is worse with gripping, batting, hitting a serve in tennis, or throwing. Patients present with medial elbow pain and often symptoms of ulnar nerve irritation. Examination reveals tenderness over the medial epicondyle and slightly distal and lateral in the tendon of the pronator teres, as well as pain with resisted pronation or wrist flexion (Figure 6-17). Careful assessment for UCL instability and ulnar nerve symptoms is required, because medial epicondylitis may occur in conjunction with these problems. Radiographs usually are normal. MRI is not usually necessary for the diagnosis of medial epicondylitis, but the changes seen are consistent with a tendinosis, or they may be more extensive and include muscular and/or bony edema.

The treatment generally is nonoperative: rest and anti-inflammatory medications with a gradual return to stretching and strengthening of the involved muscles. In more than 80% of patients, symptoms resolve with conservative treatment and the patient is able to return to the sport or activity.[19] Cortisone injections may be of benefit as an adjunct to rehabilitation.[135] Rehabilitation includes application of ice, anti-inflammatory medications, and stretching and strengthening of the flexor/pronator muscle group. A counterforce brace may be beneficial in patients who are rehabilitating but still involved in activites that may aggravate the symptoms.

If the condition does not respond to an appropriate trial of nonoperative treatment, surgery may be required. Surgical intervention involves excision of the abnormal degenerative tissue at the common flexor/pronator origin and reapproximation of the remaining healthy tissue. Unfortunately, the surgery for medial epicondylitis is not as successful as that for lateral epicondylitis. Part of the reason for decreased success is failure to recognize concomitant disease. Ulnar neuropathy is present 40% to 60% of the time. The success of medial epicondylitis debridement is significantly reduced when concomitant ulnar neuropathy is a factor.[136,137] Vangsness and Jobe[138] reported 34 of

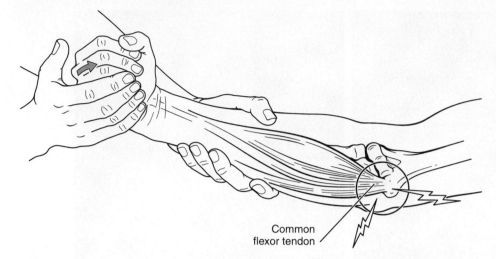

Figure 6-17

Schematic representation of the examination of a patient with medial epicondylitis. Pain in the medial elbow is reproduced by having the patient resist wrist flexion with the elbow extended. (From Esch JC, Baker CL: *Arthroscopic surgery (surgical arthroscopy): the shoulder and elbow,* p 248, Philadelphia, 199, JB Lippincott.)

Common flexor tendon

35 patients with good to excellent results after surgical debridement and reapproximation of the flexor/pronator musculature for refractory medial epicondylitis. However, Gabel and Morrey[136] showed that 96% of patients treated for medial epicondylitis without ulnar nerve symptoms had good to excellent results, compared with only 40% good to excellent results in patients with concomitant moderate to severe ulnar neuropathy requiring ulnar nerve decompression or transposition at the time of medial epicondylitis surgery. Furthermore, one needs to be suspicious of UCL instability in throwing athletes, and the appropriate workup needs to be performed in these patients.[22]

Flexor/Pronator Muscle Group Disruption

Complete disruption of the flexor/pronator muscle origin is rare. It generally occurs during the acceleration and follow-through stages of throwing in an overhead athlete, or it can occur in conjunction with dislocation of the elbow. This disruption usually occurs as a result of forceful extension of the elbow and pronation of the forearm or forceful valgus stress. Patients generally present after an acute onset of medial-sided elbow pain during a throw or pitch.[19,139,140] Clinically, disruption of the flexor/pronator muscle origin must be distinguished from a UCL injury, because the two structures frequently are injured concomitantly.[140] Patients with an isolated flexor/pronator rupture have tenderness over the anterior half of the medial epicondyle, which can be distinguished from the more posterior tenderness seen with UCL injury.[141] A muscular bulge may be present in the medial forearm from muscular contraction, as well as pain and/or weakness of wrist flexion and/or pronation. MRI usually is helpful for confirming the diagnosis (Figure 6-18). Although some authors recommend a trial of nonoperative treatment, most advocate surgical repair for complete ruptures because of the significant contribution of the flexor/pronator muscles to dynamic elbow stability and their important contributions to wrist strength. Repair

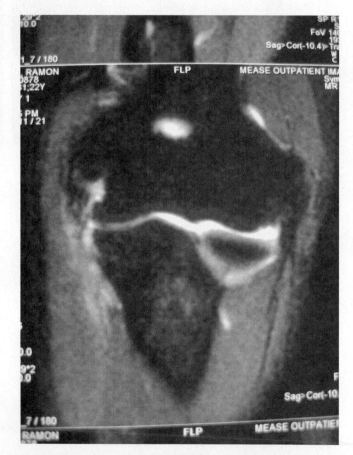

Figure 6-18

MRI scan of a patient with an acute flexor/pronator muscle strain with edema of the muscles and some edema about the tendon.

is technically difficult, and results are inconsistent. Athletes frequently cannot return to compete at the same level.[24]

Snapping Triceps

Snapping symptoms at the medial elbow can be caused by dislocation of the medial head of the triceps tendon over the medial epicondyle with elbow flexion; this often produces ulnar nerve symptoms and can be seen in association with ulnar nerve subluxation.[142,143] Underlying anatomical abnormalities generally are present.[144] Snapping of the lateral triceps tendon over the lateral epicondyle also has been described, although it is rare.[145] For persistent symptoms, operative treatment may be necessary. This most commonly involves anterior transposition of the ulnar nerve and correction of the underlying anatomical abnormality that resulted in dislocation of the tendon.

Ulnar Collateral Ligament Injury

Overhead throwing athletes subject their elbows to severe and repetitive valgus stress. The UCL, particularly the anterior band of the anterior oblique ligament of the UCL complex, which is the primary soft tissue restraint to valgus stress, is commonly injured. Chronic UCL insufficiency results from microscopic tears and attenuation.[146] Patients report pain and soreness in the medial elbow with throwing, usually in the late cocking or early acceleration phases or with ball release. Specifically, the athletes note that they are unable to throw more than 60% to 75% of maximal effort. Acute rupture can also occur with or without chronic changes. Most acute UCL ruptures (87%) occur midsubstance.[139] Ulnar and humeral avulsions are much less common. Athletes often report an episode of sudden onset of pain and "giving way" during throwing. The most common situation is an acute exacerbation of a chronically injured ligament. Associated ulnar neuropathy is quite common, and patients may report pain or numbness in the ulnar nerve distribution. Associated pathology, such as loose bodies, osteophytes, and a flexion contracture, can also produce symptoms.

Patients generally have point tenderness at the insertion of the UCL approximately 2 cm (1 inch) distal to the medial epicondyle. The UCL is the most important static stabilizer to valgus stress at 30° to 120° of flexion.[7] Therefore the appropriate position in which to assess for UCL insufficiency is the midrange of flexion. The valgus stress test has been described with the elbow at 30° flexion (Figure 6-19, A). The milking maneuver (Figure 6-19, B)[147] and its modification (Figure 6-19, C)[21] assess for valgus laxity at a higher degree of flexion. In this test, the patient's arm is stabilized proximally and the thumb is pulled laterally, imparting a valgus stress to the elbow in 70° to 90° flexion, while the examiner palpates the medial joint line for opening. O'Driscoll et al.[148] described an alternative way to assess for valgus instability, which they called the moving valgus stress test (Figure 6-19, D). In this test the elbow is brought from full flexion into extension with constant valgus force reproducing the patient's medial pain, although the pain from the UCL usually is reproducibly present between 80° and 120° flexion. The differential diagnosis includes medial epicondylitis and flexor/pronator origin rupture.

Stress radiographs can be helpful for demonstrating UCL insufficiency.[22] With the elbow flexed approximately 20° to 45°, an anteroposterior radiograph is taken while a valgus stress is applied. With UCL insufficiency, gapping at the medial joint line exceeds that of the contralateral normal side (Figure 6-20). Valgus stress is applied during these stress films either manually or with an instrumented device. Plain radiographs may also show secondary changes of chronic UCL insufficiency, such as osteophyte formation at the medial joint, loose bodies, sclerosis, radiocapitellar degeneration, or osteophytes of the olecranon. MRI can be helpful for detecting a torn UCL and for defining associated pathology. However, a MR arthrogram is even more sensitive (97%) in detecting UCL injury.[149,150] Arthroscopy is limited as a diagnostic tool because most of the anterior oblique portion of the UCL is not visualized arthroscopically; however, dynamic testing demonstrating gapping of the ulnohumeral joint when valgus stress is applied in 70° of elbow flexion and forearm pronation is consistent with UCL injury.[151,152] Ultrasonography also has been used to detect UCL injury, to demonstrate both changes within the ligament and medial joint opening with valgus stress, although it continues to be used only sparingly at this time.[153,154]

The initial treatment of UCL injury generally is nonoperative[22] and consists of rest from the overhead sport, anti-inflammatory medications, and physical therapy. One report indicates that about half of these patients can be treated successfully without surgery and are able to return to the same level of athletic activity.[155] Surgery is indicated if symptoms recur after an appropriate trial of nonoperative treatment. Surgical treatment of a UCL injury also should be considered with acute ruptures in high level throwing athletes, with significant chronic instability, and after debridement of UCL calcification.

Surgery for Ulnar Collateral Ligament Deficiency

When conservative treatment of UCL injuries fails, surgical options must be considered.[22] Surgical treatment of the UCL depends on several variables. Currently, the mainstay of surgical treatment is UCL reconstruction. Primary repair of acute ruptures of the UCL had been advocated for years; however, this has changed because of the overall consistently better results obtained with ligamentous reconstruction.[21,22] Although most tears are midsubstance (87%), some are avulsion injuries, and all have been considered amenable to suture repair.[139] This was the treatment of choice until 1992, when Conway et al.[139] reviewed their results with repair and reconstruction. They recommended reconstruction, citing the finding that overhead athletes performed significantly worse with repair than with reconstruction. They noted that repair should be considered only if the tear was a proximal avulsion, if the procedure was performed soon after injury, if the rest of the ligament was undamaged, and if no ulnar nerve symptoms were present. Repair of most injuries usually involves repair of

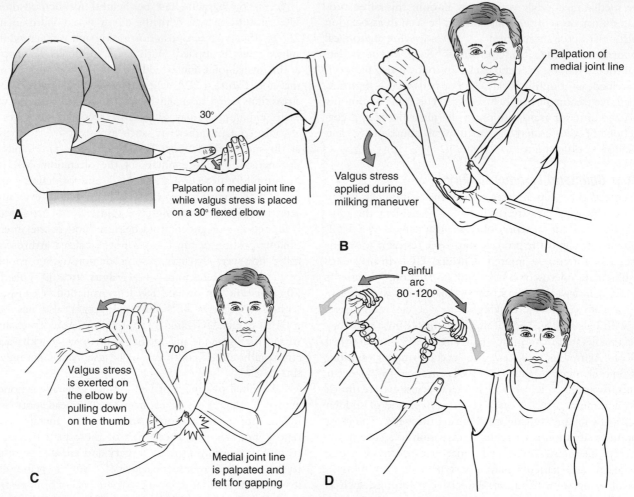

Figure 6-19

Examination of the ulnar collateral ligament (UCL). **A,** Schematic representation of the classic examination of the elbow for UCL injury. The elbow is at 30° flexion, and the hand is positioned between the examiner's elbow and body. The examiner exerts a valgus force on the elbow with one hand while palpating for medial joint opening with the other hand. **B,** The milking maneuver. The patient grabs the thumb on the arm with the affected elbow by passing the other hand beneath the affected elbow. This locks the shoulder, thereby reducing the effect of shoulder rotation and motion, which may confuse the examination. The examiner palpates the medial joint as the patient pulls on the thumb, exerting a valgus force on the elbow. Note that the elbow is in a high degree of flexion, greater than the angle at which a person throws; it also is flexed to the point that bony anatomy contributes to valgus stability of the elbow. **C,** Modified milking maneuver, in which the patient's elbow is flexed approximately 70° and the shoulder is adducted and slightly forward elevated. The examiner pulls on the patient's thumb, exerting the valgus stress with the shoulder locked in lateral rotation, and palpates the medial joint with the other hand. **D,** Schematic representation of the moving valgus stress test. The shoulder is brought into abduction and lateral rotation. The elbow is flexed and extended. The patient should reproducibly note pain in a particular degree of elbow flexion (80° to 120°). (**A** and **B** redrawn from Selby RM, Safran MR, O'Brien SJ: Elbow injuries. In Johnson DH, Pedowitz RA, editors: *Practical orthopaedic sports medicine and arthroscopy*, p 347, Philadelphia, 1007, Kluwer/Lippincott Williams & Wilkins; **C** and **D** redrawn from Safran MR: Injury to the ulnar collateral ligament: diagnosis and treatment, *Sports Med Arthrosc Rev* 11:19-20, 2003.)

tissue that frequently is chronically injured and therefore not ideal tissue. Reconstruction, therefore, has become the treatment of choice for UCL deficiency.

UCL reconstruction with a free tendon graft is the procedure usually performed for acute rupture in overhead sports athletes and for chronic UCL instability and elbow pain with UCL instability. The procedure has evolved considerably over the years.[22] Azar et al.[149] reported that 81% of patients were able to return to the same level of sports after UCL reconstruction, compared to 63% with primary repair.

Several graft options are available. A palmaris longus autograft most often is used, but other sources of autograft and even allograft also can be used for anatomical reconstruction. Sources of grafts include the ipsilateral or

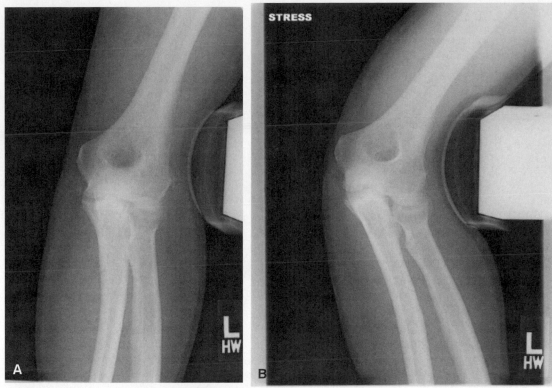

Figure 6-20
Stress x-ray films of a UCL injury. **A,** Nonstress x-ray film of a collegiate javelin thrower with chronic UCL insufficiency. Note the calcific change within the UCL, the result of attempted healing of the ligament injury. **B,** X-ray film with stress applied. Note the widened medial joint space, compared with the nonstress x-ray film.

contralateral palmaris longus, fourth toe extensor, hamstring tendon, a strip of Achilles tendon, the plantaris tendon, and allograft (hamstring and posterior or anterior tibialis tendon), although palmaris longus and hamstring grafts currently are used most often.[22] A variety of fixation techniques can be used, including bone tunnels, the docking procedure, and placement of interference screws (Figure 6-21).[156,157]

Routine ulnar nerve transposition, originally recommended with UCL reconstruction,[158] generally is not performed routinely in conjunction with UCL reconstruction, except by a few surgeons, because of the high rate of complications (21%).[139,149] If significant ulnar nerve symptoms are present, ulnar nerve transposition is performed at the same time as the reconstruction.

As the reconstruction procedure has evolved, the rate of operative success has reliably and reproducibly improved. Over the past several years, successful outcomes were reported to be 79% to 97%, with success defined as the patient returning to play at the same level or better than before the injury.[22,149,156,159-161] To achieve this level of success all sources of pathology need to be addressed. Medial epicondylitis may also be present. Also, concomitant valgus extension overload can result in olecranon osteophytes or loose bodies that need to be removed.

If clinically present, associated ulnar neuritis, as noted previously, is addressed through nerve transposition.

Ulnar Nerve Injuries

After carpal tunnel syndrome, ulnar nerve compression at the elbow is the most common compressive neuropathy of the upper extremity.[162] It is frequently seen in the general population but is even more common in overhead athletes. The medial elbow pathology seen in throwing athletes is associated with ulnar nerve symptoms approximately 50% of the time.[19] The ulnar nerve is susceptible to injury because of (1) the tight path it follows, which changes its dimensions with elbow flexion and extension, (2) its subcutaneous location, and (3) the considerable excursion required of it to accommodate the full motion of not only the elbow but also the shoulder (Figure 6-22, *A*). Proximally, the ulnar nerve can be compressed by the intermuscular septum or by a hypertrophied medial head of the triceps. At the cubital tunnel, nerve irritation and injury can result from osteophytes, loose bodies, a thickened retinaculum, or an inflamed UCL, especially with elbow flexion (Figure 6-22, *B*). The most common site of ulnar nerve compression is distal, between the two heads of the flexor carpi ulnaris (Figure 6-22, *C*).[1]

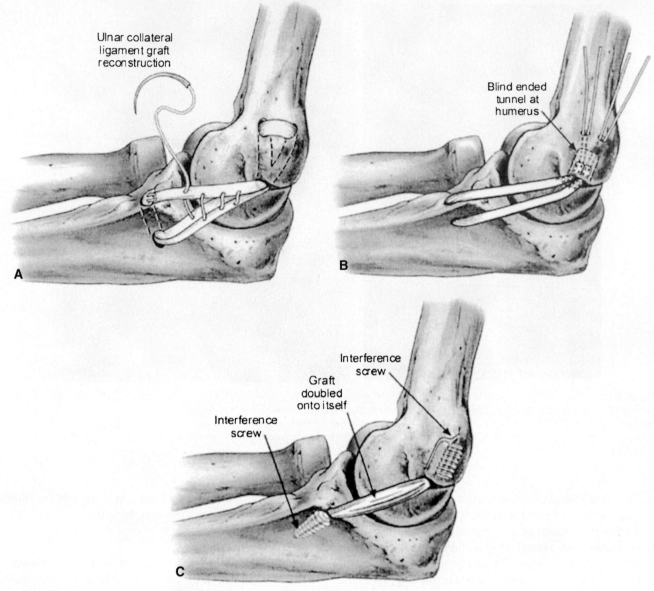

Figure 6-21

Reconstruction of the UCL. **A,** Classic three-ply UCL reconstruction. Two holes are drilled to make a tunnel in the ulna, and three holes are drilled to make two tunnels on the humeral side. This figure-of-eight appearance of the free tendon graft allows the tendon to have three strands at the medial elbow. **B,** Schematic representation of the docking technique of UCL reconstruction. The ulnar tunnel is made in the same way as for the classic technique, but a single, blind-end tunnel is used on the humeral side. This technique results in only two strands of tendon across the medial elbow, but it has two advantages: the graft is easier to tighten/tension, and the risk of medial epicondylar fracture is reduced. **C,** Interference screw technique of UCL reconstruction. Two strands are brought across the medial elbow, and both ends are fixed with interference screws in blind-end tunnels. This technique reduces the risk of tunnel fracture and, for the ulnar side, helps reduce injury to the ulnar nerve. (From Safran MR: Injury to the ulnar collateral ligament: diagnosis and treatment, *Sports Med Arthrosc Rev* 11:21-22, 2003.)

Both physiological and pathological factors contribute to irritation and compression of the ulnar nerve. Compression, either alone or in combination with other causes, can result in ulnar nerve irritation. With the elbow in full flexion, the confines of the cubital tunnel become restrictive and the retinaculum becomes taut, compressing the nerve. Flexion of the elbow and wrist extension increase the normal pressure on the ulnar nerve threefold. In overhead throwing, the pressure on the nerve has been demonstrated to be up to six times greater than normal.[163] The confines of the cubital tunnel may be reduced by scarring of the UCL (the floor of the cubital tunnel) or by osteophytes of the medial ulna at the olecranon or distal humerus (see Figure 6-22, *C*). The cumulative effect of repeated and

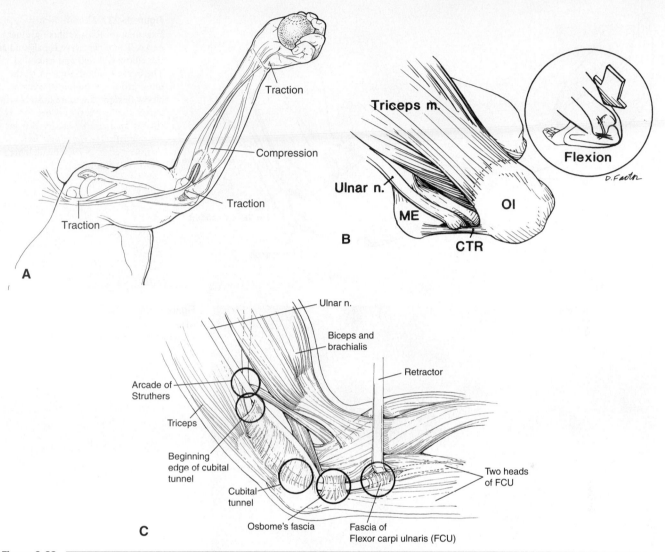

Figure 6-22

Ulnar nerve injury. **A,** Multiple sites of stress to the ulnar nerve in the throwing athlete. **B,** Elbow flexion leads to compression of the ulnar nerve within the cubital tunnel. Anything that occupies space in the tunnel (e.g., osteophytes, thickened retinaculum or ligament) can increase compression on the nerve. **C,** Multiple sites of compression where the ulnar nerve may become entrapped about the elbow. (**A** and **C** from Miller MD, Howard RF, Plancher KD: *Surgical atlas of sports medicine*, pp 397, 402, Philadelphia, 2003, WB Saunders; **B** from O'Driscoll SW, Horii E, Carmichael SW, Morrey BF: The cubital tunnel and ulnar neuropathy, *J Bone Joint Surg Br* 75:615, 1991. Copyright Mayo Foundation.)

prolonged pressure elevations is nerve ischemia and fibrosis. This pathology can be exacerbated when it occurs in association with ulnar nerve subluxation or dislocation.

The first symptoms often are medial elbow pain and clumsiness or heaviness of the hand. Subsequently, paresthesias and more significant weakness can ensue (however, these usually are not present in the athlete with ulnar neuritis). Patients may note numbness at night in the ulnar hand (the little and ring fingers) if they sleep with the elbow bent. Throwers usually note loss of control. The results of nerve conduction tests can be normal, especially in the earlier stages.[1,19,164] Symptoms may be reproduced by a Tinel's sign and/or by having the patient maximally flex

the elbow and extend the wrist and hold that position for 1 minute. Subluxation of the ulnar nerve is also common in the general population and frequently occurs without symptoms (Figure 6-23). Overhead athletes with subluxing ulnar nerves can have symptoms and may require surgery to prevent the nerve from becoming irritated as it traverses the medial epicondyle. Radiographs usually are normal, but MRI scans may reveal the ulnar neuritis (Figure 6-24).

The initial treatment is nonoperative and in the general population often is successful. Throwing athletes, however, tend to have recurrence of symptoms upon resumption of throwing, particularly those with subluxation of the ulnar nerve.

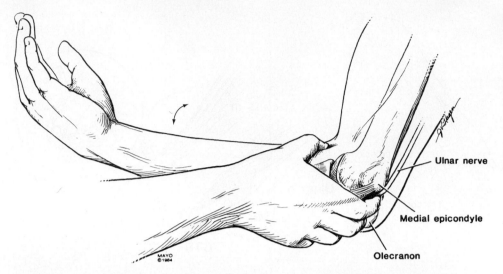

Figure 6-23
Examination for a subluxing ulnar nerve. The ulnar nerve is palpated as the elbow is flexed and extended. The nerve tends to slip out of the ulnar groove in higher degrees of elbow flexion (the more unstable the nerve, the less flexion is needed to sublux the nerve). (Modified from Morrey BF: *The elbow and its disorders*, ed 2, p 79, Philadelphia, 1993, WB Saunders.)

Ulnar nerve

Medial epicondyle

Olecranon

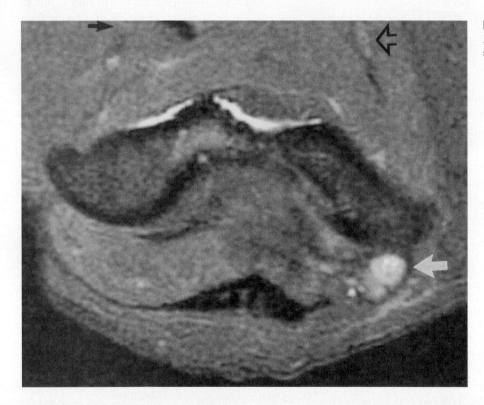

Figure 6-24
MRI scan of an inflamed ulnar nerve, showing the white nerve on T2.

Ulnar Nerve Transposition Surgery

When conservative measures fail or are deemed inappropriate, ulnar nerve neuropathy may be addressed surgically. Surgery has two goals. Decompression of the ulnar nerve at all sights of potential tightness is the primary goal. However, addressing all possible sights of decompression may result in instability of the ulnar nerve and painful subluxation of the nerve out of its groove. For this reason, transposition of the nerve to a position that would prevent instability may be necessary, particularly in athletes.

Surgical treatment most often involves either anterior subcutaneous or submuscular transposition of the nerve. The disadvantage of subcutaneous transposition is that the nerve remains vulnerable to direct injury in contact sports. Submuscular transposition requires a longer rehabilitation because of detachment and reapproximation of the flexor/pronator origin, but the nerve is protected from direct trauma. With submuscular transpositions, the wrist must be immobilized as well. The postoperative rehabilitation must be considered carefully, because early motion is encouraged to prevent scarring about the nerve, but the flexor/pronator muscle attachment must be protected until it heals.

Simple decompression and medial epicondylectomy are thought to produce poor results in the throwing athlete because of the risk of UCL injury and subluxation of the nerve.[19] However, simple decompression may be a reasonable alternative in nonthrowing athletes. Two recent prospective studies showed similar results for simple decompression and anterior submuscular decompression.[165,166] The preference of the senior author of this chapter is to perform submuscular transposition in athletes at risk for direct trauma to the area of the nerve (e.g., football and rugby players) and subcutaneous transposition in all others.

Posterior Elbow

Olecranon Apophysitis/Stress Fracture

In the adolescent athlete, the olecranon physeal plate is susceptible to injury, especially with overhead throwing.[24] The repetitive pull of the triceps tendon can lead to an apophysitis and physeal widening.[167,168] These injuries tend to occur in adolescents and may also be the result of valgus extension overload (discussed later in the chapter). These patients complain of pain on resisted elbow extension and tenderness over the olecranon. Radiographs demonstrate widening of the olecranon apophysis and should be confirmed by comparison with radiographs of the contralateral elbow (Figure 6-25, *A*). An MRI can help confirm the diagnosis when radiographs are not conclusive (Figure 6-25, *B*).

When the apophysis is widened but not separated or avulsed, the initial treatment is rest from the offending activity, gentle range of motion and flexibility exercises, and progression to strengthening. Ice and nonsteroidal anti-inflammatory medications (NSAIDs) are useful if acute inflammation is present. If the child is in severe pain, a short course of immobilization in a splint or cast may be beneficial.[169] If separation of the secondary growth center has occurred or if the adolescent has pain despite conservative management because of lack of fusion of the physis, internal fixation is recommended (Figure 6-26, *A*). Surgical intervention to promote fusion of the apophysis may require internal fixation with a screw, in addition to bone grafting, because of the high incidence of fibrous union when bone grafting is not used (Figure 6-26, *B*).[168,170,171] Left untreated, apophysitis of the olecranon may result in an incompletely fused olecranon apophysis, which may fracture as a result of direct trauma when the patient is older.[168,171-173]

In mature athletes, posterior elbow pain may represent an occult (or stress) fracture of the olecranon. This type of fracture, which is most common in baseball players, javelin throwers, shot putters, and gymnasts, can be associated with valgus extension overload syndrome (discussed later in the chapter). If radiographs are inconclusive, a bone scan or MRI may be necessary for diagnosis. Most of these

Figure 6-25

A, Olecranon stress fracture on a lateral x-ray film.

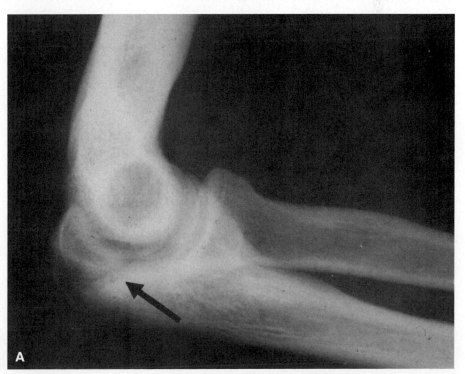

Continued

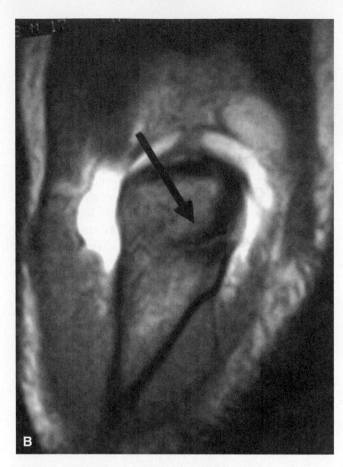

Figure 6-25 cont'd

B, MRI scan of a patient with an olecranon stress fracture.

injuries heal with rest from the offending activity. Surgery is rarely necessary.[170,174-177]

Triceps Tendonitis and Tendon Rupture

Tendonitis of the triceps insertion at the olecranon is most often seen in weight lifters. It also occurs with other sports in which large forces are required in elbow extension, such as shot put, javelin, and football. In addition, the problem has affected participants in motocross racing and BMX cycling, because the riders absorb the force of landing with the arms.[1] Patients have pain at the triceps insertion that is worsened by resisted active elbow extension and throwing. On examination, these individuals have tenderness at the tip of the olecranon and slightly proximal at the triceps insertion point. The pain may be accentuated by resisted elbow extension and full elbow flexion with shoulder flexion. This problem may be acute or chronic. Treatment is conservative. Corticosteroid injections into the tendon are contraindicated because of the risk of tendon rupture.[178]

Triceps tendon rupture is rare, the least common of all tendon ruptures in the body. It has been reported in weight lifters and football players.[179,180] In many cases it is associated with corticosteroid injections or oral anabolic steroids.[181] It commonly involves avulsion with a bony fragment as a result of a decelerating counterforce during active extension of the elbow or a direct blow. Patients with this injury usually are unable to extend the elbow against gravity and have a palpable defect in the tendon proximal to the olecranon (Figure 6-27). This injury rarely occurs

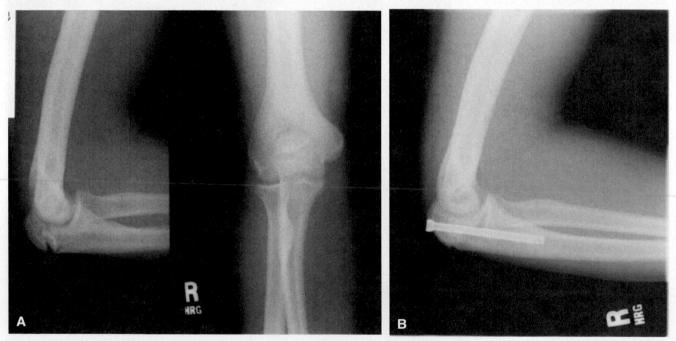

Figure 6-26

A, X-ray film of an unfused olecranon apophysis, which was treated with intramedullary screw fixation **(B).**

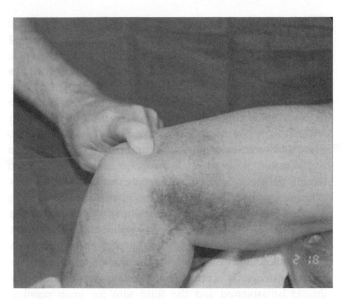

Figure 6-27
Photograph from the operating room with a patient in the prone position. This patient has a triceps tendon rupture, as evidenced by the palpable defect just proximal to the olecranon. Ecchymosis also is present, because the injury occurred only a few days before the patient underwent surgical repair.

at the musculotendinous junction. Radiographs classically show a small fleck of bone off the olecranon (Figure 6-28). MRI is rarely necessary to make the diagnosis but can confirm it. Treatment for complete ruptures is acute surgical repair, which gives consistently good results compared

to the universally poor results seen with nonoperative treatment.[179,182,183]

Valgus Extension Overload Syndrome

Overhead throwing athletes are at risk for specific elbow pathology that occurs secondary to the repetitive valgus stresses involved in throwing, which cause the olecranon to be repeatedly and forcefully driven into the olecranon fossa. A valgus stress typically causes shearing posteriorly; this results in impingement of the posteromedial olecranon against the lateral aspect of the medial wall of the olecranon fossa (see Figure 6-5, B). Ahmad et al.[184] demonstrated that UCL injury results in contact alterations in the posterior compartment that lead to osteophyte formation. This suggests that osteophyte formation may result from subtle UCL injury or increased valgus laxity as a result of increased shear forces to the posteromedial elbow. Compounding this posterior impingement is the bony hypertrophic narrowing of the olecranon fossa and hypertrophy of the proximal ulna that occur in overhead athletes who have performed since childhood. Moreover, the repeated high extension velocities may result in impaction of the olecranon tip within the fossa, resulting in localized inflammation, chondromalacia, and further osteophyte formation. With persistent impaction and shear forces, the osteophytes may break off and become loose bodies within the joint.[185,186] These loose bodies can get caught in the joint surfaces and damage the articular cartilage.

Individuals with valgus extension overload syndrome (VEOS) have posterior elbow pain, pain with extension of the elbow (especially forced extension), and occasionally locking caused by loose bodies. On examination, the patient may have a flexion contracture, swelling of the joint, and pain on forced extension of the elbow that is exacerbated by applying a valgus force to the extended elbow.[22,186] It is important that the examiner evaluate the integrity and tenderness of the UCL, because studies have shown that 42% of patients who undergo surgery for VEOS require a second operation, and 25% of these patients required reconstruction of the UCL as a result of valgus instability.[187]

Initial conservative treatment should focus on strengthening of the flexor/pronator muscle group while reducing inflammation; this is achieved through relative rest, application of ice, and NSAIDs. However, surgery is often required if loose bodies are present. Furthermore, the authors' experience has been that patients with posteromedial osteophytes on the olecranon tend not to respond to therapy and require surgery to remove the osteophytes.[21,22,186] Nonetheless, surgery usually is indicated if 6 to 12 weeks of conservative management does not lead to improvement.

Surgery for Valgus Extension Overload Syndrome

VEOS surgery involves the removal of loose bodies, which can be done arthroscopically. The osteophytes on the

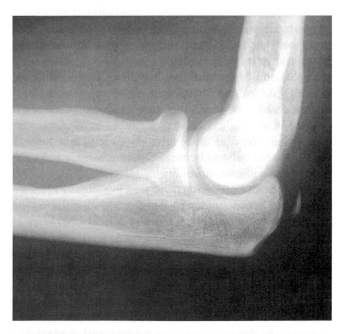

Figure 6-28
X-ray film of a patient with a triceps tendon avulsion. Note the small fleck of bone just proximal to the olecranon; this is a common finding in this rare injury.

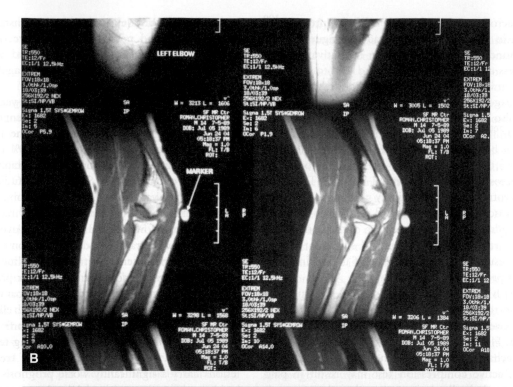

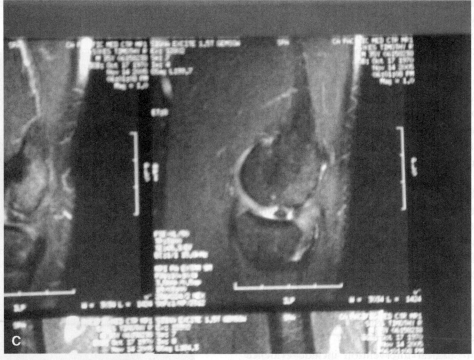

Figure 6-30 cont'd
B, MRI scan of the same boy. The lesion was partly detached and ultimately was repaired surgically.
C, MRI scan of the elbow of a 16-year-old gymnast with OCD and an apparent loose body.

to fix, some recommend debridement and microfracture of the bony bed. Others have tried osteochondral autograft plugs, particularly when the lateral column is involved in the lesion. Early experience with the osteochondral plugs is encouraging.[210,211]

Radiocapitellar Degeneration

As previously discussed, radiocapitellar degeneration most often occurs with UCL insufficiency.[22] Incompetence of the medial stabilizing structures (UCL) results in increased force at the radiocapitellar joint, which leads to softening and degeneration of the articular cartilage. Osteochondral loose bodies are common and often cause mechanical symptoms and pain.[24] Eventually, degenerative arthritis of the radiocapitellar joint may develop. Tenderness at the lateral elbow that is worsened by pronation and supination of the elbow is a common finding on examination. Arthroscopic treatment is effective for removing loose bodies but cannot reverse the changes in the articular cartilage. In athletes, the symptoms usually recur when the individual returns to the same level of throwing, especially if the UCL instability has not been corrected. For constant pain caused by radiocapitellar arthritis, radial head excision, using either open or arthroscopic techniques, often is successful. Some clinicians also advocate isolated radiocapitellar arthroplasty.

Lateral Epicondylitis

Lateral epicondylitis, or tennis elbow, is by far the most common overuse injury of the elbow; it is approximately seven times more common than medial epicondylitis.[134,212] It is commonly seen in tennis players and other athletes, although 95% of individuals with tennis elbow do not play tennis (Figure 6-31). Lateral epicondylitis or, more appropriately, epicondylosis is very common in the general population, particularly in individuals who do repetitive work, such as typing on the computer.

Nirschl and Pettrone[213] first described this condition as a degenerative more than inflammatory process involving primarily the extensor carpi radialis brevis. The extensor digitorum communis can also be involved to a lesser degree. These researchers' histological observations led them to label the condition *angiofibroblastic hyperplasia*.[213] Given the absence of inflammatory findings, the term *tendinosis* is used instead of *tendonitis*.

Lateral epicondylitis is most common in patients 35 to 50 years of age and is associated with higher levels and frequency of activity (overuse).[24] Poor conditioning and poor technique likely exacerbate the problem in many tennis players, and certainly many racquet factors have been attributed to tennis elbow, including heavy racquets, metal racquets, stiffer racquets, incorrect grip size, and tight strings. As many as half of club tennis players over age 30 have had tennis elbow.[213,214] Patients initially complain of activity-related lateral elbow pain, often a dull, aching, lateral pain, and may show weakness of grip strength. Symptoms can progress to pain at rest in the more severe stages and difficulty holding a cup, lifting a milk carton, or opening a door.[24] On examination patients have tenderness approximately 1 to 2 cm (½ to 1 inch) distal to the lateral epicondyle and pain with passive wrist flexion, resisted active wrist extension, and during grasping or lifting. Radiographs often are normal but may show a spur at the lateral epicondyle or calcification of the common extensor tendon.[1,212,214] MRI is rarely necessary but can reveal changes consistent with a tendinosis of the extensor muscles at the elbow (Figure 6-32).

Treatment initially is nonoperative; 95% of patients improve with conservative treatment.[214] Rest (i.e., avoidance of the stress or overuse) must be combined with a program that re-establishes the patient's strength, flexibility, and endurance. Counterforce bracing is thought to reduce the load at the lateral epicondyle by preventing the forearm muscles from fully expanding.[212] Corticosteroid injections can be helpful, particularly for reducing symptoms to allow rehabilitation exercises, but repeated injections (i.e., more than three in a 1-year period) are not recommended.[215] A recent randomized study showed a short-term benefit

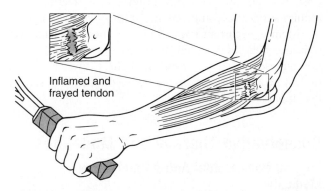

Figure 6-31
Lateral epicondylitis, a tendinosis of the wrist extensor muscles at the lateral epicondyle as a result of overuse of the wrist extensors, such as may occur in tennis players.

Inflamed and frayed tendon

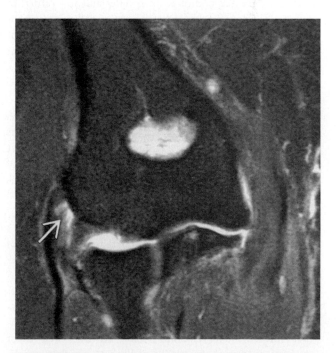

Figure 6-32
MRI scan of a patient with epicondylosis of the wrist extensors at the lateral epicondyle.

to iontophoresis of dexamethasone in patients with severe lateral epicondylitis.[216] Other research suggests that topical nitric oxide, metalloprotease inhibitors, and botulinum toxin may be beneficial.[217-219] Shock wave therapy has not been shown to be beneficial.[220] Blood injections and platelet-rich plasma recently have been shown to be beneficial in small case series.[221,222] Recreational tennis players should be encouraged to seek professional instruction, because improper technique often contributes to the problem.[24]

Surgery for Lateral Epicondylitis

If 6 months of nonoperative treatment fail to give satisfactory improvement, surgery is indicated.[1,24] Lateral epicondylitis can be treated percutaneously, by an open technique, or arthroscopically. A detailed review is beyond the scope of this chapter but can be found in the literature.[223] Only one paper in the literature compares the three main procedures for tennis elbow: percutaneous release, the open procedure described by Nirschl and Ashman,[214] and arthroscopic release; none of the three was found to be superior.[224] A systematic review of the literature also did not reveal any difference between the different procedures, but this may be due to the limited number of quality studies in the literature.[223] The principal goals generally are to remove abnormal, degenerative tissue (usually at the origin of the extensor carpi radialis brevis [ECRB]) and to encourage healing with minimal disruption of normal stabilizing structures (Figure 6-33). Outcomes after surgical treatment are excellent. According to Nirschl and Ashman,[214] 85% of patients experience complete pain relief and full return of strength. Similar outcomes have been noted with arthroscopic release; in addition, concomitant intra-articular problems may be identified and treated arthroscopically that might not be seen with an open approach.[223,225]

Extensor/Supinator Muscular Disruption

Lateral muscle disruption is rare. It has been reported in patients who have had repeated corticosteroid injections for lateral epicondylitis.[215] Patients report an acute onset of pain associated with a snap that results in weakness of wrist extension and supination. For complete or near complete injuries, surgical repair is recommended.[1]

Radial Nerve Entrapment

For some time it has been accepted that certain cases of persistent tennis elbow represent radial or posterior interosseous nerve compression, the so-called radial tunnel syndrome.[226] The radial tunnel is defined by the bony and soft tissue structures that surround the radial nerve and its posterior interosseous branch as they travel through the proximal forearm. Nerve compression in this area most commonly occurs at the arcade of Frohse, often the tendinous proximal edge of the supinator muscle. Other potential sites of compression include the proximal edge of the

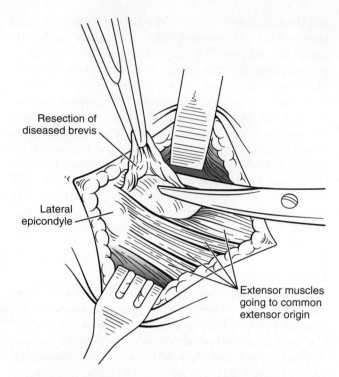

Figure 6-33

Schematic representation of open surgery for tennis elbow with excision of the degenerative tissue. (Redrawn from Safran MR: Elbow tendinopathy: surgical repair of the epicondylitides. In Craig E, editor: *Clinical orthopaedics*, p 279, Philadelphia, 1999, Lippincott Williams & Wilkins.)

extensor carpi radialis brevis, branches of the radial artery, and fibrous bands.[227,228]

When persistent forearm pain and tenderness are associated with muscle weakness in the distribution of the posterior interosseous nerve, nerve entrapment in the radial tunnel is the likely etiology. The tenderness associated with radial nerve entrapment is more distal and medial than that seen in lateral epicondylitis; that is, it is located more over the muscular area of the proximal forearm.[24] Conservative management usually is successful in treating this problem.[1] Cases that do not respond to nonoperative treatment may require surgical decompression.[24] However, many cases of persistent or recurrent tennis elbow are not associated with objective neurological deficits. These cases most likely do not represent a true entrapment neuropathy, and practitioners should be cautious about recommending surgical decompression.[228,229]

Conservative Therapy and Modalities

Ice and Nonsteroidal Anti-inflammatory Medications

Nonoperative treatment of elbow injuries usually involves multiple approaches. Ice is often recommended, especially in the acute period, because it has minimal risks and may provide symptomatic relief of swelling and pain. NSAIDs also are used as a first-line medical treatment for painful and inflammatory conditions about the elbow. They are most often administered topically or orally, although intramuscular injection is also available. For lateral elbow pain, topical NSAIDs have shown a significant effect, compared to placebo, for short-term pain relief and patient satisfaction.[230] Oral NSAIDs are also often used, although the benefit is not as well documented and the adverse effects are more significant. Long-term oral use of NSAIDs can be associated with adverse effects on the gastrointestinal and renal systems. Fortunately, these complications are uncommon with short-term use in medically healthy patients when taken with food.

Ultrasound

Ultrasound has been used as a treatment for chronic musculotendinous problems. Phonophoresis involves the addition of a gel containing a corticosteroid to the ultrasound treatment. In one study, ultrasound was shown to achieve short-term improvement in pain and pressure tolerance in patients with tendonitis, and adding phonophoresis did not provide any additional benefit.[231]

High Voltage Electrical Stimulation

Electrical stimulation frequently has been used as a treatment for various musculoskeletal conditions. Specifically, it often is used to treat nerve and tendon injuries of the upper extremity, and some evidence in animal models indicates that it may help stimulate nerve repair. However, no human clinical studies have demonstrated a significant effect in the treatment of nerve or tendon injuries.[232]

Transverse Friction Massage

Transverse friction massage has been suggested as a physical therapy modality for tendonitis pain. However, the controlled studies that have been reported have not shown a significant effect. One study looked at lateral epicondylitis and showed no difference in terms of pain relief, grip strength, or functional status compared with other physical therapy modalities.[233]

Cortisone Injections

Local corticosteroid injections are commonly used to treat a variety of chronic musculoskeletal problems. They have been used extensively to treat lateral epicondylitis. Smidt et al.[215] did an extensive review of the literature on the use of corticosteroid injections in this condition. They found a statistically significant short-term effect for pain, grip strength, and global improvement; however, no medium- or long-term effect could be demonstrated.[215]

The most commonly cited complication of corticosteroid injection is tendon rupture.[234]

General Rehabilitation Guidelines

Rehabilitation after elbow injury or elbow surgery follows a sequential and progressive multiphase approach. The ultimate goal of elbow rehabilitation is to return the patient to the previous functional level as quickly and safely as possible. The following sections provide an overview of the rehabilitation process after elbow injury and surgery. Rehabilitation protocols for specific pathologies are then presented.

Four Phases of Elbow Rehabilitation

- Phase I: Immediate motion phase
- Phase II: Intermediate phase (full ROM, minimal pain, good muscle strength)
- Phase III: Advanced strengthening phase
- Phase IV: Return to activity phase

Phase I: Immediate Motion Phase

The first phase of elbow rehabilitation is the immediate motion phase. The goals of this phase are to minimize the effects of immobilization, re-establish pain-free range of motion, reduce pain and inflammation, and retard muscular atrophy. Early range of motion activities are performed to nourish the articular cartilage and assist in the synthesis, alignment, and organization of collagen tissue.[235-243] Range of motion activities are performed for all planes of elbow and wrist motions to prevent the formation of scar tissue and adhesions. Active-assisted and passive range of motion exercises are performed for the ulnohumeral joint to restore flexion/extension, as well as supination/pronation for the radiohumeral and radioulnar joints. The re-establishment of either full elbow extension or preinjury motion is the primary goal of early ROM activities to minimize the occurrence of elbow flexion contractures.[243-245] Preoperative elbow motion must be carefully assessed and recorded. Patients should be asked whether they have had full elbow extension in the past 2 to 3 years. Postoperative ROM often is related to preoperative motion, especially with UCL reconstruction. Elbow flexion contractures can be a deleterious side effect of surgery for the overhead athlete. The elbow is predisposed to flexion contractures because of the intimate congruency of the joint articulations, the tightness of the joint capsule, and the tendency of the anterior capsule to develop adhesions after injury.[242] The brachialis muscle also attaches to the capsule and crosses the elbow joint before becoming a tendinous structure. Injury to the elbow may cause excessive scar tissue formation of the brachialis muscle and to the adjacent tissues, which may require functional splinting of the elbow.[242]

Phase I: Goals of Immediate Motion Phase

- Minimize the effects of immobilization
- Re-establish pain-free ROM
- Reduce pain and inflammation
- Reduce muscle atrophy

In addition to ROM exercises, joint mobilizations may be performed as tolerated to minimize the occurrence of joint contractures. Posterior glides with oscillations are performed at end range of motion to help regain full elbow extension. Initially grade I and grade II mobilizations are used, with progression to aggressive mobilization techniques (grade III and grade IV) at end range of motion during later stages of rehabilitation, when symptoms have subsided. Joint mobilization must include the radiocapitellar and radioulnar joints.

If the patient continues to have difficulty achieving full extension using ROM and mobilization techniques, a low load–long duration (LLLD) stretch (also called *collagen creep* or *plastic flow stretch*) may be performed to produce a deformation (creep) of the collagen tissue, resulting in tissue elongation.[245-248] The authors have found this technique to be extremely beneficial for regaining full elbow extension. The patient lies supine with a towel roll or foam placed under the distal brachium to act as a cushion and fulcrum. Light-resistance exercise tubing is applied to the wrist and secured to the table or to a dumbbell on the ground (Figure 6-34). The patient is instructed to relax as much as possible for 12 to 15 minutes. The patient is instructed to perform this type of exercise at home periodically during the day, totaling 60 minutes of stretching per day. The resistance applied should be low magnitude to enable the patient to perform the stretch for the entire duration without pain or muscle spasm; the technique should impart a low load but a long duration stretch.

The aggressiveness of stretching and mobilization techniques is dictated by the healing constraints of the involved tissues, the specific pathology or surgical technique, and the amount of motion and end feel. If the patient has decreased motion and a pathologically hard end feel without pain, aggressive stretching and mobilization techniques may be used. Conversely, a patient who has pain before resistance or an empty end feel must be progressed slowly with gentle stretching.

Another goal of phase I is to reduce the patient's pain and inflammation. Grade I and grade II mobilization techniques may also be used to neuromodulate pain by stimulating type I and type II articular receptors.[249,250] Cryotherapy and high voltage stimulation may be performed as required to further assist in reducing pain and inflammation. Once the acute inflammatory response has subsided, moist heat, warm whirlpool, and ultrasound may be used at the onset of treatment to

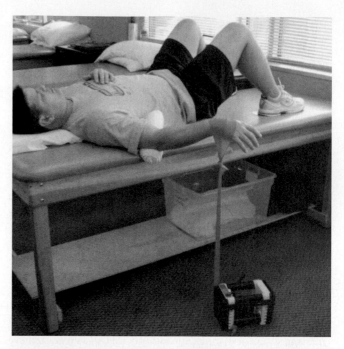

Figure 6-34

Low load–long duration stretching to improve elbow extension. A low intensity stretch is applied for 10-12 minutes. Note that the elbow is pronated and the shoulder is internally rotated to lock the humerus and prevent compensation.

prepare the tissue for stretching and improve the extensibility of the capsule and musculotendinous structures. In addition, joint mobilization glides are increased to grade III and grade IV mobilizations.

The early phase of rehabilitation also focuses on voluntary activation of muscle and the retardation of muscular atrophy. Subpainful and submaximal isometrics are performed initially for the elbow flexor and extensor, as well as for the wrist flexor, extensor, pronator, and supinator muscle groups. Shoulder isometrics may also be performed during this phase, but care must be taken to avoid internal and external rotation exercises if these are painful. Alternating rhythmic stabilization drills for shoulder flexion/extension/horizontal abduction/adduction, shoulder internal/external rotation, and elbow flexion/extension/supination/pronation are performed to begin re-establishing proprioception and neuromuscular control of the upper extremity.

Phase II: Intermediate Phase (Full ROM, Minimal Pain, Good Muscle Strength)

Phase II, the intermediate phase, is initiated when the patient exhibits full ROM, minimal pain and tenderness, and a good (4/5) manual muscle test of the elbow flexor and extensor musculature. The emphasis in this phase includes enhancing elbow and upper extremity mobility, improving muscular strength and endurance, and re-establishing neuromuscular control of the elbow complex.

Stretching exercises are continued to maintain full elbow and wrist range of motion. Mobilization techniques may be progressed to more aggressive grade III techniques as needed to apply a stretch to the capsular tissue at end range. Flexibility is progressed during this phase to focus on wrist flexion, extension, pronation, and supination. Elbow extension and forearm pronation flexibility is particularly emphasized in throwing athletes so that they can perform efficiently. Shoulder flexibility is also maintained in athletes, with emphasis on external and internal rotation at 90° abduction, flexion, and horizontal adduction. In particular, shoulder external rotation at 90° abduction is emphasized; loss of external rotation may result in increased strain on the medial elbow structures during the overhead throwing motion. Internal rotation motion also is diligently performed.

Strengthening exercises are progressed during this phase to include isotonic contractions, beginning with concentric contractions and progressing to include eccentric contractions. Emphasis is placed on elbow flexion and extension, wrist flexion and extension, and forearm pronation and supination. The glenohumeral and scapulothoracic muscles are placed on a progressive resistance program during the later stages of phase II. Emphasis is placed on strengthening the shoulder external rotators and scapular muscles. A complete upper extremity strengthening program, such as the thrower's 10 program, may be performed (Figure 6-35).

Neuromuscular control exercises are initiated in this phase to enhance the muscles' ability to control the elbow joint during athletic activities. These exercises include proprioceptive neuromuscular facilitation exercises with rhythmic stabilizations (Figure 6-36) and slow reversal manual resistance elbow/wrist flexion drills (Figure 6-37).

Phase II: Goals of Intermediate Phase (Full ROM, Minimal Pain, Good Muscle Strength)

- Enhance elbow and upper extremity mobility
- Improve muscle strength and endurance
- Re-establish neuromuscular control

Phase III: Advanced Strengthening Phase

The third phase of elbow rehabilitation involves a progression of activities to prepare the patient or athlete for high level stress situations or participation in sports. The goals of this phase are to gradually increase strength, power, endurance, and neuromuscular control to prepare for a gradual return to sports. Specific criteria that must be met before this phase is entered include full, nonpainful ROM; absence of pain or tenderness; and strength that is 70% of the contralateral extremity.

Phase III: Goals of Advanced Strengthening Phase

- Increase strength to functional levels
- Increase power to functional levels
- Increase endurance to functional levels
- Increase neuromuscular control

Criteria for Progression to Phase III

- Full, pain-free ROM
- No pain
- No tenderness
- Strength at least 70% of contralateral limb

Advanced strengthening activities during this phase include aggressive strengthening exercises that emphasize high speed and eccentric contraction and plyometric activities. Elbow flexion exercises are progressed to emphasize eccentric control. The biceps muscle is an important stabilizer during the follow-through phase of overhead throwing; it eccentrically controls the deceleration of the elbow, preventing pathological abutment of the olecranon within the fossa.[251,252] Elbow flexion can be performed with elastic tubing to emphasize slow and fast concentric and eccentric contractions. Manual resistance may be applied for concentric and eccentric contractions of the elbow flexors. Aggressive strengthening exercises done with weight machines are also incorporated during this phase. These most commonly begin with bench press, seated rowing, and front latissimus dorsi pull-downs. The triceps are exercised primarily with a concentric contraction because of the acceleration (muscle shortening) activity of the muscle during the acceleration phase of throwing.

Neuromuscular control exercises are progressed to include side lying external rotation with manual resistance. Concentric and eccentric external rotation is performed against the clinician's resistance with the addition of rhythmic stabilizations. This manual resistance exercise may be progressed to standing external rotation with exercise tubing at 0° and finally at 90° (Figure 6-38).

Plyometric drills can be an extremely beneficial form of functional exercise for training the elbow in overhead athletes.[243,253] Plyometric exercises are performed using a weighted medicine ball during the later stages of phase III to train the shoulder and elbow to develop and withstand high levels of stress. Plyometric exercises initially are performed with two hands performing a chest pass, side-to-side throw, and overhead soccer throw. These may be progressed to include one-handed activities such as 90/90 throws (Figure 6-39), external and internal rotation throws at 0° abduction (Figure 6-40), and wall dribbles. Specific

A, Diagonal pattern D2 extension: Grip the tubing handle overhead and out to the side with the hand of the involved arm. Pull the tubing down and across the body to the opposite side of the leg. During the motion, lead with the thumb. **Diagonal pattern D2 flexion:** Grip the tubing handle in the hand of the involved arm, beginning with the arm 45° out from the side and the palm facing backward. After turning the palm forward, flex the elbow and bring the arm up and over the uninvolved shoulder. Turn the palm down and reverse to take the arm to the starting position. The exercise should be performed in a controlled manner.

B, Dumbbell exercises for deltoid and supraspinatus deltoid strengthening: Stand with the arm at the side, the elbow straight, and the palm against the side. Raise the arm to the side, palm down, until the arm reaches 90°. **Supraspinatus strengthening:** Stand with the elbow straight and the thumb up. Raise the arm to shoulder level at a 30-degree angle in front of the body. Do not go above shoulder height. Hold for 2 seconds and lower slowly.

C, Prone shoulder abduction for the rhomboids: diagonal pattern D2 flexion: With the involved hand, grip the tubing handle across the body and against the thigh of the opposite leg. Starting with the palm down, rotate the palm up. Flex the elbow and bring the arm up and over the involved shoulder with the palm facing inward. Turn the palm down and reverse to take the arm to the starting position. The exercise should be performed in a controlled manner.

D, Prone shoulder extension for the latissimus dorsi: Lie on the table, face down, with the involved arm hanging straight to the floor and the palm facing down. Raise the arm straight back as far as possible. Hold for 2 seconds and lower slowly.

E, Internal rotation at 90° abduction: Stand with the shoulder abducted to 90° and externally rotated 90° and the elbow bent to 90° – this is the starting position and the tubing is held with mild tension in the tubing. Keep the shoulder abducted and rotate the shoulder forward while keeping the elbow at 90°. Return the tubing and the hand to the starting position slowly and in a controlled manner. **External rotation at 90° abduction:** Stand with the shoulder abducted to 90° and the elbow flexed to 90°. Grip the tubing handle while the other hand is fixed straight ahead. Keep the shoulder abducted and rotate the shoulder back while keeping the elbow at 90°. Return the tubing and the hand to the starting position slowly and in a controlled manner.

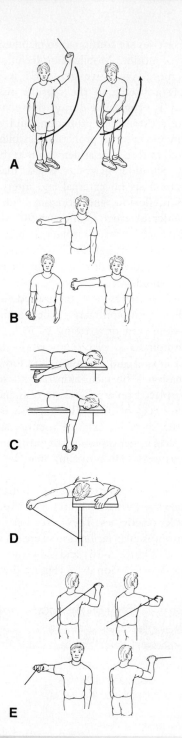

Figure 6-35

The thrower's 10 exercise program. This program is designed to exercise the major muscles necessary for throwing. The goal is to establish an organized, concise exercise program. All exercises included are specific to the thrower and are designed to improve the strength, power, and endurance of the shoulder complex musculature.

F, Biceps strengthening with tubing: Stand with one end of the tubing securely in the involved hand and the opposite end under the foot of the involved side while controlling tension. Assist with the opposite hand so that the arm is flexed through the full range of motion. Return to the starting position with a slow 5 count. Repeat 3-5 sets of 10 repetitions.

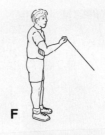

G, Dumbbell exercises for the triceps and wrist extensors/flexors: Triceps curls: Raise the involved arm overhead. Provide support at the elbow with the uninvolved hand. Straighten the arm overhead. Hold for 2 seconds and lower slowly. **Wrist flexion:** Support the forearm on a table with the hand off the edge, the palm facing upward. Hold a weight or hammer in the involved hand and lower it as far as possible, then curl it up as high as possible. Hold for a 2 count. **Wrist extension:** Support the forearm on a table with the hand off the edge, the palm facing downward. Hold a weight or hammer in the involved hand and lower it as far as possible, then curl it up as high as possible. Hold for a 2 count. **Forearm pronation:** Support the forearm on a table with the wrist in neutral position. Hold a weight or hammer in a normal hammering position and roll the wrist to bring the hammer into pronation as far as possible. Hold for a 2 count. Raise to the starting position. **Forearm supination:** Support the forearm on a table with the wrist in neutral position. Hold a weight or hammer in a normal hammering position and roll the wrist to bring the hammer into full supination. Hold for a 2 count. Raise back to the starting position.

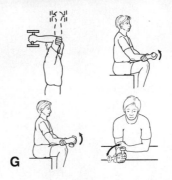

H, Serratus anterior strengthening: Start with a push-up into the wall. Gradually progress to the tabletop and eventually to the floor as tolerable.

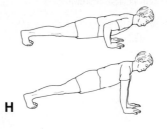

I, Press-ups: Sit on a chair or a table and place both hands firmly on the sides of the chair or table, the palm down and fingers pointed outward. The hands should be placed as far apart as the width of the shoulders. Slowly push downward through the hands to elevate the body. Hold the elevated position for 2 seconds. Repeat.

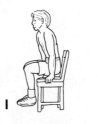

J, Rowing: Lie on the stomach with the involved arm hanging over the side of a table, the dumbbell in the hand, and the elbow straight. Slowly raise the arm while bending the elbow, and bring the dumbbell as high as possible. Hold at the top for 2 seconds, then lower slowly. Repeat.

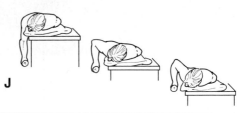

Figure 6-35 Cont'd
(From Andrews JR, Wilk KE: *The athlete's shoulder,* New York, 1994, Churchill Livingstone.)

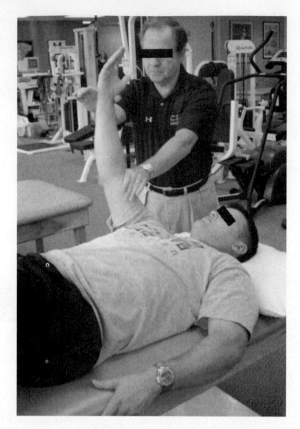

Figure 6-36
Proprioceptive neuromuscular facilitation (PNF) exercises to the elbow to enhance elbow stability.

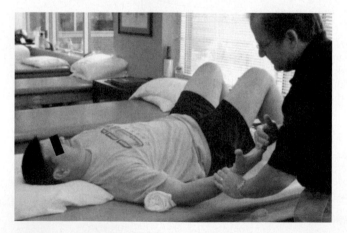

Figure 6-37
PNF exercise drills that include slow reversal of manual resistance.

plyometric drills for the forearm musculature include wrist flexion flips (Figure 6-41) and extension grips (Figure 6-42). Wrist flexion flips and extension grips are important components of an elbow rehabilitation program because they emphasize the forearm and hand musculature.

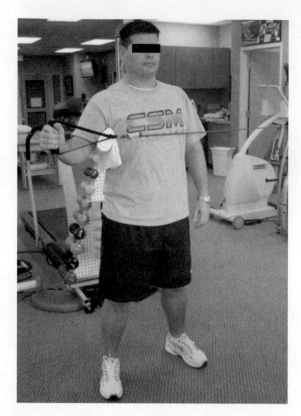

Figure 6-38
Standing external rotation with exercise tubing at 0° abduction.

Phase IV: Return to Activity Phase

The final phase of elbow rehabilitation, the return to activity phase, allows the patient progressively to return to full activity or, for the throwing athlete, to return to competition using an interval return to throwing program. Other interval programs are used for the tennis player or golfer.[254]

Phase IV: Goal of Return to Activity Phase

- Program geared to individual functional needs
- Return to full activity

Criteria for Progression to Phase IV

- Full ROM
- No pain or tenderness
- Satisfactory isokinetic test
- Satisfactory clinical examination

Figure 6-39

Plyometric drills: One-handed baseball throw at 90° abduction.

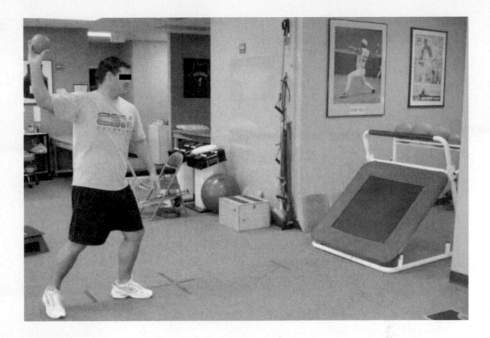

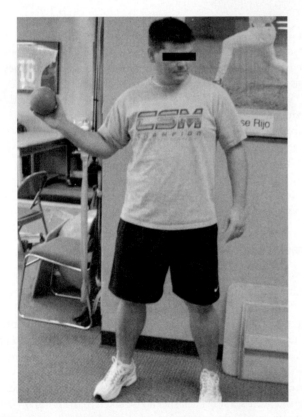

Figure 6-40

Plyometric drills: One-handed internal rotation side throws at 0° abduction.

Before being allowed to begin the return to activity phase of rehabilitation, patients must exhibit full ROM and have no pain or tenderness; they also must have a satisfactory isokinetic test and a satisfactory clinical examination.

Isokinetic testing is commonly used to determine the readiness of the athlete to begin an interval sports program.[254] Athletes routinely are tested at 180 and 300°/sec (degrees per second). The bilateral comparison at 180°/sec indicates the dominant arm's elbow flexion to be 10% to 20% stronger and the dominant extensors 5% to 15% stronger than the nondominant arm.

Upon achieving the previously mentioned criteria for returning to sports, the authors begin a formal interval sports program as described by Reinold et al.[254] For the overhead thrower, the authors initiate a long toss interval throwing program beginning at 13.7 m (45 feet) and gradually progressing to 36.6 or 54.9 m (20 or 180 feet) (player and position dependent) (Table 6-1).[254] Throwing should be performed without pain or a significant increase in symptoms. The authors believe it is important for the overhead patient or athlete to perform stretching and an abbreviated strengthening program before and after performing the interval sports program. Typically, overhead throwers warm up, stretch, and perform one set of their exercise program before throwing, followed by two additional sets of exercises following throwing.[254] This not only provides an adequate warm-up, it also ensures maintenance of necessary range of motion and flexibility of the shoulder joint. The next day, the thrower exercises the scapular muscles and external rotators and performs a core stabilization program.

After completing a long toss program, pitchers progress to phase II of the throwing program, throwing off a mound (Table 6-2).[254] In phase II, the number of throws, intensity, and type of pitch are progressed to gradually increase stress on the elbow and shoulder joints.[254] Generally, the pitcher begins at 50% intensity and gradually

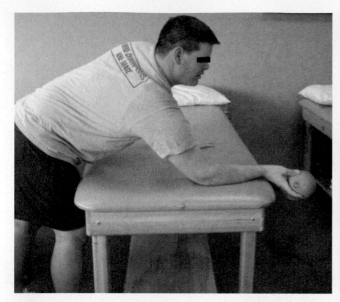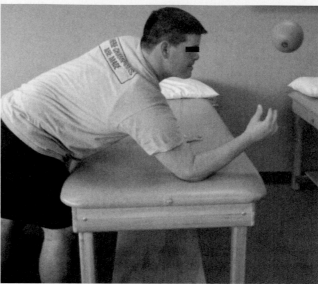

Figure 6-41
Plyometric drills: Wrist flexion ball flips.

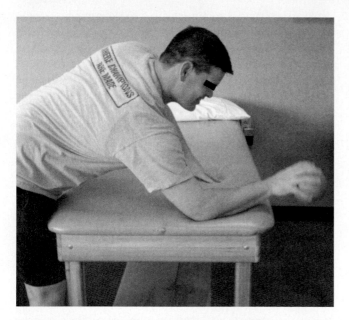

Figure 6-42
Plyometric drills: Wrist extension with ball grips.

progresses to 75%, 90%, and 100% over 4 to 6 weeks. Breaking balls are initiated once the pitcher can throw 40 to 50 pitches at at least 80% intensity with no symptoms.

Specific Rehabilitation Guidelines

Tendinopathy

The treatment of tendinopathy is based on a careful examination to determine the exact pathology present. Often practitioners diagnose patients as having "tendonitis," only to discover later that the tendon actually had undergone a degenerative process, or *tendinosis*.[213,214] The treatments for tendonitis and tendinosis are dramatically different.

The treatment for tendonitis typically is targeted at reducing inflammation and pain. This is accomplished through reducing activities, anti-inflammatory medications, cryotherapy, iontophoresis, light exercise, and stretching.

The treatment for tendinosis focuses on increasing circulation to promote collagen synthesis. This includes application of heat, ultrasound, stretching, eccentric exercises, transverse friction massage, and soft tissue mobilization.

Medial Epicondylitis

The treatment of medial epicondylitis should focus first on reducing pain and inflammation and then on increasing strength. Heat therapy followed by stretching and light strengthening is the hallmark of treatment for this condition. The session is finished with cryotherapy and electrical stimulation to decrease of inflammation and pain. A gradual increase in stretching and strengthening should be attempted, with care taken not to exacerbate the patient's symptoms. If exacerbation occurs, a step back should be taken in the program, and the patient should be progressed more slowly.

In some cases medial epicondylitis is treated with surgical debridement. Rehabilitation after surgery may be aggressive, because the flexor/pronator mass has not been stripped from the medial epicondyle. The patient is placed in a protective posterior splint for 10 to 14 days to allow the soft tissues to heal. Once the splint is removed, range of motion of the elbow is allowed immediately in all directions, including flexion, extension, supination, and pronation. Full motion

Table 6-1
Postoperative Rehabilitation After Elbow Arthroscopy

Initial phase (week 1)	*Goals:* Full wrist and elbow ROM; reduce swelling and pain; retard muscle atrophy.
	1. Day of surgery
	 • Begin gently moving elbow in bulky dressing.
	2. Postoperative days 1 and 2
	 • Remove bulky dressing and replace with elastic bandages.
	 • Immediate postoperative hand, wrist, and elbow exercises:
	  ○ Putty/grip strengthening
	  ○ Wrist flexor stretching
	  ○ Wrist extensor stretching
	  ○ Wrist curls
	  ○ Reverse wrist curls
	  ○ Neutral wrist curls
	  ○ Pronation/supination
	  ○ AA/AROM elbow ext/flex
	3. Postoperative days 3-7
	 • PROM elbow ext/flex (motion to tolerance).
	 • Begin PRE exercises with 0.5 kg (1 pound) weight:
	  ○ Wrist curls
	  ○ Reverse wrist curls
	  ○ Neutral wrist curls
	  ○ Pronation/supination
	  ○ Broomstick rollup

Intermediate phase (weeks 2 to 4)	*Goals:* Improve muscular strength and endurance; normalize joint arthrokinematics.
	1. Week 2: ROM exercises (overpressure into extension)
	 • Add biceps curl and triceps extension.
	 • Continue to progress PRE weight and repetitions as tolerable.
	2. Week 3
	 • Initiate eccentric exercises for biceps and triceps.
	 • Initiate exercises for rotator cuff:
	  ○ External rotators
	  ○ Internal rotators
	  ○ Deltoid
	  ○ Supraspinatus
	  ○ Scapulothoracic strengthening

Advanced phase (weeks 4 to 8)	*Goal:* Prepare patient for return to functional activities.
	Criteria for progression to advanced phase:
	 • Full, pain-free ROM
	 • No pain or tenderness
	 • Isokinetic test that fulfills criteria for throwing
	 • Satisfactory clinical examination
	1. Weeks 4-6
	  ○ Continue maintenance program, emphasizing muscular strength, endurance, and flexibility.
	  ○ Initiate interval throwing program phase.

ROM, Range of motion; *AA/AROM,* active assisted and active range of motion; *ext/flex,* extension flexion; *PROM,* passive range of motion; *PRE,* progressive resistance exercises.

should be obtained by 4 weeks. Light isometric exercise (i.e., 10% to 40% of the maximum voluntary contraction [MVC]) can be performed immediately after surgery. Once full motion has been obtained, strengthening may begin. Strengthening begins with isometric exercises and progresses to concentric and then eccentric exercises. Plyometric exercises are the final step.

As with all surgical procedures at the elbow, scar massage is incorporated at 2 to 3 weeks and nerve glides (i.e., neurodynamic techniques) commence when adequate motion is established. In addition, transverse massage can be performed over the debrided and released tendon.

In some cases the surgeon may choose to detach the flexor/pronator mass in the process of debridement.

Table 6-2
Postoperative Rehabilitation After Ulnar Nerve Transposition

Phase I: Immediate postoperative phase (weeks 0 to 2)	*Goals:* Allow soft tissue healing of relocated nerve; reduce pain and inflammation; retard muscular atrophy.
	1. Week 1
	  • Posterior splint at 90° elbow flexion with wrist free for motion (sling for comfort).
	  • Compression dressing.
	  • Exercises such as gripping exercises, wrist ROM, shoulder isometrics.
	2. Week 2
	  • Remove posterior splint for exercise and bathing.
	  • Progress elbow ROM (PROM 150° to 120°).
	  • Initiate elbow and wrist isometrics.
	  • Continue shoulder isometrics.

Phase II: Intermediate phase (weeks 3 to 7)	*Goals:* Restore full, pain-free ROM; improve strength, power, and endurance of upper extremity musculature; gradually increase functional demands.
	1. Week 3
	  • Discontinue posterior splint.
	  • Progress elbow ROM, emphasize full extension.
	  • Initiate flexibility exercises for wrist extension/flexion, forearm supination/pronation, and elbow extension/flexion.
	  • Initiate strengthening exercises for wrist extension/flexion, forearm supination/pronation, elbow extensors/flexors, and a shoulder program.
	2. Week 6
	  • Continue all exercises previously listed.
	  • Initiate light sports activities.

Phase III: Advanced strengthening phase (weeks 8 to 12)	*Goals:* Increase strength, power, and endurance; gradually initiate sports activities.
	1. Week 8
	  • Initiate eccentric exercise program.
	  • Initiate plyometric exercise drills.
	  • Continue shoulder and elbow strengthening and flexibility exercises.
	  • Initiate interval throwing program.

Phase IV: Return to activity phase (weeks 12 to 16)	*Goal:* Gradual return to sporting/functional activities.
	1. Week 12
	  • Return to competitive throwing.
	  • Initiate thrower's 10 exercise program. (see Figure 6-35)

ROM, Range of motion; *PROM,* passive range of motion.

In these patients, active wrist extension and flexion should be prevented for 4 weeks. Although full passive motion is allowed, it should only be done gently and in the presence of the therapist for the first 4 weeks.

Lateral Epicondylitis

A principal aspect of conservative treatment for lateral epicondylitis is therapy. Despite the misnomer, lateral epicondylitis is not a disease of inflammation, but rather a disease of degeneration. Usually little or no swelling is present, therefore heat therapy should begin each treatment session. Stretching of the extensor mass with wrist flexion is an important component of treatment. This may be done in conjunction with soft tissue mobilization. If the stretching and mobilization are well tolerated, isotonic eccentric strengthening exercises for the lateral extensor mass may be attempted. The patient also should perform shoulder and scapular flexibility and strengthening exercises during the rehabilitation program.

Conservative measures should be attempted for at least 6 months before surgical intervention is considered. Rehabilitation after surgical debridement primarily depends on whether the surgeon chooses to detach and reattach the extensor mass during surgery. If the extensor mass is detached during the procedure, active wrist extension and flexion should be prevented for 4 weeks. Although full passive motion is allowed, it should only be done gently and in the presence of the therapist for the first 4 weeks.

Caution with Elbow Surgery/Rehabilitation

- If the flexor or extensor muscle mass is detached during surgery, active wrist movement is prevented for 4 weeks to allow sufficient time for healing.

The posterior splint is removed at 10 to 14 days. Elbow flexion, extension, supination, and pronation are allowed immediately after removal of the splint. Care should be taken to perform supination and pronation gently. Cold therapy and electrical stimulation are instituted to reduce swelling and pain after sessions. Scar massage may begin at 2 to 3 weeks, and nerve glides may commence when adequate motion has been obtained. Full active motion at the elbow and wrist may begin at 4 weeks. If full motion already has been restored as a result of the passive motion instituted earlier, strengthening exercises may begin. Isometric exercises are succeeded by concentric exercises, which are followed by eccentric exercises. If the flexor mass was not detached, full motion of the elbow and wrist is allowed once the splint has been removed.

Ulnar Neuropathy

Therapy aimed at treating ulnar neuropathy depends on the pathology present. The nerve may be stretched secondary to instability at the elbow joint or may be compressed secondary to hypertrophy of surrounding soft tissue structures, or the condition may be a result of compression secondary to fibrous bands anywhere along the path of the ulnar nerve. This compression usually is observed in extremes of flexion or extension. The initial goal should be to bring the pain under control. This may involve the use of a nighttime splint with the elbow in 45° flexion to prevent recurrent compression and further damage. A full-time splint is not advised because stiffness may develop. If stability is a concern, strengthening exercises also should be performed, focusing on the flexors and extensors of the elbow. In other patients, particularly those with a large muscle mass, this may be contraindicated because the musculature may be a contributing factor.

All patients with ulnar neuropathy have nerve irritation that may result in scar formation. For this reason, nerve glides may be helpful in breaking scar tissue enveloping the nerve and possibly causing compression. The glides should be done gently at first, graduating to more aggressive treatment. This helps prevent a traction neuropraxia.

In the athlete, ulnar neuropathy often is a sequela of some other pathology and will not improve unless the underlying pathology is addressed.

Numerous theories have been advanced on the cause of ulnar neuropathy of the elbow in throwing athletes. Ulnar nerve changes can result from tensile forces, compressive forces, or nerve instability. As noted previously, any one or a combination of these mechanisms may be responsible for ulnar nerve symptoms.

Ulnar neuropathy has three stages. The first stage is marked by the acute onset of radicular symptoms. The second stage is manifested by a recurrence of symptoms as the patient attempts to return to competition. The third stage is associated with persistent motor weakness and sensory changes. If the patient presents in the third stage of injury, conservative management may not be effective.

Nonoperative treatment of ulnar neuropathy focuses on reducing ulnar nerve irritation, enhancing dynamic medial joint stability, and gradually returning the patient to previous levels and types of activities. NSAIDs often are prescribed, and rehabilitation includes an iontophoresis disposable patch and cryotherapy. With a diagnosis of ulnar neuropathy, throwing patients are instructed to discontinue throwing activities for at least 4 weeks, depending on the severity and chronicity of symptoms. The patient progresses through the immediate motion and intermediate phases over 4 to 6 weeks, with emphasis on eccentric and dynamic stabilization drills. Plyometric exercises are used to facilitate further dynamic stabilization of the medial elbow. The patient is allowed to begin an interval throwing program when full, pain-free ROM and muscle performance are present without neurological symptoms, and the individual may gradually return to activity if progression through the interval throwing program does not reveal neurological symptoms.

Ulnar Collateral Ligament Injury

Isolated UCL injuries usually are the result of chronic degeneration in repetitive-movement overhead athletes. Pain and inflammation usually are present, as well as loss of muscle strength throughout the extremity. Because instability may be present, a brace to protect against varus and valgus stresses may be helpful. The athlete must be instructed not to perform the throwing motion or to throw a ball (to control and limit valgus stress on the UCL) until adequate healing time has elapsed. The first goal of treatment is to establish a painless range of motion. The clinician begins with passive and active-assisted motion. Motion should be restored in a painless fashion to allow the ligament proper time to heal. Elbow flexion and extension range of motion does not create deleterious stress on the UCL and is actually beneficial for ligament healing. Motion begins in a pain free arc, and ROM is increased as tolerance allows. The patient progresses to active range of motion after full motion has been established with the previous measures. Elbow flexion, extension, supination, and pronation all are addressed, as are all wrist movements.

Gradual strengthening should begin with isometric exercises of the elbow and wrist. A shoulder program should be implemented to normalize range of motion and flexibility and to improve shoulder strength.

Light isotonic exercises at the elbow and wrist are started around weeks 3 to 4, after full motion has been established. The goal is to increase wrist flexor and pronator strength to assist in elbow stability. This is continued until weeks 6 to 7. At this point, plyometric exercises are initiated slowly. Once full motion, full strength, and dynamic stability have returned and the patient is symptom free, the patient may begin an interval throwing program. Upon satisfactory completion of the interval throwing program (i.e., pain-free throwing at full velocity), the patient may return to high level activity. To assist in pain-free throwing and sports, the overhead athlete should undergo a biomechanical evaluation to determine whether improper throwing mechanics are a factor or whether any biomechanical faults need to be corrected to help control the forces applied to the elbow joint.

Osteochondritis Dissecans

In OCD, conservative measures typically are reserved for nondisplaced lesions. In the painful elbow associated with this lesion, a brief period of immobilization (up to 3 weeks) can be beneficial. Used in association with cryotherapy and NSAIDs, immobilization can help limit the inflammatory process. At the end of the immobilization period, range of motion exercises can begin. When motion returns, strengthening may begin with isometric exercises. Care must be taken to avoid compressive forces on the radiocapitellar joint. Progression to isotonic exercises may begin with the same limitations. Sequential MRI and bone scans are obtained to assess the progression of healing. If healing does not progress, conservative measures should be abandoned in favor of surgical intervention. If the bone scans show evidence that the elbow is attempting to heal or is making progress, exercises that create stress in the radiocapitellar joint must be avoided, to prevent detachment or collapse of the fragment.

Medial Epicondylar Apophyseal Injury (Little Leaguer's Elbow)

A rehabilitation protocol similar to that for a UCL strain is used for medial epicondylar apophyseal injuries. Reducing pain and restoring motion are the initial priorities. When pain dissipates and motion returns, gradual strengthening may commence. One goal is to begin heavy lifting and plyometrics by 14 weeks. In milder cases, such as nondisplaced injuries, a more aggressive rehabilitation protocol may be used. An interval throwing program is the last step of the rehabilitation process.

Ulnar Nerve Transposition

The goal of rehabilitation for ulnar nerve transposition is to return motion, function, and strength while minimizing pain and preventing failure of the surgery and complications, including adhesions to the nerve. A splint is applied immediately postoperatively with flexion at 45°. This is left in place until approximately the 10th postoperative day to allow the soft tissues to heal and to enable some scar tissue to form and further secure the ulnar nerve in its new location. As with most rehabilitation around the elbow, the initial goal is to restore motion while minimizing pain.

Several techniques can be used for ulnar nerve decompression. Decompression in situ decompresses the ulnar nerve only at a specific site of compression, and no transposition takes place. In general, the ulnar nerve is quite stable and is not at risk for subluxation. For this reason, immediate active motion and passive motion are allowed. Motion should be fully restored by 4 weeks after surgery. Once motion has been restored, nerve glides are commenced to prevent scar adherence to the nerve. Isometric strengthening exercises may begin as well.

If a medial epicondylectomy or submuscular transposition is performed, active motion of the wrist should be avoided for 4 weeks to prevent flexor mass avulsion. Although full passive motion of the wrist is allowed, it should only be done gently and in the presence of a clinician for the first 4 weeks. Full active and passive motion at the elbow may begin when the splint is removed, but care should be taken to be gentle with supination and pronation. Scar massage may begin at 2 to 3 weeks, and nerve glides may commence when adequate motion has been obtained. Full active motion at the elbow and wrist may begin at 4 weeks. If full motion has already been restored, strengthening exercises may begin at 6 weeks. Isometrics may graduate to isotonic exercises. Plyometric exercises follow next. If the goal is to return a throwing athlete to his or her sport, an interval throwing program may commence by week 8. Return to competition may begin around week 12.

With a subcutaneous transposition, the flexor/pronator mass is not disrupted. The ulnar nerve is kept in place with a fascial sling. The splint is removed in 14 days, and this initial 2 weeks should be sufficient time for the soft tissues to heal. Once the splint has been removed, unlimited motion at the elbow and wrist may begin. Motion should be restored at 4 weeks. Once motion has been restored, strengthening can begin, in the same fashion as described previously. Nerve glides may begin when adequate motion has been restored. As described, scar massage may begin at 2 to 3 weeks.

Cryotherapy and electrical stimulation are encouraged in the initial stages to help minimize inflammation while motion exercises are performed; however, the nerve must be protected from thermal injury (particularly important with subcutaneous transpositions).

Arthroscopic Excision of Osteophytes

Osteophytes most often appear on the olecranon in the posterior elbow, but they also may appear anteriorly on the coronoid. Throwing athletes may develop posteromedial olecranon osteophytes associated with VEOS.

Direct posterior osteophytes on the olecranon may limit extension of the elbow. Depending on the duration and magnitude of osteophyte formation, the resultant loss of motion may cause contracture of the anterior capsule. Therefore, even with surgical excision of the osteophytes, return of full extension may be a challenge, especially if no concomitant anterior capsule release is performed. Rehabilitation focuses on return of motion, particularly extension. The general rehabilitation guidelines for the elbow should be followed. However, less emphasis is placed on strengthening and more emphasis is placed on range of motion exercises. Instability should not be expected with this procedure, therefore the clinician can be more aggressive with motion exercises, provided they do not result in more inflammation. Control of inflammation and pain is crucial to this process, because pain markedly limits the amount of stretching a patient can tolerate. NSAIDs, cryotherapy, and high voltage electrical stimulation all play roles in pain control. Once motion has been restored, strengthening may commence on a more aggressive basis. It is important to note that restoration of full extension may not be possible, therefore communication between the surgeon and clinicians is important to clarify the realistic goals of the surgical intervention.

Anterior coronoid osteophyte formation has a similar pathology. Full flexion is limited because of a bony blockage of motion anteriorly. This also results in soft tissue contractures. Therefore, even after the bone is removed, the motion in flexion is difficult to restore. Rehabilitation is similar to that described above, although more aggressive flexion exercises are instituted.

Throwing athletes can develop posteromedial osteophytes of the olecranon. This condition is different from the posterior osteophytes mentioned previously. One fourth of throwing athletes require instability surgery after excision of posteromedial osteophytes of the olecranon.[186] It is unclear whether a subtle pre-existing instability causes these osteophytes and their removal unmasks the true nature of the injury, or whether removal of the osteophytes is the primary pathology leading to instability. Regardless, this surgery is associated with instability, a factor that needs to be addressed in the rehabilitation process. Care must be taken to avoid valgus stress on the elbow. Internal and external rotation exercises of the shoulder should be avoided until 6 weeks after the operation. Thrower's isotonic exercises may begin at week 6, and an interval throwing program may begin by week 10.

Ulnar Collateral Ligament Reconstruction

Surgical reconstruction of the UCL attempts to restore the stabilizing functions of the anterior bundle of the UCL.[255]

The palmaris longus or gracilis graft source is taken and passed in a figure-of-eight pattern through drill holes in the sublime tubercle of the ulna and the medial epicondyle.[255] An ulnar nerve transposition often is performed at the time of reconstruction.[254]

The rehabilitation program the authors currently use after UCL reconstruction is outlined in Table 6-3. The patient is placed in a posterior splint with the elbow immobilized at 90° flexion for the first 7 days after surgery. This allows adequate healing of the UCL graft and soft tissue slings involved in the nerve transposition. The patient is allowed to perform wrist ROM and gripping and submaximal isometrics for the wrist and elbow. The patient is progressed from the posterior splint to an elbow ROM brace, which is adjusted to allow ROM of 30° to 100° flexion. Motion is increased by 5° of extension and 10° of flexion thereafter to restore full ROM (0° to 145°) by the end of weeks 5 to 6. The brace is discontinued by weeks 5 to 6.

Isometric exercises are progressed to include light resistance isotonic exercises at week 4 and the full thrower's 10 program by week 6. Progressive resistance exercises are incorporated at weeks 8 to 9. Emphasis again is placed on developing dynamic stabilization of the medial elbow. Because of the anatomical orientation of the flexor carpi ulnaris and flexor digitorum superficialis overlying the UCL, isotonic and stabilization activities for these muscles may assist the UCL in stabilizing valgus stress at the medial elbow.[256] For this reason, concentric strengthening of these muscles is performed.

Aggressive exercises involving eccentric and plyometric contractions are included in the advanced phase, usually weeks 9 to 14. Two-handed plyometric drills are performed at week 10, one-handed drills at weeks 12 to 14. An interval throwing program is allowed at week 16. In most cases, throwing from a mound is progressed within 4 to 6 weeks after initiation of an interval throwing program, and return to competitive throwing is permitted at approximately 9 months after surgery. The actual rate of progression of the throwing program should be individualized to each athlete and adjusted based on symptoms, mechanics, and desired goals.

Lateral Collateral Ligament Complex Reconstruction

Lateral-sided instability of the elbow usually is the result of a sudden traumatic injury rather than a chronic repetitive injury. It results in varus instability and a posterolateral rotatory instability that can be promoted with elbow supination. For this reason, special attention to elbow rotation is emphasized during the rehabilitation.

Initially, the postoperative elbow is placed in a splint with 90° of flexion and mild pronation. The splint is removed at the end of the first week (the authors immobilize for 2 to 4 weeks, depending on the type of activity to which the patient

Table 6-3

Postoperative Rehabilitation After Ulnar Collateral Ligament Reconstruction Using an Autogenous Palmaris Longus Graft

Phase I:
Immediate Postoperative
Phase (Weeks 0 to 3)
	Goals: Protect healing tissue; reduce pain and inflammation; retard muscle atrophy; protect graft site to allow healing.
	1. Postoperative Week 1
	 • Brace: Posterior splint at 90° elbow flexion
	 • Range of motion (ROM): Wrist active range of motion (AROM) extension/flexion immediately postoperative
	 • Elbow ROM: Day 1
	 • Elbow postoperative compression dressing: 5 to 7 days
	 • Wrist (graft site) compression dressing: 7 to 10 days as needed
	 • Exercises:
	  ○ Gripping exercises
	  ○ Wrist ROM
	  ○ Shoulder isometrics (no external rotation [ER] of the shoulder)
	  ○ Biceps isometrics
	 • Cryotherapy: To elbow joint and to graft site at the wrist
	
	2. Postoperative Week 2
	 • Brace: Elbow ROM 25° to 100°(gradually increase ROM by 5° extension/10deg; flexion per week)
	 • Exercise:
	  ○ Continue all exercises previously listed
	  ○ Elbow ROM in brace (30° to 105°)
	  ○ Initiate elbow extension isometrics
	  ○ Continue wrist ROM exercises
	  ○ Initiate light scar mobilization over distal incision (graft)
	 • Cryotherapy: Continue ice to elbow and graft site
	
	3. Postoperative Week 3
	 • Brace: Elbow ROM 15° to 115°
	 • Exercises:
	  ○ Continue all exercises previously listed
	  ○ Elbow ROM in brace
	  ○ Initiate active ROM for wrist and elbow (no resistance)
	  ○ Initiate light wrist flexion and stretching
	  ○ Initiate active ROM for the shoulder:
	   • Full can exercises
	   • Lateral raises
	   • External rotation/internal rotation (ER/IR) exercises with tubing
	   • Elbow flexion/extension
	 • Initiate light scapular strengthening exercises
	 • May incorporate bicycle workouts for lower extremity strength and endurance

Phase II: Intermediate
Phase (Weeks 4 to 7)
	Goals: Gradually advance to full ROM; promote healing of repaired tissue; regain and improve muscle strength; restore full function of graft site.
	1. Week 4
	 • Brace: Elbow ROM 0° to 125°
	 • Exercises:
	  ○ Begin light resistance exercises for the arm (0.5 kg [1 pound]):
	   • Wrist curls, extensions, pronation, supination
	   • Elbow extension/flexion
	 • Progress shoulder program; emphasize rotator cuff and scapular strengthening
	 • Initiate shoulder strengthening with light dumbbells
	
	2. Week 5
	 • ROM: Elbow ROM 0° to 135°
	 • Discontinue brace
	 • Continue all exercises:
	  ○ Progress all shoulder and upper extremity (UE) exercises (progress weight 0.5 kg [1 pound])

	3. Week 6 • AROM: 0° to 145° without brace (i.e., full ROM) • Exercises: ○ Initiate thrower's 10 program ○ Progress elbow strengthening exercises ○ Initiate shoulder external rotation strengthening ○ Progress shoulder program 4. Week 7 • Exercises: ○ Progress thrower's 10 program (progress weights) ○ Initiate proprioceptive neuromuscular facilitation (PNF) diagonal patterns (light)

Phase III:
 Advanced Strengthening
 Phase (Weeks 8 to 14)
	Goals: Increase strength, power, and endurance; maintain full elbow ROM; gradually initiate sports/functional activities (specificity).
	1. Week 8
	• Exercises:
	 ○ Inititate ecentric elbow flexion/extension
	 ○ Continue shoulder program (thrower's 10 program)
	 ○ Initiate manual resistance diagonal patterns
	 ○ Initiate plyometric exercise program (two-handed plyometrics close to the body only):
	  • Chest pass
	  • Side throw close to the body
	 ○ Continue calf and hamstring stretching
	
	2. Week 10
	• Exercises:
	 ○ Continue all exercises listed previously
	 ○ Advance plyometrics to two-handed drills away from the body:
	  • Side-to-side throws
	  • Soccer throws
	  • Side throws
	
	3. Weeks 12 to 14
	• Continue all exercises
	• Initiate strengthening exercises on isotonic machines (if desired):
	 • Bench press (seated)
	 • Lat pull down
	 ○ Inititate golf, swimming
	 ○ Inititate interval hitting program

Phase IV: Return to Activity Phase (Weeks 14 to 32)	*Goals:* Continue to increase strength, power, and endurance of upper extremity musculature Gradual return to sports/functional activities. 1. Week 14 • Exercise: ○ Continue strengthening program ○ Emphasize elbow and wrist strengthening and flexibility exercises ○ Maintain full elbow ROM ○ Initiate one-handed plyometic throwing (stationary throws) ○ Initiate one-handed wall dribble ○ Initiate one-handed baseball throws into wall 2. Week 16 • Exercises: ○ Initiate interval throwing program (phase I) (long toss program) ○ Continue thrower's 10 program and plyometrics ○ Continue stretching before and after throwing 3. Week 22 to 24 • Exercises: ○ Progress to phase II throwing (once phase I has been successfully completed) 4. Week 30 to 32 • Exercises: ○ Gradually progress to competitive throwing/sports ○ Functional activities

will return), and a brace is used that incorporates an extension block of 30° and a flexion block of 100°. Extension is increased by 5° per week, and flexion is increased by 10° per week. Supination encourages the radial head to sublux laterally, potentially stretching the graft. Therefore supination is restricted for 3 weeks. Active supination is allowed when the elbow passes 90° of flexion. Once supination is obtained at greater than 90° of elbow flexion, supination may be attempted in extension. Full motion about the elbow should be obtained by 6 weeks. Shoulder forward elevation and abduction may be treated aggressively for motion restriction, but internal and external rotation is limited to active motion only. Passive and active-assisted motion of the shoulder for rotation requires torque through the elbow and should be avoided until week 9.

Isometric strengthening exercises of the elbow and wrist are initiated once the splint has been removed. External and internal rotation strength exercises of the shoulder are avoided until 9 weeks after surgery, because these motions put the graft at risk. Light isotonic exercises may begin about the elbow and wrist at week 6. At week 9, an aggressive strengthening regimen may commence, including eccentric contraction exercises and plyometrics.

Nerve glides and scar massage are important to prevent pain from adherent scar after surgery. Scar massage should begin at 2 weeks, and nerve glides should commence once the appropriate motion has returned.

Total Elbow Arthroplasty

The complexity of total elbow arthroplasty depends on the disease requiring the prosthesis, the type of prosthesis to be implanted, and the presence of soft tissue constraints. Despite these variables, the rehabilitation regimens for most total elbow arthroplasties remain relative similar. The most popular prosthesis is a linked, semiconstrained prosthesis with joint stability that is quite solid. On the first postoperative day, the elbow is elevated to minimize soft tissue swelling. Motion in all directions may begin on postoperative day 1. Elbow flexion, extension, pronation, and supination may begin and can be progressed as tolerated. Lifting is limited to less than 0.5 kg (1 pound) for the first 3 months. To preserve the viability of the prosthesis, the patient is limited to lifting less than 4.5 kg (10 pounds) at one time and no more than 0.9 kg (2 pounds) repetitively in the affected arm.

Soft tissue mobilization, cryotherapy, and electrical stimulation help minimize inflammation. Scar massage and nerve glides help reduce the likelihood of problems associated with scar formation.

Arthroscopic Arthrolysis

Loss of motion is a difficult problem associated with injuries of the elbow. It can be a result of soft tissue contracture or heterotopic ossification associated with the injury. Often the motion cannot be regained through conservative measures alone, and surgical intervention is necessary. The surgeon should inform the therapist of what motion has been obtained in the operating room so that realistic goals can be set.

Motion and pain control are at the forefront of rehabilitation for this procedure. HO represents a difficult rehabilitation problem. It has been shown that passive stretching outside the painless arc of motion may cause the generation of ectopic bone in patients with burns or brain injuries.[257] Whether this literature, in a rather unique population, is relevant to other patients with HO is unclear; however, caution is advised, and aggressive passive motion exercises should not be performed. The goal is to obtain full motion by 4 weeks. The most beneficial means of achieving this goal has been the LLLD technique described earlier. As with all the motion exercises, the stretching should not cause pain.

With arthrolysis for soft tissue contractures, the clinician may be more aggressive with motion exercises. Although the risk of generating HO may be in question, other problems may arise with aggressive rehabilitation. Aggressive motion can create an inflammatory cascade and generate pain that could inhibit progress, which would be self-defeating. The goal of establishing full motion at 4 weeks does not change with soft tissue contractures.

As with the other protocols, pain should be treated with cryotherapy, high voltage electrical stimulation, and gentle soft tissue mobilization. Heat and ultrasound may be used once the initial swelling from surgery has dissipated. These are used before motion exercises to "warm up" the joint.

Strengthening exercises should begin after motion has been established. There are no contraindications to an aggressive approach to strengthening once motion has been restored. Isometric exercises are begun and progressed to plyometrics in the usual fashion.

Regardless of the origin of the contracture, stretching should be continued for 4 to 6 months after activities are resumed to prevent return of the contracture.

Fractures

The complexity of the fracture and the degree of stability after internal fixation can vary considerably in the elbow. Communication between the surgeon and all members of the rehabilitation team is essential to determine the aggressiveness of the rehabilitation process. Several different fractures about the elbow merit attention. The goal of rehabilitation after a fracture is to facilitate osseous healing, restore full motion and strength, and gradually return the individual to functional activities. With an elbow fracture (whether treated surgically or nonoperatively), the goal is to minimize immobilization to prevent loss of motion. Loss of motion is more common in adults than in children after an elbow fracture.

Radial Head and Neck Fractures

When fractures of the radial head and neck are nondisplaced, the injury may be treated conservatively and motion should be initiated immediately. Unlimited passive and active motion is the priority. This is achieved through the use of stretching techniques, as well as techniques for reducing swelling and pain, which have been mentioned earlier. The goal is to re-establish motion by 4 weeks. Strengthening about the elbow and wrist may begin once full motion has been established. Valgus stress should be avoided until the fracture has healed.

With displaced or angulated fractures, internal fixation may be necessary. In some cases the fracture is beyond repair and requires replacement with a metal implant. With stable fixation or an implant, the elbow is placed in a posterior splint at 45° to 90° of elbow flexion for 10 days. Once the splint has been removed, motion exercises are initiated without limitation. Full flexion, extension, supination, and pronation should be obtained by 4 to 6 weeks. Often patients present with mechanical blocks to motion. This often results in soft tissue contractures. With these patients, the goals for motion may be more limited. Valgus stress is avoided in patients with internal fixation until the fracture has healed. This is not necessary when a radial head prosthesis is used. Once full motion has been achieved, strengthening of the elbow and wrist may commence. If swelling and pain persist, cryotherapy and electrical stimulation may be used to limit these symptoms.

Olecranon Fractures

For most olecranon fractures, the treatment of choice is open reduction and internal fixation. Several fixation techniques yield a stable fracture, and rehabilitation should not have to be altered because of the type of fixation. Traditionally a posterior splint is placed for 7 to 10 days to allow the soft tissues to heal. The length of immobilization depends on the patient's variables (i.e., age, osseous status, health, desired goals, healing response). Once the splint has been removed, unlimited passive motion may begin. Active pronation, supination, and flexion are allowed, but active extension is avoided for 6 weeks. Full motion in all directions should be achieved by 6 weeks. Gentle active extension may be initiated, and strengthening of the elbow and wrist in all directions may begin at 8 weeks.

As with all fracture fixations at the elbow, cryotherapy and electrical stimulation should be used to reduce pain and swelling. Scar massage should be initiated at 2 weeks, and nerve glides should be used when possible.

Distal Humeral Fractures

Distal humeral fractures usually require open reduction and internal fixation. If the surgeon has difficulty with stability, a hinged external fixator that allows elbow flexion and extension may be used, although this is not common. After fixation, a splint is placed for 10 to 14 days. Once the splint has been removed, gentle passive motion at the elbow and wrist may begin. Pain and swelling are limiting factors in restoring motion to the elbow, therefore cryotherapy and electrical stimulation are crucial to this process. The clinician must take care with cryotherapy to avoid nerve injury, because ulnar nerve transposition is a routine part of distal humeral fixation.

Active motion at the elbow and wrist may begin at 6 weeks. Once full motion has been established and bony healing is apparent, strengthening may begin. Strengthening should be limited to pain-free exercises. It begins with isotonic exercises and gradually progresses to plyometrics.

Coronoid Fractures and Elbow Dislocation

After dislocation of the elbow, the patient is temporarily immobilized to allow healing of the injured capsule. The length of immobilization varies, depending on the required use of the elbow for ADL or work activities, the type of sport the patient plays, whether it is the dominant or nondominant elbow, the patient's age, and whether concomitant lesions are present. Coronoid fractures often put the patient at risk for future elbow instability. For this reason, the rehabilitation protocols for elbow dislocation and coronoid fractures are similar. The priority is to restore motion quickly while guarding against instability. The patient is placed in a posterior splint for 10 to 14 days in a position that allows no visible subluxation on radiographs. In the initial evaluation, the stable range of motion is determined. The elbow will sublux with further extension, therefore parameters are set so that the initial restrictions do not permit extension beyond this point. When the splint is removed, a dynamic elbow brace that prevents valgus and varus forces is used. This splint should also have a variable locking mechanism that blocks various degrees of extension. The clinician may work on flexion and pronation of the elbow without limitation. Passive extension may be increased by 10° every week until full extension is obtained. The patient should be closely watched for any evidence of subluxation. Often, with elbow dislocations, either the UCL or the LUCL may rupture. If the LUCL ruptures, supination should be limited for at least 3 weeks after removal of the splint. The goal is to restore motion by 8 weeks.

Motion of the wrist should be instituted immediately. Upon removal of the splint, control of pain and swelling must be established immediately to aid in the restoration of motion. As mentioned earlier, cryotherapy and electrical stimulation are beneficial. Gentle soft tissue mobilization also may help.

Strengthening may begin at 8 weeks. If the expected motion has not been achieved, strengthening should be delayed until the desired motion is obtained. Strengthening is performed in the usual fashion.

If the patient's clinical picture requires operative intervention, rehabilitation should be dictated by the procedure performed. LCL reconstruction, UCL reconstruction, and radial head fixation are common surgical procedures. If a coronoid fracture is present and fixed, this should not change the protocol; the other fixations present should guide the treatment.

Summary

The elbow is a complex joint, and our understanding of it continues to evolve. The elbow is important for positioning the hand in space and for the specialized functions demanded of athletes and the everyday requirements of the general population. Many injuries and pathological conditions can affect the elbow and its associated bony and soft tissue. The rehabilitation of these injuries, as well as conservative and surgical treatments, has been reviewed, although the depth of these discussions has had to conform to the limitations on the length of the chapter. Clearly, the anatomy and biomechanics of the elbow guide our understanding of the pathophysiology of elbow injury and pain and help direct the treatment of elbow conditions. However, the elbow's response to trauma, even iatrogenic trauma, can be tricky, because stiffness or loss of motion is a common problem after such challenges.

References

To enhance this text and add value for the reader, all references have been incorporated into a CD-ROM that is provided with this text. The reader can view the reference source and access it online whenever possible. There are a total of 257 references for this chapter.

CHAPTER 7

HAND, WRIST, AND DIGIT INJURIES

Jennifer B. Green, Helen E. Ranger, Joanne G. Draghetti, Lindsay C. Groat, Evan D. Schumer, and Bruce M. Leslie

Most of the fundamental ideas of science are essentially simple, and may, as a rule, be expressed in a language comprehensible to everyone.

Albert Einstein

Introduction

The hand is one of the pre-eminent tools of human beings. At its most basic, the hand allows the individual to touch and take hold, but the anatomy allows much more than gross grasp and coarse sensation. The structure of the hand allows a musician to play with different shades of meaning; it allows an artist to apply subtle shades of texture; it allows a parent to convey meaning by touching a child. All these emotions can be conveyed by the hand. The inability to accomplish gross grasp and coarse sensation or the subtleties in these higher functions can equally affect the ultimate outcome of the patient.

The hand's anatomy is not too difficult to understand. However, its compact nature and precision create a complexity in which subtle changes in the way tissues move in relation to one another can have a dramatic effect on function. Seemingly simple injuries that ultimately prevent tendon gliding can severely affect the ability to flex or extend the digits. Wounds that heal by secondary intention may be acceptable in some areas, but in others may greatly diminish the ability to feel and move.

Insight into hand function arises from an understanding of the ways in which anatomy, biomechanics, physiology, and wound healing work together to allow the hand to perform a myriad of tasks. This knowledge then needs to be tempered by the patient's expectations, needs, and socialization. An operation to restore hand function in one patient may be totally unacceptable to another patient. Each intervention needs to be customized to the individual patient.

Hand rehabilitation plays a critical role in restoring upper extremity function. The therapist is a crucial member of a team whose ultimate goal is to improve hand function. Not only does the therapist assist in promoting the restoration of the soft tissues to maximize function, in many cases the therapist is in the best position to recognize the patient's goals and needs. A good hand therapist is not only knowledgeable of upper extremity anatomy, but also recognizes the social and psychological implications of the original injury and subsequent treatment.

This chapter presents a fundamental approach to the diagnosis and classification of hand injuries. It also includes treatment and rehabilitation guidelines for bone and soft tissue injuries of the hand.

Fracture Injuries of the Hand

Phalangeal Fractures

General Considerations

Phalangeal and metacarpal fractures are among the most common skeletal injuries. In one large series of 11,000 fractures, these two injuries accounted for 10% of the total.[1] Unfortunately, these fractures frequently are treated as a trivial malady by both patients and health care providers. This can lead to a profound loss of digital and hand function, either from neglect or, worse still, from poorly executed treatment.

The force required to fracture one of the phalangeal bones frequently also damages the soft tissue structures of the digit. This can lead to significant scarring and fibrosis in the postinjury period. Function can best be restored with early intervention by the treating physician and by allowing the patient to begin rehabilitation of the digit as soon as stability permits. Studies have shown that immobilization for longer then 3 weeks leads to loss of total active range of motion.[2] Before the 20th century, treatment of phalangeal fractures was limited to nonoperative methods. Today, most of these fractures still can be successfully treated in this fashion, because most fractures are functionally stable either before or after closed reduction.

Indications for surgical intervention for phalangeal fractures include angulation greater than 25°, to prevent compromised digit flexion and extension;[3] bone loss; open fracture; intra-articular fracture with displacement; associated soft tissue injury (skin, vessel, tendon, nerve); and multiple trauma to the upper extremity. The treating physician must also take into consideration the patient's age, occupation, ability to cooperate with the postoperative regimen, and the surgeon's experience and skill.

Indications for Surgery for Phalangeal Fractures

- Angulation greater than 25°
- Bone loss
- Open fracture
- Intra-articular fracture with displacement
- Associated soft tissue injury
- Multiple trauma to the upper extremity

Anatomy

The proximal and middle phalanges are similar in their osseous anatomy. The distal phalanx is different in shape and in the specialized attachment of the nail bed to the dorsal periosteal surface. The soft tissue envelope can greatly affect the stability of the fracture, treatment of the injury, and the ultimate outcome. In the digits are found the osteocutaneous ligaments of Cleland and Grayson. These can serve to stabilize the bone and prevent fracture displacement. The ligaments can also prevent closed reduction of a fracture if they are interposed between the displaced fragments. The proximal interphalangeal (PIP) joint and distal interphalangeal (DIP) joint are highly constrained, hinged joints that do not tolerate even a small amount of fracture displacement. The metacarpophalangeal (MCP) joint has a less constrained configuration that allows for more lateral motion, some rotation, and slightly more forgiveness in terms of fracture displacement.

Injury Classification

Shaft fractures can be classified by their location; that is, in the neck, the shaft, or the base of the bone. They can be further classified according to the fracture geometry; for example, the fracture may be spiral, transverse, short or long oblique, or comminuted. This characteristic can predict fracture stability and can help determine the best type of surgical implant if fracture stabilization is required. The fracture can be further classified as open or closed, which is less than intuitive during the examination of a crushed distal phalanx and a nail bed injury that, for all intents and purposes, is an open injury.

Diagnosis and Medical Treatment
Fractures of the Distal Phalanx

Tuft Fractures. Tuft fractures are the most common fractures of the fingers,[4] frequently the result of a crushing injury. A crush injury may result in comminuted fractures that fail to unite. Nonunion, however, does not usually lead to instability, because the bone fragments are held tightly to the pulp tissue of the fingertip. An associated laceration of the nail matrix may be seen. Splinting for 1 to 2 weeks for comfort, with a rapid return to function, is the usual treatment course for this injury (Figure 7-1).

Repair of the nail matrix is warranted if the injury causes wide displacement of that tissue. Replacement of the nail plate, if it still exists, creates a template for the matrix to heal and provides some protection for the sensitive tissues of the fingertip. Despite adequate treatment, the end result of this injury may be some loss of motion, decreased sensation, and chronic mild pain. These unfortunate sequelae are exacerbated by prolonged immobilization. In the case of the index finger, the phenomenon of *bypassing* (i.e., using a different finger) may be observed and should be addressed early in the course of treatment.

Shaft Fractures. Shaft fractures are either longitudinal or, more commonly, transverse in orientation. If significant displacement or angulation is present, they often are easily repaired. Displacement signifies an injury of the nail matrix as well, which if left untreated leads to a nail plate deformity. If the dorsal cortex of the bone can be realigned and the overlying nail plate is also intact, the matrix will be sandwiched into the correct orientation for healing, and no further treatment likely is necessary. Displaced fractures are easily treated with a longitudinally oriented Kirschner wire (K-wire) or headless screw (Figure 7-2).

Intra-articular Fractures. Intra-articular fractures in adults usually involve either the volar or dorsal lip at the end of the bone. In children, an epiphyseal separation also

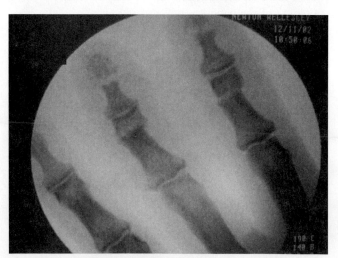

Figure 7-1

Snow blower injury, which resulted in multiple tuft fractures and fractures of the middle phalanx with overlying soft tissue trauma.

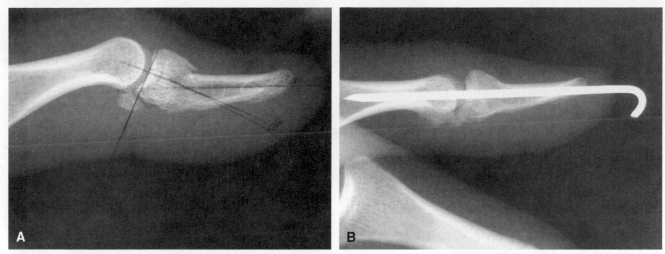

Figure 7-2
A, Angulated shaft fracture of the distal phalanx; the fracture has created a deformity of the digit that will affect the growth of the nail. **B,** Correction of the shaft fracture with a pin, which holds the bone aligned for 3 weeks. The pin subsequently was removed in the outpatient setting.

may occur. Dorsal rim fractures usually are associated with a terminal tendon avulsion injury (sometimes called a *bony mallet injury*). If the dorsal fragment of bone is small enough, no volar translation of the distal phalanx occurs at the joint surface, and the injury can be treated in the same way as a soft tissue mallet injury, only with splinting. However, the larger the fragment, the greater is the potential that the flexor digitorum profundus (FDP) tendon, which is still attached to the volar fragment, will translate the distal fragment palmarly. This can be a subtle finding on the lateral x-ray film, and the possibility must always be considered with a fracture fragment greater then 30% of the joint surface. In such cases, operative intervention to restore joint alignment is indicated (Figure 7-3).

Volar Lip Fractures. Volar lip fractures are also tendon avulsion injuries. In these fractures, the FDP tendon remains attached to the small fracture fragment. This type of injury is also known as a *rugger Jersey finger* or *sweater finger* because it commonly occurs when gripping to tackle an opponent in football or rugby. Unlike its counterpart on the extensor surface, these flexor tendon injuries frequently require surgery, because the flexor tendon retracts toward the palm after injury, pulling the fracture fragment along with it. In these cases, if the fragment is more then a few millimeters in size, it usually is caught and held in place under one of the distal annular pulleys. The fragment usually can easily be found there and reattached surgically with a screw.

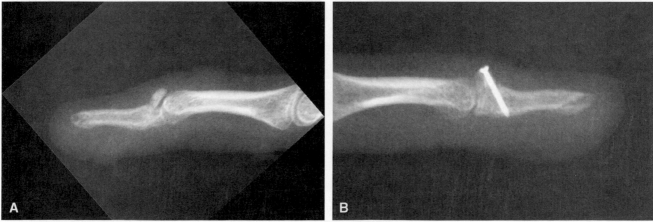

Figure 7-3
A, Bony mallet injury in which a large fracture fragment has caused volar displacement. **B,** Operative fixation is required to restore joint congruency. In the preoperative x-ray film, note that despite the splint, the joint is not congruent because of the volar translation of the distal fragment.

Fractures of the Proximal and Middle Phalanges

Shaft Fractures. A direct blow frequently causes transverse fractures to the shaft, whereas twisting injuries often cause spiral or oblique fractures. Whether displacement of the fracture occurs often is determined by the location of the fracture and the influence of the intrinsic and extrinsic forces at that specific site.

Fractures of the proximal phalanx, when displaced, fall into apex volar angulation. This occurs because the insertion of interosseous muscles on the proximal fragment flexes the MCP joint while the pull of the lateral bands and central slip extends the distal fracture fragment.

Fractures of the middle phalanx are affected more by the pull of the central slip insertion and the flexor digitorum superficialis (FDS) tendon and therefore tend to angulate apex dorsally when they are displaced.

Rotational malalignment is poorly tolerated and is best assessed with active flexion of the digit, which may require digital block anesthesia for comfort. Tenodesis is preferable to passive motion for assessment of this type of deformity. Patients sometimes use the adjacent digits to "capture" the fractured finger, thus limiting their deformity. Care must be taken to observe for this during the examination to evaluate the true extent of digital scissoring from malrotation (Figure 7-4).

The majority of proximal and middle phalanx fractures are stable or will be stable after closed reduction, which often is the first course of treatment considered for these injuries. Significant stripping of the soft tissue from the bone makes reduction easier, but the fracture will be more unstable in the long run, requiring implant augmentation. If closed reduction is not possible, the reason may be a bony spike caught on the soft tissue envelope. Most surgeons prefer to gain anatomical alignment of these fractures,[5,6] because any degree of malrotation and angulation over 25° can negatively affect hand function.[7,8] Closed treatment can be accomplished with web block anesthesia in the office or operating room. Immediate postreduction x-ray films should be obtained, before immobilization, to confirm the reduction and stability. If satisfactory alignment is achieved, the usual treatment protocol is intrinsic plus splinting for 2 to 3 weeks, with weekly confirmatory x-ray films, followed by range of motion (ROM) with the affected finger buddy-taped. Dynamic or static progressive splinting and formal therapy are initiated at week 5 if motion fails to return toward normal.

K-wire fixation is used if there is loss of reduction, comminution, or inability to hold the initial reduction. The wires can be placed down the intramedullary shaft or across the fracture to affix adjacent cortices. In this way, transverse, oblique, and spiral fractures are all amenable to this treatment. Frequently K-wire fixation can be accomplished without a skin incision if the fracture is reducible by closed means. Intraoperative fluoroscopy is essential for proper pin placement and confirmation of the reduction in multiple planes. Midlateral placement of the pin or pins prevents interference with the flexor and extensor tendons and the neurovascular structures. Two pins are required for stability unless an intramedullary pin is used. The pins usually are removed at 3 weeks, when fracture tenderness subsides, to allow resumption of motion and stretching of the scar tissue (Figure 7-5).

Open reduction may be required even in simple fracture patterns if intervening soft tissue or a hematoma prevents reduction. In addition, comminution or an open fracture with bone loss may require open reduction for bone grafting or the application of stabilizing plates. Open reduction does not have to conclude with plate or screw fixation. K-wire fixation may be an acceptable alternative in some

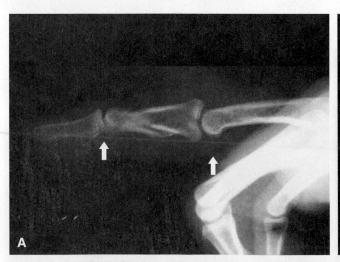
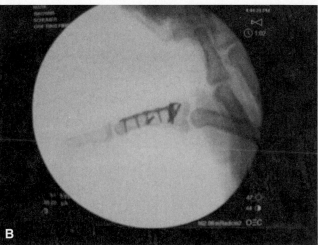

Figure 7-4

A, In the preoperative x-ray film, the distal aspect of the proximal phalanx is a perfect lateral, as evidenced by the complete overlap of the two condyles. This should also be true of the distal aspect of the middle phalanx; however, the fracture has caused a rotational deformity. **B,** A lateral fluoroscopic view obtained in the operating room shows the correction of the rotational deformity.

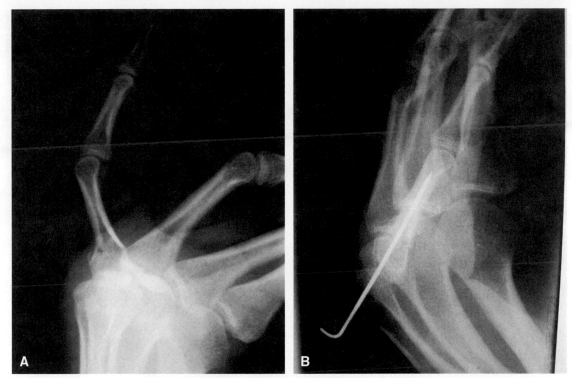

Figure 7-5

A, Low energy transverse fracture of the proximal phalanx results in volar apex angulation. **B,** This simple fracture pattern requires only closed reduction and pinning to obtain anatomical alignment of the bone and to correct the secondary deformity at the MCP and PIP joints seen in the preoperative x-ray film.

open cases. Long oblique and spiral fractures, however, are highly amenable to interfragmentary screw fixation. These fracture patterns may allow anatomical reduction and early return to motion with little interference from overlying gliding structures. Transverse and short oblique fractures cannot be treated with interfragmentary screws and must be held with a plate. Plates also can bridge gaps in the bone or secure bone graft to the reduced fracture fragments and allow early motion. The downside to plate fixation in the phalanges is that scar adherence may cause the plate to interfere with tendon gliding. Also, some patients complain of persistent pain at the plate site, requiring removal of the hardware once the fracture is healed (Figure 7-6). External fixation currently is used less often but indications for its use still exist (Figure 7-7).

Indications for External Fixation of a Fracture

- Fractures with marked comminution and soft tissue injury or that have been contaminated
- Fractures with significant soft tissue injury in which further dissection may compromise digit viability
- Fractures with a segmental defect in which length needs to be preserved until formal open reduction and internal fixation (ORIF) is done
- Temporary stability in a patient with multiple injuries

Articular and Periarticular Fractures

Unicondylar Fractures. Unicondylar fractures of the phalanges occur from a shearing force and tend to be unstable, falling into a shortened and malrotated position. This injury, although subtle, causes pain, deformity, and loss of motion. The collateral ligament remains attached to the fragment, causing it to rotate, creating an angular deformity and intra-articular incongruity. Often the fracture malalignment is best appreciated on a true lateral or oblique x-ray film, because on an anteroposterior (AP) x-ray film it may appear only mildly gapped (Figure 7-8).

Unicondylar fractures are treated surgically, because open reduction and fragment stabilization are required. Often the size of the fragments prevents the use of anything but a K-wire for fixation (Figure 7-9), but occasionally a larger fragment can be fixed with a screw.

Bicondylar Fractures. A bicondylar fracture occurs when a compressive load to the digit splits the head of the phalanx into two pieces and further separates it from the shaft. Each condylar piece is held by the collateral ligament, which tends to separate and rotate them apart. These injuries usually require open reduction and internal fixation (ORIF); K-wires often are used, but they do not allow early motion. Newly devised plates allow early motion but can be difficult to use.

Pilon (hairline) fractures occur with an axial load to the digit. Fracture of the dorsal and volar lip of the middle

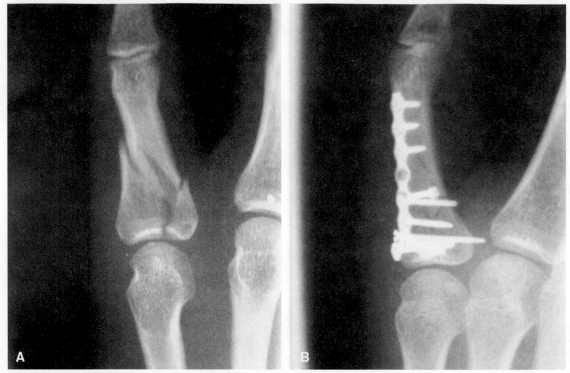

Figure 7-6
A, Markedly unstable, comminuted, intra-articular fracture of the proximal phalanx. **B,** Plate fixation was
required to obtain alignment and stability. Active range of motion was started on postoperative day 5.

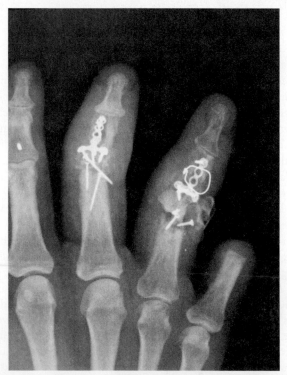

Figure 7-7
Roller crush injury with extensive soft tissue and bony damage. The
patient was a poor candidate for internal fixation; he presented with
open wounds, infection, and unstable fixation. External fixation was
the ideal treatment in this case, because it allowed the soft tissues to
heal and the infection to resolve, and it permitted eventual bone
grafting and stabilization, which facilitated bony union.

phalanx occurs, with loss of congruency and stability of the
PIP joint. Dynamic external fixation uses ligamentotaxis
(i.e., the use of the ligament to reduce the fracture) to
restore overall joint alignment. The dynamic nature of the
fixator allows early motion to promote joint congruency
and cartilage health (Figure 7-10).

Rehabilitation Principles and Considerations for Hand Fractures

Fracture healing is the regeneration of mineralized tissue,
which results in the restoration of bony mechanical
strength. The primary concern during rehabilitation and
before motion is initiated is the stability of the fracture.
The ultimate goals of rehabilitation are (1) to produce
pain-free, functional motion and strength and (2) to restore
and optimize soft tissue balance and glide without disrupting the healing tissues.

The progression of rehabilitation is based on the stages
of soft tissue and bony healing. Two well-documented
progressions of fracture healing, described as primary and
secondary healing, have been classified based on both the
approximation and motion between the bone fragments.

Progression of Fracture Healing

• Primary healing
• Secondary healing

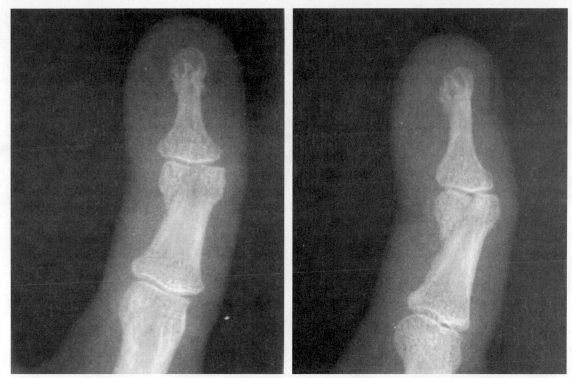

Figure 7-8
The displacement seen with a unicondylar fracture of the phalanx is not as easily appreciated in the AP view as in the oblique view. The articular incongruity and instability of the fracture require operative treatment.

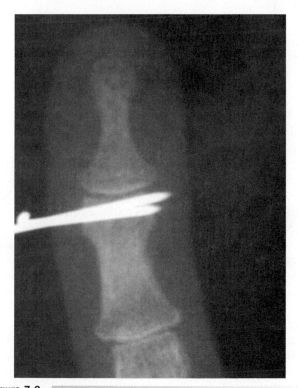

Figure 7-9
Fixation of a unicondylar fracture with K-wires.

Primary Healing. Primary healing occurs when the fracture fragments are aligned and compressed so that no motion is allowed between the fragments. Motionless fixation of the fracture fragments is achieved through open reduction and internal fixation. The fixation hardware acts as a support matrix to provide immediate strength at the fracture site. Calcification and remodeling of the tissues, which are required for true fracture strength, generally take 6 weeks. Primary healing allows for early therapeutic intervention to initiate motion and soft tissue glide, to control edema, to address wounds, and to restore normal neurological input to prevent guarding or avoidance of use. Primary healing does not allow for early strengthening, because true fracture strength is not achieved until week 6 or later.[9,10]

Secondary Healing. Secondary healing takes place when the fracture fragments are approximated but not compressed, leaving a slight gap and/or potential for motion. Bone healing occurs through progressive stages in which callus formation is a precursor to bone.[9,10] Fractures primarily managed by closed reduction heal in these stages. Closed reduction is achieved through casting and semirigid fixation, such as K-wires, external fixators, and intramedullary pins.

Secondary healing progresses in three stages. The first stage, which lasts approximately 2 weeks, is the inflammatory stage. During this stage high cellular activity occurs, which is

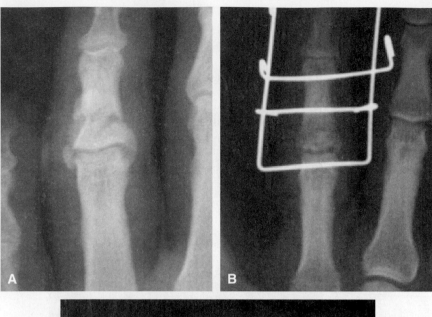

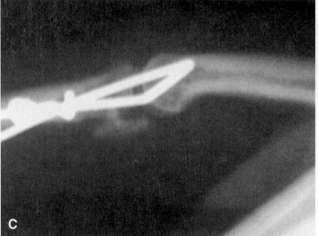

Figure 7-10
A, Pilon fracture with loss of volar and dorsal bony stability of the middle phalanx at the PIP joint. **B** and **C**, It is critical to obtain PIP joint alignment and to begin motion early. This can be accomplished with dynamic fixators through ligamentotaxis.

required for ultimate healing. The healing tissues are at their weakest and are vulnerable to mechanical disruption. The fracture site requires protection by means of splinting or casting immobilization during the inflammatory stage.[9,10]

The second stage, the repair stage, occurs during weeks 2 through 4. During this stage soft callus forms and stabilizes the fracture site. Splint protection continues, and controlled motion, tendon gliding, and edema management are initiated.[9,10]

During the third stage, which can last from weeks 4 to 6 up to 2 years, remodeling of the fracture progresses. During this stage, restoration of bone strength occurs. At this point, the tissues have regained enough strength to tolerate passive range of motion (PROM), stretching, splinting for motion, strengthening, and return to preinjury function. In general, as with primary healing, fractures progressing through the stages of secondary healing should not be

subjected to strengthening exercises until weeks 6 to 8, when healing is confirmed (Figure 7-11).

Factors that can impede healing should be considered before increased demand is placed on a fracture through stretching, strengthening, or high demand activity. These include infection, prolonged steroid use, diabetes, anemia, osteopenia, and use of alcohol, nicotine, or caffeine.[11-15] Fracture healing is a dynamic process in which healing stages are progressive but overlap. Special care must be taken with patients with multiple trauma, in whom multiple fixation methods are used and who may have fractures that are progressing through both primary and secondary healing. Multiple trauma also causes significant soft tissue damage. Attention should be given to soft tissue healing, which takes place in a well-documented, staged healing process.[10,16-20] In devising a therapeutic approach and initiating therapy, clinicians involved in the rehabilitation of

Figure 7-11

Algorithm for therapeutic management of a fracture. (From LaStayo PC, Winters KM, Hardy M: Fracture healing: bone healing, fracture management and current concepts related to the hand, *J Hand Ther* 16(2):90, Copyright @ Paul LaStayo, PhD, PT, CHT. 2003.)

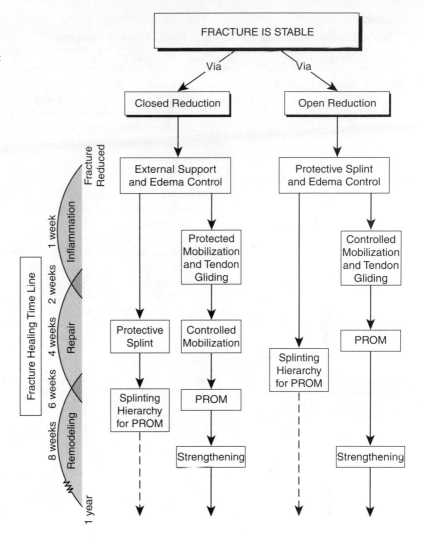

patients with these types of fractures should pay close attention to differences in the healing time frames for the various tissues involved.

The combined impact of soft tissue injury and the effects of immobilization creates challenges for both the treating physician and the therapist. Immobilization can cause a reduction in spacing and lubrication among collagen fibers, leading to reduced soft tissue gliding, shortening, and contracture development.[21] Muscle atrophy, with decreased extensibility and motion loss, is another documented effect of immobilization.[22]

Effects of Prolonged Immobilization

- Reduced soft tissue glide
- Soft tissue contracture
- Muscle atrophy
- Motion loss

The importance of direct communication between the surgeon and the therapist cannot be overstated. The most important information that determines the rehabilitation strategy is the stability of the fracture. Additional information that is significant for determining a therapeutic approach includes the type and location of the fracture and the fixation method or methods used to stabilize it.

Fractures of the Distal Phalanx. Rehabilitation guidelines for fractures of the distal phalanx can be found in Table 7-1. Therapeutic considerations are presented, taking into account the stage of healing and whether the fracture has been fixated (Figure 7-12).

Mallet Finger. Treatment of a bony mallet injury consists of continuous splinting immobilization of the DIP joint in extension for 6 to 8 weeks (Figure 7-13). Care should be taken to avoid skin blanching on the dorsum of the finger with forced hyperextension. The remaining joints of the finger are left free. Immobilization promotes healing and scarring of the terminal tendon. Skin checks

Table 7-1
Rehabilitation Guidelines for Tuft and Distal Phalanx Fractures[23-26]

Healing Stages	Fractures Without Fixation	Fractures with Fixation
Stage I: Inflammatory stage (weeks 0 to 2)	Wound care and dressing changes: If the nail bed has been repaired, sterile dressing changes may be required every 24 hours using a gauze-covered petroleum or nonstick dressing (e.g., Xeroform or Adaptic) over the injury site Static and resting splint with DIP immobilization AROM of PIP and MCP joints	Fixation for 3 weeks Static resting splint to protect the fixation
Stage II: Fibroplasia and repair stage (weeks 2 to 4)	AROM of DIP joint Edema management is required Light functional tasks may be performed Splint is discontinued Protective padding with silicone is used Desensitization: Because of the high number of nerve endings in this region of the finger, patients often complain of cold sensitivity and hypesthesia for a prolonged period after this type of injury Blocking exercises for DIP joint	AROM of uninvolved joints Week 3: Progress as stage II of tuft fracture without fixation
Stage III: Remodeling and maturation stage (weeks 4 to 6+)	Functional progression Strengthening Splinting to increase motion	Functional progression Strengthening Splinting to increase motion

DIP, Distal interphalangeal; *AROM,* active range of motion; *PIP,* proximal interphalangeal; *MCP,* metacarpophalangeal.

should be performed during the immobilization period to prevent complications from skin breakdown.

Active motion is initiated at weeks 6 to 8, and splinting is continued when the patient is not exercising. Blocking exercises (limited movement of one joint) should be avoided until week 10 to protect the oblique retinacular ligament (ORL)

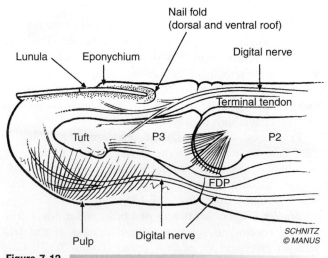

Figure 7-12
Schematic of the distal phalanx. The distal phalanx often is referred to as *P3,* the middle phalanx as *P2,* and the proximal phalanx (not shown) as *P1.* (From Cannon NM: Rehabilitation approaches for distal and middle phalanx fractures of the hand, *J Hand Ther* 16(2):105-116, 2003.)

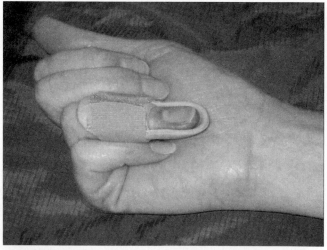

Figure 7-13
Custom splint for mallet finger. Similar prefabricated splints are available in a variety of designs and in the choice of thermoplastic materials used. A variation of the design shown is a simple clamshell splint in which thin, perforated splinting material is brought up and around the tip of the finger, providing both dorsal and volar support to the DIP in extension. Although the middle phalanx is enclosed in the splint, the PIP joint is left free to move. If splinting materials are not available, a similar splint can be formed using aluminum strips covered with foam. In each case, strapping or tape around the middle phalanx portion of the splint is required for stability. Maintaining skin integrity is a prime concern with any type of splint.

from stretching (the ORL assists in DIP extension with the PIP in extension) (Figures 7-14 and 7-15). Stretching and strengthening to increase motion are initiated at week 12. If a lag greater than 10° persists at weeks 6 to 8, continuous static splinting can be continued through week 16.[23]

Fractures of the Proximal and Middle Phalanges

Shaft Fractures. Table 7-2 presents details and considerations the clinician can follow and should keep in mind when working with patients who have sustained proximal and middle phalanx fractures (Figures 7-16 to 7-18).

Articular and Periarticular Fractures. Initiation of motion after ORIF or percutaneous pinning of unicondylar and bicondylar fractures depends on the stability of the fragments after surgery.

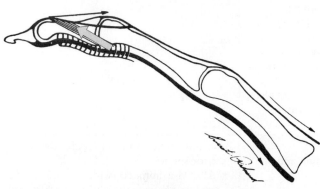

Figure 7-14

The ORL *(arrow)* arises from the volar lateral ridge of the distal tip of the middle phalanx and courses distally and dorsally to attach to the terminal tendon. (From Aulicino PL: Clinical examination of the hand. In Hunter JM, Mackin EJ, Callahan AD, editors: *Rehabilitation of the hand: surgery and therapy,* ed 4, p 53-75, St Louis, 1995, Mosby. Modified from Tubiana R: *The hand,* Philadelphia, 1981, WB Saunders.)

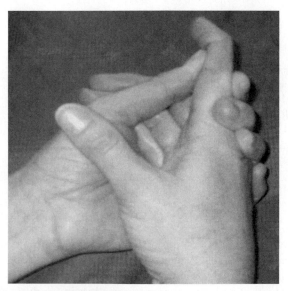

Figure 7-15

Blocking in which the PIP is extended and the DIP is flexed places a stretch on the ORL.

With an early active range of motion (AROM) program, a forearm-based dorsal block splint is fabricated for protection and worn for up to 6 weeks. Positioning within the splint may vary, depending on the injured structures and the surgical repair procedure. An AROM program begins on postoperative days 3 to 5, with the affected finger buddy-taped to the adjacent finger or fingers to prevent lateral or rotary stresses to the joint. Motion parameters differ, depending on the stability of the fracture and bony fixation. Limitations in both terminal flexion and extension may be necessary to protect the healing structures. Advancement in 10° increments per week should be done if the initial motion has been restricted. PROM, stretching, splinting for motion, and strengthening occur at 8 weeks or when healing is confirmed.[28]

With hinged external fixation of a pilon fracture, motion is initiated within 3 to 5 days. If the external fixator does not lock into extension, a static resting extension finger splint is fabricated, and the patient wears it at all times when not exercising. The resting splint is removed for AROM exercises in the clinic and 3 to 5 times daily as a home program (Figure 7-19). External fixators generally are removed at week 6. Gentle strengthening and splinting for motion begin at week 8 or when healing is confirmed.

Traction splinting may also be used in the treatment of unicondylar, bicondylar, and pilon fractures. In some cases ORIF to restore articular congruency is used in combination with traction splinting. The traction splint is fabricated using an outrigger. Outriggers can be custom fabricated or prefabricated. The finger then is attached to the outrigger designed to provide consistent traction to the PIP joint through an arc of motion. The traction reduces the fracture fragments through ligamentotaxis and restores optimal joint space for tissue healing and gliding (Figure 7-20). The optimum traction and motion parameters vary, depending on the fracture. Imaging and a tension gauge are used to measure appropriate traction on the tissues within a safe range. The splint usually is removed at week 6. After removal of the splint, a program of edema management, AROM and PROM exercises, differential tendon gliding, and stretching is initiated. Gentle strengthening and splinting for motion begins at week 8 or when healing is confirmed.[28] Management of fractures with external fixators or traction splinting requires direct, consistent communication with the physician. The risk of infection is a complication with external fixation or traction splinting.

Complications off fractures of the proximal and middle phalanges include soft tissue adherence of the flexor and extensor tendons. Moreover, the imbalance in strength between the flexor and extensor tendon forces creates an initial extensor lag (inability to fully extend actively). This lag can lead to a chronic flexion contracture of the PIP joint (Figure 7-21).[28]

Table 7-2

Rehabilitation Guidelines for Fractures of the Proximal and Middle Phalanges[26-29]

Healing Stages	Fractures with Rigid Fixation	Fractures with Semirigid Fixation
Stage I: Inflammatory stage (weeks 0 to 2)	AROM is initiated on post-op day 5 (pain level should be kept under 5 on a 1-10 pain scale) Edema management Soft tissue mobilization Splinting is done in the intrinsic plus position and includes the adjacent finger or fingers for added stability (hand or forearm based, depending on the fracture's site and stability and the patient profile) (Figure 7-16) In the intrinsic plus position (MCP joint: 70° flexion; IP joints, straight): • Intrinsic muscles are placed at rest, reducing forces to the proximal phalanx • The extensor hood glides distally, providing compressive stability to a fracture of the proximal phalanx • The IP joints are held in extension, reducing force imbalances, which can lead to flexion contracture • The periarticular structures, including the MCP collaterals, the IP collaterals, and the PIP volar plate, are held in the optimum position for preventing flexion contracture	Fixation usually is removed at 3 to 4 weeks; midshaft fractures of the proximal or middle phalanx may take 1 to 2 weeks longer to heal Casting or splinting may be used for 3 to 6 weeks, depending on the stability of the fracture in the intrinsic plus position Forces should not disrupt, loosen, or dislodge wires or pins. The surgeon should be contacted if any change in the hardware occurs
Stage II: Fibroplasia and repair stage (weeks 2 to 4)	Tendon gliding exercises Blocking for differential flexor tendon gliding and extensor tendon excursion (Figure 7-17) Light functional tasks begin at week 4 Protective splinting continues until week 6 Protective splinting or buddy taping for sports or high level activity may be indicated until week 8, depending on the stability of the fracture	After 3 to 6 weeks of immobilization in a cast or splint: • AROM is initiated (with fractures of the middle phalanx, the pull of the FDS can put stress on the fracture fragments; therefore *gentle* AROM is indicated) • Protective splint in the intrinsic plus position is fabricated for wear between exercises and is used until week 6-8 • Light functional tasks are begun at week 4
Stage III: Remodeling and maturation stage (weeks 4 to 6+)	Functional progression Stretching Strengthening begins after fracture healing is confirmed at 6-8 weeks Splinting to increase motion (Figure 7-18) Dynamic and/or static progressive splinting can be initiated at week 6 when healing is confirmed. Studies have shown the positive effects of prolonged stretching of a stiff joint, and presented considerations for choosing dynamic versus static progressive splinting[30-33]	Functional progression Stretching Strengthening begins after fracture healing is confirmed at 6 to 8 weeks Splinting to increase motion

AROM, Active range of motion; *MCP*, metacarpophalangeal; *IP*, interphalangeal; *PIP*, proximal interphalangeal; *FDS*, flexor digitorum superficialis.

Metacarpal Fractures

General Considerations

The metacarpals support the phalanges, ensuring the proper length for optimal function and balance between the extrinsic and intrinsic tendons of the hand. They also provide for the origin of the intrinsic muscles and the mobility obtained at the carpometacarpal and metacarpophalangeal joints. A change in the normal length and alignment of the metacarpals as a result of injury must be recognized and treated to prevent a loss in hand function. Fractures of the metacarpals account for up to one third of hand fractures, and fifth metacarpal fractures account for

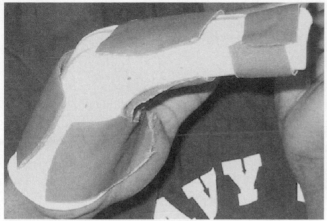

Figure 7-16

Hand-based ulnar gutter static resting splint in the intrinsic plus position: MCP joints in 70° flexion; PIP and DIP joints, extended.

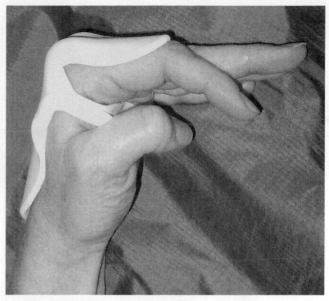

Figure 7-17

An MCP extension block splint promotes isolated IP extension.

more than 50% of metacarpal fractures.[34] The goal of treatment is to regain stability with enough osseous length for correct tendon balance and to prevent the complications of soft tissue injury, tendon adhesion, and malalignment.

Anatomy

The anatomy of the metacarpals, specifically their articulations and muscle attachments, directly affects the injury pattern and the management of these fractures. The index and middle finger metacarpals articulate with the trapezoid and capitate bones respectively. These carpometacarpal (CMC) joints have very little motion. The ulnar two metacarpals articulate with the hamate bone which, with its relatively flat articular surface, allows for substantial motion both in flexion and extension and to a lesser degree in rotation. Because these metacarpals align with a joint allowing considerable motion in the plane of flexion and extension, more fracture malalignment can be accepted on this side of the hand. Deformity is much more obvious and difficult to compensate for in the two radial metacarpals, where little to no motion occurs at the CMC joints.

The deforming forces that displace metacarpal fractures are related to the crossing extrinsic tendons and the attachments of the intrinsic musculature. The intrinsic hand muscles, including the palmar and dorsal interossei, originate on the metacarpal shafts. The lumbrical muscles, originating from the tendons of the flexor digitorum profundi and the interossei, are the primary flexors of the MCP joint. The metacarpal bones act as a fulcrum for digital motion by stabilizing the phalanges against the pull of the flexor and extensor tendons. When these bones are fractured, the resulting disruption causes an imbalance in these forces, leading to specific patterns of deformity.

Diagnosis

Fractures of the metacarpal shaft generally are caused by a fall or a direct blow to the hand. Neck fractures, particularly those of the fourth and fifth metacarpals, are the result of an axial load, such as when a fist strikes a hard surface. Areas of edema, ecchymosis, and tenderness should alert the examiner to the potential for an underlying fracture and should be thoroughly examined. Clinical suspicion should be increased if the patient has a gross deformity over the dorsum of the hand, loss of normal knuckle height or contour, and an alteration in the rotational alignment of the digits.

Rotational malalignment is best appreciated in digital flexion, and the injured finger or fingers should be examined under active range of motion, with use of a digital block if pain is limiting the evaluation (Figure 7-22). Passive range of motion is not reliable, because the examiner may inadvertently alter the digital rotation while flexing the digit. Tenodesis active motion is better than passive range of motion for an uncooperative patient who cannot actively range the digits. The clinician also must make sure the patient does not use an adjacent finger to "capture" and hold the affected digit "in alignment." The results of the examination should be compared to the findings for the contralateral hand. Plain x-ray films, including AP, lateral, and oblique views, are necessary to evaluate most metacarpal fractures, and special views occasionally are required (e.g., Brewerton, 20° pronation).

Injury Classification and Medical Treatment

General Principles. Metacarpal fractures usually are discussed in terms of the location of the fracture, the

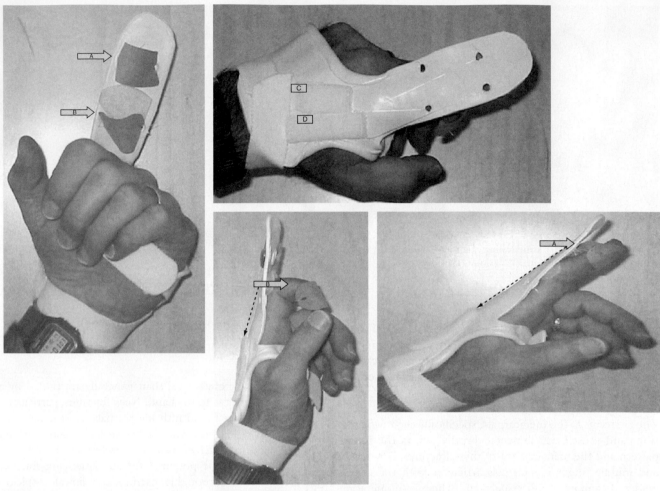

Figure 7-18
Static progressive splinting to regain PIP extension and IP flexion. Leather slings (*A* and *B*) are attached
to fishing wire, which is brought through holes drilled in the splint. The fishing wire is attached to sticky back
Velcro loop tape (*C* and *D*), which is folded over and attached to the Velcro hook side of the tape, which has
been affixed to the splint. The Velcro loop is pulled, tightening the slings to patient tolerance, which provides
a static progressive stretch. The patient alternates between flexion and extension stretches during the day.

pattern of the fracture, and the resulting deformity. Fractures can occur at the level of the metacarpal base, shaft, neck, or head. The pattern that results usually is secondary to the mechanism of injury; the fracture may be transverse, oblique, spiral, or comminuted (Figure 7-23). A direct blow usually produces a transverse fracture, whereas torsion of the digit causes a spiral or oblique fracture. Comminuted fractures result from higher energy injuries. Fracture deformity is described relative to changes in angulation, rotation, or length. Malrotation is problematic because if not corrected, it may interfere with flexion of the adjacent fingers (referred to as *scissoring*). Malrotation of as little as 5° may cause 1.5 cm (0.6 inch) of digital overlap with flexion of the fingers[35,36] An uncorrected angular deformity of the metacarpal shaft (usually a flexion deformity) not only results in a cosmetic concern; if severe enough, it may cause hyperextension at the MCP joint (e.g., clawing) (Figure 7-24). Metacarpal

fractures with significant shortening may cause an imbalance of the intrinsic and extrinsic tendons.

Management Approach. The management of a patient with a metacarpal fracture depends on a variety of factors. The location of the fracture, degree of displacement, angulation, and rotation all influence the acceptability of fracture alignment and also predict the likelihood that the injury will proceed to further displacement. The patient's age, occupation, general health, and concomitant injuries also must be considered.

Transverse fractures with minimal displacement usually have little potential for further displacement and are relatively stable. Treatment usually is nonoperative, consisting of immobilization in a plaster splint or cast for 3 to 4 weeks.[37] Displaced and unstable transverse fractures can be treated with closed reduction and splinting or closed reduction and percutaneous pin fixation, depending on the perceived fracture stability at the time of evaluation and reduction.

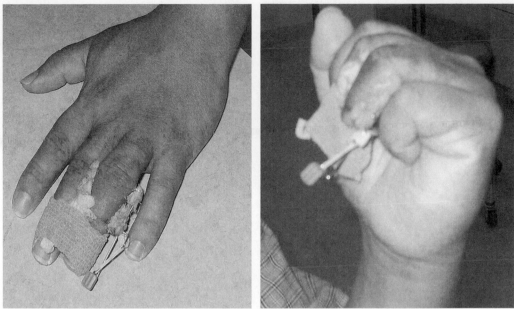

Figure 7-19

A pilon fracture of the ring finger is stabilized with finger-based dynamic external fixation, which allows for active PIP flexion and extension at day 3. The ring finger is buddy-taped to the long finger to provide increased stability to the PIP joint.

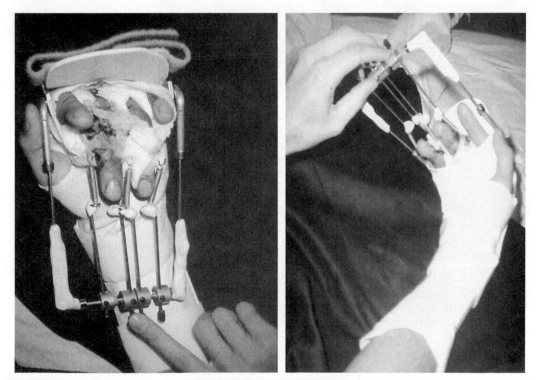

Figure 7-20

Custom-fabricated traction splint for traumatic PIP intra-articular fractures of the middle and ring fingers. This type of splint allows flexion and extension of the PIP joints. The fingers are attached to a custom-made outrigger by means of springs, which are hooked to surgically placed K-wires that exit through the skin from the middle phalanx, providing consistent traction through the available ROM. The patient rests at night against the dorsal protective hood with the PIP and DIP strapped into extension. (External finger dressings have been taken down for clarity.)

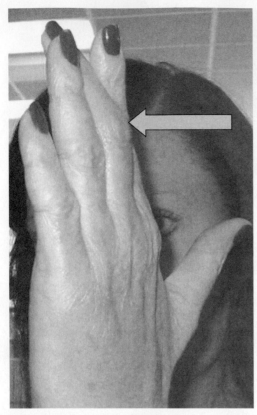

Figure 7-21
Flexion contracture of the long finger PIP joint.

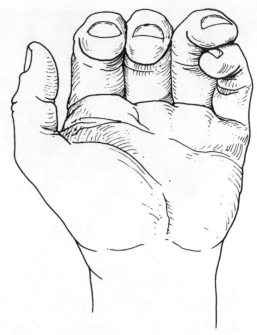

Figure 7-22
Malrotation of the ring finger, caused by a metacarpal fracture, is best appreciated during active finger flexion. (From Hunter JM, Mackin EJ, Callahan AD et al, editors: *Rehabilitation of the hand and upper extremity,* ed 5, p 383, St Louis, 2002, Mosby.)

Oblique and spiral fractures with a minimal amount of shortening and no malrotation can be treated nonoperatively with casting or splinting. If any malrotation or significant shortening is present, open reduction and fixation with interfragmentary lag screws is indicated. Short fracture lines may need the additional stability of a dorsal plate for resistance to torsional and bending stresses. Fractures of the index and small finger metacarpals have less inherent stability because they lack the suspensory effect of the intermetacarpal ligaments; therefore these fractures may benefit from the added stability of plate fixation.

Specific Metacarpal Fractures

Metacarpal Head Fractures. Fractures of the metacarpal head are a rare injury. They often are the result of an axial load or direct trauma, and they generally are intra-articular. These fractures can be classified in terms of their descriptive characteristics: epiphyseal, ligamentous avulsion, osteochondral, comminuted, and compression fractures. Treatment of metacarpal head fractures is individually based on the type of fracture and the degree of displacement. Nondisplaced fractures are stable and can be treated with a short course of immobilization. Noncomminuted fractures with more than 1 mm of articular displacement or with joint surface involvement greater than 25% likely will require operative fixation in the form of ORIF using K-wires

or interfragmentary screws.[38] Fractures that involve ligamentous avulsion and displaced osteochondral fragments can also be treated with open reduction and internal fixation (Figure 7-25). Comminuted intra-articular metacarpal fractures usually are the result of a higher energy injury. This makes them difficult to manage because of the surrounding soft tissue injury, the degree of bone loss, and the presence of small bony fragments. Treatment options include immobilization, ligamentotaxis through placement of an external fixator, or primary or secondary joint arthroplasty if the degree of bone loss and fragmentation prevents adequate reduction and stabilization.

Metacarpal Neck Fractures. Fractures of the metacarpal neck are common and usually occur in the ring and small fingers. The mechanism of injury commonly involves a flexed MCP joint striking a solid object, causing a neck fracture with apex dorsal angulation. This pattern of angulation occurs because the traumatic impact causes volar comminution at the level of the neck and also because the intrinsic muscles maintain the metacarpal head in a flexed position, leading to apex dorsal angulation. The CMC joints in the ring and small fingers allow more mobility than the CMC joints in the index and middle fingers, and they therefore compensate for a larger degree of angular deformity. The amount of angulation that can be tolerated without functional impairment varies throughout the orthopedic literature, ranging from 20° to 60° in the small metacarpal and 10° to 40° in the ring metacarpal.[39-41]

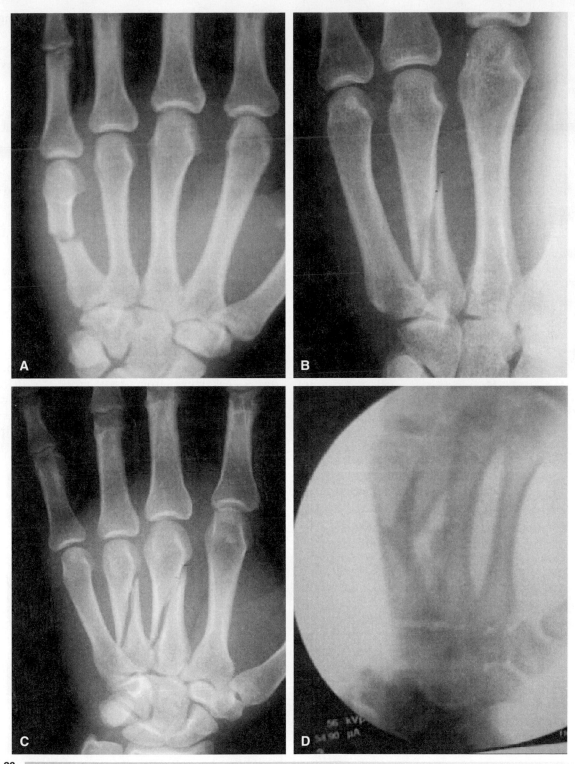

Figure 7-23

Types of metacarpal fractures. **A**, Transverse. **B**, Spiral. **C**, Oblique. **D**, Comminuted.

Malrotation of a metacarpal neck fracture cannot be tolerated, because it will affect the flexion ability of the other fingers and impair the ability to grip.

Treatment of metacarpal neck fractures depends on the stability of the fracture and whether a reduction will hold the fracture within the acceptable range of alignment. Closed reduction may be attempted, with subsequent immobilization. If the fracture remains reduced and stable and has no associated malrotation, immobilization may be the definitive treatment. If the reduction cannot be

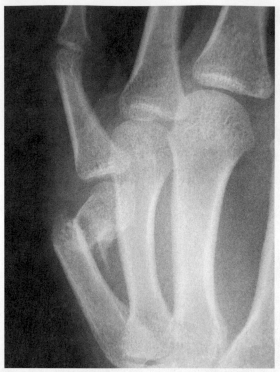

Figure 7-24
Oblique x-ray film showing the secondary claw deformity that occurs at the MCP joint as a result of a flexion deformity of the metacarpal shaft at the site of the fracture.

maintained because of fracture instability or comminution or if an unacceptable degree of angulation or rotation is present, closed reduction and fixation with K-wires or open reduction with plate and screw constructs may be necessary (Figure 7-26).

Metacarpal Shaft Fractures. Fractures of the metacarpal shaft are common injuries, and the management of these fractures must take into account several factors, including the fracture pattern, the degree of displacement, and the overall stability of the fracture.

Transverse fractures usually are caused by a direct blow or an axial load. Because of the deforming force of the intrinsic muscles, these fractures tend to fall into apex dorsal angulation. As with metacarpal neck fractures, a certain degree of angulation can be tolerated without compromising hand function. More deformity is tolerated in the small and ring finger metacarpals because of the larger degree of motion at their CMC joints. Angulation of the index and middle metacarpal shafts is not as well tolerated because of the limited motion at these CMC joints. The acceptable degree of angulation is the subject of debate in the orthopedic literature. The acceptable degree of angulation for the ring and small finger metacarpals ranges from less than 20° to 40°, whereas the acceptable angulation for the index and middle metacarpals ranges from 0° to 10°.[37,42,43] Excess angulation causes prominence of the metacarpal head in the palm,

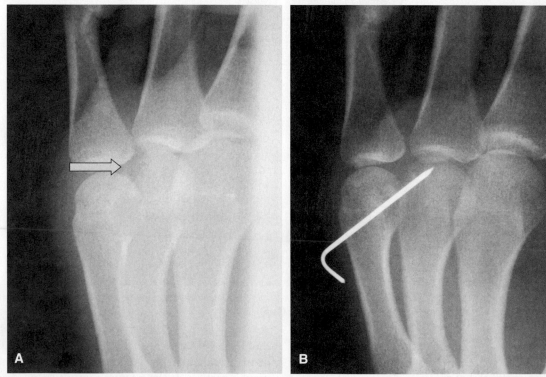

Figure 7-25
Osteochondral avulsion fracture (**A**) involving the ulnar collateral ligament and part of the articular surface in a thin section of bone fixed with a K-wire (**B**).

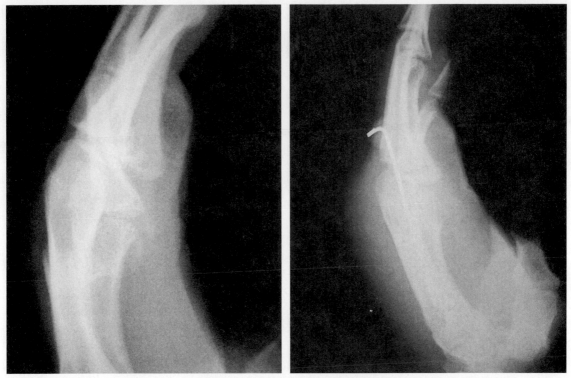

Figure 7-26

Preoperative and postoperative lateral x-ray films of a transverse displaced fracture of the fifth
metacarpal. Note that in the preoperative view *(left)*, the metacarpal head does not align with the other
metacarpals nor along the shaft of the fifth metacarpal, as it does in the postoperative view *(right)* after
reduction and pinning.

which can make gripping uncomfortable; it also results in
hyperextension of the MCP joint, causing limited MCP
joint flexion and loss of grip.

Oblique and spiral fractures typically are caused by a
torsional load. If these fractures are unstable, they tend
to cause a rotational deformity. The presence of any
degree of malrotation, regardless of the specific metacarpal
involved, warrants reduction and stabilization, otherwise
the fingers will overlap, causing problems with digital
flexion.

Comminuted fractures usually are caused by a high
energy force and often are associated with significant soft
tissue injury. The clinician must include the integrity of
the skin and soft tissue envelope as part of the treatment
algorithm when determining management options.
Comminuted fractures tend to cause shortening of the
metacarpal because of the multiple small bone fragments
and the overall unstable fracture pattern. Shortening of
the metacarpals results in an imbalance of forces and
compromised function of the flexor and extensor
mechanisms. For every 2 mm of shortening, a 7° extensor lag of the MCP joint results.[44] The degree of acceptable shortening for metacarpal fractures is somewhat
controversial, ranging from 3 to 6 mm in the orthopedic
literature.[45-47]

Management of metacarpal shaft fractures is based on the
degree of displacement, including angulation, malrotation,
and shortening, and the stability of the fracture. In essence,
the clinician needs to determine whether the fracture is
acceptably aligned and whether it is likely to remain that
way if treated by closed techniques.

For minimally displaced, stable fractures, nonoperative
management with cast or splint immobilization is adequate
treatment. However, surgical intervention is warranted if
the fracture is unstable, if the resulting deformity compromises function, and in some cases when the concomitant
injury necessitates correction. The surgical options for shaft
fractures include transosseous percutaneous or open K-wire
fixation, cerclage wires, intramedullary wire fixation, interfragmentary screws, plate fixation, and external fixation
(Figure 7-27).

Transverse fractures with minimal displacement usually
have little potential to further displace and are relatively stable. Treatment usually is nonoperative, consisting of immobilization in a plaster splint or cast for 3 to 4 weeks.[37] If the
degree of angulation is unacceptable or the reduction cannot be maintained by nonoperative methods, operative fixation is warranted.

Oblique and spiral fractures with a minimal amount of
shortening and without malrotation can be treated

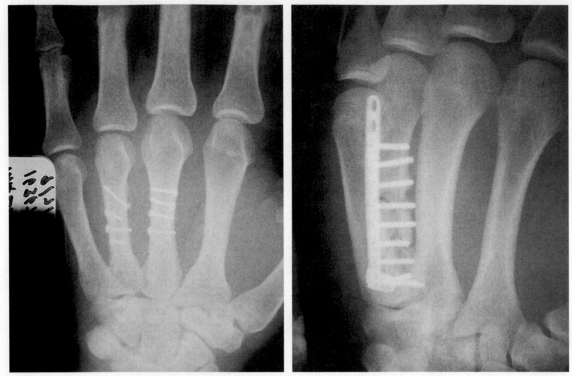

Figure 7-27

Previously seen as Figures 7-23C and 7-23D, these oblique and comminuted fractures were treated with different operative techniques. The long oblique fractures *(left)* are amenable to interfragmentary screw fixation, which allows early ROM with little interference from hardware. The more unstable comminuted fracture *(right)* requires the plate for rigidity. This allows early ROM, but the hardware sometimes interferes with gliding structures.

nonoperatively with casting or splinting. If malrotation, significant shortening, or instability is present, open reduction and fixation are necessary.

Metacarpal shaft fractures with significant displacement, angulation, rotation, or shortening that are still unstable after reduction attempts require either closed reduction with percutaneous pin placement or open reduction and internal fixation. Fractures may be closed, reduced and pinned directly through the fracture site, or pins may be placed transversely through the metacarpal bone, with at least one proximal and one distal to the fracture site. Flexible intramedullary nail fixation is also an option, in which special rods or K-wires are placed through a small incision near the base of the metacarpal. The closed reduction and fixation technique is beneficial because it is less invasive than open management; however, controlling the rotation of the distal fragment is difficult with this method. Open reduction allows direct control of the bone and the potential for perfect anatomical restoration, albeit at the cost of increased trauma to the soft tissue envelope in the surgical approach. Also, rigid fixation may be obtained with interfragmentary compression screws or a plate and screw construct, allowing for earlier return to motion. With an open fracture or an injury with

significant bone loss or contamination of the soft tissue envelope surrounding the metacarpal shaft, the best course of action is to rigidly stabilize the skeleton with the least trauma to the surrounding soft tissues. Often this can be accomplished most readily with external fixation.

Metacarpal Base Fractures. Fractures of the base of the metacarpal are often intra-articular and frequently are associated with subluxation or frank dislocation of the CMC joint. This fracture pattern is far less common in the index and middle finger metacarpals because of the tight bony geometry and firm ligamentous support at these CMC joints. On the ulnar side of the hand, an axially directed force causes a fracture of the metacarpal base, along with a proximal and dorsal subluxation of the fourth and fifth metacarpals relative to their articulation with the hamate. This fracture-dislocation can be difficult to visualize on plain AP or lateral x-ray films, and suspicion for this injury should alert the clinician to the need for 30° rotated x-ray views, or possibly a computed tomography (CT) scan. This fracture is inherently unstable, and if it goes unrecognized or ignored, it may result in articular surface incongruity and possibly weakened grip strength and arthrosis.[48] These fractures may be treated with closed reduction and

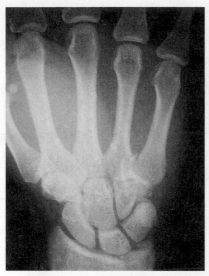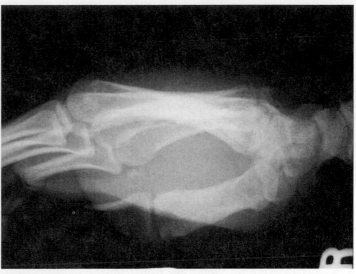

Figure 7-28
AP and lateral x-ray views of a fracture-dislocation of the fifth CMC joint. On the AP view, note the
inability to see the joint space between the base of the metacarpal and the hamate, as well as the loss of the
normal height cascade of the metacarpals. The lateral view shows the dorsal displacement of the base of
the fifth metacarpal compared to the rest of the hand.

percutaneous pinning, but if reduction is difficult or inadequate, ORIF is indicated (Figure 7-28).

Thumb Metacarpal Fractures. Fractures of the
thumb metacarpal are common, accounting for 25% of all
metacarpal fractures.[49] Thumb metacarpal fractures have
the same type of classification and management options
as the other types of metacarpal fractures, and the treatment
of head, neck, and shaft fractures usually is similar to that for
the digits. More angulation and rotation are tolerated in
thumb metacarpal shaft fractures because of the large degree
of compensatory motion at the thumb CMC joint.

Fractures of the thumb metacarpal base deserve
unique consideration because of the frequency of intra-
articular extension and the association of these fractures
with CMC joint subluxation or frank dislocation.
In order of increasing fracture fragmentation and instability, these fractures are Bennett's fracture, Rolando's
fracture, and intra-articular comminuted fractures. The
mechanism of injury is the same; all are the result of an
axial load applied through a partially flexed metacarpal
shaft. Bennett's fracture is a two-part fracture involving
an avulsion of the thumb metacarpal from the volar ulnar
aspect of the metacarpal base. The ligament attached to
this fragment, the volar oblique ligament, keeps the small
avulsed fracture fragment aligned to the joint while
the remainder of the metacarpal shaft is subluxed. The
deforming forces that create the subluxation include
the thumb extensors, the abductor pollicis longus and
the adductor pollicis longus. The pull of these muscles
results in a dorsal, radial, and proximal subluxation of

the thumb metacarpal shaft. Rolando's fracture is similar
to Bennett's fracture except that the metacarpal is broken
into three pieces instead of two. An intra-articular comminuted fracture has additional fracture components
and therefore is more difficult to treat. Because of strong
deforming forces and bony instability, these injuries tend
to displace and therefore require operative fixation. The
disrupted articular congruity may hasten the onset of
post-traumatic arthritis, which can lead to pain and functional compromise.

Thumb metacarpal fractures often are difficult to manage because of the degree of displacement and the involvement of the articular surface. The degree of articular
incongruity that is acceptable without predisposing a
patient to symptomatic post-traumatic arthritis is the subject of controversy. Some authors believe that the articular
surface must be restored as anatomically as possible (within
1 mm),[50,51] whereas others believe that good outcomes
result with articular surface incongruity up to 2 mm.[52]
When closed reduction can produce restoration of the
articular surface, K-wires may be used to secure the reduction. If the articular surface remains significantly displaced
after attempted reduction, open reduction and fixation
is indicated to maintain length, using lag screws, plates,
K-wires, or possibly an external fixator.

Rehabilitation of Metacarpal Fractures
Therapeutic intervention for metacarpal fractures differs,
depending on the location and stability of the fracture.
The progression of rehabilitation is determined by bony

healing (see Figure 7-11). The major complication of these fractures is adherence of soft tissues as a result of injury, immobilization, and persistent edema. Soft tissues can adhere to extrinsic tendons, intrinsic muscles, and periarticular structures. Reduction of soft tissue glide can result in a lag and contractures at the MCP joint and secondarily at the PIP joint. The primary goals of rehabilitation are to restore and optimize soft tissue balance and glide, allowing pain-free motion and strength, while protecting the healing tissues (Tables 7-3 and 7-4).

Splinting Guidelines. Splinting is an essential element of the optimum management of metacarpal fractures. Guidelines for appropriate splinting vary, depending on the particular metacarpal fractured.

Table 7-3
Rehabilitation Guidelines for Fractures of the Second Through Fifth Metacarpals[26,29,53-55]

Healing Stages	Fractures with Rigid Fixation*	Fractures with Semirigid Fixation†
Stage I: Inflammatory stage (weeks 0 to 2)	AROM tendon gliding exercises are initiated on post-op day 5 (pain level should be kept under 5 on a 1-10 pain scale) Edema management Soft tissue mobilization Scar management with silicone Splinting	Casting or splinting for 3 to 6 weeks, depending on fracture stability, in the forearm-based intrinsic plus position
Stage II: Fibroplasia and repair stage (weeks 2 to 4)	Gentle blocking for flexor and extensor pull through, including isolated EDC exercises Soft tissue mobilization of the scar	After 3 to 6 weeks of immobilization in a cast or splint: • AROM and tendon gliding are started • Gentle blocking and isolated EDC pull-through exercises are started • Protective hand-based splint in the intrinsic plus position (IP joints may or may not be included) is fabricated for use between exercises and is worn until week 6 to 8 • Hand-based ulnar gutter or radial gutter splint that leaves the MCP joints free is indicated for stable shaft and base fractures
Stage III: Remodeling and maturation stage (weeks 4 to 6+)	Week 4: Splint is reduced to a hand-based, protective splint for use between exercises; it is worn until week 6 Protective splint for sports or high level activity may be worn until week 8: • Protective, hand-based ulnar gutter or radial gutter splint with MCP joints included at 70° to 90° flexion, IP joints free • Hand-based ulnar gutter or radial gutter splint with MCP joints free is indicated for stable shaft and base fractures Light functional tasks are initiated Functional progression: high level activities may be limited until week 8 Stretching begins for all tissues, including the intrinsics Strengthening begins after fracture healing is confirmed at weeks 6 to 8 Splinting to increase motion begins at weeks 6 to 8	Protective splint for sports or high level activity may be worn until week 8 Light functional tasks begin at week 4 Functional progression: high level activities may be limited until week 8 Stretching, including intrinsic stretching Splinting to increase motion begins at week 6, when healing is confirmed Strengthening begins after fracture healing is confirmed at weeks 6 to 8

*Fixation may or may not be removed.
†Fixation is removed at 3 to 4 weeks.
AROM, Active range of motion; *EDC,* extensor digitorum communis; *IP,* interphalangeal; *MCP,* metacarpophalangeal.

Table 7-4

Rehabilitation Guidelines for Fractures of the First Metacarpal[26,29,53–55]

Healing Stages	Fractures with Rigid Fixation*	Fractures with Semirigid Fixation†
Stage I: Inflammatory stage (weeks 0 to 2)	Head and shaft fractures: AROM of the thumb IP joint and tendon gliding exercises of the FPL and EPL are initiated on post-op day 5 if the surgeon has confirm the stability of the fracture by the surgeon. The pain level should be kept under 5 on a 1-10 scale IP joint should not be moved if the fracture is unstable Base fractures: IP joint is immobilized for 2 weeks to prevent stress force to the CMC joint unless stability is confirmed by the surgeon Splinting (see splinting guidelines for thumb metacarpal fractures)	Casting or splinting for 3 to 6 weeks, depending on fracture stability, in a forearm-based opponens splint or thumb spica cast
Stage II: Fibroplasia and repair stage (weeks 2 to 4)	AROM of IP joint continues or is initiated, based on fracture stability and stress-loading considerations for the CMC joint (with base fractures)	After 3 to 6 weeks of immobilization with a cast or splint: • AROM and tendon gliding: Blocking and isolated EPL and FPL pull-through exercises • Protective, hand-based short opponens splint with the IP joint free, to be used between exercises and worn until weeks 6 to 8
Stage III: Remodeling and maturation stage (weeks 4 to 6+)	Stable fractures: Splint may be reduced to a hand-based short opponens protective splint that is used between exercises and worn until weeks 6 to 8 Protective splinting for sports or high level activity may be indicated until week 8 Light functional tasks are initiated Splinting for motion begins at week 6 Strengthening begins when healing is confirmed at approximately weeks 6 to 8 Functional progression	Light functional tasks begin at week 4 Functional progression Stretching Splinting to increase motion begins at week 6 Strengthening begins after fracture healing is confirmed at weeks 6 to 8

*Fixation may or may not be removed.
†Fixation is removed at 3 to 4 weeks.
AROM, Active range of motion; IP, interphalangeal; FPL, flexor pollicis longus; EPL, extensor pollicis longus; CMC, carpometacarpal.

Guidelines for Splinting Fractures of the Second through Fifth Metacarpals[25,29,54,56]

- The splint design is based on the location and stability of the fracture and the patient profile, including the individual's compliance with fracture healing precautions and activity level (Figures 7-29 and 7-30)
- The adjacent digit is included for added stabilization and to prevent rotational forces
- A circumferential splint is used (e.g., ulnar or radial gutter splint)
- For fractures of the metacarpal head, the forearm-based intrinsic plus position is used (i.e., wrist, 20° extension; MCP joints, 70° to 90° flexion; interphalangeal (IP) joints, 0° extension)*

- For fractures of the metacarpal neck, shaft, or base, a forearm-based splint is used with the wrist in 20° extension, the MCP joints flexed 70° to 90°, and the IP joints left free[29,54]
- For a stable shaft fracture, a three-point stabilization splint is used. This is a hand-based circumferential splint with counterforces that stabilize the fracture site. The involved finger is buddy-taped to the adjacent finger to prevent rotational forces to the fracture site.[56]

*The intrinsic plus position (MCP joint flexed 70°, IP joints in 0° extension) allows the intrinsic muscles to relax, reducing forces to the proximal phalanx. The extensor hood glides distally, providing compressive stability to the metacarpal head fracture. The IP joints are held in extension, reducing force imbalances, which can lead to flexion contractures. The periarticular structures, including the MCP joint collaterals, the IP collaterals, and the PIP volar plate, are held in the optimum position to prevent a flexion contracture.[25]

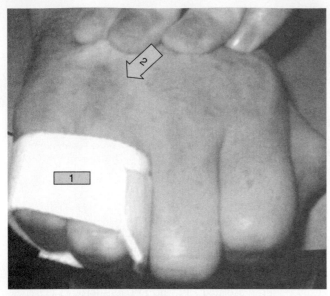

Figure 7-29

1, A flexion strap can be made to hold the IPs in flexion. The patient is asked to extend the MCP joints, which encourages isolated pull through of the extensor digitorum communis (EDC). *2,* Applying pressure on the dorsum of the hand, pushing distally, while the exercise is performed encourages further separation from the scar tissue.

> ### Guidelines for Splinting Fractures of the First Metacarpal[25,29,53,54]
>
> - The splint design is based on the location and stability of the fracture and the patient profile, including the individual's compliance with fracture healing precautions and activity level
> - The design should prevent first web contracture
> - The splint is circumferential, passing around the thumb, and is forearm based, as in a long-opponens splint
> - For fractures of the head, shaft, or base, a long-opponens splint that includes the IP joint is used. IP motion is allowed after fracture stability has been confirmed by imaging

Ligament Injuries of the Hand

Ligament Injuries of the Digits

General Considerations

Stretching and tearing of the soft tissue constraints of the PIP joint are the most common ligamentous injuries in the hand. Sports, industrial mishaps, falls, and motor vehicle accidents account for most of these injuries.

Complete digital dislocations are quite painful, and the deformity is obvious enough that patients usually seek

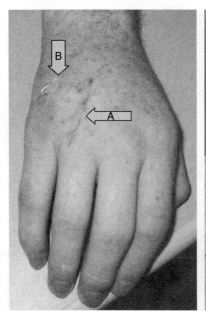 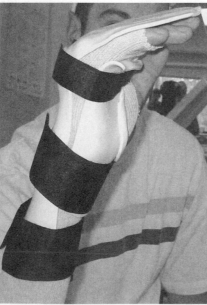 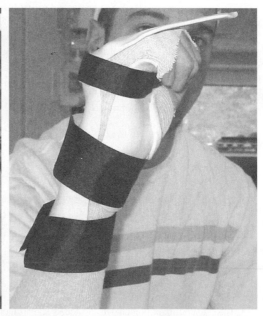

Figure 7-30

Postoperative management of *(A)* open reduction and internal fixation of a fourth metacarpal neck fracture and *(B)* pinning of a fifth metacarpal head fracture on day 5 after cast removal. A custom-made, protective, forearm-based splint is fabricated to put the long, ring, and little fingers in the intrinsic plus positions; this allows active flexion and extension within the splint and prevents adherence of soft tissue structures. The design of this splint provides circumferential, maximum protection for healing fractures. The patient straps the fingers into the hood or roof of the splint for sleeping. A similar, hand-based version can be fabricated if less protection is needed.

acute treatment; however, follow-up care for these injuries is surprisingly limited. Often patients are seen months later with chronic joint contractures, loss of tendon excursion, and swelling. By this time, they may require extensive therapy or even surgery. In the more acute stage, therapeutic intervention for these injuries is far simpler and more effective. Prompt treatment and immediate follow-up care are particularly important in a patient with an injury to the ulnar collateral ligament to the thumb (see later discussion). In the acute stage, the thumb may be quite swollen and ecchymotic, but no obvious deformity may be present, and in these injuries the acute symptoms improve over several days to a week. Unfortunately, if the ligament remains incompetent and untreated, a chronic painful condition develops perhaps months to years later, as does the potential for arthritis at the MCP joint.[57]

Anatomy

The PIP joint is a constrained hinge joint with tight articular congruency. The proximal phalanx is cam shaped and composed of a bicondylar head with a central groove. The double concave middle phalanx is divided in the midline by a bony tongue that guides the joint through its eccentric arc of motion (Figure 7-31).

The main lateral stabilizer of the joint is the proper collateral ligament, which is 2 to 3 mm thick. This ligament originates at the head of the proximal phalanx and inserts into the base of the middle phalanx. The proper collateral ligament is connected to the volar plate by the shroudlike

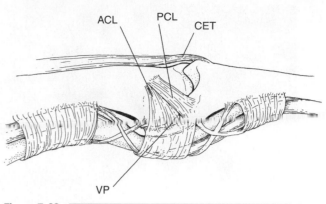

Figure 7-32

Lateral view of the PIP joint. The proper collateral ligament (*PCL*), accessory collateral ligament (*ACL*), volar plate (*VP*), and dorsal capsule with the central extensor tendon (*CET*) provide support to the PIP joint. Note that the ACL inserts into the volar plate, and the PCL travels distally and volarly to insert onto the bone of the middle phalanx. (From Campbell PJ, Wilson RL: Management of joint injuries and intraarticular fractures. In Hunter JM, Mackin EJ, Callahan AD et al, editors: *Rehabilitation of the hand and upper extremity*, ed 5, St Louis, 2002, Mosby.)

fibers of the accessory collateral ligament. The collateral ligaments and the volar plate combine to act as a three-sided box that stabilizes the PIP joint through its arc, resisting both hyperextension and lateral forces (Figure 7-32). In extension, the volar plate is tight and the collateral ligaments are relatively lax. As the joint flexes, the collateral ligaments are tightened over the bulge of the condyles; as a result, the base of the middle phalanx is firmly seated against the proximal phalanx.

The MCP joint has less bony constraint than the PIP joint because it does not have an intercondylar groove. The PIP joint is considered a "sloppy hinge" joint with only a small amount of motion outside of the sagittal plane (flexion/extension). Far more motion exists in the MCP joint for coronal plane (radioulnar deviation) and transaxial motion (pronation/supination). Despite the lack of bony constraint, the MCP joint is dislocated less frequently than the PIP joint. Its location at the base of the fingers and its surrounding supporting structures serve to protect the joint. The overall ligamentous arrangement of the MCP joint is similar to that of the PIP joint with certain subtle differences. Radial and ulnar proper and accessory collateral ligaments prevent lateral joint movement. These ligaments connect to a volar plate ligament that forms the stabilizing element to hyperextension on the volar portion of the joint.

The main differences in the ligamentous support structures of the MCP and PIP joints are (1) the volar plate of the MCP joint is highly mobile and does not become contracted, unlike the volar plate of the PIP joint, which easily

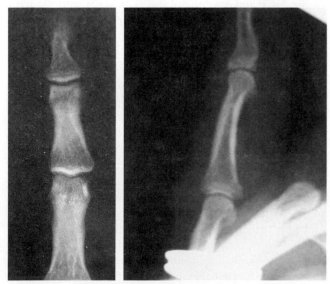

Figure 7-31

AP and lateral x-ray films of the PIP joint. The cam shape of the proximal phalanx is apparent on the lateral view. The tight, bony geometry of the joint can be appreciated on both views.

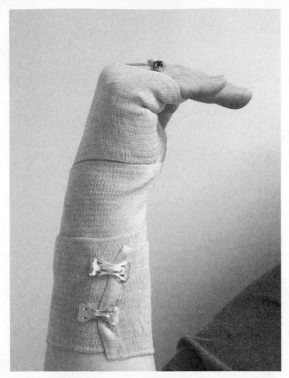

Figure 7-33

The intrinsic plus position of splinting. Positioning the IP joints in extension and flexing the MCP joints to 70° or more prevents the development of contractures.

becomes contracted over time, and (2) the distal insertion of the volar plate at the PIP joint is the weakest attachment, whereas in the MCP joint the weakest area of attachment is the proximal portion. Both of these points are clinically relevant. The first is that the position in which patients are splinted to prevent contractures is flexion of the MCP and extension of the PIP joints (Figure 7-33). The second is that dorsal dislocations of the PIP joint rarely interpose the volar plate into the joint, whereas this is more of a concern in the MCP joint.

Injury Classification

Displacement of the MCP or PIP joint can occur in any of three directions, which are referenced by the position of the distal bone: volar, lateral, or dorsal. The direction of displacement aids the classification of the injury.

Diagnosis

Radiographic analysis of the injured digit is instrumental in the diagnostic evaluation of a joint dislocation or subluxation. Standard AP and lateral views of the digit are always warranted. Because the lateral view often is the most helpful, it is important to avoid overlap of the other digits in obtaining this view. Loss of concentric reduction of the joint can be subtle and can be seen only on a perfect lateral view of the joint; therefore the clinician must not settle for inferior

x-ray films, particularly in type III injuries (Table 7-5), in which treatment might be affected by joint reduction.

It is important that the examiner first determine whether the digit is currently reduced. If the joint is anatomically located, the examiner should determine whether active range of motion in flexion and extension causes joint instability, and if so, at what point in the arc of motion. If the joint is stable throughout active range of motion, passive stability is tested. Each collateral ligament is gently stressed, and the examiner looks for pain and instability.

Medical Treatment

Volar dislocation of the PIP joint is an extremely rare injury. The mechanism usually involves rotation and axial loading of a partly flexed digit. This results in the rupture of at least one of the collateral ligaments and part of the volar plate. The middle phalanx then displaces volarly, causing the distal aspect of the proximal phalanx to move dorsally through the extensor mechanism. This most often occurs with the proximal phalanx rupturing through the interval between the central slip and one of the lateral bands. Less often, the proximal phalanx moves directly dorsally, disrupting the attachment of the central slip on the base of the middle phalanx (Figure 7-34). The latter mechanism produces loss in continuity of the extensor mechanism, which results in a closed boutonniere deformity. After reduction of the joint, the clinician must be sure to evaluate the extensor function at the PIP joint and treat any loss accordingly with extension splinting, as a closed boutonniere injury would be treated. Closed reduction of a volar dislocation can be difficult, especially when the proximal phalanx protrudes through the interval between the central slip and the lateral band. Flexion of the MCP and interphalangeal (IP) joints with the wrist held in extension to relax the extensor apparatus may allow manipulation and closed reduction; otherwise, an open reduction may be required. Once the joint has been reduced, assuming that the extensor mechanism is intact, the ligaments should fall back into anatomical alignment without the need for surgical intervention. Management therefore is aimed at regaining motion and limiting scar formation while protecting the joint from additional injury.

Lateral dislocation of the PIP joint constitutes a rupture of one of the collateral ligaments and at least a partial tearing of the volar plate. The diagnosis is confirmed with stress testing of the joint that indicates more then 20° of deformity.[58] With reduction of the joint, the collateral ligaments and volar plate return to their anatomical locations. By virtue of its bony congruency, the joint should allow for active range of motion without instability that enables the patient to begin a protected therapy program. The most common complication of this injury is not late instability, but rather arthrofibrosis with loss of joint motion. Therefore it is imperative to begin regaining motion, reducing swelling, and manipulating the scar process early to achieve the best possible outcome for the patient.

Table 7-5
Nonoperative Rehabilitation Guidelines for Dorsal Dislocation of the PIP Joint[26-28,67,68]

	Type I	Type II	Type III (Stable)	Type III (Unstable)
Pathology	Disruption of the volar plate from the middle phalanx Minor disruption of collateral ligaments Joint is stable	Avulsion of the volar plate Major disruption of collateral ligaments Bayoneting of middle phalanx dorsally on top of proximal phalanx Joint is unstable	Fragment is less than 30% to 40% of the articular surface Collateral ligament remains attached to larger shaft of middle phalanx but is not attached to small fracture fragment After reduction joint is stable	Fragment is more than 30% to 40% of the articular surface Collateral ligament remains attached to smaller shaft of the volar fracture fragment No ligament support to the dorsally displaced midphalanx With concentric reduction, PIP joint is stable in flexion
Healing Stages				
Stage I: Inflammatory stage (weeks 0 to 2)	Static IP extension splinting	Static IP extension splinting Alternative: Dorsal block splint at 30° flexion, progressed 10° weekly to week 3 to 4 Adjacent digit is included and buddy-taped Full motion within the splint is allowed	Hand-based dorsal block splint at 10° to 45° PIP flexion (usually 30°) for 4 weeks, progressed 10° of extension weekly Adjacent digit is included and buddy-taped to prevent lateral stress to the joint Buddy-taping ROM within the splint	Hand-based dorsal block splint with PIP joint in flexion to weeks 4 to 6 When x-ray films confirm a stable PIP flexion position, 5° to 10° is added to the flexion angle to protect the reduction Adjacent digit is included and buddy-taped to prevent lateral stress to the joint Buddy-taping ROM within the splint
Stage II: Fibroplasia and repair stage (weeks 2 to 6)	Buddy taping for 2 to 6 weeks to protect against hyperextension AROM Blocking exercises Edema management with Coban or a compression sleeve Soft tissue mobilization	Buddy taping for 2 to 12 weeks to protect against hyperextension and lateral stress AROM Blocking exercises to maintain ORL length and tendon gliding exercises Edema management with Coban or a compression sleeve Soft tissue mobilization Static IP extension splint is worn at night	Dorsal block splinting continues Edema management techniques should not place lateral stress on the PIP joint If Coban wrap is used, use 5 cm (2 inches) and make a sleeve that can be removed easily	Dorsal block splinting continues Edema management techniques should not place lateral stress on the PIP joint If Coban wrap is used, use 5 cm (2 inches) and make a sleeve that can be removed easily
Stage III: Remodeling and maturation stage (weeks 6 to 8+)	Strengthening as tolerated at weeks 6 to 8	Splinting for motion as tolerated at weeks 6 to 8 Strengthening as tolerated at weeks 8 to 12 Night static splint continues	Buddy taping for up to 12 weeks for protection Blocking exercises to maintain ORL length Tendon gliding exercises Edema management with Coban or a compression sleeve Soft tissue mobilization Static IP extension splint is worn at night Strengthening is begun at week 12+ as tolerated	Buddy taping for up to 12 weeks for protection Blocking exercises to maintain ORL length Tendon gliding exercises Edema management with Coban or a compression sleeve Soft tissue mobilization Static IP extension splint is worn at night Strengthening is begun at week 12+ as tolerated

PIP, Proximal interphalangeal; *IP,* interphalangeal; *ROM,* range of motion; *AROM,* active range of motion; *ORL,* oblique retinacular ligament.

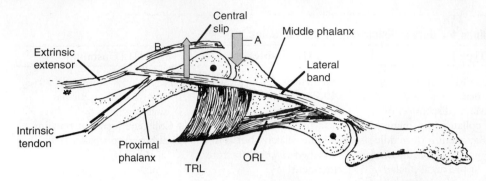

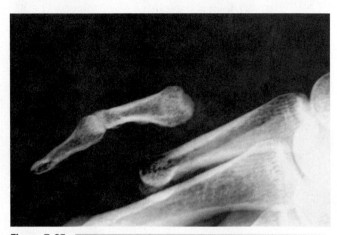

Figure 7-34
Volar PIP dislocation. *A,* Volar translation of the middle phalanx. *B,* Proximal phalanx gets caught between the central slip and the lateral band, which usually is not disrupted from the middle phalanx as depicted here. *TRL,* transverse retinacular ligament; *ORL,* oblique retinacular ligament. (From Coons MS, Green SM: Boutonniere deformity, *Hand Clin* 11 (3):389, 1995.)

Dorsal dislocation is the most common of the three types of PIP injuries and occurs when a longitudinal force coupled with some extension is applied to the digit. Basketballs and footballs are frequently the culprits in this injury mechanism. The distal aspect of the volar plate is disrupted, and the interval between the accessory and proper collateral ligaments is torn, allowing the middle phalanx to ride dorsally up on the proximal phalanx. The injury is further classified into three categories that depict increasing energy and further damage and instability of the joint.

In a type I injury (see Table 7-5), hyperextension results in the avulsion of the volar plate from the middle phalanx and a minor longitudinal split in the collateral ligaments. In severe cases, the middle phalanx may be locked in 70° of hyperextension.

A type II injury involves an avulsion of the volar plate plus a major bilateral collateral ligament tear that allows complete bayoneting (overriding) of the middle phalanx on top of the proximal phalanx (Figure 7-35).

When the longitudinal force is great enough to produce shearing of the volar rim of the middle phalanx, a fracture-dislocation occurs. This is a type III injury, which differs from the previous two patterns. As the middle phalanx begins to ride dorsally over the proximal phalanx, the volar rim is fractured off. This type III injury is subclassified simply into two types, stable (type IIIA) and unstable (type IIIB) (Figure 7-36). In a stable dorsal fracture-dislocation of the PIP joint, the fracture fragment is small (i.e., less then 30% to 40% of the articular contour of the joint). In this case,

Figure 7-35
Lateral x-ray film of a type II dorsal dislocation of the PIP joint, showing complete overlapping of the bones. This often is an open injury.

the collateral ligaments are not attached to the small fracture fragment but remain attached to the larger shaft fracture. An unstable dorsal fracture-dislocation involves a disruption of greater then 40% of the joint. In this instance, the collateral ligaments remain with the volar fracture segment. The dorsally displaced shaft no longer has any soft tissue constraint or bony buttress to contain the joint (Figure 7-37).

Type I and type II dorsal PIP dislocations are stable injuries (type II requires reduction). The patient may be splinted for comfort for up to 2 weeks and must take care to avoid excessive flexion of the IP joints, which could promote the

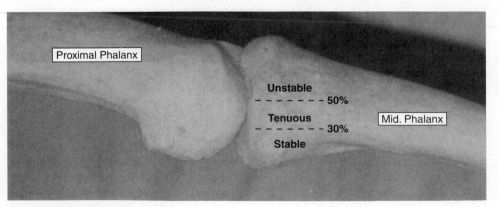

Figure 7-36
The level of the fracture determines the stability of the joint. A large fracture fragment causes a loss of volar support at the PIP joint. With a large volar fragment of bone, the insertions of the collateral ligaments are still attached to the fragment. This leaves the shaft of the middle phalanx without the support of the collateral ligaments or the volar bone at the PIP joint.

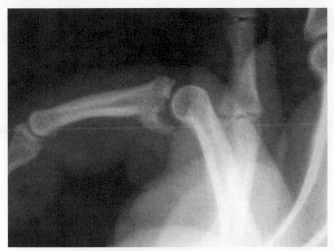

Figure 7-37
Clinical example of a type IIIB fracture-dislocation of the PIP joint. In this case, because the fracture fragment is large, the joint no longer remains congruently aligned. This can be appreciated by the V shape formed by the intact middle phalanx and the proximal phalangeal head.

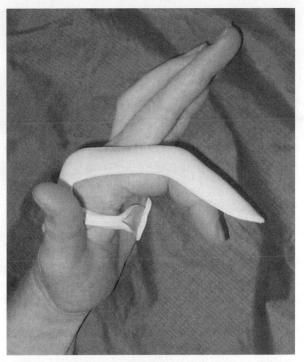

Figure 7-38
A dorsal block splint can be used to allow motion within the stable range for types IIIA and IIIB dorsal fracture-dislocations at the PIP joint.

formation of a flexion contracture. ROM with the affected finger buddy-taped is then begun, and therapy is initiated to control edema, reduce scar formation, and gain motion.

Type III dorsal dislocations with fracture of the volar rim of the middle phalanx are higher energy injuries. In the stable subtype (type IIIA), the joint is congruent on a lateral x-ray film. The patient is treated with 2 to 3 weeks of immobilization. If a small amount of joint incongruence is present, the joint can be flexed slightly to obtain alignment in a dorsal block splint. ROM with the finger buddy-taped for protection is begun after the period of immobilization.

Multiple treatment options are available for type III dorsal dislocations with a large, unstable fracture fragment (type IIIB). These include a dorsal block splint, ORIF, a dynamic external fixator, volar plate arthroplasty, fusion, silicone arthroplasty, and reconstruction of the joint using bone obtained from the patient's joint between the hamate and the metacarpal.

A dorsal block splint is used if the dislocated joint can be concentrically reduced by some degree of flexion. Beyond this, the joint remains stable in any amount of further flexion. The clinician confirms the position of the stable concentric reduction and creates a splint adding 5° to 10° of further flexion for safety. Extension to this point is allowed with full active flexion. Each week, the splint is adjusted to increase the extension 10°, and x-ray films are taken to confirm that the reduction is maintained (Figure 7-38).

Open reduction and internal fixation is a technically demanding procedure, because the bone fragment to be fixed is quite small and frequently more comminuted than it appears on x-ray films. However, if the fragment can be fixed with a screw, rehabilitation can be started much sooner, and the best results are obtained (Figure 7-39).

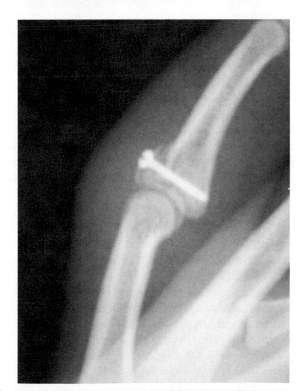

Figure 7-39
In this rare case of a volar fracture-dislocation, the insertion of the central slip has avulsed, which allows the middle phalanx to sublux on the proximal phalanx. Screw fixation allows concentric joint reduction and immediate return to motion.

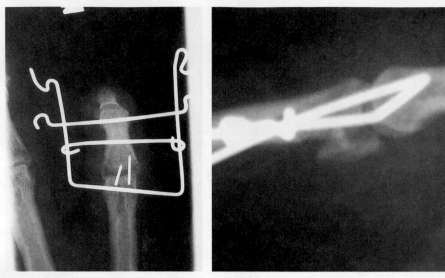

Figure 7-40

Ligamentotaxis can be used to regain joint congruency and allow for motion. This prevents joint subluxation and allows fractures of the middle phalanx to remodel using the intact proximal phalanx as a template during the healing process.

Dynamic external fixation uses forces to counteract those that displace the interarticular fracture.[59] By attaching rubber bands or other dynamic traction forces to pins implanted temporarily into the bone, the joint is reduced, yet allowed to move through an arc of motion to prevent contracture and to facilitate healing of the cartilage (Figure 7-40).[60] Therapy is provided throughout the immediate postoperative period to prevent tendon adherence and joint contracture. The device usually is removed 4 to 6 weeks later, when the joint is stable enough to move without fear of late dislocation.

Volar plate arthroplasty is a technique for inserting the torn distal end of the volar plate into the fractured base of the middle phalanx to re-establish ligamentous attachment to the base of the middle phalanx. The volar plate serves to prevent hyperextension of the joint and to provide a smooth contour for the joint for motion; also, over time, it has been shown to metaplase (convert) into a more normal-appearing bony joint surface.[61] In the immediate postoperative period, the joint must be protected from extension, which can tear the repair apart. To regain motion, AROM of extension can be attempted at 4 weeks and PROM of extension at 6 weeks (Figure 7-41).

Silicone arthroplasty is a viable primary option for an older patient with an already arthritic PIP joint who has sustained an unstable fracture-dislocation of the PIP joint.[62] In this case, rehabilitation, return to function, and pain issues are greatly simplified by a primary arthroplasty of the joint (Figure 7-42). The caveat with this procedure is the index finger; in this digit, forces from lateral pinch with the thumb are too great for a silicone arthroplasty, which will fail. In this unique situation, a primary fusion of the PIP joint might be the better course, if the patient's

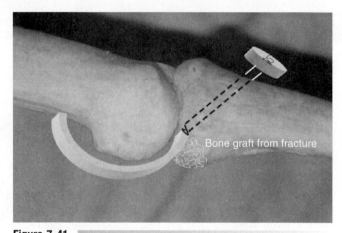

Bone graft from fracture

Figure 7-41

Representation of a volar plate arthroplasty. In this operation the volar plate is detached distally and reinserted into the fracture site to re-establish the smooth contour of the joint. The fibrocartilage of the volar plate metaplases into bone, re-establishing a bony joint with a concentric rim for the phalangeal head.

MCP function is adequate. Therapy proceeds as for a primary arthroplasty performed from the volar approach (the extensor mechanism is spared, but the collateral ligaments have been resected or in this case torn).[62]

Collateral Ligament Injuries of the Thumb

General Considerations

Injury to the ligaments of the thumb occur most commonly at the MCP joint in ball-handling sports and, even more frequently, from falls during skiing; this injury therefore generally is called *skier's thumb*. In the 18th and 19th centuries, tearing of the ulnar collateral ligament was an

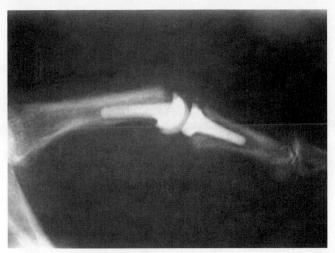

Figure 7-42
Replacement arthroplasty. Newer materials recently have become available that may outlast silicone, particularly for higher demand patients. (Courtesy B.M. Leslie, MD.)

attritional injury attributed to the work of Scottish game wardens and was known as *gamekeeper's thumb*. This often is now a single radial deviation event that occurs with ball contact or a fall with a ski pole in the hand that allows

the thumb to strike directly into the ground with the weight of the body forcing the thumb radially. Radial collateral ligament injuries occur less regularly, usually in ball-handling sports, and are easily overlooked. Either type of injury, if severe, causes significant bruising and swelling. The patient also may have considerable pain that lasts several days. The pain usually resolves, as does the swelling, with local anti-inflammatory treatment. The rapid resolution of swelling and pain has lead many patients to believe that this is a trivial injury that does not require treatment. Unfortunately, this belief can lead to poor outcomes, including chronic laxity, pain, and the onset of MCP joint arthrosis (Figure 7-43).[57]

Anatomy

The MCP joint of the thumb is primarily designed to allow flexion and extension. However, some degree of abduction and adduction, as well as rotation, can occur. The shape of the joint is condyloid, with the proximal phalanx behaving like an inverted golf tee sitting on a golf ball (i.e., the metacarpal head). Some people have far more round metacarpal heads than others; therefore the amount of flexion and extension at the joint varies considerably from patient to patient. Radial and ulnar deviation (abduction/adduction)

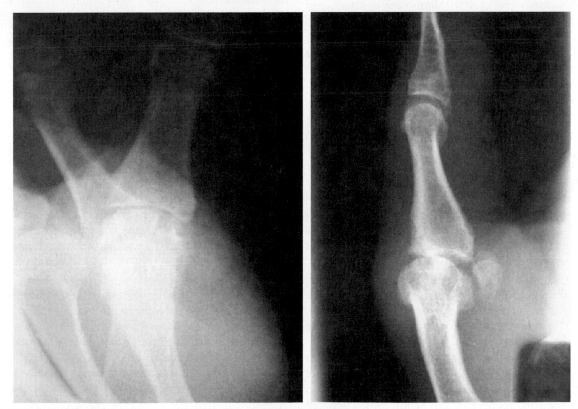

Figure 7-43
AP and lateral x-ray films showing chronic laxity of the ulnar collateral ligament of the thumb at the MCP joint. Note the radial deviation of the thumb at rest, as well as the volar subluxation of the joint. These factors, in addition to some rotational malalignment, have created the incongruence that has caused joint destruction.

and rotation are limited by both static and dynamic constraints. The primary stabilizers to ulnar and radial motion are the proper collateral ligaments, which originate at the lateral condyles of the metacarpal head dorsal to the axis of rotation. These ligaments pass obliquely and distally to insert on the proximal phalanx volar (anterior) to the axis of rotation. Along the volar aspect of the proper collateral ligament is a shroudlike attachment, the accessory collateral ligament, that connects the proper collateral ligament to the volar plate of the joint. This arrangement creates a three-sided box configuration between the two collateral ligaments and the intervening volar plate, similar to that seen at the PIP joint in the digits (see Figure 7-32). Dynamic support of the joint is created by the adductor pollicis muscle, which inserts into the ulnar sesamoid at the base of the MCP joint, and the flexor pollicis brevis and abductor pollicis brevis muscles, which insert onto the radial sesamoid bone at the base of the MCP joint. These muscles are intrinsic to the thumb, and they flex the MCP joint and extend the IP joint by way of attachments to the extensor mechanism. They also create dynamic stability to radial and ulnar stress, respectively.

Injury Classification

Collateral ligament injuries of the thumb can be classified in the same way as ligamentous injuries to other parts of the body, such as the ankle and knee. Grade I injuries consist of stretching of the collagen fibers within the ligaments without macroscopic fiber tearing. Grade II injuries involve further deformity of the collagen fibers, with tearing of some portion of the ligament, but overall continuity remains. Grade III injuries are the most severe and show macroscopic disruption of the collagen fibers that results in discontinuity of the ligament.

In addition to the tearing of the collateral ligament, the dorsal capsule and the volar plate on the same side as the ligament injury usually are also partly disrupted. Furthermore, the ligament may avulse a portion of the proximal phalanx at its insertion. The fracture fragment usually does not represent a large segment of the articular surface, but on rare occasions it may be as large as 10% of the joint. The clinician cannot assume that the ligament is attached to the small fragment of bone. The presence of a nondisplaced small fracture fragment does not exclude the possibility of a displaced ligament; studies have shown that the two can be present simultaneously.[63]

When the injury involves the ulnar collateral ligament (UCL) at the MCP of the thumb, a unique situation can arise with grade III injuries. As was first described in 1962, the adductor aponeurosis can be interposed between the distal end of the ligament and the proximal phalanx holding it in a displaced position.[64] This is known as a *Stener lesion,* and it has important implications in both diagnosis and treatment (Figure 7-44).

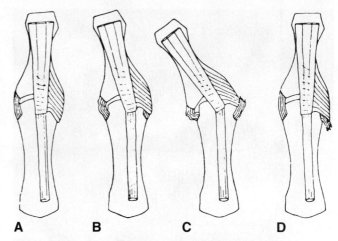

Figure 7-44

Stener lesion: Diagram of the displacement of the ulnar collateral ligament of the thumb metacarpophalangeal joint. **A**, Normal relationship, with the ulnar ligament covered by the adductor aponeurosis. **B**, With slight radial angulation, the proximal margin of the aponeurosis slides distally, leaving part of the ligament uncovered. **C**, With major radial angulation, the ulnar ligament ruptures at its distal insertion. With this degree of angulation, the aponeurosis has displaced distal to the rupture, allowing the ligament to escape from beneath it. **D**, As the joint is realigned, the proximal edge of the adductor aponeurosis sweeps the free end of the ligament proximally and farther from its insertion. This is the Stener lesion. Unless surgically restored, the ulnar ligament will not heal properly and will be unstable to lateral stress. (From Stener B: Displacement of the ruptured ulnar collateral ligament of the metacarpo-phalangeal joint of the thumb: a clinical and anatomical study. In Green DP, Hotchkiss RN, Pederson WC, Wolfe SW, editors: *Green's operative hand surgery,* ed 5, Philadelphia, 2005, Churchill Livingstone.)

Diagnosis

Diagnosis begins with the history and careful attention to the mechanism of injury. The amount of swelling and ecchymosis can alert the examiner to the degree of damage to the soft tissues. If the injury is more chronic and the swelling has receded, the resting posture of the thumb (i.e., both its angle and its rotational alignment) provides clues to the amount of ligamentous disruption.

With a grade III UCL injury, the thumb rests in radial deviation. Also, because of the loss of the ulnar ligament and dorsal capsular support, the thumb tends to rotate around the intact radial collateral ligament in a supinated position. In a complete tear of the radial collateral ligament, the opposite is found.

Tenderness to palpation is noted over the torn ligament, and swelling and induration are present at the site of the ligament injury. With a Stener lesion, a palpable hard mass is felt that is asymmetrical to the patient's other thumb; this is the displaced distal end of the UCL (Figure 7-45). If x-ray films have confirmed that no fracture is present, gentle stress testing should be performed to assess ligament competence. It is imperative to differentiate a grade III injury from either a grade I or grade II tear. A grade III

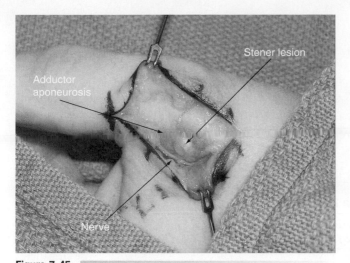

Figure 7-45

Surgical view of a Stener lesion. The ulnar collateral ligament has been torn from its distal insertion on the proximal phalanx. It now is reflected back on itself, resting superficial and proximal to the adductor aponeurosis (it normally is located deep to this structure). Note the nerve encountered during this surgical approach; injury to or irritation of this nerve can result in postoperative symptoms.

injury shows 30° more instability to radial stress testing than is seen on the patient's opposite side. In addition, usually no firm end point is noted in the stress test[65,66] Testing should be done with the joint in full extension and in 30° flexion. Clinicians should practice on normal thumbs to get an idea of what a normal end feel is like. Patients often contract the muscles to guard against the pain of stress testing. The clinician must be alert for this, and if the patient is too uncomfortable to reliably relax for the examination, a local anesthetic injected around the torn ligament usually suffices to allow stress testing. Stress x-ray films have little use in the diagnostic process. Alternative imaging studies, including ultrasound and magnetic resonance imaging (MRI), can be performed to delineate the position of the ligament.

Medical Treatment

Differentiation of partial and complete ligament tears is critical. With grade I and II injuries, the ligament remains in its anatomically correct position. In this situation, protection of the ligament with a thumb spica cast for 4 to 6 weeks, followed by a return to motion rehabilitation program, generally leads to excellent results. In the case of complete ligament disruption, the question arises whether the ligament is anatomically positioned and will heal under conservative management. Clearly, if a Stener lesion can be felt, the answer is no, and some clinicians believe that it is best to surgically fix all grade III injuries so that a displaced ligament is never missed.

In a ligament tear, the torn tissue generally avulses from the bone and can be directly repaired with sutures through drill holes or with the use of small bone anchors. The volar plate and dorsal capsule are repaired at the same time. A pin is placed across the MCP joint to hold it in a flexed and slightly overcorrected position to allow the ligament to heal without tension for the first 3 weeks. The pin is easily removed in the outpatient setting, and 6 weeks of casting is completed before therapy commences.

If a fracture fragment is associated with the avulsion, the surgeon may choose to discard the fragment and repair the ligament into the cancellous bony bed. However, if the fracture fragment represents a substantial portion of the joint surface, direct repair of the bone with small screw fixation is preferable. It is critical that the tiny sensory nerve branches be protected in the dissection, because these can be a source of debilitating pain postoperatively. Even under the gentlest of circumstances, therapists frequently must spend time desensitizing these nerves from the traction endured during the procedure.

Rehabilitation of Proximal Interphalangeal Joint Injuries and Ulnar Collateral Ligament Injuries of the Thumb

Proximal Interphalangeal Joint Injuries

Both the tight articular congruency of the PIP joint and the soft tissue constraints that surround it contribute to the joint's stability. The soft tissue stabilizers include the joint capsule, the proper and accessory collateral ligaments, the volar plate, and the flexor and extensor tendons.

The rehabilitation treatment strategy takes into consideration the direction and type of fracture-dislocation, which soft tissue structures are implicated, and whether the joint is stable or unstable. Patients often can assist the clinician by describing the mechanism of injury and PIP joint positioning immediately after injury. The direction of the dislocation is based on where the middle phalanx sits in relation to the proximal phalanx.

Rehabilitation strategies are geared toward maintaining joint stability while mobilizing the soft tissues. Restoring and optimizing soft tissue gliding and mechanics are prime considerations. The goal of treatment is to regain and preserve soft tissue and joint mobility while preventing the development of adhesions, joint flexion contractures, deformities, and loss of function. Progression of the treatment program depends on the healing stages of both the soft tissue and bony structures; edema management, soft tissue mobilization, joint mobilization, and splinting are key elements of the program. Strengthening is initiated only when the tissues have fully healed, no instability is present, and the program does not provoke pain. Residual enlargement and stiffness of the PIP joint is common. The clinician should explain to the patient that management of these injuries can take 6 months to 1 year.

Determinants of Treatment Progression

- Tissue healing (bone and soft tissue)
- Amount of edema
- Degree of stability
- Soft tissue mobility
- Joint mobility
- Pain

Dorsal Dislocation. Rehabilitation guidelines for dorsal dislocations are based on the stability of the joint, the classification type, and nonoperative and postoperative treatment. Soft tissues injured in dorsal dislocations include the collateral ligaments and the volar plate (Table 7-6).

Lateral Dislocation. Rehabilitation for lateral dislocations is based on the degree of injury to the collateral ligaments and volar plate. The Bowers classification system divides soft issue injuries into three grades.[68]

Table 7-6
Postoperative Rehabilitation Guidelines for Dislocation of the PIP Joint[26-28,67,68,69]

	Open Reduction and Internal Fixation	External Fixation/Traction Splinting (Weeks 0 to 6)	Volar Plate Arthroplasty
Special considerations	Hand therapy may or may not be initiated until weeks 4 to 6, depending on the stability of the reduction	A risk for infection exists with the use of external fixators. A variety of devices can be used for external fixation: • Commercially available finger-based hinge devices • Surgeon-fabricated finger-based fixators using K-wires and elastics • Traction splinting fabricated by a hand therapist. Designs vary. Forearm based. Finger is attached to an outrigger providing consistent traction through a safe arc of motion Positioning in the splint varies, depending on the injury classification or the direction of dislocation and implicated structures[70]	The torn distal end of the volar plate is inserted into the fractured base of the middle phalanx to re-establish ligamentous attachment to the base of the middle phalanx
Healing Stages			
Stage I: Inflammatory stage (weeks 0 to 2)	Immobilization is achieved in a forearm-based dorsal protective cast or splint that includes the full hand. Gentle AROM with buddy-taping may be initiated only if the reduction is stable. Positioning in the splint may vary, depending on the implicated structures and surgical procedure	*External fixation:* • Immobilization for 3 days • At days 3 to 5, AROM is initiated within a safe range determined by the physician • Static protective splinting at night if the device does not lock • Resting PIP position is determined by the physician *Traction splinting:* • Initiation of motion varies from day 1 to week 3, depending on the stability of the fracture and the implicated structures • AROM of the PIP joint within a safe arc of motion is begun, and DIP blocking exercises are initiated • Dorsal block splint is worn, resting the finger in MCP flexion, the PIP joint in the safe amount of extension as determined by the physician, and the DIP joint in extension, until AROM is initiated and also at night until week 6 • Patient is taught to monitor for signs of infection and to modify activities	Immobilization in a cast for 2 to 4 weeks

Table 7-6
Postoperative Rehabilitation Guidelines for Dislocation of the PIP Joint[26-28,67,68,69]

	Open Reduction and Internal Fixation	External Fixation/Traction Splinting (Weeks 0 to 6)	Volar Plate Arthroplasty
Stage II: Fibroplasia and repair stage (weeks 2 to 6)	Gentle AROM with the finger buddy-taped to the adjacent finger Edema management techniques should not put lateral stress on the PIP joint If Coban wrap is used, use 5 cm (2 inches) and make a sleeve that can be removed easily Gentle tendon gliding exercises	*External fixation:* • AROM within the device continues • Blocking initiated with emphasis on DIP flexion *Traction splinting:* • AROM of the PIP joint within a safe arc of motion and DIP blocking exercises are begun or continued	Hand-based dorsal block splint with the PIP joint in 30° flexion is fabricated at weeks 2 to 4, and extension is increased 10° per week *Or* the digit may remain immobilized, depending on the stability of the repair The finger is buddy-taped to the adjacent digit Edema management techniques should not put lateral stress on the PIP joint If Coban wrap is used, use 5 cm (2 inches) and make a sleeve that can be removed easily Blocking, full tendon gliding, and stretching are initiated at weeks 4 to 6
Stage III: Remodeling and maturation stage (weeks 6 to 8+)	PROM Stretching Blocking and tendon gliding Splinting for motion Functional progression Gentle strengthening at week 8, respecting tissue tolerance and pain	Device is removed Edema management Full tendon gliding and blocking exercises are initiated The finger is buddy-taped to the adjacent digit to protect soft tissue healing Strengthening begins at weeks 8 to 12, respecting tissue tolerance and pain Splinting for motion Functional progression	Buddy taping continues. Splinting for motion is done, respecting tissue tolerance Strengthening begins at weeks 8 to 12, respecting tissue tolerance and pain Functional progression

AROM, Active range of motion; *PIP,* proximal interphalangeal; *DIP,* distal interphalangeal; *MCP,* metacarpophalangeal; *PROM,* passive range of motion.

Grade I injuries, which involve a sprain to the collateral ligaments without instability, require immobilization up to 1 week in a finger-based extension splint to reduce inflammation. After immobilization, the affected finger is buddy-taped to the adjacent digit for 2 to 4 weeks, depending on the degree of pain and the patient's activity level. Buddy taping provides stability and prevents lateral stresses to the finger. AROM and blocking exercises are also initiated at 2 to 4 weeks.

In grade II injuries, the volar plate remains attached but may be injured, and the collateral ligaments are completely disrupted. Treatment varies, depending on the amount of disruption to the volar plate. Treatment consists of immobilization for 1 to 2 weeks with the finger splinted in 10° to 20° of PIP flexion for pain tolerance. Buddy taping for 8 to 12 weeks follows, and AROM and blocking exercises are initiated at 2 to 4 weeks. If greater disruption of the volar plate is present and the joint is unstable, an extension block splint is fabricated at 0° to 45° flexion. The degree of flexion depends on the stability of the joint, which is determined by imaging. The extension block splint is advanced into extension by 10° per week, and joint reduction should

be confirmed by x-ray films. Active flexion and extension into the block is completed after an initial week of immobilization. After removal of the extension block splint, the finger is buddy-taped for 8 to 12 weeks to protect the joint.

Grade III injuries are associated with complete disruption of both the collateral ligaments and volar plate; these injuries may require surgical intervention for stabilization. Postoperative rehabilitation is similar to that for grade II injuries (see Table 7-6).

Volar (Anterior) Dislocation. Volar dislocation injuries are rare. The soft tissue structures injured in volar dislocations are the collateral ligaments, the volar plate, and the extensor mechanism, including the central slip and lateral bands. Bony involvement can include middle phalanx dorsal lip fractures at the insertion of the central slip.[28,71]

Initial rehabilitation for nonoperative volar dislocations consists of immobilization in a finger-based extension splint with the DIP free for 6 to 8 weeks to protect soft tissue healing (Figure 7-46). AROM of the DIP maintains soft tissue gliding and appropriate positioning of the lateral bands dorsal to the joint axis. The PIP joint is then mobilized at 6 to

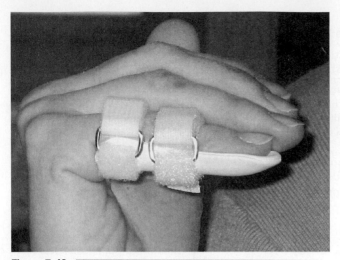

Figure 7-46
Static PIP and DIP extension splint.

8 weeks. Buddy taping is used for 6 to 12 weeks to protect the joint.[28] A PIP extension splint can be worn at night to prevent periarticular soft tissue shortening and can be used for up to 3 to 6 months. An extension block splint with the MCP joints in flexion can help the patient perform blocking exercises to promote pull through and glide of the extensor mechanism. If the collateral ligaments and volar plate have been completely disrupted, surgical intervention is necessary.

Ulnar Collateral Ligament Injuries of the Thumb

The rehabilitation strategy for the thumb is based on the degree of injury to the ulnar collateral ligament and/or the volar plate, which renders the joint stable or unstable. The degree of ligamentous injury has been classified into three grades. Rehabilitation strategies are geared toward maintaining thumb MCP joint stability while mobilizing the soft tissues to prevent the development of adhesions, flexion contractures, and loss of function. Progression of the therapy program depends on the stages of healing. Emphasis is placed on avoiding lateral and radial stresses to the MCP joint in the initial stages of healing. Terminal thumb abduction should be avoided initially. Force transmission to the MCP joint through pinching and pulling activities, in which the thumb tip is engaged, should also be modified and/or avoided to reduce demands on the healing tissues.

Consideration should be given to protecting the IP joint from hyperextension, which can place a stress on the MCP joint. Edema management, soft tissue mobilization, joint mobilization, and splinting are key elements of the program. Care should be taken with cast or splint designs to protect the ligament while preventing a thumb adduction contracture. Strengthening of the thumb is initiated only when the soft tissues have fully healed, no instability is present and the program does not provoke pain and/or an inflammatory response. Residual problems include stiffness at both the MCP and IP joints (Table 7-7).

Tendon Injuries of the Hand

Flexor Tendon Injury

General Considerations

Tendon injuries are common, although the exact incidence is unknown. Patients with a tendon injury face months of profound physical, emotional, and socioeconomic hurdles. These hurdles arise under the best of circumstances, such as when the injury is recognized early and treated appropriately. Unfortunately, many pitfalls can lead to a poor result after a tendon injury, with profound repercussions that can affect the patient's ability to return to gainful employment and to use the hand for activities of daily living.

Tendon injuries often are the result of a sharp instrument coming into contact with the digit, hand, or wrist. This can occur accidentally at work or in the home, or sometimes deliberately, as in an altercation or self-inflicted wound. In the case of an accidental injury, the nondominant hand frequently is hurt because the individual is wielding the knife in the dominant hand when the accident occurs. The opposite is true for a person who uses the hand to protect himself or herself from an assailant; these individuals reflexively use the dominant limb to ward off the knife assault.

Spontaneous tendon ruptures can occur without any preceding trauma. The most common cause of this type of tendon injury is rheumatoid arthritis, although other conditions, such as chronic tenosynovitis, partial flexor tendon lacerations, and attrition of the flexor tendons over bony prominences or hardware from previous surgery, may result in the same type of atraumatic tendon rupture (Figure 7-47). Timely recognition, diagnosis, and direct repair are important to increase the chances of restoring function.

Avulsion injuries to the flexor tendons usually are caused by a closed traumatic injury to the finger. These tend to occur during athletic events, and unfortunately, the diagnosis often is missed initially, which can lead to permanent disability. Avulsion injuries of the flexor digitorum superficialis tendons are rare compared to disruption of the flexor digitorum profundus tendons.

The ability of a tendon to heal and the degree to which adhesions develop in the area of the healing tendon depend on factors that relate to the injury and the surgical repair. The goal of tendon repair is based on establishing a strong enough repair to enable the patient to begin early protected motion, while achieving the repair without inducing excessive scarring. Crush injuries and aggressive handling of the tendon sheath and tendon during surgery increase the chances of scar formation. Tendon ischemia, tendon immobilization, and gapping at the repair site also contribute to the formation of excursion-restricting adhesions.

After tendon repair, healing progresses through several stages. The first stage involves an inflammatory response.

Table 7-7
Rehabilitation of Ulnar Collateral Ligament Injuries of the Thumb[26,54,63-65]

	Grade I	Grade II	Grade III
Description	Ligamentous stretching without tearing	Ligamentous tearing without complete disruption	Ligamentous disruption Surgical repair or reconstruction
Healing Stages			
Stage I: Inflammatory stage (weeks 0 to 2)	Splinting at all times for weeks 0 to 4 Splint design may vary, depending on the surgeon's preference: • Hand-based short opponens splint with MCP joint in slight flexion, with or without a dorsal hood extending to the thumb tip that allows IP flexion while restricting hyperextension • Thumb spica cast or splint	Weeks 0 to 4: Thumb spica cast or splint at all times; IP joint may be included or free	Weeks 0 to 6: Casting
Stage II: Fibroplasia and repair stage (weeks 2 to 6)	Splint immobilization continues until weeks 4 to 6 Functional use is progressed, with modifications to avoid heavy pinching, pulling, and grasping	Weeks 4 to 6: Thumb spica cast is reduced to a hand-based short opponens splint that leaves the IP joint free; a dorsal hood prevents hyperextension of the IP joint. The splint must be worn between exercises. Splinting time frames vary, depending on stability and pain at the MCP joint; the splint can be worn up to week 12 for protection Week 6: • AROM • Soft tissue mobilization • Edema management	Weeks 0 to 6: Casting
Stage III: Remodeling and maturation stage (weeks 6 to 8+)	Week 8: Strengthening to tissue tolerance, focusing on the abductor pollicis brevis, flexor pollicis brevis, and adductor pollicis brevis	Splinting continues Blocking exercises for tendon gliding Light functional tasks Joint mobilization, respecting tissue tolerance Strengthening begins at week 12, respecting tissue tolerance and pain Full pinching and pulling activities at weeks 12 to 16, as tolerated	Progression to hand-based thumb splint with IP joint free; worn between exercises Splint worn up to weeks 8 to 12 Straight plane flexion and extension AROM Radial stress (terminal abduction) to the MCP joint must be avoided. Soft tissue and scar mobilization Edema management Blocking for tendon excursion. Weeks 8+: Unrestricted AROM, PROM, gentle stretching Strengthening and return to full pinching and pulling activities at weeks 12 to 16

MCP, Metacarpophalangeal; *IP,* interphalangeal; *AROM,* active range of motion; *PROM,* passive range of motion.

During this stage, the strength of the tendon repair relies primarily on the strength of the sutures in place, with the fibrin clot (between the tendon ends) offering a small contribution. The second stage is the fibroblast-producing stage. The strength of the tendon increases rapidly during this stage as granulation tissue forms at the site of the repair. The final stage is the remodeling stage, in which collagen synthesis continues and the repaired tendon becomes progressively stronger. This restorative progression is important, because it is the physiological basis for the protected therapy program, which prevents the formation of adhesions while caring for the still mending tendon.[72,73]

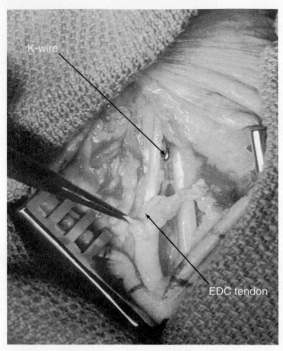

Figure 7-47

Rupture of a tendon from attrition over prominent hardware. The EDC to the index finger ruptured over the K-wire when the wire backed out of the bone. Side-to-side tendon repair produced an excellent result.

Anatomy

The tendons for the flexor muscle groups insert distally on the metacarpals and phalanges to provide wrist and finger flexion. The forearm flexor muscles that power these tendons originate on the medial aspect of the elbow and are divided into three anatomical layers. The superficial layer of muscles consists of the pronator teres, flexor carpi radialis, flexor carpi ulnaris, and palmaris longus. The intermediate muscle group is the flexor digitorum superficialis. The deep muscle group consists of the flexor digitorum profundus and the flexor pollicis longus (FPL). The FDS tendons arise from individual muscle bundles and act independently to provide flexion of the PIP joints. This is in contrast to the FDP tendons, which arise from a common muscle, simultaneously flexing the DIP joints of the four digits. Each digit therefore has two flexors that originate in the forearm, and the thumb has one. Every one of these nine tendons travels through the forearm and enters the wrist through the carpal tunnel beneath the transverse carpal ligament. The tendons continue in the palmar aspect of the hand, with the FDS tendons traveling anterior to the FDP tendons. They remain in this configuration until they enter their individual digits, through the digital sheath at the A1 pulley (Figure 7-48). At this point, the FDS tendon divides into two slips, traveling dorsally and on either side of the FDP tendon. The split FDS fibers rejoin, now dorsal to the FDP tendon, and insert along the proximal half of the middle phalanx, functioning to flex the PIP joint.

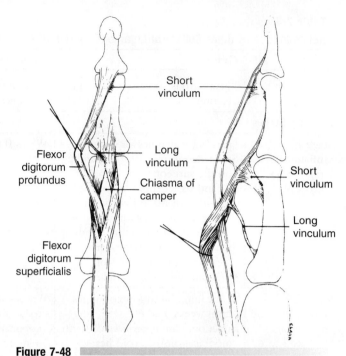

Figure 7-48

Anatomy of the flexor tendon. (From Schneider LH: *Flexor tendon injuries,* Boston, 1985, Little, Brown.)

The FDP tendons pass through the FDS bifurcation (Camper's chiasm) and insert on the distal phalanx, providing flexion of the DIP joint (Figure 7-49).

In the digits, the flexor tendons are enclosed in synovial sheaths. These sheaths provide a smooth synovial lining for tendon nutrition and to reduce the work of gliding. An intricate pulley system exists to create an efficient flexor mechanism by maintaining the tendons in close contact with the phalanges and preventing bow-stringing of the tendons with the flexion motion. The A1, A3, and A5 annular pulleys arise from the volar plates of the MCP joints, the PIP joints, and the DIP joints, respectively. The A2 and A4 pulleys are functionally the most important pulleys, arising from the periosteum of the proximal half of the proximal phalanx (A2) and the midportion of the middle phalanx (A4). Also present are the thinner, less substantial cruciate pulleys: C1 (between A2 and A3), C2 (between A3 and A4) and C3 (between A4 and A5). These pulleys allow the annular pulleys to approximate each other during flexion (see Figure 7-49).

Injury or disruption of these tendons anywhere along their course causes functional impairment of the distally involved joints.

Injury Classification

Flexor tendon injuries have been divided into zones over the volar aspect of the hand and wrist, based on differing anatomical characteristics. Zone I, the most distal zone, includes the area distal to the insertion of the FDS on the

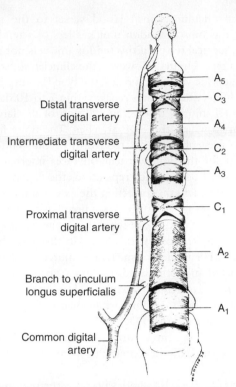

Figure 7-49
Pulley system of the finger, which includes five annular pulleys (A1-A5) and three cruciform pulleys (C1-C3). (From Schneider LH: *Flexor tendon injuries,* Boston, 1985, Little, Brown.)

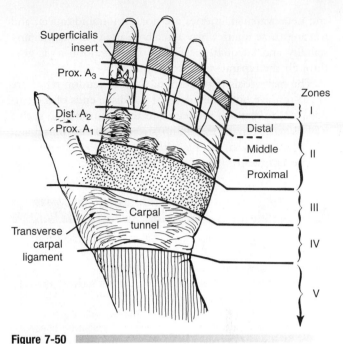

Figure 7-50
Flexor tendon zones. (From Chase RA: *Atlas of hand surgery,* vol 2, Philadelphia, 1984, WB Saunders.)

proximal phalanx. Zone II encompasses the area from the proximal border of zone I to the level of the distal palmar crease, which is the beginning of the flexor tendon sheath. This zone has been known historically as "no man's land" because of the complexity of the flexor tendons and fibro-osseous sheath anatomy in this region, which has led to poorer outcomes after tendon repairs. Zone III represents the area between the start of the fibro-osseous tendon sheath and the distal edge of the transverse carpal ligament. This also happens to be the area of the lumbrical muscle origin. The carpal tunnel region is zone IV, and proximal to the transverse carpal ligament is zone V. The thumb has its own zone distribution; zone T-I is distal to the DIP joint, zone T-II is between the MCP and IP joints, and zone T-III is proximal to the MCP volar flexion crease (Figure 7-50).

Diagnosis

A complete examination of the involved extremity must be performed to evaluate the extent of injury. In the inspection of the upper extremity, the examiner should note the posture of the hand. The presence of an abnormal cascade because of a digit resting in extension and an inability to perform specific flexion motor tests should alert the examiner to possible tendon injury. Specifically, when examining for a potential FDS injury, the examiner must hold the other digits in extension at the tips to prevent flexion of

the injured digit through its possibly intact FDP tendon. Likewise, when examining for a FDP injury, the examiner must allow the patient to flex all the fingertips freely, because the muscle for DIP flexion is not independent. Sensory evaluation can identify injuries to the digital nerves, which may accompany trauma to a flexor tendon. It is important that the clinician recognize concomitant nerve injuries, because nerve and vascular injuries affect the approach to operative management.

Medical Treatment

Before surgery is performed on an injured flexor tendon, relevant factors such as timing, prognosis, and concomitant injuries must be considered, because they may affect the approach to surgical management. In the past, a flexor tendon injury was considered a surgical emergency. This is no longer true, given current evidence that delayed primary flexor tendon repair leads to results that are equal to or better than those obtained with immediate repair.[74] With increasing delay, however, repair of the tendons at the appropriate length becomes more difficult, because the tendon ends begin to deteriorate, and the flexor tendon/muscle system shortens.[74] The preferable course, therefore, is to perform the repair within a reasonable period. In most cases, the time elapsed before myostatic contraction makes primary repairs technically difficult or impossible to achieve is thought to be 3 weeks.

Any concomitant injuries must be taken into consideration at the time of surgery. A contaminated wound or an injury with significant skin loss usually is a contraindication to repair of an injured flexor tendon. Associated fractures and neurovascular injuries are not a contraindication, and treating these injuries may actually be useful in maintaining stability and adequate perfusion of the tendon as it goes through the reparative process.

The main goals in performing a flexor tendon repair are (1) to retrieve both the proximal and distal ends of the tendons, (2) to reattach the segments to one another in such a way as to maintain maximum strength of the repair and allow easy tendon gliding within the tendon sheath, and (3) prevent the formation of adhesions as much as possible.

Principles of Flexor Tendon Repair[75,76]

- Repair strength is proportional to the number of strands that cross the repair site
- Repairs usually rupture at the suture knots
- The preferable course is to have as few suture knots as possible and to keep the knots away from the repair site
- Gapping at the repair site should be avoided, because it is a major contributor to adhesion formation and negatively affects the strength and stiffness of the tendon repair
- Tension across all suture strands should be equal
- Equal tension prevents asymmetrical loading across the repair site, which can weaken the repair
- Use of a peripheral circumferential suture in addition to the core sutures across the repair increases the strength of the repair

---

Zone Considerations in Flexor Tendon Injuries

Zone I. In zone I injuries, only the FDP is cut, and locating the proximal end of the FDP tendon is relatively simple. A primary end-to-end suture repair can be performed if adequate length of the distal portion of the tendon is left. If the distal portion is short or nonexistent, the proximal tendon end may be attached directly to the bone of the distal phalanx either by a suture anchor within the bone or by sutures pulled through the bone and tied over a button on the dorsal aspect of the distal phalanx.

Avulsion of the FDP usually results from forced extension of a flexed digit, which causes the profundus tendon to pull away at its insertion on the distal phalanx (sweater finger). This injury has a high incidence among young, male athletes, and the ring finger is involved in more than 75% of cases.[77] This injury should be suspected if a patient has tenderness and swelling over the volar aspect of the finger and is unable to flex the DIP joint.

Three types of avulsion injuries can occur at the level of the profundus tendon.[78] In type I injuries, the proximal portion of the tendon retracts into the palm. This end should be retrieved and reattached to the distal segment before muscle contracture occurs, resulting in shortening of the flexor system and making primary repair impossible. Surgical repair should take place within 7 to 10 days.

With type II injuries, the proximal segment of tendon retracts to the level of the PIP joint and is held in place by an intact vinculum (small blood vessel to the tendon). Because this muscle-tendon unit has less of a tendency to shorten, surgical repair of this tendon injury is not as emergent as a type I injury. However, the clinician must keep in mind that if the vinculum breaks, the type II injury becomes a type I injury and requires repair within 7 to 10 days.

Type III injuries involve an avulsion of the large bony fragment to which the FDP attaches. The bone fragment tends to prevent proximal retraction of the tendon, and treatment for this injury usually involves internal fixation of the avulsed bone, which repositions the flexor tendon at its appropriate length, correcting the extension deformity.

Zone II. Zone II injuries were previously referred to as "no man's land" because of the difficulty involved in repairing the flexor tendons at this level. In this zone both the FDP and FDS tendons usually are injured, and the ends are retracted in both the distal and proximal directions. Surgical repair to achieve flexor function involves retrieving both ends of both tendons while maintaining the pulley system, realigning the FDP and FDS tendons anatomically, and repairing the tendons with the strength to maintain the repair without generating increased formation of adhesions.

Zone III. Zone III injuries occur in the region just distal to the carpal tunnel. Both the FDP and FDS tendons travel in this region, and either one or both tendons may be injured. Primary repair of the tendon ends has a good prognosis in this region.

Zone IV. In zone IV, the carpal tunnel, the FDP and FDS tendons travel together, along with the median nerve. Laceration at this level may result in injury to one or multiple tendons and to the median nerve. A thorough neurovascular examination must be performed to determine the extent of tendon and nerve damage, and primary repair should be performed before muscle contractures occur.

Zone V. In zone V (the wrist and forearm), the tendons originate from their musculotendinous junctions and travel together toward their insertion sites. They are less constrained in this region, and tendon repair tends to have a favorable prognosis. However, these injuries may be complicated by multiple tendon lacerations or accompanying neurovascular injury.

Flexor tendon repair of the thumb follows the same principles as tendon injury in the digits, even though the thumb has only one flexor tendon and three pulleys. The lacerated proximal portion of the FPL may be located within the thumb, or it may have retracted into the thenar eminence or the carpal tunnel, making retrieval more complicated. The proximal section should be located, retrieved, and then sutured to the distal section of tendon.

Complications

Surgical repair of flexor tendons often is successful at restoring tendon function; however, the procedure is not without associated complications. The most significant complication is rupture of the flexor tendon at the repair site. If this is recognized, treatment involves re-exploration of the area and repair at the earliest possible time. Flexion contractures at the DIP or PIP joints are frequent complications of repair of flexor tendon injuries. If noted early, alteration of therapy strategies may help reverse these contractures. The development of tendon adhesions is another frustrating complication of flexor tendon repairs. The formation of adhesions prevents functional excursion of the tendon within the sheath, resulting in decreased motion of the involved digit. A tenolysis procedure may be performed to remove adhesions once a plateau has been reached in therapy.

Extensor Tendon Injury

General Considerations

The extensor mechanism of the hand is a unique system that relies on an intricate link between the radial nerve–innervated extrinsic extensor system, which originates in the forearm, and the ulnar nerve–innervated intrinsic system, which originates in the hand.

Injury to the extensor tendon mechanism occurs more frequently than flexor tendon injury because of the more superficial anatomical location of these tendons. This injury should be recognized and taken seriously, because a very delicate balance is achieved within the extensor mechanism. Injury that compromises length, alignment, or stability disrupts this equilibrium, and repair must be meticulous to re-establish the balance of function.

Anatomy

The extrinsic extensor muscles located in the forearm and inserting into the phalanges include the extensor pollicis longus, extensor pollicis brevis, extensor indicis proprius, and extensor digiti minimi. The tendons arising from these muscle bellies have an independent origin and action. The extensor digitorum communis is the common origin of four independent tendons. These become the primary extensor component of the four digits. The intrinsic muscle contribution to the extensor system consists of four dorsal interossei, three palmar interossei, and four lumbrical muscles. These intrinsic muscles function to flex the MCP joints of the four digits and extend the PIP and DIP joints.

The extensor tendons leave the forearm and enter the hand through six dorsal compartments at the level of the wrist and are secured by the extensor retinaculum. This retinaculum functions to prevent bow-stringing of the tendons, causing close approximation of the tendon to the bone and allowing efficient extension. As the tendons enter the hand and travel dorsal to the metacarpals, the extensor digitorum communis tendons, despite originating as independent tendons, become interconnected by the juncturae tendinum. This interconnection results in some codependence and shared extensor activity by these four digits. As the tendons

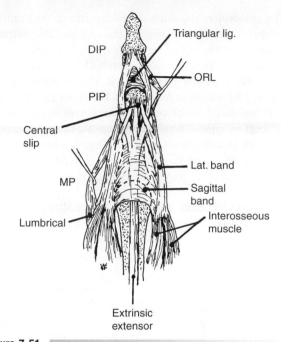

Figure 7-51

Dorsal view of the extensor mechanism. (From Coons MS, Green SM: Boutonniere deformity, *Hand Clin* 11(3):387-402, 1995.)

continue to travel distally toward the fingers, they become centrally located over their respective metacarpal heads. They extend the proximal phalanx by way of a sling mechanism and are stabilized in this central position by the sagittal bands, which run on both sides of the tendon and insert on the volar plate of the MCP joint. As the tendons travel distally along the proximal phalanx (never inserting into that bone), they divide into three slips. The central slip crosses the PIP joint and inserts on the proximal portion of the middle phalanx. The lateral slips travel along both sides of the PIP and the middle phalanx (Figure 7-51).

In the region of the proximal phalanx, the intrinsic muscle tendons begin their contribution to the extensor mechanism. The lumbrical and the palmar and dorsal interossei tendons converge to form the lateral bands, which travel on either side of the proximal phalanx. A portion of the lateral bands joins with the extensor tendon at the PIP joint to insert as a central slip. The remainder contribute fibers that travel on both sides of the middle phalanx and insert into the dorsum of the distal phalanx as the terminal tendon. Because the intrinsic tendons are located volar to the axis of rotation of the MCP joints and dorsal to the axis of rotation of the PIP and DIP joints, the intrinsic muscles function to flex the MCP joint and extend the PIP and DIP joints. In summary, the central slip insertion on the middle phalanx is a convergence of the extrinsic extensor tendon, lumbrical tendon. and interossei tendon. Portions of these tendons travel distally to form the lateral bands, which then converge to form the terminal tendon, inserting on the proximal aspect of the distal phalanx.

The anatomy of the extensor mechanism of the thumb is somewhat different than that of the fingers. The extrinsic tendons enter the hand via the extensor retinaculum in the wrist. The extensor pollicis brevis (EPB) inserts at the base of the proximal phalanx, and the extensor pollicis longus (EPL) inserts at the base of the distal phalanx. The EPL is stabilized in its central position over the thumb MCP joint by sagittal bands. The intrinsic extensor component to the thumb comes from the ulnar nerve–innervated adductor pollicis, which functions to adduct the thumb, flex the thumb MCP joint, and extend the thumb IP joint.

Injury Classification and Medical Treatment

Zone Considerations. The extensor tendon mechanism can be divided into eight zones based on the differing physical characteristics of the tendons and their insertions. The even-numbered zones occur over bones, and the odd-numbered zones are positioned over joints. Zone I represents the most distal aspect of the extensor mechanism, where the lateral bands on either side of the digit converge to form the terminal tendon, inserting on the distal phalanx. The terminal tendon functions to extend the DIP joint in concert with PIP joint extension. Moving proximally, zone II covers the middle phalanx, the area where the two lateral bands join together and are held in place by the triangular ligament just before forming the terminal tendon. Zone III is at the PIP joint, the area where the central slip inserts; it functions to extend the PIP joint. Zone IV covers the region of the proximal phalanx, where the extrinsic extensor system converges with the intrinsic system. Zone V covers the region over the MCP joint, where the extensor tendons lie centrally over the joint, stabilized by the sagittal bands. Zone VI exists over the metacarpal bones, where the extensor communis tendons are interconnected by the juncturae tendinum. In zone VII, at the level of the wrist joint, the tendons lie within the tenosynovium, covered by the extensor retinaculum. Zone VIII is the most proximal zone, containing the extensor tendons at their musculotendinous junctions. Zone IX consists of the proximal one half of the forearm above the musculotendinous junction (Figure 7-52).

Zone I (Mallet Finger Deformities). Zone I injuries create a mallet finger deformity. These injuries result in a disruption of the extensor tendon at the level of the DIP joint, caused by a closed avulsion injury, an open skin and tendon injury, or a fracture of the proximal portion of the distal phalanx, where the terminal tendon of the extensor system inserts. Closed injuries occur more often, usually when sudden flexion of the extended digit ruptures the tendon from its bony insertion; or, the bony insertion site, with the tendon attached, may avulse from the distal phalanx. Open injuries may be lacerations or crush injuries that disrupt the extensor tendon.

Upon physical examination, the distal phalanx is found to be in some degree of flexion, and the patient is unable

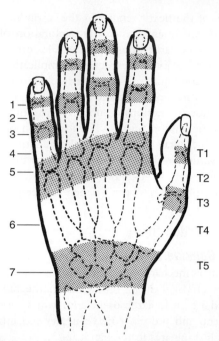

Figure 7-52

Extensor tendon zones. (From Kleinert HE, Schepel S, Gill T: Flexor tendon injuries, *Surg Clin North Am* 61:267-286, 1981.)

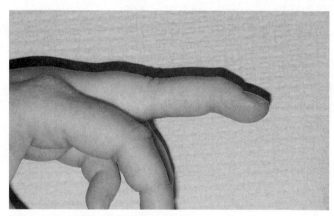

Figure 7-53

Mallet injury. Note the extensor lag at the DIP joint and the mild hyperextension at the PIP joint.

to actively extend the distal portion of the injured finger. Hyperextension of the PIP joint may be present, secondary to the unopposed tension of the central slip combined with volar plate laxity, resulting in a swan neck deformity (Figure 7-53).

Mallet finger deformities have been classified according to the cause of the deformity, because this assists in the determination of the treatment plan. The goal of management is to restore tendon continuity with maximum return to function.

A type I mallet finger injury is the result of closed or blunt trauma, with or without a small avulsion fracture. This is the most common type of injury, and splinting of the DIP in extension is the optimum treatment option.

Hyperextension should be avoided, because this may cause ischemia of the thin dorsal skin. The patient wears a splint continuously for a minimum of 6 weeks, followed by 2 weeks of nighttime splinting.[79] This usually results in excellent recovery. On rare occasions, if a patient is unable to wear a splint, a K-wire may be placed across the DIP joint to maintain the joint in extension.

A type II mallet deformity results from a laceration at the level of or just proximal to the DIP joint, causing disruption of the extensor tendon. Given the numerous attachments of the extensor tendon to the digit, very little retraction of the proximal end occurs, and in this situation the tendon should be primarily repaired. The extensor tendon at this level is broad and thin, and repair should consist of a running suture that reapproximates the skin and tendon simultaneously. After repair, a splint should be worn to maintain the DIP in an extended position for 6 weeks.

A type III mallet deformity is caused by a deep abrasion to the distal aspect of the finger, resulting in loss of skin, subcutaneous tissue, and tendon substance. Given the nature of this injury, reconstructive surgery is needed for soft tissue coverage, and tendon reconstruction with a free tendon graft should be the treatment of choice. The loss of tendon substance, resulting in loss of extensor tendon length, impairs the surgeon's ability to restore function of the extensor mechanism using primary repair.

Type IV mallet deformities are further subdivided into three groups. Type IV-A deformities result from a transepiphyseal plate fracture in children. Because the extensor tendon is attached to the epiphysis, a mallet finger deformity results secondary to the fracture. Closed reduction of the fracture corrects this deformity. Continuous splinting of the DIP in extension for 3 to 4 weeks usually produces union of the fracture and resolution of the deformity. Type IV-B deformities are caused by a hyperflexion injury with a fracture that compromises 20% to 50% of the dorsal articular surface. A hyperextension injury that causes a fracture with a bone fragment larger than 50% of the dorsal articular surface results in a type IV-C mallet finger deformity. Because of the largely compromised articular surface in these injuries, they often are associated with volar subluxation of the distal phalanx relative to the proximal phalanx. In both type IV-B and IV-C injuries, the mallet deformity results because the extensor tendon remains attached to the fractured segment of bone.

For fractures that have subluxed anteriorly, operative management is recommended to achieve an accurate reduction of the fracture and to restore articular congruity (see Figure 7-3). Surgery restores the extensor tendon length and resolves the mallet deformity. For fractures that are not subluxed, splinting of the DIP in extension for 6 weeks results in fracture union and remodeling of the articular surface, with subsequent resolution of the mallet deformity.

Mallet thumb, or injury to the extensor mechanism of the thumb in zone I, at the level of the IP joint, is a rare injury. It may be caused by a closed rupture of the EPL insertion or a laceration of the tendon at this level. A closed injury should be treated with IP extension splinting for 6 to 8 weeks. An open laceration is best treated by primary repair, with sutures incorporating both skin and tendon.

Zone II. Zone II injuries of the fingers and thumb occur at the level of the middle phalanx and usually result from a laceration or crush injury that leads to disruption of the extensor tendon. Partial lacerations, in which less than 50% of the tendon is disrupted, are common in this region because of the broad, curved shape of the tendon as it lies against the phalanx. If a partial laceration occurs, treatment involves wound care and splinting for 7 to 10 days. If the laceration causes more extensive tendon damage, the distal and proximal tendon ends should be primarily repaired, followed by extension splinting.

Zone III. Zone III injuries occur at the level of the PIP joint, with disruption to the central slip. If allowed to progress, these injuries cause the classic boutonniere deformity (i.e., hyperflexion of the PIP joint and subsequent hyperextension at the DIP joint). Loss of extension at the PIP joint may not result immediately because the lateral bands retain the ability to extend this joint. However, over time, the head of the proximal phalanx buttonholes through the defect created by the ruptured central slip, and the lateral bands migrate anteriorly below the axis of rotation of the PIP joint, converting them from PIP extensors to PIP flexors. This causes loss of extension at the PIP joint, and a flexion deformity results. At the same time, the more anterior position of the lateral bands at the level of the PIP joint causes increased tension along these bands, which is transmitted to the terminal tendon and leads to hyperextension of the DIP joint. This injury may result from either a laceration of the central slip or closed trauma with acute forceful flexion of the PIP joint, causing avulsion of the central slip. Correction of this deformity requires reestablishment of the tendon balance and the tendon length relationship between the central slip and the lateral bands. If a closed rupture has occurred, the PIP can be splinted, gradually progressing to full extension. This allows reapproximation and healing of the ends of the central slip. A K-wire across the extended PIP joint can achieve the same goal. If the central slip is injured by an acute laceration, primary repair of this tendon should be performed.

Zone III injuries of the thumb at the level of the MCP joint may involve one or both of the thumb extensor tendons. If only the EPB is injured, thumb extension at the MCP joint likely will be retained, because the EPL remains functional. If the EPL is disrupted, an extension lag across both the MCP and IP joints results. Primary repair is usually indicated for laceration injuries within this zone.

Zone IV. Zone IV injuries occur at the level of the proximal phalanx. In this region, the lateral bands contribute significantly to the extensor function and offer protection against complete lacerations of the central tendon. Therefore injury in this zone usually results in partial lacerations; however, this diagnosis can be made only under direct visualization of the tendon. If the tendon is partly lacerated, splinting the PIP for 3 to 4 weeks is adequate treatment.[80] If laceration of a lateral band is diagnosed, primary repair may be performed, followed by early protected motion. For complete lacerations of the extensor tendon, primary repair should be undertaken, followed by 6 weeks of PIP extension splinting. Preserving appropriate tendon length during this repair is crucial, so that the balance between the central tendon and the lateral bands is maintained.

Zone V. Many types of injuries involving the extensor mechanism can occur in zone V, at the level of the MCP joint. Open wounds often occur at this level and are of special concern given the proximity of the MCP joint to the surface of the skin. If a patient uses a fist to strike someone in the mouth, a fight bite may result, which is a contaminated open wound most likely communicating with the MCP joint. Immediate debridement, irrigation, and antibiotic therapy must be started. Partial tendon injuries usually are associated with this type of wound, but a complete tendon injury does occur, and either a primary or secondary repair may be performed, depending on the status of the wound. If a clean laceration occurs at the level of the MCP joint, primary repair of the tendon may be performed.

The sagittal bands, which are found on both sides of the extensor tendon at the level of the MCP joint, are vulnerable to injury in zone V. The sagittal bands centralize the extensor tendon over the MCP joint. Injuries to these bands may be caused by a laceration, or the bands may be ruptured by a forceful blow of the clenched fist against a hard surface. Prompt recognition of this injury allows for treatment by extension splinting. If this is not successful, repair of the sagittal bands may be undertaken at a later date to prevent subluxation and to improve extensor function at the MCP joint.

Zone V injuries of the thumb occur at the level of the CMC joint and commonly involve lacerations of the EPB and abductor pollicis longus (APL) tendons. Injuries in this region must be carefully evaluated for possible compromise of the radial artery and the radial nerve sensory branches. The proximal segment of the APL may retract in this region, therefore retrieval of this tendon and primary repair should be performed.

Zone VI. Injuries in zone VI occur at the level of the metacarpals, where the tendons for the extensor digitorum communis, extensor indicis proprius, and extensor digiti minimi are located. Tendon lacerations, either partial or complete, are difficult to diagnose at this level, because full active extension may not be completely lost; extensor action may be transmitted through the juncturae tendinae,

or redundant tendon function may be present (in the case of the index and small fingers). To test for independent tendon function on the physical examination, the examiner should hold all digits except the one being examined in flexion at the MCP joints to prevent any possible contribution of the juncturae tendinum from confounding the examination.[81] Ideally, the diagnosis for this injury should be made under direct visualization. Tendons in this region are thicker and more oval and can support a stronger core suture for use in primary repair. After repair, postoperative management includes splinting for 4 to 6 weeks. If an extensor digitorum communis tendon is involved, all fingers should be splinted; if an extensor indicis propius tendon was injured, only the specific index finger needs splinting.

Zone VII. Zone VII injuries occur at the level of the wrist and usually involve injury to the extensor retinaculum. The wrist and finger extensor tendons coexist in this region, and the chance of multiple tendon injuries is high. Injury may result from lacerations, tendon ruptures after fracture, or tendon dislocation after injury to the retinaculum. The distal and proximal ends of the injured tendons retract in this area, making primary repair of these injuries more complicated. If multiple tendons are lacerated, the appropriate proximal and distal regions must be retrieved and anatomically matched and then primarily repaired. Damage to the retinaculum also complicates injury in this zone. This structure is necessary to prevent bow-stringing of the extensor tendons as they function to extend the wrist and the fingers. Part of the retinaculum may be resected to allow adequate exposure and retrieval of the tendons, but the retinaculum should not be fully excised, and its function should be preserved. However, tendon healing at this level is often associated with the formation of adhesions to the overlying retinaculum.[82] Measures attempted to prevent adhesion formation include early dynamic splinting.

Zone VIII. Tendon injuries in the distal forearm, zone VIII, usually occur at the musculotendinous junction and may be caused by a laceration or rupture. Primary repair of these injuries is difficult, because although the distal tendon segment retains suture well, the proximal muscle region does not. Options for restoring adequate extensor function in this type of injury are side-to-side suture repairs or tendon transfers.

Zone IX. Zone IX injuries occur in the proximal forearm and usually are due to a penetrating wound. Injury at this level is complicated by the multiple structures present and vulnerable. Muscle transection or nerve injury may result in functional impairment. A careful, thorough physical examination must be performed, and often surgical exploration is undertaken for diagnosis. If the muscle is found to be damaged, it is repaired primarily or, if the muscle defect is too extensive, tendon grafting may be performed.

Rehabilitation Principles and Considerations for Tendon Injuries

Flexor Tendon Injuries of the Hand

Numerous articles and studies have been written about the rehabilitation of flexor tendon injuries. Despite the wealth of information available to clinicians, determining which approach to choose can be confusing and difficult.

Effects of Early, Controlled Force on a Repaired Flexor Tendon

- More rapid recovery of tensile strength
- Fewer adhesions
- Improved tendon excursion
- Less gapping at the repair site

Several studies provide evidence that incremental stress and tendon excursion increase the rate at which the repair site achieves normal tensile strength and reduce the amount of scar adhesion. A variety of postoperative flexor tendon protocols have been designed to provide the optimum amount of tension loading at the precise time in the patient's treatment.[9,84]

Early mobilization, either passive or active, starting within the first week of the repair, has been shown to produce excellent results compared to postoperative immobilization. Early passive mobilization (EPM) consists of passive flexion with active extension within the confines of a protective splint. Early active mobilization (EAM) consists of active flexion and extension of the involved finger within certain parameters of a protective splint.[84-86]

Despite the benefits of these early mobilization programs, questions remain as to how much motion should be allowed and when to begin. If early active motion is too aggressive, it may cause gap formation or even rupture the repaired tendon. However, traditional early passive motion protocols may not provide enough tendon gliding within the tendon sheath to prevent scar adhesions.[87]

Selection of a Treatment Protocol. The postoperative treatment protocol and guidelines chosen to guide rehabilitation decisions and interventions are critically important. Surgical repairs and treatment protocols can vary greatly. Communication between the surgeon and therapist is vital to ensure the most successful outcome for the patient. It is important that the therapist know the type of flexor tendon repair and suture technique performed before initiating a rehabilitation protocol. The combination of advanced suture techniques and immediate passive mobilization has reduced adhesions and repair site gaps and increased tendon excursion. Recent methods of core suture techniques offer greater tensile strength to the tendon at the time of the repair and improve strength up to 6 weeks postoperatively.[88] Stronger suture techniques

designed for active motion have also been developed, but it is critical that the therapist know what type of repair was performed before initiating early EAM protocols.

Several factors can affect the strength of a flexor tendon repair, such as the suture caliber, the number of strands crossing a repair, and the type of suture loops used. A suture caliber of 3-0 is recommended over 4-0, and a four-strand repair is thought to be better than a two-strand repair. Also, some surgeons believe that locking suture loops that hold the tendon on either side are best for enhancing the strength of the repair.[89,90] It has become accepted that four- or six-strand flexor tendon repair methods, combined with a strong epitendinous suture, should be sufficiently strong to withstand light active forces through healing.[91]

Factors Affecting the Strength of a Tendon Repair

- Suture caliber (e.g., 3-0)
- Number of suture strands that cross the repair (four to six)
- Type of suture loops

Another important consideration for therapists treating patients with flexor tendon repairs is how much friction is present and how well the tendon glides. In an injured finger, joint stiffness caused by diffuse swelling or soft tissue restrictions becomes a major factor, and significant tendon force is needed to overcome it. Other sources that cause resistance to motion within the tendon sheath include damage to the pulley system, tendon sheath, or gliding surfaces of the tendon, all of which can cause adhesions to form later during the healing process.[89]

Sources of Resistance to Tendon Motion

- Swelling
- Scarring (adhesions)
- Joint stiffness (hypomobility)
- Damage to the pulley system
- Damage to the tendon sheath
- Damage to the tendon gliding surfaces

The effects of drag and other viscous effects on a joint significantly affect the outcome of a tendon repair. Gentle passive motion of the involved finger joints should be performed at slow speeds to eliminate the potential for viscoelastic forces. Passive motion serves to release and reduce fluid around a joint, which reduces the resistance to motion.[91] Passive joint motion also enhances the motion of the tendons with respect to one another. Passive flexion of the DIP joint produces excursion of the FDP in relation to the FDS of 1 to 2 mm for every 10° of motion, and passive flexion of the PIP joint produces 1.5 mm of tendon excursion between the two tendons for every 10° of joint flexion.[92]

An extremely swollen finger will have a significant increase in friction, which can affect tendon gliding. Any degree of joint excursion will require significantly more force, posing the danger of gapping at the tendon repair site. Discrepancy in the literature exists about the acceptable amount of gapping at the repair site. Gaps also cause increased friction, and gaps of 3 mm or more can block tendon motion, causing the tendon to rupture or adhesions to form.[89,92]

Most protocols developed for both EPM and EAM recommend that treatment begin 24 to 48 hours after surgery to prevent adhesion formation and joint contracture. Recently some experts have said that starting passive motion the day after surgery may hurt the final result, because the gliding resistance of the tendon is high during this time because of swelling. Starting early motion the day after surgery can be associated with an increased risk of inducing fresh bleeding, which can lead to adhesions; therefore some recommend waiting 3 to 5 days before initiating treatment to prevent joint stiffness and scar formation. The consensus for all tendon rehabilitation is that treatment should begin early, no later than 3 to 5 days after surgery, to prevent joint stiffness and adhesions.[89,93] One of the benefits of early mobilization is an increase in tensile strength, which is achieved by stimulating maturation of the tendon wound and remodeling the scar tissue. This process prevents "softening" of the tendon, which can occur after day 5 if the tendon has been immobile, causing the tendon to be weaker during this time frame.[83,94] Clinicians must evaluate each patient and determine with the patient's surgeon the most appropriate time to begin treatment.

A third consideration in treating flexor tendon injuries involves the position of the wrist and its relationship to the finger flexors. Internal flexor tendon loading is greatly influenced by wrist position. Tendon loading occurs during wrist flexion, because passive finger extension causes the tendon to move distally. Internal tendon loading also occurs during wrist extension with passive finger flexion as the tendon is pulled proximally. The tenodesis effect of wrist extension with finger flexion and wrist flexion with finger extension enhances tendon excursion. This concept has been incorporated into both EPM and EAM tendon rehabilitation protocols.[95,96] A study by Savage[97] has shown that a position of wrist extension and MCP joint flexion produces the least tension in a repaired flexor tendon during active finger flexion.

It also is important that the therapist know the zone or location of the injury and repair, because this affects the patient's treatment. The flexor tendons are divided into five zones, which were described previously. Treatment protocols vary, depending on the zone of the injury and repair.

The literature primarily focuses on zone II flexor tendon injuries. This zone has the highest probability of developing adhesions, because the FDP travels through the FDS at Camper's chiasm, and the two tendons are located within one flexor tendon sheath.

Other important considerations are associated injuries, patient compliance, and the timing of surgery.

The presence of associated injuries, such as digital nerve or artery lacerations, significant soft tissue loss, and dislocations or fractures, also influences the course of treatment for a flexor tendon injury. Clinicians may need to alter rehabilitation protocols to accommodate these injuries. The patient's ability to understand a rehabilitation program and to follow it faithfully is critical to a successful recovery. Rehabilitation protocols are valuable guidelines, but each patient must be evaluated independently to determine the most suitable treatment regimen and the ways it might need to be altered to best serve the individual.

Early Passive Mobilization. Immobilization protocols have largely been abandoned in favor of early mobilization programs, which have resulted in much better motion and greater function. Occasionally a very young child or patient who is unable to participate appropriately with an early mobilization program is a candidate for an immobilization program, which usually consists of 4 weeks of immobilization in a plaster cast or protective splint before initiation of passive and active range of motion exercises. Patients can begin gentle resistance at 8 weeks and progress with a strengthening program at 10 weeks, with no restrictions by 12 weeks. Unfortunately, some patients treated with immobilization programs may not achieve full motion and have some residual limitations, depending on the location and nature of the injury.

One of the original controlled motion protocols developed by Kleinert for flexor tendon repairs consisted of a dorsal block splint with the wrist positioned at 40° flexion and the MCP joints in 40° to 60° flexion. The injured finger was held in flexion by a rubber band attached from the fingernail to a bandage or strap at the wrist level. Patients were instructed to actively extend against the rubber band up to the dorsal hood of the splint and then relax the finger, allowing the rubber band to passively flex the digit. Active flexion of the finger was not permitted for 4 weeks. After 4 weeks in the dorsal protective splint, patients were instructed to begin active flexion and extension exercises.[98] Modifications of the Kleinert traction approach include a palmar bar with pulley to increase DIP joint flexion. Although results using the rubber bands, or Kleinert method (Figure 7-54), were much better than the immobilization programs, some patients developed flexion contractures at PIP joint from being held in flexion by the rubber band traction.

In the 1970s Duran and Houser presented a controlled passive motion method that has been modified over the years. It has become the basis for EPM protocols used

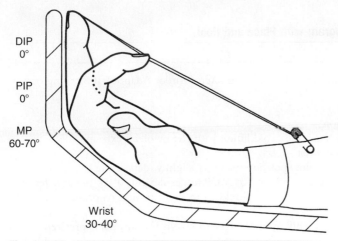

Figure 7-54
Kleinert splinting protocol. (From Randall WC, Taras JS: Primary care of flexor injuries. In Hunter JM, Mackin EJ, Callahan AD et al, editors: *Rehabilitation of the hand and upper extremity,* ed 5, p 425, St Louis, 2002, Mosby.)

today by many clinicians and surgeons. Duran used a dorsal block splint similar to that described previously, but instead of a rubber band positioning the finger in flexion, the fingers were held in the splint with the PIP and DIP joints held in neutral (0°) with a Velcro strap, up against the hood of the dorsal block splint. The patient was instructed to remove the Velcro strap and perform three passive exercises within the confines of the splint. The first exercise was isolated passive DIP flexion, which allowed the FDP to independently glide from the FDS. The second exercise was passive flexion and extension of the PIP joint with the MCP in flexion in the splint, which allowed the FDS and FDP to move away from the damaged tendon sheath.

The third exercise was full composite passive flexion of the MCP, PIP, and DIP joints, alternated with passive extension of the IP joints while the MCP joint was blocked in flexion (Figure 7-55).[99]

Modified Duran protocols incorporate active finger extension to meet the confines of the dorsal block splint, after passive flexion and extension of the finger. Active flexion of the finger is contraindicated for 3½ to 4 weeks following surgery. Proponents of the modified Duran method feel that it is less likely to cause flexion contractures at the IP joints than the Kleinert method and that the involved finger is protected better with a Velcro strap when the patient is not exercising. In recent years clinicians have combined some components of early active motion with the modified Duran protocol.[91,100,101] Modified Duran flexor tendon protocols are used to treat zone I and zone II flexor tendon injuries and may vary slightly among clinicians, surgeons, and clinics; this is the reason good communication with the surgeon and a thorough knowledge of the patient's injury and repair are important. (The modified Duran program with place and hold guidelines are presented in Table 7-8.)

Early Active Mobilization. Early mobilization programs originally focused on early passive mobilization. It now is widely accepted that tensile strength at the repair site increases when tendons are mobilized early. Despite improved results with EPM, some patients with zone I and zone II flexor tendon repairs still fail to achieve normal range of motion. This led to the desire for rehabilitation algorithms that would allow for safe, early active mobilization. Recently, new suture techniques have been designed to minimize repair site gapping, which can lead to adhesions and tendon rupture but allow some early active motion. Repair site strength is directly related to the

Figure 7-55
Duran protocol. (From Strickland WJ: Biologic rationale, clinical application, and results of early motion following flexor tendon repair, *J Hand Ther* 2:78, 1989.)

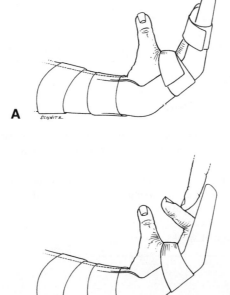
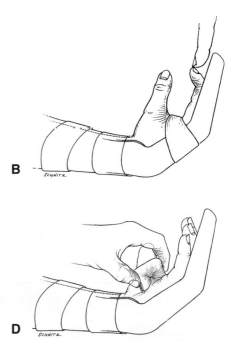

Table 7-8

Flexor Tendon Repairs in Zones I and II: Modified Duran Program with Place and Hold

Time Frame	Program Considerations
0 to 5 Days	Inspect the wound. Apply a nonrestrictive sterile dressing (e.g., Xeroform or Adaptic); if bleeding occurs, combine with light gauze Instruct the patient in all precautions: • Avoid all active finger or wrist flexion • Avoid functional use of the injured hand and avoid lifting with the involved extremity • Avoid fully extending the fingers and wrist *Splint:* Fabricate a dorsal block protective splint (position may vary slightly, depending on surgeon's preference): 20° to 30° wrist flexion, 50° to 70° MCP finger flexion, 0° IP finger extension. (If a digital nerve repair was performed, the PIP joint should be in slight flexion to protect the nerve repair) *Exercise program:* The protocol may vary, depending on the type of repair, the surgeon's preference, and the patient's age and compliance. The following is a modified Duran protocol with a place and hold component (four strand repair): • Instruct the patient in *gentle passive flexion* of each digit at the MCP joint, the PIP joint, and the DIP joint, and in *active extension* within the confines of the splint. The splint should be worn at all times and during exercises; only the top strap is removed to complete the exercises. The exercises should be performed 10 times for each digit once an hour if the patient is very restricted in passive flexion; otherwise, they should be performed 5 to 6 times a day for 3½ weeks after surgery • Apply compressive wrap (e.g., Coban) to reduce swelling: instruct the patient in edema management, ice packs, and elevation. The patient should be assisted by another person in applying the Coban *Early AROM/place and hold:* In addition to the previous program, the following can be initiated within 5 days after surgery *only* with reliable patients who have full passive flexion and decreased edema. The therapist needs to know whether the procedure was at least a four-strand repair of the flexor tendon before initiating place and hold: • Place and hold should be done after passive flexion of the digits within the confines of the splint. Passively place the patient's finger in a partly flexed position and have the patient hold this position with minimum tension for 3 seconds. During weeks 2 and 3, place and hold can progress with the finger held in more flexion, again using minimum tension to hold Sutures generally are removed within 10 to 15 days; the patient can begin gentle massage to the scar once the wound has closed
3½ to 4½ Weeks	Initiate gentle active flexion and extension of the digits within the confines of the splint after passive flexion of the digits Continue with edema and scar management as needed. Fabricate an Otoform or elastomer mold for nighttime wear if the wound has closed Straighten the wrist position of the splint to neutral and increase MCP flexion, if needed, to 60° to 70° At 4 to 4½ weeks, begin active flexion and extension out of the splint with the wrist in neutral after passive flexion of the digits. The splint is removed only for exercises. Tendon gliding exercises with a hook fist and full composite fist are initiated Apply foam padding to the dorsal part of the splint as needed to assist with PIP extension of the digits if a flexion contracture is forming Begin active wrist flexion and extension exercises; start with tenodesis wrist motion Continue to reinforce the frequency of the home exercise regimen: every 1 to 2 hours, 10 repetitions of each exercise Begin light, nonresistive activity to encourage finger flexion and extension while in therapy Begin gentle blocking exercises, emphasizing no resistance, and avoid blocking to the DIP joint of the little finger. Gentle, supervised, passive IP extension can be performed with the tendon on slack (with the wrist and MCP joint flexed) Ultrasound may be initiated at weeks 4 to 6

Table 7-8
Flexor Tendon Repairs in Zones I and II: Modified Duran Program with Place and Hold

Time Frame	Program Considerations
6 to 8 Weeks	Depending on the patient's judgment and activity level, the dorsal block protective splint may be discharged. The patient may need the splint for protection only in certain situations; otherwise, it should be kept off The patient can begin to use the injured hand for light ADLs (e.g., buttoning a shirt, washing the face) *Emphasize:* • No heavy gripping or squeezing • No lifting • No using the hand for pushing or pulling (e.g., opening doors) Begin light resistive exercises and activities (e.g., squeeze soft putty, sponge, or light grippers) Some patients may benefit from a resting splint at night to gradually increase finger and wrist extension. Aggressive scar management is continued Gradually increase resistance for strengthening program (moderate resistance) Dynamic or static progressive PIP extension splinting or casting may be necessary Evaluate grip strength at weeks 8 to 10 after surgery, depending on the level of scar tissue present
10 to 12 Weeks	Continue with strengthening program and progress as tolerated or as needed The patient can return to all normal activities, including heavy work or sports, as tolerated. Most patients should be on a home program by week 12; however, treatment may vary for patients with complex injuries or complications

MCP, Metacarpophalangeal; *IP,* interphalangeal; *PIP,* proximal interphalangeal; *DIP,* distal interphalangeal; *AROM,* active range of motion; *ADLs,* activities of daily living.

number of suture strands crossing the tendon laceration; however, as the number of sutures increases, so does repair site volume and the work for tendon gliding. The suture technique used by surgeons may vary, and debate continues as to whether four-strand, six-strand, or eight-strand repairs are best.[88-90] Strickland[92] has determined that a four-strand core suture plus a strong peripheral suture can withstand the stress of gentle early active motion.

Trends over the past decade have been moving toward early active mobilization programs that allow active flexion and extension of the involved fingers within the first 3 to 5 days. A concept known as *place and hold* is included in this category of EAM, in which the involved finger is passively flexed to a certain position and the patient is asked to hold it there through active contraction of that muscle. Evans and Thompson[91] studied the forces applied to a tendon with minimal active muscle-tendon tension (MAMTT) and developed guidelines for joint angles and force application with an adequate safety margin. Their study showed that as the angle of joint flexion increases, the amount of force required also increases. They devised a protocol for treating flexor tendon repairs, recommending a position of place and hold with the wrist in 20° extension, the MCP joint in 83° flexion, the PIP joint in 75° flexion, and the DIP joints in 40° flexion, using a Haldex pinch gauge and string held perpendicular to the digit to measure external force during the active hold position. According to this protocol, the patient should apply only 15 to 20 g of force to hold the position.

This method of treatment has been modified by various clinicians and treatment centers, and EAM protocols have emerged with varying degrees of motion involving the

digits and wrist. Incorporating tenodesis, wrist and finger motion has become standard treatment along, with decreasing the degree of wrist flexion in the dorsal block splint. The Indiana Hand Center[102,103] has devised an EAM protocol using a tenodesis wrist hinge splint that allows wrist flexion but blocks wrist extension at 30°; the MCP joints are blocked with a dorsal hood at 60° flexion. The patient wears this splint for exercise only and wears a dorsal protective block splint when not exercising. The patient is instructed to passively flex the involved finger into full composite flexion and then to bring the wrist up to extension. The patient is instructed to actively hold the flexed position of the finger with a minimal amount of tension for a few seconds. The patient then relaxes the muscle contraction and allows the wrist to drop into flexion and the fingers to extend to the dorsal hood of the splint (Figure 7-56).[102,103] This method should be used only by an experienced clinician who can evaluate a patient to determine whether the individual is an appropriate candidate for this type of synergistic protocol. EAM programs should be used with patients who are very compliant and can fully understand the program and its precautions.

Zones I and II. Gratton[101] described an uncomplicated method of splinting and an EAM program for the treatment of zone I and zone II flexor tendon repairs that took place in Great Britain. This protocol was devised with the goal of producing a treatment program that could be used for difficult cases and for patients who were less compliant or unable to attend therapy on a regular basis. Immediately after surgical repair, patients were placed in a dorsal block plaster splint with the wrist in 20° flexion, the MCP

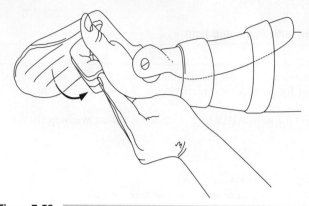

Figure 7-56
Indiana protocol with a hinge splint allows for active wrist extension combined with passive finger flexion. (From Cannon N: Post flexor tendon repair motion protocol, *Indiana Hand Center Newsletter* 1:13, 1993.)

joints in 80° to 90° flexion, and the IP joints in neutral (0° in extension). No other splints were fabricated. The patients were admitted to the hospital for up to 3 days, and they wore a sling to prevent edema. Patients began motion 24 to 48 hours after surgery. The program consisted of passive flexion, active flexion, and two repetitions of active extension in the plaster splint every 4 hours. If joint stiffness was present, the patient increased the exercises to every 2 hours. The plaster splint was removed at 5 weeks after surgery, and the patients were allowed active range of motion; they worked toward active loading of the tendon at 8 weeks after surgery and returned to heavy work at 12 weeks. With this approach, 49% of the patients achieved an excellent outcome, 36% achieved a good outcome, and 7% had tendon ruptures.[101]

Protocols vary from clinic to clinic, because each clinic develops an individualized approach, which often depends on the surgeons' and therapists' preferences and expertise. A survey of 191 therapists revealed that 33% used some type of active finger flexion exercise within the first operative week. Only 5.5% of the therapists used the tenodesis hinge splint, but most of the therapists reported using a Kleinert type or Duran type of protocol, and 89.6% used some type of dorsal protective splint. More than half of those surveyed reported that their patients had experienced a tendon rupture, but this was less likely to occur in patients whose therapists saw them more frequently.[104]

Hold for Flexor Tendon Repairs in Zones I and II. Evans[105] has devised a postoperative program for treating FDP injuries in zone I that have undergone tendon to tendon or tendon to bone repair, using a technique consisting of limited DIP extension and active flexion. In addition to the dorsal block splint, the patient wears an individual static dorsal splint that positions the DIP joint in 40° to 45° flexion. This prevents the loss of DIP joint flexion that commonly occurs with zone I lacerations. The splint is taped in place to hold the DIP securely flexed, but the PIP joint is not included.

Evans' protocol includes the use of passive flexion/active extension exercises and an active exercise component known as *immediate active short arc motion (SAM)*. After gentle passive exercises, the therapist removes the patient's splint and positions the patient with the wrist in 20° extension, the MCP joints in 75° to 80° flexion, the PIP joints in 70° to 75° flexion, and the DIP joints in 40° flexion (SAM position). The patient is instructed to gently hold this position to create minimum active tension in the flexor system. The force of flexion is measured with a Haldex pinch gauge, as described earlier with the MAMTT program. The therapist also performs wrist tenodesis exercises with the patient by passively holding the digits into a composite fist and simultaneously extending the wrist to 30° to 40°. The wrist then is passively flexed to 60° while the digits are allowed to extend through tenodesis action. The patient follows this exercise regimen for 3 to 4 weeks before full active range of motion and traditional tendon gliding exercises are begun. This protocol was developed with a defined safety margin for the active short arc motion.[105] Many clinicians and clinics have incorporated these concepts and modified them, depending on their level of experience, the surgeon's preference, and the individual patient's status. Table 7-9 details this type of protocol.

Zones III to V. Injuries in zones III to V are also treated with the modified Duran protocol or early passive mobilization. Flexor tendon repairs in zone IV and proximally, which include the wrist and forearm, generally result in better range of motion in the digits than repairs distal to this area. Peritendinous scar adhesions are less likely to form in these regions. The tensile strength of repaired tendons in zone IV and proximally is substantial enough to tolerate AROM exercises starting at 3 weeks after surgery. Active range of motion of the digits can begin in the dorsal block splint at 3 weeks after surgery and gentle blocking exercises of the PIP and DIP joints at 4 weeks. Unrestricted AROM of the wrist and fingers can begin at 4 to 4½ weeks after surgery, and gentle resistance can be initiated at 6 weeks, progressing with strengthening at 8 to 10 weeks; most patients are discharged at 12 weeks after surgery. Patients may develop extrinsic flexor tightness with repairs in these zones. The dorsal block splint is discontinued at 6 weeks, and a full extension resting splint may be indicated if extrinsic flexor tightness is present.[106,107]

Anatomical structures that may be involved with a laceration to the wrist and forearm include the FDS, FDP, FPL, palmaris longus (PL), flexor carpi radialis (FCR), flexor carpi ulnaris (FCU), the medial nerve, the ulnar nerve, the radial artery, and/or the ulnar artery. All of these structures must be repaired to ensure a positive functional outcome for the patient.[106] If an injury in zone IV or V involves a median and/or ulnar nerve repair, the wrist should be positioned in approximately 30° flexion in the dorsal block splint and, starting at 3 weeks after surgery, the amount of wrist extension should be increased by 10°

Table 7-9
Flexor Digitorum Profundus Repairs in Zone I (Tendon to Bone): Modified Early Mobilization Program

Time Frame	Program Considerations
0 to 5 Days	*Splint:* Fabricate a static dorsal block splint: Wrist, 20° to 30° flexion; MCP joints, 30° to 50° flexion; IP joints extended. The DIP joint may be positioned in flexion up to 45° by the surgeon to prevent stress on the repair. Based on the surgeon's guidelines, the dorsal block splint may be padded, or a separate finger splint may be taped dorsally over the involved digit, positioning the DIP joint in flexion *Exercise program:* Instruct the patient in the following: passive flexion of all finger joints within the splint; passive DIP flexion to 75° within a static finger splint and dorsal block splint; active extension of the IP joints within the splint with the MCP blocked in full passive flexion. Exercises are performed as 10 repetitions, 5 to 6 times a day Initiate edema management
1 to 2 Weeks	In addition to the previously described exercises, DIP extension is progressed in the splint weekly to tissue tolerance or to the surgeon's guidelines. Begin scar management when appropriate Begin passive modified hook position (hook with the MCP joints resting on the hood of the splint with full IP flexion to tolerance) Begin modified place and hold within the splint once edema had decreased and full passive motion has been achieved. Passively flex the PIP joint of the affected finger while holding the uninvolved fingers to the hood of the splint to encourage differential FDS gliding from the FDP. Instruct the patient to gently contract to hold the PIP joint in this flexed position with minimum tension for 3 seconds These exercises should be performed in the clinic by the therapist: Remove the patient's splint. Passively extend the patient's wrist to 30° to 40° with the fingers passively held in composite flexion. Passively flex the wrist to 60° with passive hook fisting of the fingers
3 to 4 Weeks	Continue as previously described. The individual finger splint or DIP extension block can be discarded. The patient can begin full composite flexion with place and hold with the wrist positioned in slight flexion to neutral Begin active finger flexion and extension with the wrist in slight flexion to neutral; also begin active hook fisting with the wrist in slight flexion to neutral Instruct the patient in active tenodesis wrist exercises
4 to 6 Weeks	Gentle blocking exercises are initiated, with care taken not to apply resistance during flexion while blocking. Instruct the patient in full active wrist flexion and extension Begin passive finger extension with the MCP joints flexed and then progress to stretching and splinting to restore motion if needed Low-intensity ultrasound (3 MHz) is initiated if appropriate
6 to 8 Weeks	The dorsal block splint is discharged unless the patient needs splinting for protection in certain environments. Instruct the patient to use the affected hand for light ADLs but to avoid lifting, gripping, or heavy activities. Begin gentle resistance
8 Weeks	Progress with the strengthening program as needed and tolerated. The patient can begin resisted blocking exercises to increase IP flexion

MCP, Metacarpophalangeal; *IP,* interphalangeal; *DIP,* distal interphalangeal; *FDS,* flexor digitorum superficialis; *FDP,* flexor digitorum profundus; *PIP,* proximal interphalangeal; *ADLs,* activities of daily living.

each week. If the ulnar nerve has been repaired, the MCP joints must be positioned in flexion to prevent hyperextension and clawing of the digits. If the median nerve has been repaired, adding a thumb component to the dorsal block splint is recommended to prevent shortening of the first web space and to maintain abduction.[108] If repairs in zone V are the tendon to tendon type, early active motion can be initiated and can follow the zone II protocol. However, if repairs in zone V are at the musculotendinous junction, active motion should be delayed until 3 to 4 weeks after surgery.

Flexor Pollicis Longus Injuries of the Thumb

Surgical repairs of the FPL tendon can be challenging because the proximal end of the lacerated FPL tendon retracts more proximally than a lacerated digital flexor tendon, which is restrained by its interconnections. Delaying surgery even up to 48 hours can make pulling out the proximal tendon to its original length difficult, because muscle shortening can occur quickly. Unfortunately, increased tension of the FPL tendon from muscle shortening puts the patient at risk of rupturing the tendon and/or of developing thumb IP flexion contractures. Tendon retraction can be addressed during surgery by lengthening the FPL tendon within the muscle with transverse divisions or Z-lengthening of the tendon at the musculotendinous junction, which reduces FPL tension.[109]

Factors that affect the outcome of FPL injuries include retraction of the proximal tendon, the zone of injury, and postoperative management. Patients with proximal stump retraction have a higher incidence of unsatisfactory results. FPL lacerations in zone II can involve the A1 pulley, which is important for FPL function because it prevents the tendon from bow-stringing. Excessive scarring in this area can lead to loss of tendon gliding. A study by Kasashima et al.[110] showed that passive flexion and active extension exercises using rubber band traction significantly reduced the risk of unsatisfactory results in patients with FPL repairs, particularly in those with a zone II laceration or retraction of the proximal tendon stump.

Many of the concepts and methods discussed for post-operative management of finger flexor tendon repairs apply to repairs of the FPL. Therapists and surgeons may use immobilization or EPM or EAM protocols, depending on their experience, preference, the type of repair, and the patient's age and compliance. Splint position and treatment protocols can vary, therefore communication is essential between the surgeon and the therapist.

Young children or patients who are noncompliant may benefit from an immobilization program. Cooperation is reported to be poor in children under 5 years of age, and some advocate immobilizing these injuries in an above the elbow cast (with the wrist and the MCP and IP joints in flexion and the thumb abducted) for 4 to 6 weeks, at which time motion can begin. No significant formation of adhesions was found using this method with this age group.[111] Older children and adults involved in an immobilization program after FPL repair generally are splinted with a forearm-based dorsal protective splint with the wrist in approximately 15° to 25° flexion, the thumb abducted, the CMC joint in 10° flexion, and the MCP joint in 20° to 30° flexion.

The thumb IP joint is in neutral, although this position could vary, depending on the type of repair and the amount of tension on the FPL tendon (Figure 7-57). If tendon shortening occurred or if approximating the tendon ends was difficult, the IP joint may need to be positioned in slight flexion.[107] Patients are immobilized for 4 weeks and then can begin gentle active range of motion exercises.

Proponents of the Kleinert method use rubber band traction to position the thumb in flexion for active extension/passive flexion exercises for the first 3 to 4 weeks before starting active thumb flexion.[110] The modified Duran protocol is also used for FPL repairs, and the patient is instructed to passively flex the thumb and then actively extend to the confines of the dorsal block splint for the first 3 to 4 weeks after surgery. As described earlier, with finger flexor tendon rehabilitation, some protocols treating FPL repairs combine elements of the modified Duran method

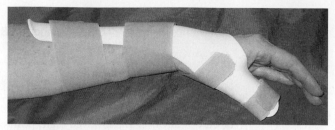

Figure 7-57
Dorsal protective splint for a flexor pollicis longus repair. The wrist is held in flexion, and the thumb is also placed in flexion to protect the healing tendon repair.

with a place and hold component. The Evans MAMTT technique recommends using an active hold component with the thumb positioned in 15° of CMC joint flexion, 45° of MCP joint flexion, and 40° of IP joint flexion with an external force of 15-20 g, measured with a Haldex pinch gauge and string held perpendicular to the thumb.[91] Table 7-10 details the guidelines and most widely used protocols for the postoperative management and rehabilitation of FPL injuries in zones I and II.

Elliot and Southgate[109] have reported an EAM regimen for FPL repairs in zones I and II performed with a four-strand core suture with a Silfverskiöld circumferential suture. They recommended splinting the patient with the wrist in 10° extension and 10° ulnar deviation, the thumb abducted to 30°, the CMC joint flexed to 10°, the MCP joint flexed to 30°, and the IP joint at 0° extension. The patient is positioned in ulnar deviation at the wrist to reduce the turning angle of the FPL as it passes from the carpal tunnel into the thenar muscles. All remaining digits are also strapped into the dorsal hood of the splint with the fingers in neutral. The rationale for splinting the fingers is to prevent inadvertent increased strain on the FPL tendon with free finger motion.[109] This protocol is detailed in Table 7-11.

Extensor Tendon Injuries of the Hand

Extensor tendon rehabilitation involves many of the same concepts that apply to flexor tendon rehabilitation. Communication between the surgeon and the therapist is crucial, and the therapist must have a thorough understanding of the patient's injury and the type of surgical repair performed. Just as flexor tendon management has moved from immobilization toward early passive mobilization and early active mobilization, so has the management of extensor tendons. A variety of early motion protocols have been developed for zones III through VII, including thumb zones T-I to T-III.

The strength of the repaired tendon, the ability of the tendon to glide, and tendon excursion in relation to the position of the wrist all affect the treatment of extensor tendon repairs. The extensor tendon is smaller and flatter than the flexor tendon and therefore is not as suitable for more complicated, multistrand suture techniques. However, some suture techniques have been developed for extensor tendon repairs that allow for early controlled motion.[112]

Table 7-10

Flexor Pollicis Longus Repairs in Zones I and II: Guidelines for Kleinert, Modified Duran, and Place and Hold Programs

Time Frame	Program Considerations
0 to 1 Week	*Splint:* Fabricate a dorsal protective splint: wrist, 15° to 30° flexion; CMC joint, 0° to 10° flexion; MCP joint, 20° to 30° flexion; IP joint, 0° (unless otherwise specified by the physician) to position in flexion *Exercise program:* Begin postoperative day 2 to 5; communicate with surgeon to determine the most appropriate program for the specific patient: • Modified Duran: Begin passive flexion of the IP, MCP, and CMC joints and allow active extension to meet the confines of the splint • Kleinert traction: Begin passive flexion with a rubber band and active extension against the rubber band traction to meet the confines of the splint • PROM and AROM to all noninvolved digits, with care taken not to actively flex the thumb. Instruct the patient to avoid all functional use of the injured thumb at this time (i.e., no lifting or gripping with the noninvolved digits). Instruct the patients to do the exercises frequently (i.e., 10 repetitions every 1 to 2 hours) • Place and hold should begin only with the physician's orders and once edema has diminished and the patient demonstrates good passive thumb flexion. Instruct the patient to place the thumb in limited flexion, exert a minimum amount of tension, and hold the position for 2 to 3 seconds. The degree of restriction of motion may be determined by the surgeon Begin edema management and scar management when the incision has healed
3 to 4 Weeks	Discharge Kleinert rubber band traction unless the patient does not have full passive flexion. Continue with modified Duran exercises. Progress to place and hold with full range of motion Begin active thumb flexion in the splint with caution, because FPL repairs have a higher rate of rupture. The wrist position of the splint may be changed to neutral
4 to 6 Weeks	AROM of the thumb out of the splint, AROM of the wrist No resistance or gripping is allowed; light, functional, nonresistive activity of the thumb is allowed at week 6 Ultrasound can be used at weeks 4 to 6 if indicated Gentle IP joint blocking with no resistance can begin
6 to 8 Weeks	Dorsal block splint is discontinued unless protection is needed in a high risk environment or circumstance Minimal resistance with a soft sponge or putty can begin Light functional use but no forceful pinching or gripping is allowed Progress with strengthening activities over 8 to 12 weeks

CMC, Carpometacarpal; *MCP,* metacarpophalangeal; *IP,* interphalangeal; *FPL,* flexor pollicis longus; *PROM,* passive range of motion; *AROM,* active range of motion.

Factors That Affect the Strength of a Repaired Extensor Tendon

• Ability of the tendon to glide
• Tendon excursion in relation to wrist position
• Wrist position
• Metacarpophalangeal joint position

Studies done by Newport and Tucker[112] have shown that finger extension strength varies significantly, depending on the wrist and MCP joint positions, because of the tenodesis effect the wrist has on the extensor tendons. The extensor tendons have less excursion than the flexor tendons because of the linkage between them known as the *juncturae tendinae.*[112] Evans and Burkhalter[113] have determined that 5 mm of extensor digitorum communis excursion is generated when the MCP joints of the index and middle fingers are flexed to 30° and when the MCP joints of the ring and little fingers are flexed to 40°. This amount of gliding is considered to be sufficient to prevent the formation of adhesions after an extensor tendon repair.[113]

Zones I and II (Mallet Finger Injuries). Mallet finger injuries involve a disruption of the terminal tendon and are treated with immobilization by splinting the DIP joint of the finger in 0° extension. The length of time in the splint depends on the classification of the injury (see previous descriptions of the four types of mallet injuries). Closed mallet injuries without fractures are treated by splinting the DIP joint in extension with a stack splint, a custom-molded thermoplastic splint, or aluminum foam splint. The splint should not interfere with PIP flexion and should be checked regularly to ensure proper positioning, especially if the swelling in the patient's finger is declining. Proper alignment at 0° extension is important because it prevents hyperextension of the DIP joint, which

Table 7-11
Flexor Pollicis Longus Repairs in Zones I and II: Guidelines for the Elliot and Southgate Program[109]

Time Frame	Program Considerations
Week 1	Instruct the patient to actively flex and extend the fingers only 25% of their full motion Limit active flexion of the thumb to touching the tip of the middle finger After 1 week the patient can passively flex the fingers fully
Week 2	Increase finger active range of motion to 50% Limit active flexion of the thumb to touching the tip of the ring finger Begin passive flexion of the thumb
Week 3	Full active range of motion of the fingers is allowed Full active flexion of the thumb is allowed*

*The authors did not discuss resistive activity, strengthening exercises, and functional activity; however, they concluded that the repair they chose was strong enough to allow early active mobilization and to avoid the risk of rupture.

can cause blanching of the dorsal skin and lead to skin necrosis. The patient wears the splint continuously for 6 to 7 weeks, then gentle active range of motion can begin. If an extension lag occurs at the DIP joint, the splint may need to be applied for an additional 2 to 4 weeks. Patients are gradually weaned out of the splint during the day, although they may need to continue with night splinting if a lag persists. Open lacerations to a terminal tendon or those with associated fractures may be repaired and the DIP joint pinned in extension with a K-wire. Patients are instructed in AROM at approximately 6 weeks after surgery but continue to wear a static extension splint for several more weeks between exercises and at night.[114]

Swan neck deformities, which cause hyperextension of the PIP joint with flexion of the DIP joint, can occur if a significant mallet injury goes untreated. This deformity occurs as a result of unopposed tension of the central slip, dorsal migration of the lateral bands, and laxity of the volar plate. Swan neck deformities can be treated with a figure-of-eight splint that allows for PIP flexion but blocks hyperextension of the PIP joint. Splinting helps with functional grasp and prevents the finger from locking in hyperextension, but this is not a long-term or permanent solution for severe deformities, which may require surgical intervention (Figure 7-58).

Figure 7-58

Figure-of-eight splint for a swan neck deformity prevents PIP hyperextension while allowing full PIP and DIP flexion.

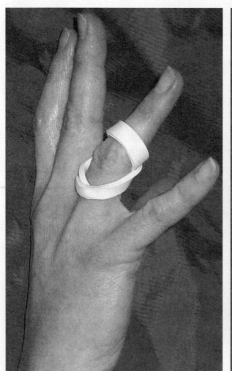
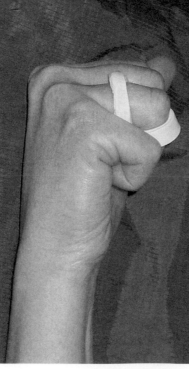

Zones III and IV. Zone III extensor tendon injuries occur at the PIP joint and involve the central slip. Zone IV extensor tendon injuries occur at the level of the proximal phalanx and involve the lateral bands. If these injuries go untreated, a boutonniere deformity can develop, causing flexion of the PIP joint and hyperextension of the DIP joint. Early intervention is important to prevent a flexion contracture of the PIP joint. If a closed rupture has occurred, the recommended course is to splint only the PIP joint in full extension and leave the DIP joint free to move. The patient is instructed to passively and actively flex the DIP joint with the PIP splint on. This allows the lateral bands, which have migrated anteriorly, to return to their proper anatomical position and also assists the central slip in moving distally to heal in the correct position. Closed boutonniere injuries are splinted anywhere from 2 to 6 weeks, depending on the severity of the injury. Patients should be checked frequently and should be instructed to remove the splint to perform gentle active range of motion, with active-assistive extension exercises. Passive PIP joint flexion should be avoided for 6 weeks. The patient may be weaned out of the splint gradually, to wearing it at night as needed.[114]

Complete extensor tendon lacerations in zones III and IV are treated with surgical intervention. Postoperative treatment consists of immobilization (Table 7-12), early controlled motion (Table 7-13), or EAM protocols.

Immobilization After Extensor Tendon Repair. Immobilization is considered the "safest" treatment because it limits motion altogether, thereby minimizing tension on the repaired tendon; however, it unfortunately leads to adhesion formation, loss of joint flexion, and extensor tendon lag. Despite these disadvantages, immobilization

programs may be most appropriate for young children or for patients who are unable to comply with early controlled motion methods.[112]

Effect of Immobilization on a Repaired Extensor Tendon

- Limit movement
- Lead to the formation of adhesions
- Decrease joint tension on the tendon
- Lead to extensor tendon lag

Early Controlled Motion After Extensor Tendon Repair. Early controlled motion (ECM) programs that incorporate various combinations of dynamic splinting and tendon gliding, when used after extensor tendon repair, have resulted in significant improvements in the outcome of these injuries. ECM programs for extensor tendon repairs limit active flexion but allow passive extension of the digit, provided by rubber band traction attached to an outrigger (Figure 7-59). Based on the same rationale as that for flexor tendon studies, controlled stress combined with early motion has been shown to have a positive outcome on the healing extensor tendon.[115] Studies have shown that the protocol presented in Table 7-13, using a hand-based dynamic splint with early controlled motion for repairs in zones III and IV, provides excellent results with fewer treatment visits and a shorter duration of treatment.[116,117]

Extensor tendon repairs in zones III and IV can also be treated with a dynamic extension assist splint with a spring coil, referred to as a modified Wynn Parry splint or Capener

Table 7-12
Extensor Tendon Repairs in Zones III and IV: Immobilization Protocol

Time Frame	Program Considerations
0 to 1 Week	*Splint:* PIP joint in 0° extension; if only zone III was repaired, leave the MCP and DIP joints free If zone IV repair or lateral bands were involved, include the DIP joint in the splint at 0° extension for 4 to 6 weeks. *Exercise program:* Begin 10 to 14 days after repair. If zone III was repaired, instruct the patient to actively flex the DIP joint every 2 hours Manage edema
3 to 6 Weeks	Isometric extensor exercises can begin with the splint on; continue with DIP flexion exercises At weeks 4 to 6, remove the splint to begin gentle AROM exercises (hook and composite fist) but instruct the patient to wear the splint between exercise sessions Begin scar management if needed
6 to 8 Weeks	Progress with gentle AROM and AAROM to increase flexion; progress to gentle flexion exercises Incorporate a dynamic flexion splint, if needed, and alternate with the extension splint Begin resistive activity and progress as needed

PIP, Proximal interphalangeal; *MCP,* metacarpophalangeal; *DIP,* distal interphalangeal; *AROM,* active range of motion; *AAROM,* active-assisted range of motion.

Table 7-13
Extensor Tendon Repairs in Zones III and IV: Early Controlled Motion with Dynamic Splinting

Time Frame	Program Considerations
0 to 1 Week	*Splint:* • Fabricate a dorsal hand-based splint with the wrist free, the MCP joint in 0° to 20° flexion (surgeon's preference), and a Velcro strap around the proximal phalanx • Apply dynamic traction to hold the PIP joint in 0° extension or slight hyperextension (surgeon's preference). The DIP joint is left free • Apply a stop bead to the dynamic traction to limit PIP flexion (which is determined by surgeon) (Figure 7-59) *Exercise program:* • Allow the patient to actively flex the PIP joint against the rubber band traction, with limited flexion because of the stop bead (generally 30° if the repair is strong) and with passive extension back to neutral through dynamic traction • Zone III repairs: If the patient is reliable, in the clinic the therapist can remove the strap around the proximal phalanx and perform limited MCP flexion with the PIP joint held in 0° extension • Active DIP flexion can be performed with the PIP joint positioned or held in 0° extension. Begin edema management if indicated • Week 2: With the physician's approval, adjust the stop bead to allow 40° of active PIP joint flexion. Continue with active flexion, passive extension, and previous exercises Begin scar management when incision heals
3 Weeks	With the surgeon's approval, adjust the stop bead to allow 50° of active PIP flexion. Continue with previous exercises
4 to 6 Weeks	Discharge dynamic traction. Instruct the patient to begin active extension and full active flexion exercises (composite fist, hook fist). Educate the patient about light use of the hand for functional, nonresistive, light tasks at week 6 Begin blocking exercises to increase PIP flexion. Continue use of the static extension splint at night and for protection between exercises if needed
6 to 8 Weeks	Begin PROM or dynamic flexion splinting or strap to increase flexion only if no extensor lag is present. Continue use of the night extension splint if needed Begin resistive flexion exercises and progress with strengthening program

MCP, Metacarpophalangeal; *PIP,* proximal interphalangeal; *DIP,* distal interphalangeal; *PROM,* passive range of motion.

splint. The advantages of this splint are that it is finger based and low profile, and it allows the MCP joint to be free.[118] The disadvantages are that it requires a longer splinting period before AROM out of the splint begins; it can be difficult to fit, especially if edema is present; it can cause pressure sores; and the duration of the treatment is longer than with dynamic splinting.

Early Active Motion for a Zone III Extensor Tendon Repair. Evans and Thompson[119] have defined the parameters for an early active SAM protocol for a repaired central slip. The patient begins controlled active finger extension and limited flexion within 24 to 48 hours immediately after surgery. These researchers showed that 30° of PIP active motion allows 3.75 mm of extensor digitorum

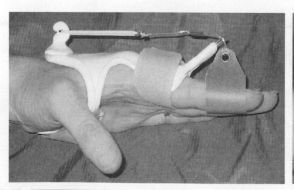
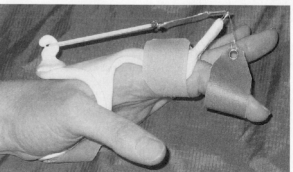

Figure 7-59
Hand-based dynamic extension splint for extensor tendon repairs in zones III and IV.

communis (EDC) excursion. This provides enough gliding to allow healing but prevents the formation of adhesions in zones III and IV. The patient is splinted with the PIP and DIP joints in 0° extension and wears the splint at all times except when exercising. The patient uses two other static volar splints for an exercise program. One splint limits PIP flexion to 30° and DIP flexion to 20° to 25°. The patient is allowed to perform active extension of the digit and then flexes to meet the splint, but the MCP joint must be positioned in 0° extension and the wrist in 30° flexion. The second exercise splint positions the PIP joint in extension and allows DIP flexion. If the lateral bands have been repaired, DIP flexion is limited to 30°; if the lateral bands are not involved, the DIP is allowed to flex fully. The patient is instructed to perform each exercise 20 times every hour.[119,120]

Two weeks after surgery, if no extensor lag is present, the exercise splint that limits PIP flexion is adjusted to limit PIP flexion to 40°; 3 weeks after surgery, it can be adjusted to 50°; by the end of the fourth week, it can be adjusted up to 70° to 80° of PIP flexion if no extension lag exists. Patients can begin composite flexion exercises and gentle strengthening at 5 weeks after surgery, and some are discharged at 6 weeks after surgery. If the PIP joint is stiff, intermittent flexion splinting is recommended at approximately 4 weeks, alternating with night static extension splinting, which may need to continue for 5 to 6 weeks after surgery.[119,120] Evans[91] also recommended the MAMTT technique combined with dynamic splinting for more proximal extensor tendon zones.

Early Protected Motion with Passive Flexion.
Crosby and Wehbe[121] advocate an early protected motion program that combines dynamic splinting with early passive flexion. This method is recommended for extensor tendon repairs in zones III to VII and all thumb zones (T-I to T-III), as well as in zones VI and VII. Their study includes incomplete, complete, and complex extensor tendon lacerations. Surgical repairs were performed with mattress, figure-of-eight, or modified Kessler sutures, depending on the level of repair and the thickness of the tendon. Repairs in zones III and IV were treated with a dorsal hand-based dynamic splint with the MCP joint at 0° extension and the PIP joint held in 0° extension with traction from the splint. Some patients were allowed to flex the PIP joint with no limitations in the splint. In other patients, PIP flexion was limited with a block, as determined by the surgeon based on the integrity and status of the repair. Patients were instructed to perform, on an hourly basis, active hook fisting within the confines of the splint, allowing the dynamic traction to passively extend the finger back to extension.[121]

This protocol introduced the concept of tendon mobilization, performed by the clinician, which involves holding the affected digit and the wrist in maximum extension while passively ranging only one joint at a time. The PIP joint is passively flexed to its specified block while the MCP and DIP joints and the wrist are all held in maximum extension. If there is no flexion block, the clinician applies gentle gradual force until full range of motion is obtained or until resistance or pain is encountered.[121]

Dynamic splinting and tendon mobilization are initiated 1 to 5 days after surgery. After 4 weeks, the patient is instructed in AROM and tendon gliding exercises and weaned out of the splint over a few days. If an extension lag is present, the patient uses a static volar splint for extension. After removal of the splint, the patient begins a gentle, graded strengthening program. Grip and pinch strength are measured at 8 weeks after surgery with a Jamar Dynamometer and pinch meter. A flexion strap is used at 8 weeks if IP flexion is limited.[121]

This method is used with extensor tendon repairs performed in zones V through VII. These patients are splinted with a dorsal forearm-based dynamic splint that positions the wrist in 20° extension and holds the MCP joints at 0° extension with dynamic traction. The use and degree of MCP joint flexion blocks are determined at the time of surgery, depending on the strength of the repair and how well the tendon is able to glide without tension. These zones are also treated with an early protected mobilization program, and excellent to good results have been reported.[121]

Zones V to VIII
Immobilization Program. Zone V involves the area over the MCP joint, and zone VI is located over the dorsal aspect of the metacarpals. Zones VII and VIII, which are found at the extensor retinaculum and the musculotendinous junction, often are associated with scar adhesions that lead to extrinsic tightness and loss of finger flexion. Debate exists over whether patients treated with immobilization in zones V to VIII may not do as well as with early controlled motion, resulting in extensor tendon lag and limited flexion. Proponents of immobilization programs for extensor tendon zones V to VIII report that equally good functional results can be achieved using static splints that are simpler, less labor intensive, and less expensive than programs that use dynamic splinting.[122] Many experts seem to agree that immobilization methods may be indicated for young children or noncompliant patients.

The position for immobilization depends on the level and complexity of the injury and whether other associated structures have been involved. The patient generally is splinted with the wrist in 30° extension and the MCP joints in 20° to 30° flexion. The IP joints may be included at neutral or left free to move. Patients who are allowed to actively flex and extend the IP joints without compromising the repair do better than patients whose IP joints are splinted.[122] Three to 4 weeks after surgery, the patient can remove the splint only for gentle AROM exercises, with the wrist extended during finger flexion and care taken to avoid full wrist and finger composite flexion. Tenodesis exercises for the wrist can begin 4 to 6 weeks after surgery, with composite AROM of the wrist and fingers at 6 weeks after surgery. Gentle passive finger flexion can be initiated at 4 to 6 weeks after surgery, or gentle dynamic splinting alternating with extension splinting may be used if needed. A gentle strengthening program can begin at 6 weeks and progress to 8 weeks after surgery.[120]

Early Controlled Motion. Early motion protocols consisting of dynamic splinting and tendon gliding have become widely accepted and successful in treating zones V to VIII (Table 7-14). Protocols for treatment vary, depending on the position of the wrist and the MCP joints; they also may be determined by the surgeon at the time of surgery based on the status of the repair. More proximal zones often can tolerate more composite flexion within the confines of the dynamic splint, especially if the wrist is extended beyond 20° extension (Figure 7-60). However, excessive wrist extension may cause the extensors to buckle in the more proximal zones and interfere with tendon gliding.[112]

Chow et al.[115] presented a study of early controlled motion for extensor zones IV through VII. They used a dorsal forearm-based splint with dynamic traction to passively extend the MCP joint to 0° extension, allowed limited MCP flexion, and provided unrestricted active flexion of the PIP and DIP joints. During the first week after surgery, the MCP joint of the involved finger was allowed to flex to 30°; during the second week, this was increased to 45°; during the third week, to 60°; and during the fourth and fifth weeks, full flexion was allowed with the splint on. Patients were instructed to actively flex within the confines of the splint 10 times every hour. The splint was discontinued by the end of the fifth week, and AROM out of the splint was initiated. Resistive exercises and strength were not discussed in this study, but patients had no restrictions after 8 weeks.[115]

Table 7-14
Extensor Tendon Repairs in Zones V to VIII: Early Controlled Motion with Dynamic Splinting

Time Frame	Program Considerations
0 to 1 Week	*Splint:* • Fabricate a dorsal forearm-based dynamic splint with the wrist in 20° extension and the MCP joints in 0° to 20° flexion (depending on the surgeon's preference and the repair performed) • The surgeon may order a MCP flexion block, or the MCP joint may be allowed to flex fully. The IP joints may be unrestricted, or the surgeon may request that loops from dynamic traction support them in neutral position. Adjacent fingers may or may not be included, depending on the level and location of the injury • Some surgeons may request a separate volar resting splint that blocks MCP flexion and supports the IP joints in extension. This splint is worn with the dorsal dynamic splint for exercises (Figure 7-60) • Some patients may find sleeping while wearing the dorsal forearm-based dynamic splint difficult; these patients may benefit from wearing a volar static resting splint at night, which positions the wrist and fingers in extension. (The IP joints may or may not be included in the splint, depending on the repair zone and the surgeon's orders) *Exercise program:* • Begin active MCP flexion within the confines of the splint with passive MCP extension through the dynamic traction of the splint. If loops are not restricting IP motion, the patient is instructed to perform active flexion and extension of the PIP and DIP joints in the splint (i.e., active hook fisting) 10 times every hour Begin edema management
2 to 3 Weeks	Continue with the previous exercises. The therapist can begin gentle passive IP flexion with the MCP joints and wrist in extension Begin scar management when appropriate
4 to 6 Weeks	The patient can begin AROM and tendon gliding out of the splint, taking care with full composite wrist and finger flexion. Instruct the patient to keep the wrist extended with gentle finger flexion The patient can also begin tenodesis wrist and finger motion. Continue use of the night static extension splint if extension lag is present. Gradually wean the patient out of the dynamic extension splint for daytime
6 to 8 Weeks	Full wrist and finger composite flexion and extension can performed. The patient should wean out of the dynamic splint and continue with a night static splint if needed Instruct the patient in gentle PROM exercises. A dynamic flexion splint or strap can be used if flexion is limited Begin a gentle strengthening program and progress as needed. No restrictions are necessary after 10 to 12 weeks

MCP, Metacarpophalangeal; *IP,* interphalangeal; *PIP,* proximal interphalangeal; *DIP,* distal interphalangeal; *AROM,* active range of motion; *PROM,* passive range of motion.

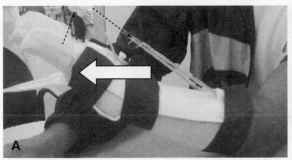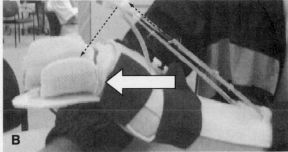

Figure 7-60

A, Dynamic forearm-based extension splint with elastic band assistance for passive finger extension. **B,** This splint allows active MCP flexion into a volar resting splint, blocking MCP flexion to approximately 30° for zone V extensor tendon repairs in the index, long, ring, and little fingers. The injuries, caused by a table saw accident, required open reduction and internal fixation of metacarpal fractures in the index, ring, and long fingers. The PIP and DIP joints are held in extension in finger troughs, which are attached to the elastics by opaque fishing line *(dotted lines and arrows)*.

Some protocols advocate positioning the MCP joint in 0° extension, whereas others suggest blocking the MCP joints at 5° to 10° flexion to prevent hyperextension and extensor activity, which has been detected through electromyographical (EMG) studies when the extensor tendons are at rest in 0° extension.[112] Active MCP flexion may also be limited with early motion protocols, depending on the repair and the ability of the tendon to glide freely.[121]

Immediate Controlled Active Motion for Zones IV to VII After Extensor Tendon Repair. Early mobilization programs vary among clinicians, surgeons, and clinics, depending on their experience level, the patient's presentation, and the extent of the injury. Just as there are trends toward early active flexion with flexor tendon rehabilitation, a trend has arisen for early active extension after extensor tendon repairs.

Immediate controlled active motion (ICAM) has been used to treat extensor tendon repairs in zones IV to VII. Howell et al.[123] designed an EAM program that consists of three phases and uses a low profile, two-part splint. The patient wears two static splints. One is a static volar wrist cock-up splint that positions the wrist in 20° to 25° extension. The second splint, called the ICAM yoke splint, links the injured digit to the noninjured digits to unload the repair and harness extension forces during active motion. The yoke is positioned across the proximal phalanges of the fingers and allows active flexion and extension of the fingers but positions the involved MCP joint in 15° to 20° more extension relative to the uninjured MCP joints (Figure 7-61).[123] The EAM program consists of three phases (Table 7-15). The authors had a 30% noncompliance rate, but they did not know of any complications or ruptured tendons. 140 patients completed the program. Categorization of an excellent outcome was based on the occurrence of no extensor lag or loss of terminal flexion. Of the 140 patients, 81% of the patients had no extensor lag and 79% of the patients had no loss of terminal flexion. The timing of strengthening and resistive exercises was not discussed, but grip strength was reported to be 85% of the opposite, uninjured hand at the time of discharge, which averaged 7 weeks after surgery.[123]

Rehabilitation of the Extensor Pollicis Longus in the Thumb

Immobilization Program After Extensor Pollicis Longus Tendon Repair. EPL tendon repairs can be treated with immobilization or early controlled motion programs. Treatment programs vary, depending on the level of injury, the clinician's expertise, and the individual patient. Injuries in zone T-I are referred to as a *mallet thumb* and can be treated by splinting the IP joint of the thumb in 0° extension for 6 to 8 weeks for a closed injury or 5 to 6 weeks for an open repair. Gentle AROM can begin after the immobilization period, using caution if an extensor lag is present, and the patient continues to wear a static extension splint between exercises and at night. Patients can progress in active IP joint flexion slowly and begin resistive exercises at 6 to 8 weeks.[120]

Zone T-II injuries are also treated by immobilizing the MCP and IP joints in 0° extension in a hand-based splint with the thumb in radial extension. Limited active range of motion begins at 3 to 4 weeks, and over the next 3 weeks, the patient can increase joint motion gradually. If an extension lag is present, an extension splint should be used. Patients should use the splint for protection between exercises for a total of 6 weeks.[120]

EPL repairs in zones T-III and T-IV are treated by splinting the thumb MCP joint at 0° extension and slight abduction with the wrist in 30° extension for 3 to 4 weeks before starting AROM exercises. The MCP joint may become restricted from hyperextension or from prolonged splinting in extension, requiring dynamic flexion splinting at 4 to 6 weeks. Injuries in zone V are susceptible to the

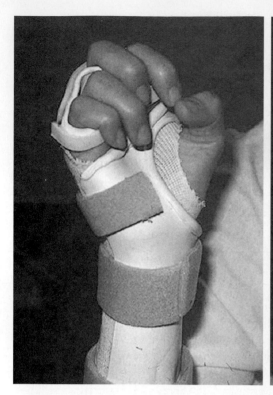
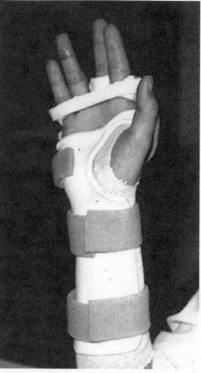

Figure 7-61

Splinting for immediate controlled active motion. (From Howell JW, Merritt WH, Robinson SJ: Immediate controlled active motion following zone 4-7 extensor tendon repair, *J Hand Ther* 18:185, 2005.)

Table 7-15

Extensor Tendon Repairs in Zones IV to VIII: Immediate Controlled Active Motion

Time Frame	Program Considerations
Phase 1 (0 to 21 days)	Within 48 to 72 hours after surgery, splints are fabricated and the ICAM program begins The patient begins full active composite finger flexion and extension within the confines of the splint The splint must be worn at all times The patient is instructed in edema and scar management
Phase 2 (22 to 35 days)	Before the patient can begin phase 2, full active motion must be achieved within the limits of the ICAM splint. The patient continues to wear the ICAM yoke splint, but the wrist splint is removed to begin AROM exercises to the wrist with the finger held in a relaxed position The patient is instructed to wear the wrist splint and yoke if doing medium to heavy activity. If no extension lag is present, the patient progresses to wrist flexion with finger fisting in the yoke and wrist extension with finger extension Once the wrist is moving freely, the patient can discontinue the wrist splint for light tasks but should be instructed to wear the wrist splint and yoke if performing medium to heavy tasks
Phase 3 (36 to 49 days)	The wrist splint is discharged To prepare the patient for yoke-off activity, the yoke is removed for AROM of the digits The finger yoke or a buddy strap is worn during activities Full composite wrist and finger flexion and extension without the splints should be achieved during phase 3

ICAM, Immediate controlled active motion; *AROM,* active range of motion.

formation of dense adhesions, which can limit the excursion of the EPL at the retinacular level. Extension contractures of the thumb MCP joint, thumb web space contracture, and restrictions in the joint capsule and on tendon gliding are all problems that can occur at this level with immobilization.[120]

Immobilization programs can result in loss of thumb motion after repair of the EPL tendon. Scar tissue causes the extensor tendon to adhere to bone or skin. In addition, the scar tissue causes a thickening of the dorsal joint capsule. Even if no actual injury has occurred to the dorsal joint capsule, it can play a role in the loss of motion at these levels.

The potential for loss of IP joint motion is greatest for zone T-I injuries, and loss of MCP joint motion is greatest for zone T-III injuries, which can be caused by tendon tethering. Scar tethering of the small branches of the superficial radial nerve of the thumb not only results in loss of thumb IP motion, but also can cause dorsal thumb pain.[109]

Early Mobilization Programs After Extensor Pollicis Longus Tendon Repair. Early mobilization programs have been designed to reduce the potential for loss of thumb motion caused by scar formation and decreased tendon gliding. Most early mobilization programs used to treat EPL tendon repairs involve the use of a dynamic extension splint that allows for active flexion and provides passive extension of the thumb to neutral. This splint is used for approximately 4 weeks and then can be removed so that the patient can begin AROM out of the splint. Graded strengthening exercises begin at 6 to 8 weeks after surgery, and a static extension splint may be necessary if an extensor lag is present. The amount of active thumb IP or MCP flexion may be determined at the time of surgery and may depend on the level of injury. Protocols can vary among clinicians, surgeons, and clinics, depending on the surgical repair, the clinician's experience, and the patient's presentation.

Elliot and Southgate[109] have described an early mobilization program for EPL repairs in zones T-I to T-IV that allows the IP joint to be free in zones T-II to T-IV and to partly flex in zone T-I. Patients underwent primary repair, and splinting and exercises began 3 to 4 days after surgery using the protocol (Table 7-16).[109]

Early Active Motion to Zones T-IV to T-V After Extensor Tendon Repair. For extensor tendon repairs in zones T-IV and T-V, Evans[120] described the use of a dorsal forearm-based dynamic extension splint and a volar component that supports the MCP joint in neutral and the wrist in extension, with a cutaway at the IP joint that enables the dynamic traction to support it in neutral (0° extension) but allows the IP joint to flex only 60°. She added the component of active hold (MAMTT), which is done after protected passive exercise. The patient's wrist is placed in 20° flexion while the CMC, MCP, and IP joints are held in extension, and the patient is asked to gently maintain this position. The patient can come out of the splint for exercises during the third and fourth weeks but continues to wear the splint for protection. Composite thumb flexion and opposition exercises are initiated by the fifth week, and resistive exercises can begin at 6 to 8 weeks.[120]

Specific Injuries of the Wrist
Radial Fractures
General Considerations
Distal radial fractures account for about 17% of all fractures treated in the emergency department. In the United States, 1 person in 500 is treated each year for a distal radial fracture. These also are the most common physeal fractures in children. There is a bimodal preponderance of immature patients with physeal injuries and older patients with osteoporotic bone (6 to 10 and 60 to 69 years of age).[124]

The alignment requirements for a good functional outcome are still the subject of controversy for the fracture named after Abraham Colles, who said, "[despite] the distortion...the limb will at some remote period again enjoy perfect freedom in all its motions and be completely exempt from pain.It is remarkable that this common fracture remains one of the most challenging of all fractures [with] no consensus regarding description, outcome, or treatment."[126]

Anatomy
The distal radius consists of two intra-articular surfaces with three concave facets. The resting plateau for the carpal bones is the radiocarpal joint, which consists of two concave surfaces, the scaphoid and lunate fossae (Figure 7-62). The scaphoid fossa is a concave triangular space with the radial styloid as its apex. A ridge running dorsally to palmarly separates it from the lunate fossa. The lunate fossa is concave in both dorsal to palmar and radial to ulnar directions, making it more of a quadrangular space than the scaphoid fossa. The lunate therefore is nearly always congruently aligned within the joint, unlike the scaphoid, which can easily become incongruent within its fossa when it is rotated out of position.

The second intra-articular component, which is often overlooked in the evaluation of distal radial fractures, is the distal radioulnar joint. It consists of a concave fossa, the sigmoid notch, which has well-defined distal, dorsal, and palmar margins. This joint allows the radius, along with the attached hand, to rotate about the stationary ulnar head in pronation and supination.

Injury Classification
Any classification system ought to accomplish several tasks. It should make organizing data and communicating the information to other health care providers simple; in addition, it should provide insight into the treatment of and prognosis for the injury. At best, the system enables the user to better understand the injury by clearly explaining the mechanism, graphically depicting the fracture fragments, or revealing the concomitant injuries.

Over the years, multiple systems have been devised to categorize wrist fractures. Some are based on historical eponyms (a person's name), others on the mechanism of injury, and still others on the number of fracture fragments and the location of the fracture. Many of these systems remain in use today, and each has its strengths and weaknesses. Although it is tempting to choose one that works well, clinicians should examine and develop an understanding of several to gain the knowledge that each imparts.

Of all the fracture classification systems, those based on eponyms impart the least insight; they require the health care provider to memorize a fracture pattern and assign a name to

Table 7-16
Extensor Pollicis Longus Repairs in Zones T-I to T-IV: Early Controlled Motion with Dynamic Splinting

Time Frame	Program Considerations
0 to 1 Week	*Splint*: • Zones T-II to T-IV are splinted with a forearm-based dynamic extension splint with the wrist in 30° extension and the thumb MCP joint held in neutral by the dynamic traction with the loop supporting the proximal phalanx. The IP joint is free to move. Only partial MCP flexion is allowed in the splint • Zone I is splinted in the same way except the traction loop should support the IP joint in neutral; it also should restrict full IP active flexion slightly but allow passive extension of the MCP and IP joints with dynamic traction *Exercise program:* • Injuries in zones II through IV allow partial MCP active flexion with the IP joint held in extension within the confines of the splint. Full MCP flexion is restricted for the first 2 weeks. The dynamic traction passively extends the MCP joint back to neutral. Instruct the patient to perform exercises 10 times every hour • Also instruct the patient to manually support the MCP joint in neutral and actively flex and extend the IP joint of the thumb 10 times every hour • Rehabilitation of zone I repairs follows the same regimen of active MCP flexion except that the patient is allowed only slight flexion of the IP joint Begin edema management
2 Weeks	Patients with repairs in zones II through IV are allowed to synchronously flex both the MCP and IP joints of the thumb in the splint to oppose the tip of the middle finger. Patients with a zone I repair do the same, but full IP flexion is restricted Continue previous exercises Begin scar management if needed
3 Weeks	Patients with repairs in zones II through IV are allowed to flex and oppose the thumb MCP and IP joints in the splint to oppose the tip of the ring finger The regimen for zone I repairs is the same, although with limited IP flexion
4 to 5 Weeks	Patients with repairs in zones II through IV are allowed to flex and oppose the thumb MCP and IP joints in the splint to the base of the little finger. The regimen for zone I repairs is the same, although with the IP joint restricted from full flexion The splint is worn at all times until the end of the fourth week. The patient then can begin AROM of the MCP and IP joints out of the splint Ultrasound is initiated at 4 weeks if needed The patient can wear the splint only for protection during the fifth and sixth weeks at night and in crowded places
6 to 12 Weeks	PROM can begin at 7 weeks. Begin gentle resistive flexion exercises and progress to 8 weeks. Patients can return to driving at 8 weeks No restrictions are necessary at 12 weeks

MCP, Metacarpophalangeal; *IP*, interphalangeal; *AROM*, active range of motion; *PROM*, passive range of motion.

it. Frequently, misnamed by the casual user, the systems impart limited information as to prognosis and treatment.

The most common eponyms used to describe distal radial fractures are Colles' fracture, Barton's fracture, Smith's fracture, and Chauffeur's fracture. Colles' fracture is a transverse metaphyseal fracture with dorsal comminution that results in radial shortening, dorsal tilt, and loss of radial height. Classically it does not enter the radiocarpal joint but may enter the distal radioulnar joint. Barton's fracture is a shear-type fracture that involves either the volar or dorsal rim of the radius. Smith described three fractures that are in essence either Colles' or Barton's fractures.

Archetype classification systems work by organizing known fracture patterns from simple into more intricate models with a concomitantly worse prognosis and more complex treatment algorithms. The Frykman classification system is an excellent example.[127] This system, which was based on biomechanical and clinical studies, was presented in 1967 (Figure 7-63). It distinguishes between extra-articular radial fractures and three types of intra-articular radial fractures (radiocarpal, distal radioulnar, and radiocarpal–distal radioulnar fractures). This leads to four possible fracture patterns; however, each pattern is further differentiated based on whether the ulnar styloid is also fractured. The fractures get more intricate as the system progresses from type I to type VIII, with worsening prognoses. The strength of this system is that it reveals multiple intra-articular fracture patterns and the importance of the ulnar

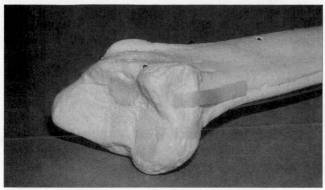

Figure 7-62
Model of the distal radius showing both the distal radioulnar joint and the radiocarpal joint. The radiocarpal joint has a fossa for the lunate and one for the scaphoid.

styloid (and ulnar carpal ligaments) to the prognosis for the injury. Its weakness lies in the fact that not all fractures within one class behave the same way. In other words, the treatment and prognosis for a minimally displaced intra-articular fracture of the radiocarpal joint are very different from the treatment and prognosis for a fracture in the same location that is massively comminuted and displaced.

Melone's classification system,[128] introduced in 1984, identifies four possible major fracture fragments of the radius: the radial styloid, the radial shaft, and the medial aspect of the radius (the lunate facet), which frequently is split coronally into two fragments (Figure 7-64). Fractures can have one component or all four, and they become more complex and worsen prognostically as the number of fragments increases. This system of categorizing complex fractures has regained popularity with the advent of newer, more aggressive open fixation techniques. Its strength lies in its accurate depiction of complex fracture patterns and

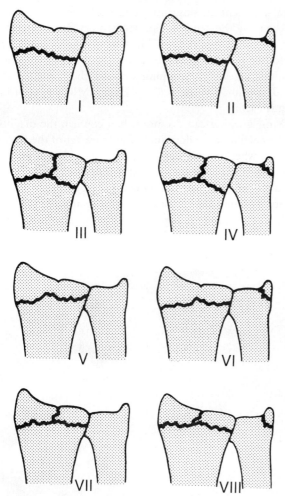

Figure 7-63
Frykman classification of distal radial fractures: types I to VIII. The higher numbers in the classification system indicate a poorer prognosis. (From Fernandez DL, Wolfe SW: Distal radius fractures. In Green DP, Hotchkiss RN, Pederson WC, Wolfe SW, editors: *Green's operative hand surgery*, ed 5, Philadelphia, 2005, Churchill Livingstone.)

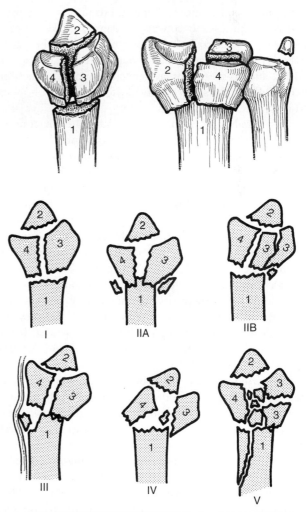

Figure 7-64
Melone's classification of distal radial fractures. (From Fernandez DL, Wolfe SW: Distal radius fractures. In Green DP, Hotchkiss RN, Pederson WC, Wolfe SW, editors: *Green's operative hand surgery*, ed 5, Philadelphia, 2005, Churchill Livingstone.)

its emphasis on the lunate facet fragments, which affect the distal radioulnar articulation and therefore subsequently affect forearm rotation.

Fernandez[129] described a fracture classification system based on the mechanism of the injury. This system links the pattern of the break to the forces that caused it to occur. For instance, a shearing mechanism results in an unstable, oblique fracture off the volar or dorsal rim of the radius that requires open reduction and internal fixation. Although this system can be cumbersome, it relates the force that caused the injury to the relative stability of the fracture and makes treatment recommendations. This train of thought should start the clinician thinking about what other soft tissue injuries occurred with the osseous insult that will affect the overall outcome for the patient.

Diagnosis

The diagnosis of wrist fractures begins with a careful history to discover the mechanism of damage to the bone and the surrounding soft tissue envelope and to uncover any previous wrist injuries and concurrent damage. Likewise, it is important to get to know some things about the patient that will help determine the approach to this specific wound and to treatment in general. Important questions include: What does the patient do for work and hobbies? Which is the dominant hand? Does the patient live alone or with family and friends? What other health concerns does the patient have that may affect treatment?

The physical examination is conducted not only on the fractured wrist but on the entire upper extremity and any other body part the patient may have injured. Special consideration is warranted with patients who have fallen without an obvious reason (e.g., they can not remember slipping on ice or tripping). This should alert the examiner to the fact that the patient may have passed out briefly because of cardiac or neurological reasons that require further workup. Patients often are not forthcoming with this information. For them, it is a momentary blank out of memory, often filled in with the assumption that they simply tripped over something but cannot recall what it was. At this point, it is frequently helpful to note whether anyone else witnessed the injury.

The extremity then should be gently examined to evaluate the skin integrity, the overall alignment of the hand on the forearm, and the amount of swelling and discoloration. All these factors give insight into the amount of energy absorbed by the soft tissue and bone as a result of the trauma. Vascular and neurological examinations need to be performed carefully to verify brisk capillary refill in each digit and subjectively normal sensation. Wrist fractures have been known to cause injury to the median nerve or to worsen or create carpal tunnel syndrome. This possibility should be carefully evaluated. Tendon function for the digital flexors and extensors should be checked as well. The patient may be reluctant to move the digits, because the

gliding of the tendons past the injury zone is painful; however, the clinician must remember that tendon rupture can occur even with nondisplaced fractures, especially rupture of the long extensor to the thumb.[130] Displaced wrist fractures frequently have a similar appearance. The classic "silver (or dinner) fork" deformity has been used to describe the dorsal tilt created by the fracture. In addition, the clinician might note the loss of normal ulnar deviation of the hand at rest and a slightly pronated position of the hand on the forearm compared to the opposite side. If the swelling is not substantial, the distal ulna will look much more prominent, because the radius has shortened and the ulna has not (Figure 7-65). Gentle palpation causes pain at the fracture site, and a palpable area of cortical incongruity and crepitus often is noted.

Imaging of the wrist usually confirms the diagnosis. Plain x-ray films taken in at least two planes, AP and lateral, should show most fractures. Oblique views can show additional fragments. Special x-ray views have been created to highlight joint incongruity, and these can be useful in determining the need for operative intervention. Occasionally, x-ray films are not sufficient to find an occult fracture or to depict the damage of a complex fracture accurately. In these cases, CT scanning can aid the clinician. If an occult fracture is suspected, a CT scan, MRI study, or bone scan is useful.

X-ray imaging can do more than confirm the diagnosis. The x-ray films help determine the character of the fracture, such as whether it is displaced or nondisplaced, stable or unstable, intra-articular or extra-articular; and, if intra-articular, whether joint alignment is acceptable or a incongruity is present that must be managed surgically. Determination of all these factors leads to the proper treatment.

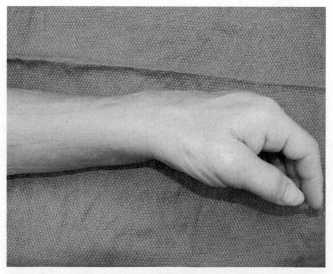

Figure 7-65

Displaced distal radial fracture with a classic "silver fork" deformity. Note the pronation and dorsal angulation of the hand on the forearm.

Medical Treatment

Wrist fractures range from stable and nondisplaced to intra-articular, displaced, comminuted injuries. The treatment modalities chosen must reflect this continuum, as well as consider the patient's requirements of the hand and the skill of the surgeon and rehabilitation team.

Myriad treatment options are available for distal radial fractures. Splinting and casting, percutaneous pinning with x-ray or arthroscopically assisted reduction, external fixation, and internal fixation with plates or fragment-specific fixation devices are all currently in use. Recent advances in fragment-specific fixation and plate design, with the introduction of locking plates, has allowed hand surgeons to surgically repair extremely comminuted fractures in which such repair might not have been previously attempted.

When the clinician is deciding among this variety of options, clearly experience, preference, and the availability of equipment have an impact; however, certain principles guide treatment. The clinician must first determine whether the fracture is acceptably aligned. Knirk and Jupiter[131] showed that 90% of patients who had a healed intra-articular distal radial fracture with greater than 1 mm of stepoff went on to have symptomatic arthritis in the radiocarpal joint.[131] Multiple studies of extra-articular fractures have been done to determine the biomechanical changes that result from displacement. One study found that a 12° loss of palmar tilt increases the ulnar load by 35%.[132] Another study showed that a loss in radial length of 2.5 mm increases the load on the ulna by almost 45%.[133] Increased ulnar loading is presumed to lead to an increased incidence of ulnar-sided wrist pain. Other effects of radial malunion include secondary midcarpal alignment changes and the possibility of early onset of degenerative joint changes in both the radiocarpal and distal radioulnar joints.[134]

If the fracture currently is acceptably aligned, the clinician must try to determine whether it is likely to stay in that satisfactory position as it heals. Good epidemiological studies are available describing what usually constitutes a stable fracture. The amount of displacement and comminution of the fracture and the patient's age are excellent predictors of subsequent redisplacement despite what initially might be a perfect closed reduction.[135–137]

If an injury requires operative intervention, either to prevent loss of reduction or to treat bony incongruence that cannot be resolved by closed methods, the surgeon must choose the method of treatment. Surgeons must have in their arsenal as many tactics or techniques as possible from which to choose. The surgeon must perform the appropriate surgery for the fracture *and the patient* to obtain the best outcome.

Pin Fixation. Pin fixation is percutaneous surgery that requires no dissection and causes very little additional soft tissue swelling. It relies on relatively good bone to hold the fixation around the pins and cannot correct extensively comminuted intra-articular fractures, nor can it reliably correct all of the volar tilt. This technique is most useful in older patients with shortened, dorsally tilted, minimally comminuted fractures, because it holds better than a cast and does not require formal surgical dissection. Pin fixation also is very useful in young patients with open growth plates who require reduction. With careful application of the pins, the growth plate can be avoided, and the small amount of volar tilt correction can usually be counted on to remodel with normal bone growth over time. Intrafocal dorsal pin application corrects length and volar tilt, and the addition of supplemental radial styloid K-wires provides stability. Pins require casting for supplemental stability, therefore motion cannot begin for 6 weeks or longer until the bone unites and the cast is removed. Pins are easily removed in the office and leave little scarring (Figure 7-66).

External Fixation. External fixation is a technique that uses ligamentotaxis to pull the fracture fragments into better alignment. The surgeon dissects and drills threaded pins into the radius proximal to the fracture and into the index finger metacarpal distal to the fracture and spanning the carpal joint. The surgeon attaches to these pins a mechanical frame with gears, which can be used to apply traction in different directions to pull on the hand to reduce the fracture fragments. Still a popular technique, it recently has begun to fall out of favor among hand surgeons as improved internal fixation technologies have become available. It still has a variety of indications that make it the procedure of choice. For fractures with extensive bone disruption, plate application may not be possible. Also, crush injuries may damage the soft tissue envelope such that the surgeon does not want to dissect extensively to apply a plate and screws to obtain rigid fixation. In this case, an external fixator is the ideal choice. Finger motion should be started early, because a potential drawback of the technique is stiff fingers as a result of overdistraction with the device. However, wrist motion must wait for removal of the device.

Internal Fixation. Internal fixation with a single locking plate and screws or with multiple small fragment-specific fixation components has been the most recent advance in the treatment of distal radial fractures. Previous attempts to apply plates to the distal radius had not been entirely successful because of the poor quality of the distal bone and the subsequent inability of the screws to obtain purchase and any type of holding strength. The new designs have successfully addressed these concerns and enabled anatomical repair of markedly comminuted unstable fractures in a stable configuration. The techniques differ in dissection and complexity, with the locking plate being far simpler to apply. However, in some instances the single locking plate will not obtain anatomical fixation of the joint surface, and the individual fracture fragments need to be addressed and repaired with the fragment-specific

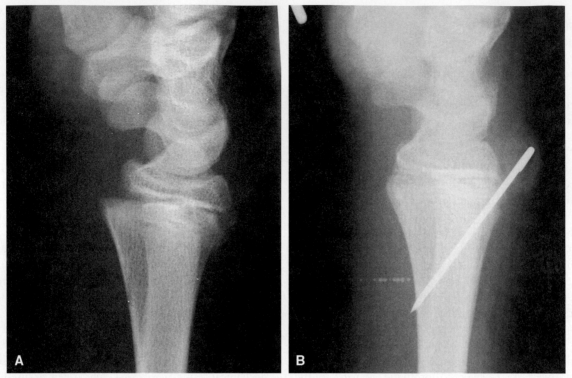

Figure 7-66

A, X-ray film of a displaced Salter II fracture. **B**, The fracture was treated with closed reduction and percutaneous pin fixation. The pin avoids the growth plate but helps maintain alignment while healing occurs in a cast over a few weeks.

technique. These approaches require a surgeon who is experienced and comfortable with operating around the wrist. They should result in a stable reduction that allows motion in the early postoperative period. Ideally, because both the dissection and the initial injury will cause scarring, aggressive therapy to obtain mobility should be started in the first 7 to 10 days (Figures 7-67 and 7-68).

As the operative techniques evolve, so must the rehabilitation protocols. New expectations for recovery of function in these injuries are being developed. Along the way, pitfalls and setbacks undoubtedly will be encountered and must be overcome. Hand surgeons and therapists must work more closely than ever to accomplish these tasks.

Scaphoid Fractures

General Considerations

Fractures of the carpal bones are relatively common injuries, and scaphoid fractures are the most common, accounting for nearly 80% of all wrist bone injuries.[138] The mechanism usually is a fall onto an outstretched hand (FOOSH injury), which creates a forced dorsiflexion of the wrist. The injured person may not have much pain, thinking the injury is little more then a sprain. Frequently little swelling or ecchymosis is present except in the anatomical snuffbox. Young men are the most frequently affected. The injury can be associated with ligamentous injuries of the wrist, particularly scapholunate dissociations[139] or perilunate dislocations.[138]

Anatomy

The carpus consists of eight bones that are best thought of biomechanically as existing in two rows. The scaphoid traverses and links the two rows. This unique feature makes fractures of the scaphoid particularly important, because the injury in essence unlinks the two rows, allowing them to function independently. It has been shown that, over time, chronic scaphoid fracture nonunions produce arthritis of the wrist in a reproducible and predictable pattern.[140,141]

The scaphoid is the most mobile bone in the wrist, bridging the midcarpal joint and providing three planes of motion. It is subject to the same deforming forces that cross the midcarpal joint, which in the fractured state causes the distal pole to flex with the distal carpal row, whereas the proximal pole tends to extend with the lunate and triquetrum. This creates foreshortening of the bone and the "humpback," or flexion, deformity. Simulated wrist motion has shown that healing of a 5° flexion deformity of the scaphoid leads to a 24% loss of wrist extension.[142]

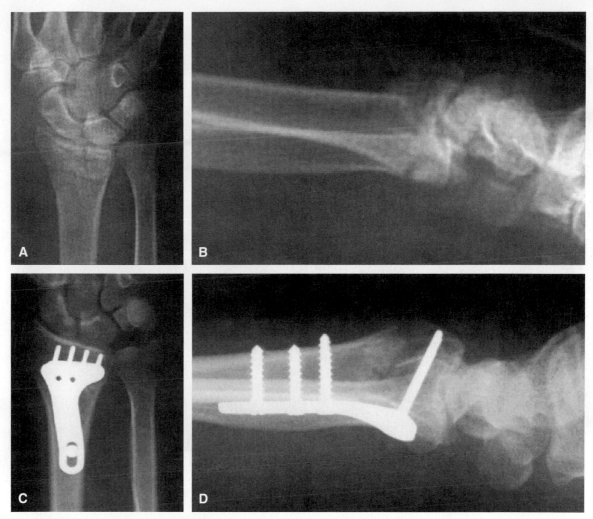

Figure 7-67

A and **B**, Comminuted intra-articular radial fracture. **C** and **D**, The fracture is repaired with a fixed-angle locking plate.

The shape of the scaphoid is complex, and its orientation makes visualizing fracture lines with plain x-ray films difficult. The bone is described in thirds: the distal tubercle; the midportion, or waist; and the proximal pole. The scaphoid has multiple ligamentous attachments, both intrinsic (within the carpus) and extrinsic (between the radius or metacarpals and carpus). The scaphoid is nearly entirely covered with articular cartilage, which means that few areas are available for vessels to enter the bone. The blood supply is quite tenuous, which directly affects the bone's ability to heal. The scaphoid receives blood through a set of dorsal and volar arteries. The most important of these is the scaphoid branches of the radial artery, which enter the bone dorsally through foramina at the scaphoid waist. These dorsal ridge vessels supply blood to the proximal half of the bone. Because they enter the waist or distal third of the scaphoid, retrograde flow is required for blood to reach the proximal portions of the bone. This means that the proximal one third of the scaphoid is analogous to the femoral head or the talus in that it has little or no direct vascular input and it receives its blood through intraosseous flow. A fracture that displaces the waist or especially the proximal pole can disrupt this blood supply and prevent fracture healing or cause avascular necrosis of the proximal portion of the bone. The second group of vessels arises from the palmar branches of the radial artery and enters the distal end of the scaphoid. The scaphoid tubercle and the distal 20% to 30% of the bone are perfused by this arterial leash. The increased supply of blood at the distal pole of the scaphoid helps account for its more rapid fracture healing (Figure 7-69).

Injury Classification

The Russe classification system[143] is relatively straightforward and is based on the relationship of the fracture line to the long axis of the scaphoid bone. The horizontal

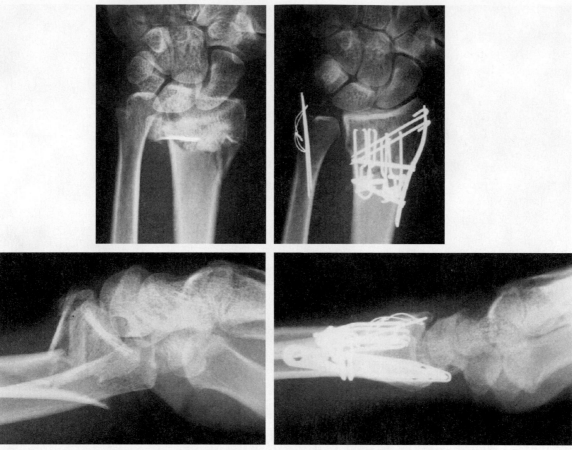

Figure 7-68

Complex intra-articular distal radial fracture. The fracture is treated with fragment-specific fixation. Anatomical restoration can be obtained, but this technique requires more extensive dissection than the fixed angle volar plate.

Figure 7-69

Blood supply to the scaphoid bone.

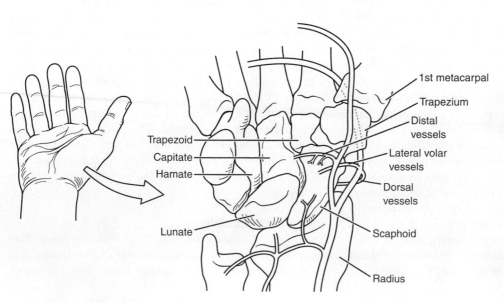

oblique and transverse fracture types are considered stable and are not expected to displace with immobilization. The third type, the vertical oblique fracture, is considered far more unstable and requires longer immobilization with a higher potential for late instability.

Critical Elements in the Classification of a Scaphoid Fracture

- Location of the fracture
- Chronicity of the fracture
- Type of fracture (i.e., displaced or nondisplaced)
- Fracture pattern (i.e., stable or unstable)

The Herbert classification[144] is a more complex alphanumeric system that rates the injury based on fracture anatomy, stability, and history (e.g., delayed union, fibrous union). By combining these several factors, a prognostic grade can be assigned to each injury.

Diagnosis

Scaphoid fractures can easily be missed, often with serious consequences; therefore it is imperative that clinicians have a high index of suspicion for this fracture in making the diagnosis. The patient's age (the fracture is uncommon in very young patients) and the mechanism of trauma should alert the clinician to the possibility the injury exists. Any tenderness on careful examination at the anatomical snuffbox should be presumed to indicate a scaphoid fracture until proven otherwise.

Radiographic imaging is the mainstay in confirming the diagnosis. However, plain films frequently can fail to detect acute nondisplaced fractures. Initial x-ray films should include a posteroanterior (PA) view, a PA view with ulnar deviation to extend the bone in a plane more parallel with the x-ray film, and lateral and oblique views (Figure 7-70). If the clinical examination leads to a high level of suspicion for a fracture but the plain films are negative, the patient should be treated with cast immobilization and the plain films repeated in 2 to 3 weeks. At that time, resorption of bone around the fracture line may be sufficient to allow positive identification of the injury on plain x-ray films. If not, a bone scan is a good alternative to screen for a possible occult fracture. If an urgent need exists to rule out the fracture before 2 to 3 weeks has elapsed (e.g., professional athletes), imaging with MRI or a thin slice CT scan can be performed. The cost of these imaging modalities may make them prohibitive for routine applications.

CT scanning gives the highest resolution images of the bone and the trabeculae and is very useful for evaluating the healing of treated fractures. It frequently is used after surgery or cast immobilization to confirm that bridging trabeculae are crossing the fracture site, indicating healing. In chronic nonunion, CT scanning is useful preoperatively to plan for bone grafting of deformities that are frequently encountered.

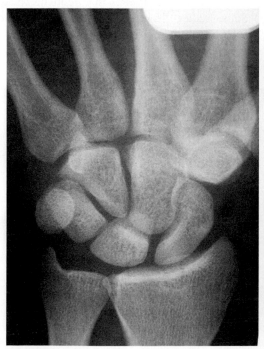 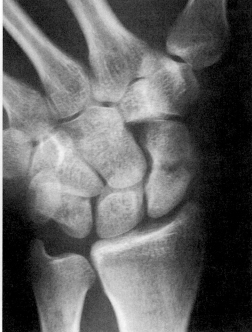

Figure 7-70
An AP x-ray film may fail to show a scaphoid fracture. Ulnar deviation extends the bone and may help reveal the fracture.

MRI does not depict the cortical bone well, but it gives an excellent image of the cancellous bone. It is both a highly sensitive and specific method of detecting occult scaphoid fractures. It also is the best means of evaluating the blood supply to the proximal pole of the scaphoid if avascular necrosis is suspected.

Medical Treatment

For an acute, nondisplaced scaphoid fracture, treatment traditionally has consisted of cast immobilization. Healing time depends on the level of the fracture; distal fractures heal most quickly, and those that are most proximal take longest. Proximal fractures sometimes require 3 to 6 months of immobilization to heal, whereas fractures of the distal third generally heal in 6 to 8 weeks. Studies have shown a slightly faster time to union if the initial casting done is above the elbow for the first several weeks.[145]

More recent techniques have become available that allow limited incision or even percutaneous compression screw placement in the scaphoid (Figure 7-71), which can obviate the need for prolonged cast immobilization while the fracture heals.[146] This has the obvious benefit of returning patients to work or sports much more quickly.

In one study in which 12 athletes were treated for minimally displaced or nondisplaced fractures, the average time for return to sports was within 6 weeks. One fracture in the study failed to unite.[147]

Fractures that are unstable and/or displaced are associated with a nonunion rate of 50% and an avascular necrosis rate of 55%; these fractures therefore need to be treated operatively.[148,149] Displacement (and subsequent instability) is considered present if a gap greater than 1 mm is present at any point along the fracture; if the scapholunate

angle exceeds 60°; or if the radiolunate angle is greater then 15°.[150] If the fracture is acute and does not require bone grafting, a limited approach (i.e., manipulation of the fragments into alignment and placement of a compression screw) can be used. However, if the fracture requires bone grafting or cannot be manipulated into alignment, a more traditional open reduction and internal fixation should be performed. For waist and midthird fractures, a volar approach generally is favored (Figure 7-72). With proximal third fractures, a dorsal approach allows the screw to be placed for optimum compression of the small proximal fragment.[151]

Nonunions of the scaphoid that have not progressed to arthritis and do not require any type of salvage surgery require operative treatment to create a bony union. The fracture needs to be opened, bone grafted, and then rigidly fixed so that it can heal.[152,153] With fractures of the proximal third of the scaphoid or if sclerosis of the proximal pole of the bone is seen on plain x-ray films, the surgeon must consider that the blood supply to the proximal fracture fragment may have been disrupted. A preoperative MRI scan should help determine whether this is the case (Figure 7-73). If in fact the bone is avascular, a vascularized bone grafting procedure may be chosen in an effort to increase the likelihood of successful union.[154,155] This procedure is more technically demanding than traditional fracture repair. A dorsal approach is used, and a segment of bone with its intact blood vessel is elevated from the radius and directly inserted into the scaphoid.

The treatment of scaphoid fractures that have gone unrecognized is a problem that frequently plagues clinicians. Some studies[156] have suggested that a scaphoid fracture that is left untreated for longer then 4 weeks is at increased risk

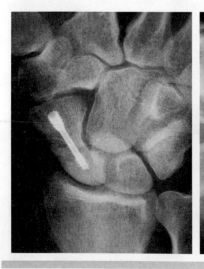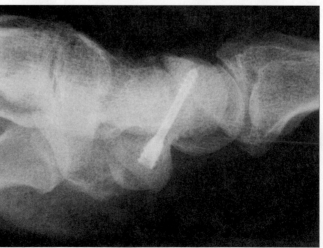

Figure 7-71
Percutaneous compression screw fixation of a scaphoid fracture. This allows early removal from a cast and return to function.

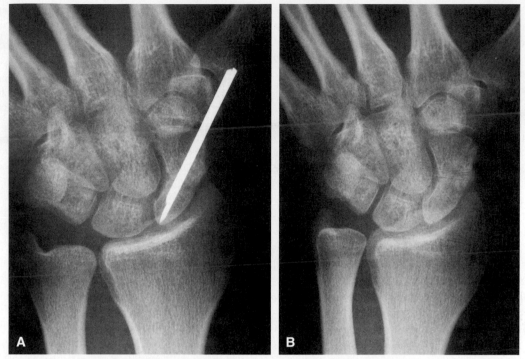

Figure 7-72
A, AP x-ray films of a chronic scaphoid nonunion that was treated with bone grafting and pins. **B**, After the fracture healed, the pins were removed.

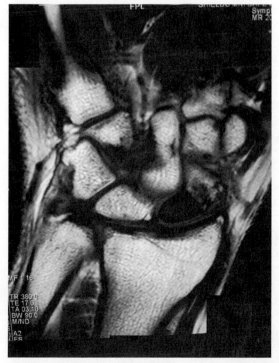

Figure 7-73
MRI scan of the scaphoid showing avascular changes in the proximal pole.

of nonunion. For this reason, fractures of the scaphoid that are delayed in coming to treatment should be considered more readily for operative repair.[156]

Triangular Fibrocartilage Complex Injuries

General Considerations

A common problem clinicians encounter in patients is ulnar-sided wrist pain. Previously considered the "low back pain" of the upper extremity, this is an area of exciting new developments and understanding. Although still a significant diagnostic challenge, a better understanding of the anatomy and biomechanics of the ulnar side of the wrist has enabled clinicians to more accurately screen and treat patients with injuries that previously might have meant vocational retraining or limited sports activity.

The triangular fibrocartilage complex (TFCC) is one of several structures on the ulnar side of the wrist that can be injured, leading to debilitating pain and mechanical changes. Discussion of the more than three dozen recognized causes of ulnar-sided wrist pain is beyond the scope of this text. However, by understanding the function and pathology of the TFCC, the clinician can develop an appreciation of one common cause of ulnar-sided wrist pain and gain knowledge of some of the other structures in which injury can lead to pathology on the ulnar side of the wrist.

Anatomy

The TFCC is described as a composite of ligaments and fibrocartilage that originates from the ulnar border of the distal radius at the articular surface. It inserts onto the base of the ulnar styloid and the fovea of the ulnar head.[157] This horizontal portion, considered the TFCC, or the articular disc proper, is fibrocartilagenous and relatively avascular. The periphery of this horizontal portion is composed of highly vascular ligaments, both dorsally and volarly, that connect the distal radius and ulna. These radioulnar ligaments are oriented perpendicular to the long axis of the forearm. In contrast with this are additional ligaments still considered part of the TFCC that arise from the base of the ulnar styloid to insert on the lunate, triquetrum, hamate, and base of the fifth metacarpal (Figure 7-74).[158] The distinct anatomical structures composed of differing biomaterial and oriented in several planes should alert the reader that the TFCC is both complex and multifunctional.

As the forearm moves through pronation and supination, the TFCC ligaments stabilize the distal radioulnar joint. As it arcs over the ulna in pronation, the radius becomes shorter relative to the ulna, resulting in positive ulnar variance. While in supination the radius is out at its maximum length relative to the ulna, resulting in a relative negative ulnar variance. These changes in relative ulnar height in relation to the carpus produce significant changes in the load borne by the TFCC.[159–166]

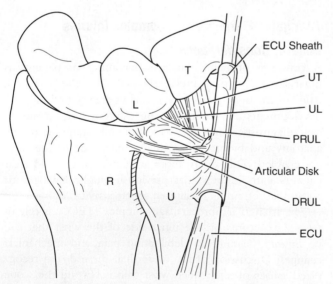

Figure 7-74

Ulnocarpal joint and TFCC, triquetrum *(T),* lunate *(L),* ulna *(U),* radius *(R),* extensor carpi ulnaris *(ECU),* dorsal radioulnar ligament *(DRUL),* ulnotriquetral ligament *(UT),* palmar radioulnar ligament *(PRUL)* and ulnolunate ligament *(UL).* The volar radioulnar ligament and ulnar collateral ligaments are not shown. (From Trumble TE, Budoff JE, Cornwall R: *Hand, elbow and shoulder: core knowledge in orthopaedics,* Philadelphia, 2006, Mosby.)

Major Roles of the Triangular Fibrocartilage Complex

- The triangular fibrocartilage complex (TFCC) creates a shock absorber for the ulnar carpus. The ulnar side of the lunate and the triquetrum do not articulate with the ulna, as the scaphoid and lunate do with the radius. The TFCC transfers about 20% of the axial load between the hand and the forearm.
- The dorsal and volar radioulnar ligaments are the primary stabilizers of the distal radioulnar joint. This arrangement allows stable pronation and supination of the forearm. The ligaments become taut at the end range of rotation in either direction.
- The ligaments that arise from the ulna and insert onto the lunate, triquetrum, hamate, and fifth metacarpal serve as stabilizers for the ulnar carpus. Their function is similar to that of the extrinsic wrist ligaments on the radial side of the wrist.

Injury Classification

In 1989 a classification system was devised that described TFCC lesions based on the mechanism of injury, the location of the injury, and the involvement of surrounding structures. This system is widely accepted as the standard for describing these injuries.[167]

Lesions of the TFCC are divided into two major types, traumatic and degenerative (Table 7-17). Traumatic (type I) lesions have four subtypes based on the location of the injury in the TFCC. Degenerative lesions are the result of chronic loading on the ulnar side of the wrist (ulnar carpal impaction syndrome). This leads to destruction of the TFCC and surrounding structures. These lesions therefore are subclassified by the extent of injury to the surrounding bones and ligaments.

Table 7-17

Classification of Triangular Fibrocartilage Complex (TFCC) Tears

Type	Subclassification
Type I: Traumatic	IA: Central perforation IB: Ulnar avulsion (with or without a styloid fracture) IC: Volar tear ID: Radial avulsion
Type II: Degenerative	IIA: TFCC wear IIB: TFCC wear plus lunate or ulnar articular wear (chondromalacia) IIC: TFCC perforation plus lunate or ulnar chondromalacia IID: TFCC perforation plus chondromalacia plus LT ligament tear IIE: TFCC perforation, chondromalacia, lunotriquetral ligament tear, and ulnocarpal arthritis

Classification of Traumatic Lesions of the Triangular Fibrocartilage Complex

- *Type IA* lesions consist of a perforation of the horizontal portion of the triangular fibrocartilage complex (TFCC) in its avascular region. The tear usually is 1 to 2 mm wide, anterior to dorsal in orientation, and about 3 mm ulnar to the radial side attachment of the TFCC proper. These lesions cause mechanical pain on the ulnar side of the wrist but are not usually associated with instability (Figure 7-75).
- *Type IB* tears represent injury to the dorsal aspect of the TFCC or its insertion into the ulna. These tears may be accompanied by an ulnar styloid fracture, and they are frequently seen with displaced distal radial fractures. Type IB lesions can cause instability at the distal radioulnar joint.
- *Type IC* injuries are tears of the anterior aspect of the TFCC at its periphery. The lesion often occurs with avulsion of the attachment of the TFCC to the lunate or the triquetrum. This can result in ulnocarpal instability, which is manifested as palmar translocation of the ulnar carpus.
- *Type ID* lesions are traumatic avulsions of the ligament proper from its origin at the radius just distal to the sigmoid notch (Figure 7-76).

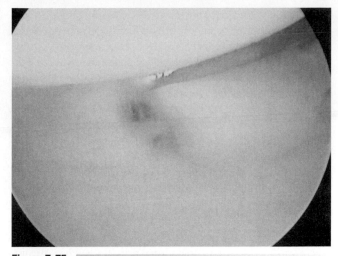

Figure 7-75

Arthroscopic view of a type IA tear in the TFCC (indicated by the probe).

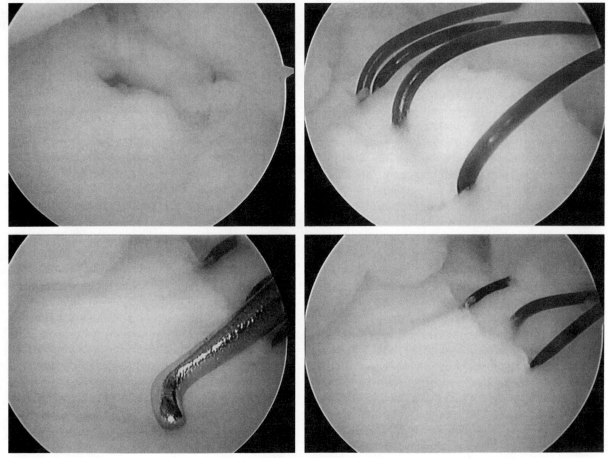

Figure 7-76

Peripheral TFCC tear (i.e., type ID lesion). Tears such as this cause instability and require fixation, which can be done arthroscopically.

Diagnosis

Patients often are seen months after the initial symptoms started. They frequently cannot remember any specific trauma. When an injury is recalled, it is regularly a fall onto a pronated and outstretched hand or a traction or rotation injury. The authors have treated several patients injured by rotating power tools that became bound and forcibly rotated the forearm. They also have treated several golfers who injured the nondominant wrist when they inadvertently struck a tree root or made a deep divot.

Patients generally complain of ulnar-sided wrist pain, although not all can readily localize the pain to the ulnar side of the wrist without the prompting of an examination. Clicking and mechanical symptoms are sometimes encountered but are not nearly as reliably as pain. The symptoms seem most evident with rotational activities such as turning a key or the steering wheel of a car.

Pain can be elicited in the ulnar-sided snuffbox, the space just beyond the distal ulna between the extensor carpi ulnaris (ECU) and FCU tendons. This is a sensitive area to palpate, and the patient's opposite wrist should be used for comparison. The **TFCC load test** is used to detect ulnocarpal abutment or TFCC tears. It is performed by ulnarly deviating and axially loading the wrist while rotating the forearm. A positive test elicits pain, clicking, or crepitus.[168] The **ulnomeniscal dorsal glide test** increases the motion between the ulna, the TFCC, and the triquetrum to elicit symptoms. The examiner places the thumb of the right hand on the dorsum of the right ulnar head of the patient; the radial aspect of the examiner's right index finger PIP joint then rests on the patient's pisiform. The examiner compresses the pisotriquetral joint dorsally while pushing the ulnar head volarly by reproducing a key pinch maneuver. This increases the stress on the TFCC and ulnocarpal ligaments and should produce pain if a lesion or laxity is present in this region.[169] Evaluation of the distal radioulnar joint for laxity may reveal torn ligaments of the TFCC. This can be accomplished by moving/gliding the distal ulna head while stabilizing the radius in neutral rotation, pronation, and supination and comparing the findings to those of the patient's opposite wrist.

Imaging studies should always be part of the workup of ulnar-sided wrist pain. These begin with a series of plain x-ray films, including a PA and a gripping PA view taken in neutral rotation, as well as lateral views. These films aid the evaluation for distal radioulnar joint arthritis, ulnar variance, lesions consistent with ulnar abutment syndrome, ulnar styloid fractures, and wrist instability consistent with intrinsic ligament lesions.

However useful x-ray films are, they fail to visualize the ligaments of the wrist. Therefore other diagnostic imaging modalities are used if questions remain as to the diagnosis of the patient's ulnar-sided wrist pain. Wrist arthrography is useful for assessing the integrity of the TFCC complex and the other intrinsic ligaments of the wrist, including the lunotriquetral joint. Arthrography is accomplished by injecting dye into the radiocarpal joint and radiographically looking for leaks of the contrast material into the other compartments of the wrist, each of which should be watertight. If no contrast is seen to leak, the examination is repeated by injecting dye into the distal radioulnar joint and then the midcarpal joint and looking for dye leaking back into the radiocarpal joint. This three-phase arthrogram is more sensitive than a single phase study for detecting small ligament tears (Figure 7-77).

MRI, both with and without arthrographic dye injection, has also been used to visualize the ligaments of the wrist, including the TFCC. It has proven to be a highly sensitive modality, with up to 95% correlation with arthroscopic findings when positive.[170] However, it is not as useful in patients in which the MRI is found to be normal. In this case, Skahen et al.[171] found its sensitivity to be 44% and the specificity only 75%. These same authors found that the clinical examination could be more sensitive than MRI, with up to a 95% correlation with arthroscopic findings. Therefore a patient with a strongly positive clinical examination should not be assumed to have an intact ligament if the MRI is normal. As the clinician gains more experience and confidence in wrist examination, the need for MRI for correlation diminishes.

Medical Treatment

The treatment of acute TFCC lesions initially is conservative. Long arm cast immobilization is used if the patient does not have a fracture of the ulnar styloid or instability

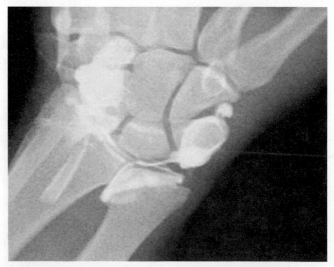

Figure 7-77

Arthrogram showing dye leaking between the radiocarpal joint and the distal radioulnar joint, an indication of a TFCC tear.

of the distal radioulnar joint. If the tear is peripheral and acute, the highly vascular tissue is likely to scar together over a 4- to 6-week period. If the tear is more central, it is not expected to heal, although the synovitis associated with it may diminish and the symptoms of wrist pain may abate. Central tears do not cause instability and only require treatment if they are painful. Patients who present acutely but have instability of the distal radioulnar joint should undergo ligament repair.

When conservative treatment fails or a patient presents months after the onset of injury, arthroscopic evaluation is the gold standard for diagnosis of TFCC pathology. This modality also affords the possibility of treatment. Open treatment of TFCC tears is possible but creates more scarring postoperatively, and visualization of the ligament structure may not be as good as can be obtained arthroscopically.

Central (type IA) tears of the TFCC do not cause instability as long as the outer third of the TFCC remains intact. In patients with ulnar neutral or negative variance, debridement of the central tear to a stable rim of tissue (leaving at least 2 mm of the volar and dorsal ligaments of the TFCC) should resolve the pain. Several studies have shown that with ulnar positive variance, simple ligament debridement will fail to give long-term pain relief in many patients, and the procedure should be combined with ulnar recession either in the form of a wafer-type procedure or formal ulnar shortening.[172,173] Postoperatively, no immobilization is required, and patients are encouraged to begin using the hand and wrist immediately. Pain relief is fairly rapid, usually within a few weeks.

Peripheral TFCC tears can cause instability and a change in the load distribution between the hand and the forearm. These injuries need to be repaired to restore normal mechanics and reduce pain. TFCC tears can be best visualized through the arthroscope. Small instruments are used to remove inflamed synovium and scar and debride torn ligaments to fresh, healing tissue. Also, sutures are placed arthroscopically in one of several described methods to recreate the preinjury anatomy (see Figure 7-76). In the case of ID-type tears in which the ligament is avulsed from the radius, sutures are passed through drill holes made in the radius to reattach the TFCC to its point of origin. IC-type tears can be difficult to repair arthroscopically and may require a small open incision to safely place sutures. After suture repair of a peripheral TFCC lesion, patients are immobilized for the first 3 to 4 weeks in a long arm cast, followed by a well-molded short arm cast that limits forearm rotation for an additional 2 to 3 weeks. Pain relief is not as rapid as it is with treatment of IA-type tears. Immobilization can lead to stiffness and loss of strength, which respond well to therapy. Studies show that 95% of patients who undergo surgery for a torn TFCC return to work and sports, and grip strength can be expected to return to 85% of normal.[173]

Scapholunate Dissociation

General Considerations

Instability of the scaphoid and lunate secondary to a traumatic ligamentous disruption has been described many times, beginning with Vaughan-Jackson and Russell in 1949.[174,175] The characteristic symptoms of pain, clicking, and loss of motion at the radioscaphoid joint, along with the radiographic findings of scaphoid flexion, pronation, and lunate extension, have been well documented. Despite this, patients frequently fail to be diagnosed with this injury until months or often years after the onset. This can have unfortunate consequences in that the instability, given enough time, causes arthritic changes. This has been clearly borne out in the hand literature and is referred to as **scapholunate advanced collapse**.[176,177] With an understanding of the relevant anatomy, common mechanisms of injury, and clinical signs and symptoms, clinicians can be more prepared to make the diagnosis in patients at an earlier stage, perhaps preventing or at least delaying the onset of painful arthrosis of the wrist.

Anatomy

The wrist joint is made up of eight bones, best thought of biomechanically to exist in two rows. The lunate is located in the center of the proximal carpal row and articulates distally with the capitate, which is in the center of the distal carpal row. The scaphoid bone articulates with the radial side of the lunate and is the single bone in the wrist that bridges the proximal and distal rows. Both scaphoid and lunate bones move on the radius in their respective fossae. What is important to note is that the lunate fossa has a spherical shape, and the scaphoid has an elliptical shape.

The ligaments of the wrist are considered intrinsic ligaments if they both begin and end on carpal bones. In contrast, extrinsic wrist ligaments attach on one side to the carpal bone and on the other side to the radius, the ulna, or one of the metacarpal bones of the hand. The scapholunate ligament complex is thought to have both intrinsic and extrinsic components.

The intrinsic portion of the complex consists of the scapholunate interosseous ligament, which connects the radial side of the lunate to the ulnar side of the scaphoid. It is composed of three distinct regions. The thick dorsal portion is the strongest and is composed of short transverse fibers that are biomechanically the most important for stability. The proximal section is composed primarily of fibrocartilage and is the least important stabilizer of the three sections. The volar ligament is thinner than the dorsal ligament, and consists of obliquely oriented fibers that allow some movement to account for the differences in the arcs of motion between the scaphoid and lunate. Isolated cutting of the scapholunate ligament in cadaver models has not caused instability patterns that mimic those seen clinically, which has lead clinicians to believe that more than an isolated injury to the intrinsic ligament is needed to produce a scapholunate dissociation.[178]

The extrinsic portion of the scapholunate ligament complex is made up of ligaments that originate from the radius and insert on various carpal bones. The radioscaphocapitate (RSC) ligament extends from the radial styloid through a small groove on the volar aspect of the scaphoid to insert onto the palmar portion of the capitate. It serves as a rotational fulcrum around which the scaphoid can revolve. The long radiolunate ligament runs parallel and just ulnar to the RSC ligament from the radius to the volar radial portion of the lunate. The short radiolunate ligament originates from the palmar portion of the radius and inserts onto the palmar portion of the lunate. Both the intrinsic and extrinsic ligaments described can be partly visualized during routine wrist arthroscopy.

On the dorsal surface of the wrist capsule are some thickenings considered to be ligamentous that provide additional stability to the wrist; these are not easily seen during routine wrist arthroscopy. The dorsal radiocarpal (DRC) ligament originates on the dorsal radial portion of the radius and runs ulnarly and distally to insert onto the lunate, lunotriquetral ligament, and dorsal portion of the triquetrum. The dorsal intercarpal (DIC) ligament originates from the triquetrum and runs radially and distally to insert onto the lunate, scaphoid, and dorsal aspect of the trapezium (Figure 7-78).

The importance of understanding the complexity of the extrinsic ligaments is twofold. First, these ligaments are used or reconstructed in the soft tissue operations that have been developed to treat scapholunate dissociation injuries. Second, some have reported that injury to the extrinsic ligaments is required to produce the radiographic results seen clinically in patients with scapholunate dissociation patterns.[179]

Injury Classification

Classification of scapholunate dissociative injuries can be based on several factors: the time since the injury, the presence or absence of radiographic abnormalities, the extent of ligamentous disruption, and the presence of additional carpal abnormalities or arthritic changes.

Injuries sustained within 6 weeks of diagnosis are classified as acute. Those that have happened beyond 6 weeks but before degenerative changes in the wrist have occurred are considered to be subacute. After degenerative changes have taken place within the wrist, the injury is best thought of as chronic and the treatment options differ considerably.

The chronic condition of scapholunate dissociation is referred to as **scapholunate advanced collapse,** or a **SLAC wrist.** It is a progression of arthrosis that occurs in the wrist because of the scapholunate instability and rotatory subluxation of the scaphoid. The arthritic changes begin at the radial styloid and progress into the radioscaphoid articulation. Over time, the midcarpal joints become arthritic, specifically in the scaphocapitate and lunocapitate joints. The radiolunate joint is spared in all but the most severe cases of pancarpal arthritis.

The injury is also classified according to whether it is apparent on x-ray films at rest or requires some provocative maneuver. With a less severe ligament injury, a stress x-ray

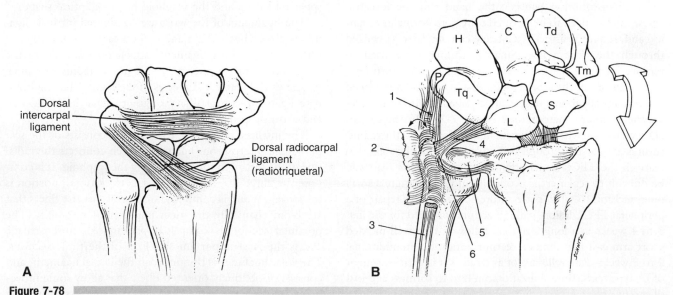

Figure 7-78

A, Dorsal aspect of the wrist. **B,** Volar aspect of the wrist. *1,* Ulnar collateral ligament; *2,* retinacular sheath; *3,* tendon of extensor carpi ulnaris; *4,* ulnolunate ligament; *5,* triangular fibro-cartilage; *6,* ulnocarpal meniscus homologue; *7,* palmar radioscaphoid lunate ligament. *P,* Pisiform; *H,* hamate; *C,* capitate; *Td,* trapezoid; *Tm,* trapezium; *Tq,* triquetrum; *L,* lunate; *S,* scaphoid. (From Fess E, Gettle K, Philips C, Janson J: *Hand and upper extremity splinting principles and methods,* ed 3, St Louis, 2005, Mosby.)

film is required to uncover the changes caused by the instability. The stress can be created by asking the patient to tightly grip and/or ulnarly deviate the hand on the PA view. A wrist that can be seen to be unstable at rest is classified as having static instability, whereas a wrist that requires stress to uncover the instability is considered dynamically unstable. A third group is thought to exist: those that are predynamically unstable. In this case the wrist cannot be shown to be unstable radiographically by any means, but the patient is clinically believed to have the beginnings of instability secondary to ligamentous injury.

Diagnosis

The typical patient describes the mechanism as a FOOSH injury, which causes a dorsiflexion and pronation injury at the wrist. A less common mechanism of injury is a rotational injury to the hand and wrist from a twisting force. Pain and swelling often are not severe and generally subside with rest after a few days. Frequently, little ecchymosis or edema is present, and no obvious deformity makes the diagnosis clearer to the patient, sports trainers, or coaches or to the uninitiated health care worker. Because these patients often do not seek treatment in the acute phase, they may not recall the inciting injury when, at some later time, they present for evaluation of the wrist pain.

Physical findings are related to the degree of instability of the scaphoid. In the least severe cases, pain is present over the dorsal scapholunate ligament and the radioscaphoid joint. Dorsal wrist pain usually can be elicited by applying dorsal pressure to the volar pole of the scaphoid. In addition, pain often is elicited at the anatomical snuffbox secondary to synovitis of the radial side of the wrist joint.

The stability of the scaphoid can be checked in the manner described by Watson et al;[180] dorsal pressure is applied to the volar pole of the scaphoid while the wrist is moved from ulnar to radial deviation in an effort to sublux the proximal pole of the scaphoid out over the dorsal rim of the radius. This is known as a **scaphoid shift test,** and it can produce pain either from the instability or from compression of the scaphoid in its fossa in the presence of chronic synovitis. In a patient with an unstable injury, a discernable, painful clunk occurs when the examiner releases pressure on the scaphoid, allowing the subluxed proximal pole to reduce back into the scaphoid fossa of the radius.

A patient with long-standing instability who has progressed to arthritis of the joint may have a fixed subluxation of the scaphoid. This can be palpated as a firm dorsal prominence at the distal edge of the radius. Severe limitation of wrist motion and significant tenderness are indicative of the degenerative changes that have occurred at the radiocarpal joint. Osteophyte formation on the radial side of the wrist can lead to a deformity that is observable and palpable.

Plain x-ray films are the most important imaging study and should accompany the history and physical examination whenever a ligamentous injury of the wrist is suspected. Many articles have been devoted to the way the x-ray films should be obtained. It has been the authors' practice to obtain a PA, a clenched fist PA, and a lateral view. In obtaining the PA films, a foam block is used that elevates the ulnar side of the wrist 10° to 15° which allows a more perpendicular view of the scapholunate articulation. Abnormalities seen on the PA films include a widened scapholunate gap, usually greater then 3 mm in adults. The clinician can see signs of the flexed scaphoid by noting its loss of length and the appearance of the "signet ring sign," indicative of the cortical projection of the distal pole seen through the long axis of the bone as it becomes more vertical (Figure 7-79).[181]

The lateral projection views require more experience to read but generally provide even more information than the PA views. The scaphoid flexes and creates a bigger angle in relation to the long axis of the radius. In addition, the lunate tends to extend, pointing dorsally and translating volarly. The angle between the axial long axis of the lunate and scaphoid normally is 30° to 60°, with the average being 47°. As the scaphoid flexes and the lunate extends, that angle increases to greater than 60° and often approaches 90° (Figure 7-80).

Clinicians occasionally can see the proximal pole of the scaphoid sitting dorsal to the center of its fossa on the

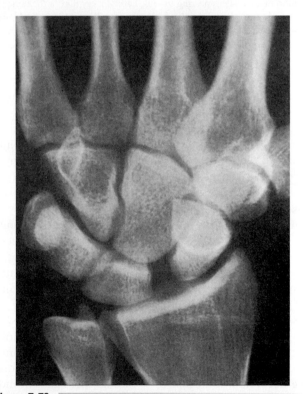

Figure 7-79

AP and lateral x-ray films of a wrist with a scapholunate tear. The scaphoid is flexed and shortened, and the lunate is extended. A gap is created between the scaphoid and the lunate as the scaphoid rotates away from the lunate. The scaphoid no longer lies correctly in its fossa in the radius, and over time this will cause joint degeneration.

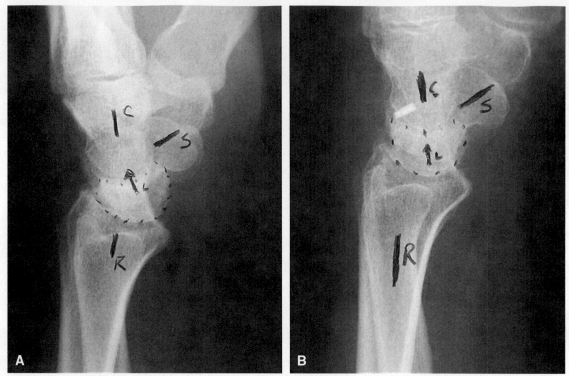

Figure 7-80
A, Lateral x-ray film of a patient with a scapholunate dissociation. The lunate is tilted dorsally, and the scapholunate angle is nearing 90°. **B,** Lateral x-ray film of the same patient after repair of the ligament and capsulodesis of the scaphoid. The lunate is no longer tilting backward, and the scaphoid is more extended. This creates a more normal angle between the two (approximately 45°).

radius. As the lunate extends, the capitate translates proximally and dorsally, and the normal collinear relationship of the radius, lunate, and capitate is disrupted.

Arthrography can confirm loss of the watertight compartment between the midcarpal and radiocarpal joints. This indicates a tear of some portion of the scapholunate interosseous ligament. Communication can be seen if a small perforation exists in the membranous portion of the ligament; this perforation is not biomechanically important, but it increases the potential for false positive results. In addition, some tears flow only unidirectionally; therefore, if the dye is injected into only one compartment, it may fail to reveal a substantial tear, leading to false negative results. Detection can be improved by injecting dye into all three compartments of the wrist over the course of the test.[182]

MRI can visualize the different sections of the scapholunate ligament. Edema, thickening, tortuosity (twisting), and lengthening of the ligament indicate injury and possible disruption. Joint fluid flow through the ligament indicates a tear as much as arthrography does, without the need for an injection before the examination. In addition, the MRI can help visualize the bony alterations between the radius, capitate, lunate, and scaphoid that occur with scapholunate instability.

Medical Treatment

With acute or subacute injuries in which the scaphoid flexion deformity is still flexible and no joint destruction has occurred, the preferable course is to attempt a soft tissue reconstruction of the wrist. This retains the most mobility of the radiocarpal and midcarpal joints while attempting to regain stability. By restoring appropriate carpal alignment and improving the kinematics of the wrist, the surgeon attempts to prevent or delay the onset of arthritic changes that would occur if no treatment were given.

Many surgical solutions have been proposed for acute and subacute scapholunate dissociation. Many begin to restore the normal anatomy by repairing the scapholunate interosseous ligament back to the ulnar side of the scaphoid from which it usually detaches. This can be done through bone tunnels drilled into the scaphoid or with various suture anchors. However, this repair does not address the flexion and rotation deformity of the scaphoid. To do so, ligamentous tissue from the dorsal capsule of the wrist is rerouted to the distal pole of the scaphoid to act as a tether that prevents the scaphoid from flexing and rotating.

Additional soft tissue repairs have been created using various tendons, including the extensor carpi radialis longus

(ECRL) and FCR ligaments. Tunnels are drilled through the scaphoid in a dorsal-volar direction, allowing one of these tendons to be passed through the bone and create a tenodesis effect, keeping the scaphoid in the correct posture in relation to the lunate.

The alternative to soft tissue procedures is partial wrist fusion or proximal row carpectomy. The scaphotrapeziotrapezoid (STT) fusion has been advocated in cases that have not progressed to arthritis at the radiocarpal joint. The scaphoid is brought out of its flexed position and locked in place by its fusion across the midcarpal row. This allows motion to continue at the radiocarpal joint. Criticism of this procedure relates to the increased load borne on the radial side of the wrist between the scaphoid and radius after the fusion, in the area at risk for arthritic changes secondary to the initial injury.

If arthritis has injured the radiocarpal joint but left the midcarpal joint intact, a proximal row carpectomy can be considered. In this instance, the scaphoid, lunate, and triquetrum are excised, allowing the capitate to articulate in the lunate fossa of the radius. This changes the wrist from a complex link joint to a simple hinge joint with concomitant loss of motion. This procedure is criticized for the fact that the capitate is not an exact fit in the lunate fossa of the radius and that the relative shortening of the wrist leads to some weakness of grip.

As arthritis progresses in chronic scapholunate instability, the midcarpal joint between the scaphoid, lunate, and capitate is affected. In many surgeons' eyes, this midcarpal arthrosis, especially of the proximal capitate, is a contraindication to the proximal row carpectomy. In this case they favor removal of the arthritic scaphoid and fusion of the ulnar midcarpal joint (four-corner fusion). This stabilizes the midcarpal joint in the absence of the scaphoid. Again, the link joint has been turned into a hinge joint, with subsequent sacrifice of 30% to 50% of flexion and extension, as well as radioulnar deviation. The operation succeeds because as bad as the arthritis becomes with scapholunate advance collapse, the surface between the lunate and the radius usually is preserved. This occurs because, as mentioned previously, the radiolunate articulation is spherical; therefore, when the lunate tips backward because of ligament instability, the congruency between the two bones is maintained. This is not true of the radioscaphoid fossa, which is elliptical and becomes incongruous as the scaphoid flexes and pronates.

Rehabilitation Principles and Considerations for Wrist Injuries

Rehabilitation of wrist injuries requires an understanding of carpal anatomy, force distribution, and wrist kinematics.[183] An optimally aligned, stable but mobile wrist is capable of the precise interaction needed between bone and soft tissues to produce pain-free, functional motion. Restoration of alignment, stability, and pain-free motion poses a challenge to the treating clinician.

Key Therapeutic Considerations in Management of Wrist Injuries

- Soft tissue injury accompanies bony injury[134]
- Disruption of ligaments can lead to altered mechanics, instability, degenerative changes, and pain[134,176,177]
- Nerve irritation or injury contributes to pain syndromes[184–188]
- Motor and sensory loss can occur as a result of nerve injury

Distal Radial Fractures

Understanding normal force distributions at the wrist and the impact of altered mechanics is essential in initiating therapy regimens. When the distal ulna is equal in length to the distal radius, this is termed **ulnar neutral variance.** Changes from ulnar neutral variance can occur as a result of injury, and they alter the mechanics of the wrist joint (Figure 7-81). Shortening of the distal radius during fracture healing, with no change in the position of the ulna, results in **ulnar positive variance.** This change increases the force distributed to the ulna and potentially results in ulnar-sided wrist pain.[165,189-192]

In a typical ulnar neutral wrist, 80% of the force is borne by the radius, with only 20% through the ulnocarpal joint. However, even a small change in height results in the ulna absorbing 40% of the load if the ulna is 2 mm ulnar

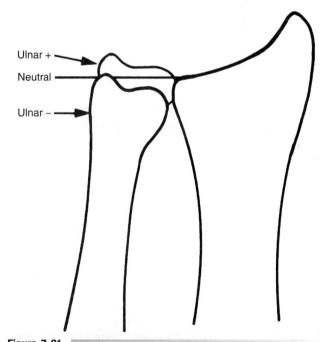

Figure 7-81

Differences in ulnar variance. (From Frykman GK, Krop WE: Fractures and traumatic conditions of the wrist. In Hunter JM, Mackin EJ, Callahan AD, editors: *Rehabilitation of the hand: surgery and therapy,* ed 4, p 325, St Louis, 1995, Mosby.)

positive or 4% of the load if it is 2 mm ulnar negative.[133,165,192-194] Loading the wrist, which occurs during weight bearing and gripping, places stress on the primary ligamentous stabilizers of the wrist. Evaluation for ligamentous injury should be considered in the event of persistent pain with loading of the wrist.[195] For the clinician charged with the rehabilitative management of a patient with a wrist injury and pain, the key considerations regarding force distribution at the wrist are summarized below.

Key Therapeutic Considerations in Force Distribution at the Wrist

- Ulnar-sided wrist pain may result from a change in mechanics and may not be limited to a healing ulnar styloid fracture. For example, a radial compression fracture that shortens the radius changes the relationship between the radius and the ulna, causing ulnar-sided wrist pain from ulnar positive variance.
- Care must be taken when loading the wrist to protect healing structures on the radial side of the wrist (e.g., with scaphoid fractures) or the ulnar side of the wrist (e.g., with tears in the triangular fibrocartilage complex).
- Loading the wrist stresses many of the carpal ligaments. Care must be taken when loading a wrist known to have or suspected of having a ligament tear. Wrist and grip strengthening may not be appropriate in patients with ligamentous instability. Appropriate diagnosis of the source of wrist pain is paramount in preventing further injury or degenerative changes of the carpus.
- Forearm position affects force distribution at the wrist. Activity modification, taking into account forearm position, should be considered in patients with persistent ulnar-sided wrist pain. Pronation shortens the radius and increases ulnar variance; this can increase ulnar-sided wrist pain.

The dynamics of wrist motion are important for the rehabilitation strategy. Wrist kinematics is described by the direction in which the proximal carpal row moves.[196,197] Normal kinematics and wrist motion are detailed in Table 7-18.

Table 7-18
Normal Wrist Kinematics and Motion

Physiological Motion	Carpal Movement
Wrist flexion	The proximal carpal row shifts dorsally in relation to the radius
Wrist extension	The proximal carpal row shifts volarly in relation to the radius
Ulnar deviation	The proximal carpal row extends and shifts radially
Radial deviation	The proximal carpal row flexes and shifts ulnarly

Table 7-19
Degrees of Normal Active Range of Motion Compared to Active Motion Used in Light Activites of Daily Living (ADLs)[200,201]

Active Motion	Normal (degrees)	Light ADLs (degrees)
Wrist flexion	80	30-40
Wrist extension	70	30-40
Ulnar deviation	30	20
Radial deviation	20	20
Pronation	80-90	40-50
Supination	80-90	60

Normal values for active range of motion at the wrist compared to what is needed for light activities of daily living (ADL) tasks are presented in Table 7-19. Of note, 40% to 60% of wrist flexion and extension occurs at the radiocarpal joint, and the remaining motion occurs at the midcarpal joint. As well, 60% of radial and ulnar deviation occurs at the midcarpal joint and 40% at the radiocarpal joint.[198,199]

Key Therapeutic Considerations for Wrist Kinematics and Wrist Motion

- Optimization of motion depends on restoration of wrist kinematics. Specific joint mobilization techniques can be used to improve wrist kinematics.[202]
- Surgical procedures or conditions in which the midcarpal joint is fused or significantly limited reduce motion 40% to 60% (except pronation/supination, which remains unaffected).
- Light activities of daily living can be performed without restoration of full motion.
- Optimization of pain-free motion is essential and should be based on individual activity requirements and realistic goals. The goals should consider the status of the joints comprising the wrist, including alignment.

In a postoperative or postinjury therapy regimen, the clinician should consider the ultimate goals for motion and strength. Joint mobilization should focus on restoring normal kinematics.[202,203] Surgical procedures with any partial fusion of the wrist reduce motion 40% to 60%. However, most ADLs can be completed without full motion. Optimizing pain-free motion is essential. The clinician must perform a realistic evaluation of the patient's needs and expectations.

In summary, the wrist is a complex structure with key specific considerations for the treating clinician. Direct communication between the surgeon and the therapist is essential. The overall rehabilitation strategy must account for the type and location of injury, possible concomitant ligament disruption, fixation methods used for fracture stabilization, overall fracture stability, and joint alignment (Figure 7-82). Table 7-20 presents rehabilitation strategies the clinician can use with patients who have suffered a wrist injury. Successful therapeutic intervention and its progression must incorporate all stages of the healing process.

Scaphoid Fractures

Rehabilitation of scaphoid fractures depends on the location and healing of the fracture. General casting guidelines for nondisplaced fractures at the distal pole is 4 to 8 weeks in a thumb spica cast. Midscaphoid (waist) fractures are immobilized longer, for 6 to 12 weeks. Proximal pole fractures are protected the longest, for 12 to 20 weeks.[145] During the casting phase, emphasis is placed on maintaining normal ROM of the fingers. After the cast is removed, the goals of therapy are joint mobilization and strengthening at the wrist and fingers.

Compression screw fixation of scaphoid fractures allows for earlier motion and return to activities. Generally, the thumb and wrist are immobilized for 1 to 3 weeks after

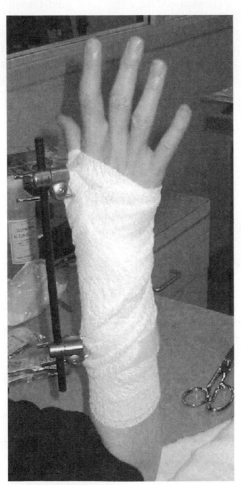

Figure 7-82

Use of an external fixator to stabilize a distal radial fracture.

compression screw fixation. After the cast has been removed, gentle motion is initiated. Weight bearing, gripping, and loading of the wrist should be avoided for the first 3 weeks. Between weeks 3 and 6, return to sports with casting or splinting is possible. Strengthening is initiated at week 8, after fracture healing allows for an increased demand. After 8 weeks, return to normal activities generally is permissible.

Displaced fractures that require ORIF are immobilized for 4 to 12 weeks, depending on the type of fixation. After the cast has been removed, active motion begins. If the scaphoid vascular supply is a concern, no weight bearing or strengthening can begin until CT scanning has confirmed fracture healing. Return to sports usually begins at 4 to 6 months.

Complications from scaphoid fractures include nonunion and malunion. Either of these causes kinematic disturbance within the wrist that can cause pain, instability, loss of motion, and eventually arthritic degeneration.[145,207,211–213]

Triangular Fibrocartilage Complex Injuries

Splinting in an ulnar gutter splint for stable TFCC sprains and strains to prevent ulnar deviation can be helpful for reducing inflammation and preventing repetitive stress to the region. Activity modification is essential. Activities that require ulnar deviation or forceful gripping should be avoided. Splinting during these activities prevents the incriminating wrist motions of ulnar deviation with or without terminal wrist flexion and extension. The splint often acts as a reminder to the patient to avoid the positions or activities that irritate the TFCC. Weight bearing, such as yoga or cycling, should be avoided regardless of the wrist position used. A splinting approach is used until the pain diminishes (approximately 4 to 6 weeks), at which time a strengthening to tolerance regimen can be initiated in all wrist positions. As previously mentioned, if pain persists after a 4-week period of splinting and activity modification, the patient should return to the referring physician.

Cast immobilization in a long arm cast as an initial treatment for peripheral and central tears has been reviewed previously and is used for 4 to 6 weeks. After cast immobilization, the goal of therapeutic strategies is restoration of pain-free motion and function. Strengthening is initiated when full AROM has returned. Weight bearing is avoided for 6 to 12 weeks and should be pain free before the patient returns to aggressive weight-bearing activities. If pain limits progression of the rehabilitation course, further evaluation is required.

Debridement of the central portion of the TFCC requires little or no immobilization. The patient wears a wrist or ulnar gutter splint for 1 week when not exercising. Occasionally the splint time is extended to respect patient comfort. AROM is initiated during the first week to pain tolerance. At 2 to 4 weeks, light functional tasks can be resumed with limited ulnar deviation and weight bearing.

Table 7-20
Rehabilitation Guidelines for Wrist Fractures[26,204-210]

	Closed Reduction	External Fixation	ORIF with Plate and Screws	ORIF with Fixed-Angle Locking Plate
Description	Fracture is manually reduced Reduction is maintained in cast support for 6 weeks	Fracture is reduced through distraction provided by external fixation in which pins are inserted in the radial shaft proximal to the fracture and distal to the fracture in the second metacarpal Fixation is removed at 6 weeks	Fragments require internal stabilization to hold reduction and achieve alignment Plate and screws still allow slight motion at the fracture site Casting is required for additional stability for 6 weeks	Fragments require internal stabilization to hold reduction Technique provides optimum anatomical realignment and stabilization of the fracture fragment Procedure allows for early motion
Healing Stages				
Stage I: Inflammatory stage (weeks 0 to 2)	Casting; elbow may or may not be included in the cast AROM of the uninvolved joints: emphasis on the fingers and shoulder Tendon gliding exercises Blocking exercises to maintain flexor tendon gliding and encourage extensor tendon gliding. Edema management of the fingers with Coban Soft tissue mobilization of the fingers	AROM of the uninvolved joints; emphasis on the fingers and shoulder Tendon gliding exercises Blocking exercises to maintain flexor tendon gliding and encourage extensor tendon gliding Edema management with Coban or a compression sleeve Soft tissue mobilization	Casting AROM of the uninvolved joints; emphasis on the fingers and shoulder Tendon gliding exercises Blocking exercises to maintain flexor tendon gliding and encourage extensor tendon gliding Edema management of the fingers with Coban	Splinting between exercises and at night AROM of the wrist and forearm (per physician guidelines) AROM of the uninvolved joints; emphasis on the fingers and shoulder Tendon gliding exercises to prevent adhesions Blocking exercises to maintain flexor tendon gliding and encourage extensor tendon gliding Scar management Soft tissue mobilization Edema management Activity modification: No lifting, pulling, or pushing
Stage II: Fibroplasia and repair stage (weeks 2 to 6)	As above *Nerve symptoms, color changes, and extreme swelling should be reported to physician, because they may indicate that the cast is too tight*	As above Stretch to thumb web space *Median nerve symptoms or findings should be reported to the physician. Distraction placed by the fixator may compromise the nerve*	As above *Nerve symptoms, color changes, and extreme swelling should be reported to physician because they may indicate that the cast is too tight or that an infection may have developed*	As above Stretch to thumb web space Progress to PROM, gentle stretching at weeks 3 to 4 Progress to light activities

Table 7-20
Rehabilitation Guidelines for Wrist Fractures[26,204-210]

	Closed Reduction	External Fixation	ORIF with Plate and Screws	ORIF with Fixed-Angle Locking Plate
Stage III: Remodeling and maturation stage (weeks 6 to 8+)	Joint mobilization Stretching Splinting for motion Static wrist splint for comfort during the day and support at night, worn for 2 weeks Strengthening as tolerated at weeks 6 to 8 Functional progression	Joint mobilization Stretching Splinting for motion Strengthening at weeks 8 to 12 as tolerated Static wrist splint for comfort, to be worn during the day and at night as necessary Functional progression *After removal of the fixator, structures shift slightly because the distraction from the fixator has been removed. The patient's performance may be reduced as the tissues adjust*	Joint mobilization Stretching Splinting for motion Strengthening at weeks 8 to 12 as tolerated Static wrist splint for comfort to be worn during the day and at night as necessary Functional progression *New onset of pain with active finger or thumb flexion and extension may be a sign of soft tissue shearing against the hardware and should be reported to the physician*	Joint mobilization Stretching Splinting for motion Strengthening at weeks 8 to 12 as tolerated Static resting splint usually is discontinued Functional progression *New onset of pain with active finger or thumb flexion and extension may be a sign of soft tissue shearing against the hardware and should be reported to the physician*

ORIF, Open reduction and internal fixation; *AROM,* active range of motion; *PROM,* passive range of motion.

Strengthening and functional progression begin at 6 to 8 weeks, during which a gradual return of ulnar deviation and weight-bearing activities is initiated. If pain limits progression of the therapeutic intervention, a mechanical issue (e.g., positive ulnar variance) may be contributing to the patient's pain and TFCC irritation.

Repair of the peripheral portion of the TFCC is treated with an initial casting period of 3 to 4 weeks in a long arm cast, followed by a short arm cast for an additional 2 to 3 weeks. Casting times can vary. At 6 to 8 weeks, restoration of motion begins with the initiation of AROM. Ulnar deviation and forearm rotation are avoided. A wrist or ulnar gutter splint is worn between exercises and at night for comfort. Progression of motion, including forearm rotation and ulnar deviation, occurs between 8 and 12 weeks. Strengthening is initiated at week 12, with a gradual return to sports and weight-bearing activities as tolerated.[214,215]

Scapholunate Dissociation

As noted, surgical solutions for scapholunate dissociation include both soft tissue repairs or reconstructions and fusions. The period of cast immobilization after soft tissue repairs or reconstructions varies and can last up to 12 weeks.[198]

After cast immobilization, an AROM program is initiated, as well as scar management, edema control, and activity modification, avoiding weight bearing and gripping. At 12 weeks, gentle stretching and strengthening and functional progression are begun. A wrist splint can be worn for comfort. Taking care to avoid stretching out the repair is a prime postoperative concern. Motion limitations of

approximately 30° of flexion and 50° of extension are to be expected in procedures such as the Blatt technique,[216] in which a portion of the dorsal wrist capsule is used to correct the rotation and flexion deformity of the scaphoid (Figure 7-83). Return to high demand activities and/or competitive sports occurs at 6 to 9 months after surgery.[198,216]

The surgical fusion procedures (proximal row carpectomy, STT fusion, and four-corner fusion) follow a similar rehabilitative course (Figure 7-84). The wrist is immobilized for up to 6 to 12 weeks. After immobilization, AROM is initiated, along with scar management, edema control, and activity modification and splinting for comfort. At 12 weeks, stretching, strengthening, and functional progression begin. A reduction in motion is to be expected. Return to high demand function and competitive sports may occur at 6 to 9 months after surgery. Persistent problems with scapholunate dissociation can include wrist pain despite surgical intervention to correct the instability.

Tendonitis, Tenosynovitis, and Entrapment

Trigger Finger or Thumb (Stenosing Tenosynovitis)

General Considerations

Stenosing tenosynovitis of the digits and thumb, also known as *trigger finger* and *trigger thumb,* is a common cause of hand pain and dysfunction. The problem arises from a size disparity between the flexor tendon and the annular pulley portion of the tendon sheath through which

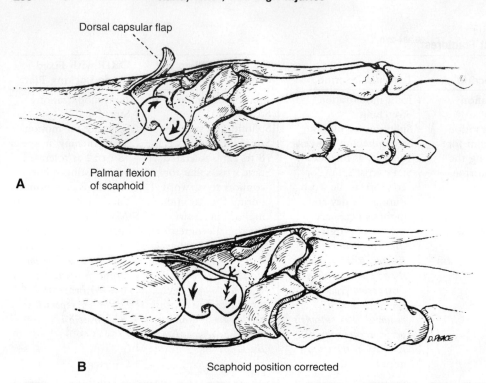

Dorsal capsular flap

Palmar flexion
of scaphoid

A

Scaphoid position corrected

B

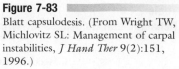

Figure 7-83
Blatt capsulodesis. (From Wright TW, Michlovitz SL: Management of carpal instabilities, *J Hand Ther* 9(2):151, 1996.)

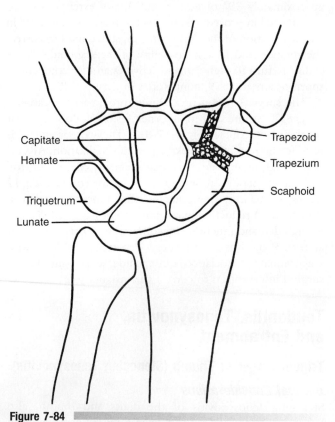

Capitate

Hamate

Triquetrum

Lunate

Trapezoid

Trapezium

Scaphoid

Figure 7-84
STT joint fusion with pinning and bone grafting. (From Frykman GK, Krop WE: Fractures and traumatic conditions of the wrist. In Hunter JM, Mackin EJ, Callahan AD, editors: *Rehabilitation of the hand: surgery and therapy,* ed 4, p 330, St Louis, 1995, Mosby.)

the tendon should glide smoothly. The two types of stenosing tenosynovitis are nodular stenosing tenosynovitis and diffuse stenosing tenosynovitis. Patients present with a catching or snapping sensation (which often is quite painful) that occurs with finger or thumb motion. If this problem progresses, the affected finger or thumb may become locked in flexion and the patient may lose the ability to actively extend the digit. Treatment of this disability ranges from conservative nonoperative management to surgical release of the constrictive A1 pulley.

Anatomy

The flexor tendons are enveloped in a synovial sheath that glides through a series of pulleys, which function to keep the tendon closely apposed to the bone during bending. Damage to critical portions of the pulley system leads to bow-stringing of the tendon away from the bone, which causes finger flexion contracture and loss of motion (Figure 7-85). The two types of pulleys in the flexor system are the annular pulleys and the cruciate pulleys. Two annular pulleys (A2 and A4; see Figure 7-49) cover the flexor tendons over the proximal and middle phalanges and are the most critical in preventing bow-stringing. The three remaining annular pulleys (A1, A3, and A5) are closely associated with the volar plates of the MCP joint, the PIP joint, and the DIP joint, respectively. The three cruciate pulleys (C1, C2, and C3) provide additional support to the flexor tendon as it crosses the MCP, PIP, and DIP joints, but they are more flexible by design than the annular pulleys (Figure 7-86).

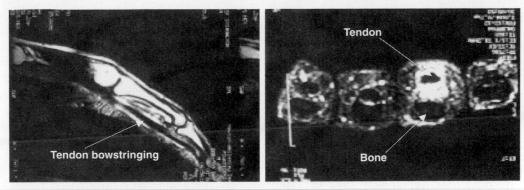

Figure 7-85

MRI scan of a closed rupture of the A2 pulley over the proximal phalanx. This injury led to bow-stringing of the flexor tendon *(black structure)* away from the bone.

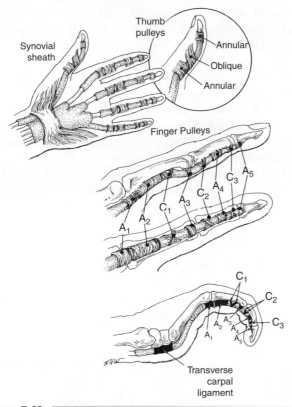

Figure 7-86

Synovial sheaths and retinacular and annular pulleys of the fingers and thumb. (From Chase RA: *Atlas of hand surgery,* vol 2, Philadelphia, 1984, WB Saunders.)

Pathophysiology

During finger flexion, the annular pulleys are under the greatest degree of stress from the flexor tendons. Flexion of the proximal phalanx, especially with power gripping, induces high angular loads across the most proximal pulley (the A1 pulley). Hypertrophy of the A1 pulley occurs in response to the increased stress. Microscopic examination of an A1 pulley involved in trigger digits shows degeneration, cyst formation, fiber splitting, and the presence of inflammatory cells. Inflammation and thickening also occur in the associated area of the flexor tendon. In nodular stenosing tenosynovitis, the thickening of the flexor tendon occurs in a localized area, just distal to the A1 pulley, where the increased friction between the pulley and tendon causes a thickened nodule to form. In diffuse stenosing tenosynovitis, the inflammation in the flexor tendon is not localized, but rather extends beyond the region of the A1 pulley. No discrete nodule develops in this form of trigger finger. In both types of stenosing tenosynovitis, because of the inflammation noted in both the A1 pulley and the flexor tendon, a size disproportion develops, and the flexor tendon is no longer able to glide smoothly through the pulley. The patient experiences this as a snapping sensation when attempting to extend the affected finger. The etiology of this process is unclear, but it may be associated with repetitive activity that causes trauma to the hands. Activities that require increased finger flexor activity, such as cutting or sewing, may exert excessive stress across the A1 pulley, resulting in the inflammatory process of stenosing tenosynovitis. However, in most cases of trigger finger or thumb, no inciting activity can be identified.

Diagnosis

Patients with a triggering finger or thumb may feel a click or snapping sensation as they attempt to extend the affected digit from a flexed position. Although the pathology of this process usually occurs at the A1 pulley, at the level of the MCP joint, the patient generally feels as if the mechanical problem exists at the level of the PIP joint. Initially this triggering may not be painful. As the stenosis becomes worse, the patient may report increased pain and decreased ability to actively extend the affected digit. The digit may become locked in a flexed position, and the use of the other hand to passively extend the digit may be required to "unlock" the flexed digit. The thumb is the most frequently affected digit, followed in declining order by the ring finger, the middle finger, the small finger, and the index finger.

The medical history and physical examination can assist with the diagnosis of stenosing tenosynovitis. Trigger digits have been associated with other medical conditions, including rheumatoid arthritis, diabetes, gout, carpal tunnel syndrome, De Quervain's tenosynovitis, Dupuytren's contracture, and hypertension.[217] On the physical examination, the patient has tenderness at the level of the A1 pulley over the palmar aspect of the MCP joint. A catching sensation may be felt over the A1 pulley when the patient is asked to extend the affected digit from a flexed position. In severe cases, the patient is unable to extend the digit. A tender nodule sometimes may be palpable on the flexor tendon at the level of the A1 pulley. This is associated with the nodular type of stenosing tenosynovitis. Usually the diagnosis of trigger digit can be based on the history and physical examination.

Medical Treatment

Treatment for stenosing tenosynovitis ranges from nonoperative management to splinting and cortisone injections to surgical management, including release of the A1 pulley. If a patient presents with a mild form of trigger finger or thumb, initial management may consist of splinting the MCP joint of the involved digit. The splint should allow free motion at the PIP and DIP joints.[218] Splinting has been successful, mostly in the four fingers, excluding the thumb, and in fingers that have mild triggering. However, the patient may need to spend up to 4 months in the splint. Because of this, patients may be less compliant with this treatment regimen. This method is an alternative for patients with mild disease who are hesitant to accept a steroid injection.

Steroid injections into the flexor tendon sheaths can be a successful treatment option for some patients with trigger fingers. Studies have shown that corticosteroid injections into the flexor tendon sheath tend to be more successful in women with trigger fingers, in patients who have had symptoms for less than 6 months, in patients who have the nodular rather than the diffuse form of tenosynovitis, and in patients in whom only one digit is involved.[219,220] Up to three corticosteroid injections may be given for an attempt at successful therapy; if triggering symptoms continue or recur after three injections, operative management should be considered, because the efficiency of further injections seems to decrease.[219]

Surgical management of stenosing tenosynovitis involves release of the A1 pulley, resulting in the return of the smooth gliding mechanism of the flexor tendon. By opening the pulley, the size disproportion between the pulley and the flexor tendon is resolved. Two different techniques are used for this purpose, percutaneous release and open release.

Percutaneous release of a trigger digit can be done in the office with administration of a local anesthetic. A needle or other cutting device is used to transect the A1 pulley longitudinally. The needle is placed through the skin into the A1 pulley at the level of the metacarpal head. The pulley is opened by sweeping the needle or cutting device back and forth in a longitudinal direction. After the cutting utensil is removed, the patient is asked to flex and extend the affected digit. Release of the pulley is confirmed when the patient can demonstrate this motion without any triggering.

Open release of a trigger digit typically is performed in the operating room and involves a skin incision proximal to the palmar digital crease. Blunt dissection is carried out by moving the neurovascular structures out of harm's way. The A1 pulley then is longitudinally transected with a scalpel or scissor tips under direct visualization.

Possible complications associated with surgical release of the A1 pulley include injury to the closely associated digital nerves. These nerves travel parallel to the flexor tendon on either side of the A1 pulley in the fingers. In the thumb, however, the radial digital nerve crosses from the ulnar to the radial side of the digit at the level of the palmar digital crease, just proximal to the A1 pulley. The proximity of these digital nerves to the A1 pulley, especially in the thumb, puts the nerves at risk during pulley transection. Inadvertent release of the A2 pulley, resulting in bowstringing of the flexor tendon, has been reported with both open and percutaneous techniques.[221] Incomplete release of the A1 pulley and injury to the underlying flexor tendon can occur and seem to be more prevalent with the percutaneous technique.[222]

For the most part, surgical management of this problem results in successful resolution of symptoms, and the chance of recurrence is low.

De Quervain's Disease
General Considerations
De Quervain's disease is a stenosing tenosynovitis of the first dorsal compartment in the wrist. It causes pain over the radial aspect of the wrist that worsens with thumb motion.

Anatomy
Extension of the wrist, fingers, and thumb is controlled by a group of muscles which that originate in the proximal half of the forearm. The tendons of these muscles course over the dorsal aspect of the wrist and hand before inserting on their target of motion. As these tendons approach the wrist, their outer covering forms a synovial sheath, which provides lubrication for the tendons as they move back and forth. As the extensor tendons cross the dorsal aspect of the wrist, they are covered by the extensor retinaculum, a ligamentous structure that prevents bow-stringing of the extensor tendons, allowing the tendons to stay closely approximated to the bones despite changes in wrist position.

The extensor retinaculum also organizes the tendons into six distinct anatomical compartments. The first compartment lies over the radial aspect of the wrist and contains the multiple slips of the APL and EPB tendons, both of which control thumb motion (Figure 7-87). The APL

Figure 7-87

First dorsal extensor compartment of the wrist. (From Wolfe SW: Tenosynovitis. In Green DP, Hotchkiss RN, Pederson WC, Wolfe SW, editors: *Green's operative hand surgery,* ed 5, Philadelphia, 2005, Churchill Livingstone.)

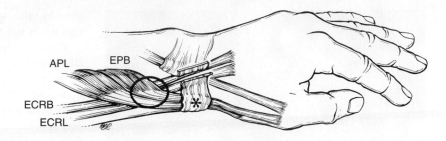

inserts on the dorsal base of the thumb metacarpal. The EPB inserts at the proximal dorsal aspect of the first phalanx of the thumb. Disease of these tendons is the cause of De Quervain's tenosynovitis. The second dorsal compartment contains the extensor carpi radialis longus (ECRL) and extensor carpi radialis brevis (ECRB) tendons, which provide wrist extension and radial deviation of the hand. The third compartment contains the EPL tendon, which extends the distal joint of the thumb. This tendon runs ulnar to Lister's tubercle and can be ruptured in distal radial fractures, particularly those that are nondisplaced. The fourth compartment contains the EDC and extensor indicis tendons, which control finger extension. The fifth compartment contains the extensor digiti minimi tendon, which extends the small finger. The sixth compartment contains the ECU tendon, which extends and ulnarly deviates the wrist and hand.

Also relevant to the anatomy of the dorsal wrist is the presence of the radial artery and branches of the radial sensory nerve that travel close to the first dorsal compartment. The radial artery travels from the volar to the dorsal wrist through the anatomical snuffbox. The tendons of the first dorsal compartment (APL and EPB) form the volar border of this space, and the EPL tendon forms its dorsal portion. The radial artery lies deep to these tendons as it moves to pass between the heads of the first dorsal interosseous muscle on its way to become the deep palmar arch. Branches of the radial sensory nerve lie superficial to the first dorsal compartment, providing sensation in this region. Just volar to the first dorsal compartment tendons in this subcutaneous layer lie the terminal branches of the lateral antebrachial cutaneous nerve. Either nerve can easily be injured in the surgical approach to release the first extensor compartment, resulting in a painful neuroma.

Pathophysiology

Normally the extensor tendons glide smoothly through the fibro-osseous compartments of the extensor retinaculum with finger and thumb motion. De Quervain's disease is a stenosing tenosynovitis that occurs because of a thickening of the tendons in the first dorsal compartment and a narrowing of the compartment itself. This disproportion in size between the tendon and the canal results in the loss of the smooth gliding motion, which leads to significant pain with any thumb movement. The cause may be repetitive thumb abduction and ulnar deviation motions, leading

to increased tension on the first dorsal compartment tendons. This increases the friction at the extensor retinaculum sheath, causing swelling of the tendons and narrowing of the compartment. Anatomical variations of the first dorsal compartment may also contribute to the development of De Quervain's disease, as well as to the success or failure of the treatment of this disorder. In up to 80% of patients, the first compartment may be divided by a longitudinal septum, resulting in separate canals for the APL and EPB tendons.[223,224] Separate canals may even be present for the multiple tendon slips of the APL. The possibility of these variations must be recognized, because it may influence management.

Diagnosis

Patients present with increasing pain of insidious onset. The tenderness generally is described as involving the thumb and wrist, and on examination may be localized to the area of the radial styloid. This pain radiates in a longitudinal fashion along the first extensor compartment from the metacarpal or proximal phalanx of the thumb onto the distal third of the forearm. Aching usually accompanies thumb motions, as well as grasping with the thumb and ulnar deviation of the wrist.

Examination of a patient with De Quervain's disease may demonstrate tenderness with palpation at the radial styloid and pain with active or passive stretching of the APL and EPB tendons. Finkelstein's test is pathognomonic for the diagnosis of De Quervain's tenosynovitis. This test is performed by passively adducting the patient's thumb into the palm of the patient's hand and then providing an ulnar deviation force to the wrist. Replication of the patient's pain with this action is a positive Finkelstein's sign and leads to the diagnosis of De Quervain's disease (Figure 7-88). The clinician must take care to rule out arthrosis of the thumb as the primary source of pain, because this condition can easily mimic or even create a secondary De Quervain's tenosynovitis.

Medical Treatment

The management of De Quervain's stenosing tenosynovitis ranges from immobilization to steroid injection therapy to an operative procedure. Immobilization in a cast may be attempted for a patient who is hesitant about having an injection or undergoing an operative procedure. This may alleviate symptoms for a short period, but pain tends to

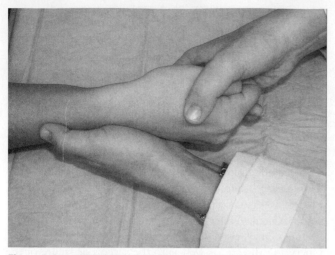

Figure 7-88
The Finkelstein maneuver is performed by placing the patient's thumb inside the palm and then gently deviating the wrist ulnarly. This maneuver causes severe discomfort in a patient with De Quervain's tenosynovitis.

recur after the cast is removed. Overall, the failure rate for immobilization alone is 70%.[225]

A corticosteroid injection is a beneficial treatment option for patients with De Quervain's tenosynovitis. An injection is given into the two separate tendon sheaths of the first dorsal compartment, which is located approximately 1 cm (0.4 inch) proximal to the radial styloid. It is important to recognize that subdivisions may be present in the first dorsal compartment, therefore some of the injection solution should be redirected in a more dorsal direction to permeate a separate EPB sheath. The success rate for alleviating De Quervain's disease with corticosteroid injections can be as high as 80% after two injections.[223]

If nonoperative management has been unsuccessful for a patient with De Quervain's tenosynovitis, a surgical procedure may be necessary to release the stenotic fibro-osseous canal and restore smooth gliding of the tendons through the first dorsal compartment. The procedure involves incising the extensor retinaculum that covers the first dorsal compartment, and allowing decompression of the residing tendons. It is important to visualize the compartment fully and to incise any septa that may be subdividing the compartment. Each tendon slip should be identified and proven to glide smoothly before the procedure is completed. Some surgeons elect to widen and repair the extensor retinaculum, whereas others simply leave the compartment open after the release. A tenosynovectomy of the tendons is routinely performed at the time of surgery.

Complications

Both the operative and nonoperative management of De Quervain's disease can have complications. Corticosteroid injections have been associated with depigmentation in the area of the injection, fat necrosis, and subcutaneous atrophy. Also, the risk of infection or nerve injury, although remote, is still present.

Operative treatment for De Quervain's disease risks the lateral antebrachial cutaneous or superficial sensory branch of the radial nerve, because they both lie close to the tendons and can easily be injured in the surgical approach. If these branches are not identified and preserved, injury may result in a painful neuroma. Incomplete release of the first dorsal compartment leads to ongoing painful symptoms. Incomplete release most often is due to failure to recognize a septum separating the APL and EPB tendons into separate compartments or multiple compartments for the slips of the APL tendons. The pain also may be due to a secondary diagnosis (e.g., arthritis of the CMC joints) that was overlooked during the patient's workup. A devastating complication of surgical release of the first compartment without its repair is the painful volar subluxation of the tendons from their usual position with thumb abduction and wrist volar flexion. This causes a painful snapping of the tendons as they slip volarly away from the radius. This generally requires reconstruction of a retinacular sling for tendon stabilization.

Carpal Tunnel Syndrome

General Considerations

According to Kerwin et al., carpal tunnel syndrome is the most frequently encountered peripheral compressive neuropathy.[226] Due to the frequency of this condition in the United States, approximately 500,000 operations to decompress the median nerve are performed each year.[227]

To understand carpal tunnel syndrome, it is necessary to appreciate the response of a peripheral nerve to injury, specifically the effect of compression and ischemia. Then the clinical manifestations that enable diagnosis and treatment will become clear.

Peripheral Nerves. Peripheral nerves consist of cell bodies that project axons to the extremities. The cell body resides in the anterior horn of the spinal cord for motor neurons and in the dorsal root ganglion for sensory neurons. Axons are surrounded by an outer layer, called *myelin*, which is produced by Schwann cells. Together the axon and the surrounding Schwann cells constitute what is commonly referred to as a nerve.

The myelin sheath produced by the Schwann cells functions as insulation so that the axons can more efficiently transmit electrical impulses, a phenomenon known as *saltatory conduction*. These nerve fibers transfer sensory information from the periphery to the cell body in the dorsal root ganglion (i.e., afferent conduction). They also conduct motor orders from the brain and spinal cord to the extremities to dictate muscle function (i.e., efferent conduction).

Microscopically, the smallest unit of the nerve is a fiber called a *fascicle*. These fibers are often bundled together in groups that are surrounded by a strong connective tissue layer called the *perineurium*. Groups of fascicles, each bundled within its perineurial sleeve, travel together within a loose connective tissue known as the *internal epineurium*. This material is believed to function as a mechanical insulator to shock and pressure, and different nerves have various amounts of internal epineurium. The groups of fascicles lying in the internal epineurium are ultimately surrounded by the external epineurium, which defines the periphery of the nerve (Figure 7-89).

The blood supply to the peripheral nerves runs from superficial epineurium to the deep endoneurial layer. A plexus of vessels runs longitudinally with the nerve at the level of the epineurium. These vessels send perforating arterioles into the perineurium. At the level of the endoneurium is a thin capillary network that is supplied by the vessels of the perineurial matrix. For the median nerve, the blood supply arises from branches from the radial and ulnar arteries. Nutrient vessels from these two major arteries accompany the median nerve through the carpal tunnel.

Peripheral nerves are subjected to different types of injury mechanisms, including compression, ischemia, stretching, chemical injury, and complete transection. Injuries to peripheral nerves are commonly classified by one of two systems. The simpler system, devised by Seddon,[228] describes three levels of nerve injury: the neuropraxia, the axonotmesis, and the neurotmesis. Sunderland[229] subsequently devised a more complex classification that describes injuries in terms of degrees, ranging from first degree (least severe) to fifth degree (most severe). Sunderland's system, although more involved to learn, appears to correlate better with clinical and pathological findings.

A first-degree injury (classified as a neuropraxia by Seddon) is localized damage to the myelin sheath without injury to the axon. In this situation, the electrical impulses carrying the sensory and motor information are temporarily interrupted, but the nerve fiber architecture remains intact. This is a reversible injury, with full recovery of nerve function anticipated within 3 months. Most patients with carpal tunnel syndrome fall into this category.

A second-degree injury (Seddon classification, axonotmesis) involves injury to the axon. Traction or a severe crush to the nerve disrupts the axonal fibers; however, the endoneurial tubes in which they travel remain intact. In this situation the axon undergoes degeneration (i.e., wallerian degeneration) at the time of the injury and will therefore must regenerate if function is to be regained. Surgical intervention is not required. and return of function is anticipated, although it may not be complete.

In third-degree nerve injuries, both the axon and endoneurium are disrupted, which increases the difficulty of regeneration. Therefore recovery of nerve function usually is incomplete.

In a Sunderland fourth-degree injury, the perineurium is disrupted along with the axon and endoneurial tubes, and in a fifth-degree injury (Seddon classification, neurotmesis), the nerve is completely transected and the epineurium is cleaved. Degeneration occurs, and regeneration is limited because of the large amount of scar tissue that forms and, in the case of complete transection, the physical separation of the cut nerve ends. In these cases, nerve damage is irreversible and surgical nerve repair is necessary to regain function.

Figure 7-89

Cross section of a peripheral nerve and its blood supply. (In Magee DJ, Zachazewski JE, Quillen WS, editors: *Scientific foundations and principles of practice in musculoskeletal rehabilitation*, p 178, St Louis, 2007, Saunders.)

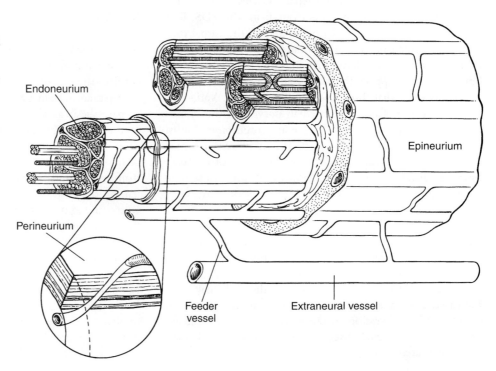

Endoneurium

Epineurium

Perineurium

Feeder vessel

Extraneural vessel

Compression Injury. Carpal tunnel syndrome is a chronic compressive injury to the median nerve caused by increased pressure within the carpal canal at the wrist. Acute compression causes mechanical deformation of the nerve. Chronically this pressure compromises the neural blood flow, resulting in nerve ischemia. This creates an inflammatory response within the nerve. The connective tissue of the endoneurium and perineurium becomes edematous and eventually fibrotic. Demyelination occurs, resulting in less efficient signal conduction and compromised nerve function. If compression continues, axonal degeneration can occur. This manifests itself clinically on a continuum, depending on the degree of nerve damage. Initially a patient may complain of pain and sensory disturbances ranging from intermittent paresthesia to constant numbness. With progression of the compression, the patient loses the ability of two-point discrimination. Symptoms of motor disturbance may begin as pain and progress to muscle atrophy as more diffuse nerve damage occurs.

Anatomy

The carpal tunnel is a relatively rigid structure, open ended at both the proximal and distal margins, which allows structures to pass through it from the forearm to the hand. The carpal bones border the tunnel on the dorsal, radial, and ulnar sides. The ulnar border consists of the hook of the hamate, triquetrum, and pisiform. The scaphoid and trapezium make up the radial border. The volar surface or roof of the tunnel is the flexor retinaculum, which extends from the distal radius to the metacarpal bases. The flexor retinaculum is made up of three structures: the deep forearm fascia, the transverse carpal ligament, and the aponeurosis between the thenar and hypothenar muscles. The median nerve, along with nine tendons (four from the FDS, four from the FDP, and the FPL) pass through the carpal tunnel. The median nerve usually branches at the distal edge of the flexor retinaculum, forming the recurrent motor branch, which supplies the thenar muscles and the digital nerves to the radial three and one-half fingers. Variability in the anatomy of both the median nerve and the branch point of the recurrent motor nerve are common and must be considered during surgical treatment of carpal tunnel syndrome. In most cases the recurrent motor nerve branches distal to the distal edge of the flexor retinaculum (extraligamentous), putting it at low risk during carpal tunnel releases.

Etiology

Several possible reasons can account for the development of increased pressure within the carpal tunnel.

Conditions that alter fluid balance in the body may cause increased edema and pressure within the carpal tunnel, resulting in compression of the median nerve. Pregnancy, hypothyroidism, renal disease, and hemodialysis all have been associated with the onset of symptoms. Inflammatory conditions, such as rheumatoid arthritis, lupus, and infection, may also cause increased pressure within the carpal tunnel. Traumatic injuries such as distal radial fractures or carpal dislocations can directly injure the nerve and lead to increased pressure in the carpal tunnel. Space-occupying lesions, arthritic spurs, or ganglions also can compress the median nerve at the wrist.

Neuropathic factors, such as diabetes, alcoholism, or nutritional deficiency, may affect the median nerve directly without ever altering the fluid pressure within the carpal canal. It is imperative that, during the workup, the clinician differentiate these intrinsic nerve processes from extrinsic pressure that is compromising median nerve function.

Despite this list of multiple etiologies, which is far from complete, most cases of carpal tunnel syndrome are idiopathic. Patients with this type of carpal tunnel syndrome usually are women between the ages of 40 and 60, and in half of the cases, the carpal tunnel syndrome is bilateral.[230] Currently, the cause of the nerve compression in this situation is unclear. It may be associated with hormonal factors, or changes in the tenosynovium in a person with an anatomically small tunnel, or vascular sclerosis.

Determining the etiology of the carpal tunnel syndrome is important, because the etiology influences the treatment options. If carpal tunnel syndrome is due to an underlying disorder, resolution of the condition sometimes can alleviate the median nerve dysfunction. For example, if carpal tunnel syndrome results from the fluid shifts induced by pregnancy, operative treatment usually can be avoided. Delivery of the child frequently resolves the compression quite quickly; therefore, steps to alleviate symptoms during the pregnancy may be all that is required.

Diagnosis

The diagnosis of carpal tunnel syndrome is made primarily on the patient's experience of symptoms. However, a number of physical examination findings, if positive, can help confirm the diagnosis.

A patient usually presents with a complaint of pain and/or paresthesia along the median nerve sensory distribution in the hand. This encompasses the palmar aspect of the thumb, index finger, middle finger, and the radial border of the ring finger. Symptoms increase insidiously over time from activity-related paresthesia and pain to constant, unrelenting numbness. Patients complain that these usually are worse at night, and this is believed to be related to the flexed position of the wrists during sleep, resulting in narrowing of the carpal tunnel and increased pressure on the median nerve.[231] Patients report worsening of symptoms during activities that cause prolonged wrist flexion or wrist extension, such as driving and talking on the telephone. If compression continues, weakness and atrophy of the thenar muscles may develop, resulting in loss of dexterity, difficulty grasping and holding objects, and an overall compromise in hand function.

The patient's history is critical in making the diagnosis. Provocative clinical tests, such as **Durkan's carpal compression test** (compression directly over the carpal tunnel), **Phalen's wrist flexion test** (wrist flexion for 60 seconds), and **Tinel's nerve percussion test** (tapping along the course of the median nerve), attempt to reproduce symptoms in the median nerve. Reproduction of the pain, numbness, or tingling is considered a positive finding and supports the diagnosis of carpal tunnel syndrome. However, if the tests are negative, this does not rule out the condition. Threshold sensory tests using Semmes-Weinstein monofilaments can elucidate the degree of sensibility the patient has lost secondary to nerve compression.

Electrodiagnostic tests (e.g., nerve conduction) and electromyographic studies provide objective evidence of impaired nerve conduction and intrinsic muscle function, which can be useful adjuncts to the clinical examination. These tests establish nerve conduction velocity, latency, and intrinsic muscle activity. They are helpful in isolating the location of a nerve lesion or injury and the degree of conduction block. This is important in cases in which the compression of the median nerve occurs at a level more proximal than the carpal canal.

Medical Treatment

Treatment options for carpal tunnel syndrome are varied, ranging from noninvasive splinting and cortisone injections to operative release of the transverse carpal ligament either by open or endoscopic techniques. Initially, attempts at nonoperative management are emphasized. The use of splints to maintain the wrist in a neutral position, which reduces the pressure in the carpal canal, is a standard option for patients with low grade symptoms. The patient may wear the splint at night while asleep or during activities that provoke symptoms.

If wrist splints are unsuccessful, a steroid injection into the carpal tunnel is another treatment option. This reduces the inflammation in the carpal tunnel, creating more space for the median nerve. In a select group of patients this results in complete alleviation of symptoms; however, 50% to 70% of patients have a return of their symptoms months after the injection. Care must be taken during the procedure to avoid needle injury or, even worse, injection into the nerve, which has long-term negative effects.

Surgical management of carpal tunnel syndrome is useful for patients who have thenar muscle weakness, who have failed nonoperative therapy, or who have numbness and tingling that is constant and no longer intermittent. Operative management consists of opening the roof of the carpal tunnel by incising the flexor retinaculum. This allows the carpal canal to increase its volume, relieving the pressure on the median nerve. Currently two major surgical options are available. The first is the traditional open procedure, and the second is the relatively newer endoscopic procedure. Both accomplish the same goal, incising the transverse retinacular ligament to release the carpal tunnel.

The open carpal tunnel release begins with a vertical skin incision at the proximal aspect of the palm. Dissection continues through the subcutaneous tissue and the palmar fascia, ultimately leading to transection of the transverse carpal ligament. Care must be taken to preserve all cutaneous nerve branches and to visualize and preserve any branches of the median nerve, specifically the recurrent motor branch, which innervates the thenar muscles. Possible postoperative problems associated with open carpal tunnel release are scar tenderness and pillar pain. Pillar pain, which is discomfort that extends along the thenar and hypothenar borders of the hand, may be related to the release of the thenar-hypothenar fascia, which is necessary to reach the transverse carpal ligament through the open approach.

With endoscopic carpal tunnel release, the large palmar incision and dissection are avoided. Instead, an endoscope and cutting instrument are used to visualize and transect the transverse carpal ligament from its undersurface (Figure 7-90). During this procedure, care must be taken to avoid injury to the recurrent motor branch of the median nerve, because this nerve occasionally has an anomalous course. The procedure is technically demanding and, in the hands of an inexperienced surgeon, poses risks to neurovascular and tendinous structures. Postoperatively, patients have fewer complaints of discomfort, and they return to work sooner than with the open procedure.[232]

Each technique has its advocates. However, the final result with either procedure, the transection of the transverse carpal ligament, releases the pressure within the canal and alleviates the patient's symptoms of pain and paresthesia.

Rehabilitation Principles and Considerations for Tendonitis, Tenosynovitis, and Entrapment

Trigger Finger

Rehabilitation for trigger digit begins after the involved digit is splinted in extension and if the patient experiences pain or stiffness, or both. It is important that the splint allow free motion at the PIP and DIP joints, with a hooked flexed position and full extension (Figure 7-91). Flexion of the IP joint with the MCP joint extended allows the flexor tendon to glide without stressing the A1 pulley. Splinting in extension prevents PIP flexion contractures and assists maximal glide of the flexor tendons.[218] The splint should be hand based and can be limited to the involved digit. The splint can rest dorsally or volarly, according to the patient's preference. Patients should be educated to avoid prolonged grasping.

Postoperative referral for therapy is indicated if pain, diminished motion, and reduced soft tissue mobilization, including scar adhesion, persist. After inflammation has diminished, night extension splinting is implemented to aid in prolonged stretching of the flexors, if shortening has occurred. Emphasis is placed on differential flexor

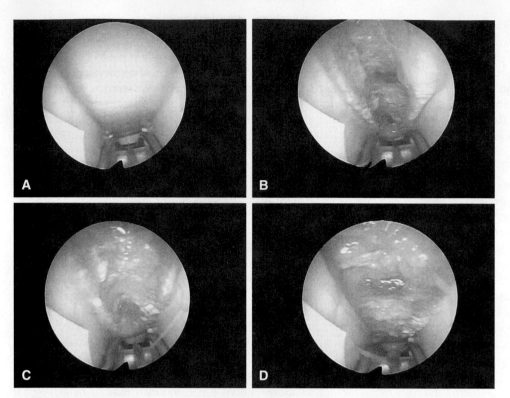

Figure 7-90
Endoscopic carpal tunnel release. **A**, Intact ligament. **B**, Partly incised ligament. **C** and **D**, Ligament is completely divided and "pops" widely apart. The overlying normal muscle and fascia are left intact.

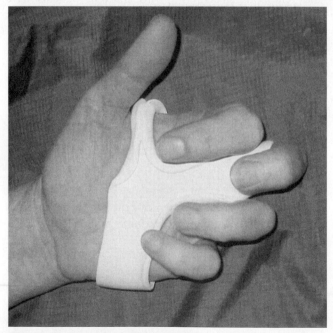

Figure 7-91
Volar-based trigger finger splint. The MCP is supported in extension, allowing PIP and DIP flexion. An alternative dorsal splint can be made, depending on the patient's preference.

tendon gliding with blocking exercises. Edema and scar management, to improve gliding of the soft tissues, is often necessary. Strengthening and prolonged grasp activity are avoided until full healing and the return of pain-free motion have been achieved.

De Quervain's Disease

In the early treatment of De Quervain's disease, intervention through immobilization may be initiated in the acute inflammatory cycle. In this case, a thumb spica splint with the IP joint free reduces stress to the tendons by resting the tissues. Soft tissue mobilization may help reduce inflammation and tissue guarding. Extensive patient education is essential to protect the tissues from overuse. Splinting can be attempted for 2 to 4 weeks.

Patients should be advised to modify activities after a corticosteroid injection for 1 to 2 weeks. These patients may also benefit from wearing a thumb spica splint for 1 to 2 weeks after the injection.

Postoperatively, emphasis should be placed on differential tendon gliding, edema and scar management, and modalities to improve soft tissue glide. Desensitization for nerve irritability is often also needed. Strengthening and prolonged pinching are avoided until healing is complete and the patient is pain free.

Carpal Tunnel Syndrome

Nonsurgical intervention for carpal tunnel syndrome consists of splinting the wrist in a neutral position and extensive patient education, including activity and work site modification, to prevent irritation of the median nerve. Splints are worn at night to prevent the wrist from resting in flexion and/or extension.[231] Splinting may also be recommended for day use. Patients may benefit from wearing a splint for 1 to 2 weeks after a corticosteroid injection.

Postoperative referral to therapy is indicated if pain, hypersensitivity, motion deficits, and reduced soft tissue mobilization, including scar tissue, persist. Emphasis is placed on scar management and modalities to improve the glide of soft tissues. Desensitization is included if nerve irritability is present. Activity modification (e.g., avoiding prolonged grasping) is indicated if inflammation is present.

References

To enhance this text and add value for the reader, all references have been incorporated into a CD-ROM that is provided with this text. The reader can view the reference source and access it online whenever possible. There are a total of 232 references for this chapter.

CHAPTER 8

INTEGRATED, MULTIMODAL APPROACH TO THE THORACIC SPINE AND RIBS

Linda-Joy Lee and Diane Lee

Introduction

Clinicians widely recognize that the thorax (the thoracic spine, ribs, costal cartilage) is an important area to assess and treat, not only in patients with thoracic pain and dysfunction, but also in those with lumbopelvic and cervical pain.[1-3] The upper thoracic spine has been implicated in disorders such as T4 syndrome, a collection of symptoms that includes upper extremity pain and paresthesia, along with neck and head symptoms.[4-6]

In contrast to other areas of the spine, research on the thorax is significantly lacking. The multiple articulations and anatomical complexity of the region create challenges in biomechanical studies. Cadaveric and animal studies on load capacity and other biomechanical features have primarily been performed on specimens without an intact rib cage, which limits how well they accurately reflect the in vivo state.[7-11] In 1993 Lee[12] proposed a biomechanical model, based on in vivo observations, that has not yet been validated or disproved. In terms of muscle function and motor control, studies have investigated erector spinae strength in relation to kyphosis,[13,14] the effects of postural exercises in patients with osteoporosis,[14-17] and electromyographic responses of the erector spinae in patients with scoliosis;[18,19] however, few studies have investigated the patterns of timing and activation of the multiple layers of muscles in the thorax. The treatment approach presented here, therefore, is based on the current evidence, a clinical biomechanical model, and exercise rehabilitation approaches modeled from research on muscle function and motor control in the lumbopelvic and cervical regions. As yet, no clinical trials have been done to evaluate treatment protocols in the thorax. Clearly more evidence is required to validate the approach presented here, but for now, this is our "best evidence"—an approach based on current research and on clinical experience from treating patients with pain and dysfunction of the thorax.[20]

The aim of this chapter is to present an integrated, multimodal approach for treating the thorax, with a clinical reasoning framework to guide the clinician in making decisions about *which* type of treatment technique to use (manipulation, mobilization, muscle energy, exercise) and *when* to use each kind of treatment. Careful assessment is required to design an effective treatment program.[21]

Functions of the Thoracic Spine and Ribs and the Integrated Model

The thorax is an important region of load transfer between the upper body (the head, cervical spine, and upper extremities) and the lower body (the lumbopelvic region and lower extremities).[22] The thorax also functions to protect the heart and lungs and facilitates optimum respiratory function. The rib cage gives the thorax more passive stability than the neighboring cervical and lumbar regions. Indeed, when the rib cage is transected, the stiffness of the thorax is significantly reduced.[9,23,24] However, multiple articulations at each level (13 per typical thoracic ring) allow movement in all planes, which requires appropriate activation (timing) and modulation of activity (amount of force) of the myofascial system for control of motion. In terms of range of motion for trunk rotation, the thorax provides most of the movement, with 4 to 9 degrees of movement (in one direction) per segment,[25] as compared to the lumbar spine, which has 3 degrees of rotation available per segment.[26] Optimum function of the thorax, therefore, as in other areas, requires a balance of mobility and stability,

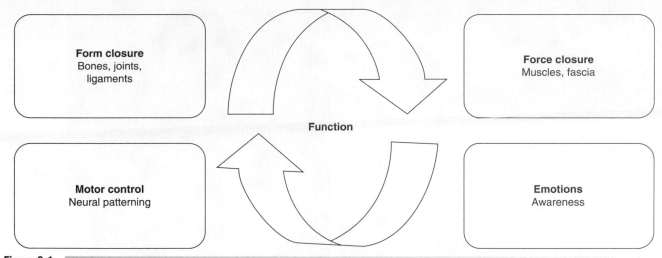

Figure 8-1

The integrated model centers on function and has four components: form closure (the role of the bones, joints, and ligaments), force closure (the forces produced by myofascial action), motor control (specific timing, modulation, and co-ordination of muscle action and inaction), and emotions. (From Lee DG, Lee LJ: An integrated approach to the assessment and treatment of the lumbopelvic-hip region – DVD, 2004.)

which is modulated according to the specific demands of the task (load, predictability, threat value) without compromising respiratory function or creating excessive increases in intra-abdominal pressure. This balance is provided by interaction among the passive, active, and control systems.[27] Panjabi's model of stability has been expanded into an integrated model,[28] which is introduced elsewhere in this text (see Chapter 14). The integrated model (Figure 8-1) provides the framework for assessment and treatment of the thoracic spine, with the ultimate goal of restoring optimum function.

rather than load sharing among structures. For example, lumbopelvic pain can change patterns of recruitment and activity in muscles that span the thoracic spine,[29-32] and if this occurs unilaterally, the resulting asymmetrical muscle activity creates rotation and side-bending curves in the thorax both at rest and during loading (Figure 8-2). Excessive, repetitive unilateral compression can result in thoracic pain and breakdown of structures over time. Excessive or poorly controlled mobility of the thorax (Figure 8-3) may result in local pain, as well as pain and dysfunction in the shoulder,

Functions of the Thoracic Spine and Ribs

- To transfer loads
- To protect the heart and lungs
- To facilitate optimum respiratory function

The integrated model is not a pain- or structure-based model that focuses only on identifying the pain-generating structure. This is not to say that pain is ignored; rather, the model seeks to help the clinician understand *why* a structure has become painful. Often nonpainful but dysfunctional components contribute to excessive tensile, compression, and/or shear forces on other structures. These structures then become a source of nociception (pain) and may show signs of degeneration on imaging tests. Local treatment can temporarily address the painful structure, but an examination of all components of the model (form closure, force closure, motor control, and emotions) can reveal *why* load transfer has failed, resulting in a concentration of forces

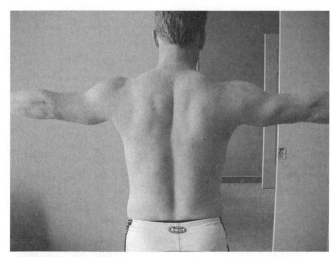

Figure 8-2

During bilateral arm abduction, this individual shows asymmetrical activation of muscles that span the thorax, resulting in side-bending and rotation. (Courtesy Diane G. Lee Physiotherapist Corporation and Linda-Joy Lee Physiotherapist Corporation.)

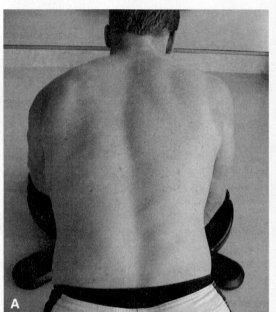
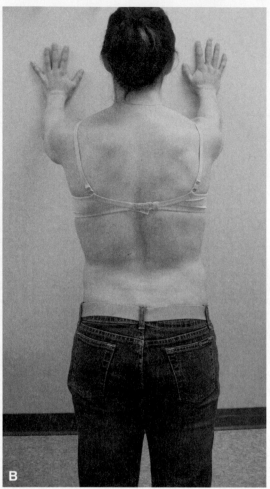

Figure 8-3

A and **B**, These individuals show poor control of the thorax during bilateral upper extremity weight bearing. This is considered loss of rotational control, because the symmetrical loading task results in rotation at several levels of the thorax. (Courtesy Diane G. Lee Physiotherapist Corporation and Linda-Joy Lee Physiotherapist Corporation.)

neck, and low back, because many of the muscles that span the low back and neck and control scapulohumeral movement have their origins in the thorax. Conversely, insufficient mobility of the thorax (Figures 8-4 and 8-5) increases the movement requirements of the cervical and lumbar regions and may result in neck and/or low back pain coupled with a painless, stiff thorax.

The goal of treatment, therefore, is to optimize load transfer and the sharing of forces throughout the thorax, the spine, and the entire body. This requires restoration of mobility to restricted areas, restoration of muscle control and the capacity to stabilize poorly controlled areas, and consideration of the emotional components that may alter posture and increase sensitization to pain. Ultimately, all techniques need to be incorporated into an overall approach that increases awareness of postural habits and movement patterns in order to change the way the patients live and move in their bodies, so that

pain-free, effortless movement is restored. The clinician's goal is to empower patients through knowledge, movement, and awareness to help regain control and achieve their optimum potential.

Goals of Treatment: Creating Optimum Load Transfer

- Remove non-optimum strategies
- Restore mobility in restricted areas
- Restore segmental and inter-regional control
- Coordinate movement and postural strategies with respiratory function
- Restore muscle capacity according to required load demands
- Retrain optimum strategies for posture and movement
- Create program according to patient goals and psychosocial context

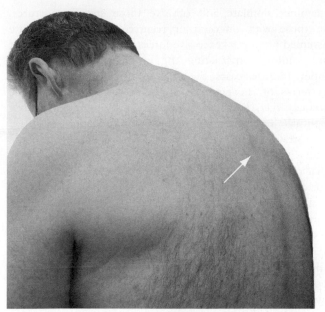

Figure 8-4

This individual shows loss of segmental flexion mobility at T5-6 *(arrow)*. (Copyright Diane G. Lee Physiotherapist Corporation and Linda-Joy Lee Physiotherapist Corporation.)

Effective management of pain and dysfunction in the thorax requires a multimodal program derived from a careful examination of form closure, force closure, and motor control. The examination includes tests for functional load transfer, joint compression (mobility), and motion control (stability). Joint mobility can be affected by factors intrinsic to the joint itself (i.e., the capsule and ligaments) or by factors extrinsic to the joint (i.e., overactivation or underactivation of muscles, which compresses the joint). Motion control of the joints requires timely activation of various muscle groups (neuromuscular function) such that co-activation patterns occur in a balanced manner around the joint axes and at minimal cost to the musculoskeletal system. Analysis of neuromuscular function requires tests for both motor control (i.e., the timing, modulation, and coordination of muscle activation) and muscular capacity (i.e., strength and endurance), because both are required for control between the segments of the thorax, regional control (i.e., between the thorax and pelvis, thorax and shoulder girdle, and thorax and head), as well as maintenance of whole body equilibrium during functional tasks. Effective management of thoracic pain should include techniques to reduce joint compression where necessary (i.e., joint manipulation, joint mobilization, muscle release techniques), techniques to align the thorax where necessary (i.e., muscle energy techniques and postural re-education), exercises to increase joint compression where and when necessary (i.e., motor control and muscle capacity [strength and endurance] training), and patient education to help patients understand both the mechanical and emotional components of their experience.

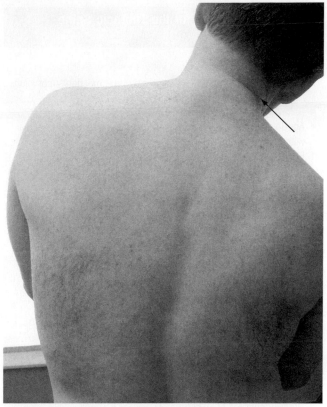

Figure 8-5

This individual presented with complaints of right-sided neck pain, but he had no thoracic pain. He shows loss of right side-bending mobility at several levels of the thorax; this painless restriction is a contributing factor in the development of cervical pain caused by excessive movement at C5-6 *(arrow)*. The decreased thoracic mobility may be due to joint stiffness or altered patterns of muscle recruitment (poor motor control); further testing is required to determine the cause of the restriction. (Copyright Diane G. Lee Physiotherapist Corporation and Linda-Joy Lee Physiotherapist Corporation.)

Goals for Treating the Thoracic Spine and Ribs

- To reduce joint compression
- To align the thorax
- To control articular compression
- To educate the patient in proper movement of the thoracic spine

Assessment of the Thoracic Spine and Ribs

Implementation of the appropriate technique at the appropriate time in a treatment program requires a clinical reasoning approach that is based on careful assessment and ongoing reassessment.[21] New assessment tests have been developed; some of these tests currently are being studied for their reliability and validity. Pertinent assessment tests are presented here in the context of the integrated model: tests of functional load transfer, form closure, and force closure/motor control.

Assessment Process for the Thoracic Spine and Ribs

Patient History
- Insidious onset of pain or history of trauma – mechanism of injury
- Aggravating postures and activities
- Relieving postures and activities
- Any relationship to breathing – sense of difficulty breathing, pain with breathing, etc.
- Sympathetic nervous system symptoms – altered temperature, non-dermatomal paresthesias
- Paresthesias or abnormal sensations, vascular changes
- Visceral symptoms – changes in digestion, relationship of pain to eating

Observation
- Kyphosis
- Scoliosis
- Disordered breathing patterns
- Chest deformities

Examination
- Active movements (forward flexion, extension, side flexion, rotation, costovertebral expansion, rib motion)
- Passive movements
- Resisted isometric movements
- Functional assessment
- Special tests:
  - Slump test
  - Reflexes and cutaneous distribution
  - Joint play movements
  - Palpation (anterior, posterior)
  - Diagnostic imaging

Static Tests of Functional Load Transfer

Postural Analysis

Posture is one of the first observations the clinician makes. Indeed, the way patients hold themselves in space can provide insight on many levels, including habitual patterns, the degree of pain, and the patient's emotional status. Analysis of posture is more than an observation of how joints are aligned. It is an assessment of the ability of multiple joints and structures to transfer load in a static loading environment; that is, a test of functional load transfer. Therefore, in the analysis of posture, two components are of interest: alignment and strategy. How is the spine aligned, what muscles are being used, and how does the muscle activity relate to the resultant posture? Why are those muscles being used? What is the impact of the resultant forces (line of gravity, compression from muscle activity) on the joints as a result of the combination of alignment and muscle strategy? How does this relate to the pain-generating structure?

If the individual identifies particular postures as painful or aggravating to their symptoms, it is important that the examiner simulate and observe those specific postures. In those with ongoing or recurrent pain, the posture assumed often puts excessive forces through structures that are painful, perpetuating the generation of nociceptive input. In other cases, the alignment assumed may be ideal in terms of the position of the bones, but the muscle strategy (i.e., *how* they attain the ideal alignment) is not optimal, resulting in excessive compression, repetitive microtrauma, and pain (Figure 8-6). Conversely, in acute pain states, the posture the patient chooses often is one that results in the most relief and unloading of the painful structure or structures.

In the thorax, individuals often rely on the passive structures for stability, either by using the posterior ligamentous system in full flexion (Figure 8-7) or by using the erector spinae muscles to close-pack the spinal joints into extension (Figure 8-8). Neither of these strategies is optimal, because both result in excessive stress on different structures. Optimum postural strategies place the joints in a neutral position (Figure 8-9), where compression forces are best distributed; however, the ability to maintain this position relies on complex feedback and feedforward mechanisms to modulate and maintain muscle activity at multiple levels.

Optimum spinal alignment has been described in detail in many texts; in volume 1 of this series (*Orthopedic Physical Assessment*), several categories of deviation from optimum alignment are described.[21] In addition to excessive thoracic kyphosis (see Figure 8-7), a loss of thoracic kyphosis can occur. This is a reversal of the normal curvature in the thoracic spine, which can occur segmentally or multisegmentally (Figure 8-10); the areas appear flat or extended at rest. If this loss of kyphosis is present in the upper thoracic spine, the scapulae may appear to wing, but they actually are in an optimum position. The scapulae appear nonoptimal because the spine has moved into extension away from the scapulae. Further tests are needed to determine *why* the spine is held in this nonoptimum position (i.e., articular, myofascial, neural, or emotional factors, or a combination of these).

Postural Analysis: Segmental Alignment

In addition to observing the multisegmental curves, the examiner should specifically palpate the thoracic spine to determine whether any alterations in segmental alignment are present in static standing, sitting, or other positions identified as aggravating the patient's pain. The clinician palpates the spinous processes and notes whether one vertebra is sitting relatively ventral or dorsal, compared to the vertebra above and the one below, to identify extension (ventral position) (Figure 8-11) or flexion (dorsal position) loss of segmental alignment. Rotation of the vertebra also is noted. Bony anomalies of the spinous process are common, therefore the transverse processes of the corresponding vertebra should be palpated to confirm the position indicated by the spinous process. Malaligned segments should then

Figure 8-6

A, This individual shows nonoptimum postural alignment and strategy. The thorax is flexed and displaced posteriorly relative to the pelvis and head, and the pelvis is displaced anteriorly relative to the feet and thorax. **B**, The same individual in corrected postural alignment but using a nonoptimum muscle strategy to achieve the posture. The positions of the head, thorax, pelvis, and feet are improved (note the position relative to a vertical line), but excessive activity is present in several muscles, including the sternocleidomastoid and external obliques. (Copyright Diane G. Lee Physiotherapist Corporation and Linda-Joy Lee Physiotherapist Corporation.)

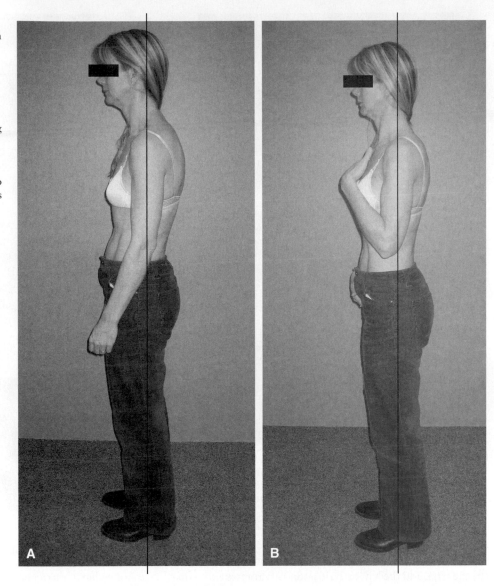

be assessed (1) during active movements, to determine whether limited or excessive motion is present, and (2) during passive segmental stability tests, to determine whether any loss of passive structural integrity is contributing to the altered alignment (Figures 8-12 and 8-13). An altered resting position of a segment does not necessarily mean that a loss of passive support and stability has occurred; however, over time, continued loading in that position may result in stretching of the passive supports, hypermobility, and instability. Alternately, trauma can result in loss of passive support and stability and may be the initiating cause of the altered position. The altered segmental position can be thought of as a "buckle" in the spine; further tests of form closure, force closure, and motor control are required to determine the forces and deficiencies causing the buckle.

Dynamic Tests of Functional Load Transfer

Active Thoracic Rotation with Palpation and Correction

Rotation is a primary movement of the thoracic spine and a key component of functional activities. It therefore is one of the essential movements to assess in patients with thoracic pain or dysfunction. One thoracic ring is defined as two vertebrae and the intervening disc, the right and left ribs connected between the vertebrae, and the interconnecting ligaments, including the anterior attachments of the ribs to the sternum.

It has been proposed that the following biomechanics occur between the third and seventh thoracic rings.[12] During right rotation of the sixth ring, the entire complex translates to the left. Specifically, the T5 vertebra rotates and side flexes

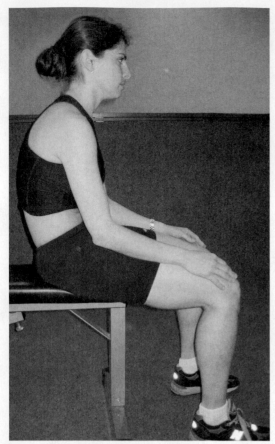

Figure 8-7

Slump sitting is a passive sitting posture that uses full thoracic flexion to create tension in the posterior ligamentous system for stability. (Copyright Diane G. Lee Physiotherapist Corporation and Linda-Joy Lee Physiotherapist Corporation.)

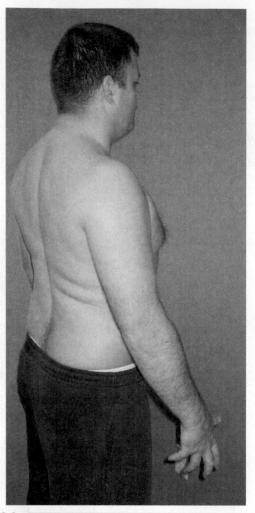

Figure 8-8

This individual uses increased activity in the erector spinae muscles as a postural stabilization strategy. Observation and palpation of the thoracic curvature reveals extension of the zygapophyseal joints (close-packed position), which provides passive stability, along with active stability from the muscle contraction. (Copyright Diane G. Lee Physiotherapist Corporation and Linda-Joy Lee Physiotherapist Corporation.)

to the right and translates to the left relative to T6; the right sixth rib posteriorly rotates and translates anteromedially (to the left); and the left sixth rib anteriorly rotates and translates posterolaterally (to the left) (Figure 8-14). These movements are osteokinematic (movements of the bones) and require concurrent accessory movements at all joints (arthrokinematics) of the functional thoracic ring. It is important to note that these biomechanics require intact form closure to occur. If trauma disrupts the passive structures (vertebral body, disc, ligaments, cartilaginous or synovial joints) anteriorly, posteriorly, or both, the body's ability to produce these physiological movements is affected. In these situations, nonphysiological biomechanics may be observed, especially in the middle to end ranges of movement.

In addition to assessing overall range of rotation motion in each direction, the examiner should note whether asymmetry of range is present. The different regions of the thorax can then be more specifically analyzed, through palpation of various rings as the patient repeats the rotation movement. Initially the clinician's hands are spread along the bodies of several ribs bilaterally (at the lateral rib cage) to assess the small amount of translation between the rings.

A dysfunctional pattern or positive test result is identified when one (or more) thoracic ring(s) (1) does not move to the contralateral side in synchrony with the rings above and below, (2) moves to the ipsilateral side, (3) does not move in either direction, or (4) moves excessively into contralateral translation. These are examples of **failed load transfer** of the specific level during trunk rotation. Note that the definition of failed load transfer can be applied to any static position, movement of the thorax (i.e., flexion, extension, rotation, lateral bending), or task requiring load transfer through the thorax (i.e., movements of the neck, lower extremity, or upper extremity). Failed load transfer in any specific test thus is defined as loss of the optimum alignment or biomechanics during the specific task being assessed (Tables 8-1 and 8-2; see Figures 8-2 to 8-8, 8-10, and 8-11).

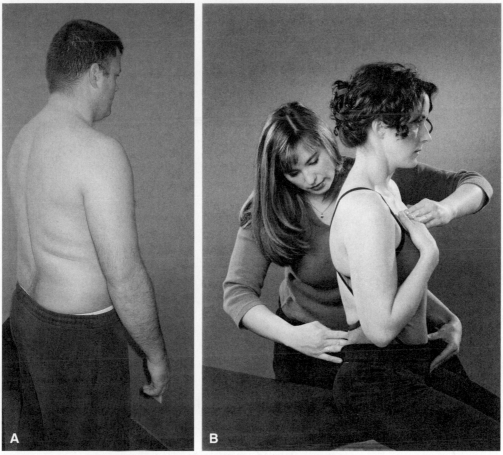

Figure 8-9

A, The same individual as in Figure 8-8 after treatment to change postural awareness and strategy. Note the more neutral thoracic alignment (thoracic kyphosis) and improved postural strategy. **B,** Neutral spine alignment. The clinician uses manual and verbal cues to facilitate a gentle, even thoracic kyphosis and lumbar lordosis; this is followed by correction of the head position to create a cervical lordosis. (Copyright Diane G. Lee Physiotherapist Corporation and Linda-Joy Lee Physiotherapist Corporation.)

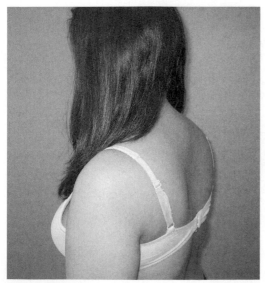

Figure 8-10

Multisegmental loss of kyphosis is indicated by the flat area from T5 to T8. On palpation the spinous processes sit vertically aligned instead of in a gentle posterior curve. (Copyright Diane G. Lee Physiotherapist Corporation and Linda-Joy Lee Physiotherapist Corporation.)

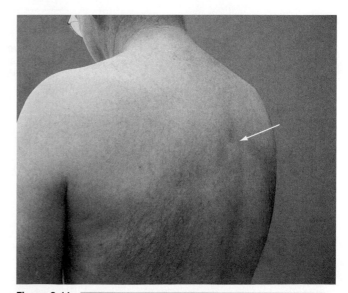

Figure 8-11

This individual has a segmental loss of the thoracic kyphosis at T5-6 *(arrow)*. On palpation, T5 feels anterior (ventral) relative to the levels above and below. (Copyright Diane G. Lee Physiotherapist Corporation and Linda-Joy Lee Physiotherapist Corporation.)

Postural analysis – Segmental alignment
Clinical reasoning: analysis of the flexed T4 segment

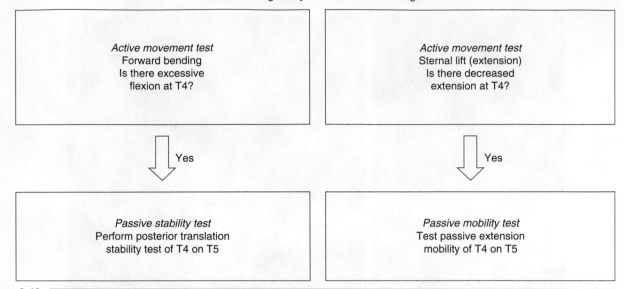

Active movement test Forward bending Is there excessive flexion at T4?	Active movement test Sternal lift (extension) Is there decreased extension at T4?
↓ Yes	↓ Yes
Passive stability test Perform posterior translation stability test of T4 on T5	Passive mobility test Test passive extension mobility of T4 on T5

Figure 8-12

Postural analysis: segmental alignment. This clinical reasoning process is used when the T4 segment is found to be flexed on postural assessment.

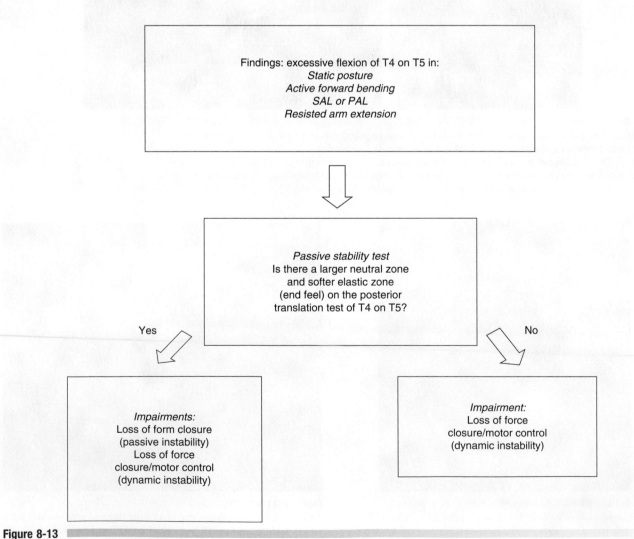

Findings: excessive flexion of T4 on T5 in:
Static posture
Active forward bending
SAL or PAL
Resisted arm extension

Passive stability test
Is there a larger neutral zone
and softer elastic zone
(end feel) on the posterior
translation test of T4 on T5?

Yes

No

Impairments:
Loss of form closure
(passive instability)
Loss of force
closure/motor control
(dynamic instability)

Impairment:
Loss of force
closure/motor control
(dynamic instability)

Figure 8-13

Postural analysis: segmental alignment. This clinical reasoning process is used when the T4 segment is excessively flexed during load transfer tests.

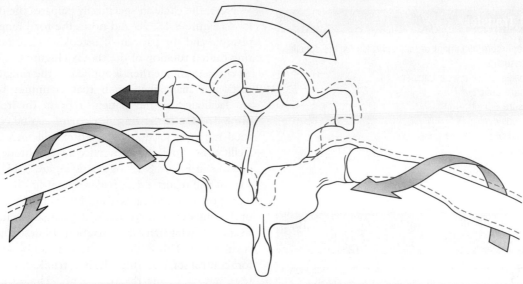

Figure 8-14
Osteokinematic and arthrokinematic motions proposed to occur during right rotation of the thorax.
(Copyright Diane G. Lee Physiotherapist Corporation and Linda-Joy Lee Physiotherapist Corporation.)

Table 8-1
Possible Causes of Failed Load Transfer

Form Closure Deficit	Force Closure/Motor Control Deficits
Disc disruption	Insufficient muscle bulk or resting tone
Ligament strain	Nonrecruitment
Capsule strain	Altered timing and coordination of recruitment
Cartilaginous disruption (anterior joints)	Increased resting tone
Altered vertebral body height or shape	Decreased threshold to recruit (overactivity)
	Altered modulation of force generation
Form closure deficits present with concurrent force closure/motor control deficits	Force closure/motor control deficits can exist without form closure deficits

Table 8-2
Biomechanics of T5-6 During Right Trunk Rotation

Physiological Optimum Load Transfer	Nonoptimum Biomechanics (Failed Load Transfer)
Right rotation and left lateral translation of T5	Decreased or no movement or excessive right rotation/left lateral translation of T5
Posterior rotation and anteromedial translation of the right sixth rib	Left rotation and right lateral translation of T5
Anterior rotation and posterolateral translation of the left sixth rib	Decreased or no posterior rotation of the right sixth rib, excessive posterior rotation, or anterior rotation
Ring complex translation to the left	Decreased or no anterior rotation of the left sixth rib, excessive anterior rotation, or posterior rotation
	Ring translation to the left but not in synchrony with the rings above and below; excessive ring translation to the left; ring translation to the right; no movement of the ring

Failed Load Transfer

- Absence of optimum alignment or biomechanics for the specific task being assessed
- Possible causes of failed load transfer:
  - Form closure deficit
  - Force closure deficit
  - Altered motor control
  - Combination of any of the above

Non-physiological Biomechanics Require a Form Closure Deficit

- Excessive mobility in one or more directions, with a translation component that is opposite to that of normal biomechanics (e.g., excessive posterior translation of the vertebra during flexion)
- Lack of any mobility, with concurrent marked positional findings in a pattern that is opposite that of normal biomechanics (e.g., the sixth ring is fixated in left lateral translation, but the T5 vertebra is left rotated, the right sixth rib is anteriorly rotated, and the left sixth rib is posteriorly rotated)

Next, the clinician specifically palpates the dysfunctional level (Figure 8-15, *A*) and notes the total range of motion possible and the pattern of osteokinematic motion of the ring during rotation of the thorax (Figure 8-15, *B*). A gentle corrective force then is applied to the ring, and this correction is maintained such that optimum biomechanics are facilitated as the patient repeats the rotation (Figure 8-15, *C*). If the ring movement can be corrected, the total range of motion of rotation will increase with this facilitation (note the difference in amplitude of rotation possible in Figure 8-15, *B* versus Figure 8-15, *C*), and the patient will report a decrease of symptoms if the symptoms were present on initial testing. Furthermore, if the motion of the ring can be corrected with manual facilitation, a joint fixation (lateral translation fixation, as described by Lee[12]) is ruled out. This finding suggests a nonoptimum strategy for control of the ring during trunk rotation. Further tests can determine the treatment techniques required to change this pattern, but the clinician has confirmed that one specific ring needs to be addressed to restore full functional thoracic rotation.

Correction of ring motion may not be possible for several reasons, including joint fixation, fibrosis that causes stiffness in one or more joints, and/or excessive muscle tone, resulting in excessive compression and loss of mobility in one or more joints.

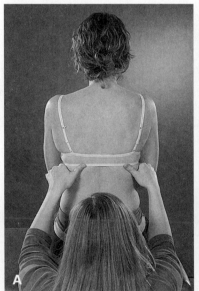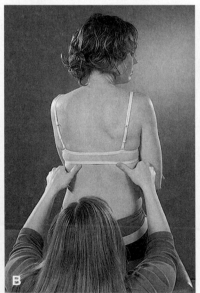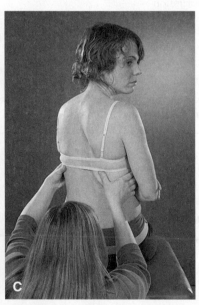

Figure 8-15
Active thoracic rotation with palpation and correction of the ring. **A,** Clinician's hand position for palpation of the eighth thoracic ring. The index fingers rest along the lateral borders and the thumbs along the posterior borders of the right and left eighth ribs. **B,** The patient right rotates; the clinician notes the range of motion and the osteokinematic movements of the right and left ribs, as well as the whole ring complex, during the movement. The patient then returns to neutral. **C,** Right rotation with correction of the eighth ring position, which facilitated correct osteokinematics. Note the increased range of motion resulting from this ring correction. (Copyright Diane G. Lee Physiotherapist Corporation and Linda-Joy Lee Physiotherapist Corporation.)

Sitting Arm Lift and Prone Arm Lift Tests

The sitting arm lift (SAL) and the prone arm lift (PAL) are two tests that were originally developed for the thorax[33,34] based on the principles of the active straight leg raise (ASLR) test,[35-37] a validated test of failed load transfer in the pelvic girdle in pregnancy-related pelvic girdle pain. The SAL and PAL tests have been further developed to identify the site or sites of failed load transfer in the thorax, cervical spine, scapula, and glenohumeral joint, and these tests should be performed in all patients with upper quadrant symptoms. The results of the tests guide the clinician in determining which area should be the focus of treatment. This is especially useful for patients with pain in multiple areas, and it highlights the value of assessing loss of effective load transfer in all areas involved in a movement, not just the painful structures.

Sitting Arm Lift Test

Patient Position. Sitting, hands resting on the thighs. Initially no postural correction is given, because the goal is to assess the patient's habitual pattern. The test is repeated with a variety of modifications; postural correction can be one of these modifications if indicated.

Test Procedure. The clinician instructs the patient to lift one arm (usually the pain-free side first if ipsilateral symptoms are present), with the arm straight and the thumb up, into elevation through shoulder flexion and then to lower the arm (Figure 8-16). Next, the patient is instructed to lift the other arm and lower it. The patient then is asked, "Does one arm feel heavier to lift than the other or different to lift than the other?" The clinician notes whether symptoms are produced and also observes which arm looks as if it requires more effort to lift. With regard to effort, the key part of the range to note is from the initiation of movement to the first 70° to 90° of flexion. If one arm is heavier or requires more effort to lift, the SAL test result is positive. The remainder of the test is performed using the positive (heavy) arm.

Palpation for Areas of Failed Load Transfer.

1. *Thorax:* The ribs are palpated as described previously (see Figure 8-15, *A*). The clinician should note whether any levels are not in neutral alignment; that is, whether any of the rings are resting in a laterally translated position relative to others. The patient then repeats the SAL on the positive side, and the clinician notes any translation of the ring, especially with the initiation of movement (see Figure 8-16). It is well understood that movement of a limb results in perturbation to the spine, and the central nervous system prepares for this perturbation by activating trunk muscles before or shortly after the primary mover for the limb.[38-41] If this principle is applied to the thoracic spine, then ideally, as the patient prepares to lift the arm, the muscles of the thorax should be activated such that no intersegmental translation occurs in any part of the thorax, and the relationship of the thorax to the head and to the pelvis should be maintained (maintenance

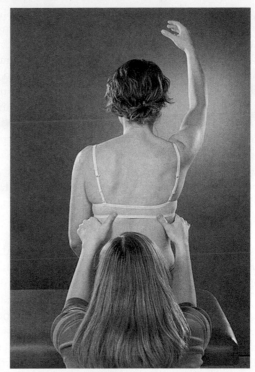

Figure 8-16

Thoracic assessment: SAL test. The patient first performs elevation through flexion of the right and left arms and identifies which arm feels more difficult to lift or to initiate movement. Elevation of the heavy arm then is repeated, and the clinician palpates the osteokinematic motion of each thoracic ring (here, the eighth ring) as the patient performs active elevation through flexion. A positive test result for failed load transfer through the thorax occurs when (1) a thoracic ring (or more than one) translates along any axis or rotates in any plane or (2) any component of the ring (vertebra or rib) translates or rotates along any axis or plane. (Copyright Diane G. Lee Physiotherapist Corporation and Linda-Joy Lee Physiotherapist Corporation.)

of the spinal curves). A positive test result for failed load transfer through the thorax occurs when one (or more) of the thoracic rings translates along any axis or rotates in any plane, or when any component of the ring (vertebra or rib) translates or rotates along any axis or plane, during the SAL. The clinician should note the level and direction of the loss of control. Because the SAL creates a rotational perturbation force to the thorax, the common pattern of failed load transfer is loss of rotational control of one or more of the rings, with concurrent lateral translation either to the same side as the arm lift (ipsilateral) or to the contralateral side. Loss of control usually is observed in the early to middle range of arm elevation and is different from the normal biomechanics that occur at the end of arm elevation. During the last stage of full arm elevation, all levels of the thorax should move into extension, ipsilateral rotation, and side-bending; this occurs more in the upper thorax than in the lower portion.

2. *Scapula:* The medial border and spine of the scapula are observed for normal scapulohumeral rhythm during the SAL movement. The clinician can palpate the medial border and inferior angle to confirm what is observed. Several patterns of abnormal scapular movement can occur, and these are defined as failed load transfer of the scapula during the SAL. Common patterns include downward rotation, insufficient upward rotation, insufficient elevation, insufficient posterior tilt, and medial border winging. If the scapula is in a nonoptimum position to start (before the arm is lifted), such as downwardly rotated and depressed (i.e., the "dumped" scapula), this also is noted. In the next stage of the SAL test, the clinician must correct these faults. (See volume 1 of this series, *Orthopedic Physical Assessment,* Chapter 5, for further details on scapular assessment.[21])

3. *Glenohumeral joint:* The humeral head is palpated anteriorly and posteriorly just inferior to the acromion. The position of the humeral head is noted at rest and during the SAL. The humeral head should remain centered with respect to the glenoid fossa throughout full elevation of the arm. Failed load transfer of the glenohumeral joint is defined as a loss of the centered position; often the humeral head is displaced anteriorly or translates anteriorly (or both) during the SAL. The clinician should note where in the range of motion the humeral head loses its centered position. If the starting position is excessively anterior, when forward flexion is initiated, the humeral head should move back into a centered position and remain centered throughout the shoulder flexion range of motion.

4. *Cervical spine (C2-C7):* The lateral aspect of the articular pillars are palpated bilaterally for any loss of intersegmental position during the SAL (Figure 8-17). Failed load transfer is defined as one vertebra moving into anterior translation, posterior translation, or lateral translation/rotation relative to the vertebra below during the initiation of or through range of forward arm flexion. As with the thorax, a small amount of extension/rotation/lateral bending occurs at the very end of arm elevation, but this should be shared throughout the midcervical spine rather than occur excessively at one level. The level and direction of loss of segmental control are noted. Commonly, the poorly controlled segment translates ipsilaterally (to the side of the moving arm during the SAL), with concurrent contralateral rotation of the vertebra.

Correction of Areas of Failed Load Transfer and Assessment of the Impact on the Test Result.

1. *Thorax:* Using a hand position that allows a specific force to be applied to the poorly controlled thoracic ring or rib, the clinician applies a gentle corrective force that aligns the dysfunctional ring into a neutral starting position. For example, if the patient demonstrates a positive right SAL and the seventh ring is translated to the right at rest, a gentle left translation of the seventh ring is applied, along with a gentle posterior rotation of the right (ipsilateral) seventh rib and an anterior rotation of the left

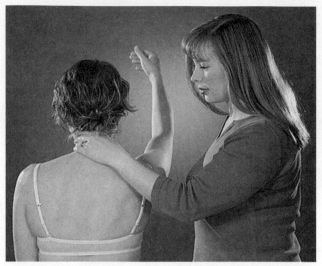

Figure 8-17

Cervical assessment: SAL test. To assess for failed load transfer in the cervical spine, the sitting arm lift is repeated as the clinician palpates the articular pillars of the cervical spine. Failed load transfer is defined as the movement of one vertebra into anterior translation, posterior translation, or lateral translation/rotation relative to the vertebra below during the initiation of or through the range of forward arm flexion. (Copyright Diane G. Lee Physiotherapist Corporation and Linda-Joy Lee Physiotherapist Corporation.)

(contralateral) seventh rib. Often the correction is more successful if the clinician asks the patient to relax the chest and then gently applies vertical traction (decompression) to the ring before attempting the lateral correction. This correction is maintained as the patient repeats the SAL; any difference in effort or change in symptoms is noted by both the clinician and the patient.

2. *Scapula:* If the scapula is in a nonoptimum starting position, the clinician corrects the scapular position and maintains this correction while the patient repeats the SAL. Again, the impact on the SAL is noted (i.e., easier, harder, or no change). If a nonoptimum scapular pattern occurs through the range of motion, the clinician uses manual support to facilitate the optimum pattern as the patient performs the SAL, and the impact of the manual support is noted as described previously.

3. *Humeral head:* The clinician palpates the humeral head and uses gentle pressure to correct the starting position and/or to maintain a centered humeral head position during the SAL. The impact of this correction is assessed and noted.

4. *Cervical spine:* The clinician palpates the specific level that was identified with failed load transfer during the SAL. Gentle manual traction is applied, along with pressure, to maintain optimum alignment of the vertebra (usually a lateral translation force to the contralateral side) while the SAL is repeated.

5. *General postural alignment:* The clinician corrects the patient's postural alignment, making sure that no excessive effort or use of the thoracic erector spinae is required to

attain the new position. The SAL is then repeated on the positive side. If the arm is easier to lift, this indicates that postural re-education will improve functional load transfer when the arm is used. This often is a good way to impress upon patients the effects of poor postural habits.

Clinical Reasoning for the Sitting Arm Lift Test. The goals of the SAL test are (1) to identify areas of failed load transfer in the upper quadrant and (2) to determine how correction and addition of compression (increased control) affect the patient's ability to perform the load transfer (SAL) test. If the manual correction improves the person's ability to perform the SAL (the arm is easier to lift, symptoms are diminished), this is an indication that treatment interventions should be directed toward optimizing motor control and stability in that area (thorax, scapula, glenohumeral joint, cervical segment, or general postural alignment). If correction of an area has a negative effect on the SAL result (the arm is harder to lift, symptoms are increased), this is an indication that the area is already under excessive compression, and treatment interventions should be directed at reducing compression through release of excessive muscle tone and increasing joint mobility in that area (Figure 8-18). Further tests are required to determine which muscles to facilitate or release and which joints to mobilize. In most situations both release and facilitation of optimum patterns of movement is required.

Prone Arm Lift Test. The prone arm lift (PAL) is a variation of the SAL test in a higher load position (prone). It assesses the ability to initially take the load of the arm in a greater amount of shoulder flexion. It is particularly important to assess this ability in patients who require this position functionally (e.g., overhead workers, swimmers) or who complain of difficulties with higher loads. It can also be used as a test at later stages of treatment. The starting position is prone, with the arms overhead in approximately 120° flexion and fully supported on the treatment plinth (the head of the plinth needs to be dropped down). The clinician instructs the patient to lift one arm 2 cm (about 1 inch) and then lower it. This movement is repeated on the other side. The arm that tests positive is the arm that is heavier to lift. The palpation and correction techniques described previously are applied and the results evaluated.

Tests of Form Closure

To date few studies have been done to validate the use of passive accessory joint mobility testing in the thoracic spine. However, such testing remains a valuable clinical technique. These techniques are described in detail elsewhere.[21,42]

In addition to passive mobility testing, passive stability tests[43] are indicated when there is a loss of optimum segmental alignment noted on postural assessment (excessively

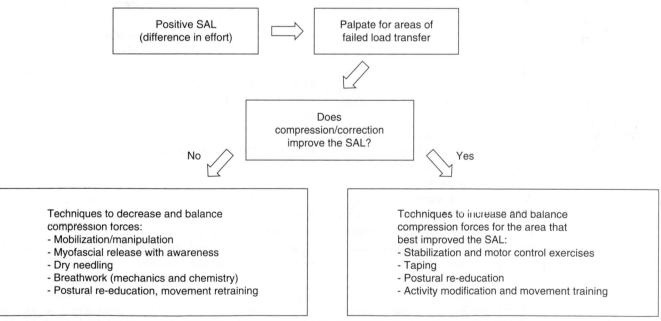

Figure 8-18

Clinical reasoning for the SAL test. Note that after any treatment technique, the SAL test should be repeated to assist in the next stage of treatment planning. For example, the patient initially may present with excessive global muscle tone; applying compression during the SAL test makes the arm harder to lift. Treatment techniques therefore should focus on myofascial release to reduce and balance compression in the affected region. After this, the SAL movement often is easier, and compression of the area of failed load transfer now makes the arm even easier to lift; this indicates that techniques to increase and balance compression are appropriate (e.g., taping, segmental control exercises).

flexed or extended, lateral translation of one ring) and/or excessive movement on active and passive mobility tests (see Figures 8-12 and 8-13). An analysis of the amplitude and quality of both the neutral and elastic zones of motion is performed with the joint initially in a neutral position (not flexed nor extended). An increase in the size of the neutral zone combined with a soft end feel are characteristic of a joint with a loss of integrity in the passive system (see volume 2 of this series, *Scientific Foundations and Principles of Practice in Musculoskeletal Rehabilitation,* chapters 19 and 24). The specific structures affected depend on the direction of the translation applied. The specific stability tests are described elsewhere.[42,43] If an increased neutral zone and soft end feel are noted with the joint in a neutral position, the tests can be repeated with the joint in the close packed position (full extension or flexion), in which the size of the neutral zone should be minimal and the end feel firm. The presence of an increased neutral zone and soft end feel in full extension or flexion confirms that some degree of laxity exists in the ligamentous (and connecting fascial) support system (i.e., a loss of form closure).

A dynamic component can be added to the passive stability tests in several ways. In the sitting position, the patient can be asked to lift the arms against the clinician's resistance. The stability test is repeated while the muscles are active. If the segmental local and superficial global muscles are working synergistically, the stability test result is negative (translation is controlled). If the local muscles are not working appropriately, even with contraction of the global muscles the stability test result is positive (translation is not controlled). Once the patient has been taught how to recruit the local segmental stabilizing muscles, the stability test can be repeated with a precontraction of the segmental muscles in any position. With a low force contraction of the local stabilizing muscles (i.e., 10% to 20% of the maximum voluntary contraction [MVC]), the neutral zone should be reduced to zero and produce a solid resistance to the translation applied in the stability test. This suggests a good prognosis for recovery of dynamic control.

If the neutral zone does not change with the segmental muscle contraction, the clinician has several scenarios to consider. First, the patient may not be sufficiently recruiting the segmental muscles. Second, the segmental muscles (e.g., multifidus) may have insufficient bulk to produce a sufficient increase in tension in the fascial system to change the resistance to translation. Change in fascial tension is one mechanism by which the muscle system changes compression across joints.[40,44,45] In this case, a palpable decrease in the bulk and resting tone of the segmental muscles will be noted. As the exercise rehabilitation program is progressed and muscle bulk increases, the resultant increased fascial tension may increase passive support sufficiently to produce a negative result on the stability test.

Finally, significant ligamentous and other passive support deficiencies may require remediation, potentially with tools such as prolotherapy. In these cases, the clinician can advise the patient on activities to avoid and when to use support, such as taping. These patients are likely to have recurrent episodes of pain, depending on their activities and postures, and intermittent treatment may be necessary to settle flare-ups.

Surgical intervention in the thorax is indicated only in extreme and severe cases when cord compromise is a risk.

Tests of Force Closure/Motor Control

The ability of the spine to withstand intersegmental shearing forces, multisegmental buckling forces, and challenges to postural equilibrium depends on finely tuned coordination of activity between the deep and superficial muscles of the trunk.[40,46-51] A significant body of evidence has established that, in the lumbar and cervical spines, specific patterns of muscle recruitment occur in healthy controls, and these patterns are disrupted in patients with low back, pelvic girdle, and neck pain.[29,30,39-41,49,52-79] Based on these studies, muscle training and exercise rehabilitation assessment and treatment approaches have been developed for patients with lumbopelvic and cervical pain and dysfunction.[2,46-49,51,60,63,70,80-84] The clinical approach presented here for restoring force closure and motor control has been developed based on this evidence, combined with clinical experience in treating thoracic pain and dysfunction. Specific studies of muscle function in the thorax are required to establish how the brain controls the muscle system for optimum stability and mobility of the thorax while meeting the requirements for optimum respiration. This section describes tests of muscle function that have been found clinically useful for decision making about treatment planning and exercise prescription.

Muscle Assessment: Segmental Stabilizers

In patients with low back pain, studies have demonstrated a loss of cross sectional area in the lumbar multifidus.[85-88] Investigations of muscle timing and activation patterns have identified differential activity between the deep and superficial fibers in people without back pain.[64,65,89] In patients with low back pain, changes in muscle activity occur specifically in the deep fibers of the multifidus rather than in the superficial fibers.[64] Clinical approaches have been developed for the training of isolated recruitment of the deep fibers, followed by the integration of these recruitment strategies into functional movements,[2,47,80,82-84,90] and these methods have been shown to be effective at reducing pain, disability,[84,90] and the recurrence of low back pain[80] and also for improving quality of life.[90]

Like the lumbopelvic region, the thorax has a complex arrangement of deep and superficial muscles; however, few studies have investigated the function of these muscles and how their function is affected by pain. Deep segmental muscles of the thorax that are anatomically situated to be classified as local stabilizers include the deep fibers of the multifidus/rotatores, the levator costarum, the intercostals, and the diaphragm (lower thorax). Although no studies of the cross sectional area have been done, recent electromyographic studies have shown that differential activity occurs between the deep multifidus/rotatores and the longissimus thoracis muscles during seated rotation[91] and fast perturbations to trunk stability.[92] This early evidence supports the theory that the paraspinal muscle group cannot be considered as a single unit; rather, the component muscles should be assessed and treated specifically.

Clinically, it has been noted that loss of resting tone or atrophy can occur segmentally in the thoracic spine, similar to the changes seen in the lumbar spine.[42,93] This may occur unilaterally or bilaterally. Loss of resting tone or atrophy of the deep multifidus/rotatores can be palpated close to the spinous processes as a softening in the deep muscle tissue or a loss of resistance to pressure (Figure 8-19). A similar loss of tone or atrophy can occur segmentally in the intercostal muscles, usually at the level correlating to an area of poor segmental control (see later discussion). Palpation of both the multifidus/rotatores and the intercostal muscles requires that the patient be positioned such that the superficial muscles are as relaxed as possible. If hypertonicity is present in the superficial muscles (i.e., spinalis thoracis, longissimus thoracis, iliocostalis thoracis,

semispinalis thoracis, rhomboids, and trapezius), the loss of tone in the deep muscles often is not evident until techniques to reduce the excessive tone have been performed. Tone should be palpated and compared to levels above and below the area of interest, as well as between the right and left sides. In addition to palpating the muscle, the clinician should use verbal cues to assess the patient's ability to cognitively activate the muscle at a segment and to assess the symmetry of this activation between the left and right sides. These palpation and activation tests should be correlated with areas of failed load transfer revealed by dynamic tests (rotation, SAL and PAL tests) and areas of passive instability. The function of the diaphragm is assessed by examining breathing parameters in multiple positions (see *Orthopedic Physical Assessment*[21] and Lee[34]).

Palpation of Tone and Muscle Bulk: Superficial Muscles

Different patterns of excessive activity in the superficial muscles have been observed in patients with low back pain.[29,30,32,47,94] Muscles that commonly tend to become hypertonic in patients with thoracic pain or dysfunction include (unilaterally or bilaterally): specific fascicles of the erector spinae, latissimus dorsi, rhomboids, trapezius, rotator cuff muscles, serratus anterior, scalenes, levator scapulae, pectoralis minor and major, quadratus lumborum, internal and external obliques, rectus abdominis, and superficial lumbar multifidus. These muscles should be palpated for tone and muscle bulk and the results compared to those on the other side; they also should be assessed for their ability to decrease in tone during functional movements. For example, during trunk rotation, the contralateral longissimus should decrease in activity.[91] If muscle activity increases or remains the same during this task, treatment should include techniques to reduce and inhibit the muscle's tone. In addition, movement strategy retraining for synergistic muscle activation during rotation is required. Although the intercostal muscles have been classified as segmental stabilizers for the thorax, the authors have also observed that the intercostals on one side of a ring may be hypertonic and have poor recruitment in response to verbal cueing. It is not possible with manual palpation to distinguish the internal and external intercostals. In these cases restoration of optimal ring control requires releasing the hypertonic intercostals, followed by techniques to recruit the muscles in a more optimum pattern.

Neurodynamics and Ring Position

Slump Test. The slump test is described in *Orthopedic Physical Assessment*,[21] and by Butler.[95,96] Because of the connections of the nervous system, restrictions in the thoracic region can play a role in distal symptoms in the legs or arms. To assess the impact of the thoracic spine on distal symptoms, the authors propose a variation of the slump

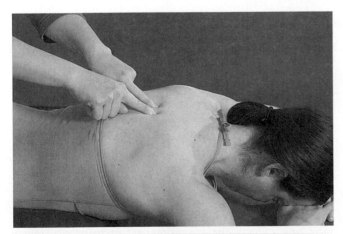

Figure 8-19

Palpation of the thoracic multifidus/rotatores. The clinician assesses the tone and resistance to sinking pressure of the muscle just lateral to the spinous processes. This is compared from side to side and between levels above and below. In the thoracic spine, the multifidus lies deep to the global multisegmental muscles. If hypertonicity is present in these more superficial muscles, atrophy in the deep multifidus/rotatores is not evident until this global hypertonicity is released. (Copyright Diane G. Lee Physiotherapist Corporation and Linda-Joy Lee Physiotherapist Corporation.)

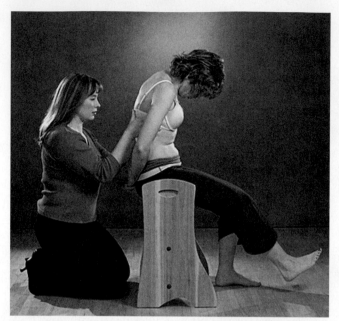

Figure 8-20
Neurodynamics and ring position: Slump test. The clinician palpates a specific thoracic ring as the patient performs the slump test. The overall range of motion of the slump test (the amount of leg extension) is noted, as is the osteokinematic motion of the ring as the components of the slump test are performed. Nonoptimum osteokinematics of the ring and when they occur are noted. The clinician then repeats the slump test while correcting and facilitating optimum osteokinematics; the impact on the range of motion of leg extension and on the patient's symptoms is noted. (Copyright Diane G. Lee Physiotherapist Corporation and Linda-Joy Lee Physiotherapist Corporation.)

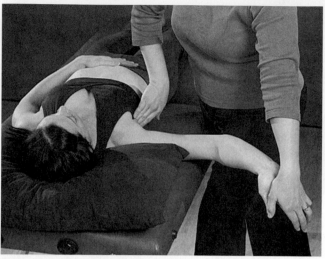

Figure 8-21
Neurodynamics and ring position: Upper limb neurodynamic test. The clinician palpates one thoracic ring at the lateral border of one rib during the upper limb neurodynamic test (median nerve). The clinician then performs the variations of the upper limb neurodynamic test to determine which variation is positive for symptom reproduction and restricted motion compared to the other side. The thoracic rings are then palpated in the midaxillary line while the positive test is repeated. If movement of one or more rings is palpated during the test, the clinician returns to the start position and applies manual compression to correct and maintain ring position while the test is repeated. An increase in the range of motion and/or decrease in symptoms indicates that the thoracic ring is a component of the restriction in the neurodynamic test. (Copyright Diane G. Lee Physiotherapist Corporation and Linda-Joy Lee Physiotherapist Corporation.)

and upper limb neurodynamic tests as originally proposed by Butler.[95,96] Using the ring palpation as described previously, the clinician assesses the thorax and identifies any rings that translate laterally as the patient moves into the slump position while extending the knee and then dorsiflexing the ankle (Figure 8-20). The side of knee extension/ankle dorsiflexion that reproduces the patient's symptoms is noted, along with any asymmetry or restriction of range of leg movement. If one ring translates laterally during any component of the slump test, the patient is asked to return to the neutral starting position. The clinician then corrects and stabilizes the dysfunctional ring (with gentle traction, lateral translation, and rib rotations as described previously) as the patient repeats the slump test and lower extremity movements that reproduced the symptoms. If correction of the thoracic ring reduces the symptoms and increases the range of motion of the lower extremity movements, treatment of the thoracic ring should be included to alleviate the distal symptoms.

Upper Limb Neurodynamic Test. The upper thorax is often involved when the upper limb neurodynamic test result is positive, although all rings should be assessed.

The upper limb neurodynamic test as described by Butler[95,96] and in *Orthopedic Physical Assessment*[21] is performed. The clinician then repeats the positive variation of the test (ULNT1 [median], ULNT2 [median], ULNT2 [radial], ULNT3 [ulnar]) while palpating the lateral border of the ribs to feel for any lateral translation (Figure 8-21). The ideal response is no movement of the thoracic rings (until very end range movement) and specifically no movement of one level compared to the rest of the rib cage. The arm is returned to the starting position, the clinician corrects and stabilizes the ring with a gentle posterior rotation of the ipsilateral rib and contralateral lateral translation, and the neurodynamic test is repeated. If correction of the thoracic ring reduces the symptoms and increases the range of motion of the arm movements, treatment of the thoracic ring should be included to alleviate the distal arm symptoms.

In both the slump test and the upper limb neurodynamic tests, if the clinician is unable to correct the ring position or maintain the correction, excessive compression exists in the thorax that needs to be assessed and treated to complete the neurodynamic test and evaluate the impact of the thorax on the distal symptoms.

Management of Thoracic Pain and Dysfunction

Treatment of the impaired thorax must be prescriptive, because every individual has a unique clinical presentation. Ultimately, the goal is to teach the patient a healthier way to live and move so that sustained compression and/or tensile forces on any one structure are avoided. The clinician uses manual skills to facilitate this process; however, the primary role is to educate and coach the patient through the recovery process, because only the patient can make the changes necessary for optimum function. Rarely is only one dysfunction present (e.g., one stiff joint or one poorly controlled joint). More commonly, multiple problems coexist; therefore, the most effective treatment consists of a combination of techniques and exercises that are patient specific.

For patients presenting with stiff or compressed joints, the clinician may decide to use manual techniques and exercises that decompress the joints (increase mobility) and follow this with an exercise plan that establishes optimum movement and stabilization strategies. For patients presenting with poorly controlled joints, the clinician may decide to start a program that emphasizes retraining of the stability muscle system and then later add decompression techniques and exercises (to increase mobility) as necessary. In the most common scenario, a combination of concurrent decompression and stabilization is required. In these cases, the clinician uses techniques to decompress specific areas while prescribing exercises and/or support (taping) for increased stability in other areas. It is not uncommon in the thorax to have to release the tension and compression forces creating a non-optimal ring position, and then to train control and stability of the same ring. The clinician makes decisions about where and when to use techniques to reduce or increase compression based on the findings from the combination of assessment tests. The common findings and recommended treatment techniques are described in this section (Boxes 8-1 and 8-2; Figures 8-22 to 8-24).

Principles for Reducing Articular Compression: Restoring Mobility

Excessive articular compression in the thorax can occur as a result of factors intrinsic to the joint, such as capsular fibrosis secondary to a joint effusion or joint ankylosis in a pathological condition such as ankylosing spondylitis. Excessive articular compression can also occur as a result of factors extrinsic to the joint, such as increased tone in muscles at rest that span the joints. In both cases, the excessive compression results in reduced mobility of the joint, but the treatment techniques used to restore mobility are quite different, based on the different reasons for the restriction.

Joint fibrosis commonly occurs secondary to a traumatic event, but habitual poor postures over time also can result in multisegmental joint stiffness. Whereas an acute zygapophyseal or costotransverse joint sprain produces localized pain over the involved joint, chronic restrictions often are pain free and are identified on assessment as restriction on active and passive mobility testing. The neutral zone of the joint is reduced, and the end feel is early with increased firmness. The pain-free restricted

---

Box 8-1 Treatment Principles for Form Closure Deficit

Goals of Treatment
- Relieve pain
- Reduce loading and stress to injured structure or structures
- Support the healing process (acute phase)
- Train the force closure/motor control system to compensate for form closure deficits
- Prevent the development of nonoptimum movement patterns that can contribute to recurrence and chronicity

Treatment Techniques
- Articular techniques are graded according to the stage of healing and irritability:
  - Specific traction (especially for disc injury) and oscillatory mobilizations to relieve pain and increase joint lubrication and circulation
  - Oscillatory and sustained mobilization to hypomobile segments above and below the injured structure
- Myofascial release with awareness techniques to reduce tone and activity in muscles that compress the injured structures /or create altered movement patterns
- Muscle energy techniques to facilitate optimum alignment
- Taping of injured structure for support and/or to facilitate optimum biomechanics
- Postural education to ensure unloading of injured structures
- Activity modification to prevent further injury and patient education about positions and activities that can unload injured structures
- Assessment and treatment of force closure/motor control deficits (see Box 8-2)

Box 8-2 Treatment Principles for Force Closure/Motor Control Deficit

Goal
- Remove the old movement strategy

Treatment Techniques
- Reduce resting tone and activity of hypertonic and dominant muscles (usually superficial global muscles):
  - Breath work, with attention to focusing the breath into restricted areas of the thorax
  - Soft tissue mobilization and myofascial release techniques
  - Muscle energy techniques
  - Trigger point techniques
  - Dry needling or intramuscular stimulation
  - Release with awareness techniques
  - Retraining of postural patterns and restoration of ability to find neutral spine
  - Surface electromyographic (EMG) recordings or real-time ultrasound imaging to foster relaxation of the targeted muscle
  - Manual therapy techniques (oscillatory joint mobilization, manipulation) to facilitate neurophysiological relaxation of the affected muscle
- Use muscle energy techniques and postural education to create optimum alignment

Goal
- Teach a new movement strategy in order to:
  - Create optimum static and dynamic motor control patterns so that compression and tensile forces are balanced through all structures in the kinetic chain
  - Create adequate force closure/motor control to compensate for underlying form closure deficits, if present

Treatment Techniques
- Facilitate and train local muscle control for segmental and inter-ring stability
- Integrate local muscle activation and segmental/inter-ring control into:
  - Functional postures (sitting, standing, upper extremity weight bearing)
  - Functional movements (integrate with scapula, arm, and neck movement)
  - Sport-specific and work-related tasks
- Start endurance training while motor patterns are established and progress to strength and power training for specific tasks and muscles as identified on assessment and as related to the patient's goals
- Tape to increase proprioceptive input and awareness and to facilitate optimum control and biomechanics
- With a form closure deficit: Monitor the level and direction of instability by palpation through all stages of treatment to ensure dynamic control of the specific passive instability

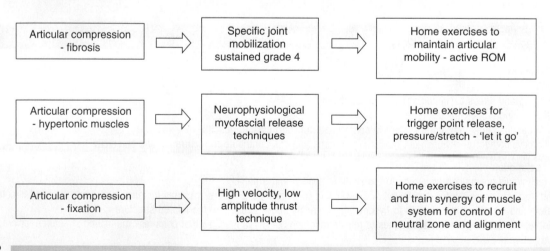

Figure 8-22

Treatment of a compressed/hypomobile joint. Treatment techniques vary, depending on the cause of the excessive articular compression. For a stiff, fibrotic joint, the most effective technique is a specific, grade 4, sustained passive articular mobilization that is held for up to 3 minutes. Numerous techniques are effective for a neuromyofascially compressed joint; any technique that targets a change in the neurophysiology of the impaired, overactive muscles can be used. Note that home exercises also vary, depending on the cause of the excessive articular compression.

Treatment principles

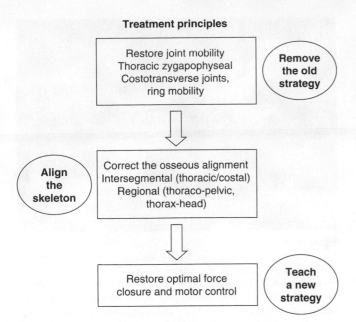

Figure 8-23

Treatment principles for pain and/or dysfunction in the thorax.

joint tends to produce symptoms elsewhere, either on the contralateral side or at levels above and below the restriction. The joint that is compressed because of fibrosis is most effectively treated with specific passive articular mobilization techniques. The technique is graded according to the irritability of the articular tissues, but generally long-standing fibrosis requires a sustained grade 4+ passive mobilization (see Chapter 10) (Figure 8-25).

Home exercises are designed to promote use of the new mobility gained in the specific joints from the passive mobilization technique. For example, a home exercise that produces focused right side-bending of the midthoracic spine is indicated if the inferior glide of the right T6-7 zygapophyseal joint was restricted. The clinician should palpate the right T6-7 zygapophyseal joint while the patient performs the exercise to make sure that movement occurs at the desired level.

In a joint that is compressed as a result of overactivation or increased resting tone of muscles, many neuromuscular techniques can reduce the hypertonicity and restore joint mobility. Distinguishing a neuromyofascially compressed joint from a fibrotic joint requires attention to the differences in the feel of the neutral zone during passive mobility testing. Like a fibrotic joint, a neuromyofascially compressed joint has a reduced neutral zone, but the quality of the neutral zone is different. In a fibrotic joint, the neutral zone is smaller but clearly present and does not require increased force to produce movement until the end feel is reached. In contrast, a neuromyofascially compressed joint produces increased resistance throughout the neutral zone; the joint can be moved, but more force is required (much like the feel of moderate hamstring guarding when trying to apply Lachman's test to the knee). In the case of neuromyofascial compression, palpable bands of hypertonicity are present in specific muscles, and usually in specific fascicles of these muscles, of the thorax. These hypertonic muscle bands are evident during active range of motion, functional load transfer tests, and palpation. Effective treatment of a neuromyofascially compressed

Figure 8-24

Treatment principles for pain and/or dysfunction in the thorax.

Treatment principles

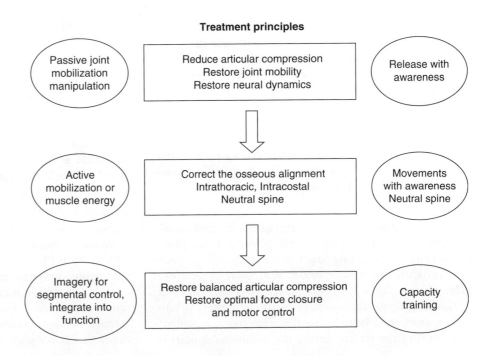

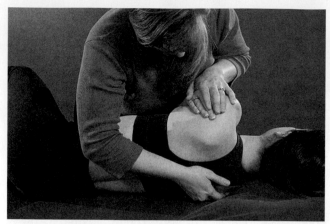

Figure 8-25

Therapist's posterior hand position for restoring unilateral flexion of the left T4-5 zygapophyseal joint. The therapist's scaphoid stabilizes the left transverse process of T5, and the flexed third finger stabilizes the right transverse process of T4. The motion barrier for flexion/side flexion is engaged through the patient's thorax as the patient is rolled back toward the table. The mobilization is localized and specific to the left T4-5 segment, and a sustained grade 4 mobilization is then performed. (Copyright Diane G. Lee Physiotherapist Corporation and Linda-Joy Lee Physiotherapist Corporation.)

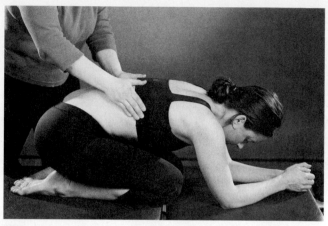

Figure 8-26

Use of breathing for neuromyofascial release in the thorax. When the thoracic erector spinae are hypertonic, this position (child's pose) or prone over a ball is a good position to use because the thorax is flexed and open posteriorly. The clinician palpates the rib cage during several breath cycles to identify areas of decreased expansion during inspiration. Subsequently, manual and verbal cues are used to create awareness in the areas of less expansion. The patient is encouraged to breathe into the restricted regions. The clinician asks the patient to breathe into the tight muscle and provides the patient with cues to "open" into the clinician's fingers and to "make the muscle melt." As the patient breathes in and the clinician feels the spine/rib start to move, the clinician provides a gentle lateral pull on the portion of the rib cage he is holding. This pressure is released as the patient breathes out, and the clinician lets his hands go soft and heavy to encourage relaxation of the rib cage during expiration; the clinician cues the patient to "let the chest go heavy" as the individual breathes out. Breathing into an area requires relaxation of muscles that restrict the rib cage and thus facilitates neuromyofascial release and increased mobility over several breath cycles. The patient can do this exercise at home to perform self-release and to control pain. (Copyright Diane G. Lee Physiotherapist Corporation and Linda-Joy Lee Physiotherapist Corporation.)

joint involves identifying the key muscles responsible for the compression and applying one or more neuromuscular techniques, such as the following:

1. Breath work, with attention to focusing the breath into restricted areas of the thorax[34] (Figure 8-26)
2. Soft tissue mobilization and myofascial release techniques[97] and muscle energy techniques[98]
3. Trigger point techniques[99]
4. Dry needling or intramuscular stimulation[100]
5. Release with awareness techniques[2] (see discussion later in the chapter) (Figures 8-27 and 8-28)
6. Retraining of postural patterns and restoration of the ability to find neutral spine (see Figure 8-9, *B*)[2,34,101,102]
7. Surface electromyography or rehabilitative ultrasound imaging to foster "relaxation" of the targeted muscle[47,102]
8. Manual therapy techniques (oscillatory joint mobilization, joint manipulation) to facilitate a neurophysiological relaxation in the affected muscle (see Figure 8-25)[2,102]

Neuromyofascial release techniques for hypertonic muscles are not new. Osteopathic physicians and physical therapists have long used these techniques, which are also known as *counterstrain, functional* or *positional release techniques,* and *trigger point techniques.* However, performing these techniques on a patient appears to have only a short-term benefit, whereas engaging the patient's awareness of the release during the technique appears to

have a more lasting effect. The latter approach gives patients control over the state of hypertonicity and strategies for self-treatment. It empowers them to take control and to choose whether to brace or not. This technique is called *Release with awareness,*[102] and it is clinically applicable whenever hypertonicity is present. Using patient awareness is felt to alter neural drive to the hypertonic muscles from higher centers.

Clinical Example

A common nonoptimum strategy for stabilizing the thorax is overactivation of the thoracic erector spinae, a strategy referred to as "back gripping" (see Figure 8-8). This strategy impairs optimum respiratory function and the function of the joints of the thorax. It also affects lumbopelvic function and can occur with co-activation of the internal and external obliques ("chest gripping"). Also common in the upper thorax is "scapular gripping," in which the muscles

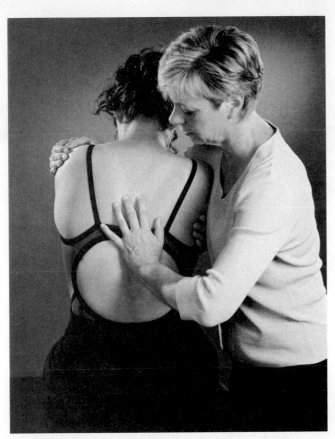

Figure 8-27

Release with awareness technique for restoring optimum resting tone of the longissimus thoracis. Hypertonicity of the global muscles can limit both segmental and multisegmental mobility and inhibit the deeper stability system. Release of these hypertonic bands is essential before the local muscle system can be trained. The clinician supports the patient's thorax and positions the segment or segments in a combination of extension/side flexion/rotation until the best relaxation response is felt. Further release is achieved by bringing awareness into the technique. The clinician cues the patient to "sense the tender spot; find this place in your brain" and then to "let go." Various words, images, and tactile support cues are used to facilitate this learning process. When the patient is successful at establishing an awareness of the hypertonic fascicle and can "let it go," the clinician feels the muscle soften under her fingers, and the resistance to motion of the thorax is immediately reduced. An alternative strategy for segmental and multisegmental motion control must then be taught. (Copyright Diane G. Lee Physiotherapist Corporation and Linda-Joy Lee Physiotherapist Corporation.)

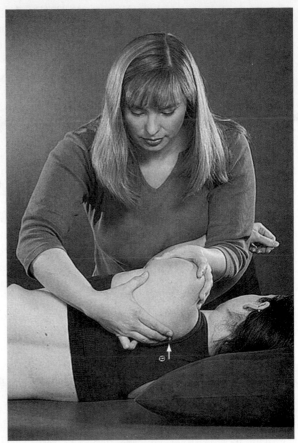

Figure 8-28

Release with awareness technique for the rhomboids. Hypertonicity of individual fascicles of the rhomboids is common in patients with poor thoracic ring control. Release of these hypertonic bands is essential before the local muscle system can be trained. With the patient's arm completely supported, the clinician palpates the hypertonic fascicle *(arrow)*. The scapula is positioned in varying degrees of retraction/ elevation and downward rotation until the fascicle is felt to relax. Further release is obtained by bringing awareness into the technique. The clinician cues the patient to "sense the tender spot; find this place in your brain" and then to "let go." Various words, images, and tactile support cues are given to facilitate this learning process. When the patient is successful at establishing an awareness of the hypertonic fascicle and can "let it go," the clinician feels the muscle soften under his fingers, and the resistance to motion of both the scapula and thoracic ring is immediately reduced. (Copyright Diane G. Lee Physiotherapist Corporation and Linda-Joy Lee Physiotherapist Corporation.)

of the scapula (i.e., rhomboids, levator scapulae, serratus anterior, trapezius, rotator cuff, and latissimus dorsi) are overactive to brace the upper rib cage. This strategy creates additional impairment of scapulothoracic and glenohumeral function. In all of these nonoptimum strategies, the deeper stability system of the thorax (i.e., thoracic multifidus, intercostals, levator costarum, and diaphragm) may be impaired, as is the stability system for the scapula and the lumbopelvic region (i.e., transversus abdominis, diaphragm, pelvic floor, and deep fibers of the lumbar multifidus).

Release with Awareness Technique for the Thoracic Erector Spinae and Scapula

The principles of the release with awareness technique, as they are applied to the thorax and scapula, are as follows:

1. The area of increased tone (hypertonic fascicle or trigger point) is palpated with gentle pressure.

2. To release the erector spinae, the spine and/or ribs are positioned so as to shorten the origin and insertion of the specific fascicle of the erector spinae muscle that is hypertonic (e.g., spinalis, longissimus, iliocostalis) (see Figure 8-27). For scapular release, the scapula is

moved to shorten the origin and insertion of the hypertonic muscle (see Figure 8-28). As the clinician passively shortens the muscle, the afferent input from the primary annulospiral ending in the intrafusal muscle spindle decreases, and the spinal cord responds by decreasing the efferent output to the extrafusal muscle fiber. This is felt as a "softening of tone" in the trigger point. The clinician waits for this to occur (30 to 45 seconds).

3. The clinician cues the patient to "release," or soften, the muscle with verbal and manual cues to "let go." This step is critical to the awareness training, and it is the point where learning occurs.

4. The scapula or spine/rib is moved in various combinations to maximally release the muscle as the clinician cues the patient (with words and touch) to be aware of the softening and release. The key is to use words that encourage the patient to "let go" and stop holding rather than to "do something."

5. The patients' homework is to recreate this sensation of letting go. As they practice at home, they quickly remember and learn how to stop bracing. They also learn that they can control and reduce the pain when the bracing is decreased. This is positive reinforcement for changing the bracing strategy.

Once the muscle hypertonicity has been treated, it is essential that the clinician reassess the load transfer tests that initially were positive (e.g., rotation, SAL test). Often the release of the global hypertonicity improves the results of the load transfer tests (i.e., increased range of motion and decreased effort), but levels with poor segmental control will still be present, especially on repetition of the movement. When correction/compression is performed at that segment, the load transfer test becomes even easier, indicating that the next treatment component should involve techniques to increase segmental support and control (see Figure 8-18). This combination of excessive global muscle tone and poor segmental control is a common presentation. The global muscle hypertonicity creates forces that inhibit and restrict the ability of the local system to control the dysfunctional segment. By releasing the hypertonicity (e.g., an external oblique that pulls the rib anteriorly), the findings of the load transfer test improve as a result of the removal of the anterior pull on the rib; then the local system can work to stabilize the rib and move it posteromedially.

When a patient seeks treatment early, before the problem becomes chronic and movement patterns become habitual, removing the global hypertonicity often is enough to allow the local segmental system to return through normal movement. However, most patients wait until the problem has been present for some time, and the clinician must use specific techniques to retrain the local stabilizing system and increase articular control (see following section) after releasing the global tone; otherwise, the compensatory global pattern of neuromyofascial compression will return and again need to be treated.

Home exercises for a neuromyofascially restricted joint must include a self-release exercise. Using breath work (i.e., breathing into areas of restriction) while focusing on relaxing and "letting go" of tight restricted areas, as described previously, is one example. Another useful technique involves using small balls or other equipment to apply pressure to trigger points as the patient focuses on releasing and relaxing specific muscles.

The clinician must assess static loading habits (i.e., sitting, standing, and sleeping), as well as posture (dynamic and static), during any activities that aggravate the patient's symptoms to determine whether the muscles being treated are excessively recruited in these activities. To prevent recurrence of muscular hypertonicity, the patient must become aware of the postures and activities that are causal. Once aware of poor habits, the patient has the choice of making a change and using the new postural and movement strategies.

When a force is applied to the joints of the thorax sufficient to stretch or tear the articular ligaments, the muscles respond to prevent dislocation and further trauma to the joint. The resulting spasm may fix the joint in an abnormal resting position, and marked asymmetry may be present. This is an unstable joint under excessive compression, and the clinician will note marked altered positional findings and joint restriction. On passive mobility testing, the neutral zone of movement cannot be felt, and a hard, nonbony end feel is present. This type of articular "fixation"[93] can occur in any movement direction. It is common with trauma involving excessive rotation of the unrestrained thorax or when rotation of the thorax is forced against a fixed rib cage (seat belt injury).

Another common scenario is an impact force to a specific rib, such as can occur in contact sports. This results in a fixation of the costotransverse joint. Treatment of this individual that focuses on exercise without first addressing the fixation of the joint tends to be ineffective and commonly increases symptoms. Conversely, if treatment includes only manual therapy (i.e., joint mobilization, manipulation, or muscle energy techniques), relief tends to be temporary, and dependence on the health care practitioner to provide the manual correction is common. Fixation impairments require a multimodal therapeutic approach to management that includes manual therapy to decompress and align the thorax (specific articular manipulation technique) (Figure 8-29), followed by exercises and patient education to restore optimum motor control, strength, and endurance for functional tasks (see later discussion of controlling articular compression principles).

Anteriorly, the costochondral and sternochondral joints can be a source of localized anterior chest pain when the capsuloligamentous support is damaged by a blunt force injury. Acute management of these injuries is essential to

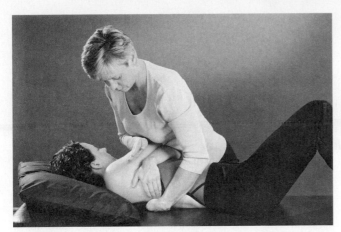

Figure 8-29

A high velocity, low amplitude thrust technique (grade 5 manipulation) is used to restore a fixated, left-translated ring. This is an articular instability under excessive muscular compression. The manipulative technique must be specific both segmentally and directionally to correct the fixation. Subsequently, motor control retraining is essential. (Copyright Diane G. Lee Physiotherapist Corporation and Linda-Joy Lee Physiotherapist Corporation.)

prevent a chronic passive instability. These joints may be fixated or subluxed as a result of the trauma, but they are not treated with manipulation. Instead, myofascial release techniques are used both anteriorly and posteriorly to align the thoracic ring, and tape is used to support the joints and ring in optimum alignment to reduce stress on the injured structures and optimize the formation of a functional scar.

Principles for Restoring Segmental Thoracic Ring Neurodynamics

When the neurodynamic tests described previously are positive, mobilization techniques for this system should be included in the treatment program. The reader is referred to *The Sensitive Nervous System*[95] for a more complete description of the guidelines and parameters for treatment.[95,96] To create thoracic ring–specific neurodynamic mobilization techniques, the clinician uses the patient position and palpation points described previously in the assessment section (see Figures 8-20 and 8-21). The basic principle is to correct and stabilize the dysfunctional ring in a neutral position while taking movement up to the point of the first resistance in either the slump or variation of the upper limb neurodynamic test that is positive. At this first barrier, the upper extremity position is maintained and a gentle, oscillatory corrective force/mobilization is applied to the ring. Moving in and out of the barrier is most effective, and the number of oscillations is graded according to irritability and symptom response (very little symptom provocation should occur). Because latent responses are common in the treatment of the neural system, the clinician should begin with as few as 4 or 5 oscillations and then

reassess. The clinician should be sure to inquire about post-treatment symptom provocation on subsequent visits to avoid increasing neural sensitivity.

Principles for Correcting Alignment

Loads are transferred more effectively through joints that are properly aligned, such that the compression and tension forces induced are shared among all structures. Malalignment can create excessive stress on individual structures (i.e., tension or compression) and ultimately leads to tissue breakdown, resulting in inflammation and pain. It is the authors' observation that that if patients have been previously prescribed motor control and stabilization exercises when malalignment is present, the resultant muscle contractions are asymmetrical and suboptimal, and asymmetrical breathing patterns persist. Therefore, techniques that correct alignment are necessary in most treatment plans.

Malalignment resulting from a joint fixation of the zygapophyseal or costotransverse joints or entire ring requires a manipulative technique for correction (addressed previously). Malalignment that is the result of muscle imbalance often is corrected when the neuromyofascial hypertonicity in the muscles responsible is addressed (i.e., myofascial release with awareness technique, described previously); however, it sometimes needs to be followed with a specific muscle energy technique[98] for the remaining malaligned joint or joints. In both cases (i.e., fixation and myofascial malalignment), treatment must be followed by postural re-education so that the patient learns how to find a neutral spine position both within the thorax and between the thorax and head, and thorax and pelvis[34] (see later discussion of principles for changing movement strategies). An exercise program is also required to restore motor control, strength, and endurance if optimum alignment is to be maintained (see the following section).

Principles for Controlling Articular Compression: A New Approach to Exercise for the Thoracic Spine and Ribs

Historically, little attention has been paid to the importance of segmental stability in the thorax. Because of the presence of the rib cage and sternum, the thorax has been considered relatively stable. Indeed, cadaveric studies suggest that significant anatomical disruption is required to produce passive instability in the thoracic spine.[103,104] Thus, recommended treatment approaches often have focused primarily on restoring mobility to the thorax and correcting postural faults.[105-107]

Until recently, exercise programs for the thoracic spine have focused on training the large, superficial muscles of the thorax, primarily targeting the thoracic erector spinae and the scapular retractors to correct excessive thoracic kyphosis and shoulder protraction. Exercises promote co-contraction of the trunk flexors and extensors to increase control of postural orientation and equilibrium.[107,108] Unilateral trunk muscle exercises for scoliosis have also been proposed,[105,107,108] in which the focus again has been on the superficial abdominal muscles (i.e., internal and external obliques) and the thoracic erector spinae. Although more passively stable than the neighboring cervical and lumbar regions, intersegmental movement exists both within and between the rings of the thorax, and this movement needs to be controlled for optimum function. As defined by Panjabi, requirements for stability do not merely depend on the passive structures, but also on the ability to control movement in the neutral zone of each joint, which is dependent on muscle contraction.[27] The multiple articulations at each level of the thorax provide the ability for multiple planes of movement, and optimum function requires not only the ability to move at these joints, but also the ability to *control movement* at these joints. For this reason, the authors have previously proposed that segmental control between each level in the thorax is required and is just as important as regional control between the head and thorax, the thorax and arms, the thorax and lumbopelvis, and the trunk and legs.[34]

Insufficient or inappropriate activation of the myofascial system (i.e., force closure/motor control deficit) results in insufficient or imbalanced compression of the joints of the thoracic spine. Depending on the deficit, the insufficient/imbalanced compression may occur primarily during static loading (in prolonged positions) or during a variety of dynamic loading situations. Patients commonly report difficulty with both static and dynamic loading tasks and often with tasks involving use of the upper extremity or neck. Complaints of vague arm weakness without thoracic pain and of thoracic pain during arm loading can both be caused by insufficient/imbalanced compression of specific joints in the thorax.

Treatment for this impairment requires the restoration of both motor control and muscle capacity (i.e., strength and endurance) with specific exercises that initially train an optimum recruitment strategy for control of the thorax, followed by exercises that challenge stability during functional tasks. Several different types of exercise are required to address these different control requirements and to restore optimum muscle function and motor control for the thorax. These exercise components are summarized in Figures 8-30 to 8-32. The temporary application of tape

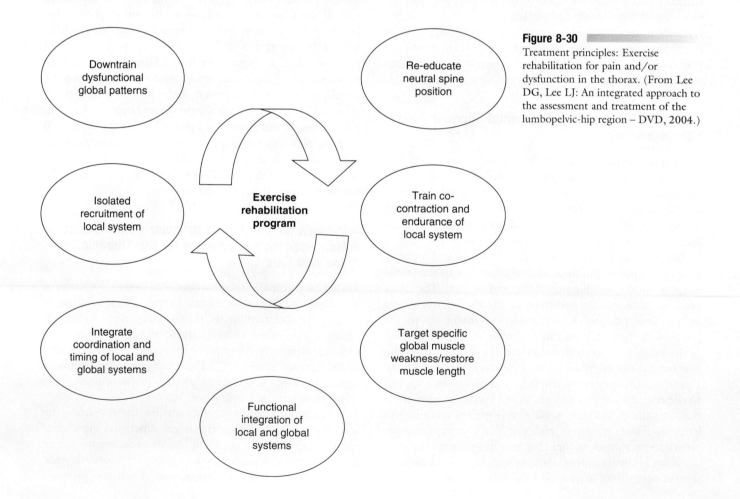

Figure 8-30

Treatment principles: Exercise rehabilitation for pain and/or dysfunction in the thorax. (From Lee DG, Lee LJ: An integrated approach to the assessment and treatment of the lumbopelvic-hip region – DVD, 2004.)

Downtrain dysfunctional global patterns

Re-educate neutral spine position

Isolated recruitment of local system

Exercise rehabilitation program

Train co-contraction and endurance of local system

Integrate coordination and timing of local and global systems

Target specific global muscle weakness/restore muscle length

Functional integration of local and global systems

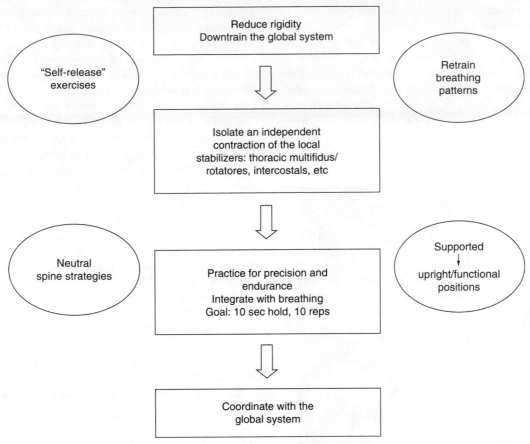

Figure 8-31

Program for stabilization and motor control of the thorax. (From Lee LJ: Restoring force closure/motor control of the thorax. In Lee DG, editor: *The thorax: an integrated approach,* White Rock, BC, 2003, Diane G. Lee Physiotherapist Corporation, www.dianelee.ca.)

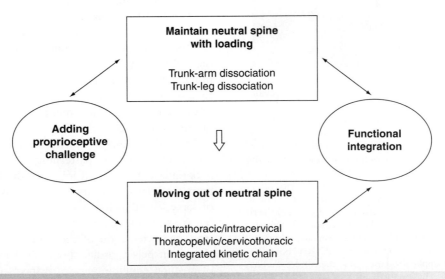

Figure 8-32

Program for stabilization and motor control of the thorax: Coordinating the local and global systems. (From Lee LJ: Restoring force closure/motor control of the thorax. In Lee DG, editor: *The thorax: an integrated approach,* White Rock, BC, 2003, Diane G. Lee Physiotherapist Corporation, www.dianelee.ca.)

can be used to augment force closure during this stage of rehabilitation (Figure 8-33).

When treatment is planned, exercises should be prescribed as part of a multimodal approach. If exercise is prescribed before joint and neurodynamic mobility have been restored, the patient's pain and dysfunction often worsen. This may lead to the conclusion that certain exercises are "bad" or unsuccessful for treating back pain, when in fact, the problem may merely be one of *inappropriate*

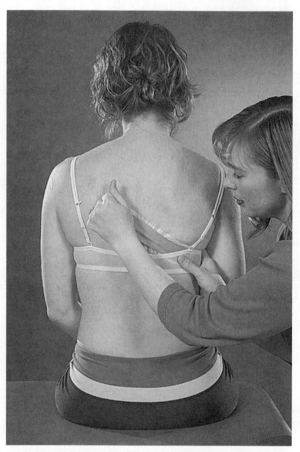

Figure 8-33

Supportive tape can be applied in a variety of directions to provide both proprioceptive input and mechanical support to a dysfunctional rib/ring. Here, the eighth ring complex is corrected from a right lateral translation/left-rotated position via the right eighth rib. The entire ring can be corrected only in this way in the absence of a significant form closure deficit in one of the articulations of the ring. The clinician's right hand provides a gentle force to translate the ring to the left while positioning the right eighth rib into posterior rotation and craniomedial compression. Tape is applied to support the rib in this position. It is essential that the osteokinematic position of the rib/ring be corrected before the tape is applied; otherwise, the wrong information will be conveyed to the nervous system, and optimum movement behavior will not be facilitated. The SAL test should be repeated after the tape is applied to ensure that the correct level has been taped and that sufficient support has been provided (the SAL movement should be easier after application of the tape). (Copyright Diane G. Lee Physiotherapist Corporation and Linda-Joy Lee Physiotherapist Corporation.)

timing of exercise intervention. In addition, the *type* of exercise prescribed is of utmost importance. For patients with pain, studies of the cervical and lumbopelvic regions support the correction of motor control deficits before focusing on the strength and power of individual muscles. Clinically, it is evident that patients who go through a routine of exercises without awareness often have limited success in retraining motor patterns. When poor patterns and control are reinforced with exercise, symptoms often worsen, because this may result in irritation of nociceptive structures. The problem is not which exercise was prescribed, but how the exercise was performed.

With respect to the low back and pelvic girdle, evidence[29,109] indicates that individuals with pain develop strategies that make them more rigid and stiff and that these strategies occur at a functional cost (e.g., loss of mobility, loss of ability to control postural equilibrium, and ineffective load transfer).[47,59,72,73,110] There is also evidence that these strategies affect the deep stability system such that it becomes inhibited or delayed in activation and/or atrophies very quickly.[47,52,53,55,59,64,87,111] In addition, recovery of optimum motor control is not spontaneous,[87] and this nonresolution is linked to higher recurrence rates for low back pain.[80]

Clinically, the authors have found that restoring optimum motor control and stabilization strategies is facilitated by first releasing the nonoptimum bracing strategy (i.e., releasing the hypertonicity in the superficial system (covered previously in Principles for Reducing Articular Compression: Restoring Mobility).[2,34,42,102] After the superficial system has been released and the patients learn how to do this themselves, the deeper stability system is "reminded," through sensorial cues and images (feeling optimum force vectors), how to activate the deep system in isolation from the superficial one. Then, a more efficient way to stabilize and move can be trained and integrated into functional tasks. In short, the principles are to remove the old strategy (release techniques and manual therapy), align the skeleton (muscle energy techniques and neutral spine/pelvis postural retraining) and then teach the patient a new way to move and live in their body (stabilization/movement control exercises and integration into functional tasks) (see Figure 8-23).

Exercises for motor control are aimed at retraining strategies of muscular patterning so that load transfer is optimized through all joints of the kinetic chain. Optimum load transfer occurs when there is precise modulation of force, coordination, and timing of specific muscle contractions, ensuring control of each joint (segmental control), the orientation of the spine (i.e., spinal curvatures, thorax on pelvic girdle, thorax under head), and control of postural equilibrium with respect to the environment. The result is stability with mobility, marked by stability without rigidity of posture, without episodes of collapse, and with fluidity of movement. Optimum coordination of the myofascial system produces optimum stabilization strategies. These patients will then have:

1. The ability to find and maintain control of neutral spinal alignment both within the thorax and in relationship to the cervical and lumbosacral curves (see Figure 8-9, *B*).
2. Optimum lumbopelvic function.
3. The ability to consciously recruit and maintain a tonic, isolated contraction of the deep stabilizers of the thorax to ensure segmental control and then to maintain this contraction during loading (Figure 8-34).
4. The ability to move in and out of neutral spine (i.e., flex, extend, laterally bend, rotate) without segmental or regional collapse (Figure 8-35).
5. The ability to maintain all of the above in coordination with the rest of the spine and the extremities in functional, work-specific, and sport-specific postures and movements (Figure 8-36).

For further information on the specific exercises that address each component of this type of program, the reader is referred to Lee.[34] The purpose of this chapter is not to describe these exercises in detail, but rather to outline the key principles of an integrated multimodal treatment program for the thorax. From this section, the clinician is encouraged to reconsider how to prescribe exercises for patients with thoracic dysfunction and/or pain. Specifically, cues, images, and facilitation techniques are needed to address deficits in the function of the deep stabilizing muscle system. Because information on the

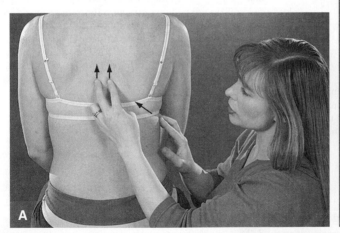
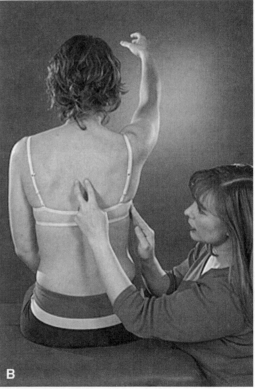

Figure 8-34

A, Facilitation of a contraction of the local system for the eighth ring. The clinician monitors the segmental muscle response and the change in ring position as various cues are given. For example, here the clinician palpates T8-9 and the eighth rib in the midaxillary line. The patient is instructed to "imagine a guy wire that runs from this finger (at the lateral aspect of the right eighth rib) diagonally up and medial to connect to my fingers at your spine (at the T8 vertebra), and this wire then suspends your vertebra vertically." Along with these verbal cues, the clinician provides manual sensory cues by applying gentle pressure to the lateral rib in a craniomedial direction (along the body of the rib *[arrow]*), as well as a gentle cranial force to T8 (suggestive of suspension) *(small arrows)*. Optimum contraction of the local system is felt as a swelling of the segmental muscles; however, note that the patient is not asked to make the muscles swell. The eighth rib also should be felt to move craniomedially as the patient finds the correct muscles. **B,** While maintaining this local system contraction and connection, the patient elevates the right arm to add further load to the task. The arm lift should feel light and effortless, and the thoracic ring should not translate to the right during this task. (Copyright Diane G. Lee Physiotherapist Corporation and Linda-Joy Lee Physiotherapist Corporation.)

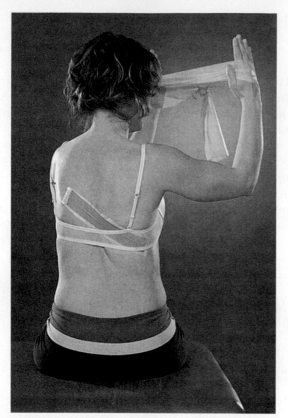

Figure 8-35

Exercise for retraining rotation out of the neutral spine position. The supportive tape provides a proprioceptive cue, as well as mechanical support (similar to that provided by the clinician in Figure 8-15C), to the right eighth rib. A low resistance band is wrapped between the hands, and before lifting the arms into flexion, the patient uses her local system image to achieve segmental ring stability; she then raises the arms while applying a gentle abduction force to the band (5% of the maximum voluntary contraction [MVC]). She then rotates to the right while maintaining the local system connection and the tension in the band. The Thera-Band facilitates an integrated connection between the arms and the thorax; the motion should feel light and effortless. (Copyright Diane G. Lee Physiotherapist Corporation and Linda-Joy Lee Physiotherapist Corporation.)

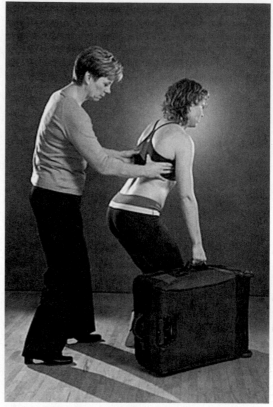

Figure 8-36

During this lifting task, the clinician monitors the segmental control of the thoracic ring as well as the total body strategy used for optimum load transfer. This task requires optimum function of the upper extremity, head and neck, thorax, lumbopelvic region and lower extremities. Many sites of failed load transfer can be observed and corrected during this functional task. (Note the clinician in this picture; she needs some postural correction!) (Copyright Diane G. Lee Physiotherapist Corporation and Linda-Joy Lee Physiotherapist Corporation.)

deep stabilizing system for the thorax is limited, the goal of the images, cues, and facilitation techniques is to create a response that results in control of the dysfunctional segment, which may be the result of several local muscles co-contracting (e.g., segmental intercostals, segmental multifidus/rotatores, segmental levator costarum, diaphragm). Depending on the position and task, these local muscles may not be easily or reliably palpated for a contraction (deep swelling), but if the dysfunctional segment exhibits control with the cue when a passive stability test or functional load transfer test is applied, without activity in the global muscle system on the initial cue for the local recruitment, then the clinician can be confident the appropriate muscles are being recruited.

Subsequently, exercises that are patient specific according to the person's functional, work, and recreation demands need to be integrated into the program. For most patients with thoracic pain, this requires education and exercises that address an optimum sitting posture (Figure 8-37), driving position, lifting strategies (see Figure 8-36), and functional integration of the upper extremity and neck.

Proprioceptive challenges, such as exercises on a half foam roll, gym ball, rocker board, or SitFit® (Figure 8-38), are added to help the patient learn how to use the new strategies in situations requiring focus on multiple factors simultaneously, and seems to facilitate the automatic recruitment of the segmental control system. These challenges also prepare the patient for unanticipated changes in base of support that commonly occur in daily life. During the introduction of all new exercises, the clinician should monitor the stability of the dysfunctional thoracic segment (i.e., vertebra, rib,

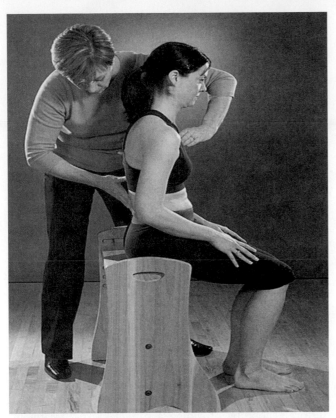

Figure 8-37
Restoration of a neutral spine position begins with setting the optimum base of the pelvis. Once the pelvic girdle has been set into neutral (see Figure 14-23, *A*), the clinician can use manual and verbal cues to facilitate the optimum strategy for aligning the thoracolumbar spine. A key element is teaching the patient how to find this new position independently; to do this, the clinician has the patient practice the repositioning activity with fewer tactile and verbal cues on subsequent repetitions. (Copyright Diane G. Lee Physiotherapist Corporation and Linda-Joy Lee Physiotherapist Corporation.)

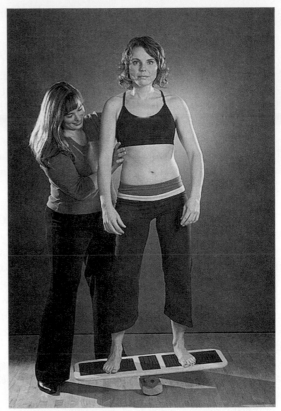

Figure 8-38
During this proprioceptive exercise, the patient's base of support is challenged in the coronal plane. The patient must maintain segmental ring control, thoracopelvic control, and postural equilibrium while maintaining balance; movement can be introduced as a higher level of challenge. The therapist monitors closely for loss of segmental and/or regional control. (Copyright Diane G. Lee Physiotherapist Corporation and Linda-Joy Lee Physiotherapist Corporation.)

or ring), watching and palpating for movement into the direction of loss of control and/or passive instability, to ensure that the patient is ready for the new load challenge.

Principles for Changing Movement Strategies: A New Way to Live in the Body

Many physical, emotional, and psychosocial factors influence and affect the static (posture) and dynamic movement strategies that patients exhibit. The body and the mind collect experiences, some good and some bad. The cumulative effects of these experiences are reflected in our posture, movements, and attitudes toward ourselves and others. Pain in many places in the body often arises as a consequence of these experiences. A natural response to pain is to embrace the body part, to protect it from further injury, and to render it motionless, possibly in an attempt to avoid the pain. This strategy of bracing can

be useful for an acute soft tissue injury; however, it becomes nonoptimal when perpetuated as a habit. Thus most patients present with altered and nonoptimum postural and movement strategies. The challenge for the clinician is to determine when altered movement strategies is a contributing factor to abnormal tissue loading and ongoing symptoms. In acute stages of injury, what normally would be considered nonoptimum movement patterns are usually necessary and beneficial in reducing loads on injured tissues, and correction of these patterns leads to symptom exacerbation in this stage. However, if these patterns become habitual past the acute and subacute healing stages, the nonoptimum movement patterns can lead to excess loading through other structures and can become the cause of pain in areas distal or proximal to the initial injury site. Alternately, poor postural habits and movement strategies that have been learned over time can result in ongoing microtrauma to tissues, which eventually exhaust their adaptive potential and become the source of pain in an insidious onset. In both of these cases, successful treatment requires that movement strategies be specifically addressed in the treatment program.

To correct movement strategies, it is important that the clinician use the treatment techniques already described to create an easier path to better movement. Therefore, if there are hypertonic muscles that have not been released, they will create resistance to changing posture and muscle recruitment patterns during movement. Similarly, stiff fibrotic joints will prevent movement, and no amount of motor learning instructions or cues will change movement through those joints. It is the combination of addressing the specific form and force closure impairments and then retraining movement strategies that results in lasting change. In some cases, manual treatment creates the option for a different movement pattern, and simply educating the patient to move freely and perform activities without fear is enough to restore optimum movement patterns. More commonly, especially with recurrent or chronic pain states, manual treatment is not sufficient to change movement strategies, and specific exercises must be given to retrain patterns.

To decide which movement strategies to target in treatment, the clinician uses information from the assessment. The clinician should inquire as to which postures and activities aggravate the patient's symptoms and then observe and analyze the patient's strategies during these events to determine their efficacy and impact on pain. Relieving postures and movements should be similarly analyzed. The breathing pattern and, in some cases, breathing chemistry should also be analyzed, and if these are faulty, strategies to train optimum breathing should be included early in the treatment program.

Movement and breathing patterns are retrained using tactile (both clinician and patient), verbal, and visual (mirrors) cueing during many repetitions. For in-depth cues and techniques to retrain breathing and neutral spine posture, the reader is referred to other sources that focus on a movement retraining approach.[2,34,101,102,112] More general movement approaches include Pilates, Feldenkrais, and Aston patterning. The clinician can ask patients to rate their pain or degree of difficulty, or the clinician can note the lack of range of motion in the performance of a task (1) during the patient's habitual nonoptimum pattern and (2) during the new position or movement pattern. If correctly done, the optimum pattern results in less pain, increased ease (decreased difficulty), and/or increased range of motion. and these differences positively reinforce the importance of retraining these patterns to the patient.

Changing behavior is not easy, but neither is it dauntingly difficult. The goal is to educate patients about the mechanical and neurophysiological processes that led to the nonoptimum movement strategies or pain and then teach them to let go of the strategies that are nonoptimal

for their needs. Manual techniques facilitate this process, but used alone, they are not sufficient to change behavior. Release techniques with awareness, described previously, cannot be "done to" a patient; rather, they should be "done with" the patient so that the patient learns how to "let go" of muscle bracing and can apply this new skill in functional tasks. This learning component is the key to changing postural and movement strategies and to long-term success.

For both myofascial release and training isolation of the deep stability system, the language used appears to make a significant difference. In addition, engaging patients to be aware of the different sensations each strategy produces in their bodies and the immediate response of the body (effort and efficiency of movement) to these different strategies empowers them to take control both of what they are doing and how they are doing it.

Principles for Integrating the Emotional Component

The patient's emotional state can maintain a detrimental motor pattern and prevent a successful outcome. The clinician can help relieve patients' anxiety about their current physical status and the future by explaining the possible causal factors, as well as the physiology of pain.[113-117] Restoring hope by providing a patient-specific treatment plan often is motivational and helps to build trust. When positive changes in function occur, the treatment plan is reinforced, and this builds patients' commitment to and confidence in both the treatment plan and their own abilities. In the end, it is critical that clinicians teach people to accept responsibility for their health through education, awareness, and motivation.

Summary

It has long been recognized that physical factors affect joint motion. The integrated, multimodal approach to the management of thoracic pain suggests that multiple factors influence joint mechanics, some intrinsic to the joint itself and others produced by muscle action that in turn is influenced by the emotional state. More studies are required to identify subgroups of patients with thoracic pain according to specific impairments, recognizing that not all patients have the same impairments. Clinical tests for motion and load transfer need to be further developed and evaluated for reliability, validity, sensitivity, and specificity. More studies on muscle control and function are required to elucidate the changes that occur in patients with thoracic pain. Clinicians then will be able to develop better studies (randomized and controlled) to test the efficacy of treatment programs specific to each subgroup of impairment. Until then, the best evidence-based treatment involves a multimodal approach that takes into consideration the patient's biomechanical, neuromuscular, and emotional needs.

This chapter has introduced assessment tests for the thorax and outlined principles for multimodal management of patients with pain and dysfunction of the thorax. Effective management of thoracic pain and dysfunction requires restoration of all four components of the integrated model: form closure, force closure, motor control, and emotions. The goal is to use manual techniques and exercise in a process that educates and inspires patients to make changes in postural and movement strategies, which ultimately will result in a healthier way to live and move in their bodies.

References

To enhance this text and add value for the reader, all references have been incorporated into a CD-ROM that is provided with this text. The reader can view the reference source and access it online whenever possible. There are a total of 117 references for this chapter.

Low Back Pain: Causes and Differential Diagnosis

Steven Z. George and Mark D. Bishop

Introduction

This chapter presents a current and practical approach to the diagnosis of low back pain (LBP). It discusses the etiology, epidemiology, course, and societal impact of LBP so as to give the clinician a context for understanding the importance of effective LBP management. The chapter also presents a diagnostic model for differential diagnosis of LBP that emphasizes a classification approach. This approach involves the identification of red and yellow flags, as well as specific subgroups of patients with LBP.

Etiology of Low Back Pain

Definitive causes of LBP represent a "holy grail" for clinicians and researchers working in spine care. Current evidence indicates that identifiable causes exist for specific lumbar conditions. The most notable of this work is the line of research involving intervertebral disc degeneration. However, current evidence also suggests that single, definite causes of clinical LBP remain elusive.

Cross sectional studies involving LBP are commonly reported in the peer-reviewed literature. However, although cross sectional studies give an indication of how certain factors are associated with LBP at one point in time, they do not directly address whether the factor *causes* LBP. Instead, the ideal study design to determine the cause of LBP would involve a prospective cohort of symptom-free subjects without a prior history of LBP who were followed until they developed LBP. Unfortunately, these studies are extremely difficult to perform and consequently are rarely reported in the peer-reviewed literature. The authors have made every attempt to identify and include prospective studies whenever possible in this review of factors that may cause LBP.

It is more common for researchers to use study designs that are less than ideal but that still address specific factors that are likely to cause LBP. The authors emphasize results from two commonly implemented study designs that are used to investigate causes of LBP: epidemiological and monozygotic twin studies. In epidemiological studies, cause can be inferred if the proposed causative factor meets all five criteria presented in Table 9-1.[1,2] If the proposed causative factor does not meet all five criteria, it is not likely to cause LBP. In this chapter, the authors have limited the review to factors that have a theoretically plausible link to the development of LBP.

Monozygotic twin studies can also be used to infer causes of LBP because they control for potential confounding factors by matching participants on gender, age, genotype, and childhood environments.[3] Using this methodology, groups of twins who have discordance on the factor of interest are recruited and statistically compared for differences in the prevalence of LBP. For example, in this type of study design, LBP prevalence would be compared in monozygotic twins who differed in smoking status to determine whether smoking was a likely cause of LBP.[4]

Genetics

When genetic causes of LBP are considered, research has focused on allele (one of two or more alternative forms of a gene) variations that adversely affect the quality of the intervertebral discs. A direct pathway involves polymorphisms that affect intervertebral disc composition, resulting in an increased probability of disc degeneration. Polymorphisms in the collagen IX,[5,6] aggrecan,[7] vitamin D receptor,[8,9] and matrix metalloproteinase-3[10] genes all have been associated with the development of intervertebral disc

Table 9-1

Determining the Cause of Low Back Pain from Epidemiological Studies

Criteria	Definition
Theoretically plausible	The factor of interest has a reasonable biological, anatomical, biomechanical, or physiological causal link with low back pain
Significant and meaningful association	The factor of interest has a consistent, statistically significant, and strong association (i.e., odds or relative risk ratios greater than 2) with low back pain as reported across several studies
Monotonic dose-response relationship	Low back pain increases in prevalence as the factor of interest increases in magnitude
Temporality	The factor of interest is present before the onset of low back pain
Reversibility	Low back pain decreases in prevalence when the factor of interest is stopped or is no longer present

Data from Leboeuf-Yde C: Body weight and low back pain: a systematic literature review of 56 journal articles reporting on 65 epidemiologic studies, *Spine* 25:226-237, 2000.

degeneration in humans. For example, one case-control study found that a specific variation in one of three collagen IX genes was present in 12.2% of patients with intervertebral disc degeneration but in only 4.7% of control patients. This difference was statistically significant (p < 0.001) and suggested that a polymorphism in one of the collagen IX genes increased the risk of disc degeneration by about three times.[6] Another study demonstrated that patients with a specific polymorphism in the vitamin D receptor gene were more likely to experience annular tears.[8]

An indirect pathway for a genetic cause of LBP involves polymorphisms that adversely affect the inflammatory cascade by creating excessive amounts of proinflammatory cytokines (i.e., interleukin-1, interleukin-6, interleukin-8, and tumor necrosis factor α) and/or creating limited amounts of cytokines that mediate the inflammatory response (i.e., interleukin receptor antagonists). Proinflammatory cytokines are produced when intervertebral discs are damaged,[11,12] and these substances can irritate nerve roots without concurrent mechanical compression.[13,14] Therefore it has been hypothesized that polymorphisms in genes that produce proinflammatory or inflammatory-mediating cytokines have the potential to cause intervertebral disc degeneration, LBP, and/or sciatica.[15-17] Recent research supports this hypothesis, because a cluster polymorphism in the interleukin-1 gene locus has been associated with increased odds of disc degeneration.[17] Specifically, patients who were heterozygous (odds ratio [OR], 2.2; 95% confidence interval [CI], 1.1-4.5) or homozygous (OR, 3.5; 95% CI, 1-11.9) for the interleukin-1αT[889] allele were more likely to have a specific sign of degeneration (disc bulge) compared to patients who were homozygous for the interleukin-1αC[889] allele.[17]

Monozygotic twin studies corroborate these findings by investigating the broad role that heredity plays without investigating the effect of specific genes. Heredity for lumbar disc degeneration has been estimated at about 74% (95% CI, 64% to 81%).[18] In a study by Battie et al.,[19]

heredity explained the largest amount of variance in disc degeneration in a multivariate model that included age and physical loading. In the prediction of variance in disc degeneration from monozygotic twins at levels T12 to L4, the addition of physical loading explained 7% of the variance, age explained 9% of the variance, and familial aggregation explained 61%, and a similar pattern was noticed for levels L4 to S1.[19]

Collectively, the studies suggest that genetic factors play an important role in the development of lumbar disc degeneration. However, the clinician must interpret these studies with caution, because the presence of lumbar disc degeneration does not automatically preclude clinical presentation of LBP.[3] In fact, a monozygotic twin study published in 1989 suggested that the overall genetic influence on clinical LBP may be low.[20] In this study, the heredity estimates for LBP were low: 20.8% for sciatica and 10.6% for hospitalizations caused by disc herniation.[20] Studies linking specific genetic factors to LBP have recently been reported in the literature, and cluster polymorphisms in the aforementioned interleukin-1 gene locus were associated with an increased prevalence of LBP in the past year, an increased number of days experiencing LBP, and increased pain intensity with LBP.[15] Another study involving a single polymorphism of the interleukin-6 gene locus demonstrated that a specific genotype was more likely to be associated with sciatica (OR, 5.4; 95% CI, 1.5-19.2).[16] The studies demonstrate a promising start in confirming a genetic link to the clinical presentation of LBP, but these results should be viewed with caution, because they conflict with the results reported in the better controlled twin study,[20] and they involved small sample sizes with imprecise estimates of the influence of genetic factors on LBP.

Genetic factors, therefore, seem to play an important role in the development of disc degeneration, but their role in the cause of clinical LBP is unclear (Table 9-2). This is an area of current interest in the scientific literature, and many advances are likely in the next few years. The clinician

Table 9-2

Summary of Possible Causative Factors in Low Back Pain

Criteria	Genetics	Physical Loading	Smoking	Obesity	Psychological and Psychosocial	Alcohol
Significant and meaningful association	?	?	N	N	?	N
Monotonic dose-response relationship	?	?	N	N	?	N
Temporality	Y	?	N	N	Y	N
Reversibility	?	N	N	N	N	N

?, Preliminary or inconsistent evidence supporting this factor.
Y, Consistent evidence supporting this factor.
N, Consistent evidence against this factor.

should realize that genetic factors do not appear to play a purely Mendelian role in the development of LBP. In fact, already some evidence in the literature indicates how complex the relationship may be among genetic factors, nongenetic factors, and clinical LBP. A monozygotic twin study by Hestbaek et al.[21] modeled the influence of genes and the environment to predict the strongest component in the development of LBP. The results suggested that shared environment was the strongest component until age 15; after age 15, the effect of nonshared environment increased, as did nonadditive genetic effects. These researchers estimated the age-adjusted heredity for LBP to be 44% (95% CI, 37% to 50%) for males and 40% (95% CI, 34% to 46%) for females, and they concluded, "As people grow older, the effect of the nonshared environment increases and nonadditive genetic effects become more evident, indicating an increasing degree of genetic interaction as age increases."[21] Another study demonstrated that a polymorphism in the collagen IX gene was more likely to be associated with lumbar disc degeneration for obese subjects.[22] Clearly, more research is needed to elucidate the relationships between genetic factors and nongenetic factors, as well as their role in the development of LBP.

Physical Loading

In the peer-reviewed literature, the relationship of physical loading factors, intervertebral disc degeneration, and LBP has been investigated extensively. Common examples of physical loading factors that have been studied include materials handling, postural loading, vehicular vibration, and type and/or amount of exercise. The common way these factors are theorized to cause LBP is that excessive or repeated loads cause macro or microtrauma (respectively) to tissues of the spine. This tissue damage accelerates degenerative changes to spinal structures, eventually causing LBP. For example, basic studies have suggested that intervertebral disc degeneration results from increased intradiscal pressure and/or ligamentous creep after physical loading.[23-27]

The clinical evidence presented on physical loading factors and lumbar disc degeneration is paradoxical, because some studies have shown a positive association between the two factors,[28-32] and other studies have not.[33-35] In these studies, many potential confounding factors were not adequately controlled, which limits their comparison and interpretability. As a result, this review focuses on studies of monozygotic twins who differed in amounts of physical loading. In a study of monozygotic twins who differed in occupational and leisure time activities, Battie et al.[19] found that physical loading explained only small amounts of variance in disc degeneration, 7% (occupational physical loading) and 2% (leisure time physical loading) for the upper and lower lumbar spine, respectively. In other monozygotic twin studies, no difference in lumbar disc degeneration was seen for twins who differed in resistance or endurance training.[29] However, it should be noted that the same study found evidence of increased disc degeneration in the lower thoracic spine (T6 to T12) for twins who participated in resistance training.[29] Twins who differed in whole body vibration through lifetime exposure to motorized vehicles did not have measurable differences in lumbar disc degeneration.[30] Therefore, physical loading appears to have a minimal effect on lumbar disc degeneration when these better controlled clinical studies are considered.[3]

In contrast to the association for disc degeneration, the evidence presented on physical loading factors and the clinical presentation of LBP suggests a positive association between the two.[36-42] However, whether this is a causal relationship is not clear. For example, a study in a machinery manufacturing plant compared the prevalence of LBP in 69 workers involved with manual handling with its prevalence in 51 workers involved in machinery operation.[39] The workers involved with manual handling were more likely to have experienced LBP in the past year (63.8% versus 37.3%, p < 0.01).[39] However, whether the jobs caused the difference in the prevalence of LBP cannot be determined, because the study was cross sectional and lacked the necessary temporal requirement for inferring cause.

Other examples in the literature that meet the temporal requirement for causality appear to have inconsistent results. A 3-year study of LBP incidence and prevalence in a cohort of 288 scaffolders found that none of the physical loading factors (i.e., high manual handling of materials, high strenuous arm movements, and high awkward back postures) were associated with the onset of LBP.[40] In contrast, another study found that policemen who wore body armor (weighing approximately 8.5 kg [18.7 lbs]) were more likely to have LBP than those who did not wear body armor.[41] A likely reason for the inconsistency in the literature is that these studies often did not adequately control for confounding factors with the potential to influence associations between physical factors and LBP. Another likely reason for the inconsistency is that many different occupations have been studied, and standard definitions for job demands are not universally applied. Therefore, more rigorous studies appear to be needed to determine whether physical factors definitively cause LBP (see Table 9-2) or whether the causality of physical factors is occupation specific.

Smoking

Smoking has been hypothesized to be a causative factor in LBP. One theory suggests that smoking adversely affects the blood supply to the lumbar spine (i.e., the abdominal aorta, lumbar artery, and middle sacral artery) through functional vasoconstriction (immediate effect) and cardiovascular disease (long-term effect).[43,44] It has been suggested that either of these mechanisms could cause LBP. For example, functional vasoconstriction could cause LBP through ischemia, and cardiovascular disease could cause LBP by limiting the blood supply to lumbar structures, accelerating degeneration of the lumbar intervertebral disc and/or spinal structures. The importance of an oxygen gradient for the intervertebral disc was confirmed in a statistical model,[45] and an acute smoking test has been shown to adversely affect the diffusion of nutrients into the disc in an animal model.[46] Another way smoking has been linked to lumbar disc degeneration is through nicotine exposure. In basic studies, direct nicotine exposure to intervertebral discs caused morphological changes (i.e., disruptions in cell proliferation and architecture) indicative of early degenerative changes.[47,48]

Support for a link between the effects of smoking, disc degeneration, and LBP is consistently found in smaller scale studies (n < 200) involving postmortem examinations of patients.[49-51] In one study, atherosclerosis of the abdominal aorta and stenosis of the ostia of the lumbar and middle sacral arteries were significantly associated with lumbar disc degeneration, which was independent of the age of the subject.[50] Also, lumbar and middle sacral arteries were significantly more likely to be missing or occluded in patients who had reported a history of low back symptoms during their lifetime.[51] Occluded lumbar and middle sacral arteries were more common in those with a history of LBP that lasted 3 months or longer, with an OR of 8.5 (95% CI, 2.9-24), adjusted for age and gender.[49]

Support for a link between the effects of smoking, disc degeneration, and LBP can also be found in population-based studies. For example, a prospective cohort of 606 subjects was followed, and those who developed calcifications in the posterior wall of the abdominal aorta were twice as likely to develop intervertebral disc degeneration (OR, 2; 95% CI, 1.2-3.5).[52] In the same study, subjects with grade 3 (severe) posterior aortic calcification were more likely to report LBP during adult life (OR, 1.6; 95% CI, 1.1-2.2).[52] In a different population-based study of 29,244 subjects, 57% of habitual smokers (defined as having at least one cigarette a day) reported having LBP in the past year, whereas only 40% of nonsmokers (defined as never having smoked) reported LBP in the past year (OR, 2; 95% CI, 1.9-2.1).[43] Habitual smoking was also associated with a longer duration of LBP, with an OR of 1.4 (95% CI, 1.3-1.6) for 1-7 days of LBP and increasing to an OR of 3 (95% CI, 2.8-3.3) for LBP that lasted longer than 30 days.[43]

However, support for a smoking link to LBP diminishes when studies of monozygotic twins are considered. Differences in LBP were either minimal or not observed when monozygotic twins who smoked and did not smoke were compared.[4,19,43] In one specific twin study, 53% of the smokers and 52% of the nonsmokers reported LBP, a difference that was not statistically significant.[43] Further evidence against smoking as a cause of LBP was demonstrated in this same study, which reported no clear dose-response association between smoking and LBP for the number of cigarettes smoked or the number of years smoked; smoking cessation was not associated with a lower prevalence of LBP; and no difference in LBP was seen for smokers based on body mass index (BMI).[43] A 1999 systematic literature review of 47 epidemiological studies reached similar conclusions, finding statistically significant associations between LBP and smoking in only 51% of the studies, and rate ratios reported generally were below 2 (indication of a noncausal association).[44] In addition, the systematic literature review found no clear evidence of a dose-response association between smoking and LBP and no true data supporting temporality or reversibility of smoking and LBP.[44] Therefore, no substantive evidence appears to support smoking as a definitive cause of LBP (see Table 9-2).

Obesity

Obesity has been hypothesized to act as a cause of LBP by increasing the mechanical demands (i.e., via compressive or shear forces) on the lumbar anatomy.[1,53] Obesity also has been hypothesized to be an indirect cause of LBP, because it may represent a proxy measure for another, more difficult to measure factor (i.e., lifestyle) that is actually the "true cause" of LBP.[1,53]

A study involving a multivariate model for predicting LBP found that obesity (measured by BMI) was a significant predictor of LBP when gender, age, educational level, and living conditions were controlled.[54] However, it should be noted that many studies report no association between obesity and LBP. In fact, a systematic review of the literature in 2000 indicated that, in 65 studies published from 1965 to 1997, fewer than 25% had a positive statistically significant association between measures of body weight and LBP variables (Figure 9-1).[1] Another issue of concern is the fact that the reported associations between obesity and LBP are also weak, with event rates not large enough to be considered a causative factor. For example, compared to a normal weight category, the OR for experiencing LBP in the past year was 0.6 (95% CI, 0.5-0.6) for an underweight category, 1.3 (95% CI, 1.2-1.4) for an overweight category, and 1.1 (95% CI, 0.9-1.3) for a heavy overweight category.[53]

Further evidence against obesity as a cause of LBP is demonstrated in a study that investigated monozygotic twins who differed in BMI.[53] In that study, no association was found between obesity and LBP in the past year, with the OR for LBP being 0.9 (95% CI, 0.7-1.2) for an underweight category, 1.1 (95% CI, 0.8-1.5) for an overweight category, and 1.1 (95% CI, 0.5-2) for a heavy overweight category. The lack of a consistent dose-response curve is

another indication that obesity is not a cause of LBP. Positive monotonic dose-response curves (higher weight associated with more LBP) have been reported in the literature,[55,56] but other shaped dose-response curves also have been reported.[53,57] Furthermore, no studies have been reported in the literature that suggest that temporality or reversibility exists with regard to obesity and LBP.[1] Collectively, the peer-reviewed literature does not appear to support obesity as a definitive cause of LBP (see Table 9-2).

Obesity, therefore, does not appear to be causative of LBP, but some evidence suggests that obesity is associated with a longer duration of LBP. In one study, LBP that lasted longer than 30 days was consistently associated with BMI categories; for example, the OR for the underweight category was 0.7, the OR for the overweight category was 1.6, and the OR for the heavy overweight category was 1.7.[53] The authors did not report the 95% CI for the ORs in the text, but they indicated that a significant difference was seen between the underweight and the heavy overweight categories.[53] In a separate study in an occupational setting, obesity was a significant prognostic factor (OR, 1.68; 95% CI, 1.01-2.81) in a multivariate model for determining patients receiving compensation 3 months after a low back injury.[58] This evidence is preliminary, but it suggests that, *although obesity may not cause LBP, it may have a meaningful impact on how long LBP persists.*

Psychological and Psychosocial Factors

Psychological and/or psychosocial distress is thought to be causative of LBP through two pathways.[59] The first pathway involves the notion that psychological distress can lead to a situation in which the nervous system is "sensitized," making it more likely to perceive a non-noxious peripheral stimulus as painful. The second pathway relates to the notion that patients with psychological distress also have a tendency to somatize their symptoms.[60] Certain patients who are distressed, therefore, may express their psychological symptoms as LBP. Extensive literature exists describing cross sectional relations between psychological factors, psychosocial factors, and LBP, but a review of those studies is beyond the scope of this chapter. Instead, evidence is presented from prospective studies that considered whether psychological and/or psychosocial factors were associated with or causative of LBP.

In a U.K. study of 1638 adults who were not currently experiencing LBP, a validated measure of psychological distress (the General Health Questionnaire, which primarily focuses on symptoms of anxiety and depression) was predictive of new episodes of LBP during the next 12 months.[59] Specifically, the OR for those with higher psychological distress (patients in the upper third of the General Health Questionnaire versus those in the lower third) was 1.8 (95% CI, 1.4-2.4).[59] This factor remained predictive even when

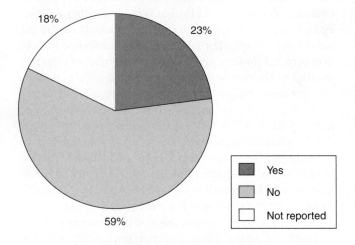

18% 23% 59%

- ■ Yes
- ▨ No
- □ Not reported

Yes = Significant, positive association between body weight and LBP variable

No = No significant, positive association between body weight and LBP variable

Not reported = No association reported in study

Figure 9-1

Statistically significant associations reported in the literature between body weight measures and variables related to low back pain. (Adapted from Leboeuf-Yde C: Body weight and low back pain: a systematic literature review of 56 journal articles reporting on 65 epidemiologic studies, *Spine* 25:226-237, 2000.)

potential confounders were considered, such as poor physical health, history of LBP, employment status, age, gender, and social status.[59] A prospective study of 403 volunteers with no prior history of "serious" LBP showed that psychological distress (a combination of somatic perception and depressive symptoms) was significantly predictive of a "serious" first time episode of LBP, whereas only somatic perception was predictive of "any" first-time episode of LBP.[61]

In another U.K. study of 1412 workers not currently experiencing LBP, psychosocial factors related to the workplace were predictive of new episodes of LBP.[62] Patients who were slightly dissatisfied (OR, 1.7; 95% CI, 1.2-2.4) or severely dissatisfied (OR, 2; 95% CI, 1.2-3.3) with their job were more likely to experience an episode of LBP in the 12-month study period. Patients who perceived their income to be severely inadequate were also more likely (OR, 3.6; 95% CI, 1.8-7.2) to experience an episode of LBP during the 12-month study period.[62] The psychosocial factors remained predictive, even after controlling for the potential confounder of general psychological distress.[62] Further evidence suggesting that psychological factors precede LBP can be found in an intriguing study that reported that discography in asymptomatic patients with psychological distress resulted in reports of significant back pain for at least 1 year after injection, whereas subjects with normal psychometric test results reported no long-term back pain after discography.[63]

This smaller body of literature suggests that psychological and psychosocial factors are associated with new episodes of LBP.[59,61-63] The influence of these factors has been estimated to account for about 16% of new episodes of LBP in the general population[59] and up to 25% of new episodes in the working population.[62] However, these factors still cannot be seen as causative of LBP because the number of prospective cohort reports remains relatively small, the magnitude of the reported associations is not consistently higher than 2, a clear monotonic dose-response curve has not been reported, and studies of reversibility have not been reported (see Table 9-2).

Therefore, psychological and psychosocial factors may not cause LBP but, like obesity, they appear to have a meaningful effect on the duration of LBP. Several prospective studies have documented that psychological and/or psychosocial distress during acute LBP episodes significantly increases the probability of chronic LBP.[64,65] The OR for high levels of psychological distress predicting chronic LBP was 3.3 (95% CI, 1.5-7.2) in a group of 180 patients followed for a year in the United Kingdom.[65] *The identification of psychological and/or psychosocial distress factors (i.e., yellow flags) is an important part of the differential diagnosis of LBP because of their strong link to the development of chronic LBP.* A strategy for identifying specific psychological factors is discussed later in the chapter.

Alcohol

Alcohol has been hypothesized to contribute to LBP by a direct route, involving uncoordinated movements that damage spinal structures, or by indirect routes, involving the development of comorbidities that cause LBP.[66] Alcohol has not been thoroughly investigated as a cause of LBP in the peer-reviewed literature. For example, a systematic review identified only nine potential studies that focused on alcohol and LBP, and none of them were prospective in nature.[66] When these studies were reviewed collectively, none reported statistically significant associations between increased alcohol consumption and LBP.[66] For example, one study found similar LBP rates between moderate (OR, 0.88; 95% CI, 0.79-0.99) and excessive (OR, 0.72; 95% CI, 0.62-0.85) alcohol consumption.[56] Because of the limited number of reports and concerns with the methodology of the studies that were reported in the literature, the author of the systematic review concluded that alcohol did not appear to be a cause of LBP (see Table 9-2).[66]

Epidemiology of Low Back Pain

Expert opinion has likened the frequency of LBP among members of modern society to an "epidemic,"[67] and reports in the literature consistently support this view. A Dutch postal questionnaire study demonstrated that LBP was the most prevalent form of musculoskeletal pain reported by adults 25 years of age or older.[68] Specifically, the point prevalence of LBP in the study was 26.9% (95% CI, 25.5-28.3), which was significantly higher than the point prevalence of the next two most common categories: shoulder pain, at 20.9% (95% CI, 19.6-22.2) and neck pain, at 20.6% (95% CI, 19.3-21.9).[68] Although it is clear that individuals in all strata of society commonly experience LBP, its prevalence does appear to vary based on factors such as gender, age, occupation, and socioeconomic status.

Women tend to have a higher prevalence of LBP than men, although the differences reported vary in magnitude.[54,68-71] For example, in the previously mentioned Dutch study, the point prevalence was 28.1% (95% CI, 26.1-30.1) for women and 25.6% (95% CI, 23.5-27.7) for men. In a study of Arabic subjects, the difference in overall prevalence was larger, reported as 73.8% for females and 56.1% for males. An increase in age is also associated with a higher prevalence of LBP. In a Greek population–based study, the odds of experiencing any LBP in the past month were significantly higher for the age groups 46-65 (OR, 1.82; 95% CI, 1.38-2.38) and 66+ (OR, 2.7; 95% CI, 1.85-3.93) compared to the group age 45 or younger.[72] In a Danish study of individuals 12 to 41 years old, the prevalence of LBP in the past year increased from 7% for 12-year-olds to 56% for 41-year-olds.[70] A separate epidemiological review suggests that this trend in increasing

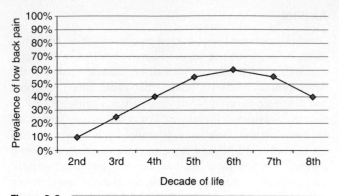

Figure 9-2

Qualitative composite of 1-year LBP prevalence through the 2nd to 8th decades of life.[68,70,73]

prevalence of LBP continues past 41 and peaks in the 6th decade of life.[73] After the 6th decade, the prevalence of LBP appears to level off, and it eventually declines in the later decades (Figure 9-2).[68]

Occupational differences in the prevalence of LBP were demonstrated in a study of Chinese workers.[36] A 50% annual prevalence rate of LBP (defined as lasting 24 hours or longer) was reported, but the rate was significantly higher for garment workers than teachers (74% versus 40%).[36] In a study involving 1562 Canadian utility workers, lifetime and point prevalence of LBP was 60% and 11%, respectively.[38] In this same sample, LBP prevalence was significantly higher in workers who had jobs that were physically demanding or involved heavy lifting.[38] In a group of 288 scaffolders who were followed for 3 years, 60% experienced LBP in the past year, and the prevalence was significantly associated with high material handling or job demand.[40] Interestingly, although differences exist between different occupational groups, similar LBP prevalence rates have been reported for working and nonworking groups.[69]

Specific socioeconomic factors appear to be associated with the prevalence of LBP. In the previously mentioned Greek study, being married resulted in an OR of 1.53 (95% CI, 1.15-2.03) for experiencing LBP in the past month.[72] The study of Canadian utility workers found a similar association between LBP and marriage.[38] Lower educational levels also have been linked with a higher prevalence of LBP,[54,68] and social classes involving unskilled occupations have been weakly linked with a higher prevalence of LBP.[62]

The differences in reported LBP prevalence rates for specific factors (e.g., gender and age) can be confusing to interpret. It is important that the clinician realize that these prevalence estimates vary in large part because of methodological differences between studies.[74] For example, epidemiological studies commonly differ on sampling methods, populations sampled, response rates, definitions of LBP, and measurement techniques. All of these factors have the potential to influence the prevalence estimate reported in a study. This fact is best demonstrated when systematic

reviews of prevalence studies are attempted. One systematic review of LBP prevalence found that only 30 of 56 identified studies were homogenous and methodologically sound enough for pooling.[74] Once pooled, the prevalence estimates continued to have wide intervals; for example, the LBP point prevalence was estimated at 12% to 33%, the 1-year prevalence was estimated at 22% to 65%, and the lifetime LBP prevalence was estimated at 11% to 84%.[74] Although LBP clearly is a common experience, improving the precision of prevalence estimates is a goal of future epidemiological research.

Given the overall prevalence of LBP, it is not surprising that the disorder is a common reason people seek health care. In a Finnish study, pain was the primary reason for visiting a physician in 40% of reviewed cases, and LBP was the most common source of pain.[75] In the United States, LBP is the second most common reason given for visiting a physician, behind the common cold.[76] Patients commonly seek health care from traditional medical providers, such as general practice (primary care) physicians, orthopedic physicians, and physical therapists.[76-78] LBP is also one of the most common reasons people seek health care from complementary and alternative medicine (CAM) providers.[79] In fact, a 1997 study indicated that 30.1% of Americans with LBP saw a CAM provider, and 39.1% saw a CAM and traditional medical provider for LBP.[79] Studies published in 2003-2005 suggest that the current rates of CAM are consistent with the 1997 report and that the CAM treatments most commonly used for LBP are chiropractic, massage, and relaxation techniques.[80-82]

The clinician should be aware that a patient with LBP could be using some form of CAM treatment during the episode of care. This issue is relevant, because the evidence suggests that only 38.5% of patients discuss their CAM treatment with their traditional medical provider, and 46% use a CAM treatment for a principal medical condition without input from either type of provider.[79] The clinician who diagnoses a patient with LBP should determine whether and what type of CAM treatments are currently being used, because this allows appropriate coordination of the patient's subsequent therapy.

Clinicians must also recognize that not all who experience LBP seek health care. In fact, several studies in general practice and occupational settings reported that only 25% to 50% of individuals who experienced LBP actually sought health care.[68,77,83] These studies found that high levels of disability and pain were the primary differences between patients seeking health care and those who did not seek health care.[68,77,83,84] Specifically, women and men with high disability were more likely to seek health care for LBP than individuals of the same gender with low disability, with the odds ratios being 7.4 (95% CI, 5-11) and 4.9 (95% CI, 3.3-7.1), respectively.[84] Women and men with high pain intensity were also more likely to seek health care for LBP compared to individuals of the same gender with low pain intensity, with the odds ratios being 3.7 (95% CI, 2.2-6) and 1.7 (95% CI, 1.1-2.8), respectively.[84] Another study suggested that patients from unskilled, manual occupations (OR, 4.8; 95% CI, 2-11.5) were more likely to seek health care for LBP compared to those who perceived their income to be inadequate (OR, 3.6; 95% CI, 1.8-7.2).[62]

Course of Low Back Pain

The course of LBP has been described as consisting of acute, subacute, and chronic phases, with temporal definitions typically associated with each phase. Different operational definitions have been reported in the literature, but the commonly accepted definitions are: acute phase, 0 to 1 month since the episode of LBP; subacute phase, 2 to 3 months since the episode of LBP; and chronic phase, longer than 3 months since the episode of LBP. The prognosis for LBP appears to be favorable, predictable, and static when these temporal definitions are used (Figure 9-3, *A*). For example, up to 90% of patients with LBP are expected to be pain free or to show dramatic improvement during the acute phase, and only about 10% of patients are expected to report LBP that continues into the chronic phase.

Because LBP often is recurrent, exclusive use of temporal definitions to describe its course has been challenged in the literature.[85,86] The primary argument is that when LBP is recurrent, the time to improvement from a single episode does not accurately describe its outcome. This issue is perhaps best summarized by Von Korff et al.:[86] "For example, a person experiencing recurrent episodes of back pain on half the days in a year might appear to have a favorable outcome of each episode, but an unfavorable outcome across episodes. For this reason, the outcome of a recurrent pain condition is more appropriately assessed by the total time with pain across episodes and the characteristic severity of those episodes than by the duration of a single episode."

This is not a purely academic issue, because the prognosis of LBP changes when the influence of recurrence is considered. Of patients with acute LBP who were followed for 1 year, 65% reported one or more additional episodes.[87] In that same study, 2 months was the median time to another episode of LBP, and 60 days was the median time to experience LBP in the year. Other studies have reported lower but still substantial recurrence rates, ranging from to 20% to 35% (6 to 22 months)[88] to 45% (4 years). Von Korff[85] suggested operational definitions to standardize the description of the course of LBP for clinicians and researchers (Table 9-3). Although these definitions have not been universally adopted, preliminary evidence supports their construct validity; patients classified with chronic LBP

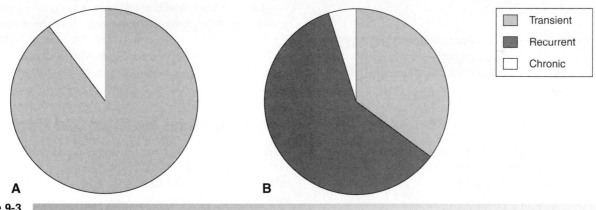

Figure 9-3

A, Traditional course of LBP. **B,** Evidence-based course of LBP.

Table 9-3
Standard Definitions for Manifestations of Low Back Pain

Descriptor	Operational Definition for an Episode of Low Back Pain
Transient back pain	Present for no more than 90 consecutive days and does not recur over a 12-month period
Recurrent back pain	Present for fewer than half the days in a 12-month period and occurs in multiple episodes over the year
Chronic back pain	Present for at least half the days in a 12-month period in single or multiple episodes
Acute back pain	Recent and sudden in onset and does not meet the previously defined criteria for recurrent or chronic pain
First onset	First occurrence in the patient's lifetime
Flare-up	Distinct phase of pain (with definable beginning and end points) superimposed on a chronic or recurrent course; a period when the pain is markedly more severe than is usual for the patient

Data from Von Korff M: Studying the natural history of back pain, *Spine* 19:2041S-2046S, 1994.

had higher pain scores and higher social disability and were more likely to use medication to treat LBP.[89]

When these other factors are considered, the prognosis for LBP becomes less favorable and more variable (Figure 9-3, *B*). At a 1-year follow-up of primary care back patients, 69% of patients with recent onset of LBP (within the past 6 months) reported having pain in the last month.[86] Only 21% of these patients were pain free at 1 year, with 55% reporting low disability and pain intensity, 10% reporting low disability and high pain intensity, and 14% reporting high disability with varying pain intensity.[86] Similar trends were noted for the 82% of patients with prevalent LBP (onset longer than the past 6 months) who reported having pain in the last month.[86] At 1-year follow-up, only 12% were pain free, with 52% reporting low disability and pain intensity, 16% reporting low disability and high pain intensity, and 20% reporting high disability with varying pain intensity.[86]

This line of research suggests that the clinician obtaining a history from a patient with LBP must ask the patient to describe its course in more than just temporal terms associated with the most recent episode that led to the current episode of health care. Other pertinent historical factors include the number of previous episodes, the severity of the current episode, the number of days with LBP in the past year, and the extent to which the condition interferes with daily activities.[85,90]

Important Historical Questions Related to the Course of Low Back Pain[85,90]

- How long has the present episode of low back pain bothered you?
- How many previous episodes of low back pain have you experienced?
- How many days have you had low back pain in the past year?
- How severe is your present episode of low back pain?
- How much does low back pain interfere with your daily activities?

Societal Impact of Low Back Pain

Given that LBP is a common experience that can be chronic or recurrent, it is not surprising that it is a significant cause of disability and cost to society, and this cost seems to be increasing exponentially.[67,91-93] One study found that in the general population, 53% of adults had experienced some disability from LBP during a 6-month period.[92] Chronic LBP substantially affects the capacity to work and has been associated with the inability to obtain or maintain employment[93] and to reduced productivity at work.[94]

LBP is included in a top 10 list for most costly physical ailments.[73] LBP related to occupational settings appears to have had an especially large impact on society. Estimates

are that LBP accounts for at least 33% of all health care and indemnity costs under workers' compensation.[95] The cost of lost work productivity from the most common chronic pain conditions (including LBP, headache, arthritis, and an "other" category) has been estimated at $61.2 billion per year.[94] Of specific pain categories studied, chronic LBP accounted for the most lost productivity time (5.2 hours/week).[94]

Other estimates of annual health care expenditure for chronic LBP are excessive, especially when compared to other chronic pain conditions. For example, the 1993 direct health care cost estimates were $1 billion for headache[96] and $33 billion for LBP.[97] Indirect cost estimates showed a similar discrepancy, with estimates exceeding $13 billion for headache[96] and $50 billion for LBP.[97] Interestingly, the excessive costs associated with disability from LBP did not appear to be evenly distributed.[98] For example, Williams et al.[99] found that health care costs were disproportionate, with 20% of the claimants disabled for 16 weeks or longer accounting for 60% of the health care costs. Other authors have reported similar disproportionate patient/cost associations in LBP.[100-102]

Therefore, the excessive and increasing societal cost of LBP does not appear to be due to an increase in the condition; a study that used consistent methodology showed similar prevalence rates over different time periods.[103] Instead, the increased cost seems to be associated with the way LBP has been traditionally been managed.[67] Clinicians working in progressive environments must be aware that a priority of their treatment is the effective reduction of LBP for the minority of individuals who eventually experience chronic symptoms and accrue exorbitant health care costs.[104-109]

Biopsychosocial Model of Low Back Pain

Currently, very little evidence supports a single, "magic bullet" cause of LBP (see Table 9-2). The conceptualization of the disorder as a distinct and specific disease may be the most direct explanation for difficulty identifying causative factors of LBP.[108] Instead of a specific disease, LBP may best be conceptualized as an illness characterized and influenced by input from different factors across multiple domains.[108] This realization has led to the implementation of a comprehensive model that describes the development of LBP.

In 1987, Gordon Waddell proposed a model that considered the simultaneous influence of physical, psychological, and social factors in the development of LBP.[108] The exact parameters of this "biopsychosocial" model have been modified over time, but it remains the currently accepted model of LBP for research and clinical practice (Figure 9-4). The advantage of using this model in clinical practice is that it accounts for all the previously described considerations relating to the etiology, epidemiology, course, and societal impact of LBP. Quite simply, a biopsychosocial model regards LBP as an illness, which is a more accurate

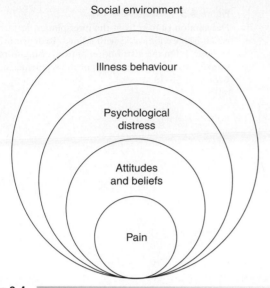

Figure 9-4

Biopsychosocial model of low back pain. (From Waddell G: 1987 Volvo Award in Clinical Sciences: a new clinical model for the treatment of low-back pain, *Spine* 12:632-644, 1987.)

Potential Generators of Low Back Pain[110-112]

- Muscles
- Ligaments
- Dura mater
- Nerve roots
- Zygapophyseal joints
- Annulus fibrosus
- Thoracolumbar fascia
- Vertebrae

Table 9-4

Percentage of Patients Reporting Pain and Pain Location After Stimulation of Different Lumbar Tissues

Anatomical Structure	Number Tested	Percentage Reporting Pain	Pain Location
Lumbar fascia	193	17%	Back
Paravertebral muscle	193	41%	Back
Supraspinous ligament	193	25%	Back
Lamina	193	10%	Back
Facet capsule	192	30%	Back, buttock
Ligamentum flavum	167	0	—
Posterior dura	92	23%	Buttock, leg
Compressed nerve root	167	99%	Buttock, leg, foot
Normal nerve root	55	11%	Buttock, leg
Central annulus	183	74%	Back
Lateral annulus	144	71%	Back
Nucleus	176	0	—
Vertebral end plate	109	61%	Back

Data from Kuslich SD, Ulstrom CL, Michael CJ: The tissue origin of low back pain and sciatica: a report of pain response to tissue stimulation during operations on the lumbar spine using local anesthesia, *Orthop Clin North Am* 22:181-187, 1991.

representation of the clinical presentation. Therefore, a biopsychosocial model of LBP is this chapter's framework for discussing the differential diagnosis of LBP.

Differential Diagnosis of Low Back Pain

The tasks of the clinician are straightforward when a biopsychosocial model is used for differential diagnosis and classification of patients with LBP. The specific tasks are described in detail, after a brief review of anatomical causes of LBP and diagnostic imaging of the lumbar spine.

Potential Pain Generators in the Lumbar Spine

Any innervated structure in the lumbar spine can cause symptoms of low back pain and referred pain into the extremity or extremities. For example, in a study by Kuslich et al.,[110] 193 consecutive patients with back pain were progressively anesthetized and the structures of the lumbar spine were stimulated either by blunt mechanical force from a surgical tool or by low power cautery. In this investigation, only stimulation of the posterior dura and nerve roots by mechanical or thermal stimuli gave patients the sensation of leg pain (Table 9-4). In comparison, after Kellgren[111] injected the intraspinous ligaments with saline, subjects reported aching pain in the buttock and leg from a variety of segmental levels, which implies that somatic musculoskeletal structures can also refer pain into the extremity (Figure 9-5).

The quality of pain reported by the patient may help differentiate whether the source of the pain is related to a somatic musculoskeletal structure or the pain is radicular in origin. Radicular pain is a sharp, shooting pain in the leg in a defined band less than 4 cm (1.6 inches) wide,[113] either superficial or deep in the leg,[113,114] whereas somatic pain is poorly localized and reported as aching. However, compression of the nerve root is unlikely to be the primary causative mechanism. Compression of nerve root tissue causes radiculopathy; that is, radiating paresthesia, numbness, and weakness, or a combination of symptoms, but not pain.[113] The characteristic pain is elicited only when

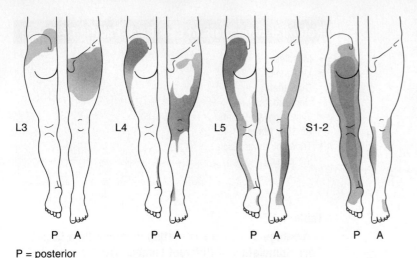

L3   L4   L5   S1-2

P A   P A   P A   P A

P = posterior
A = anterior

Figure 9-5

Distribution of pain from the interspinous ligament, which has been injected with saline. (Redrawn from Kellgren J: On the distribution of pain arising from deep somatic structures with charts of the segmental areas, *Clin Sci* 4:35-46, 1939.)

a previously damaged nerve root is compressed.[110,113] Consequently, a patient may not always present with radiculopathy *and* radicular pain.

Radicular Pain, Radiculopathy, and Somatic Pain

- *Radicular pain:* Sharp, shooting, superficial or deep pain into the leg in a defined band less than 4 cm (1.6 inches) wide
- *Radiculopathy:* Radiating paresthesia, numbness in a dermatome, weakness (myotome), or a combination of these; however, the patient does not experience pain
- *Somatic pain:* Poorly localized, aching pain

Inflammation of the dural sleeve and nerve root is implicated in the genesis of the initial radicular symptoms. Although the source of the inflammation is not obvious, exposure to nuclear material of the intervertebral disc may cause a chemical inflammatory response in the dural and nerve root tissue and eventual fibrosis of the perineural tissues.[113,115] Subsequent compression of the damaged neural tissue generates radicular symptoms. For example, Kuslich et al.[110] demonstrated that mechanical deformation of perineural scar tissue evoked no pain response, but stimulation of the nerve root at the point of compression produced radicular symptoms.

In the absence of extrusion of nucleus pulposus material into the spinal canal, a precursor inflammatory response may result from traumatic compression.[116] Animal models also suggest that compression of the nerve root tissue eventually generates local edema and ischemia of the nerve root and ganglion.[117,118] Therefore, any of the pathologies that cause prolonged nerve root compression eventually may result in damage to the nerve root or ganglion. After this damage occurs, further compression may then result in complaints of radicular pain.

Specific Somatic Pain Generators
Contractile Tissue

The available literature suggests that paraspinal muscles of patients with LBP are dysfunctional. Studies have demonstrated muscle atrophy,[119-121] reduced activity during trunk movements,[122,123] decreased muscle strength,[124,125] and increased trunk muscular fatigability[126,127] in patients with LBP. The studies that demonstrate decreased muscle performance associated with LBP support a model of muscle deficiency in lumbar dysfunction rather than a muscle spasm model.[128] Atrophy of the paraspinal muscles has been documented in patients with short duration[120] and chronic[119] LBP. The atrophy appears specific to the multifidus, which suggests a mechanism other than disuse to explain the atrophy.[128] Hides et al.[120] have suggested that reflex inhibition is a likely cause of atrophy in lumbar paraspinal muscles. Experimental support for this theoretical construct is offered in a porcine model in which rapid inhibition of the deep paraspinal muscles occurs after distention of the zygapophyseal joints by injection with saline solution.[129]

Characteristics of Paraspinal and Trunk Muscles in Patients with Low Back Pain

- Atrophy
- Reduced activity during trunk movements
- Decreased muscle strength
- Increased fatigability
- Change in percentage of fiber types

In addition to deep muscle atrophy, patients with LBP have a significantly higher proportion of type IIB (fast twitch glycolytic) fibers than type I slow twitch fibers[127] in the posterior trunk muscles. The duration of LBP symptoms was shown to be significantly associated with a higher proportion of type II fibers, such that the longer the duration of pain, the more glycolytic the paraspinal fiber composition.[127] This finding may provide some explanation for the increase in fatigability noted in patients with LBP. These muscular performance changes may contribute to LBP by reducing the muscular support of the lumbar spine, resulting in increased stress on the noncontractile structures.

Muscles of the lumbar spine have been demonstrated to act as primary sources of back and buttock pain in experiments using saline distention of a muscle[112] and mechanical stimulation.[110,111] The disorders that affect predominantly the musculature of the lumbar spine include muscle strain injury, spasm or guarding, and myofascial complaints, such as trigger points.

Evidence that increased activity occurs in the muscles in response to pain has been shown in patients with temporomandibular dysfunction,[130] healthy subjects chewing gum,[131] and patients with cervical dysfunction.[132,133] Subjects with pain and a history of cervical soft tissue injury have lower blood flow in the muscles on the painful side, relative to the pain-free side, compared with control subjects.[134] The differences in blood flow were pronounced at low level muscle contractions. The impaired circulation probably contributes to muscle pain by causing metabolites to accumulate, producing pain and a further disturbance of the circulation in a vicious circle.[135] Although this phenomenon has not been demonstrated in the lumbar spine, similar increases in muscle activity and changes in circulation conceivably might occur.

Noncontractile Tissue

Kellgren[111,112] demonstrated that noncontractile tissue such as fascia, ligaments, and the periosteum are viable sources of LBP. Work by the Kuslich et al.[110] supports these early observations and provides additional insight into components of the intervertebral disc as direct sources of pain (see Table 9-4).

Discogenic Pain

Mechanical stimulation of the outer annulus fibrosus causes central back pain, not leg pain,[110,113] and the innervation of the outer annulus fibrosus has been well documented. Therefore, the intervertebral disc should be considered a cause of back pain. In addition, changes in the intervertebral disc contribute to other conditions that subsequently result in somatic or radicular pain.

Only the outer third of the annulus is innervated. Torsional injury is thought to occur to the outer annulus fibrosis, particularly when the torsion is coupled with lumbar flexion.[136,137] Bogduk[138] has suggested that this mechanism should be considered similar to a ligamentous

sprain injury, because fibers of the outer annulus might be traumatized.

Alternatively, a pain response from the outer annulus fibrosus may be elicited with exposure of nociceptive endings in the annulus fibrosus to material from the nucleus pulposus or breakdown products from nuclear degradation. The specific mechanism of degeneration is not well understood but may be related to genetic factors (see previous section). In vitro evidence suggests that changes in compressive stress on the disc within the nucleus (such as occur with disruption of the annulus or minor vertebral body damage) disrupt cellular metabolism throughout the disc, progressively deteriorating the matrix.[139] Radial fissures that develop in the inner two thirds of the annulus eventually reach the innervated outer third.[137,140,141] As the innervated outer third of the annulus becomes disrupted or comes into contact with nuclear material, or both, the patient will complain of backache but is not likely to have radicular pain or signs of radiculopathy because no prolapse or herniation of disc material has occurred.

Disc prolapse can occur gradually when discs are subjected to repetitive compression and flexion loading,[139] but radial fissuring in the annulus must precede disc prolapse.[142] Milette et al.[143] report that disc bulges and disc protrusions do not differ significantly in internal architecture, based on the findings of discography. A bulge in the disc that occurs as the annulus weakens may impinge on neural structures within the spinal canal. Eventually disc material herniates; that is, when the radial fissures reach the periphery of the disc, nuclear material may be herniated into the spinal canal.[139,140] The chemical irritation of the nerve root or ganglion leads to subsequent radicular pain. However, not only nuclear material is herniated. Lebkowski and Dzieciol[144] examined specimens of herniated disc material from 187 patients and reported that in 29% of the cases, the herniation was primarily annular material. This finding may explain the lack of radicular symptoms in some cases of disc herniation in which the nerve root is predominantly exposed to annular material.

Ligament and Fascia

Kuslich et al.[110] demonstrated that both the supraspinous and interspinous ligaments can be a source of central LBP, and Kellgren[111] reported back and leg pain in subjects in whom the interspinous ligament had been injected. However, the prevalence of specific sprain injury to the interspinous ligament is likely to be very low. The common tendon of the longissimus thoracis,[145,146] and the long dorsal sacroiliac ligament[147] are also ligamentous sources of pain, particularly pain on palpation around the posterior iliac spine. The thoracolumbar fascia also might be a source of pain. Little data have been identified regarding the diagnosis of ligamentous or fascial injury in the low back; however, it might be speculated that sprain injuries to these structures would have a similar mechanism of injury in the trunk as in the extremities. Alternatively, pain might arise after prolonged stress on ligamentous tissue related to postural changes or movement impairments.[148]

Zygapophyseal Joints (Facet Joint Syndrome)

The prevalence of zygapophyseal involvement in the genesis of LBP may be as high as 25%.[149] The zygapophyseal joints have been identified as a source of back and leg pain by generating pain in healthy subjects,[150] by reproducing pain in patients,[112] and by relieving pain with injection in certain patients.[151]

El-Bohy et al.[152] demonstrated the potential for capsular sprain injury of the zygapophyseal joint, and fractures, capsular tears, and damage to the articular cartilage have been documented in postmortem studies.[153] Degenerative arthritis of the zygapophyseal joints is another possible cause of pain. However, not all arthritis is painful; radiographic changes of osteoarthritis are equally common in patients with and without LBP.[154] Other theories regarding the genesis of lumbar pain from the zygapophyseal joint include meniscoid entrapment,[155] synovial impingement,[151,155] and mechanical injury to the joint's capsule.[156] Unfortunately, no definitive means exists to identify the zygapophyseal joint as the source of LBP and lower extremity pain from the history or clinical findings.[151,157,158] For example, Marks[159] reported that pain radiating to the buttock or trochanteric region occurred mostly from the L4 and L5 levels, and groin pain was produced from L2 to L5; however, no consistent pain pattern has been identified related to the joints. Diagnosis of the zygapophyseal joint as the source of LBP is based on controlled diagnostic blocks of the joint or its nerve supply.[151,157,158]

Vertebrae

The vertebral body is involved in several painful conditions, such as Paget's disease,[160] primary or secondary tumors,[160,161] and fractures. The posterior elements of the vertebrae can be affected similarly to the vertebral body; however, several lesions are peculiar to the posterior elements. Increased lumbar lordosis or hyperextension trauma may result in impact of the spinous process or lamina of articulating vertebrae. This may result in periostitis of the spinous process or lamina or inflammation of the interspinous ligament.

Spondylolysis is a defect of the pars articularis often related to fatigue fracture,[162] although some predisposition to development of the condition may be related to weakness in the pars interarticularis.[163] The location of a pars defect is related to the activities in which the patient is involved. For example, fast bowling in cricket is associated with unilateral defects, whereas soccer players develop more bilateral defects.[162] Likewise, the incidence of spondylolysis is related to activity. In gymnastics, the incidence of a pars defect is 11% in females,[164] and the incidence in university-aged athletes playing American football may be as high as 15%.

The prevalence of spondylolysis in asymptomatic adult subjects ranges from 6%[165] to 9.7%.[166] Libson et al.[166] compared 938 asymptomatic individuals to 662 with LBP and determined the overall incidence of spondylolysis to be equivalent (9.7%) for both groups. However, these authors indicated that a bilateral defect is more likely to be associated with a complaint of pain. These data suggest that a pars defect itself may not be the source of pain. Rather, the defect compromises the arthrokinematics of intervertebral motion such that increased stress is placed on other structures of the posterior vertebral arch, such as the ligaments or paraspinal muscles.

Spondylolisthesis is anterior displacement of one vertebra over another.[167] Spondylolisthesis usually results from spondylolysis after the normal resistance to forward displacement of the vertebra is disrupted because of fracture or elongation of the pars interarticularis.[168] Narrowing of the spinal canal occurs if posterior elements also slide forward. Szypryt et al.[169] demonstrated that a pars defect was associated with a prevalence of disc degeneration greater than that seen in a normal aging population.

With enough anterior slippage, the central spinal canal and the structures within may become compromised. However, slips present in juvenile or adolescent patients may autofuse or ankylose once the patient reaches skeletal maturity and remain asymptomatic throughout life.[170] Frennered et al.[171] performed follow-up with juvenile patients with spondylolisthesis after a mean time of 7 years. Thirty percent of the patients had surgery after 3.7 years, and results in 83% of the patients treated without surgery were rated excellent or good. These authors were unable to predict the progression of the slippage or the need for future operative treatment from the findings at the initial consultation.[171] Beutler et al.[172] followed juvenile patients in whom lesions of the pars had been identified radiographically for 45 years. Patients with unilateral defects never experienced slippage over the course of the study, and 30% of the defects healed. Of the patients with bilateral defects, 81% progressed to spondylolisthesis. Progression of spondylolisthesis was greatest in the 1st decade after identification (teens) with subsequent slowing with each subsequent decade. There was no association of slip progression and low back pain.[172]

Other vertebral anomalies, such as transitional lumbar vertebrae (TLV) or spina bifida occulta (SBO), have been associated with increased severity of LBP,[173] but the overall evidence for such an association is equivocal.[174] In a series of 4000 individuals, Tini et al.[175] demonstrated no association between LBP and the presence of a TLV. More recently, Peterson et al.[176] found similar results; 352

patients with LBP had no difference in self-report of pain or disability based on TLV status.

Other reports indicated that TLV increased nerve root symptoms, whereas SBO did not.[173] Patients with nerve root symptoms and a TLV have a greater incidence of disc prolapse than those without a TLV for the vertebral level directly above the TLV.[177] In addition, spinal stenosis in the absence of spondylolisthesis is more likely to occur at the level above a TLV.[177] However, it is important to note that radiographic evidence of a vertebral anomaly does not necessarily indicate a greater likelihood of LBP.

Dilemma of Lumbar Spine Imaging

The advent of stronger magnets used in magnetic resonance imaging (MRI) has resulted in finer resolution of subsequent image reconstructions of the target tissue. For example, researchers at the University of Florida have successfully obtained MR images and spectra from single neurons.[178] Improvement in the resolution of imaging technology might be expected to increase the likelihood of detecting a link between pathology and pain in the lumbar spine. Realistically, the determination of a pathoanatomical origin for LBP is complicated by the rate of false positive findings on imaging studies; that is, subjects without LBP showing abnormal findings.

The reported rates of these false positive findings appear to vary. For example, Stadnik et al.[179] reported that 81% of asymptomatic patients have evidence of a bulging disc, and radial annular tears might be found in 56% of asymptomatic patients. Jensen et al.[180] reported that 52% of subjects without pain had a bulge at one level, 27% showed disc protrusion, and 14% had evidence of disruption of the outer annulus. Evidence of herniation of disc material was seen on computed tomography (CT) scans,[154] MRI scans,[181] and myelography[182] in 20% to 76% of individuals with no sciatica.

Nondisc pathology also is often identified in patients without back pain. Some 13%[182,183] to 19%[180] of asymptomatic patients have evidence of Schmorl's nodes. Spina bifida occulta (26%) and osteophyte formation (47%) may be present in individuals without the symptoms of back pain,[183] as can stenotic change.[184] In addition, the prevalence of all identified conditions increases with age. Autopsy studies on a large number of subjects have found disc degeneration, facet joint osteoarthritis, or osteophytes in 90% to 100% of subjects over age 64.[185] Using MRI, researchers have identified central stenosis in as many as 21% of asymptomatic subjects over age 60 and 80% of subjects over age 70.[184] Likewise the prevalence of disc bulges increases, but not that of protrusions.[180] Other vertebral anomalies, such as SBO and TLV, also occur in people without pain. For example, 12% of high school and college-aged males without LBP have evidence of SBO without LBP,[186] and the incidence of TLV may be as high as 30%, regardless of whether the person has LBP.[187]

Thus the association between clinical complaints and concurrent "pathological" radiological findings must be considered cautiously. This association also appears to apply to the predictive ability of imaging. Savage et al.[188] reported that 32% of asymptomatic subjects had had "abnormal" lumbar spines (i.e., evidence of disc degeneration, disc bulging or protrusion, facet hypertrophy, or nerve root compression). To obfuscate matters, an abnormality was identified in only 47% of subjects experiencing LBP.[188] When the subjects without LBP but with abnormal findings on imaging were followed for 12 months, 13 experienced LBP for the first time; however, no changes occurred in the MRI appearance of their lumbar spines that these authors could identify as accounting for the onset of LBP.[188] Pain, therefore, developed in the absence of any associated change in the radiographic appearance of the spine.

In contrast, Elfering[189] reported that, over the course of 5 years, identified disc herniations progressed to degenerative disc disease although the patients remained asymptomatic, indicating that pathology progressed in the absence of any associated pain response. Boos et al.[190] followed asymptomatic patients with a disc herniation for 5 years and determined that physical job characteristics and psychological aspects of work were more powerful than MRI-identified disc abnormalities in predicting the need for medical consultation related to LBP.

Multiple potential pathoanatomical pain generators have been identified in the lumbar spine by diagnostic imaging. The reality, however, is that the ability of the clinician to identify specific anatomical lesions causing the pain is limited, even with the best available imaging studies. In fact, it has been estimated that the specific anatomical lesion causing LBP is unidentifiable 80% to 85% of the time.[191] However, the utility of imaging of the lumbar spine increases when the clinician is suspicious of a serious pathology or nerve root compression. For example, radiography is indicated when the clinician suspects a compression fracture or neoplasm. Likewise, ultrasound of the abdomen is the currently accepted gold standard for identification of abdominal aneurysm.[192] Imaging studies may also be appropriate if the patient fails to improve with conservative therapy or shows progression of neurological involvement. These assertions of focused imaging in the diagnostic process of LBP are supported by a longitudinal study that found limited accuracy of "common" MRI findings (i.e., disc desiccation, bulges, loss of height), but improved accuracy when less common MRI findings (i.e., central stenosis and nerve root compression) were considered.[193]

Differential Diagnosis and Classification of Low Back Pain Subgroups

Figure 9-6 summarizes the specific differential diagnosis and classification process presented in this chapter. The

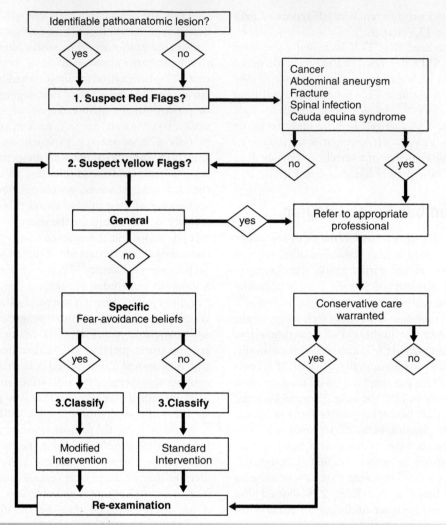

Figure 9-6
Overview of the differential diagnosis and classification process for low back pain.

primary task of the clinician is to identify red flags that may indicate a serious pathology, mimicking the symptoms of LBP, that should be referred to a specialist. Red flag identification is accomplished through the patient history or appropriate laboratory studies. Once systemic pathology has been eliminated as a potential source of LBP, the secondary task is to identify yellow flags that are predictive of the development of chronic LBP. Once factors that affect the prognosis have been identified, the tertiary task is to recognize the subgroup classification associated with the optimum treatment outcome.

Identification of Red Flags

The clinician must first determine whether the LBP symptoms arise from a serious pathology of another source (see Figure 9-5). This procedure should take little time for most

patients, and a high number of "positive" findings is not expected. However, the clinician must remain diligent in performing this part of the diagnostic process, because the consequences of failing to identify serious pathology are potentially severe for the patient.

Deyo et al.[194] have suggested a set of historical questions that can be used in screening for serious pathology in patients with LBP. These cover topics such as a history of cancer, unexplained weight loss, failure of rest to relieve pain, and a history of fevers or chills, intravenous drug use, and/or recent urinary tract infection.[194] Additional screening questions should be specific for urinary retention and saddle anesthesia, osteoporosis, and/or history of compression fracture.[194] If necessary, a review of pertinent medical history in first-order relatives may give insight into possible spondyloarthropathies if these are suspected in a particular patient.

Red Flags for Low Back Pain

- Abdominal aortic aneurysm
- Kidney disease
- Liver disease
- Duodenal ulcers
- Pancreatitis
- Endometriosis
- Cancer
- Cauda equina syndrome
- Spondyloarthropathies
- Fractures
- Infection

Abdominal Aortic Aneurysm

An abdominal aortic aneurysm (AAA) is a pathological dilation of the abdominal aorta below the renal arteries to a diameter greater than 3 cm (1.2 inches). Abdominal aortic aneurysms are found in 4% to 8% of older men and 0.5% to 1.5% of older women.[195-198] Fielding et al.[199] reported

that the most common symptoms reported by patients on the first presentation with AAA are abdominal pain and backache. Age, smoking, gender, and family history are the most significant risk factors for AAA. In fact, Laderle et al.[196] indicated that the greater prevalence associated with smoking (100 cigarettes lifetime) accounted for 75% of all abdominal aortic aneurysms 4 cm (1.6 inches) in diameter or larger. Table 9-5 lists the odds ratios associated with these individual risk factors for AAA.

Fielding et al.[199] found that the diagnosis could be made by careful routine palpation. The clinician should perform deep, careful palpation to the left of the midline, keeping the hands steady in one position until the aortic pulse is felt and then carefully evaluating the lateral extent of the pulse with the pads of the fingers.[200] Physical findings may include a tender, palpable, pulsatile abdominal mass.[199] However, the reported sensitivity and specificity of palpation varies dramatically.[201] For example, detection of AAA by palpation improves in thinner patients[200] and when recognizable risk factors are present.[192,200]

Despite the support for palpation, abdominal ultrasound remains the gold standard for identification of AAA.[192]

Table 9-5
Red Flag Pathology and Associated Likelihood and Odds Ratios Indicative of Serious Disease

Condition	Findings	LR	OR (95% CI)
Cancer[161]	Previous history of cancer	14.7	
	Age over 50	2.7	
	Failure to respond to conservative intervention	3.0	
	ESR ≥ 20 mm/hr	2.4	
	ESR ≥ 50 mm/hr	19.2	
	ESR ≥ 100 mm/hr	55.5	
Aneurysm (≥4 cm [1.6 inches])[195]	Smoking (100 cigarettes lifetime)		5.07 (4.13-6.21)
	Female		0.18 (0.07-0.48)
	Non-Caucasian		1.02 (0.77-1.35)
	Age		1.71 (1.61-1.82)
	Family history		1.94 (1.63-2.32)
Aneurysm[199]	Positive palpation examination: Abdominal girth ≤100 cm (39.4 inches) Each 1 cm (0.5 inch) increase in AAA diameter	3.2	1.95 (1.06-3.58)
Compression fracture[161]	Age ≥50	2.2	
	Age ≥70	5.5	
	Corticosteroid use	12.0	
Spinal infection[161,212,228]	Fever: tuberculous osteomyelitis	13.5	
	Fever: pyogenic osteomyelitis	25.0	
	Fever: spinal epidural abscess	41.5	
General red flag history[229]	Sleep problems (wakes from sleep, uses medication, cannot sleep)	3.8	
	Unable to urinate	3.0	
	Unable to hold urine	1.4	
	Current smoker	3.3	

LR, Likelihood ratio; OR, odds ratio; CI, confidence interval; ESR, erythrocyte sedimentation rate; AAA, abdominal aortic aneurysm.

Specifically, the clinician should consider the possibility of rupture of an abdominal aortic aneurysm in a male patient over age 60 who smokes and who presents with sudden onset back and/or loin pain.[202]

Back pain is a common historical complaint in a variety of conditions affecting the kidney. Low back pain (71.3%) was the most common discomfort reported by patients with polycystic kidney disease (PKD) during the course of the disease, and abdominal pain was the second most common. These complaints were recorded by 42% of patients before diagnosis of PKD.[203] Also, in a study by Bajwa et al.,[203] 26% of patients with PKD reported back pain radiating to the hips or legs. Central back and flank pain has been described by patients in renal failure[204] and with a viral infection.[205]

Massive liver cysts may also cause low back pain through the effect of changes in posture as the cysts grow, enlarging the abdomen.[203] Duodenal ulcers[206] may refer pain into the upper lumbar spine, and abdominal pain and low back pain are the primary historical complaints of patients with pancreatitis[207] and endometriosis.[208]

Cancer

Although spinal cord compression is a complication of malignancy that affects the quality of life of an estimated 12,700 new patients each year,[209] the prevalence of cancer related to back pain is likely to be low in primary care settings. Deyo and Diehl[161] reported a prevalence of cancer-related back pain in primary care patients of 0.66%. This is similar to the prevalence reported for academic multidisciplinary spine centers (0.69%) and higher than the prevalence noted in private practice multidisciplinary spine centers (0.12%).[210] Deyo and Diehl[161] have presented several historical and laboratory findings associated with cancer-related back pain. These authors outlined a strategy in which key historical findings (i.e., age over 50, previous history of cancer, unexplained weight loss, and failure to respond to conservative intervention) are supported by key laboratory tests (erythrocyte sedimentation rate [ESR]).[161] Subsequent investigation has supported the key historical findings of night pain, aching character of symptom manifestation, and unexplained weight loss originally reported.[210] Cancers of the skin may also be implicated in local tenderness over the tissues of the lumbar spine. Ogboli et al.[211] found that six different types of common skin tumors may present as areas reported as tender by the patient when palpated.

The positive likelihood ratios for cancer screening using selected historical and laboratory findings are presented in Table 9-5. It has been suggested that prompt spinal imaging may be indicated for patients with two or more historical findings and an ESR of 20 mm/hr or higher.[161] It should also be noted that Hollingworth et al.[212] indicated that the benefits of using MRI for screening, rather than x-ray films, did not justify the increased costs of doing so.

Cauda Equina Syndrome

Compression of the cauda equina of any cause (e.g., trauma, central disc protrusion, hemorrhage, or tumor) requires immediate surgical referral.[194] Fortunately, the incidence and prevalence of this condition are very low. Johnsson et al.[213] reported the population incidence of the syndrome to be 0.03% in Denmark and 0.005% in Sweden.[214,215]

The most consistent findings in cauda equina syndrome are urinary retention and sensory changes on the buttocks, thighs, and peritoneum (i.e., saddle anesthesia).[216] Loss of anal sphincter tone occurs in 60% to 80% of cases.[217] Urinary retention is also common in simple nerve root compression syndromes with no relation to true cauda equina syndrome.[217]

Spondyloarthropathies

Spondyloarthropathies are related inflammatory spinal arthropathies characterized by sacroiliac involvement and a relationship to HLA-B27 but distinct from rheumatoid arthritis. This group of conditions includes ankylosing spondylitis, reactive arthritis (including Reiter's syndrome), psoriatic arthritis, arthritis associated with bowel disease (enteropathic arthritis), juvenile spondyloarthropathy, and a set of unspecified spondyloarthropathies. The diagnostic criteria recommended by the European Spondyloarthropathy Study Group are listed in Box 9-1.[218]

Ankylosis spondylitis (AS) is considered the most common of the spondyloarthropathies. Connective tissue changes occur as subchondral tissue thickens and eventually is replaced by fibrocartilage and, finally, bone. AS affects men more than women, beginning with complaints of back pain and stiffness in early adulthood. The final diagnosis often is not made until the patient is older because the earlier symptoms are minimal. Neck pain and stiffness are associated with advanced disease. Historical findings include reports of insidious onset back pain that is worse with inactivity and improves with exercise. These complaints are not particularly specific; however, association with a family history of spondyloarthropathy, acute anterior uveitis (iritis), and impaired trunk mobility or chest expansion strengthens the clinical picture. Clinical diagnosis is further supported by radiographic evidence of sacroiliitis, which is considered the hallmark of AS. MRI can be helpful in detecting early change in the spine, but the increased cost may limit its routine use.

Reactive arthritis is an episode of aseptic, acute, asymmetrical peripheral arthritis that occurs within 1 month of a primary infection elsewhere in the body. It frequently is associated with one or more extra-articular features, including conjunctivitis or acute iritis, enthesitis at the Achilles tendon or plantar fascia, mucocutaneous lesions, urethritis, and carditis.[219] The combination of arthritis, conjunctivitis, and urethritis has been labeled Reiter's syndrome, but most patients with reactive arthritis do not present with this triad.[219]

Box 9-1 European Spondyloarthropathy Study Group Criteria

Criterion: Inflammatory spinal pain with at least four of the following components:

- At least 3 months in duration
- Onset before 45 years of age
- Insidious (gradual) onset
- Improved by exercise
- Associated with morning spinal stiffness

or

Synovitis (past or present asymmetrical arthritis or arthritis predominately in the lower limbs) *plus* at least one of the following:

- Family history (first- or second-degree relative with ankylosing spondylitis, psoriasis, or acute iritis)
- Reactive arthritis or inflammatory bowel disease
- Psoriasis
- Ulcerative colitis or Crohn's disease
- Pain alternating between the buttocks
- Spontaneous pain or tenderness on examination of the site of the insertion of the Achilles tendon or plantar fascia (enthesitis)
- Episode of diarrhea that occurs within 1 month before the onset of arthritis
- Nongonococcal urethritis or cervicitis that occurs within 1 month before the onset of arthritis
- Bilateral grades 2-4 sacroiliitis, or unilateral grade 3 or grade 4 sacroiliitis

Data from Dougados M, van der LS, Juhlin R et al: The European Spondylarthropathy Study Group preliminary criteria for the classification of spondylarthropathy, *Arthritis Rheum* 34:1218-1227, 1991.

Psoriasis is a common skin disease in Caucasian adults (1% to 3% prevalence)[220,221] that affects men and women equally. The disease is less common in other ethnic groups, such as Native Americans (0.3%).[221] Some 10%[221] to 30%[222,223] of patients with psoriasis have associated inflammatory arthritis. Skin lesions usually appear before the arthritis in about 50% of patients with psoriatic arthritis. The arthritis usually begins at age 30 to 50, but it can also begin in childhood. When searching for psoriasis, the examiner should not limit the skin check to the extremities but should also include the scalp, ears, umbilicus, pelvic area, perineum, natal cleft, palms, soles, and nails. Nail involvement often is a useful clue in the diagnosis of psoriatic arthritis.[220] Gladman[224] suggested that psoriatic arthritis may be distinguished from the other spondyloarthropathies by the presence of asymmetrical, peripheral arthritis, asymmetrical spinal involvement, and a lower level of pain.

Enteropathic arthritis is a term for inflammatory arthritic conditions associated with bowel disorders such as Crohn's disease and ulcerative colitis. De Vlam et al.[225] reported that 39% of consecutive patients with ulcerative colitis or Crohn's disease had enteropathic arthritis, and 90% met the criteria for spondyloarthropathy. Peripheral arthritis tends to be more frequent in enteropathic arthritis than in AS.[225]

Fractures

Compression fractures usually occur in osteoporotic bone, most frequently at T8, T12, L1, and L5.[226] Historical findings that increase the probability of a compression fracture are presented in Table 9-5. The patient often is older and does not have a history of specific spinal trauma but may have other clinical features of osteoporosis, such as kyphosis or a previous history of wrist or hip fractures.[226] The patient often reports pain after a seemingly simple maneuver, such as coughing or opening a window. Some compression fractures occur spontaneously while the patient is lying in bed.[226] Deyo et al.[194] recommended that a patient on long-term corticosteroid therapy who complains of spinal pain should be considered to have a fracture until proven otherwise, because this historical finding greatly affects the probability of a compression fracture (see Table 9-5).

Spinal Infections

Fever of unknown origin is defined as a temperature higher than 38.3 °C (101 °F).[227] Urinary tract infections, indwelling urinary catheters, skin infections, and injection sites for intravenous drugs have been identified as potential sites from which a spinal infection develops in about 40% of patients with osteomyelitis.[228] Fewer than 2% of patients with back pain at a primary care clinic presented with fever,[161] indicating that very few false positives are seen when associating fever with infection in patients with LBP (see Table 9-5).

Red Flag Summary

Roach et al.[229] collected demographic and clinical information from 174 patients with LBP to examine the sensitivity and specificity of historical questions to identify patients with serious pathology in the lumbar spine. These authors classified serious pathology to include osteoporotic fracture, tumor, infection, and surgical management of spinal stenosis or disc herniation. The historical questions with the best positive likelihood ratios were related to the inability to urinate or to hold urine, sleep disturbances, and current smoking history (see Table 9-5).[229] It should be noted that although these questions had very high specificity (high true negative), they also had a very low true positive rate. The implication of this relationship is that many of the patients with serious pathology (as defined by Roach et al.[229]) did not answer "yes" to the historical questions.

Identification of Yellow Flags

After red flags have been considered, the clinician may decide that referral to another specialist is necessary before conservative rehabilitation is deemed appropriate. This outcome must always be considered, but it is not a frequent outcome for most practice areas. More often, the clinician proceeds to screen for yellow flags, the second step of the differential diagnosis and classification approach (see Figure 9-6).

Yellow Flags for Low Back Pain

- Depression
- Fear-avoidance beliefs
- Pain catastrophizing

In general terms, the identification of yellow flags allows the clinician to determine the potential for a psychological influence on a patient's clinical presentation of LBP. The rationale for considering yellow flags in the differential diagnosis and classification of LBP is summarized in the *New Zealand Acute Low Back Pain Guide*.[230] "The goal of identifying yellow flags is to find factors that can be influenced positively to facilitate recovery and prevent or reduce long-term disability and work loss. This includes identifying both the frequent unintentional learning or emotional barriers and the less common intentional barriers to improvement."

A variety of yellow flag screening methods have been reported in the literature. In our clinical experience, a common way to screen for yellow flags is through assessment of nonorganic signs. Waddell et al.[231,232] first described the signs believed to be associated with aspects of distress and abnormal illness behavior that could lead to increased amounts of disability. The specific nonorganic signs assessed during the physical examination have been thoroughly described in other sources and are not reviewed here.[231-233] The presence of nonorganic signs does not have any obvious medicolegal implications, and these signs are not diagnostic of lack of sincere effort or psychopathology.[234] Nonorganic signs are simply a way to investigate the potential for psychological influence during the physical examination.

Nonorganic signs have been investigated in prospective studies predicting return to work status. Several studies have demonstrated that the presence of nonorganic signs was predictive of a delayed return to work,[235-238] whereas other studies have reported that nonorganic signs were not predictive of return to work.[239,240] Several explanations are possible for these conflicting reports. For example, nonorganic signs may have been investigated in patients with a wide range of acuity, including those who already had chronic LBP. Also, the studies used different definitions of what constituted a positive nonorganic sign and different definitions for determining return to work status.

Fritz et al.[241] investigated nonorganic signs as a screening tool for predicting return to work at 4 weeks in a homogenous cohort of patients with acute, work-related low back pain. Cutoff values were calculated for the number of nonorganic signs that minimized false negative findings. The best cutoff value was two or more signs (negative likelihood ratio [−LR], 0.75; 95% CI, 0.51-1.1).[241] However, even this optimum cutoff value was not sufficient for accurate screening in clinical settings because of the associated high false positive rates. Fritz et al.[241] presented strong evidence from other studies indicating that high false positive rates are a consistent problem with nonorganic signs (Table 9-6). For example, even under the best condition reported in the literature (−LR, 0.48), the post-test probably only decreases from 50% to 32% for predicting inability to return to work based on two or fewer nonorganic signs. Collectively, this evidence suggests that clinicians should consider methods other than nonorganic signs when screening for yellow flags.

Other yellow flag screening methods focus on identifying specific psychological factors involved in the maintenance and development of chronic LBP. A comprehensive

Table 9-6
Lack of Evidence for Use of Nonorganic Signs to Screen for Return to Work

Author	Sample Description	Nonorganic Signs for Positive Finding	Outcome Determination	Negative LR
Bradish et al.[239]	Work-related LBP	Three or more	Return to at least part-time work	0.60
Werneke et al.[240]	Nonworking or partly disabled patients with LBP	One or more	Return to work or improved work status	0.59
Kummel[236]	Work-related LBP	Three or more	Return to at least part-time work	0.48
Karas et al.[235]	Work-related LBP	Three or more	Return to at least part-time work	0.77
Fritz et al.[241]	Work-related LBP	Two or more	Return to full-time work	0.75

LR, Likelihood ratio; *LBP,* low back pain.
Data from Fritz JM, Wainner RS, Hicks GE: The use of nonorganic signs and symptoms as a screening tool for return-to-work in patients with acute low back pain, *Spine* 25:1925-1931, 2000.

review of such psychological factors is beyond the scope of this chapter; interested readers are referred to reviews by Pincus et al.[242,243] Typically, self-report questionnaires are used to screen for psychological factors. Some questionnaires reported in the peer-reviewed literature considered a variety of psychological factors,[244,245] but in the approach presented here, the clinician screens for psychological influences involved with LBP that are general (depression) or specific (fear-avoidance beliefs, pain catastrophizing) in nature.

Depression

Depression is a commonly experienced illness or mood state with a wide variety of symptoms, ranging from loss of appetite to suicidal thoughts.[246] Depression is common in the general population, but it appears to be more commonly experienced in conjunction with chronic low back pain (CLBP).[247-249] A recent Canadian population-based study estimated the general rate of major depression to be 5.9% for pain-free individuals and 19.8% for individuals with CLBP.[247] Depression is associated with increased pain intensity, disability, medication use, and unemployment for patients with LBP.[250] Based on this epidemiological information, the authors feel that routine screening for depression should be part of the clinical diagnosis of LBP.

Despite this evidence of its deleterious influence on LBP, depression does not appear to be adequately screened for in practices that commonly examine patients with LBP. For example, depressive symptoms were not identified in 35% to 75% of patients seeking treatment from primary care physicians;[246,251] 63% of spine surgeons indicated that they only occasionally or never screened for depression using psychological tests;[252] and surveys of physical therapy practices do not mention psychological screening as part of the normal practice patterns.[253-255]

Effective screening for depression involves more than just generating a clinical impression that the patient is depressed. Separate studies involving spine surgeons[252] and physical therapists[249] have demonstrated that clinical impressions are not sensitive enough to detect depression in patients with LBP. A more effective approach is to use self-report questionnaires (e.g., Beck's Depression Inventory or the Depression Anxiety Stress Scales). However, these questionnaires often have more than 20 items, which may put a burden on the patient and clinician.

Evidence suggests that using two specific questions from the Primary Care Evaluation of Mental Disorders patient questionnaire can effectively screen for depression in primary care settings.[256] The questions are (1) "During the past month, have you often been bothered by feeling down, depressed, or hopeless?" and (2) "During the past month, have you often been bothered by little interest or pleasure in doing things?" The patient responds to the questions with "yes" or "no," and the number of yes items are totaled, giving a potential range of 0-2. A recent study involving LBP suggested that these two questions also accurately identified depression in patients seeking physical therapy treatment for LBP (Table 9-7).[249] The resultant dialogue between mental health and spine clinicians should determine whether depressed patients should be treated concurrently. In our opinion, examples of **inappropriate treatment** of a depressed patient by a spine clinician include (1) a patient in whom low back symptoms represent only somatic complaints, without associated physical impairment, and (2) a patient whose depressive symptoms are severe or extreme and include suicidal thoughts.

Fear-Avoidance Beliefs

Fear-avoidance beliefs are a measure of patients' beliefs and attitudes toward LBP.[257] Specifically, fear-avoidance beliefs are a composite measure of the patient's fear related to LBP, how physical activity and work affect LBP, and how LBP should be managed.[257-259] Theoretically, patients with elevated fear-avoidance beliefs are more likely to use

Table 9-7

Accuracy of Screening for Depression Using Two Questions from the Primary Care Evaluation of Mental Disorders Patient Questionnaire

	Mild Depression	Moderate Depression	Severe Depression	Extreme Depression
One Question Result				
Positive LR	3.40 (2.40, 4.82)	2.76 (2.10, 3.62)	2.44 (1.91, 3.12)	2.25 (1.71, 2.96)
Negative LR	0.37 (0.26, 0.51)	0.29 (0.18, 0.49)	0.25 (0.11, 0.55)	0.23 (0.06, 0.84)
Two Questions Result				
Positive LR	5.40 (3.10, 9.42)	4.61 (3.0, 7.0)	4.32 (3.0, 6.1)	3.89 (2.80, 5.40)
Negative LR	0.55 (0.44, 0.67)	0.43 (0.30, 0.60)	0.28 (0.14, 0.53)	0.18 (0.05, 0.66)

LR, Likelihood ratio.
Modified from Haggman S, Maher CG, Refshauge KM: Screening for symptoms of depression by physical therapists managing low back pain, *Phys Ther* 84:1157-1166, 2004; and Whooley MA, Avins AL, Miranda J, Browner WS: Case-finding instruments for depression: two questions are as good as many, *J Gen Intern Med* 12:439-445, 1997.

an avoidance response to their LBP, resulting in the development of an exaggerated pain perception and chronic disability.[257] Prospective studies have supported the validity of fear-avoidance beliefs, because they are predictive of the development of chronic LBP.[260-263]

As a result of this evidence, identification of elevated fear-avoidance beliefs has been suggested as an important component in the diagnosis of LBP. The Fear-Avoidance Beliefs Questionnaire (FABQ) is commonly used to assess fear-avoidance beliefs in patients with LBP.[259] The FABQ has 16 items, which are scored on a scale ranging from 0 (strongly disagree) to 6 (strongly agree). The individual items are then summed to generate an estimate of fear-avoidance beliefs; higher numbers on the FABQ indicate increased levels of fear-avoidance beliefs. The FABQ has two subscales: a seven-item (items 6, 7, 9-12, and 15) work subscale (FABQ-W; score range, 0-42) for fear-avoidance beliefs about work, and a four-item (items 2-5) physical activity subscale (FABQ-PA; score range, 0-24) for fear-avoidance beliefs about physical activity. Several studies indicate that the FABQ is a reliable, valid, and/or responsive measure[259,264-266] that is appropriate for use in clinical settings.

Evidence suggests that the FABQ-W can be used to screen effectively in occupational LBP. A study of patients with acute, work-related LBP who were evaluated for demographic, physical, and psychosocial factors found that the FABQ-W was the strongest predictor for return to work at 4 weeks.[260] Patients who scored higher than 34 on the FABQ-W were less likely to return to work by 4 weeks (positive likelihood ratio [+LR], 3.33; 95% CI, 1.65-6.77). In contrast, patients who scored lower than 29 on the FABQ-W were less likely to return to work (−LR, 0.08; 95% CI, 0.01-0.54).

Unfortunately, similar cutoff scores have not been reported for the FABQ-PA, making screening for fear-avoidance beliefs in nonoccupational settings difficult. It has been suggested that a score higher than 15 indicates an elevated FABQ-PA,[259,261-267] but likelihood ratios have not been reported in the peer-reviewed literature; therefore, clinicians do not know by how much an FABQ-PA score higher than 15 alters post-test probabilities. The authors' own unpublished data suggest that the FABQ-W is also an effective screening tool for general orthopedic populations when a cutoff score of 33 is used (+LR, 3.7). The authors' own unpublished data also suggest that the FABQ-PA can be used to screen general orthopedic populations, but the cutoff score of 19 (+LR, 1.7) is not as accurate as the corresponding FABQ-W cutoff score.

Pain Catastrophizing

Pain catastrophizing is a negative cognition related to the belief that the experienced pain will inevitably result in the worst possible outcome.[268] Pain catastrophizing is believed to be a multidimensional construct comprised of rumination, helplessness, and pessimism.[268] A practical example might help to illustrate the concept of pain catastrophizing. A patient with elevated pain catastrophizing would expect to have severe pain for the rest of his life, even if his LBP was mild and was being treated appropriately.

Pain catastrophizing has also been linked to the development and maintenance of chronic pain. Most of the literature documenting the unique influence of pain catastrophizing on chronic pain is cross sectional,[269-272] but some prospective studies provide supporting evidence. For example, frequent pain catastrophizing during acute LBP was predictive of self-reported disability 6 months[273] and 1 year later,[274] even after select historical and clinical predictors were considered.

Pain catastrophizing can be measured by the Pain Catastrophizing Scale (PCS), a 13-item scale that assesses the degree of catastrophic cognitions a patient experiences while in pain.[275] The scale ranges from 1 (not at all) to 4 (always), and an example of an item is, "I worry all the time about whether the pain will end." Psychometric studies suggest acceptable levels of reliability and validity.[270,275] Factor analysis suggests a hierarchical factor structure, with three individual subscales of the PCS (rumination, magnification, and pessimism) contributing to an overall factor of pain catastrophizing.[270,275] In clinical settings, the PCS is commonly reported as a whole number by summing all 13 items (range, 0 to 52).

No cutoffs have been reported in the peer-reviewed literature for use of the PCS to predict the clinical outcome of LBP. However, normative data on the PCS are available through a Canadian pain disability prevention Web site (http://pdp-pgap.com/en/pdp/index.html). According to the Web site, the median PCS score is 20, and the 75th percentile score is 31. This pain disability program suggests that a score exceeding the 75th percentile indicates a patient at risk for having chronic disability from musculoskeletal pain, although the degree of risk cannot be quantified with this data.

Yellow Flag Summary

The consideration of yellow flags is an important part of the diagnostic process of low back pain because it alerts the clinician to patients who may be appropriate for referral because of depression or who have an increased risk of experiencing chronic disability. For example, early identification of elevated fear-avoidance beliefs allows identification of patients with a poor prognosis, as well as appropriate treatment modifications. Specific education and exercise philosophies have been proposed to address elevated fear-avoidance beliefs.[258] A detailed discussion of these philosophies is beyond the scope of this chapter; however, they have been described in the literature,[276] and results from randomized trials have demonstrated their efficacy in reducing fear-avoidance beliefs.[267,277]

Identification of Low Back Pain Subgroups

At this point in the process, the clinician has already considered systemic causes (red flags) and psychological influences (yellow flags) in LBP. The third task is to assign the patient to the most appropriate LBP subgroup (i.e., the one that maximizes the probability of a favorable outcome) (see Figure 9-6). In this section, the authors describe a focused, evidence-based clinical examination to confirm the appropriate subgroup classification.

This approach represents a philosophical shift from determining a specific anatomical diagnosis, which was favored by spine care clinicians in the past. The authors feel that the best available evidence supports a classification approach that de-emphasizes the importance of identifying specific anatomical lesions. To support this opinion, the authors cite (1) the previously outlined concerns related to the plethora of lumbar spine pain generators and the dilemma of imaging lumbar anatomy and (2) recent reports in the literature that suggest that interventions based on nonanatomical subgroup classification are an effective strategy for the management of LBP.[278-283]

A variety of LBP classifications are described in the literature. An individual review of each classification system is beyond the scope of this chapter. Readers interested in more detailed information are referred to a critical review by Riddle.[284] This review included LBP classification systems that were previously described in the literature, widely taught in continuing education seminars, and commonly used in clinical practice; it also used terms familiar to rehabilitation professionals. Table 9-8 presents the four classification systems that met these criteria and were included in the review.[284]

The reported evidence to support these four classification systems varies in quality. Available peer-reviewed reports of the systems' reliability, discriminant validity, predictive validity, and prescriptive validity is used to briefly summarize the evidence supporting each system. To ensure the quality of the evidence presented, information on prescriptive validity is limited to randomized trials. The Bernard and Kirkaldy-Willis classification[285] was not included in this summary because the authors of this chapter found no reports in the peer-reviewed literature regarding its reliability and/or validity.

No reliability reports were available for the Quebec Task Force on Spinal Disorder (QTFSD) system, but its discriminant and predictive validity have been reported in the peer-reviewed literature.[286-288] QTFSD classification has been associated with baseline symptom severity for patients with spinal stenosis[286] and baseline symptom severity and functional status for patients with work-related LBP.[287,288] The QTFSD has demonstrated its predictive validity for patients with sciatica by determining whether surgical treatment was more likely to be an eventual outcome and being associated with improvement in functional status after

1 year of nonsurgical treatment.[286] In patients with work-related LBP, subjects with higher QTFSD classifications were more likely to have lower functional status and more pain and to not to return to work at 1 year.[287] Specifically, baseline QTSFD classification associated with symptom radiation increased the likelihood of lower functional status (OR, 5.72; 95% CI, 1.18-36.01) and higher pain scores (OR, 7.84; 95% CI, 2.25-32.07) at 1 year.[287] The prescriptive validity of the QTFSD has not been reported in the literature, because it is not meant to be a treatment-driven classification approach.

The reliability of the Delitto et al.[289] treatment-based classification (DTBC) has been investigated in two studies, one reporting moderate reliability ($\kappa = 0.56$)[6] and another reporting low reliability ($\kappa = 0.14$-0.41).[290] The discriminant, predictive, and prescriptive validity of the DTBC has also been reported in the peer-reviewed literature.[278,280,291-293] Baseline differences in age, history of LBP, and presence of leg pain for specific DTBC groups were observed in 120 consecutive patients seeking outpatient physical therapy.[291] Another study suggested that DTBC groups differed on clusters of clinical examination factors.[293] For example, one DTBC classification (stabilization) was more likely to have patients with low pain intensity, a previous history of LBP, and longer duration of LBP, whereas another DTBC classification (specific exercise) was more likely to have patients with higher pain intensity and lower amounts of lumbar flexion.[293] The DTBC has demonstrated its predictive validity for patients with acute LBP; 4-week outcomes for patients differed among two of the three most common classifications.[291] Furthermore, the DTBC has also demonstrated its prescriptive validity in several randomized trials. Specifically, DTBC-guided physical therapy intervention was found to be more effective than generic exercise prescription in short-term follow-up[278,279] and guideline-based intervention[280] or assigned physical therapy intervention[292] in short- and long-term follow-up. No studies have been done to investigate the validity of DTBC for patients with chronic LBP.

The reliability of the McKenzie treatment-based classification (MTBC) has been investigated in several studies, with high ($\kappa = 0.7$-1),[294,295] moderate ($\kappa = 0.4$-0.6),[294,295] and low ($\kappa < 0.4$)[294-296] reliability reported in the literature. The authors could not find any studies that specifically addressed the discriminant or predictive validity of the MTBC, but numerous reports had investigated its prescriptive validity. For patients with acute LBP, the MTBC was more effective than a back school program in the short term but equally effective in the long term.[297,298] The MTBC was also equally as effective as chiropractic manipulation or an educational pamphlet for short- and long-term follow-up times.[299] For patients with chronic LBP, the MTBC was compared to a flexion exercise protocol, and no significant difference was found between the two groups in short-term follow-up.[300] The MTBC was also compared to a comprehensive lumbar-pelvic strength training program; it was more

Table 9-8
Four Common Classification Systems Reviewed in Critical Appraisal

	Bernard and Kirkaldy-Willis[285]	Delitto and Colleagues[289]	McKenzie[294,295,301,311]	Quebec Task Force[286,288]
Professional or discipline orientation of system developer	Orthopedic surgery	Physical therapy	Physical therapy	Many medical and nonmedical disciplines
Type	Status index	Clinical guideline index	Clinical guideline index	Mixed index
Method of development*	Judgment approach	Judgment approach	Judgment approach	Judgment approach
Purpose	To determine the pathology causing the problem	To determine the appropriate treatment	To determine the appropriate treatment	For clinical decision making, establishing a prognosis, quality control, and research
Setting	Not specified	Not specified	Not specified	Occupational health
Domain of interest	All patients with LBP	All patients with LBP	Most patients with LBP	All patients with LBP
Patients excluded	None	None	Patients with severe sciatica and neurological deficits and those whose symptoms cannot be reduced or centralized	None
Categories	23 categories: *Group A* Herniated nucleus pulposus Lateral stenosis Central stenosis Spondylolisthesis Segmental instability *Group B* Sacroiliac joint syndrome Posterior joint syndrome Maigne syndrome Muscle syndromes (6) *Group C* Chronic pain syndrome Pseudarthrosis Nonspecific Postfusion stenosis Ankylosing spondylitis Infection Tumor Arachnoiditis Lateral femoral nerve entrapment	Three levels of classification (not all categories have been described): *Stage 1:* Extension Flexion Lateral shift (2) Immobilization (4) Traction (5) Mobilization (5)	13 categories: Postural syndrome Four dysfunction syndromes (flexion, extension, side-gliding, adherent nerve root) Seven derangement syndromes Hip joint or sacroiliac joint problem	11 categories with two axes: Pain without radiation Pain with radiation proximal Pain with radiation distal Pain with radiation with neurological signs (<7, 7-49, >49 days) (working, idle) Presumptive root compression + image Spinal stenosis Postsurgical < 6 months Postsurgical > 6 months Chronic pain syndrome Other (working or idle)

LBP, Low back pain.
From Riddle DL: Classification and low back pain: a review of the literature and critical analysis of selected systems, *Phys Ther* 78:708-737, 1998.
*A statistical approach to developing a classification system relies primarily on statistical procedures to guide decisions about how to group patients. A judgment approach relies primarily on the clinical experience of the developer or on commonly accepted clinical knowledge to assign patients to groups.

effective at the short-term follow-up but not at the long term.[301] In a study that involved patients with acute and chronic LBP, MTBC-recommended intervention was more effective than recommendations that countered the MTBC for short-term follow-up.[282]

As this summary indicates, no consensus exists for any one particular classification approach in the management of patients with LBP. The chapter authors, therefore, consider a synthesis of these classification approaches by highlighting particular subgroups of LBP that have high levels of evidence supporting their identification. The classification subgroups discussed in this chapter are for manipulation, stabilization, centralization phenomenon, lumbar spinal stenosis, neural tension, and adverse mechanical tension.

Classification of Specific Low Back Pain Subgroups

- Manipulation group
- Stabilization group
- Centralization phenomenon group
- Lumbar spinal stenosis group
- Neurodynamic tension group

Manipulation Classification

Spinal manipulation is a common treatment for LBP. Historically, diagnosis or classification of a patient appropriate for manipulation was determined from two potential sources. The first source was opinion and/or authority, based primarily on clinical experience that had not been substantiated in the peer-reviewed literature. The second was the detection of lumbar asymmetries and limitations through static and dynamic clinical tests that involved the pelvis and/or lumbar spine. The use of these tests was primarily based on biomechanical theories or studies. Unfortunately, neither of these approaches truly encompass an evidence-based approach.[302] The problem with the first source is not that it relies on expert opinion, but rather that the opinion has not been appropriately tested through well-designed studies. The problem with the second approach is that many clinical tests commonly used to classify patients with LBP lack the reliability[303-305] or validity[306-308] required for effective clinical use.

Recent research has identified a clinical prediction rule that accurately identifies characteristics of patients who should be classified for manipulative treatment when a specific technique is used.[283,306] This prediction rule started with a study that considered a wide range of examination procedures and found five that accurately predicted patients experiencing at least a 50% improvement in disability at 1 week.[306] Then, a clinical prediction rule (defined as at least four out of five positive examination findings) was developed.[306] This rule was then tested and validated in a

Table 9-9
Validated Clinical Prediction Rule* for Manipulation Classification[2,283]

Examination Finding	Positive Definition
Duration of current low back pain episode	Less than 16 days
Presence of leg pain	Symptoms proximal to knee
Fear-avoidance beliefs questionnaire (work scale)	Less than 19/42
Lumbar spine mobility testing (prone)	One or more hypomobile segments
Hip internal rotation	At least one hip with internal rotation greater than 35°

*At least 4/5 positive examination findings constitute a positive clinical prediction rule (+LR = 13.2) and fewer than 3/5 positive examination findings constitute a negative clinical prediction rule (−LR = 0.10).
LR, Likelihood ratio.

separate clinical trial (Table 9-9).[284] Patients receiving manipulation who were positive on the clinical prediction rule fared significantly better (+LR, 13.2; 95% CI, 3.4-52.1) than those receiving exercise; this provided strong evidence that the clinical prediction rule was a valid way to classify patients.[283] Further evidence supporting the validity of this clinical prediction rule is found in a study that supported the validity of a negative clinical prediction rule (defined as less than three positive examination findings). The negative clinical prediction rule was also significantly associated with an unsuccessful clinical outcome (−LR, 0.1; 95% CI, 0.03-0.41) after manipulation.[2]

Stabilization Classification

Lumbar strengthening and stabilization exercises are another commonly used treatment for LBP. Theoretically, these exercises are prescribed for patients who are diagnosed with lumbar instability. Lumbar instability can be determined by measuring excessive amounts of sagittal plane translation or rotation. For example, instability criteria for sagittal plane translation have been suggested to be 4.5 mm or more than 15% of the vertebral body width of sagittal plane translation during flexion/extension x-ray films. However, lumbar instability is a difficult anatomical diagnosis to make, because a clear gold standard for diagnosing lumbar instability exclusively with radiography has not been established.[309] Therefore, the determination of patients appropriate for stabilization classification has many of the same problems as those already outlined for manipulation, and the clinician must rely on clinical examination findings in addition to radiographic findings.

A preliminary clinical prediction rule for stabilization classification has recently been proposed, which can assist the clinician in accurately identifying patients who appear

Table 9-10

Preliminary Clinical Prediction Rule* for Stabilization Classification[310]

Examination Finding	Positive Definition
Age	Less than 40 years old
Lumbar flexion observation (standing)	Aberrant movement pattern noted
Straight leg raise range of motion (supine)	Average (R + L)/2 is greater than 91°
Prone instability test	Decrease in pain when posteroanterior pressure is applied during muscle contraction

*At least 3/4 positive examination findings constitute a positive clinical prediction rule (+LR = 4.0) and at least 1/4 positive examination findings constitutes a negative clinical prediction rule (−LR = 0.20). *LR,* Likelihood ratio.

Table 9-11

Factors That Account for Differences in Operational Definitions of the Centralization Phenomenon

Factor for Determining Centralization Phenomenon	Source of Variation
Type of lumbar spine movement	Repeated
	Single
	Sustained
Direction of lumbar spine movement	Sagittal (flexion or extension)
	Frontal plane (side glide or rotation)
Criterion for "positive" centralization	Decrease in symptoms
	Abolishment of symptoms
	Physical change in location of symptoms
Time frame for centralization to occur	Single visit
	Multiple visits

to be appropriate for stabilization classification.[310] The clinical prediction rule for stabilization classification was developed using methodology similar to that for the manipulation rule. First, multiple examination variables were considered in a univariate setting, and then variables that significantly predicted a 50% improvement in disability from LBP at 4 weeks in a multivariate setting were retained for the clinical prediction rule (Table 9-10).[310] Four examination findings were identified, and a positive clinical prediction rule for stabilization was defined as the presence of at least three of these four findings (+LR, 4; 95% CI, 1.6-10); a negative clinical prediction rule was defined as the presence of at least one of the findings (−LR, 0.2; 95% CI, 0.03-1.4).[310]

Centralization Phenomenon Classification

Lumbar exercises that emphasize direction-specific end range lumbar movements (i.e., flexion, extension, side glide or rotation in flexion) are commonly used to treat patients with LBP. Patients are identified for these types of exercises primarily through identification of the centralization phenomenon (CP). Robin McKenzie originally described CP from clinical observations by noting that some patients with LBP reported changes in symptom location during lumbar movement testing.[311] Classically, CP occurs when a patient reports symptoms moving from an area more distal or lateral (i.e., in the buttocks and/or lower extremity) to a location nearer the midline position in reference to the lumbar spine.[311]

The reader must keep in mind that no uniform definition of CP exists, because different operational definitions have been reported in the literature and a recent report has even introduced the term *directional preference.*[282,312-318] The different factors that account for variations in the definition of CP are summarized in Table 9-11.

In contrast to some of the examination techniques routinely used by clinicians, ample evidence supports the inclusion of CP as an identified subgroup classification for LBP. For example, the tests used to determine the directional preference of the lumbar spine are repeatable.[312,319] Several studies have documented the prognostic value of CP; for example, patients who experienced symptom centralization returned to work sooner and showed greater improvement in pain and function than patients who were unable to centralize symptoms.[288,313,316,320] Conversely, inability to centralize symptoms has been predictive of a decreased chance of returning to work and of the likelihood of chronic pain and disability at 12 months.[235,317]

Evidence for subgroup classification by response to lumbar spine movements is also found in a randomized trial comparing patients experiencing CP who were randomly assigned to exercise that matched their directional preference, exercise that was opposite to their directional preference, and exercise that was guideline based.[282] Patients randomly assigned to receive matched exercise were significantly more likely to say at 2 weeks that their back pain had resolved, compared with the other two groups.[282] One relative risk (RR) ratio calculated from data presented in the paper indicated that patients were seven times more likely to say that their back pain had resolved when lumbar exercise matched the direction of CP, compared with exercise opposite the direction of CP (RR, 7.08).[282] The same study compared lumbar exercise that matched directional preference to a guideline-based program (multidirectional, midrange lumbar exercises and lower extremity stretching exercises). In that comparison, patients were almost 2.5 times more likely to say that their back pain had resolved when the lumbar exercise matched the direction of CP (RR, 2.42).[282] Collectively, these results provide strong evidence suggesting that CP should be used to identify a specific subgroup of patients with LBP.

The clinician must base decisions on centralization on the patient's response to lumbar movements, not on the theoretical effect lumbar movements have on the lumbar intervertebral discs. A study by Adams et al.[321] that investigated degenerated discs in cadavers found a high variability in the direction of nucleus pulposus movement in response to flexion and extension moments. These researchers succinctly summarized their findings: "Comparisons between living and cadaveric discs should not be taken too far, but the variability of the response of the cadaveric discs makes it clear that exercise therapy cannot be justified by a single theoretical model."[321]

Lumbar Spinal Stenosis Classification

Lumbar spinal stenosis (LSS) has a consistent anatomical component, which makes it an exception to the other LBP subgroup classifications described in this chapter. LSS is a pathological condition caused by compression of the neural and vascular structures, which occurs because of narrowing of the lateral or central spinal canals.[322] LSS typically is classified as primary or secondary. Primary stenosis results from developmental or congenital flaws of the vertebral body or posterior elements.[160] Degenerative changes are by far the most common cause of secondary LSS.[322] Degenerative changes include posterior disc protrusion, zygapophyseal joint and ligamentum flavum hypertrophy, disc degeneration, and spondylolisthesis.[323] Systemic processes potentially involved in secondary stenosis include Paget's disease, neoplasm, and ankylosing spondylitis.

Hallmark clinical symptoms of LSS are complaints of back and leg pain with erect postures or prolonged ambulation. This collection of symptoms is called *neurogenic claudication,* and anatomical studies provide insight as to why patients with LSS are likely to experience neurogenic claudication. The cross sectional area of central and lateral spinal canals decrease with lumbar extension movements and/or compression of the lumbar spine.[324-326] Porter and Ward[327] proposed that neurogenic claudication is caused by venous pooling subsequent to impairment of venous drainage at the root level and occurs only if the lumbar stenosis (central and/or lateral canal) is present at two adjacent levels of the spine.

LSS is frequently seen in elderly patients, and classification in the stenosis subgroup is based on the patient's age and on key historical findings consistent with neurogenic claudication (i.e., increased symptoms with erect postures, symptoms relieved with sitting, and leg pain with walking). Although LSS appears to have a strong anatomical component, the role of imaging in confirming LSS is the subject of debate. For example, Szpalski et al.[322] found that LSS is primarily a clinical condition, not a radiological finding or diagnosis. Herno et al.[328] demonstrated a poor correlation between radiological stenosis

Table 9-12
Positive Likelihood Ratios for Differentiating Neurogenic and Vascular Claudication[330]

Clinical Treadmill Test Result	Positive LR
Onset of symptoms occurs earlier during level walking	4.1
Longer total time is spent walking on incline than on level	6.5
Both results are observed	14.5

LR, Likelihood ratio.

and symptoms, and the ability to predict future spine-related problems from asymptomatic patients with LSS on MRI is limited.[329]

An important component of the differential diagnosis of LSS is establishing that the lower extremity claudication arises from neurological sources and not vascular sources. Fritz et al.[330] presented a clinical treadmill test to differentiate neural from vascular claudication for patients who report leg pain with activity. The clinical treadmill test is performed under two different conditions. The patient first walks on a level treadmill and then on a 15-degree incline. Both phases are performed for a maximum of 10 minutes, with 10 minutes of rest in between. Patients with neurogenic claudication will typically be able to walk for a longer time on an inclined treadmill than on level ground as the lumbar spine should be more flexed when on the incline. Patients with vascular claudication will walk for a longer time on the level treadmill as the vascular demand of the lower extremities should be elevated when walking up on incline. Fritz et al.[330] reported that the best classification is based on the time to onset of symptoms and recovery time; the associated positive likelihood ratios are presented in Table 9-12.

Neurodynamic Classification

Adverse mechanical tension in the nervous system has been defined as an abnormal physiological and/or mechanical response produced when structures of the nervous system exceed their normal range of movement.[331,332] It has been theorized that neurodynamic limitation (e.g., adverse mechanical tension, neurobiological mechanisms) in the nervous system can generate pain when decreased neural mobility occurs with movement.[331,332] A detailed discussion of this theory is beyond the scope of this chapter; interested readers can refer to the information presented in the original sources.[331-336]

Various examination techniques have been described for testing for neurodynamic limitation in the neuromusculoskeletal system. Specific to this chapter, the slump test has been advocated as such a test for the lower quarter.[331,334,336] Anatomical studies confirm that components of the slump test put extra stress on neural structures.[337-341] For example, full flexion of the cervical, thoracic, and lumbar regions of the spine lengthen the vertebral canal[338] and are associated with stretching of the spinal dura mater and lumbosacral nerve roots.[337-342] However, it is important to note that other anatomical structures, in addition to nervous tissue, are stressed by components of the slump test.[343,344]

Despite the widespread use of the slump test in clinical settings, limited evidence suggests that it is a useful examination technique.[336,345,346] Other than a positive response to the slump test, previous reports do not sufficiently describe other factors that may distinguish patients who might be treated appropriately with interventions that address neurodynamic limitations. Relying on the result of a single diagnostic test to make treatment decisions is a matter of concern, especially when several authors have noted that a false positive response may be a common occurrence with the slump test.[347,348]

A case report and series outlined several clinical criteria used to identify patients with a neurodynamic classification (Table 9-13).[349,350] These criteria were associated with positive outcomes for six patients treated with a specific technique believed to address neurodynamic limitations (slump stretching). For example, all of the patients had a decrease in pain intensity, and four of the six had favorable changes in pain location (more proximal to the lumbar spine).[349]

Higher quality evidence supporting the existence of a neurodynamic classification was reported in a randomized clinical trial from Cleland et al.[351] This trial used the same clinical criteria presented in the case report and series from George.[349,350] Cleland et al.[351] enrolled only patients who met the proposed criteria for neural tension (see Table 9-13),

and the subjects were randomly assigned to lumbar spine mobilization and exercise or slump stretching with lumbar spine mobilization and exercise. At short-term follow-up, patients receiving the slump stretching had significantly less pain (p < 0.01) and disability and were more likely to have a favorable change in symptom location (more proximal to the lumbar spine).[351]

Summary of Subgroup Classification Process

The LBP subgroup classifications described in this chapter are summarized in Table 9-14. The authors acknowledge that these subgroups do not account for every single LBP syndrome, but they appear to be subgroups that have the best supporting evidence from the peer-reviewed literature. However, the quantity and quality of supporting evidence for each classification group varies. For example, the evidence supporting the manipulation classification is strong, because the clinical prediction rule confirming the classification has been validated in a second clinical trial. In contrast, only one rigorously designed study supports the neurodynamic classification; therefore, the evidence supporting that classification is less compelling.

Case Examples for Diagnosing Low Back Pain

Case Example 1

A 62-year-old patient presents with complaints of nonspecific central low back pain. He is unable to describe a mechanism of injury but relates that the pain has gradually worsened over several months. Furthermore, he describes his current pain as a constant, deep ache. During the history, the patient indicates that he has a previous history of cancer.

Cancer is a potential cause of low back pain for this patient. The likelihood ratios from Table 9-5 are used to estimate the probability that this patient has cancer. In general, a 0.66% probability exists that cancer is a source of back pain (this estimate is based on a previously reported prevalence study[161]). The +LR that a patient over age 50 has cancer as a source of LBP is 2.7. Figure 9-7 shows a graphic method used to estimate the effect the patient's age has on the probability that cancer is a source of LBP. The Y-axis on the left side of the graph is the pretest probability in percent. The line begins at 0.66%, crosses the central Y-axis (representing the LR) at 2.7 and, as a result, intersects the right axis at approximately 2% (see Figure 9-7, *A*). Two percent is the new (post-test) probability that the patient has cancer (the actual calculated value is 1.8%). The previous history of cancer (+LR, 14.7) is considered in Figure 9-7, *B*, and the resultant post-test probability of cancer has increased to 22%. Blood work is ordered for this patient, and it shows an ESR of 60 mm/hr (+LR, 19.2) (Figure 9-7, *C*); the resultant post-test probability of cancer has increased to greater than 80%. At this point,

Table 9-13

Proposed Criteria to Confirm Neurodynamic Classification in Patients with Lower Quarter Symptoms[349,350]

Criterion	Finding Appropriate for Neural Tension Classification
Symptom location	Lumbar spine and unilateral/bilateral lower extremity
Repeated lumbar movements	No centralization of symptoms
Slump test	Reproduces patient's symptoms
	Symptoms decrease with cervical extension
Neurological examination	Negative straight leg raise test
	Muscle testing normal in L2-S1 dermatomes
	Sensory testing normal in L2-S1 dermatomes
	Deep tendon reflex testing normal in patellar and Achilles tendons

Table 9-14

Summary of Low Back Pain Subgroup Classifications

Classification	Manipulation	Stabilization	Centralization Phenomenon	Lumbar Spinal Stenosis	Neurodynamic
Potential anatomical causes	Zygapophyseal joint Sacroiliac joint	Disc disruption Lumbar instability Spondylolysis Spondylolisthesis Poor dynamic muscle control	Nerve root inflammation Mechanical deformation of a damaged nerve root Irritation of the dural sleeve Movement impairment Ligamentous creep from postural positioning	Degenerative change Osteophyte Zygapophyseal joint arthropathy Ligamentum flavum hypertrophy High grade spondylolisthesis Paget's disease	Adverse mechanical tension Neurobiological mechanisms
Relation between radiological findings and clinical syndrome	Inconsistent	Inconsistent	Inconsistent	Consistent but weak	Unknown
Key preliminary examination findings	Variable age Shorter duration of symptoms Local pain	Younger age Multiple, recurrent episodes Longer duration of symptoms Local pain Spontaneous resolution of previous episodes Symptoms worsened by prolonged postures Symptoms relieved by changing posture	Variable age Leg pain Symptoms worsened with flexed postures and improved with extended postures or Symptoms worsened with extended postures and improved with flexed postures	Older age Symptoms worsened with erect postures Leg pain, especially with walking Symptoms relieved with flexed postures	Variable age Leg pain Symptoms worsened with combined movements (neck or ankle) Normal neurological examination
Classification confirmed	Clinical prediction rule	Clinical prediction rule	Centralization phenomenon	Treadmill test	Jump test

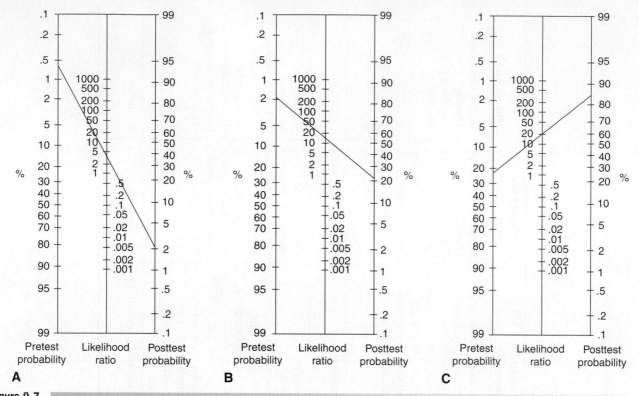

Figure 9-7

A, The probability of cancer for this patient increases from 0.66% to approximately 2% because he is over 50 years of age. **B,** The probability of cancer for this patient increases from 2% to approximately 22% because he has a previous history of cancer. **C,** The probability of cancer for this patient increases from 22% to greater than 80% based on ESR results.

the most appropriate course of action for this patient is referral to an oncologist.

This example also provides specific detail on how to estimate the influence of examination findings on pretext to post-test probabilities using likelihood ratios.

Case Example 2

A 45-year-old patient presents to a clinic with complaints of low back pain. Patients examined in this clinic are routinely screened for depression with the two previously described questions from the Primary Care Evaluation of Mental Disorders patient questionnaire.

The likelihood ratios from Table 9-7 were used to estimate the probability that this patient has severe depression. In general, about a 20% probability exists that patients with back pain also have major depression (this estimate is based on a previously reported prevalence study[247]).

The −LR that a patient with one negative response has severe depression is 0.29. Figure 9-8 shows a graphic method used to estimate the effect one negative response has on the probability of having severe depression. The Y-axis on the left side of the graph is the pretest probability in percent. The line begins at 20%, crosses the central Y-axis

(representing the LR) at 0.29 and, as a result, intersects the right axis at approximately 5% (see Figure 9-8, *A*). Five percent is the new (post-test) probability that the patient has severe depression (the actual calculated value is 5.8%). The most appropriate course of action in this scenario would be to continue the examination of this patient, with lowered suspicion of severe depression.

In contrast, the +LR that a patient with two positive responses has severe depression is 4.32 (see Table 9-5). Figure 9-8, *B* demonstrates that two positive responses raise the post-test probability of having severe depression from 20% to approximately 50% (the actual calculated value is 51.9%). The most appropriate course of action in this scenario would be to consider the patient for referral or further workup for depression, depending on the expertise of the clinician.

Case Example 3

A 34-year-old patient injured his back at work and is examined 7 days after the injury. As part of the examination process, the clinician has the patient complete the FABQ. Then, estimates of whether the patient will return to work in 4 weeks can be generated.

Figure 9-8

A, The probability of severe depression decreases from 20% to approximately 5% with one negative response to the two-question depression screening instrument. **B,** The probability of severe depression increases from 20% to approximately 50% with two positive responses to the two-question depression screening instrument.

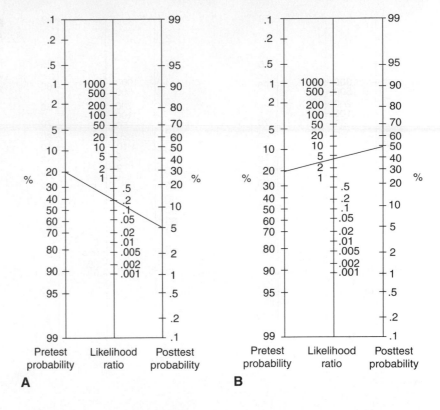

Pretest probability   Likelihood ratio   Posttest probability

A   **B**

The likelihood ratios from the study[260] cited in the text were used to estimate the probability that this patient would *not* return to work. The clinician estimates that a 25% probability exists that patients with back pain will not return to work (this estimate is based on a clinic's database).

In the first scenario, the patient has an FABW-W score of 38, and the associated +LR is 3.33. Figure 9-9 shows a graphic method used to estimate the effect this FABQ score has on the probability of not returning to work in 4 weeks. The Y-axis on the left side of the graph is the pretest probability in percent. The line begins at 25%, crosses the central Y-axis (representing the LR) at 3.33, and, as a result, intersects the right axis at approximately 52% (see Figure 9-9, *A*). Fifty-two percent is the new (post-test) probability that the patient will not return to work in 4 weeks (the actual calculated value is 52.6%). The most appropriate course of action in this scenario would be a management strategy that optimized the likelihood of returning to work. For example, interventions that addressed elevated fear-avoidance beliefs and/or early involvement of case management might be considered.

In the second scenario, the patient has an FABQ-W score of 17, and the associated −LR is 0.08. Figure 9-9, *B* shows that the post-test probability of not returning to work has decreased from 25% to approximately 2.5% (the actual calculated value is 2.6%). The most appropriate course of action in this scenario would be to continue the examination process in anticipation of a favorable outcome.

Case Example 4

A clinician is considering a 27-year-old patient for appropriate LBP subgroup classification. During the examination process, information is collected about the duration and location of complaints, FABQ scores, hip range of motion, and segmental mobility of the spine. This information can be used to generate an estimate of whether this patient is appropriate for manipulation classification.

The likelihood ratios from Table 9-9 were used to estimate the probability that this patient was appropriate for manipulation classification. Based on the results of a previous study, this clinician estimated that manipulation classification can be expected approximately 35% of the time.[291]

In the first scenario, the patient has four positive examination findings from the clinical prediction rule, and the associated +LR is 13.2. Figure 9-10 shows a graphic method used to estimate the effect these examination findings have on the probability of the patient being considered for manipulation classification. The Y-axis on the left side of the graph is the pretest probability in percent. The line begins at 35%, crosses the central Y-axis (representing the LR) at 13.2, and, as a result, intersects the right axis at approximately 88% (see Figure 9-10, *A*). Eighty-eight percent is the new (post-test) probability that the patient is appropriate for manipulation classification (the actual calculated value is 87.7%). The most appropriate course of action in this scenario would be to recommend a management strategy that included spinal manipulation.

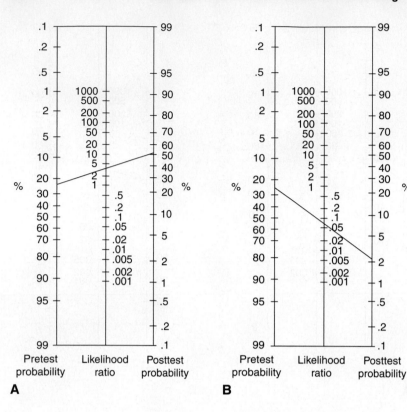

Figure 9-9

A, The probability of not returning to work increases from 25% to approximately 52% with a positive FABQ-W. **B,** The probability of not returning to work decreases from 25% to approximately 2.5% with a negative FABQ-W.

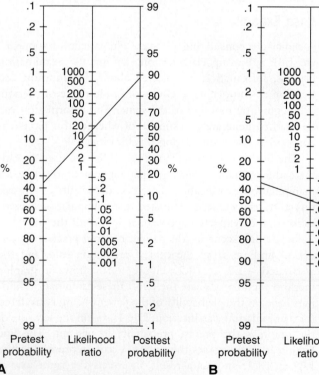

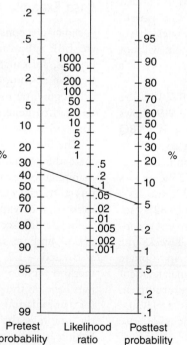

Figure 9-10

A, The probability of manipulation classification with a positive result on the clinical prediction rule increases from 35% to approximately 88%. **B,** The probability of manipulation classification with a negative result on the clinical prediction rule decreases from 35% to approximately 5%.

In the second scenario, the patient has only two positive examination findings from the clinical prediction rule, and the associated −LR is 0.1. Figure 9-10, *B* shows that the post-test probability of manipulation classification has decreased from 35% to approximately 5% (the actual calculated value is 5.1%). The most appropriate course of action in this scenario would be to consider this patient for classification in some other LBP subgroup.

Case Example 5

A clinician is considering a 38-year-old patient for appropriate LBP subgroup classification. During the examination process, information is collected about the patient's age, straight leg raise range of motion, movement pattern, and prone instability test. This information can be used to generate an estimate of whether this patient is appropriate for stabilization classification.

The likelihood ratios from Table 9-10 were used to estimate the probability that this patient was appropriate for stabilization classification. Based on the results of a previous study, the clinician estimated that stabilization classification can be expected approximately 57% of the time.[352]

In the first scenario, the patient has three positive examination findings from the clinical prediction rule, and the associated +LR is 4. Figure 9-11 shows a graphic method used to estimate the effect these examination findings have on the probability of the patient being considered for manipulation classification. The Y-axis on the left side of the graph is the pretest probability in percent. The line begins at 57%, crosses the central Y-axis (representing the LR) at 4, and, as a result, intersects the right axis at approximately 82% (see Figure 9-11, *A*). Eighty-two percent is the new (post-test) probability that the patient is appropriate for stabilization classification (the actual calculated value is 84.2%). The most appropriate course of action

in this scenario would be to recommend a management strategy that includes lumbar strengthening or stabilization exercises.

In the second scenario, the patient has only one positive examination finding from the clinical prediction rule, and the associated −LR is 0.2. Figure 9-11, *B* shows that the post-test probability of manipulation classification has decreased from 57% to approximately 19% (the actual calculated value is 20.9%). The most appropriate course of action in this scenario would be to perform other tests to determine whether this patient was appropriate for classification in another LBP subgroup.

Case Example 6

A 70-year-old patient presents to a spine clinic with complaints of low back and leg pain. He reports a long history of low back pain but says that the leg pain has gradually worsened over the past several months. He notices that his leg hurts more when he is walking and that the pain is relieved by sitting. During the history, the patient states that he has no previous history of heart or vascular disease. An MRI scan shows moderate to severe lateral and central canal stenosis at L4-L5.

Even with the radiographic evidence of LSS, the clinician realizes that either vascular or neurogenic claudication

Figure 9-11
A, The probability of stabilization classification with a positive clinical prediction rule increases from 57% to approximately 82%. **B,** The probability of stabilization classification with a negative clinical prediction rule decreases from 57% to approximately 19%.

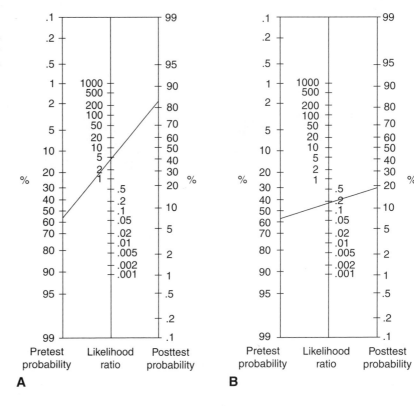

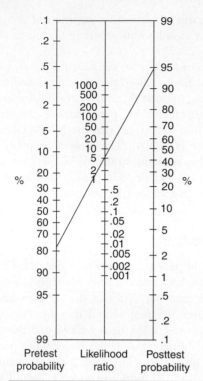

Figure 9-12

The probability of neurogenic claudication, based on results from a clinical treadmill test, increases from 75% to 95%.

could be a potential cause of the leg pain. The likelihood ratios from Table 9-12 can be used to estimate the probability that this patient has neurogenic claudication. From previous clinical experience, the clinician estimates that a 75% probability exists that the leg pain is from a neurogenic source. This pretest estimate is based on the radiographic evidence and the lack of a cardiovascular history. The clinician has the patient perform the clinical treadmill test described by Fritz et al.,[330] and the patient has a longer walking time on the incline portion of the test (+LR, 6.5).

Figure 9-12 shows a graphic method used to estimate the probability that the leg pain is neurogenic, considering the results of the treadmill test. The Y-axis on the left side of the graph is the pre-test probability in percent. The line begins at approximately 75%, crosses the central Y-axis (representing the +LR) at 6.5, and, as a result, intersects the right axis at approximately 95%. Ninety-five percent is the new (post-test) probability that the patient has neurogenic claudication. This information effectively rules out vascular claudication as a source of the leg pain.

References

To enhance this text and add value for the reader, all references have been incorporated into a CD-ROM that is provided with this text. The reader can view the reference source and access it online whenever possible. There are a total of 352 references for this chapter.

CHAPTER 10

Lumbar Spine: Treatment of Hypomobility and Disc Conditions

Jim Meadows and David J. Magee

Introduction

Manual therapy techniques (spinal mobilization and spinal manipulation) play a major role in the treatment of low back pain. This chapter discusses the use of manual therapy, particularly specific and semispecific segmental techniques for lumbopelvic pain. *Mobilization* is defined as a series of rhythmical or nonrhythmical movements of the joints' articular surfaces, applied by the clinician, that are within the patient's control to stop (through muscle contraction). *Manipulation* is defined as a single, high velocity, low amplitude thrust technique, intended to abolish the barrier to movement, that is not within the patient's control (i.e., it happens too quickly for the patient to react).

Characteristics of Hypomobility Dysfunction

- Altered patterns of movement
- Decreased range of motion
- Tissue or joint swelling
- Altered joint play
- Abnormal end feel
- Tight, short muscles
- Inhibition of antagonists

For the most part, the manual therapy techniques applied in the treatment of lumbar hypomobility are used to reduce pain and increase range of movement. They also may be used to reduce reflex inhibition of the musculature that supports the spine. The exact mechanism of these effects is unknown. However, two primary models are used to explain the effects of spinal mobilization and manipulation: the neurophysiological model and the pathomechanical model.

Neurophysiological Model

According to the neurophysiological model, segmental hypomobility occurs as a result of a neurophysiological processing problem in the control system; this processing problem is caused by pain, which produces protective muscle spasm and instability. In this context, the term *control system* refers to the concept set forth by Panjabi[1-3] and involves neural control (the central and peripheral nervous systems) as well as the passive structures around the joints (ligaments, capsules, and discs) and the active components (muscles). It also refers to control of the arthrokinematic movements (e.g., spin, slide, roll). Inadequate control of the joint leads to changes in muscle tone, which in turn result in more pain and reduced range of motion, a somewhat circuitous model.

According to the neurophysiological model, manual therapy techniques such as mobilization and manipulation provide a sensory stimulus that affects one or more of the joint mechanoreceptors, muscle spindle systems, or Golgi tendon organs, resulting in reduced muscle tone, increased range of motion, and decreased pain. These changes are produced through neurophysiological pain and mechanoreceptor modulation at the spinal cord level (summation or gating) and/or by activating descending pathways.

Pathomechanical Model

The pathomechanical model is based on the premise that the primary dysfunction is essentially the result of a structural breakdown of one or more spinal segments, which allows the articulations to jam, fixate, lock, or sublux. In this context, a *spinal segment* is the trijoint complex (two vertebrae, the zygapophyseal joints, and the disc). The result of the structural breakdown is a pathomechanical hypomobility that limits movement in one or more directions. Pain is caused by mechanical stress; this stress can occur to the affected joint, or it may occur at another location as a result of excess stress on some other, remote tissue, possibly resulting in hypermobility of the remote tissue because of the pathomechanical hypomobility of the specific segment in question. In the pathomechanical model, manual treatment mechanically mobilizes the hypomobile joint to relieve the stress on the painful structure while protecting the hypermobile structures.

Both the neurophysiological and pathomechanical models are able to explain clinical observations (pain, restricted or excessive movement), and each of the two models can be used in isolation. However, they are more useful to clinicians if they are combined.

Manual therapy techniques have been shown to produce both neurophysiological and mechanical effects on the segmental tissues.[4-12] In acute pain states, particularly with spasm or nonreflexive muscle guarding, overly aggressive manual therapy techniques (e.g., Maitland's grade 3+ and grade 4+) can and usually do aggravate the condition by exacerbating existing inflammation (see volume 2 in this series, *Scientific Foundations and Principles of Practice in Musculoskeletal Rehabilitation,* Chapter 24). In these cases, more gentle manual therapy techniques (e.g., Maitland's grade 1 and grade 2) are used to reduce the pain through neurophysiological modulation.[13] These gentle techniques do not (or should not) directly engage the pathological or anatomical barrier (end of range of motion) or cause any discomfort; they can be considered pain-dominant techniques. If pain is not the predominant clinical feature and if its onset follows the clinician's perception of the pathological barrier to passive movement (restriction-dominant condition), a technique that directly stresses the pathological barrier (e.g., Maitland's grade 3+ and grade 4+ and minithrusts) is the treatment of choice. For pathomechanical or pericapsular hypomobility (i.e., stiff, inextensible articular tissues), manipulation and mobilization, respectively, may be more efficient and effective.

For the purposes of manual therapy, pathological barriers can be divided into muscle, collagen, or inert tissue related, as well as neurological barriers. Muscle barriers occur as a result of injury to contract out tissue (i.e., muscle), or they are the result of protective muscle spasm. Examples of a muscle barrier include hypertonicity of a muscle, muscle spasm, and adaptive shortening of the muscle. In these cases, the end feel is muscle spasm or, as Cyriax described it, a "vibrant twang" or "mushy" tissue stretch (i.e., a tight muscle).[14-17] Collagen and inert tissue barriers occur as a result of injury to inert tissue (e.g., the capsule and ligaments) and other collagen in or adjacent to the joint, including scar tissue. In these cases, the end feel is capsular (e.g., a capsular pattern), soft capsular (e.g., synovitis or soft tissue edema), springy block (e.g., meniscus), or bone to bone (e.g., osteophyte formation). Inert tissue barriers may be articular or periarticular. Neurological barriers are primarily the result of pain causing an empty end feel or one with neurological signs (e.g., tingling, numbness, pins and needles, painless weakness).

Manual Therapy for Lumbar Intervertebral Disc Herniation

In addition to addressing pain and segmental pathomechanics, manual therapy techniques, especially manipulation, may be used as an intervention for lumbar intervertebral disc herniation. Probably the greatest proponent of manipulative therapy for the treatment of disc herniation was James Cyriax.[14-17] However, his advocacy of this approach was not based so much on existing pathology but on the clinical model he proposed. This model essentially held that facet joint syndrome (and other, similar pathomechanical conditions) and sacroiliac joint dysfunction were extremely rare and that most low back pain was caused by varying degrees of disc pathology (i.e., protrusion, prolapse, extrusion, or sequestration).

Currently spinal manipulation in the treatment of disc herniation is used primarily by chiropractors and tends to be avoided by the medical, osteopathic, and physical therapy professions. The contention that manipulative techniques affect the intervertebral disc is not controversial; what is open to question is whether the effect is beneficial or harmful. In a cadaveric study, Sheng et al.[18] found that rotation manipulation combined with compression increased intradiscal pressure, and rotation manipulation combined with traction reduced it. Two magnetic resonance imaging (MRI) and clinical outcome studies of patients with lumbar disc herniation found that spinal manipulation combined with traction, physical therapy (undefined), and exercises,[19] or spinal manipulation alone,[20] resulted in a significant improvement in clinical symptoms, function, and MRI findings.

Most of the evidence for the efficacy of manipulation in the treatment of disc herniation is anecdotal or comes from case reports; however, the use of spinal manipulation for lumbar disc herniation appears to have some degree of effectiveness. Chiropractic reports provide examples of cases of lumbosacral disc herniations that were more lateral, causing back and leg pain with sensory deficit (confirmed by MRI), that were treated successfully by manipulation.[21-23] Some case reports even indicate the successful use of manipulation in patients with established cauda equina lesions, a condition most clinicians consider an absolute contraindication to manual therapy.[24-27]

Many other reports show harmful effects from spinal manipulation with a disc herniation. According to Assendelft,[28] disc herniation, aggravation of disc herniation, and cauda equina syndrome are the most common serious complications of lumbar spinal manipulation, accounting for more than 20% of all serious complications of manipulation in all spinal regions, making possible disc herniation the second most serious complication after neurovascular injury subsequent to manipulation of the cervical spine.

A literature review by Haldeman and Rubinstein[29] that covered the years 1911 to 1989 found only 10 cases of cauda equina syndrome after spinal manipulative therapy (SMT). Their review also reported on three new cases that were related at least temporally to SMT. In the three new cases, neither the treating clinician nor the emergency department physician recognized the onset of the problem.[29] A number of other cases of cauda equina syndrome have been reported since 1989. In an unusual case, the disc fragment did not fragment but bulged onto the artery that supplied the conus (caudal narrowing area of the spinal canal).[30] Li[31] reported five cases of cauda equina syndrome (CES) or conus medullaris syndrome (CMS), all of which occurred after spinal manipulation, some of them immediately after the manipulation. Powell et al.[32] listed six risk factors for spinal manipulation, one of which was the presence of a herniated nucleus pulposus.

It cannot be argued, therefore, that SMT does not result in CES or CMS syndrome in some cases; however, the incidence of these syndromes as adverse effects of SMT is believed to be very low, somewhere in the range of 0.5-1 per 1 million manipulations.[27,33]

For most clinicians, the risk, however low, of very serious complications; unproven efficacy; and inexperience in the use of manipulation for disc herniation are factors that cause them to avoid using these techniques. Most clinicians also have the advantage of working in a system that encourages referral of difficult cases for further investigation and the availability of other treatment methods that do not carry the same degree of risk. Consequently, for the most part, clinicians tend to view the presence of an established disc herniation as a contraindication to most forms of manual therapy.

Traction for Disc Herniations (Vertebral Axial Decompression Therapy)

In contrast to manipulation, spinal traction is used quite frequently in the treatment of disc herniation. Since the age of Hippocrates, practitioners have known about the application of longitudinal force to the axis of the spine to provide facet joint distraction, reduction of disc protrusion, soft tissue elongation, muscle relaxation, and patient mobilization. Spinal traction has been heavily explored as a therapeutic option in musculoskeletal medicine since the late 18th century. It enjoyed a renewed popularity in the 1950s and 1960s based on James Cyriax's findings on the efficacy of spinal traction for the treatment of discogenic back and leg pain.[15] Saunders[34] further popularized the use of intermittent spinal traction in the 1980s and 1990s through the development of improved stabilization belts and split table technology. Today, as a result of improved pneumatic instrumentation, an enhanced form of vertebral axial spinal decompression (VAX-D) is being widely used in the management of disc conditions. Advances in imaging and microinstrumentation have fueled a growing body of clinical evidence that spinal decompression and/or traction should be considered a front-line intervention for these conditions.[35-37]

Vertebral axial decompression therapy uses a computer-driven table to apply traction to the lumbar spine. It is postulated that this traction technique may effect decompression of the disc. Experimental results have been encouraging,[38,39] but the lack of scientific evidence based on well-designed studies has led several groups to question its effectiveness.[38-42]

Selection of a Lumbar Spine Manual Therapy Technique

The primary use of manual therapy is in the treatment of segmental dysfunction or hypomobility. In this context, "segmental dysfunction" means injury or abnormal movement in the trijoint complex, which consists of the two zygapophyseal joints and the disc. The technique selected must be specific to the pathological barrier associated with the dysfunction. If pain, spasm, or hypertonicity (or all three) is the principal problem, a neurophysiological technique is indicated; however, if inextensibility of pericapsular tissues or pathomechanical hypomobility is the chief problem, a restriction-dominant technique is the preferred choice. If the joint must be stretched or if it is fixed (jammed or subluxed) and the hypomobility is pathomechanical, the joint needs to be manipulated with a sudden, low amplitude force.

A number of factors must be considered in the selection of a manual technique. Two of these have already been discussed: the level of pain (pain dominant or restriction dominant) and the condition itself (disc herniation, pericapsular restriction, pathomechanical hypomobility). In addition, the dose of the treatment must be selected; this is actually a subset of the previous considerations.

Causes of Hypomobility

Myofascial Causes
- Adaptive shortening or hypertonicity of muscles
- Post-traumatic adhesions
- Scarring

Pericapsular Causes
- Damage to capsule or ligament
- Adhesions
- Scarring
- Arthritis/arthrosis
- Fibrosis
- Tissue adaptation

Pathomechanical Causes (Joint Trauma)
- Macrotrauma
- Microtrauma

Causes of a Pathological (Restrictive) Barrier

- Trauma (macrotrauma or microtrauma)
- Inflammatory response
- Muscle spasm
- Edema
- Pain
- Tissue alterations (e.g., adaptive shortening)

Important Factors in the Mobilization Process

- Presenting condition or tissue disorder (contractile, inert (collagen), neurological)
- Quality of the movement present
- Resistance felt (type of barrier, end feel)
- Pathological state of the tissues (acute, subacute, chronic; stage of healing)
- Symptoms elicited before, during, and after treatment (pain dominant, restriction dominant)
- Indications for treatment (pain dominant, restriction dominant)
- Treatment parameters (e.g., grade of technique, positioning of patient)
- Cautions and contraindications to use of certain techniques
- Patient's use of any medications (e.g., nonsteroidal anti-inflammatory medications [NSAIDS]) that may affect treatment
- Methods of testing for instability and vascular insufficiency
- Need for adjunctive treatment (e.g., exercise, electrophysical agent)
- Need to reassess

Probably the most common method used to discuss doses of manual treatment is Maitland's grading system.[13,43,44] This system has undergone many refinements over the years; however, for the purposes of this chapter, the grades can be divided into two categories: those that have mainly a neurophysiological effect and those that have a mechanical effect on the pathological barrier. Figure 10-1 depicts the simplest interpretation of this system. Purists may take issue with this interpretation, but it presents all that is required to discuss grading techniques for the purposes of this chapter.

As the diagram in Figure 10-1 shows, grade 1 and grade 2 techniques are unquestionably neurophysiological in effect, because they do not approach the end of the available range of movement, and they should not produce pain or discomfort. Technically, grade 3 and grade 4 techniques are also sub-barrier, because they should reach the end of range but not stress the tissues at end range. Minithrusts and grade 5 (manipulation) techniques would be applied at the barrier. If pain is experienced before or at the same time tissue resistance is encountered, a sub-barrier technique is indicated. If any attempt at reaching the pathological barrier produces or increases pain, the condition is in a subacute stage or almost certainly in the acute phase. However, in clinical practice, clinicians commonly tend to push into the barrier; when this happens, these techniques more properly should be labeled grade 3+ and grade 4+ techniques. Regardless of the grade of technique used, all mobilizations include an oscillatory component, which prevents neurophysiological accommodation to the input from attenuating the pain reduction effect of the technique.

Clinicians commonly use terms such as *acute, subacute,* and *nonacute* in nontemporal terms to depict how painful and irritable (i.e., acute) the condition is. Semantics, definitions, and communication, as well as a common level of understanding, are critical among clinicians, and this is often a problem in manual therapy. Terms must be standardized to some extent, and associating the onset of pain with the onset of the symptoms can do this. Table 10-1 is an attempt to "quasi-quantify" the relationship of pain to the end feel to enable the clinician to determine whether the problem is pain dominant or restriction dominant.

True constant pain must be considered to possibly indicate visceral or certain types of bone pathology that are not usually amendable to manual therapy techniques. Pain that is unrelieved by rest and generally considered an indication of inflammation should actually be called *variable pain,* because it is affected by varying mechanical stresses and therefore variable rather than constant. In actuality, this is high level, continuous pain that may be treated by manual therapy techniques (see Table 10-1).

To summarize, the choice of manual therapy techniques depends on the dominant barrier. In addition, whether pain or restriction predominates, whether the problem is pericapsular or pathomechanical, the clinician must consider

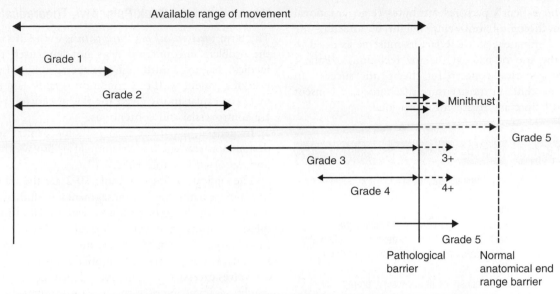

Figure 10-1

Maitland's grades of movement used in lumbar mobilization techniques. As the diagram shows, grade 1 and grade 2 techniques are definitely neurophysiological, because they do not approach the end of the available range of movement, and they should not produce pain or discomfort. Technically, grade 3 and grade 4 techniques are also sub-barrier, because they should reach the end of the available range but not stress it. However, in clinical practice, clinicians commonly tend to push into the barrier. When this happens, these techniques are more properly labeled grade 3+ and grade 4+. Regardless of the grade of the technique, all mobilizations have an oscillatory component. Oscillation prevents neurophysiological accommodation to the input, which would attenuate the pain reduction effect of the technique. (Data from Maitland GD: *Vertebral manipulation*, London, 1986, Butterworth.)

Table 10-1

Relationship of Pain to End Feel, Presumptive Pathology, and Treatment

Pain and Tissue Resistance (End Feel)	Acuteness or "Irritability" Level	Presumptive Pathology	Treatment	
All pain, no resistance	Hyperacute	Almost always serious pathology	Refer to physician	Pain Dominant
Constant pain*	Hyperacute	Significant inflammation or serious pathology	No manual treatment	
Pain before resistance	Acute	Inflammation, very irritable	Low dose sub-barrier techniques (grade 1)	
Pain simultaneous with resistance	Subacute	Moderate or mild inflammation, moderately irritable	Higher dose sub-barrier techniques (grade 2)	
Pain after resistance	Nonacute	Mechanical pathology; may be slightly irritable	Barrier techniques (grade 3 or grade 4), either mobilization or manipulation, depending on end feel	Restriction Dominant
No pain, all resistance	Stiff or jammed	Mechanical pathology with no irritability	Barrier techniques (grade 3 or grade 4), either mobilization or manipulation, depending on end feel	

*Constant pain implies pain that is always present and does not change with movement or weight bearing.

whether the patient's personal attributes (e.g., emotional liability, psychological well-being) might be affecting the condition. Ultimately, all these factors must be assessed to optimize the use of manual therapy techniques. Patient selection is a critical concern for therapeutic success. In addition, the clinician must ensure that informed consent is obtained before any treatment is provided.

Informed Consent Process

- Discuss the proposed technique and the reason it is deemed the best choice
- Discuss possible alternatives
- Discuss both the benefits and the risks of the technique
- Have information sheets available for the patient, or note how the information was given; include the time and date it was provided (documentation)
- Allow the patient to ask questions (if necessary, prompt the person)
- Obtain the patient's written consent

Patient Selection

Not all patients are suited for manual therapy. The list of patients who fall into this category is longer for some professions than for others. For example, physical therapists in general lack enthusiasm for manual treatment of a disc herniation, whereas chiropractors frequently use manipulation for this condition. For most physical therapists, the patients suited for manual therapy are those suffering from a biomechanical segmental dysfunction (or its peripheral equivalent). For the purposes of this chapter, manual therapy as described is used for a very specific type of mechanical low back pain.

Mechanical Low Back Pain: Two Theoretical Models

The term *mechanical low back pain* is a way of saying that the problem encountered does not lend itself to a true medical diagnosis. Although the average clinical presentation of a patient with this condition is fairly easy to recognize, the explanations given for the underlying pathology are controversial and contentious.

In general, a patient with pathomechanical segmental dysfunction (caused by hypomobility) displays the clinical findings listed in Table 10-2.[44-46]

The clinical findings in Table 10-2 are the criteria used to diagnose pathomechanical segmental dysfunction (hypomobility), which can be addressed with mobilization techniques. In contrast, neurophysiological segmental dysfunction (instability), which often accompanies or results from hypomobility, is not amenable to mobilization therapy, because it involves excessive motion, not reduced motion. However, conditions involving excessive motion are amenable to stabilization training (see Chapter 11 of this book and volume 2 of this series, *Scientific Foundation and Principles of Practice in Musculoskeletal Rehabilitation*, Chapter 19).

Two primary theories have been proposed for this apparent dichotomy. One theory holds that in patients with the clinical profile previously described, two distinct dysfunctions are present at different joints or different segments, one being hypomobile and the other unstable. According to the other theory, only one dysfunction is present, but its characteristics change from time to time, with painful episodes interrupting longer periods of pain-free function. The affected segment undergoes a form of phase transition. A *phase transition* can be defined as a clinical episode in which a profound change occurs in symptom behavior and manifestation with little change in the physical composition of the segment. Regardless of which theory

---

Table 10-2

Signs and Symptoms of Segmental Dysfunction

Neurophysiological Segmental Dysfunction (Hypermobility/Instability)	Pathomechanical Segmental Dysfunction (Hypomobility)
Asynchronous movement	Altered patterns of movement
Increased range of motion	Decreased range of motion when joint is painful
Joint swelling	Tissue or joint swelling
Altered joint play	Altered joint play
Late muscle spasm	Abnormal end feel
Abnormal end feel	Tight (hypertonic) muscles (postural)
Pain localized to back	Inhibition of antagonists
Seldom pain referral	Moderate non-neuropathic pain
Painful episode related to load, speed of movements, muscle fatigue	Possibly referral of pain to buttock
No incapacitation deformity	Minor or unknown trigger to painful episodes
Possible instability jog (muscle twitch)	

is preferred, it must be understood that a theory or explanation is not required to be the "truth"; rather, its function is to offer a conceptualization of what is happening so that the user of the model can visualize events. Theories are used, consciously or unconsciously, all of the time. The following model of phase transition fits the observations concerning the presentation of biomechanical back pain and its response to various treatments at least as well if not better than most other models, but it is not necessarily true.

As mentioned, a phase transition is considered to have occurred when a radical change in the behavioral characteristics of a substance or system occurs without a similar change in the composition of the substance or system. This concept has been taken from physics; it describes a major change in the thermodynamics of a system in which essentially the same substance has completely different behavioral characteristics. Consider, for example, the change from water to ice; ice cannot put out fire until it changes to water; ice is extremely slippery, water considerably less so. Although in the strictest sense the term *phase transition* is used to describe fundamental property changes in a thermodynamic system, it might be used to good effect to describe a model of biomechanical dysfunction of the lumbar spine.

If the patient is experiencing a "phase" that may best be described as a lack of spinal stability and control, this phase is relatively painless and mobile, and it leaves the patient fully functional but with symptoms indicating that the patient cannot control the movement. Assessment during this unstable phase reveals abnormally pliable tissue compliance (instability) and hypermobility. If a phase transition occurs, passive physiological mobility tests will demonstrate hypomobility and will be painful; however, all the characteristics of subluxation/fixation and the stability test results will be negative. In effect, the segment goes from the matrix of instability to hyperstability and from a painless state to a painful state. It undergoes transition from one phase to another and back again as effective forces are applied. Therefore, using the phase transition model for segmental dysfunction, an unstable segment oscillates between a pain-free phase, which is its unstable ground state, and a painful phase, in which its very instability allows the joint to fix at one end of its range and either become painful itself or cause pain at another joint that is stressed by the hypomobility. Treatment, therefore, focuses on the phase in which patients find themselves at the time of treatment. If the painful, hypomobile phase is encountered, manual therapy to move the joint and relieve the pain is required. If the unstable phase is to be treated, stability therapy and movement re-education can be used.

To determine the motion state dysfunction at the segment, the clinician must perform a detailed biomechanical examination. This examination must determine four important factors:

1. Is a movement dysfunction present?
2. If a movement dysfunction is present, is it one of hypomobility, hypermobility or instability?
3. If the dysfunction is a hypomobility dysfunction, is it articular or extra-articular in origin?
4. If the hypomobility dysfunction is articular in origin, is it pericapsular or pathomechanical?

Only after these determinations have been made can a specific treatment be applied to a specific segment in a specific direction. Some schools of thought hold that it is unnecessary to be specific about the segment to be mobilized. The intervention discussion in this chapter focuses on specific treatments. However, some discussion of the nonspecific approach is needed, because it is rapidly becoming *the* method of treatment, especially in the United States.

The use of nonspecific manual treatment by physical therapists was first popularized by Cyriax in the 1950s, and this approach still has its adherents.[15] A disc herniation model was used, and it was thought that large amplitude regional techniques using strong traction would have a beneficial effect on the disc lesion. The differential diagnostic examination afforded limited specificity as to the segment requiring treatment, and absolutely no attempt was made to make the treatment technique specific. Recently Flynn et al.[47] resurrected this idea, using clinical prediction rules to determine which patients would benefit from manipulative therapy of the lumbar spine. The study came up with a five-point clinical prediction rule that gave a likelihood of success of 45% to 90% if four out of five points were evident.

Flynn's Clinical Prediction Rules[47]

- Recent onset of symptoms (<16 days)
- No fear-avoidance beliefs (Fear-Avoidance Beliefs Questionnaire [FABQ] score <19)
- Lumbar hypomobility in at least one segment
- Good medial rotation range of motion in at least one hip (>35°)
- No symptoms distal to the knee

The manipulation used in the study was not only nonspecific to any segment, it also had been used previously to manipulate the sacroiliac joint. Flynn et al.[47] further made the point that segmental specificity is not necessary for a technique to be effective (a point borne out by the longevity of the Cyriax techniques and other studies).[15-17] However, clinical reasons exist for making both the thought processes involved in the determination of treatment and the technique itself more specific. The previous discussion is entirely about effectiveness; it does not address other issues, such as safety and ways to treat patients who do not meet four of the five criteria described by Flynn et al.[47]

Nonspecific techniques do not pretend to safeguard segments that may not be able to withstand the forces involved in manual treatment if they are not specifically locked. For example, in the cervical spine, the vertebral artery is at risk unless the technique's effect is minimized throughout the neck, especially if rotational techniques are used. Although the clinical prediction rule may well help include patients in the manipulation group, it does not do much about excluding those who are marginal or who should not be manipulated because of unrelated but significant pathologies. This oversimplification of a very complex system (i.e., the patient) allows newcomers to manual therapy to assume that all that is required is that the patient match a few points on a list. As much as Flynn et al.[47] speak out against an algorithmic approach, it is the way clinicians tend to think, and it provides a stronger rationale for doing what clinicians do than simply following a clinical prediction rule.

Biomechanical Segmental Assessment

To determine whether a specific manual treatment should be performed for pathomechanical dysfunction, the clinician must perform a passive biomechanical segmental assessment that uses passive physiological intervertebral movements (PPIVMs), followed by passive arthrokinematic (accessory) intervertebral movements (PAIVMs). Figure 10-2 presents a simple algorithm of the examination.

Using PPIVMS and PAIVMS, the clinician can determine a number of findings that will guide the use of manual therapy techniques for the hypomobile joint or segment.

A pericapsular restriction is indicated by restriction on PPIVM tests associated with restriction on PAIVM tests, with both types of movements showing the hard capsular end feel of stiffness. A pathomechanical hypomobility may be determined by the PPIVM tests associated with restriction on the PAIVM tests, with both showing a pathomechanical end feel. For a hypermobile joint or segment, using the phase transition model, the presence of an instability requires treatment of the instability, because this is the phase the back condition exhibits.

Before the definitive technique can be applied, the clinician may and probably will encounter one or more pathological barriers between the initial hands-on end feel once the patient has been positioned for treatment. The end feel will vary, depending on the pathological barrier encountered. To briefly review barrier end feels: An inextensibility of the pericapsular tissues produces a predominantly hard capsular end feel, and a subluxation produces a hard, jammed end feel. Increased muscle tone can produce a variety of end feels, depending on the degree of hypertonicity and its effect. A minor degree of hypertonicity may produce only an increased drag on the way to the definitive end feel, whereas a greater amount of hypertonicity can cause an almost capsular end feel but with a "lively resilience" (Cyriax's "vibrant twang").[15] If the hypertonus alters the biomechanics of the segment by acting as an "abnormal ligament," it can cause the joint to jam, resulting in a pathomechanical end feel similar to that of a subluxed joint. In all cases, light hold/relax, contract/relax, or muscle energy techniques can reduce the hypertonus and drastically alter the end feel.

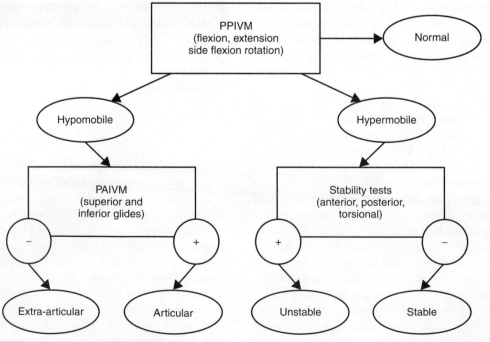

Figure 10-2

Algorithm for the passive biomechanical segmental assessment.

Another pathological barrier is soreness, which often is first encountered once the segment is positioned near its abnormal end of range. The patient may complain of soreness, or the clinician may feel the patient's reaction to the position (this is not acute pain, and certainly no spasm accompanies the pain).

For manual therapy techniques to succeed, each of these pathological barriers must be addressed as it is met. Mild degrees of soreness can be reduced or eliminated with grade 3 or grade 4 oscillatory techniques that do not produce pain; hypertonus can be addressed with muscle relaxation techniques, including hold/relax, contract/relax, and muscle energy and active release techniques; pericapsular restrictions are best treated with a grade 3+ or grade 4+ mobilization; and subluxations are treated with manipulation or with minithrusts if manipulation is not chosen. Usually multiple pathological barriers are met at each treatment. The positioning causes some minor soreness, which is relieved by a grade 3 or grade 4 mobilization, and muscle tone (normal or high) may then be encountered and reduced. Finally, the definitive pathological barrier is met and treated with a grade 3+ or 4+ mobilization or manipulation (minithrusts if manipulation is not an option). This approach is more effective, because it eliminates the inappropriate use of manual therapy techniques, such as ballistic stretching of muscle (which occurs if grade 4+ techniques are used on hypertonic muscles) and incorrect manipulative methods for extensive capsular tightening.

Positioning and Treatment

In deciding how to position the patient for the most effective use of manual therapy techniques, the clinician first must consider whether the hypomobility occurs into flexion or extension and whether it is at the right or the left zygapophyseal joint. If side flexion is considered in terms of flexion or extension of the zygapophyseal joint, rather than the segment's movement as a whole, right side flexion is seen by most authors as causing the right joint to extend and the left to flex. If rotation is considered instead of side flexion, the issue of which joint flexes and which extends becomes much more problematic; considerable controversy exists about the coupling that occurs with rotation, and there is almost no agreement on which direction of side flexion couples with a specific direction of rotation (Table 10-3). A study using live subjects found that coupling depended not only on whether it occurred at the lumbar spine, but also at which specific level;[48-50] a cadaveric study found that at L5-S1, the coupling changed, depending on whether it was initiated by rotation or by side flexion.[43]

In addition to the lack of consensus among experts and research studies on this point, the indisputable fact is that patients do not have normal or even optimum biomechanics, therefore a discussion of normal movement may be irrelevant. The most useful course is to ignore rotation and use side flexion as the coupling model, because side flexion does not interfere with the way the joint moves; it moves down with ipsilateral side flexion and up with contralateral side flexion (Table 10-4).

If the clinical requirement for treating the patient is to increase flexion of the right zygapophyseal joint, the whole segment could be mobilized into left side flexion. However, this carries the risk that the mobilization will "hypermobilize" the left joint. The clinician must also consider that if this joint has been overstressed by its hypomobile partner, it should be protected from the force of the technique. To reduce the stresses on the opposite joint, an asymmetrical technique is chosen if an asymmetrical dysfunction exists (this is determined by asymmetrical movement restriction). Therefore, flexion of the right zygapophyseal joint (where the hypomobility dysfunction exists) must be

Table 10-3

Coupled Movements (Side Flexion and Rotation) Believed to Occur in the Spine in Different Positions*

Author	In Neutral	In Flexion	In Extension
MacConnaill		Ipsilateral[†]	Contralateral
Farfan		Contralateral	Contralateral
Kaltenborn		Ipsilateral	Ipsilateral
Grieve		Ipsilateral	Contralateral
Fryette	Contralateral	Ipsilateral	Ipsilateral
Pearcy		Ipsilateral (L5-S1)	
Oxland		Contralateral (L4-5)	
		Ipsilateral (L5-S1)[‡]	
		Contralateral (L5-S1)[§]	

*Note the differences in the findings of these researchers.
[†]*Ipsilateral* implies that both movements occur in the same direction; *contralateral* implies that they occur in opposite directions.
[‡]If side flexion is induced first.
[§]If rotation is induced first.
From Magee DJ: *Orthopedic physical assessment,* ed 4, p 488, Philadelphia, 2002, WB Saunders.

Table 10-4
Positioning for Flexion and Extension of the Zygapophyseal (Facet) Joints

Position	Flexion/Extension Side	Extremity of Position
Flexion	Bilateral flexion	Moderate
Extension	Bilateral extension	Moderate
Right side flexion	Right extension	Moderate
	Left flexion	Moderate
Left side flexion	Left extension	Moderate
	Right flexion	Moderate
Flexion and right side flexion	Left flexion	End range
Flexion and left side flexion	Right flexion	End range
Extension and right side flexion	Right extension	End range
Extension and left side flexion	Left extension	End range

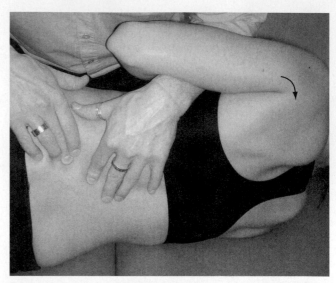

Figure 10-3
Positioning for a target segment.

combined with either rotation or side flexion to the pathological barrier of the target joint (the right zygapophyseal joint), and the opposite joint must be moved away from the end of range so that the unaffected side (the left zygapophyseal joint) is not stressed. The usual method is to select rotation as the discriminative component of the technique, but as has already been discussed, considerable controversy exists as to how rotation couples. Consequently, side flexion is the preferred method for positioning the joint at its restrictive barrier. Therefore, to increase flexion of the right zygapophyseal joint, the segment is flexed and left side flexed with the direction of the mobilization being one that increases left side flexion. To gain right zygapophyseal joint extension, the segment is extended and right side flexed, and the technique is into right side flexion. The hypomobility can be treated with the patient lying on either the right or left side.

Barriering (Locking)

If acute pain is not a factor, standard positioning can be used to mobilize a stiff or subluxed joint. When standard positioning is used, the spine is not locked specifically above and below the target segment to keep it in neutral, because there is no point in doing so; this is analogous to mobilizing the elbow to regain the last 10° of extension from the biomechanically neutral position. The effort of moving through 60° would be wasted to get to the point where treatment was needed.

If standard positioning is not used, the spine is positioned so that the target joint is moved as close to the end of its reduced physiological (or osteokinematic) range of motion as possible from above and below. This is more properly called *barriering*, rather than locking, because

the latter implies moving nontarget segments to block their motion while retaining the neutral position of the target segment. After the spine has been put in its end range of the movement to be recovered, the segments that will be levered through are "unbarriered" by passively moving them away from the end of range so that they are protected to some degree from the force of the mobilization.

Another variation in positioning is locking down to the affected segment (i.e., locking all the segments above the target joint), leaving the target joint in neutral to barrier it against the abnormal restriction. This positioning technique (Figure 10-3) is used when pain is to be treated with sub-barrier techniques (grade 1 and grade 2) or when very specific positioning is required to protect an irritable or vulnerable segment above or below the segment.

Mobilization Using the Pelvis Up or Pelvis Down Technique

The mobilization or thrust force is generated through the pelvis. Clinicians can achieve this either by using the strength of their arm (if the patient is relatively small and light) or, more usually, by exploiting gravity through the use of controlled body weight. The force is directed through the uppermost innominate, rocking the pelvic girdle on its opposite trochanter and causing side flexion of the lumbar spine. Imagine the patient lying on the left side. If the pelvis is rocked down toward the feet, left side flexion of the spine results (Figure 10-4A). If the pelvis is tipped up toward the head, right side flexion occurs (Figure 10-4B).

Rocking the pelvis upward requires positioning by arm strength and is a somewhat more complicated technique. However, it is generally a more specific technique, and the lead author's experience is that most clinicians are more

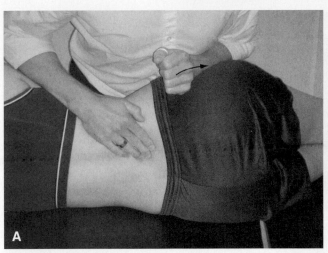 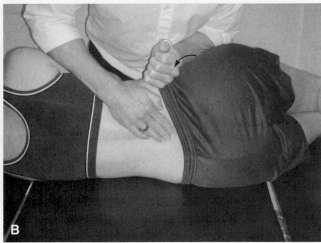

Figure 10-4
A, Pelvis down technique. **B,** Pelvis up technique.

comfortable using it to deliver the sudden, sharp thrust demanded for manipulation. The pelvis downward technique allows the clinician to use body weight, therefore it is easier to maintain for longer periods and is better used for mobilizations.

In the following treatment descriptions, the L3-4 segment is used as an example; however, these techniques may be used throughout the lumbar spine and even into the lower thoracic region.

Left Flexion Hypomobility: Pelvis Down Technique

The patient lies on the right side. The patient's hips are flexed while the target segment (L3-4) is palpated to ensure that the flexion movement goes at least through this segment (Figure 10-5, *A*). The segment is bilaterally flexed at this point. The patient's lower leg can then be extended so that the patient's thighs are not parallel; this allows rotation of the patient's pelvis when rotation locking is required for the segments below L3-4 (Figure 10-5, *B*).

The segment is now flexed and right side flexed from above; the patient's upper arm is allowed to lie forward in front of the body (this allows the side flexion to be induced into flexion), and the patient's lower arm is pulled caudally and parallel to the bed while the clinician palpates the L3-4 segment to ensure that the side flexion/flexion movement is carried through this segment (Figure 10-5, *C*). The clinician need not be concerned if the segments below are also moving, because these will be unflexed later.

The patient's upper arm can now be moved back onto the patient's side without fear of extending the spine, provided the movement is produced at the patient's shoulder and not at the trunk. The patient's lower thigh is pushed backward so that the segments below L3-4 are extended while the clinician palpates L3-4 to ensure that this segment remains in flexion (Figure 10-5, *D*). At this point, the lower segments are in side flexion but away from

their flexion barrier, whereas the target segment is fully flexed and right side flexed, meaning that the left zygapophyseal joint is fully flexed, at least as far as its restriction allows; in essence, it is at its abnormal pathological barrier and ready to be mobilized or manipulated.

To safeguard them a little more, the patient's lower segments are rotated to lock them. This is accomplished by rotating the patient's pelvis forward toward the clinician while L3-4 is palpated to ensure that the rotation does not go through this segment (Figure 10-5, *E*). If rotation in the segment occurs, coupled side flexion will alter the position and perhaps undo the previously induced side flexion, depending on the direction of coupling at this segment. The rotation should be as pure (axial) as possible to minimize the coupled side flexion, although this must occur to some degree, if not at this point then when the treatment technique is applied.

The segments below the target segment are now locked away from a flexion or extension pathological barrier (at least as much as the clinician is able to do), the segments above the target are locked in flexion and right side flexion (however, because the mobilization force going through the segments is subsequent to that going through the target segment, it should be minimal if the appropriate force is applied), and the target segment's left zygapophyseal joint is at its flexion barrier and ready to be mobilized (Figure 10-5, *F*).

The clinician "snuggles" against the patient's abdomen, linking the clinician's cranial arm with the patient's upper arm, and palpates the target segment while pulling the patient into the clinician. The flexor aspect of the clinician's caudal forearm makes contact with the soft part of the patient's innominate between the trochanter and the crest, roughly over the piriformis muscle belly, and pulls the patient's pelvis forward. The patient now is logrolled into the clinician and is stable (Figure 10-5, *G*). The patient's

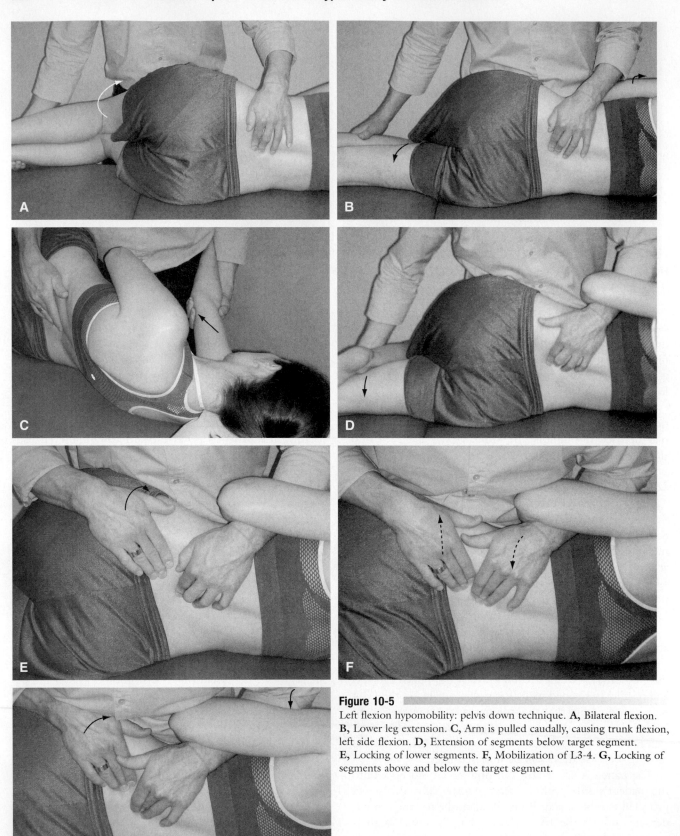

Figure 10-5

Left flexion hypomobility: pelvis down technique. **A,** Bilateral flexion.
B, Lower leg extension. **C,** Arm is pulled caudally, causing trunk flexion,
left side flexion. **D,** Extension of segments below target segment.
E, Locking of lower segments. **F,** Mobilization of L3-4. **G,** Locking of
segments above and below the target segment.

pelvis then is independently rotated forward, which sequentially rotates each spinal segment to the left (the lower vertebra is rotating to the right, of course, but the segment is rotating to the left), until slight movement is felt at the target segment. This is then undone by reversing the pelvic rotation, leaving the target segment unrotated.

The clinician's chest is then lowered onto the forearm which rests on the patient's pelvis and the clinician applies body weight onto the arm by gently lunging from the left leg. The final direction of the technique is against the worst end feel but is roughly in a sagittal plane; whether a single thrust, multiple minithrusts, or prolonged grade 3+ or grade 4+ techniques are used depends entirely on the pathological barrier to be mobilized and the clinician's decision whether to manipulate, taking into account cautions and contraindications.

Left Flexion Hypomobility: Pelvis Up Technique

The same hypomobility can be mobilized with the patient lying on the left side. One side may be chosen over the other because of the clinician's preference or the patient's requirements. For example, if a left rotatory instability is present at L5-S1 or L4-5 (or any segment below the target segment), the patient's pelvis cannot be pulled forward if the patient is lying on the left side because this would

produce right rotation; and, because of the right rotatory instability, locking could not be achieved. Similarly, if attempts at locking the lower segments with rotation produce discomfort to the point where the patient will not tolerate the attempt, an alternative position must be used.

With the patient in the left side lying position, the lumbar spine is flexed from below by flexing the patient's hips (Figure 10-6, *A*) and the patient's legs are taken from the parallel orientation by extending the lower leg in the same manner as for the previous technique. However, another method now must be used to produce flexion and right side flexion from above. The patient's upper arm is allowed to hang forward to bias the trunk to flexion in the same manner as before, but now the patient's lower arm is pulled cranially and parallel to the bed to produce right side flexion and flexion (Figure 10-6, *B*).

The clinician brings the patient's lower arm back onto the patient's side. The clinician's cranial arm is linked through and the clinician palpates the segment in the same manner as in Figure 10-5 as the patient's lower thigh is extended until the segments below the target segment are moved out of flexion and then rotated to lock them.

The patient is logrolled into the clinician in the same manner as in the previous technique, but the clinician now pulls the patient's pelvis upward, away from the

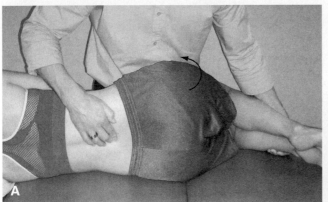
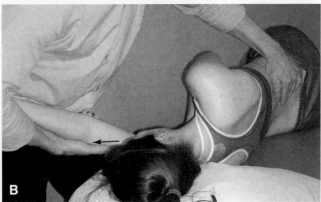
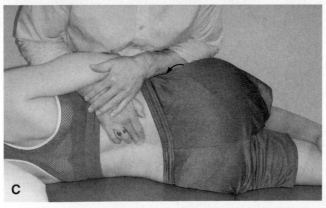

Figure 10-6

Left flexion hypomobility: pelvis up technique. **A,** Flexing the lumbar spine. **B,** Lower arm is pulled cranially. **C,** Rocking the pelvis upward.

table, rocking it onto the cranial side of the trochanter and thereby producing side flexion to the right (Figure 10-6, *C*). The clinician holds the pelvis in that position by applying controlled body weight through the forearm. The mobilization or thrust is achieved using graded amounts of body weight to the patient's pelvis. Because the pelvis is already prerocked, the clinician's "drops" (ie. the controlled body weight through the clinician's forearm to the patient's pelvis) do not have to deliberately produce side flexion but can be more or less straight downward, which is far easier.

Left Extension Hypomobility: Pelvis Down Technique

The patient lies on the left side with the hips extended as the clinician palpates the target segment to ensure that the extension movement runs through the segment (Figure 10-7, *A*). The patient's hip is then flexed to allow pelvic rotation, and the clinician makes sure that the target

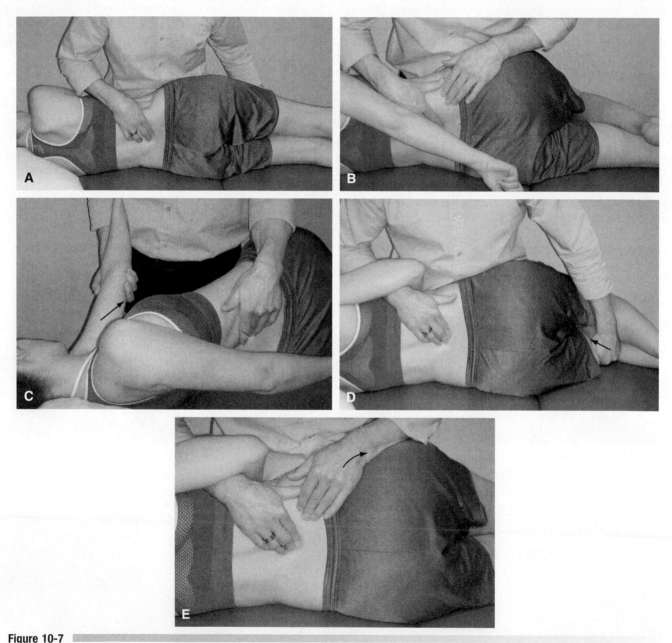

Figure 10-7

Right extension hypomobility: pelvis down technique. **A,** Extension of L3-4. **B,** Patient's arm is drawn behind to encourage extension. **C,** Lower arm is pulled caudally. **D,** Flexing segments below L3-4. **E,** Extension mobilization, pelvis down technique.

segment does not flex to take the legs out of their parallel orientation.

The patient's upper arm then is positioned behind the patient so that the side flexion is induced into extension (Figure 10-7, *B*). The patient's lower arm is pulled caudally but away from the bed to right side flex and extend the spine (Figure 10-7, *C*).

The patient's upper arm is now moved back onto the patient's side, and the patient's lower thigh is pulled forward to flex the segments below L3-4 while the clinician palpates L3-4 to make sure this segment remains in extension (Figure 10-7, *D*). At this point, the lower segments are away from their extension barrier but in side flexion, whereas the target segment is fully extended and left side flexed, meaning that the left zygapophyseal joint is fully extended at least as far as its restriction allows. The L3-4 left zygapophyseal joint is now at its abnormal pathological barrier and ready to be mobilized or manipulated.

The patient is now logrolled toward the clinician, locking the lower segments with axial rotation (Figure 10-7, *E*), and the clinician applies a caudal force to the patient's innominate with the forearm resting on the innominate to rock the pelvis downward over the trochanter.

Right Extension Hypomobility: Pelvis Up Technique

As in the previous description, the target segment needs to be extended and right side flexed; however, the patient now is lying on the left side. Again, the clinician's preference or the patient's requirements determine which side lying position is used. For example, if a left rotatory instability is present at L5-S1 or L4-5 (or any segment below the target segment), the patient's pelvis cannot be pulled forward if the patient is lying on the right side because this would produce left rotation; and, because of the left rotatory instability, locking could not be achieved. Similarly, if attempts at locking the lower segments with left rotation produce discomfort to the point where the patient will not tolerate the attempt, an alternative position must be used.

With the patient in the right side lying position, the patient's lumbar spine is extended from below by extending the patient's hips, and the legs are taken from their parallel orientation by flexing the patient's lower leg in the same manner as for the previous technique (see Figure 10-7A, which shows the opposite side). However, now another method must be used to produce extension and right side flexion from above. The patient's upper arm is positioned behind the patient to bias the trunk to extension in the same manner as before, but now the patient's lower arm is pulled cranially and upward toward the ceiling, away from the bed, to produce right side flexion and flexion (Figure 10-8, *A*).

The clinician brings the patient's lower arm back to the patient's side. The clinician's cranial arm is linked through the patient's upper arm and the clinician palpates the target segment as the patient's lower thigh is flexed until the segments below the target segment are moved out of extension. These segments are then rotated forward (right rotation) to lock them (Figure 10-8, *B*). The patient is logrolled into the clinician in the same manner as in the previous technique, but now the clinician pulls the patient's pelvis upward, away from the table, rocking it onto the cranial side of the trochanter, thereby producing side flexion to the right. The clinician holds the patient's pelvis in this position by applying controlled body weight through the forearm (Figure 10-8, *C*). The mobilization or thrust is achieved using graded amounts of the clinician's body weight to the patient's pelvis; because the patient's pelvis is already prerocked, the clinician's "drops" do not have to deliberately produce side flexion but can be more or less straight downward, which is far easier.

Superior Vertebrae Hypomobility: Rotation Lock

If a problem above the target segment must be treated (e.g., instability or discomfort with side flexion barriering such that either side flexion or the flexion or extension pathological barriers cannot be achieved), the vertebrae may be locked by means of rotation, provided the rotation does not enter the target segment. This technique is also useful when a considerable size discrepancy exists between the clinician and the patient, because rotation is easier to achieve. Side flexion requires more clinician upper body strength than does rotation, and it is not as easy to use specifically. However, care must be taken to avoid rotating through the segment (if the clinician wants to avoid issues with the coupling theory). The rotation may be combined with either flexion or extension, and the choice depends on the condition of the segments to be locked. For example, if a painful extension hypermobility exists, it can be avoided by locking the segments with rotation and flexion; because the lock does not enter the target segment, it does not matter whether flexion, extension, or right or left rotation is used.

For the lock with rotation technique, the patient lies on one side. The clinician then barriers the target segment from below through flexion or extension, as required by the dysfunction, in the manner already described. The patient's lower arm is now pulled anteriorly, away from the body, which rotates the patient's trunk around the vertical axis of the body (Figure 10-9, *A*). If the patient is lying on the left side, right rotation occurs; if the patient is lying on the right side, left rotation occurs. To bias the rotation to flexion, the patient's upper arm is allowed to hang forward in front of the body, and the patient's lower arm is pulled parallel to the bed. If extension rotation is required, the patient's upper arm is positioned behind the patient, and the patient's lower arm is pulled away from body but toward the ceiling (Figure 10-9, *B*).

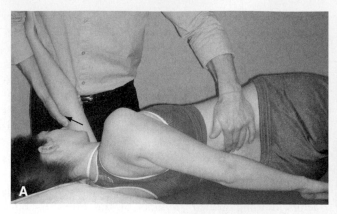
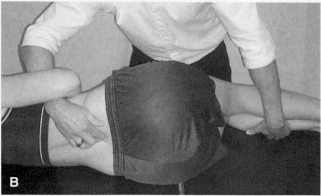
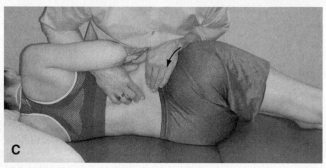

Figure 10-8

Right extension hypomobility: pelvis up technique. **A,** Arm is pulled cranially and upward. **B,** Patient's lower thigh is flexed. **C,** Right side flexion, pelvis up technique.

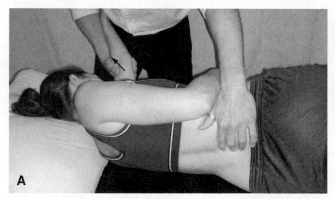
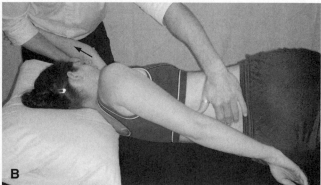

Figure 10-9

Superior vertebrae hypomobility: rotation lock. **A,** Patient's lower arm is pulled anteriorly, causing right rotation. **B,** Extension rotation.

Cautions (Yellow Flags) and Contraindications (Red Flags) to Manual Therapy

The risk of serious adverse effects from manipulative therapy (and presumably mobilization) to the lumber spine is considered very low.[27,51] However, the actual risk is not well understood. In a review of the literature, Assendelft et al.[28] found 61 cases of either cauda equine syndrome or lumbar disc herniation after manipulation, about 21% of all serious complications in this review. Another review of the literature for the years 1911 to 1989 found only 10 cases of cauda equina syndrome related to manipulative treatment.[29]

Some clinicians may believe that only one contraindication exists to manual treatment of the spine, intolerance to the technique, and that all other considerations are "detail." However, the detail is important. Presumably, manipulation carries a higher threat to the patient in that the force is sudden and not under the patient's control; therefore, any unfortunate effect occurs without warning if the detail has not been recognized before the technique is applied. This is not to say that mobilization does not carry some degree of risk. Indeed, any treatment that is completely without risk is almost certainly without benefit. Any adverse effects from mobilization are likely to be less drastic (e.g., are less likely to cause fracture and bleeding) than manipulative techniques, especially in the lumbar spine, where injuries to the arterial system seem not to occur unless a predisposition exists. Therefore, all general contraindications to manipulation and mobilization must be considered as either absolute or relative contraindications.

Absolute contraindications are those that scream "don't touch me," and this demand must be obeyed by all clinicians who care anything about the patient's and their own well-being, at least until adequate objective imaging and other medical tests have ruled out any risk. For example, multiple sclerosis produces spinal cord signs and symptoms, but it is not necessarily a contraindication to manual therapy. Examples of absolute contraindications include instability, fractures, acute pain, severe osteoporosis, bleeding disorders, acute cauda equina syndrome, spinal cord compromise, severe rheumatoid arthritis, a suggestion of cancer or visceral disease, and a truly disoriented or psychotic patient.

Relative contraindications are those that are contraindications for some clinicians, usually the newcomer to manual therapy, but not for the more experienced manual therapist; however, even these require extreme caution. Relative contraindications include pregnancy, spinal stenosis, spondylolisthesis in a nontarget segment, a patient with a past history of cancer who has had a recent clear screening test, equivocating signs of disc herniation, atypical patterns, neurological signs and symptoms, collagenous disease, and a history of poor response to manual techniques.

The main risks are misdiagnosis of cancer (especially prostatic or metastatic) and enlargement of a disc herniation with or without cauda equina compression, but other conditions must be considered. Table 10-5 lists contraindications and the possible problems that may arise if these risks are realized. However, clinicians must understand that mere lists are not the same as being faced with problematic conditions, and the clinician must be more adept at recognizing presentations that preclude manual therapy than at performing manual therapy.

For the newcomer to manual therapy, the wise course is to develop a clear understanding of the indications for manipulation and to avoid treating any patient who does not fall within these strict parameters, at least until the clinician becomes more experienced and confident with both examination and treatment techniques. The profile of the patient with mechanical back pain has been described numerous times, even in this chapter. Flynn et al.[47] looked at factors that would determine which patients would have a greater chance of a successful outcome from manipulation, and Fritz et al.[42] investigated factors that would reduce that chance. Between the two studies, a shorter duration of symptoms, minimum referred pain, restricted range of motion in the lumbar spine, and normal hip rotation range of motion indicated a better chance of a successful outcome, particularly when these factors were clustered in the individual patient. In effect, these criteria suggest the standard patient with mechanical low back pain who does not have more complex problems or contraindicating signs or symptoms. It is reasonable to suppose that these factors similarly would point to a successful outcome for mobilization and that they would also indicate patients with a greater likelihood of responding well to manual treatment in general.

High Risk Indicators in Spinal Mobilization

General indicators of high risk in the mobilization of the lumbar spine, especially manipulation, include suggestions of disc herniation and cauda equina syndrome:
- Radicular pain, especially bilateral
- Paresthesia, especially bilateral
- Severe somatic sciatica, especially bilateral
- Motor paresis, especially multisegmental and bilateral
- Sensory paresis, especially multisegmental and bilateral
- Saddle paresthesia
- Saddle anesthesia
- Segmental or multisegmental hyperreflexia or areflexia
- High frequency, low volume bladder
- Bladder incontinence
- Lack of rectal expulsive power
- L1 or L2 palsy
- Exacerbations related to diet
- Hematuria
- Severe leg pain without straight leg raising (SLR) limitation
- Severe limitation of range of motion
- Deviation with radicular pain

Signs of an Enlarging Disc Herniation
- Peripheralization of symptoms
- Bilateral symptoms
- Appearance of radicular pain
- Appearance of neurological signs
- Numbness that replaces paresthesia
- Increase in the severity of the articular signs
- Appearance of urinary retention or incontinence signs
- Decrease in the straight leg raise or prone knee bending

Table 10-5

Contraindications and Cautions to Lumbar Manipulation and Mobilization

Cautions/Contraindications	Characteristics and Potential Problems
Neoplastic disease	Medical diagnosis: Possibility of fracture
Cauda equina signs and symptoms	Bilateral, multisegmental lower motor neuron signs and symptoms, including bladder dysfunction: Possibility of serious compression damage and permanent palsy
Spinal cord signs and symptoms	Multisegmental upper motor neuron signs and symptoms: Possibility of serious compression damage and permanent deficit
Nonmechanical causes	Minimal musculoskeletal signs and symptoms: Wasted effort and delay in getting appropriate care
Trilevel segmental signs	Disc compression (can affect a maximum of two levels of the nerve root): Possibility of neoplastic disease, spondylolisthesis, or cauda equina compression
Neuropathic pain	Nerve root damage or severe inflammation
Sign of the buttock	Empty end feel on hip flexion; painful weakness of hip extension; limited straight leg raising, trunk flexion, and hip flexion; noncapsular pattern of hip restriction; swollen buttock: Possible serious disease (e.g., sacral fracture, neoplasm, infection)
Various serious pathologies	Empty end feel and severe multidirectional spasm
Adverse joint environment	Spasm: Acute inflammation, fracture
Acute fracture or dislocation	Immediate onset of post-traumatic pain and loss of function
Bone disease	Deep pain and relatively minimal musculoskeletal signs: Wasted effort and possibility of a fracture
Acute rheumatoid arthritis episode	Medical diagnosis: Possibility of increased tissue damage and severe exacerbation
Infective arthritis	Severe inflammation and reddening: Delay in getting appropriate medical care
Emotionally dependent patient	Seeks manipulation: Long-term dependency without much hope of benefit
Chronic pain/fibromyalgia–type syndromes	Inadequate signs to explain the patient's widespread symptoms: Long-term dependency without much hope of benefit
Rheumatoid arthritis	Medical diagnosis: Possibility of increased tissue damage and severe exacerbation
Osteoporosis	Medical diagnosis: Fracture
Spinal nerve (root) compression	Segmental neurological signs: Probable wasted effort and possibility of increasing the compression
Spondylolisthesis	Radiographic evidence: Exacerbation of signs and symptoms
Hypermobility	Clinical finding: Increased hypermobility and pain
Acute pain states	Onset of pain before or simultaneous with tissue resistance: Possibility of severe exacerbation
Pregnancy	Risk of ligamentous damage as a result of relaxing effect and risk of coincident miscarriage
Repeated steroid injections	Tearing of collagen tissue
Long-term systemic steroid use	Tearing of collagen tissue and fracture
History of neoplastic disease	Risk of recurrence
Distal pain on movement	Acute root compression or severe joint inflammation
Nuclear prolapse or meniscoid entrapment	Springy end feel
Central or lateral stenosis	Paresthesia that dominates pain

Summary

Manual therapy for mechanical low back pain, particularly lumbar hypomobility, is reasonably well established, both from a research perspective and as a standard of care for clinical treatment. The risk is low and the benefits, at least over the short term, are great, as long as appropriate inclusion and exclusion criteria are met. This means that before applying any technique, clinicians must have exercised competent diagnostic skills to rule out medical conditions that would contraindicate a particular type of manual treatment.

References

To enhance this text and add value for the reader, all references have been incorporated into a CD-ROM that is provided with this text. The reader can view the reference source and access it online whenever possible. There are a total of 51 references for this chapter.

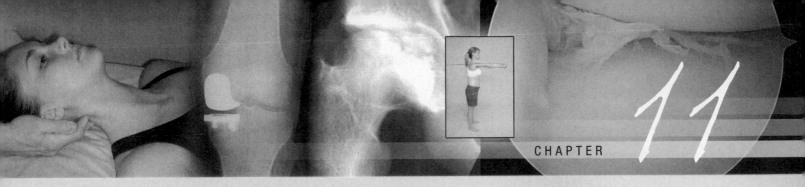

CHAPTER 11

LUMBAR SPINE: TREATMENT OF INSTABILITY AND DISORDERS OF MOVEMENT CONTROL

Paul W. Hodges, Paulo H. Ferreira, and Manuela L. Ferreira

Introduction

Control of the spine is dynamic. With this in mind, it is clear that exercise interventions aimed at rehabilitation and prevention of low back and pelvic pain should not simply maximize stability; rather, they must optimize the balance between movement and stability. Many exercise interventions have been proposed to improve control of the spine and pelvis. This chapter considers the requirements for spinal control, changes in this system that occur with low back and pelvic pain, strategies to train optimum control of the spine, and evidence for the efficacy of interventions that aim to improve motor control of the spine and pelvis.

Dynamic Control of the Lumbar Spine and Pelvis

Biomechanical Requirements for Dynamic Control of the Lumbar Spine and Pelvis

For proper function, the movement of the spine must be controlled dynamically. The requirements for dynamic control can be described in terms of a range of interdependent goals that ultimately must be integrated to meet the objectives of stability and movement. The term *stability* generally is defined as the property of a structure that allows it to return to equilibrium if perturbed.[1] In this sense, the spine is inherently unstable and depends on the contribution of muscles to maintain its stability. In vitro experiments show that without muscular support, instability can occur in any direction, and the lumbar spine without muscle buckles when loaded with as little as 9 kg (19.8 lbs) (about 90 N).[2] Buckling or instability of the spine can involve any combination of the six degrees of freedom that must be controlled

at each intervertebral segment (three rotations and three translations) and at the sacroiliac joints (Figure 11-1). Although instability can occur in any direction, static control of rotation buckling is the primary consideration in most contemporary models of spinal stability.[1-3]

If the spine can be stabilized and stiffened by muscle contraction, then greater force is required to perturb it. Controlling the movement or the "stiffness" of the trunk through the co-contraction of muscles that act on the lumbar spine is one mechanism the nervous system uses to meet the demands for stability and to control buckling. Stiffening of the spine, from the perspective of function and movement, does not involve simple co-contraction; rather, it requires carefully orchestrated patterns of muscle activity. Why does the nervous system go to so much trouble to control the unstable structure of the spine when such control could easily be achieved through co-contraction and stiffening? The answer is, to maintain the flexibility and mobility of the spine. Flexibility is necessary for healthy functioning of the spine, and it is critical for a number of reasons, not least of which is enabling movement, shock absorption, breathing, and balance control. Therefore dynamic stability/control of the spine cannot be explained by co-contraction and stiffness control alone and requires consideration of other issues.

Importance of Spinal Flexibility

Flexibility of the spine is necessary for:
- Movement
- Shock absorption
- Breathing
- Balance control

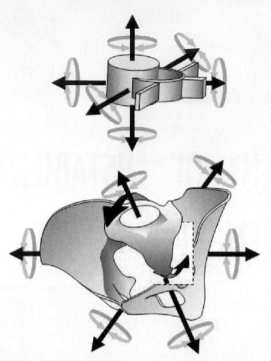

Figure 11-1

Six degrees of freedom, including rotation about and translation along each of the three orthogonal axes, must be controlled to maintain healthy spinal and pelvic function.

The notion of stability can also be applied to a trajectory of movement in which a movement is stable if the path can be maintained despite perturbation.[4] Therefore the path of the spine and pelvis must be controlled dynamically. Taken another way, it is important to consider that simple control of the static equilibrium of the spine is not sufficient; the "stable" and efficient path of moving structures of the spine must be controlled. For example, during walking, the spine is not maintained in a single position; rather, the lumbar spine and pelvis move around each axis to aid in the propulsion of the body and the control of the center of mass.

Movement can contribute to the control of stability of the spine and regulation of imposed forces. For instance, studies of arm movement suggest that when a limb is moved, the nervous system does not simply stiffen the trunk; rather, the spine and pelvis are moved in the direction opposite to the perturbation.[5,6] This dampens the impact on the spine and limits the effect of the perturbation. In addition, movement provides an element of shock absorption. If a force is applied to a stiffened structure, more force is transmitted to adjacent regions. Therefore, although coordinated movement of the spine requires more complex control strategies than simple stiffening (and hence a more complicated controller), it is likely to be more ideal in the long term.

A final consideration is that, looking beyond the demand to control buckling or potential instability and motion, other functions obviously need to be considered. For instance, the spine contributes to respiration. This is not only because of the direct contribution of spinal movement to expansion of the thorax during inspiration, but also because small amplitude motions of the spine are required to compensate for the disturbance to balance caused by breathing.[7-9] If spinal stability were maintained simply by stiffening, respiratory efficiency would be compromised by the reduced contribution of spinal movement. Similarly, balance control requires a contribution from the hips and trunk. Two basic balance strategies have been described, the "ankle" strategy and the "hip" strategy. Under conditions of quiet stance and minor perturbations, postural equilibrium can be maintained by movements about the ankle, with the body acting as an inverted pendulum (ankle strategy). When the perturbation of increased torque at the ankle is insufficient to maintain balance, movement of the hip and trunk is required (hip strategy). Movement of the spine, therefore, is essential to maintain balance. If movement is restricted, balance is compromised.[10]

Finally, movement is required to minimize energy expenditure. For instance, rotation of the spine and pelvis around each axis during gait reduces the displacement of the center of mass and the associated energy requirement to achieve this reduced displacement.[11]

Basic Balance Strategies

- Ankle strategy
- Hip strategy

In summary, healthy functioning of the spine requires a maintenance of balance between movement and stability. As such, simple attempts to stiffen the spine through co-contraction, although appropriate under some circumstances, are unlikely to be ideal for many tasks. Therefore, dynamic control of the spine requires complex control with flexible strategies to meet the multiple demands placed on the spine during function.

Guiding Principles for a Healthy Functioning Spine

- Static models are unlikely to be able to predict the ideal strategies for motor control
- Optimum stability is not the same as maximum stability
- The spine requires movement for ideal function

Guiding Principles: Requirements for Spinal Control

- Control of rotation
- Control of translation
- Control of movement trajectory
- Movement as a strategy to overcome perturbations
- Contribution of spinal movement to respiration
- Contribution of spinal movement to equilibrium control
- Contribution of spinal movement to minimization of energy expenditure

Neural Mechanisms for Dynamic Control of the Lumbar Spine and Pelvis

Panjabi[12] recognized that, in light of the demands placed on the spine, lumbopelvic stability depends not only on the passive elements (intervertebral discs, ligaments, joint capsules and facet, joints), but also on the active elements (muscles) and the controller (nervous system). When the spine is considered in a static sense, only one muscle activation strategy is required to meet the demands of stability: co-contraction of the large superficial trunk muscles to increase spinal stiffness. Observations from a number of tasks, such as lifting, are consistent with this proposal.[13] As mentioned, control of buckling is critical for maintaining healthy spinal function; however, this perspective fails to consider how *movement* of the spine is controlled or how the stability of the movement trajectory is maintained. In addition, the contribution of the trunk muscles to other homeostatic functions, such as balance, breathing, and continence, further complicates the nervous system's task of controlling the spine and pelvis. Strategies other than simple co-contraction are available and are necessary to control the movement and position of the spine and pelvis in a dynamic sense. Basic static models of stability are unlikely to be able to predict either the ideal strategies for lumbopelvic control or the ideal exercise interventions for back pain.

Controlling the spine is an immense task for the nervous system. To detect the current status of spinal stability, the nervous system must use the input from the range of mechanoreceptors in the muscles and passive structures of the spine, as well as input from the visual and vestibular systems regarding the status of the spine and the rest of the body with respect to their surroundings. The individual must consider the demands of the intended action by considering the dynamics of the intended action (built up over a lifetime of movement experience) and select an appropriate strategy of muscle activation, movement, and stability to meet the demands of the task. The appropriate muscle activation strategy must be initiated, and any appropriate adjustments must be made during the course of the activity to ensure success. The complexity of this control and the level of the nervous system involved are primarily determined by the temporal demands.

When a task is voluntarily initiated, time is available to plan and optimize movement control. In this situation, the postural adjustment precedes the movement and is referred to as *feedforward* or *preparatory adjustment*. This type of control is mediated by feedback. However, when the nervous system responds to an unexpected disturbance (e.g., a trip or a slip), the time delay must be short; therefore, the complexity of the response is usually limited, and the strategy involves a combination of reflex components and triggered components (i.e., multisegmental responses that are faster than voluntary movement but more flexible than reflexes).[6] Clearly, the simplest strategy for meeting the demands for control would be to stiffen the entire trunk by co-contraction to prevent injury and protect the spine; however, because of the need to maintain mobility, more complex strategies are involved.

A critical element in this system is the availability and accuracy of sensory information from the mechanoreceptors in the intervertebral discs, joint capsules, ligaments, and muscles of the spine and pelvis, all of which contribute to the awareness of spinal position and movement. Evidence of basic spinal mechanisms that maintain and control motion is demonstrated by the density of the proprioceptors in the deep muscles[14] and their ability to detect small intervertebral motion. Furthermore, electrical stimulation of the mechanoreceptors in the intervertebral disc[15] and joint capsule of the sacroiliac joint[15] leads to short latency responses of the paraspinal and pelvic muscles. A noteworthy fact is that deficits in sensory function are commonly reported in low back pain,[16,17] which may underlie changes in the accuracy of movement control.

One way to view movement control strategies is to consider a spectrum ranging from static/stiffening control at one end to dynamic strategies involving movement at the other (Figure 11-2). Tasks that involve high load, poor predictability, and the need to maintain the alignment of the spine are likely to involve co-contraction/stiffening strategies, because these strategies are likely to provide the greatest amount of stability. In contrast, tasks that involve lower load and greater predictability or that require greater movement are likely to involve a more complex, dynamic strategy. This simple conceptual model considers just a few of the many factors registered by the nervous system in the selection of an appropriate response; even so, it can help the clinician understand the selections made and the muscle activation patterns initiated to meet the movement demands. The nervous system has a large number of muscles available to contribute to these control strategies. Although all muscles are likely to contribute to some extent, anatomical features are likely to influence the decision to recruit specific muscles for a particular function.

Muscular Mechanisms for Control of the Spine and Pelvis

Large superficial muscles of the lumbar spine and pelvis are required for optimum control of the spine. Bergmark[18] defined the superficial muscles that ascend from the pelvis

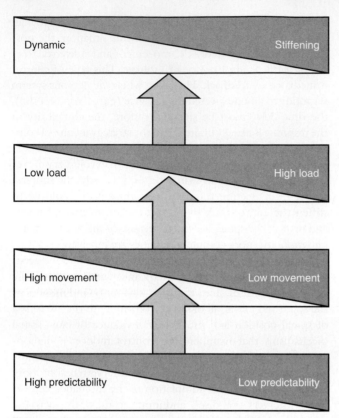

Figure 11-2

A spectrum of control strategies, ranging from dynamic control to static stiffening, is available to the nervous system, depending on task demands. The strategy used is influenced by a range of factors, including the load, movement requirement, and predictability.

to the rib cage as *global muscles.* Contraction of these muscles generates torque to oppose external forces and to move the spine, the pelvis, and the whole body. Co-contraction of these muscles on either side of the trunk provides an ideal strategy to increase the stiffness of the trunk and is common during tasks such as lifting.[13] However, during many functional activities, rather than simple co-contraction to increase trunk stiffness, the activity of these muscles is carefully timed to match perfectly the movement and stability demands. For instance, the superficial trunk muscles, such as the obliquus externus abdominis and the lumbar erector spinae, are active in alternating bursts in association with arm movements to oppose the reactive forces, creating a dynamic strategy of trunk movement rather than simple trunk stiffening.[5,6,19] Furthermore, during gait, global muscles co-contract at heel strike (the time of maximum impact to the spine) but have specific phasic bursts associated with forward propulsion of the body, displacement of the center of mass, and changes in direction of pelvic motion.[20]

Many studies have attempted to identify the global muscles with the greatest potential to maintain stability of the spine. Although muscles such as the obliquus externus abdominis and the thoracic erector spinae are often highlighted as

making a large contribution,[3] the selection of muscles for a specific function depends on a range of factors, including the direction of force. In general, the specific pattern of superficial/global muscle activity is task specific.

In addition to the essential contribution of the large superficial muscles to the control of movement and the stability of the lumbar spine and pelvis, the central nervous system (CNS) relies on the contribution of the deep muscles of the trunk. Bergmark[18] defined these muscles as local muscles with attachments directly to the lumbar vertebrae. Data from a range of biomechanical and in vitro or in vivo studies have confirmed the essential contribution of these muscles to spinal control. For instance, data from biomechanical studies,[21] animal experiments,[22] in vitro human experiments,[23] and in vivo human experiments[24] indicate that activity of the lumbar multifidus contributes to control of intervertebral motion. Likewise, animal studies[25] and in vitro[26] and in vivo human studies[5,6] indicate that activity of the transverse abdominis, the deepest abdominal muscle, contributes to control of intervertebral[6,27] and sacroiliac[28] motion, particularly translations. These muscles often are activated as a component of the control strategies in a range of tasks, early and tonically, and in a manner that generally is not specific to the direction of forces acting on the spine.

The deep muscles contribute minimally to flexion and extension of the trunk because of their anatomical location and line of action. The transversus abdominis has a minimal ability to act as a flexor, because its fibers can angle only up to 12° from horizontal. The fibers of the multifidus are close to the center of rotation of the lumbar joints and have a very small moment arm. However, by contributing to intra-abdominal pressure, tensioning of the thoracolumbar fascia, and the direct effects of contraction on the intervertebral segments, these muscles provide an additional contribution to intervertebral control. In fact, because of these muscles' limited contribution to the generation of torque at the trunk, they provide a major advantage to the nervous system: the ability to influence intervertebral control during movement without limiting motion through range.[22] A major control issue for the more superficial/global muscles is that these muscles also generate torque. This means that whenever they are recruited to provide control to the spine and pelvis, additional muscles contract to control the complex torques generated by contraction of the superficial mobilizer muscles. Therefore deep muscles provide a possible solution to simplify the control of the spine and potentially an ideal solution for maintaining dynamic control by allowing control during movement.

It is critical to note, however, that most functional tasks require coordinated activity of both the deep and superficial muscles to meet the demands for control and movement. The balance between the deep and superficial muscles is likely to be guided by the principles outlined in Figure 11-2. In this figure, tasks that lie to the right involve greater co-contraction of the superficial muscles. Tasks to the left are likely to have a greater contribution from deep muscles and fine-tuned activation of the superficial muscles to match the demands of the task exactly.

Because intra-abdominal pressure and fascial tension are important for the control of intervertebral motion, other muscles that surround the abdominal cavity provide an additional contribution. These muscles include the diaphragm and the pelvic floor muscles. Data from in vitro[29] and in vivo[9] studies confirm that activity of these muscles contributes to the control of the lumbar spine (Figure 11-3) and sacroiliac joints (Figure 11-4). Because these muscles play a dual role (i.e., they are involved in control of stability and movement of the spine, as well as respiration and continence), this introduces additional complexity for the nervous system.

Guiding Principles: Selection of a Muscle Activation Strategy

- Superficial/global muscles co-contract to stiffen the trunk during tasks with high load and poor predictability
- Phasic bursts of superficial/global muscle activity are matched to the demands of a task to overcome external and internal forces
- Deep local muscles generally are active early and tonically, in a manner less dependent on the direction of force

---

The Challenge to Coordinate the Multiple Functions of the Trunk Muscles

In addition to the control of the movement and stability of the spine and pelvis, the trunk muscles have important respiratory and continence functions. During inspiration, the diaphragm (the principal muscle of this activity) depresses the central tendon and elevates the lower ribs, increasing the lateral dimensions of the thorax. At the same time, the erector spinae and latissimus dorsi extend the spine to assist inspiration and oppose deflationary forces transmitted to the vertebral column by the rib cage articulations.[30] During strong expiration, the abdominal muscles deflate the rib cage and elevate the diaphragm to assist expiration (Figure 11-5).[31] Although many authors argue that the abdominal muscles are not active during quiet breathing and that expiration is a passive process involving elastic recoil of the rib cage and lungs, recent data suggest that some regions of the muscles are modulated with quiet breathing. Expiratory activity of the paraspinal muscles is also likely to be required to counteract the flexion moment of the expiratory abdominal muscles, especially during strong expiratory efforts. Activity of the pelvic floor muscles is required during breathing to support the abdominal contents and control continence in association with variation in intra-abdominal pressure during respiration.[32] This is necessary during both inspiration and expiration.

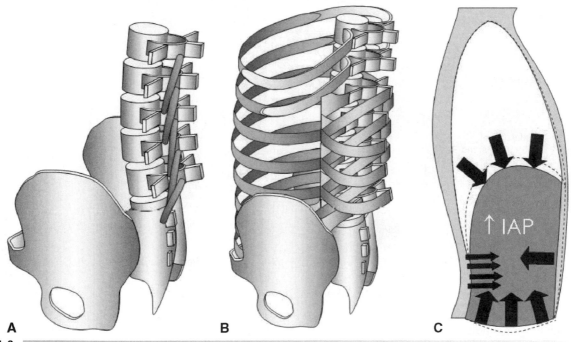

A　　　　　　　　B　　　　　　　　C

Figure 11-3

Deep muscles of the trunk contribute to control of the lumbar spine. **A,** Multifidus contributes to control of intervertebral motion by means of gentle compression between segments and control of posteroanterior translation. **B,** Transversus abdominis contributes to control of intervertebral motion by means of increased intra-abdominal pressure and tension in the thoracolumbar fascia. **C,** These effects depend on co-contraction of the diaphragm and pelvic floor muscles.

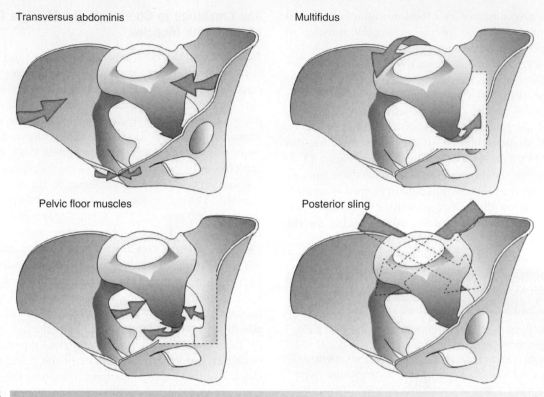

Transversus abdominis

Multifidus

Pelvic floor muscles

Posterior sling

Figure 11-4

Deep muscles of the trunk contribute to the control of sacroiliac (SI) joint stability. Contraction of the transversus abdominis and the pelvic floor muscles provides compression to the SI joint. Although contraction of the pelvic floor muscles counternutates the sacrum (rotates the sacrum posteriorly relative to the ilia), which places the joint in a less stable position, this can be counteracted by activity of the multifidus and potentially the posterior sling muscles (gluteus maximus and latissimus dorsi) that attach to the thoracolumbar fascia.

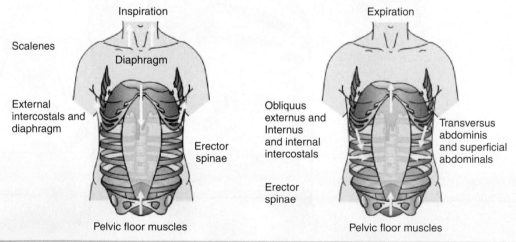

Inspiration

Expiration

Scalenes

Diaphragm

External intercostals and diaphragm

Erector spinae

Pelvic floor muscles

Obliquus externus and Internus and internal intercostals

Transversus abdominis and superficial abdominals

Erector spinae

Pelvic floor muscles

Figure 11-5

Contribution of the trunk muscles to inspiration and expiration.

The respiratory functions of the trunk muscles must be coordinated with the demands placed on these muscles to contribute to spinal control. The fact that respiratory muscles contribute to the strategies used by the nervous system to control the trunk has been well established. Activity of the diaphragm and transversus abdominis is initiated before rapid limb movements[6] and is tonic during repetitive movements of the arm[33,34] and walking.[35] Furthermore, the intercostal muscles are active during trunk rotation.[36]

The challenge for the nervous system is to coordinate the postural and respiratory functions. Under normal conditions, these functions can be easily coordinated. During repetitive arm movement, the diaphragm is tonically active, consistent with the demand to control spinal stability, but this activity is phasically modulated in conjunction with breathing to maintain airflow.[34] Similar responses of the abdominal muscles have been identified during walking.[35]

Under certain conditions, the coordination of these two functions is compromised, because a potential conflict exists in the activity of abdominal muscles during simultaneous lifting and ventilatory challenge.[37-39] Postural activity of the diaphragm is reduced during repetitive arm movement. The activity of the trunk muscles in association with spinal stability may be compromised when respiratory demand is increased; this also occurs in a person breathing with an increased dead space to induce hypercapnia (elevated CO_2 in the blood) and in people with chronic airway disease, both of which repetitively challenge spinal stability.[40,41] Reduced contribution of the trunk muscles to spinal stability during periods of increased respiratory demand may compromise control of spinal stability during exercise. Furthermore, spinal loading is increased by muscle co-contraction during lifting while breathing with increased respiratory demand.[37]

In addition to contributing to airflow, the trunk muscles also move the spine and pelvis in a manner that counteracts the body sway caused by breathing. Movement of the spine and pelvis and activity of the lumbopelvic muscles are time locked to the respiratory movement of the rib cage and abdomen[8,9] and match the displacement on the center of mass induced by breathing. Furthermore, motion of the center of pressure is increased with breathing in people with low back pain (LBP);[42,43] this is consistent with the finding that stiffness of the spine is increased in this population.

In terms of continence mechanisms, the demand to coordinate functions appears less complex. Activity of the pelvic floor muscles may contribute to lumbopelvic control in a number of ways. For instance, the pelvic floor muscles support the abdominal contents when intra-abdominal pressure is increased. This provides an indirect contribution to spinal control by means of pressure and tension in the thoracolumbar fascia.[9] The effect of pelvic floor muscle activity on the thoracolumbar fascia is due to the dependence of tension in this structure on the pressure in the abdominal cavity.[44] In addition, tension in the pelvic floor muscles increases the stiffness of the sacroiliac joints in women.[29]

Functions of the Pelvic Floor Muscles

- Control continence mechanisms
- Support abdominal contents through increased intra-abdominal pressure
- Support spine through tension and pressure in thoracolumbar fascia
- Stiffen sacroiliac joints

The demand for pelvic floor muscle activity to contribute to continence is unlikely to compete with the demands for lumbopelvic control. That is, increased activity of the pelvic floor muscles would enhance both continence and lumbopelvic control. Consistent with this proposal, recent data indicate that activity of the pelvic floor muscles contributes to postural activity associated with perturbations to the spine from arm movement.[9] However, the activity of the other muscles surrounding the abdominal cavity (i.e., the diaphragm and abdominal muscles) also influences continence. The activity of these muscles for spinal control increases intra-abdominal pressure and places increased demand on the pelvic floor muscles. In stress urinary incontinence, pelvic floor muscle activity may be compromised, and recent data suggest that women with stress incontinence often have increased activity of the obliquus externus abdominis.[45] Together, these changes may be associated with a combination of incontinence and poor dynamic control of the spine and pelvis.

It is important to consider that static models of spinal control do not take into account the interaction of spinal control, breathing, and continence. This is important because, although activation of a muscle such as the obliquus externus abdominis may provide the optimum contribution to stability in a specific task when co-contracting with the paraspinal muscles, this may restrict the person's ability to expand the rib cage to inspire. Therefore static strategies for spinal stability that stiffen the spine and prevent spinal and rib cage movement are likely to be unsustainable because of their effect on the essential demands of breathing. Because it does not take into consideration effects such as this, the static model is unlikely to accurately explain the strategies used by the CNS to control the spine. From another perspective, it is important to consider that deficits in respiration and continence may lead to compromised spinal control. Recent epidemiological studies suggest that continence and respiration are associated with an increased risk of low back pain (see the later section on changes in muscle structure as a precursor to low back and pelvic pain).

Guiding Principles for a Dynamic Spine

- Trunk muscles contribute to a range of functions in addition to their role in controlling movement and helping to maintain the stability of the spine
- Trunk muscles play a role in breathing, continence, and balance
- Incontinence and breathing disorders increase the risk for the development of low back pain
- The goal of increasing the stability of the spine may be achieved in different ways in different individuals and to different degrees

---

Changes in Dynamic Control with Lumbopelvic Pain

Dynamic Control of the Spine in Low Back and Pelvic Pain

The changes that occur in the control of the trunk muscles with LBP and pelvic pain vary considerably. An increase,[46] a decrease,[47] and no change[48,49] in muscle activity have been reported in the literature. This inconsistency and researchers' incomplete understanding of the motor adaptations in LBP and pelvic pain have led to a major controversy in clinical practice. Although recent physiological and biomechanical studies suggest that spine stability is augmented in LBP through adaptation in the activity of the trunk muscles,[50] paradoxically, clinical literature argues that exercise should aim to increase stability to compensate for spinal instability.[12] Variable trunk muscle activity in back pain and limited evaluation of stability have meant that neither view has strong support. Yet the number of exercise programs to enhance stability has exploded, despite lack of evidence that such programs reduce back pain. In contrast, strategies to restore muscle coordination improve outcomes.[51,52] Understanding the pathophysiology of trunk control changes in LBP is critical to the selection of the most effective preventive and rehabilitation strategies.

Changes in Muscle Control in Lumbopelvic Pain

Lumbopelvic pain is associated with a vast array of changes in the activity of the trunk muscles. Many of these changes are likely to affect the movement and stability of the spine and pelvis, but the nature of these changes is complicated; some changes suggest reduced stability, whereas others suggest increased stability. For instance, increased co-contraction of flexor and extensor muscles has been reported when a load is released from the trunk;[53] activity of the erector spinae muscles is increased during gait[46] and during a situp;[54] and bracing of the abdominal muscles is increased during an active straight leg raise[55] in people with chronic low back and/or pelvic pain. Furthermore, activity of the obliquus externus abdominis is increased during shoulder movements during experimentally induced pain[56] or when pain is anticipated.[57] Data presented by Radebold et al.[53] showed increased activity of at least one superficial trunk muscle in all individuals in a postural task, but the specific muscle showing increased activity varied from person to person. Although findings such as these have been used to indicate that the adaptation of muscle control during pain has no consistent goal, together these findings suggest that an increase in the static stability of the spine and pelvis is common in LBP. This is supported by findings of reduced motion of the spine in people with back pain. For instance, during rapid arm movements, people with LBP less frequently prepare the spine with movement,[10] intervertebral motion is decreased during trunk flexion,[58] and counter-rotation of the shoulders and pelvis is reduced during locomotion.[59]

In contrast, other data tend to indicate that control of the spine is compromised if pain is present. For instance, during experimentally induced back pain, activity of the transversus abdominis[60] and multifidus[61] is delayed during arm movements, and tonic activity of the transversus abdominis is reduced during walking[62] and with repetitive arm movements.[56] Furthermore, evidence exists of a decreased cross sectional area,[63] increased fatiguability,[64] and increased intramuscular fat in the paraspinal muscles.[65] These measures, although not directly indicating changes in control, do suggest functional changes in the muscle. Findings of impaired structure and behavior of the deep trunk muscles have been interpreted to suggest that control of the spine and pelvis is impaired in many individuals with LBP and pelvic pain. Although no studies have directly measured stability when activity of the deep muscles is removed, this hypothesis is based on the in vivo and in vitro evidence for a contribution of these muscles to spinal control.[22,25,66,67] Other data from specific back pain populations have provided direct evidence of impaired intervertebral control. For instance, intervertebral translation is abnormal in people with spondylolisthesis,[68] and buckling has been observed with fluoroscopy in a single subject during a weight-lifting effort.[69]

How can these findings be reconciled? Two likely explanations exist. First, it is plausible, if not likely, that while the spine may be unstable, the nervous system may respond to increase stability. Second, multiple subgroups demonstrate LBP and pelvic pain, and within these subgroups are multiple solutions to achieve a similar goal of reducing pain. Numerous researchers have proposed methods to subgroup people with LBP and pelvic pain.[70-73] Subgrouping has been based on a range of issues, including pathology,[71,74] systems (e.g., strength, sensation), and movement dysfunction.[73,75] Classification by pathology is promising but difficult because of the requirement to perform complex and often invasive tests. Perhaps the most readily accessible strategies involve assessment of movement patterns. Several approaches have been identified that consider the *direction* of movement that is provocative of symptoms and whether the patient restricts movement or moves in a less controlled manner. The ultimate test of subgrouping will be to show, with clinical trials, that the outcomes are improved when intervention is based on the subgrouping. Currently only a limited number of studies have attempted to address this question.[76]

Enormous variability is seen in the adaptation of the trunk muscles in people with lumbopelvic pain. This is often interpreted to suggest that no consistent adaptation of muscle control occurs during pain. However, a common goal may underpin the adaptations to pain. Despite the variability, it has been suggested that one underlying principle is that the CNS may adapt to pain or injury by increasing spinal stiffness to increase the "safety margin"; that is, to overprotect the part from pain and injury or reinjury. In this case, the nervous system may adopt a strategy to increase stiffness of the spine by increased co-contraction of trunk muscles. Therefore, rather than selecting a strategy of coordination of deep and superficial muscle activation that is specific to a task, the nervous system may simplify control by stiffening the spine, with reduced flexibility of movement choices. This may have a directional preference. With this strategy, the nervous system reduces the potential for error, limits the impact of unanticipated disturbances to the spine, and limits the potential for further injury. In effect, the nervous system, rather than selecting a strategy from a spectrum of dynamic possibilities that are perfectly matched to the demands of the task, may select a simple solution that provides reasonable (but perhaps not optimum) quality of control that satisfies the demands of a range of conditions. However, because many muscles can achieve the same goal (i.e., the system is redundant because multiple solutions can address the same problem), different individuals may select different combinations of muscle activity to achieve this goal, and the strategy may differ between different tasks.

To test the idea that a range of different strategies of muscle activation achieves a similar outcome for the spine, van Dieen et al.[77] undertook a modeling experiment in which they simulated a range of strategies adopted by people with back pain in a biomechanical model of stability. They found that stability was increased by each permutation of muscle activation, whether the strategy involved increased co-contraction of flexors and extensors, increased activity of the flexors alone, or increased activity of the extensors alone. Recent data from a study of experimental pain suggest that when pain is induced in healthy individuals, most subjects adopt a pattern of increased activity, but again the pattern varies from individual to individual.[78] Of note, these individuals also present with impaired activity of the deep muscles. Therefore, an individual may present with changes in the deep muscles that are consistent with compromised control, yet activity of the superficial muscles may be increased, consistent with increased stiffening of the spine. Despite the increased activity, the control of intervertebral motion may be compromised because of reduced or impaired activity of the deep muscles. (Whether the poor control of the deep muscles leads to compensation by the more superficial muscles or whether overactivity of the superficial muscles supercedes the activity of the deep muscles is considered later.) In summary, available data suggest that the goal of increasing stability of the spine may be achieved to varying degrees by different individuals. Within this large proportion of people with LBP are subgroups, which again may be categorized by the direction of pain provocation or pathology.

Mechanisms for Changes in Muscle Control in Lumbopelvic Pain

Why is control of the spine modified in people with LBP and pelvic pain? A number of key issues must be considered to answer this question. An initial consideration is which

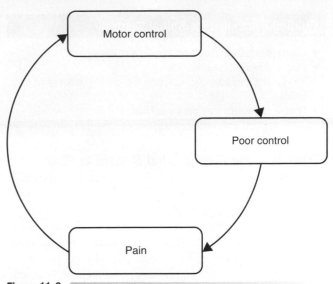

Figure 11-6
Vicious cycle of pain and motor control deficits. Although motor control deficits may lead to pain as a result of compromised control of the spine and pelvis, pain can also lead to changes in motor control. A patient who presents with pain has already entered the cycle, and where the person entered it is less important.

came first: the pain or the motor control changes (Figure 11-6). Evidence exists for both theories. Several authors argue that changes in control of the trunk muscles can lead to the development of pain. Cholewicki et al.[79] reported that delayed offset of activity of the superficial abdominal muscles is associated with the development of acute back pain in athletes. Janda[80] argued that children with soft neurological signs are at risk for the development of back pain as adults. If this is true, then the challenge is to identify factors that lead to the initial change in control. Conversely, a considerable portion of the literature argues that pain and injury lead to changes in the control and structure of the trunk muscles. For instance, experimental pain can cause changes in trunk muscle activity during gait[46] and other tasks such as arm movements; experimental injury in pigs leads to changes in the size of the multifidus,[81] and these changes are similar to those identified in people with clinical pain.[63] If pain and injury lead to changes in the structure and behavior of the trunk muscles, what is the mechanism? Pain can affect control at multiple levels of the nervous system, including all levels from motor planning to spinal mechanisms (Figure 11-7). In reality, when an individual presents with pain, whether the pain caused the changes or the changes caused the pain is somewhat academic, because the patient is already in a cycle in which pain and injury have the potential to increase or perpetuate the changes in control.

Guiding Principles for Spinal Control

- Changes in control may lead to pain and injury
- Pain and injury change control
- The system may adapt by increasing the stability of the spine and pelvis
- Control of stability may not be optimal

Changes in the Corticospinal System in Pain

Changes in the excitability of the corticospinal system at the motor cortex[82] or motoneuron,[83] peripheral effects (e.g., changes in muscle spindle sensitivity),[84] and effects upstream of the motor cortex[85] (e.g., premotor cortex) have been implicated. However, data are generally conflicting, with increased, decreased, and no change in excitability reported. For instance, transcranial magnetic stimulation (TMS) over the motor cortex has been used to assess motor cortex excitability, but reduced,[82] increased,[86,87] and unchanged[36,88] motor cortex excitability has been reported. However, the response to TMS alone is difficult to interpret, because the response is affected by other factors such as motoneuron excitability.[89] The effects of pain on motoneuron excitability have also been debated. A key issue is that techniques that have been used to evaluate corticospinal excitability have failed to control for changes at multiple sites. For instance, the response to TMS is affected not only by the excitability of the cortical cells, but also by the excitability of the motoneurons. Further work that controls for changes at multiple sites is required to clarify the changes in the corticospinal system

in pain. In contrast, strong evidence indicates that injury can lead to reflex inhibition of the motoneurons.[90] This may explain the rapid changes in the multifidus in acute LBP.

Changes in Motor Planning

Although the evidence for changes in motor pathway excitability is not clear, good evidence indicates that motor planning is changed in the presence of pain. As mentioned in the previous section, pain often is associated with activity of muscles that tend to increase the stability of the spine; that is, the nervous system appears to switch its strategy to protect the part from pain and injury or reinjury. In an acute situation, this may be an ideal strategy to prevent worsening of symptoms and provide an opportunity for tissue healing; however, when the pain is prolonged, this strategy may no longer be appropriate.

It has been argued by several authors that the CNS adopts this strategy to compensate for reduced osseoligamentous stability of the spine[12,50,77] (Figure 11-8). However, similar changes in motor control can be replicated when pain is induced experimentally by the injection of hypertonic saline;[90] that is, when osseoligamentous stability is not changed. Furthermore, similar changes may occur even when pain is anticipated but not present.[57] For example, if painful electrical shocks to the back are provided every time an arm is moved, the response of the obliquus externus abdominis is augmented and occurs earlier in association with arm movement. However, this is maintained after the painful stimulation is no longer linked to the arm movement.[91] Therefore, adaptation may occur in a number of situations when the real or perceived stability

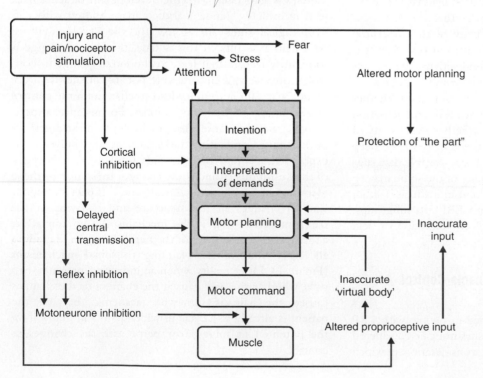

Figure 11-7

Possible mechanisms of pain that can affect the planning of movement and activation of trunk muscles.

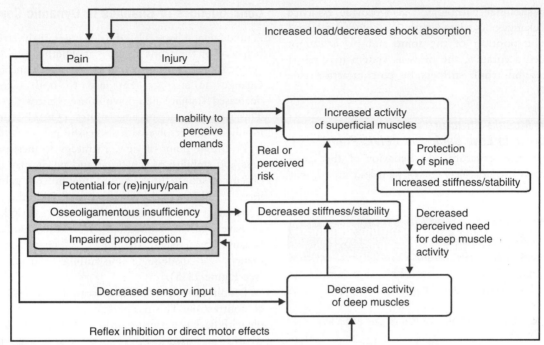

Figure 11-8

Possible factors that may explain the relationship between impaired activity of the deep muscles and increased activity of the superficial muscles. Pain and injury may lead to opposite changes in the deep and superficial muscles.

of the spine is decreased, when a real or perceived risk of further injury exists, or when there is a real or perceived risk of pain (Figure 11-9).

In dynamic control of the spine, it is important to perfectly match muscle activity to the movement demands to maintain stability of the trajectory and all other components of spinal control. However, this dynamic strategy has the potential for error. In a healthy system, which has tolerance for errors, this is not a problem. However, if the real or perceived tolerance for errors is reduced (e.g., because of osseoligamentous insufficiency, pain, or poor proprioception) the CNS may adopt a static strategy to increase spinal stiffness. Therefore, rather than using a range of control alternatives, the CNS may choose a simple solution, but with variation between individuals and tasks because of the redundancy of the system.

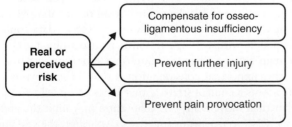

Figure 11-9

Motor control may change because of real or perceived risk to the spine as a result of instability and the risk of pain and injury or reinjury.

Sensory Changes

Motor control also may change as a result of deficits in sensation. If inaccurate sensory information is available to the nervous system, responses to external perturbations are unlikely to be accurate. Furthermore, the internal model of movement to which the nervous system refers to predict the consequence of movements and forces is unlikely to be accurate, leading to inaccurately controlled movement and stability. Considerable evidence indicates that abnormal sensory function in LBP and other musculoskeletal pain syndromes. The ability to reposition the spine to a target angle is reduced in people with chronic back symptoms,[17] and the threshold amount of displacement required to detect movement is increased.[92] Evidence also indicates that the nervous system may ignore sensory information from the lumbar spine to some degree. When vibration is applied to the back muscles in healthy individuals, there is a perception of muscle lengthening, which is interpreted as falling forward, and a postural correction occurs. A similar situation arises when vibration is applied to the ankles and neck muscles. However, when the back muscles are vibrated in people with back pain, the postural reaction is significantly reduced.[93] The postural response to vibration to the neck and ankle is not affected. One interpretation of this finding is that the nervous system has learned to ignore potentially faulty proprioceptive input from the spinal muscles. Studies of acuity for ankle movement in people with ankle sprain[94] and studies of shoulder movement detection in shoulder pathology[95] also provide evidence for sensory changes associated with musculoskeletal conditions. If the position of the spine and pelvis cannot be determined accurately, the nervous system may resort to an increase in trunk stiffness by co-contraction (see Figure 11-8).

Changes in Muscle Structure and Behavior as a Precursor to Low Back and Pelvic Pain

If changes in the structure and behavior of the trunk muscles lead to the development of pain and injury, why do the changes occur?

Mechanisms That Cause Changes in the Structure and Behavior of Trunk Muscles

- Faulty movement patterns
- Poor posture and loading patterns
- Inactivity
- Changes in control in anticipation or fear of pain and injury
- Poor proprioception
- Changes in trunk muscle function as a result of breathing difficulties or incontinence

---

Theoretically, changes in either the structure or the function of the trunk muscles may result in changes that could lead to the future development of pain and injury, but further research is required to test these theories. Two novel factors that have received some support in the literature are the potential for disorders of respiration and continence to lead to changes in control, which may lead to the development of pain. Data suggest that both of these disorders are associated with changes in control of the trunk muscles that are similar to those identified in people with LBP.[40,96] Although confirming that increased respiratory demand and incontinence reduce the capability of the trunk muscles to maintain spinal stability is difficult, data from several cross sectional[97,98] and longitudinal[99] studies suggest that the incidence of back pain is increased in populations with these disorders. Most notably, recent data suggest that breathing difficulties and incontinence are associated with increased odds for the development of LBP.[99] Future studies are required to clarify the physiological relationship between these disorders.

Summary

Multiple factors have the potential to lead to changes in the control of the trunk muscles before and after pain and injury. In most cases a range of factors likely is involved, and a key element of management is to assess the importance of each factor.

Consequences of Changes in Dynamic Control

A fundamental issue related to changes in the structure and behavior of the trunk muscles is whether the adaptations are beneficial or detrimental in the short and long term. Changes in strategy that lead to both increased and decreased stability may have consequences for the spine. This is significant, because motor control changes commonly do not resolve with successful pain treatment.[60,100]

From one point of view, a strategy to increase the stiffness and stability of the spine and pelvis may be positive because it splints the spine and may prevent pain and reinjury.[12,77] Although this may be beneficial in the short term, if the adaptation is maintained for a long period, it is likely to have negative consequences for the spine and pelvis because of increased loading,[101,102] restriction of movement,[10] and inadequate fine tuning of trunk movement (see Figure 11-8).

Loading on the spine is increased as a result of muscle co-contraction. This has been confirmed in studies of people with back pain during lifting.[101] Although debate exists whether increased loading is detrimental to the spine, some argue that a high cumulative load may lead to mechanical and physiological changes.[104,105] These conditions may accelerate degeneration[106] and potentially increase the long-term risk for recurrence of LBP.

A consequence of spinal stiffening and muscle co-contraction is reduced availability of movement as a mechanism to absorb and dissipate force. As described earlier, movement presents a range of advantages to the control of forces at the spine. Recent data confirm that people with back pain are less likely to use movement as a component of the strategy to control the spine, and this is associated with a greater perturbation to the trunk[10] and a longer time to recover balance after a perturbation.[107] Both of these factors are likely to have consequences in the long term. In addition, if spinal movement is reduced, the contribution of spinal motion to respiration and balance control is reduced. Consistent with this proposal, studies have shown that people with LBP sway more with breathing[42,43] and have increased vertical motion of the rib cage with breathing.[27] The latter finding may suggest restricted ability to use anteroposterior and lateral motion of the abdominal wall and rib cage because of increased activity of the superficial abdominal muscles. In terms of balance, increased spinal stiffness may limit the contribution of spinal movement to the control of postural equilibrium. Recent data confirm that people with LBP are less able to use a hip strategy to maintain balance when standing on a short support base.[10] Another important consideration is that if the nervous system adopts a control strategy that relies on spinal stiffening rather than movement, this adaptation may limit the ability of the CNS to perform some tasks. Although the stiffening strategy may be suitable for tasks when movement can be restricted (i.e., movement is not required, can be compensated elsewhere, or can be reduced without preventing the task from being completed) or when movement is obligatory, an appropriate strategy may not be available. For instance, when standing on one leg, shifting the center of mass over the stance leg is essential. Inappropriate control of the spine in this context, through trunk stiffening, makes the above task difficult to execute.[108]

Finally, impaired activity of the deep muscles, in conjunction with increased activity of the superficial muscles, is likely to have consequences for the control of movement and stability at the intervertebral level. As mentioned earlier, it is well accepted from a number of models that deep muscle function is important for spinal control. The contribution of the deep muscles to control of the lumbar spine and pelvis is unlikely to be completely compensated for or replicated by activity of the larger, more superficial muscles, especially in the dynamic situations. The models of Bergmark[18] and Crisco et al.[2] predict that without activity of the deeper muscles, the integrity of the spine cannot be maintained. Therefore, impaired function of these muscles is likely to leave the entire spinal system and its control vulnerable, leading to compromised quality of control. This may not be a problem in the short term, because the increased activity of the superficial muscles is likely to stiffen and protect the spine; however, in the long term, it is likely to be problematic.

For the reasons outlined previously, it could be argued that the muscle co-contraction strategy, with its short term benefit, may lead to an increased risk of the recurrence of back pain if the almost obligatory use of this strategy does not resolve after the resolution of pain. It is well accepted that previous back pain is a strong predictor of future back injury.[109] The failure of changes in trunk muscle control to resolve may be a mechanism underlying this finding. Data from numerous studies of individuals with a history of pain but no pain at the time of testing indicate that changes in motor control persist after the resolution of symptoms.[60] This implies that motor strategies do not resolve spontaneously after cessation of pain, at least in some individuals.[110] The possibility that abnormal muscle activation leads to LBP is supported by recent data that suggest that delayed onset of activity of the abdominal muscles predicts LBP.[79] However, this was a predictor not only in those with a history of LBP, but also in those with no history of pain. Furthermore, reduction in a cross sectional area of the multifidus that is not restored by the provision of specific training is associated with an increased risk of back pain recurrence, compared to individuals who received such training.[51] A key issue to consider is why some individuals go on to have a recurrence of back pain, whereas others do not. Further work is required to determine possible

factors that may contribute to the recurrence of back pain. However, recent data suggest that failure of the motor adaptation to resolve may be linked to unhelpful attitudes and beliefs about pain.[111] As persistence or recurrence of LBP[112] and pain-related attitudes are associated with changes in motor strategy,[113] this may provide a physiological link between psychological factors and the recurrence of back pain.

Guiding Principles: Consequences of Increased Stability

- Increased loading as a consequence of co-contraction
- Increased stiffness and reduced shock absorption
- Decreased quality of control of intervertebral motion

Guiding Principles: Consequences of Compromised Quality of Control

- Decreased quality of control of intervertebral motion
- Increased motion and irritation of provocative structures (i.e., sensitized tissues)

Interpretation of Motor Changes for Exercise Planning

The potential negative effects of an adaptation to increase the stability of the spine challenges the view that exercise to enhance spinal stability is appropriate for the management of LBP. In the management of a patient with LBP and/or pelvic pain, an important consideration is whether the adaptation is beneficial or detrimental; that is, whether the adaptation should be encouraged or discouraged. On the one hand, maintaining the adaptation may be necessary to increase the stiffness and stability of the spine, because the structures may be at risk as a result of osseoligamentous instability, limited ability of the tissues to tolerate load and movement, poor awareness of position and/or movement, or sensitization of the tissues (see later discussion). This point of view has been argued by several authors[12,77] and forms the basis of a range of intervention strategies that aim to increase the stiffness and stability of the spine.[103]

The alternative point of view is that maintaining a strategy to increase stability and stiffness of the spine has negative consequences for the spine and may be responsible for the persistence or recurrence of back pain and injury. From this perspective, the opinion is to reduce the overactivity of the superficial muscles and retrain the coordination of the deep and superficial muscles to restore the optimum dynamic strategy for control of the spine. In reality, both strategies likely are correct, and the approach taken depends on the individual patient. The most appropriate strategy for a particular patient can be determined only by a thorough and specific assessment.

Guiding Principles of Spinal Assessment

- In intervention planning, assessment is important to determine whether the strategy to increase stiffness and stability should be maintained or reduced
- Specific deficits in the activity of the deep and superficial muscles must be assessed

---

Motor Control and the Neurobiology of Pain

It is well known that pain is associated with changes in the nervous system, ranging from sensitization of the afferent endings in the periphery to changes in the dorsal horn and higher centers of the nervous system. In the management of LBP, it is important to consider the relationship between neurobiological changes and motor control from a range of perspectives. First, with peripheral sensitization, it may be important for control of movement and stability to be better than normal. In peripheral sensitization, the excitability of the pain afferents is increased (i.e., the threshold for causing the afferents to fire is lower) as a result of an initial chemical, thermal, or mechanical insult. These changes can persist after the danger to the tissues is removed. In this case, more refined control of the spine may be critical. Second, synaptic changes in the dorsal horn lead to changes in integration of sensory input. The provision of normal movement input is likely to be critical, again requiring control of movement and stability. Third, some have suggested that the peripheral input can maintain central sensitization (e.g., painful input from the knee can maintain secondary hyperalgesia, which is a result of central changes).[114] Therefore, peripheral input from the spine, as a result of abnormal movement control, may drive the changes centrally. A final issue that must be recognized is that pain is a complex phenomenon that is likely to be a mix of peripheral and central issues. Consequently, the contribution of these different elements requires careful consideration in the management of chronic pain. Issues such as pacing also require attention (see Moseley and Hodges[115] for review).

Biopsychosocial Model of Low Back Pain and Motor Control of the Trunk Muscles

All or most back pain involves a combination of biological, psychological, and social factors (see Chapter 9). The relevance of psychological and social issues in back pain is clear, and a range of factors has been found to be closely associated with the transition of back pain from acute to chronic pain.[111] These factors clearly must be considered in the assessment and management of back pain. An important consideration is that a person's report of pain is not simply related to the amplitude of input from the nociceptors in the periphery, but is also influenced by a range of factors, including the individual's experience and other psychological and social issues.[116]

An issue that is less well understood is the inter-relationship between psychological issues and motor control of the trunk muscles; that is, the potential for psychological factors to drive changes in control and therefore have a direct effect on biology. As mentioned previously, the fact that pain can change motor control is well known. However, motor control may possibly also be changed by psychological factors such as stress and fear of pain and injury or reinjury. Studies have shown that control of the trunk is changed during lifting under "stressful" conditions.[117] Furthermore, when a person anticipates back pain, the onset of activity of the deep abdominal muscles is delayed during arm movements,[54] and activity of the superficial muscles occurs earlier.[115] Notably, this alteration does not appear to recover rapidly in all individuals after the removal of the threat. Recent data suggest that the failure of these changes to resolve the symptoms may be linked with unhelpful attitudes about back pain.[115] In summary, biological (motor control) and psychological changes are likely to be interdependent and require co-intervention in many cases.

Summary

Clearly, optimum control of the spine and pelvis requires a carefully controlled, dynamic system. In such a system, the nervous system matches the strategy of activation of the trunk muscles to the multiple tasks that must be coordinated to achieve optimum control of the spine. On balance, data from people with low back pain indicate that in these individuals, deficits are present in the nervous system's ability to select the appropriate strategy and therefore it often prefers to activate simple strategies that involve co-contraction to stiffen the spine and increase the safety margin. These deficits are associated with changes in deep muscle control, proprioception, breathing, and continence. In view of the complex nature of these changes, comprehensive rehabilitation is likely to require a motor learning approach to restore the complex control strategies. This must be based on comprehensive assessment of the individual patient.

Clinical Strategies to Restore Dynamic Motor Control of the Spine and Pelvis

Basic Principles of Clinical Training of Dynamic Motor Control of the Spine and Pelvis

The goal of rehabilitation of motor control is to restore optimum control of the spine to meet the demands of each of the functional requirements of the spine. This is not equivalent to teaching a patient to maximize stability. Instead, the nervous system is trained to match task demands with appropriate finesse to ensure that stability is maintained and that movement is allowed as necessary for the task. Rehabilitation of motor control of the spine depends on careful assessment of movement patterns and muscle recruitment strategies. Because of the redundancy of the motor system, immense potential exists for variation in the motor control strategy adopted in individuals with LBP and pelvic pain. In addition, a large range of factors can present as barriers to rehabilitation of control. For instance, the breathing pattern and posture may be associated with the patterns of adaptation in the muscle system. These factors must be assessed and managed appropriately. A key element is identification of provocative movements and the pattern of adaptation of the trunk muscles in association with these movement patterns. This section provides a basic summary of the key elements of assessment of dynamic control of the spine and the major steps in optimizing control through clinical rehabilitation.

Assessment of Dynamic Motor Control of the Spine

Assessment of dynamic control of the spine requires consideration of all elements of the movement system. In particular, the multiple components of the lumbopelvic system must be evaluated, namely (1) the activity of the deep muscles, (2) strategies for activation of the superficial muscles, (3) posture and movement patterns, and (4) breathing and continence. Only with detailed assessment can management strategies be planned.

Assessment of the Ability to Activate the Deep Muscles of the Spine and Pelvis

Assessment of the activation of the deep muscles is inherently difficult because of their inaccessibility to conventional assessment techniques. This has required the development of new methods. These techniques involve evaluation of the structure and behavior of the deep muscles using a range of clinical tools.

Assessment of Activation of the Deep Muscles of the Lumber Spine and Pelvis

This assessment has three key parts:
1. Assessment of muscle size and quality
2. Assessment of voluntary independent muscle activation
3. Assessment of automatic muscle recruitment during specific tasks

---

Assessment of Muscle Size and Quality. The structure of the deep trunk muscles can be assessed with imaging techniques and palpation. Measurement of the size of multifidus is the most validated measure. In people with a first episode of acute LBP, the cross sectional area of the multifidus is reduced on the side affected by the back pain; this finding is confined to the level identified with manual palpation.[63] In chronic LBP, more diffuse changes have been identified, including modified areas of fat on computed tomography (CT) and magnetic resonance imaging (MRI) scans.[118-120] The thickness of the lateral abdominal muscles, including the transversus abdominis (TrA), can be measured. However, only limited evidence indicates that this measurement provides data that can discriminate between people with and without LBP or pelvic pain. Ultrasound (US) imaging can also be used to arrive at a qualitative judgment of the symmetry and position of the pelvic floor muscles. Table 11-1 provides details of the techniques for US measurement of the structure of the deep muscles.

Additional information on the structure of the deep muscles can be obtained through palpation. Because of the reduction in size of the multifidus in association with acute pain and the tendency for increased fat in the muscle with chronic pain, changes in the consistency of the muscle are likely. The muscle can be palpated at each lumbar level to identify differences in consistency between sides and between levels. For this technique, the clinician identifies the spinous process at each level of the lumbar spine and then gently sinks the thumbs or fingers into the muscle on each side at each level. Differences in the bulk and elasticity of the muscle usually can be noted. If changes are identified, they should be noted and compared with the results of the activation tests (see later discussion). Palpation of the muscle structure of the TrA is difficult because of the overlying muscles, although increased tension sometimes can be noted. Palpation of the pelvic floor muscles is possible with specialized training, but this is beyond the scope of this chapter.

Assessment of Voluntary Independent Activation. Although the deep trunk muscles are normally recruited automatically as part of complex movement patterns, and function does not involve voluntary independent activation of these muscles, the ability to contract them voluntarily, independent of the more superficial trunk muscles, appears to provide an opportunity to study the function of the muscle. For instance, the ability to activate the TrA independently from the other superficial trunk muscles is related to the timing of activation of the TrA in an arm movement task.[60] The key factor assessed is the precision of the independent activation. This is interpreted in terms of (1) which muscles are recruited, (2) the sequence, and (3) the quality. Ideal performance would involve evidence of activity of the deep muscles, minimal activation of the superficial muscles, and smooth, slow contraction with normal breathing.

Assessment of voluntary, independent activation involves teaching the patient to activate the muscle, followed by a range of assessment techniques used to evaluate evidence that contraction of the deep muscles is present and

Table 11-1

Measurement of the Structures of the Deep Muscles with Ultrasound Imaging

Muscle	Technique
Multifidus	With the patient in the prone or side lying position, a 5-7 MHz curved or linear transducer is placed transversely across the spine approximately at the level of each spinous process. The transducer is moved superiorly and inferiorly until the most obvious image of the lamina is identified. The lateral border of the multifidus can be clarified by asking the patient to gently perform an anterior pelvic tilt, which highlights the border with the adjacent longissimus. The border of the muscle is traced and the cross sectional area calculated.
Transversus abdominis	With the patient in the supine position (with or without the knees and hips flexed), a 5-7 MHz curved or linear transducer is placed transversely across the abdomen midway between the iliac crease and the inferior border of the rib cage. The medial aspect of the transducer is moved until the anterior edge of the transversus abdominis (TrA) muscle can be visualized. The thickness of the external oblique (OE), internal oblique (OI), and TrA can be measured either in the middle of the transducer or at a site 1-2 cm (0.5-1 inch) medial to the anterior edge of the TrA muscle. For consistency, measurements should be made at the end of a quiet expiration for consistency.
Pelvic floor muscles	With the patient in the supine or sitting position, a 3-5 MHz curved transducer is placed on the abdominal wall above the pubic symphysis and directed inferiorly and posteriorly to image the bladder. With the transducer placed transversely, the right and left sides of the pelvic floor can be imaged. With the transducer placed sagittally, the anterior and posterior aspects can be imaged.

evidence of substitution of the more superficial muscles. The quality and symmetry of contraction are also recorded. The typical substitution strategy is identified and recorded, because this guides management. In practice, the contraction is taught, the patient is allowed several repetitions to optimize the performance of the contraction, and then the assessment is performed. The goal is to hold the contraction for 10 seconds and repeat the contraction 10 times. The performance can be graded as shown in Table 11-2. This grading scale has been found to be reliable,[121] it can distinguish between people with and without LBP,[121] and it is related to the outcome from US measurements of TrA thickening during a leg loading task.[122] The specific cues, the ideal response, and the tools and techniques for assessment for the TrA, multifidus (MF), and pelvic floor muscles (PFM) are summarized in Tables 11-3 to 11-5, respectively. Palpation techniques for assessment of activation of the TrA and MF are presented in Figures 11-10 and 11-11. Ideally, the contractions should be performed in a number of positions so that the examiner can assess the range of substitution strategies that may be adopted by the patient. Assessment of the function of the PFM can be supplemented with additional questions to ascertain the quality of control and dysfunction of the pelvic floor (Table 11-6).

Assessment of Automatic Recruitment During Specific Tasks. Although assessment of the ability to voluntarily activate the deep muscles independently from the more superficial muscles provides useful information about

Table 11-2

Clinical Rating Scale for Assessing Quality of Contraction of Deep Muscles

Criteria	Score
Quality of Contraction	
No contraction	0
Rapid, superficial contraction	1
Just perceptible contraction	2
Gentle, slow contraction	3
Substitution	
Resting substitution	0
Moderate to strong substitution	1
Subtle perceptible substitution	2
No substitution	3
Symmetry	
Unilateral contraction	0
Bilateral but asymmetrical contraction	1
Symmetrical contraction	2
Breathing	
Inability or difficulty with breathing during contraction	0
Able to hold contraction while maintaining breathing	1
Holding	
Hold <10 seconds	0
Hold ≥10 seconds	1

Table 11-3
Assessment of the Ability to Activate the Transversus Abdominis

	Transversus Abdominis
Cues	"Relax; breathe in and then breathe out. Without breathing in, slowly and gently draw in the lower abdomen; hold the contraction and breathe; then slowly relax." "Slowly draw in the lower abdomen, away from the elastic of your pants." "Slowly pull your navel up and in toward your backbone." "Slowly pull in your abdomen to gently flatten your stomach below your navel." "Slowly move my fingers together" (examiner's fingers have been placed medial to the iliac spines).
Ideal response	Slow, gentle increase in tension under the examiner's fingers. No or little activity of the superficial muscles. Smooth and sustained action (not jerky). Symmetrical contraction. Approximately 10% to 15% effort. Able to breathe normally. 10 × 10 sec contractions.*
Confirmation of activity	*Palpation:* Examiner's fingers placed slightly inferior and medial to the anterosuperior iliac spine (ASIS). Gentle but firm pressure into the muscle. During contraction of the transversus abdominis (TrA), a gentle, deep increase in tension should be felt under the fingers. With activation of the internal oblique (OI), a swelling of muscle should occur directly below the fingers. This technique is based on the anatomy of the distal region of the abdominal muscles. Muscle fibers of the external oblique (OE) do not extend below the ASIS, TrA muscle fibers are short and deep but attach to the extensive anterior fascia. The thumbs or fingers can be used to palpate the contraction. Ideally, the contraction should be evaluated bilaterally to assess for asymmetry. Also, the contraction should be assessed with the patient in multiple postures. *Ultrasound imaging:* An ultrasound transducer (5-7 MHz curved or linear transducer) is placed transversely across the abdomen midway between the iliac crest and the rib cage. The medial edge of the transducer is positioned such that the medial edge of the muscle is visible in the image. During contraction, the TrA should slide laterally (i.e., shorten relative to the overlying oblique abdominal muscles) and thicken. The adjacent muscles should show minimal change in thickness. *Observation:* Gentle flattening or inward movement of the lower abdominal wall may be observed during contraction of the TrA.
Assessment of substitution by superficial trunk muscles	*Palpation:* Contraction of the OE can be palpated in the anterolateral aspect of the abdominal wall, where it is identifiable as an almost vertical band of muscle from the ribs to the pelvis. The muscle also can be palpated at its origin on the lower ribs. If the hands are placed on the lateral aspect of the abdomen, contraction of the OE is palpated as a broadening of the waist. The OI is best palpated as bulging in the lower abdominal wall, as described previously. Activity of the rectus abdominis (RA) is palpated as tensing of the muscle above and below the navel. In some cases, activity of the long erector spinae occurs to counteract the flexion moment generated by contraction of the flexing abdominal muscles. *Ultrasound imaging:* Although OE contraction often is not apparent with ultrasound imaging (possibly because of the stiffness of the tendon), OI contraction can be observed as a thickening of the muscle. *Observation:* Contraction of the RA/OE/OI can be observed as movement of the pelvis (posterior pelvic tilt), flexion of the thoracolumbar junction, flattening of the lower rib cage, inward movement of the upper abdomen, activation during breathing, or an inability to relax the abdominal wall. Inappropriate inward movement of the abdominal wall may also be induced by taking a deep breath and sucking in the abdominal wall. *Surface electromyography (EMG):* Surface EMG electrodes can be placed on the abdominal wall to record the activity of the RA and OE. For OE, ideal placement is over the distal edge of the ninth rib and on the abdominal wall just inferior and medial to this on an angle of about 45°. For the RA, the electrodes can be placed in a vertical direction about 2-4 cm (1-1.6 inches) lateral to the midline above or below the navel. Electrodes can be placed over the OI medial and inferior to the ASIS at an angle of about 20° to the horizontal; however, this electrode will also record activity from the TrA.

*The goal is to hold the contraction for 10 seconds and repeat the contraction 10 times.

Table 11-4

Assessment of the Ability to Activate the Lumbar Multifidus

	Lumbar Multifidus
Cues	"Relax; breathe in and then breathe out. Without breathing in, slowly and gently swell the muscle into my fingers; hold the contraction and breathe; then slowly relax." "Think about tilting the pelvis but without really doing it." "Tense a cable running from the front of the pelvis to the spine."
Ideal response	Slow, gentle increase in tension under the examiner's fingers. No or little activity of the superficial muscles. Smooth and sustained action (not jerky). Approximately 10% to 15% effort. Symmetrical contraction. Able to breathe normally. 10 × 10 sec contractions.*
Confirmation of activity	*Palpation:* Activity can be palpated as a slow, gentle increase in tension under the fingers. Palpation techniques can involve the tip of a thumb and the midphalanx of the index finger, two thumbs, or a thumb and the finger pad of the index or middle finger. Although two thumbs can be ideal for assessment of symmetry, a single hand technique may be beneficial so that the other hand can be free to palpate other muscles. During contraction of the multifidus (MF), activity of the transversus abdominis (TrA) is also commonly palpated in the anterior abdominal wall. *Ultrasound imaging:* Contraction of the MF can be best observed with the ultrasound transducer placed parasagittally about 2-3 cm (1-1.2 inches) lateral to the midline. In this image, the facet joints are observable as humps, and the muscle between the tops of the facet joints and the fascia and skin at the top of the image is the multifidus. During contraction, the fascicles of the muscle should move, and the thickness of the muscle should increase. Emphasis is placed on a slow, gentle increase in thickness, particularly in the deep fibers in the muscle. *Observation:* During contraction of the MF, minimal movement should be observed, although the contracting muscle often can be seen to push away the fingers used to palpate it.
Assessment of substitution by superficial trunk muscles	*Palpation:* Contraction of the long erector spinal muscles can be palpated, particularly lateral to the multifidus and at the thoracolumbar junction. Contraction of the superficial abdominal muscles suggests bracing. *Ultrasound imaging:* Contraction of the superficial muscles is often identified by rapid contraction on ultrasound imaging. Contraction of the long erector spinae is obvious from palpation or surface electromyography (EMG), and ultrasound imaging is not required. *Observation:* Contraction of the superficial paraspinal muscles is often accompanied by an anterior tilt of the pelvis and subtle extension of the thoracolumbar junction. A posterior tilt of the pelvis can sometimes be observed as an attempt to push the spine up into the fingers by the MF muscle. *Surface electromyography:* Surface EMG electrodes can be placed on the thoracic erector spinae and superficial abdominal muscles as described previously to assess substitution.

*The goal is to hold the contraction for 10 seconds and repeat the contraction 10 times.

the function of the deep muscles and substitution strategies, this assessment technique may be problematic because it depends on the patient's ability to learn the task and on motivation. Additional information can be gleaned from tests of recruitment of the deep muscles during movement tasks. A range of tasks has been described in the literature, including leg loading tasks (e.g., leg flexion and extension in the supine position),[125] the active straight leg raise task,[55] and partial weight-bearing tasks.[119] In each of these tasks, the activity of the deep muscles (TrA, MF, and PFM) can be assessed with ultrasound imaging. Using the US

imaging techniques described in Tables 11-3 and 11-4 and in Figures 11-12 to 11-14, activity during the performance of the movement is measured. Some initial data available suggest that changes occur in the performance of these tasks. For instance, people with LBP and/or pelvic pain show reduced thickening of the TrA during isometric flexion and extension of the leg,[124] increased thickening of the internal oblique during a simulated weight-bearing squat,[126] and descent of the pelvic floor during an active straight leg raise.[55] Further work is required to validate these techniques.

Table 11-5

Assessment of the Ability to Activate the Pelvic Floor Muscles

	Pelvic Floor Muscles
Cues	"Gently tense the pelvic floor muscles as if stopping the flow of urine." Males: "Gently lift the testes" or "Gently shorten the penis." "Gently lift the pelvic floor." "Gently pull the tailbone toward the front." "Gently pull the ischial tuberosities together."
Ideal response	Slow, gentle contraction (self-palpation, ultrasound imaging). No or little activity of the superficial abdominal muscles. Smooth and sustained action (not jerky). Approximately 10% to 15% effort. Able to breathe normally. 10 × 10 sec contractions.*
Confirmation of activity	*Palpation:* Contraction of the pelvic floor muscles (PFM) can be self-palpated as a lift of the perineum with the hand placed under the perineal body. With specialized training, physiotherapists can manually palpate the quality, quantity, and symmetry of contraction with the fingers placed in the vagina or anus. *Ultrasound imaging:* Contraction of the pelvic floor muscles can be observed noninvasively with a transducer placed suprapubically and directed in an inferoposterior direction to visualize the bladder. During contraction the pelvic floor muscle can be seen to lift slowly and gently. With the transducer placed transversely, the muscles on the right and left can be observed simultaneously, and the symmetry of the contraction can be evaluated. With the transducer placed sagittally, the anteroposterior aspect can be observed. An alternative approach involves perineal placement of the transducer to image the pelvic floor muscles transperineally. The advantage of this imaging technique is that the symphysis pubis forms a bony landmark for reference during the contraction, making objective measurement possible. This technique requires specialized training. During contraction of the PFM, activity of the transversus abdominis (TrA) is expected and can be observed with ultrasound imaging. *Surface electromyography:* Specialized surface electromyography (EMG) electrodes can be placed in the anus or vagina to record the activity of the pelvic floor muscles. Although cross talk from adjacent hip and trunk muscles may contribute to the signal during strong contractions, this is unlikely to occur during gentle contractions.
Assessment of substitution by superficial trunk muscles	*Palpation:* Palpable contraction of the superficial abdominal muscles suggests bracing. Patients can palpate the elevation of their own pelvic floor by placing a hand over the perineum on the perineal body. *Ultrasound imaging:* Inappropriate activity of the superficial abdominal muscles often causes descent of the pelvic floor muscles, which is seen as downward movement on ultrasound imaging. One caution with this technique is that bracing can push the transducer away, making the pelvic floor muscles appear to be descending. *Observation:* Activity of the superficial abdominal muscles can be observed as described previously. *Surface electromyography:* Inappropriate bracing can also be assessed with surface EMG electrodes placed over the external oblique (OE) and rectus abdominis (RA), as described previously.

*The goal is to hold the contraction for 10 seconds and repeat the contraction 10 times.

Guiding Principles: Assessment of the Deep Muscles

- Assess the structure and function of the deep muscles
- Assess the quality of control of the deep muscles
- Identify any substitution strategies that may be adopted
- Evaluate muscle symmetry
- Evaluate deep muscle activity in different postures

Assessment of the Breathing Pattern

Assessment of breathing is a critical component of the evaluation of the motor control of the trunk. Because most muscles of the abdomen and thorax contribute to respiration, respiratory activity of the trunk muscles may affect control of the spine, and changes in breathing pattern are common in low back and pelvic pain.

First, the clinician should consider the normal pattern of breathing. Breathing involves three key components:

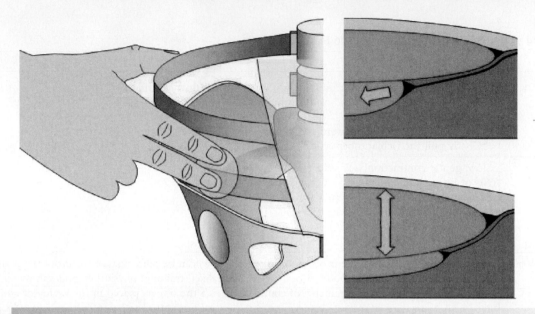

Figure 11-10

Palpation technique for the transversus abdominis. The fingers or thumbs are placed medial and inferior to the anterosuperior iliac spine. Contraction of the obliquus internus abdominis is perceived as a bulge immediately under the skin. Contraction of the transversus abdominis is perceived as a deep tensioning of the fascia,[123] because the fibers of the transversus abdominis are short and attach the strong medial fascia.

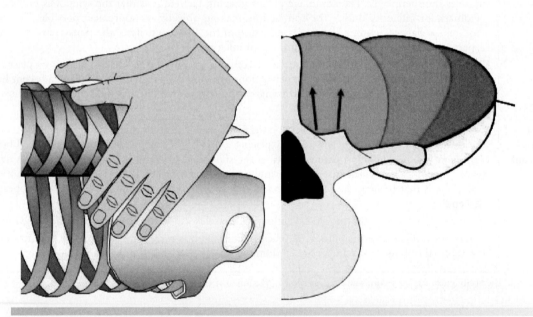

Figure 11-11

Palpation techniques for the multifidus. The thumbs (or the index finger and thumb) sink into the muscle with mild pressure. Contraction of the multifidus is perceived as a deep increase in tension in the muscle that is slow and gentle (not a sharp stiffening of the superficial fibers) close to the midline.[124]

movement of the abdominal wall, bibasal expansion of the rib cage, and upper chest motion. All three movements should be present in quiet breathing. During inspiration, activity of the diaphragm causes the central tendon to descend, which increases the vertical dimensions of the thorax and causes the abdomen to move anteriorly. When descent of the central tendon is restricted by the abdominal contents, diaphragmatic contraction causes the lower ribs to elevate, increasing the lateral dimensions of the thorax. This motion is assisted by contraction of the external intercostal muscles. As a result of the drop in intrapleural pressure, contraction of the diaphragm causes the upper chest

Table 11-6

Subjective Questions to Aid Assessment of Pelvic Floor Control*

Question	Interpretation
"Can you slow or stop the flow of urine midstream?"	Provides information about the ability to contract the pelvic floor muscles (PFM). Note: Patients should not practice this regularly or during the first void in the morning, because voiding difficulties or a urinary tract infection may develop.
"Do you have difficulty initiating urination?"	May suggest increased activity of the PFM.
"Do you have any symptoms of incontinence?"	Indicates that dysfunction of the PFM may be present.
"Is your incontinence associated with leakage of urine during exertion or coughing?"	May suggest stress urinary incontinence.
"Is your incontinence associated with sensations of an urge to urinate?"	May suggest urge incontinence.

*These questions provide a general view of PFM function. More sophisticated and invasive evaluation is required to confirm the findings. If the responses suggest abnormal function, the patient may need to be referred to a specialist for evaluation.

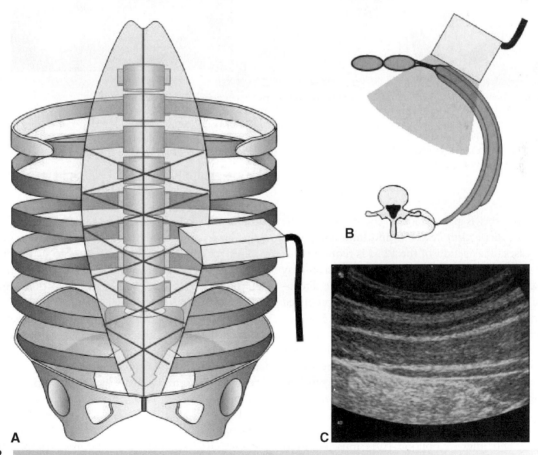

Figure 11-12

Technique for ultrasound imaging of the transversus abdominis. The transducer is placed transversely along the abdominal wall midway between the rib cage and the iliac crest; the muscles of the abdominal wall are seen as three dark layers separated by white fascia. The thickness of the muscle can be measured as described by Ferreira et al.,[123] and contraction can be quantified as shortening and thickening of the muscle.[25,121] **A,** Transducer placement. **B,** Image anatomy. **C,** Typical US image.

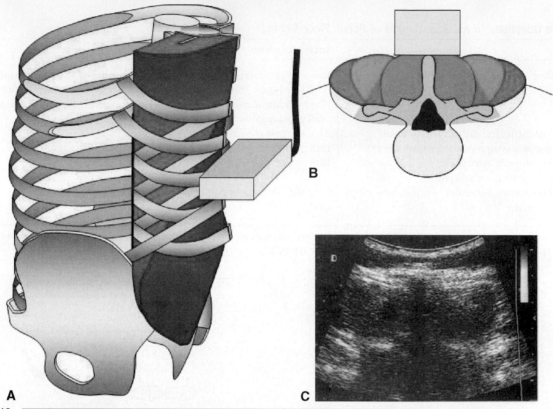

Figure 11-13

Technique for ultrasound imaging of the multifidus. The transducer is placed transversely across the spinous process at the level of the lamina; the multifidus is seen as the circular region of muscle adjacent to the spinous process surrounded by a white fascial boundary. The cross sectional area of the muscle can be measured as described by Hides et al.[124] Contraction is best observed using a parasagittal longitudinal view in which the muscle can be seen to thicken over multiple segments.[124] **A,** Transducer placement. **B,** Image anatomy. **C,** Typical US image.

to move inward; this is prevented by contraction of the scalenes.[7] As the diaphragm descends and intra-abdominal pressure increases, contraction of the PFM is required during inspiration.[127] Activity of the paraspinal muscles may also be present to extend the spine to increase the dimensions of the thorax. Quiet expiration is largely produced by the passive recoil of the chest wall and lung. However, in most positions this is assisted by gentle contraction of the TrA to elevate the diaphragm through a small change in intra-abdominal pressure.[128] Depression of the ribs is assisted by contraction of the internal intercostal muscles. As expiration increases, such as during exercise, depression of the rib cage and ascent of the diaphragm are assisted by contraction of the rectus abdominis (RA), external oblique (OE), and internal oblique (OI) muscles. PFM activity is required to control the increase in intra-abdominal pressure,[126] and erector spinae muscle activity may be present to overcome the flexion moment of the superficial abdominal muscles.

With LBP and pelvic pain, the body has a tendency to increase the vertical motion of the rib cage[27] and increase the activity of the superficial abdominal muscles to brace the abdomen.[55] Increased activity of the OE compromises the ability of the diaphragm to elevate the ribs and descend the central tendon. If basal rib cage and abdominal motion are restricted, upper chest breathing must become dominant. Alternatively, when limited tension is present in the abdominal wall, the diaphragm has limited ability to elevate the ribs (because the descent of the central tendon is not resisted), and excessive motion of the abdominal wall may occur. Careful assessment of the breathing pattern is required to identify factors that may complicate the training of ideal control of the trunk muscles.

In most patients it is important to evaluate the breathing pattern to identify any abnormal recruitment of the trunk muscles, any features that may complicate optimum control of the spine and pelvis (e.g., excessive superficial abdominal muscle activity, excessive abdominal movement), and any features that indicate inefficiency in the breathing apparatus (e.g., an upper chest breathing pattern). Components of the assessment are presented in Table 11-7.

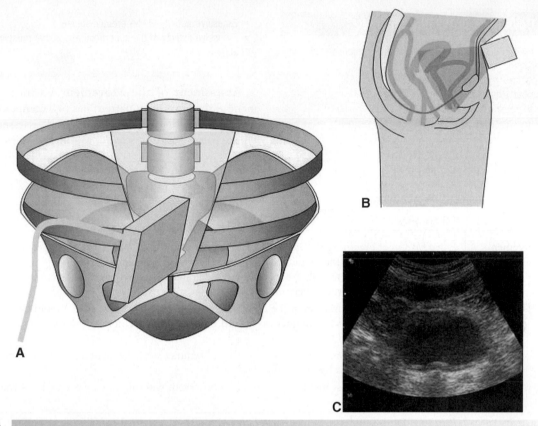

Figure 11-14

Technique for ultrasound imaging of the pelvic floor muscles. The transducer is placed sagittally in the midline in an inferoposterior direction; this allows observation of the base of the bladder. With contraction, the base of the bladder should elevate slowly and smoothly. If the patient braces the abdominal muscles, the floor may descend.[127] Symmetry of position and contraction can be observed with the transducer placed transversely across the abdominal wall just above the symphysis pubis. **A,** Transducer placement. **B,** Image anatomy. **C,** Typical US image.

Guiding Principles: Assessment of the Breathing Pattern

- Look before palpating
- Do not indicate that breathing is being evaluated
- Assess natural breathing and breathing during deep muscle contraction
- Consider whether movement is equal in each region
- Consider what movement is dominant
- Evaluate the breathing pattern in different postures
- Consider the mobility of the rib cage (stiffness may compromise the breathing pattern)
- Assess the breathing pattern during contraction of the deep trunk muscles

Assessment of Posture and Movement Pattern

Assessment of Posture. Assessment of posture involves evaluation of the spinal curves and the associated muscle activity (Figure 11-15). Assessment should include evaluation of the start and finish of curves, depth of curves, segmental changes (e.g., segmental lordosis), pelvic position, frontal curves, right and left weight bearing, activity of deep and superficial muscles (observation, palpation, US imaging, electromyography [EMG]), and ability to contract deep muscles. Rehabilitation of posture may be required to aid restoration of optimum dynamic motor control (e.g., reduction of superficial muscle activity), to help relieve pain, to reduce pain provocation, and to prevent tissue creep. Accurate assessment provides the foundation for intervention planning.

Ideal Posture in Sitting and Standing Involves:

- Neutral pelvic tilt
- Lumbar lordosis
- Thoracic kyphosis with transition at T10-11
- Cervical lordosis
- Neutral head tilt
- Minimal frontal plane curvature
- Equal weight bearing right and left
- Minimal activity of the superficial muscles
- Gentle activity of the deep muscles
- Normal breathing pattern

Common Deviations in Posture include:

- Loss of lumbar lordosis or loss of lordosis in a particular region of the lumbar spine (e.g., lower lumbar spine)
- Slumped posture with upper cervical extension
- Thoracolumbar extension
- Excessive thoracic kyphosis
- Swayback (pelvis anterior to the thorax)

- Excessive activity of the erector spinae
- Excessive activity of the superficial abdominal muscles (flat upper abdomen)

Assessment of the Movement Pattern. The assessment of the movement pattern has two components: assessment of provocative movements and assessment of the typical pattern and muscle activation strategies.

Table 11-7

Techniques for Assessment of Breathing

Parameter	Techniques
Chest wall movements	*Principle:* Quiet breathing should involve movement of the abdomen, basal rib cage, and upper chest. No region should be dominant. Basal rib cage movement is greater in positions in which tension in the abdominal wall resists abdominal displacement and therefore causes shortening of the diaphragm to elevate the lower ribs.
	Abdomen: Observe for motion in the upper and lower abdomen. Movement should be present in each region and should not be confined to inward movement of the upper abdomen with contraction of the external oblique (OE).
	Basal rib cage: Movement should be smooth and symmetrical (the symmetry of movement can be assessed by placing the hands on the lower ribs).
	Upper chest: Upper chest movement should be observed, without excessive activity of the sternocleidomastoid.
Respiratory activity of the trunk muscles	*Principle:* During quiet breathing in supported positions, minimal activity of the superficial abdominal muscles should occur during expiration. Activity of the transversus abdominis (TrA) should occur. In unsupported positions, slight activity of the external and internal obliques (OE/OI) and/or the rectus abdominis (RA) may be noted to aid elevation of the diaphragm. The diaphragm should descend smoothly during inspiration.
	TrA: Activity can be palpated in the lower abdominal wall, and sustained activity can be measured with ultrasound imaging. A slight modulation of activity should occur with breathing, particularly in positions in which the abdomen is dependent. Activity should be sustained throughout the respiratory cycle.
	OE/OI/RA: Activity can be observed, palpated, or recorded with surface electromyography (EMG) electrodes, as described previously. Some modulation of activity with respiration may be noted during breathing in unsupported positions.
	Diaphragm: Diaphragmatic activity can be monitored by evaluating abdominal and bibasal rib cage motion. A more specific assessment can be made with ultrasound imaging. Ultrasound imaging can be used to assess displacement of the diaphragm (transabdominal approach) and thickening of the diaphragm (transverse approach with the transducer placed in a rib space); it also can be used to estimate changes in the length of the diaphragm (the transducer is placed longitudinally down the lateral rib cage). For the transabdominal approach, a 3-MHz transducer is placed on the abdomen below the rib cage, and the transducer is directed upward to visualize the diaphragm, which appears as a white line at the border between with the lung and the diaphragm. The border should move caudally and cranially with breathing. To measure thickening, the transducer is placed in the eighth or ninth intercostals space; the muscle can be identified as the deepest of three muscle layers. The muscle thickens during inspiration. The length of the diaphragm can be measured with the transducer placed longitudinally down the rib cage in the anterior axillary line. The top of the diaphragm is identified by the white shadow formed by the lung, and the origin is identified inferiorly. The muscle should shorten during inspiration.
	Pelvic floor muscles: The pelvic floor muscles (PFM) should contract tonically in upright positions, but the activity can be modulated with breathing. Ultrasound imaging should show that the muscle does not descend during any respiratory phase. With surface EMG, the muscle activity may be modulated with breathing.

Basic Assessment of Lumbar Movement Patterns Includes Evaluation of:

- Provocative movements/postures (e.g., pain with early extension of the spine when returning from forward flexion)
- Any asymmetry in spine/pelvic posture, movement, and range
- Protected motions
- Limb movements that cause provocative motion of the spine/pelvis
- Excessive superficial muscle recruitment during movements (e.g., excessive activity of the erector spinae muscles during trunk flexion)

Table 11-8
Motor Control Impairment

Pattern	Features
Flexion pattern	Flexion pain and loss of segmental lordosis at the symptomatic segment; excessive flexion strain
Flexion/lateral shifting pattern	Tendency to flex and shift laterally at the symptomatic segment
Active extension pattern	Tendency to hold the lumbar spine actively into extension
Passive extension pattern	Tendency to passively overextend at the symptomatic segment of the lumbar spine
Multidirectional pattern	Multidirectional impairment

Data from O'Sullivan P: Diagnosis and classification of chronic low back pain disorders: maladaptive movement and motor control impairments as underlying mechanism, *Man Ther* 10:242-255, 2005.

A number of classification schemes have been described in the literature to characterize and subgroup movement patterns. Two contemporary approaches are the classification of motor control impairment described by O'sullivan[75] (Table 11-8), and the movement impairment syndromes described by Sahrmann[73] (Table 11-9).

Assessment of Superficial/Global Muscle Activity

Assessment of the activity of the superficial/global muscles involves a number of components, including evaluation of superficial muscle activity during assessment of activation of the deep muscles, assessment of breathing, and assessment of posture and movement pattern. Additional movement tests can be performed to assess for specific directions of force that induce either poor control or overactivity.

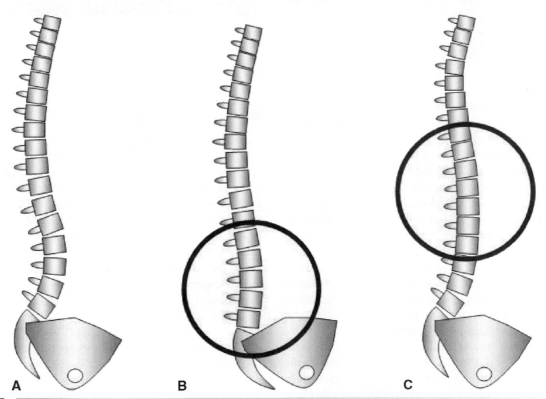

Figure 11-15
A, "Ideal" neutral spine posture with neutral pelvic tilt, lumbar lordosis and thoracic kyphosis with a smooth transition between the two, and a cervical lordosis. **B,** A common fault is a posterior pelvic tilt and reduced lordosis. **C,** Another common fault is excessive extension at the thoracolumbar junction. This may be seen over a few segments or over a long section of the spine, as shown.

Table 11-9
Movement Impairment Syndrome

Pattern	Features
Lumbar rotation/extension syndrome	Pain provocation with lumbar extension and rotation and limb movements that produce these movements Pain relief with flexion
Lumbar extension syndrome	Pain provocation with lumbar extension Pain relief with flattening of the lumbar spine, decreased hip flexor activity
Lumbar rotation syndrome	Pain provocation with rotation with or without lateral flexion. Pain relief with prevention of lumbar rotation/lumbar flexion
Lumbar rotation/flexion syndrome	Pain provocation with flexion and rotation: sitting (slump), bending, twisting Pain relief with prevention of flexion/rotation, prone lying
Lumbar flexion syndrome	Pain provocation with flexion, slump sitting Pain relief with standing, prone lying, leaning forward at the hips

Data from Sahrman S: *Diagnosis and treatment of movement impairment syndromes,* St Louis, 2002, Mosby.

Initial information on whether any of the superficial muscles are overactive and the strategy of overactivity is derived from identification of increased activity or difficulty relaxing the superficial muscles during the test of voluntary independent activation of the deep muscles. The muscles, the quality of contraction, the symmetry, and the ability to relax the muscles are recorded. During the assessment of breathing, an inability to relax and modulation of activity are recorded. Both breathing and voluntary activation of the deep muscles are undertaken in a variety of positions to facilitate identification of strategies of increased activity. Activity of the superficial muscles is also observed during static postures and during movements so that the examiner can identify evidence of excessive activity.

Comprehensive assessment of whether superficial muscle activity is sufficient to meet the demands of control of buckling can be obtained by assessing the control of the orientation of the spine and pelvis during simple movement tasks. One system of evaluating control by the superficial muscles involves assessment of the control of pelvic and lumbar position during a progression of limb loads in crook lying position (supine with the hips and knees flexed).[73]

The patient is instructed to maintain the position of the pelvis and spine during a sequence of leg movements involving abduction and external rotation of the leg and extension of one or both legs with and without support. Assessment involves evaluating for directions of motion associated with poor control of the pelvic or lumbar position. This can be done with a pressure cuff placed under the spine to evaluate the motion of the spine and pelvis. Other models are available to assess this component of the system.

Additional Factors to Assess

In many cases additional information can be gained with regard to factors likely to challenge progress in motor learning. Three key factors require consideration. First, because a patient's beliefs and attitudes about pain can hinder recovery, insight into these issues is critical. In particular, the anticipation of pain has been shown to change the control of the muscle system in a manner similar to the experience of pain.[57] For this reason, it is essential that the clinician gain some insight into the patient's fears and beliefs. Patients with more persistent and long-standing symptoms may require a more formal evaluation (see Moseley and Hodges[92] for review). Second, evaluation of the function of the adjacent segments is crucial. If restricted motion is present at the hip or thoracic spine, or both, this is likely to compromise the ability to change control at the lumbar spine. Initial insight into the function of adjacent joints is derived from the evaluation of movements. Third, evaluation of joint mobility and function can identify specific joint structures that require intervention.

Rehabilitation of Dynamic Motor Control

Rehabilitation of dynamic motor control of the spine and pelvis is guided by the assessment. At the completion of the assessment, the clinician must have a clear picture of whether motor control is altered in the patient and which components of the system are problematic. The intervention is specifically targeted to the presentation of the patient.

Rehabilitation involves a motor learning approach. Motor learning involves the acquisition and refinement of movement and coordination, leading to a permanent change in movement performance.[129] This can be achieved by drawing on the principles of motor training for skill learning.

Different researchers have defined either two or three phases of motor learning. Fitts and Posner proposed three phases.[42] The *cognitive phase* focuses on cognitively based problems, and all components of the task are organized cognitively with attention to feedback, movement sequence, and quality of performance. The *associative phase* commences once the patient has acquired the fundamentals of the movement and the focus shifts to emphasize the consistency of performance and the cognitive demands are reduced.

In the *automatic phase,* which is achieved after considerable practice, the demand for conscious intervention is reduced, and the focus shifts to transferring the task between environments. Gentile[130] proposed two phases, which parallel the phases described by Fitts and Posner. In phase one, the patient "gets the idea"; in phase two, fixation and diversification of the skill are emphasized.

Motor learning provides principles for optimum training of motor function. Motor learning of complex movements can be facilitated by practicing parts of the movement (i.e., segmentation) before practicing the whole movement. Learning can be facilitated by simplifying a task (e.g., by reduction of load) to make it easier for the patient to perform the task correctly. Feedback is critical to ensure learning. Feedback can be provided on both the quality of performances and the results of the task.

Training of motor control of the trunk, in the framework of motor learning, involves training of the components of function that were found to be deficient in the assessment. The sequence of steps is outlined in Figure 11-16. The process involves progressive steps to increase the complexity of training to manage a patient from the initial attempts to restore the coordination of the system through to high level functional training. The process presented in Figure 11-16 involves a central column that defines the progressive steps for regaining control of the system. To the left and right are factors that require consideration at all levels. For instance, regaining breathing during the early steps of training and at each progression is critical to ensure that breathing can be maintained in a controlled manner. *Functional posture* refers to the need to consider the orientation and movement patterns from the first session through to discharge. The following sections provide a description of strategies that can be used in each phase.

Activation of the Deep Muscles of the Spine and Pelvis and Reduction of Overactivity of the Superficial Muscles

In many patients, the assessment will have identified poor activation of one or more components of the deep muscle system and evidence of overactivity of one or more of the superficial muscles. Table 11-10 presents a range of strategies for dealing with these problems. At the completion of the initial session, the clinician must be able to answer three crucial questions: (1) What strategy worked best for the patient? (2) How can one be sure the patient will practice the correct task at home (e.g., strategies for feedback of contraction of the deep and superficial muscles)? (3) What will the home program be? This means the number of contractions and the duration of hold; the goal for the patient is to hold the contraction for 10 seconds and repeat the contraction 10 times (best identified through repeated contraction once a strategy has been chosen).

Rehabilitation of the Breathing Pattern

It is essential that patients are able to breathe effectively at all levels of training. In the initial phases of training,

Figure 11-16

Progression of exercise for rehabilitation of dynamic control of the spine and pelvis. The items in the grey boxes require assessment at the first session. The elements down the center of the figure relate to progressive difficulty of training. The boxes and arrows on the sides are components that need to be considered at all levels of training.

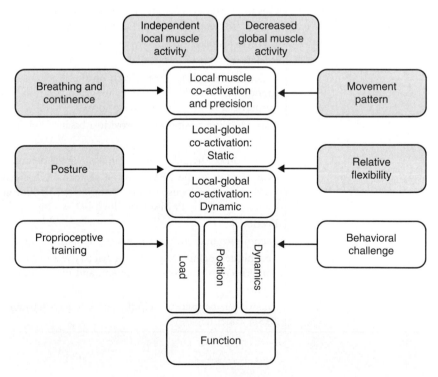

Table 11-10

Clinical Strategies to Increase Activity of the Deep Muscles and Decrease Activity of the Global/Superficial Muscles

Goal of Intervention	Clinical Strategies
Techniques to reduce activity of the superficial muscles	**Posture** Supported postures may aid in the reduction of activity of the superficial/global muscles. Supine crook lying, side lying, and lying prone over a pillow (to relax the paraspinal muscles) may be helpful Appropriate support with pillows and consideration of the position of the arms and legs Specific attention to the spinal curvature (even in the supine position); placing the patient in a more neutral position may help reduce superficial activity Consider provocative movements; correction of these may aid relaxation **Breathing** If tonic activity persists or if activity of the superficial muscles is modulated with breathing, encouraging relaxation by re-education of breathing may be helpful Focus on active inspiration using contraction of the diaphragm (movement of the abdominal wall and basal rib cage) and relaxed expiration Manual contact to encourage basal rib cage expansion Electromyographic (EMG) biofeedback on expiratory activity **Effort** Patients may require encouragement to reduce their effort such that they stop at a level below that at which the superficial muscles become active **Feedback** Feedback of contraction of the superficial muscles can be used to provide greater awareness of activation. Many options are available: palpation, observation in a mirror, surface EMG biofeedback **Imagery** Using images can help a patient "get the idea." Examples may include thinking of the sand building up in an hourglass to give the idea of the slowness required
Techniques to increase activity of the transversus abdominis (TrA)	**Instruction** Careful instruction is critical to ensure the patient understands that the task is not aimed at strength; rather, the emphasis is on control Emphasis is placed on a slow and gentle approach **Position** Positions that allow some stretch on the muscle can improve the sensation of movement of the abdominal wall; however, if a supported position is required to reduce the overactivity of the superficial muscles, that takes priority The side lying position can provide a balance between support and stretch on the muscle **Co-activation** Activation of the pelvic floor muscles (PFM) or multifidus (MF) initiates activity in the TrA Contractions of the PFM must be performed in a slow and controlled manner. Activation is best achieved if the focus is on the anterior pelvic floor and the spine is in neutral. Techniques for activation of the PFM are outlined below **Feedback** Techniques that enable patients to evaluate the quality and quantity of contractions are ideal Techniques include palpation medial to the anterorsuperior iliac spines (ASISs), observation of inward movement of the lower abdomen, and ultrasound imaging **Imagery** Images can be used to help the patient learn activation of the TrA, such as pulling the right and left ASIS together

Table 11-10
Clinical Strategies to Increase Activity of the Deep Muscles and Decrease Activity of the Global/Superficial Muscles

Goal of Intervention	Clinical Strategies
Techniques to increase activity of the MF	**Instruction** Careful instruction is critical to ensure the patient understands that the task is not aimed at strength; rather, the emphasis is on control Emphasis is placed on slow and gentle tension or swelling of the muscle **Position** Positioning the patient in neutral, with specific attention to ensure that that thoracolumbar junction is not held into extension by the long erector spinae, is critical **Co-activation** Activation of the PFM or the TrA can initiate activity in the MF Contractions of the TrA and the PFM must be performed in a slow and controlled manner **Feedback** Techniques that enable patients to evaluate the quality and quantity of contractions are ideal Palpation with the fingers placed over the muscle are ideal, as long as the patient can comfortably reach around the back Placing a small piece of tape on the skin over the muscle can help the patient find the correct level easily **Imagery** Imagining approximation of the hip into the acetabulum can activate the MF Imagining tensioning a cable from the ASIS to the spine with the hands placed on both of these points[131] Thinking about tilting the pelvis, without movement, can help, but the clinician must emphasize that the task is not about movement. This strategy is best avoided in people with pain provocation with extension
Techniques to increase activity of the PFM	**Instruction** Instructions for activation of the PFM are as follows: "Contract as if you are stopping the flow of urine. Lift the sling of muscle that runs between the front of the pelvis and the tailbone, pulling the ischial tuberosities together." (Lifting the testes or shortening the penis can be effective for men) **Position** PFM activity can be increased in a neutral position of the pelvis with lumbar lordosis **Co-activation** Activation of the TrA or MF can initiate activity in the PFM Contractions of the TrA and MF must be performed in a slow and controlled manner **Feedback** Self-palpation of lifting of the perineal body Ultrasound imaging of lifting of the bladder base using a transabdominal approach Palpable contraction of the TrA during PFM activity may provide an indirect form of feedback

breathing can be used as a strategy to help patients learn effective control strategies. Later in training, the emphasis shifts to ensuring that progression of exercise does not compromise the ability to coordinate breathing, stability, and movement. As described earlier for the assessment, optimum breathing involves movement of the abdominal wall and basal regions of the rib cage and some movement of the upper chest. Table 11-11 presents a range of potential problems in breathing control that must be assessed, along with strategies for managing these problems.

Goals of Rehabilitation of the Breathing Pattern

- Reduce activity of the external oblique, internal oblique, and rectus abdominis (OE/OI/RA)
- Change the breathing pattern to simplify control of the abdominal wall
- Optimize breathing pattern efficiency in breathing disorders
- Train control of the transversus abdominis (TrA) during breathing
- Consider posture and rib cage dynamics to optimize control of breathing
- Enable the patient to breathe efficiently at all levels of training

Rehabilitation of Functional Posture: Posture and Movement Patterns

Postural Correction. The clinician must keep a number of factors in mind when considering posture. First, although the ideal neutral posture has been argued to involve neutral pelvic tilt, lumbar lordosis, smooth transition to thoracic kyphosis, and cervical lordosis (see Figure 11-15), this may not be ideal for all patients. For instance, specific pathologies must be considered (e.g., spinal stenosis is likely to require less extension in the lumbar spine). Second, sufficient range of motion must be present to achieve the posture. This should be assessed by palpation of interspinous motion during movement. Manual mobilization techniques may be appropriate to aid the development of range. Third, it is critical that the position be comfortable and be able to be maintained with minimal activity of the large superficial muscles. The position may feel awkward, but this is reasonable. If pain occurs or the position is difficult to hold, the position must be modified within this constraint. A final consideration is that the purpose of training postural control is not to encourage the patient to hold this position statically, but to move into and out of the posture as required by a task (i.e., dynamically). A key factor is that the spine is flexible and not rigidly held in the position, therefore movement can be used to contribute to control as required. Encouraging the patient to control posture when sitting or standing for extended periods is ideal to prevent tissue creep.

Aims of Postural Correction

- Optimize posture
- Prevent provocative postures
- Optimize loading
- Reduce overactivity of superficial/global muscles
- Aid activation of deep/local muscles in functional postures
- Assist with optimization of the respiratory pattern
- Aid in optimization of control of the pelvic floor muscles

A range of techniques for correcting posture is available. The techniques chosen depend on the findings of the assessment. Key elements that often require control are the thoracolumbar junction and lumbar lordosis. Table 11-12 presents a range of factors that require consideration and strategies that can be used for training. The techniques are derived from a variety of sources, including Klein-Vogelbach[132] and Kendall and McCreary.[133] The easiest course often is to have the patient start in the sitting position with the hips flexed to about 60° to allow free movement of the pelvis. Postural correction can be undertaken by having the patient practice components before practicing the complete maneuver in subsequent sessions. Once posture has been corrected, activation of the deep muscles should be attempted to encourage functional integration of the maneuver.

Movement Patterns. Categorization of patients according to movement patterns provides guidance regarding the requirements for control of provocative postures and movements, correction of movement faults, and consideration of adjacent joints. The findings of the assessment of movement patterns will have provided essential information about the provocative movements and relieving postures. These findings also provide some guidance on the components of the muscle system that must be trained.

Treatment is directed at training muscles, movements, and postures that control the provocative movements and postures. For instance, for a patient presenting with Sahrmann's lumbar flexion syndrome,[73] the program would include training for the paraspinal muscles (particularly the superficial regions of the multifidus), training movement at the hip to reduce dependence on spinal flexion, and correction of posture (particularly control of lumbar lordosis in standing and sitting).

Relative Flexibility. If restriction of motion of the adjacent joints is a factor, it must be rectified for the spine to have normal function. The evaluation of movement patterns will have provided an initial indication of the importance of the function of the adjacent joints. In particular, Sahrmann's classification of movement impairment syndromes provides a clear indication of likely problems of flexibility.[73] Other tests of muscle length also can be considered, such as those described by Kendall[133] and Janda.[80]

Progression of Exercise

Once the initial goals of improved activation of the deep muscles, decreased overactivity of the superficial muscles, rehabilitation of the breathing pattern, and correction of posture and movement patterns have been met, progression of exercise must begin to take the patient through to functional rehabilitation. As presented in Figure 11-16, this can be achieved by progression through exercises of increasing complexity, again specific to the patient's presentation.

Table 11-11

Interpretation of Assessment and Strategies to Encourage an Efficient Breathing Pattern

Problem	Interpretation	Management
Limited basal expansion of rib cage	Increased activity of the external oblique, rectus abdominis, and internal oblique (OE/RA/OI), preventing rib elevation.	Techniques to reduce OE/RA/OI activity, such as feedback (electromyography [EMG], palpation). Encourage controlled breathing, with active inspiration and relaxed expiration. Techniques to encourage basal expansion: Manual feedback, elastic strap around the thorax to enhance awareness.
	Stiff/hypomobile thoracic spine and rib cage.	Restriction of basal expansion caused by poor flexibility of the rib cage may be managed with manual techniques and mobility exercises.
	Hyperinflation of the thorax.	This condition generally is related to respiratory disease. It may be difficult to change, but attempts to improve respiratory efficiency may help.
	Reduced potential of the diaphragm to shorten.	Restriction may be caused by fixation of the rib cage and increased intra-abdominal pressure (IAP) caused by abdominal muscle activity (use techniques as described previously to encourage diaphragmatic breathing). The condition also may be related to a primary diaphragmatic problem. Train motion of the rib cage.
Excessive abdominal displacement	May compromise ability to maintain tonic contraction of the transversus abdominis (TrA). The TrA should be tonic but modulated with breathing.	Encourage basal expansion, as described previously.
Excessive upper chest movement	Increased activity of the OE/RA/OI, preventing rib elevation and displacement of the abdominal wall.	Encourage basal expansion, as described previously.
Inability to maintain contraction of the deep muscles during breathing	Inability to hold contraction because of demand to use abdominal wall movement for breathing.	Encourage basal expansion, as described previously.
	Inability to maintain contraction during inspiration.	Enhance feedback of contraction with palpation, observation (ultrasound). Inspiratory volume training: Gradually increase inspiratory volume during successive breaths until the threshold is identified.
	Shifts breathing pattern to shallow or upper chest breathing.	Encourage basal expansion, as described previously. Inspiratory volume training: Gradually increase inspiratory volume during successive breaths until the threshold is identified.
	Poor posture prevents normal motion of rib cage, with breathing with increased demand on abdominal wall movement. Rotated positions increase demand for abdominal wall displacement.	Postural correction to reduce rotation and encourage normal basal expansion of the rib cage; neutral spinal posture.

Table 11-12
Techniques for Postural Correction

Factor to be Addressed	Cues and Techniques
Forward or backward leaning	*Feedback:* Hands placed on manubrium should be immediately over a hand placed on the anterior aspect of the pelvis.
Uneven weight bearing through ischial tuberosities	*Feedback:* Hands placed under the ischial tuberosities can be used to provide feedback of symmetry of weight bearing.
Excessive thoracolumbar extension	*Manual handling:* The therapist places a hand on the sternum and the thoracolumbar junction; the patient then is encouraged to sink to flatten the thoracolumbar junction. The patient can be allowed to roll on the pelvis temporarily but should not simply slump.
	Feedback: The thumb of one hand can be placed on the xiphoid and the little finger of the same hand in the navel; this distance reduces with thoracolumbar flexion.
	Cues: "Let your chest sink." "Open at the back." "Inspire/breathe into the midback."
	Avoid: Make sure the patient is not using scapular protraction to simulate thoracic movement. Make sure the patient does not slump the upper thorax, and take care to correct the head position by having the patient nod forward (i.e., avoid upper cervical extension).
Decreased lumbar lordosis or flexion (often in the low lumbar spine)	*Manual handling:* A hand placed on the superior aspect of the sacrum or the flexed segments can be used to provide gentle encouragement to move the spine. If the patient has difficulty dissociating lumbar and thoracic motion, an intermediate step could be to have the patient rock the pelvis without motion of the thorax in a four-point kneeling position.
	Feedback: The thumb of one hand can be placed on the xiphoid and the little finger of the same hand in the navel; this can be used to monitor and prevent thoracolumbar extension.
	Cues: "Imagine that a string is attached to your tailbone and someone is gently pulling the string up to the sky." "Grow tall from the tailbone." "Allow the ball to roll underneath you and let the pelvis fall forward." "Roll forward on your tailbone."
	Avoid: Avoid strong activation of the paraspinal muscles; the patient should be able to complete the task with gentle activity of the lumbar muscles, particularly the superficial fibers of the multifidus. Avoid extension at the thoracolumbar junction; feedback of motion at this segment can be obtained with the hand placed on the xiphoid and the little finger in the navel); this distance should not change during motion.
Increased thoracic kyphosis	*Manual handling:* The hands can be used to provide a sensation of lengthening by spreading two fingers along the spinous processes over the segments to be flattened.
	Cues: "Imagine a spot on the top of your head being gently pulled up to the sky."
	Avoid: Avoid motion simply by extension at the thoracolumbar junction.

Co-activation of Deep Muscles and Improved Precision of Training. An initial goal is to encourage co-activation of the muscles of the deep system. As discussed previously, activity of some of the deep muscles often occurs together, and this can be used as a method to initiate contraction of the other deep muscles. However, it is important to assess the degree of co-activation achieved and whether specific intervention is required to encourage this. Patients generally fall into one of three categories: those with automatic co-activation of the deep muscles, those who require emphasis on the other muscles (e.g., feedback of other muscles of the system), and those who require separate exercises for each muscle to be integrated later. The other goal of this phase of the intervention is to improve the precision and efficiency of the control of the deep muscle system. This involves increased holding time, an increased number of contractions, reduced feedback (i.e., gradual weaning from feedback), and decreased reliance on special techniques involving position and co-contraction. At the completion of this phase, the goal is for the patient to have achieved confident activation of the deep muscles. This means that the contraction should be independent of the superficial muscles (but with the deep muscles all working together); also, the patient should be able to (1) perform the contraction voluntarily, with minimal feedback and minimal effort; (2) hold the contraction for 10 seconds; and (3) breathe while holding the contraction.

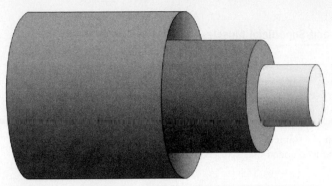

Figure 11-17
Diagram of the coordination of the deep and superficial muscles of the trunk. The deep muscles are activated first and tonically. The activity of the superficial muscles is layered over the top in a manner that is specific to the task; this activity occurs either phasically or tonically, in co-contraction or in a carefully timed sequence of muscle activity.

When this is achieved, the patient can progress to the next phase of training.

Co-activation of Deep and Superficial Muscles: Static. When the patient can confidently perform activation of the deep muscles, coordination between the deep and superficial muscle systems must be trained (Figure 11-17). The easiest way to do this is to initiate this training with static tasks. Static control training has two key goals: training of the integration between the local and global muscles and training of the control of lumbopelvic orientation and alignment. The key to this phase is to preactivate the deep muscles, hold this activation tonically, and then use load and resistance to initiate activity of the superficial muscles over the top. The underlying principle is that once load is applied to the limbs or trunk, activation of the global muscles is required to control the alignment. Many possibilities for training this level have been presented in the clinical literature. Table 11-13 presents the principles and some examples of several of the most common approaches. Many other approaches are available (e.g., TherapiMaster,[134] hydrotherapy), and the basic principles are similar to those described previously.

Co-activation of Deep and Superficial Muscles: Dynamic. Training control of the spine and pelvis in dynamic situations is more complex than static control, but it is essential for progression to function. Several

Table 11-13
Strategies to Train Static Coordination Between the Deep and Superficial Muscles

Strategy	Principles	Example Exercises
Leg loading	In the crook lying position, load is applied in a progressive manner by moving the legs in different planes of motion. The patient is instructed to maintain the position of the spine and pelvis.	Bent knee fallouts: The leg is slowly lowered to the side while maintaining the position of the pelvis and spine. The position of the spine and pelvis can be monitored with a pressure biofeedback unit. Specific directions of greater and lesser control can be identified by directions of movement associated with loss of control of alignment.
Rhythmic stabilizations (proprioceptive neuromuscular facilitation)	The patient maintains a neutral position as force is applied to the body. Force is normally low (about 30%) and the direction slowly alternates.	In the sitting position with neutral alignment, rotary force can be applied to the shoulders in alternating directions. During the change in direction, activation of the superficial muscles alternates over the top of the tonically maintained activation of the deeper muscles.
Limb loading	The neutral position of the spine is maintained in any body position as load is applied first through short levers (bent limbs) and then through longer levers (with the limbs straight).	In a quadruped position, the position of the spine is maintained in neutral as either an arm or a leg (or both) is moved to the side or in the sagittal plane. Postural preparations are required to ensure that the center of mass is placed over the new base of support.
Pilates	Load is applied though the use of limb load, springs, and other equipment as the spine is maintained in a neutral position.	On a reformer bed (sliding bed with springs adjusted to resist the motion of the bed), the patient precontracts the deep muscles and maintains the neutral position as the sliding surface is translated by extension and flexion of the bed. Although this technique often involves movement on expiration, the better course may be to train movement with both phases of breathing.
Balls	The neutral position of the spine is maintained while the body is partly or completely supported on a ball. Load can be added by addition of limb load.	The patient can sit in neutral on a large ball with the hips above 90°. Load can be applied by reduction of the base of support (lifting a leg) or by increasing the load (by movement of the arms or legs).

Table 11-14
Strategies to Train Dynamic Coordination Between the Deep and Superficial Muscles

Strategy	Principles	Example Exercises
Unstable surfaces	The patient aims to maintain balance and alignment of the trunk when placed on an unstable surface. To maintain balance, movement of the spine is necessary, because balance cannot be maintained simply by control at the ankle.	Standing on a balance board, sitting on a ball, balance shoes (Janda).
Function-specific tasks	Specific movements that are required for function are trained. The movement is segmented, simplified, and performed with reduced speed and reduced load.	Walking (progressing from side-side weight shift), trunk rotation.

strategies are available, such as tasks that involve support on an unstable surface for control during specific movements of the trunk. The key elements are to preactivate the deep muscles and to hold this tonically while movement is performed. Several examples are presented in Table 11-14.

Progression of Load, Position, and Dynamics. Although it is critical that patients do not progress too soon, it also is critical to ensure that patients are progressed to a high enough level to meet functional demands. The functional demands of the individual's work and leisure activities must be assessed, and exercise must be progressed through load, position, and dynamics to meet these demands. For instance, a patient may have to work at high levels of resistance or in unstable environments. Appropriate progression with a gym-based program may be required. Specific attention should be focused on control of deep muscle contractions during the progression, specific movement and postural faults identified in the assessment, and the patient's ability to maintain breathing during the progressions.

Functional Rehabilitation. Functional training follows principles similar to those for the preceding phases but focuses on the training of functional tasks. Again, the principles of preactivation of the deep muscles, with segmentation and simplification of the task, are followed. Ideally, the goal is automatic activation of the deep muscles with minimal requirement to activate the muscles consciously. However, it is helpful to initiate training with preactivation to ensure integration of this component. Attention to movement and postural faults and breathing are required. Progression should include practice in more challenging environments to ensure transfer of training. Practice closer to the actual functional demands is likely to lead to better transfer.

Behavioral Challenge. A final issue worthy of consideration is the requirement for behavioral training. As mentioned previously, fear of pain and injury or reinjury may disrupt control of the trunk muscles in a manner similar to the actual experience of pain. Therefore, although a patient may be able to maintain ideal control in the safe, closed environment of a clinic, this may not be the case

when the person moves in real world environments. Patients may require specific training drills to maintain control while rehearsing specific activities. This requirement is described in detail elsewhere.[91]

Evidence for Efficacy of Motor Control Exercises for Spinal and Pelvic Pain

As described in the previous sections, rehabilitation of dynamic control of the spine and pelvis involves a motor learning approach. The intervention, therefore, involves more than just exercising specific muscles. It requires the clinician's attention in assessing movement patterns and posture, detecting signs of overactivity of specific muscle groups, and evaluating breathing and continence. Because of the complexity and comprehensiveness of the intervention, the task of identifying clinical studies examining its efficacy is not always straightforward. The description of exercise interventions in clinical studies varies frequently and often is incomplete. If the description of the intervention is not clear, judging whether the study should be used to assess the efficacy of the intervention becomes difficult.

This section provides a description of the evidence of efficacy of motor control exercises for spinal and pelvic pain. The evidence considered comes from randomized, controlled studies. A typical randomized, controlled study involves patients with a specific condition who are randomly allocated to a controlled group or to a group receiving the treatment of interest. To assess the efficacy of motor control exercises, only information provided by good quality studies is used. Good quality studies usually have a score of at least 3 on the 0-10 PEDro scale. The PEDro scale assesses the quality of randomized, controlled trials based on criteria such as allocation of patients and eligibility criteria.[135]

Randomized, controlled trials that included at least one exercise intervention typically involving a motor control approach were identified. The comparison group could include no intervention, other exercise interventions, and other interventions, such as manual therapy techniques.

Motor control exercises could be delivered in isolation or in combination with other treatments.

Can Motor Control Training Help in the Treatment of Acute Low Back Pain?

Can Motor Control Training Reduce Pain or Disability in Patients with Acute Low Back Pain?

One trial, by Hides et al.,[101] has been published in the literature that addresses the issue of the efficacy of specific stabilization exercises in the treatment of pain and disability associated with acute LBP. This trial (quality score of 7 on the PEDro scale) compared motor control training plus medical management to medical management alone for acute LBP. The effect of specific stabilization exercise on pain was small and not significant. Motor control training showed no effect on disability. However, the size of the multifidus was restored only in individuals who received the motor control intervention.

Can Motor Control Training Reduce Recurrence After an Acute Episode of Low Back Pain?

Hides et al also published a follow-up study (quality score of 6 on the PEDro scale) examining the ability of motor control training to reduce the recurrence of episodes after acute LBP.[51] Motor control training plus medical management was substantially more effective than medical management alone for reducing recurrence at the 1-year and 2-year follow-up. Individuals who did not receive the motor control intervention were 12.4 times more likely to suffer a subsequent episode of LBP.

Clinical Point

Motor control training does not appear to offer substantial benefit in reducing pain or disability in patients suffering from low back pain (LBP) of less than 3 months' duration. However, research has shown that acute LBP changes the pattern of muscle recruitment, possibly leading to further back pain; therefore this approach appears to be useful in reducing the number of future episodes of LBP. Patients should be advised that the purpose of the intervention is to reduce the recurrence of back pain episodes and that the intervention is unlikely to affect pain or disability dramatically in the short term.

Can Motor Control Training Help in the Treatment of Chronic Low Back Pain?

Is Motor Control Training More Helpful in Reducing Pain or Disability Than Usual Care in Patients With Chronic Low Back Pain?

Two trials (quality scores of 6[136] and 7[52] on the PEDro scale) have examined the effects of motor control training compared to usual care (educational booklet)[136] or treatment at the discretion of the general practitioner.[52] Motor control training was substantially more effective than usual care for reducing pain at 3 months and at 6 months. Motor control training was not more effective than usual care for reducing disability at 3 months but was more effective at 6 months.

Is Motor Control Training More Helpful in Reducing Pain or Disability Than Spinal Manipulative Therapy in Patients with Chronic Low Back Pain?

Two trials (both with a quality score of 6[136,137] on the PEDro scale) have examined the effect of motor control training compared to spinal manipulative therapy. Motor control training produced reductions in pain or disability similar to those seen with spinal manipulative therapy at 3 and 12 months.

Clinical Point

Motor control training offers more benefits to patients with chronic LBP than common traditional interventions such as educational booklets or treatment at the discretion of a medical practitioner. Patients with chronic LBP have altered patterns of muscle recruitment and a high level of disability. The effects of motor control training in reducing pain and disability appear to be similar to those seen with manual therapy treatment. Some studies have attempted to identify subgroups of patients with LBP, but which characteristics mean that a patient will respond better to a particular intervention is still not known. Patients who benefit from motor control exercises show clinical patterns of spinal instability during assessment or, probably more critically, signs of altered motor control. Although this issue has not been investigated extensively, the authors recommend that clinicians assess patterns of movement and muscle recruitment to gain clinical insight into whether a patient would respond better to a motor control exercise approach or to treatment that focuses on mobilization of spinal joints. Although the idea of treating patients with chronic LBP with a combination of specific stabilization exercises and spinal manipulative therapy seems appealing, this clinical question has not yet been investigated.

What Is the Efficacy of Motor Control Training When Implemented as Part of a Treatment Package in Patients With Chronic Low Back Pain?

Two trials (quality scores of 6[138] and 8[139] on the PEDro scale) examined the effect of motor control training as part of a physical therapy treatment program (combined with spinal manipulative therapy and education) compared to either education or medical management. Physical therapy treatment that included motor control training was more effective than medical management or education for reducing pain and disability at 4 weeks and at 5 months. At 12 months, physical therapy treatment that included motor control training was more effective than medical management for reducing pain and disability and more effective than education for reducing pain but not disability. Physical therapy treatment that included motor control training marginally improved quality of life compared to education at 5 months but not at 12 months.

What Is the Efficacy of Motor Control Training Compared to Surgery for Patients with Chronic Low Back Pain?

One trial (quality score of 8[140] on the PEDro scale) examined the effect of motor control training and education compared to surgery and physical therapy treatment (advice and exercises). The two groups produced similar reductions in pain and disability at 12 months.

> ### Clinical Point
>
> Motor control training is effective when applied as part of a treatment package that usually includes sessions of manual therapy and education. Treatment packages that include motor control training produce reductions in pain and disability similar to those seen with surgical procedures, such as spinal fusion. Clinicians should keep this in mind when recommending exercises for chronic LBP, especially given the higher costs and risks involved with surgical procedures.

Is Motor Control Training Helpful in the Treatment of Pelvic Pain?

One trial (quality score of 6[134] on the PEDro scale) has compared motor control training plus a conventional physical therapy program (modalities, spinal manipulative therapy, and ergonomic advice) to a conventional physical therapy program alone for patients with pelvic pain. When added to a conventional physical therapy program, motor control training was more effective than conventional physical therapy alone for all outcomes at various assessment occasions.

> ### Clinical Point
>
> Approximately 50% of pregnant women experience lumbopelvic pain during pregnancy. It is known that specific deep abdominal and pelvic muscles maintain pelvic stability[55] . Pelvic pain has been associated with compromised control of the pelvic joints. The finding that motor control training is helpful in reducing pain and disability in patients with pregnancy-related pelvic pain[133] is important, both because of the prevalence of this condition and because of the lack of evidence of efficacy of other physical therapy interventions in its treatment.

Can Motor Control Training Change the Control of Movement and Stability and Is This Related to Outcome?

If motor control training is effective, it is important to consider whether the intervention can actually change control and, if so, whether improvements in control are associated with improvements in clinical outcomes. Recent data confirm that cognitive training of motor control of the deep muscles can change the timing of activation of the deep muscles,[141] that activation of the deep abdominal muscles is not restored after other training interventions (e.g., a situp[142]) or during abdominal bracing maneuvers,[143] and that the improvements in control persist when tested at 6 months after the intervention.[142] Other studies report increased thickening of the TrA on US imaging after a motor control intervention but not after a general exercise program or a course of manual therapy.[144] In terms of muscle structure, Hides et al.[101] reported that the cross sectional area (CSA) of the multifidus can be restored in people with acute LBP. However, Danneels et al.[145] reported that overloading was required to restore the multifidus CSA in chronic low back pain.

One recent study has assessed the association between changes in control of the TrA and clinical improvement.[144] This study investigated changes in recruitment of the TrA, measured with ultrasound, after the application of motor control training, general exercise, and spinal manipulative therapy, to examine the relationship between changes in recruitment and changes in clinical outcomes. In the study, 34 subjects with chronic LBP were assessed for ability to recruit the TrA by means of ultrasound measurement and clinical outcomes of function, disability, and pain. Patients with chronic LBP who received motor control training showed greater changes in recruitment of the TrA than did patients who received general and spinal manipulative therapy. A moderate but significant correlation was found between changes in recruitment of the TrA and changes in the clinical outcomes of global perceived effect and disability (Figure 11-18).

A final issue is whether activation of the deep muscles, before treatment, can be used to predict the potential effect of motor control training for the individual. Data from a study by Ferreira[144] suggest that people with poorer activation of the TrA before treatment have a greater response.

Summary and Directions for the Future

Although existing studies are promising, further research is needed to evaluate the efficacy of motor control training in low back pain. Critical issues that need to be addressed include the identification of subgroups that assist in the selection of the most appropriate treatment strategies and evaluation of the most appropriate clinical path for progression of exercise. Motor control training likely has a place in the management of many people with low back and pelvic pain, but the relative contribution of the intervention to clinical outcomes will vary from individual to individual.

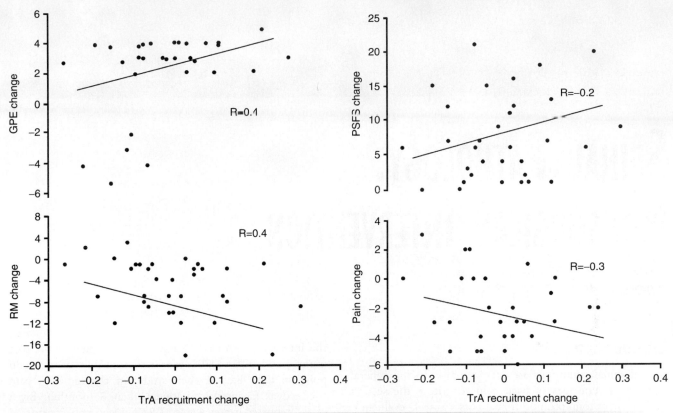

Figure 11-18

Correlation between changes in recruitment of the transversus abdominis measured with ultrasonography and changes in clinical outcomes. Lines represent R squared best of fit. *GPE,* Global perceived effect; *PSFS,* Patient Specific Functional Scale; *RM,* Roland Morris.

References

To enhance this text and add value for the reader, all references have been incorporated into a CD-ROM that is provided with this text. The reader can view the reference source and access it online whenever possible. There are a total of 145 references for this chapter.

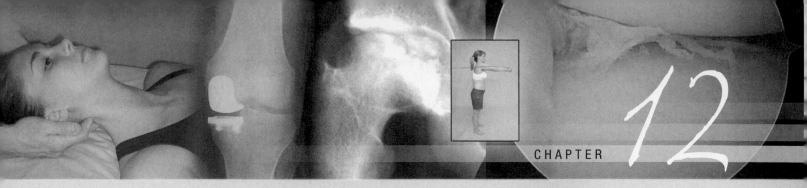

CHAPTER 12

Spinal Pathology: Nonsurgical Intervention

Omar El Abd

Introduction

Painful spinal conditions are very common in the general population. Episodes of back pain constitute the second leading symptom prompting patients to seek evaluation by a physician.[1] These conditions are responsible for a great deal of pain and physical suffering for patients and for social and financial pressures in the community. Interventional spinal techniques are a new and evolving field that combines different aspects of the medical field to manage patients with painful spinal conditions. These interventions combine various aspects of physical medicine and rehabilitation, orthopedics, pain management, radiology, rheumatology, neurology, and physical therapy. The objectives of these interventional techniques are to diagnose and efficiently treat painful spinal conditions and to minimize the persistence or recurrence of pain.

This chapter discusses painful spinal conditions and their management through interventional techniques. It provides an overview of the clinical presentations of different pathologies and, focusing on interventional spinal procedures, discusses appropriate imaging studies, indications, techniques, side effects, and complications.

Epidemiology

The incidence and prevalence of back pain have been the subjects of multiple epidemiological studies. The *incidence* is the rate at which healthy subjects report a new symptom or disease within a certain period. The *prevalence* is the number of subjects reporting certain symptoms or a certain disease at a particular period. Waddell[2] reported that 17% to 31% of patients reported back symptoms on the day of

the interview, 19% to 43% reported back pain in the past month, and 60% to 70% reported back pain at a certain point in their life. In their study on chronic back pain (defined as having lasted longer than 3 months), Blyth et al.[3] reported a prevalence of 21%. Deyo et al.[4] reported that the cumulative lifetime prevalence of low back pain that lasted at least 2 weeks was 13.8%. Lawrence et al.[5] reported an annual prevalence of low back pain of 56% and a lifetime prevalence of 70%.

With regard to the location of pain, the incidence of radiculopathy (2%) is reported to be much lower than the incidence of axial back pain (6%).[4] The percentage of patients who report an acute episode of back pain and later develop chronic pain (lasting 3 to 6 months or longer) is the subject of controversy. Several studies suggested that 90% of patients with an acute episode of back pain recover within 6 weeks.[6,7] However, recent studies have shown a higher incidence of recurrence and persistence of pain after the initial acute episode.[8] Although the findings of studies vary, clinicians encounter a number of patients who convert from acute to chronic pain.

Anatomy and Pain-Producing Structures

The human spine consists of seven cervical, 12 thoracic, and five lumbar vertebral bodies, as well as five fused sacral vertebrae and five fused coccygeal vertebrae. The spinal cord runs in the central canal and commonly ends at the L1-2 level. Nerve roots emerge from the neural foramina. There are seven cervical intervertebral discs and eight cervical nerve roots. In the cervical region, the nerve roots emerge cephalad to their corresponding vertebral bodies except for the C8 nerve root, which emerges caudal to the C7 vertebral body. In the

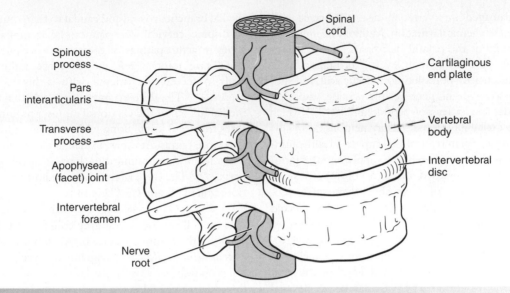

Figure 12-1
Spinal segment.

thoracic, lumbar, sacral, and coccygeal regions, nerve roots continue to emerge from the neural foramina just caudal to the corresponding vertebral bodies. The cauda equina develops at the L1-2 level; it is formed by an aggregation of lumbar, sacral, and coccygeal nerve roots. These nerve roots are present in the central canal and emerge at their corresponding neural foramina. Multiple ligaments and muscles support the spine. A spinal segment (Figure 12-1) consists of two vertebral bodies: an intervertebral disc and a set of two facets on each side (zygapophyseal joints). Pain can occur as a result of pathology involving a single element, multiple elements of a particular segment, or multiple segments.

Radicular Pain

Involvement of nerve roots causes radicular pain. Nerve roots are affected secondary to mechanical pressure, inflammation, or both. Mechanical pressure usually occurs secondary to disc protrusion (herniation) or spinal stenosis. In the case of disc herniation, the nucleus pulposus protrudes through the annulus fibrosus and causes mechanical compression of the nerve root either in the central canal or in the intervertebral foramen. Acute disc herniations are accompanied by multiple inflammatory products (listed later in the chapter), which play an important role in the production of pain. Disc herniations occur in all age groups but are predominant in the young and middle aged. Spinal stenosis, on the other hand, most often affects the elderly. This condition is a combination of disc degeneration, ligamentum hypertrophy and facet joint arthropathy, and/or spondylolisthesis, resulting in stenosis of the central spinal canal in the cervical and lumbar spine. Spinal stenosis causes pressure on and possibly dysfunction of the spinal cord (myelopathy) when it involves the central canal in the cervical and thoracic spine. In the lumbar spine, the cauda equina roots are involved, which causes neurogenic claudication.

With radiculopathy, symptoms are present along a nerve root distribution. This causes pain in the upper and lower extremities. It is worth mentioning that pain in the periscapular, pericostal, and buttocks area can be radicular in origin. Sensory symptoms include pain, numbness, and tingling that follow the distribution of a particular nerve root. The symptoms usually are accompanied by motor weakness in a myotome distribution.

Axial Pain

Axial pain occurs predominantly in the paraspinal areas and along the spinous processes. It also may be associated with pain in the extremities; however, by definition, paraspinal (axial) pain is more severe than pain in the extremities.

Disc

Degenerative disc disease is an important cause of axial pain. The pain from the intervertebral discs is located axially near the degenerated disc. The human disc is shaped like a donut and is formed of three distinct parts: the nucleus pulposus, the annulus fibrosus, and the cartilaginous end plates, which are adjacent to the vertebral bodies above and below. The nucleus pulposus is a semifluid mass of mucoid material composed of collagen fibers and proteoglycans. Water constitutes approximately 80% to 90% of the nucleus. As the disc ages, it loses its water content which is replaced by fibrocartilage. The end plates function as the nutrient pathways for the disc. They are composed of hyaline cartilage, which is located toward the vertebral body surface, and fibrocartilage, which is concentrated toward the nucleus pulposus. Degeneration of the annulus predisposes the nucleus to herniation, which occurs most often at the annulus' weakest part, its posterolateral aspect. Good evidence indicates that, in addition to the pain caused by mechanical irritation of the sensory nociceptive fibers in the damaged intervertebral disc, discogenic pain occurs secondary to chemical irritation. Multiple inflammatory products are found in the painful disc tissue. These include phospholipase A2 (present in high levels),[9] prostaglandin E, histamine-like substances, potassium ions, lactic acid, and substance P, as well as calcitonin gene–related peptide, vasoactive intestinal peptide, and other polypeptide amines,[10,11] which can increase the excitability of the sensory neurons.

The mechanism of pain referral is complex. Healthy lumbar intervertebral discs receive sensory supply into the annulus fibrosus, whereas diseased discs, according to some reports, have an in-growth of nerve fibers that express substance P into their nuclei.[11] Two extensively interconnected nerve plexuses, the anterior and the posterior plexuses, serve as the source of nerve endings within the lumbar intervertebral discs. The anterior plexus is formed from branches of both sympathetic trunks: the proximal ends of the grey ramii communicantes and the perivascular nerve plexuses of the segmental arteries. The anterior part of the disc, therefore, is innervated solely by sympathetic fibers.[12,13]

The sinuvertebral nerves constitute the vast majority of the posterior plexus. Although some consider these nerves recurrent branches of the spinal nerves, others regard them as branches of spinal nerves with a sympathetic component. Luschka first described the sinovertebral nerve as re-entering the canal and providing innervation to the posterior longitudinal ligament and annulus fibrosus.[14] It now is widely accepted that the sinovertebral nerve is the main nerve supply to all structures in the spinal canal. It enters the spinal canal through the intervertebral foramen. Once inside, it gives off multiple ascending and descending branches, which eventually combine to form a plexus along the posterior longitudinal ligament.[15,16] This plexus receives branches from the ipsilateral caudal and cephalic segments of the sinovertebral nerve and, as suggested, the contralateral side as well.[17] Because of the interaction with the sympathetic system, as well as the segmental anastomosis, somatic pain referral is extremely common; that is, pain occurs in areas that commonly feel pain, such as the skin and underlying muscles.

Facet Joint

The facet (zygapophyseal) joints can be another source of axial pain. Pain is attributed to facet joint pathology in about 30% to 50% of patients who describe axial pain.[18-21] The facets are paired synovial joints located adjacent to the neural arches. They are formed by the superior articular process of the vertebra below and the inferior articular process of the vertebra above.

Pain is located predominantly in the paraspinal area. Pain originating from the facet joints can be either unilateral or bilateral. The results of multiple studies have led to the development of specific pain referral maps for the cervical facet joints. The facet joints receive their innervations from the medial branch of the dorsal ramii, with each medial branch innervating two joints.[22] Each joint is innervated by the medial branches rostral and caudal to that joint.[22] In the cervical spine, cervical facet pain can be accompanied by headaches in arthropathies of the atlanto-occipital, atlantoaxial (C1-2 facet joint), C2-3, and C3-4 facet joints. This is especially observed in patients with a history of whiplash events.[23,24] The third occipital nerve, which is the superficial medial branch of the C3 dorsal ramus, predominantly innervates the C2-3 joint, along with articular branches from the C2 dorsal ramus. At times, a small, inconsistent contribution arises from a communicating branch of the great occipital nerve.[22,25] The C1-2 lateral joints are innervated by the anterior ramii of C1 and C2.[26] Upon entering the spinal cord, the C1, C2, and C3 nerves converge with trigeminal nerve afferents on cells in the dorsal grey column of C1 to C3. This results in the communication between both afferents known as *trigeminal volleys*. The trigeminal nerve provides superficial sensations to most of the face and anterior scalp. Therefore pain is referred in the trigeminal nerve distribution.

Compression Fractures

Acute vertebral compression fractures are becoming an increasingly common cause of axial back pain. This increase in incidence is probably due to the aging population and the prevalence of osteoporosis. The pain usually is very severe and localized, and it usually occurs in the area overlying the involved vertebral body. Vertebral osteoporotic compression fractures most often occur in the thoracolumbar junction area. The incidence of these fractures increases with age, and they affect 40% of women in their eighties.[27]

The pain usually is precipitated by trauma, although it has been reported to follow minor events, such as coughing. It also can occur spontaneously in patients with severe osteoporosis, because osteoporotic vertebral bodies are unable to withstand stress. In addition, compression fractures may be caused by malignancies involving the spine.

Sacroiliac Joint

Sacroiliac (SI) joint arthropathy also can be a cause of axial back pain. The pain is located in the lumbosacral/buttock junction with referral to the lower extremities and to the groin area. Painful conditions of the SI joint can result from spondyloarthropathies, infection, malignancies, pregnancies, and trauma, or they can even occur spontaneously.

Referred Pain

Musculoskeletal structures and organs near the spine are potential sources of pain, from which the pain can be referred to the spine and the paraspinal area. A careful, detailed physical examination is needed to assess these conditions, because various shoulder and hip conditions can mimic radiculopathies. Pelvic conditions and malignancies involving the supraclavicular area or the axilla should be considered if symptoms persist despite the absence of identifiable lesions on imaging studies, especially if the patient has constitutional symptoms (e.g., fever, chills, weight loss) or bowel and bladder changes.

Patient Evaluation

Careful history taking and a thorough physical examination are the most important aspects of the evaluation of patients with a painful spinal condition. This process is necessary so that the clinician can interpret the imaging studies accurately in context and formulate the treatment plan.

History Taking

As in any clinical encounter, the clinician inquires about the history of the painful condition, including its location, onset, character, radiation, exacerbating and mitigating factors, and accompanying symptoms. It is crucial to establish which area is the most painful; this allows the clinician to formulate the preliminary differential diagnosis and to determine whether the pain is axial, radicular, or referred from other structures. Discogenic pain originating from painful disc conditions usually is difficult to localize. On questioning, patients frequently point to a general area of pain. This pain usually is exacerbated by sitting and mitigated by a change in position. Pain may be characterized but not limited to aching or a sharp sensation. In the cervical spine, upper cervical discs refer pain to the occipital area, causing headaches.[16] In the lumbar spine, pain may be referred to the abdominal and inguinal areas.[17]

Cervical facet joint pain is usually but not explicitly exacerbated by neck extension or lateral bending. In the lumbar region, pain from facet joints usually is exacerbated by standing and walking and mitigated by sitting; however, pain from lumbar facet joints can occur on forward flexion as well. Pain from facet joints usually overlies the facet joints in the paraspinal area and is more localized than discogenic pain. Pain can be referred ipsilaterally or bilaterally.

Specific diagrams are available that show the referral patterns for cervical facet joint pain (Figure 12-2). The referral pattern for lumbar facet joint pain is not as distinct as that for cervical facet joint pain, and no pain referral maps have been described for lumbar facet joint pain.[28] To map the pain referral patterns for the cervical facet joints, researchers stimulated the joints in healthy subjects and noted the painful locations.[29-31] Different studies produced essentially very similar pain referral maps.

Patients with radicular symptoms usually describe pain predominantly in the extremities. The pain may start as axial pain (in the case of disc herniations), which is followed by the onset of limb pain as the axial pain improves. It is important to note that the buttocks and the periscapular regions are considered part of the limbs. Pain predominantly in these locations is considered radicular pain rather than axial pain. The pain often is described as shooting, stabbing, sharp, or burning, and patients often are able to localize the painful area accurately. The pain usually follows a specific nerve root distribution, with some variability.[32] Cervical radicular pain is exacerbated by cervical extension and lateral bending. The pain may be relieved by overhead elevation of the ipsilateral upper extremity, because this maneuver reduces tension on the lower nerve roots (shoulder abduction relief sign).[33] Dermatome maps are available that outline the spinal nerve root distribution (Figure 12-3). It is important to note that these maps are not 100% accurate. Nerve root distribution varies from individual to individual.

In cases of disc herniation and foraminal stenosis, lumbar radicular pain is exacerbated by sitting and mitigated by walking. In cases of spinal stenosis, pain is exacerbated by walking (spinal extension) and mitigated by sitting (neurogenic claudication). Differentiating neurogenic claudication from vascular claudication that occurs secondary to vascular insufficiency is important, because both conditions affect the same (elderly) population. Patients with vascular claudication feel relief from pain when they stop walking or when they stand rather than sit. Patients with neurogenic claudication have more pain when walking downhill (because of spinal extension) and less pain when walking with a walker or a shopping chart (because of spinal flexion). Pain from

Figure 12-2

Referral distribution of cervical facet pain. Note: Referred pain distribution shown on one side only for each example. Pattern may be the same on opposite side if same structures are involved. (Redrawn from Fukui S, Ohseto K, Shiotani M et al: Referred pain distribution of the cervical zygapophyseal joints and cervical dorsal rami, *Pain* 68:79-83, 1996.)

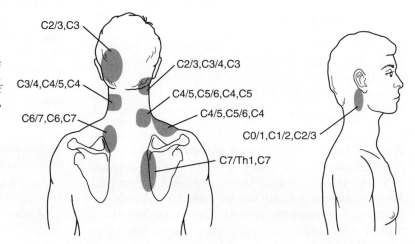

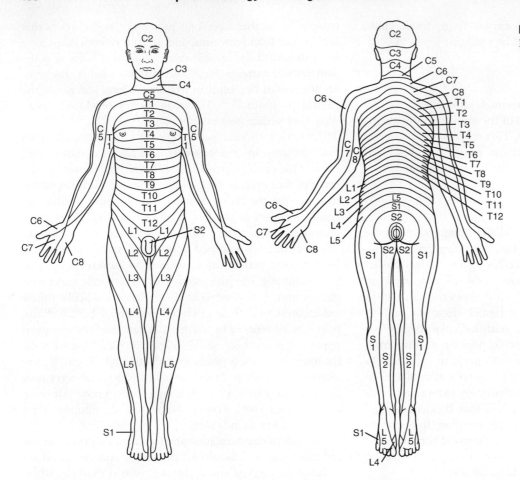

Figure 12-3
Dermatome maps.

neurogenic claudication follows a nerve root distribution, whereas pain from vascular claudication is present globally in the location supplied by specific arteries.

Pain referred from the SI joint should be suspected in patients who describe pain in the low back predominantly in the sacral sulcus area, with or without radiation to the lower extremity and the groin area. Pain occurs secondary to systemic conditions (e.g., spondyloarthropathies, repetitive shear events) and after trauma, or it can occur spontaneously.[34]

Physical Examination

A focused physical examination based on the information acquired in the patient's history establishes a working differential diagnosis. Some elements of the general physical examination are essential in the evaluation of patients with painful spinal conditions. These elements are detailed in Table 12-1.

Spinal Physical Examination Maneuvers

Specific maneuvers are used to evaluate a variety of conditions and anatomical areas that may cause a patient pain. These maneuvers are outlined in Table 12-2. Discogenic provocative maneuvers provoke pain reproduction in patients with lumbar discogenic pain. Root tension signs

in the upper and lower extremities reproduce radicular pain. Sacroiliac provocative maneuvers are used to reproduce pain in patients with SI joint syndrome. These tests are neither specific nor sensitive. (More information on these tests and others can be found in volume 1 of this series, *Orthopedic Physical Assessment.*)

The gold standard for evaluating pain that emanates from the SI joint is a fluoroscopically guided, intra-articular diagnostic injection with a local anesthetic.[35]

Sensory Examination

Pinprick, light touch, position, and vibration sensation are examined, with particular emphasis on the limb with radicular pain. The sensations of vibration and position are diminished in severe spinal stenosis, especially in the cervical spine with central canal involvement. In radiculopathy, reduced pinprick and light touch sensations are noted in specific dermatomal distribution.

Spinal Sensory Changes with Pathology

- Spinal stenosis: Sensations of vibration and position are affected
- Radiculopathy: Sensations of pinprick and light touch are affected in specific dermatomes

Table 12-1

General Physical Examination Elements That May Have Bearing on a Spinal Condition

Evaluation	Description	Rationale
Height and weight	Measurement	Height/weight ratio assessment, exercise and diet recommendations; unusual loss of weight requires medical workup
Deformity	Scoliosis, kyphosis, reduced lordosis (cervical/lumbar)	Sign of spinal pathology, postural changes, and possible causes of musculoskeletal imbalances
Muscle wasting	Inspection of the peripheral muscles	Sign of radiculopathy or other neurological disorder
Leg length discrepancy	Measurement	Postural changes and musculoskeletal imbalances
Examination of pulses	Arterial pulses in the upper and lower extremities	Peripheral vascular disease may result in painful conditions that mimic radiculopathy
Palpation of lymph nodes	Presence of lymph nodes in the neck, axilla, and inguinal area	Possible sign of occult malignancy resulting in metastasis to the spine
Palpation of tenderness	Over the spinous processes and facet and sacroiliac joints	Spine pathology, such as compression fractures and facet joint and sacroiliac joint arthropathy
Peripheral joint examination	Range of motion and specific joint maneuvers	Extraspinal source of pain with referral to the spine
Gait examination	Assessment of gait, heel walking, toe walking, and tandem walking	Good screening tool for evaluation of weakness and neurological disorders

Table 12-2

Spinal Physical Examination Maneuvers

Maneuver	Technique	Result
Pelvic rock	With the patient supine, flex the hips until the flexed knees approximate to the chest; then rotate the lower extremities from one side to the other	Provokes lumbar discogenic pain
Sustained hip flexion	With the patient supine, raise the extended lower extremities to approximately 60°. Ask the patient to hold the lower extremities in that position and release. The test result is positive with reproduction of low lumbar and/or buttock pain. Next, lower the extremities successively approximately 15° and at each point note the reproduction and intensity of pain	Provokes lumbar discogenic pain
Upper extremity: root tension signs	Perform contralateral neck lateral bending and abduction of the ipsilateral upper extremity	Reproduces cervical radicular pain in the periscapular area or in the upper extremity
Spurling's maneuver	Passively perform cervical extension, lateral bending toward the side of symptoms, and axial compression	Reproduces cervical radicular pain in the periscapular area or in the upper extremity
Straight leg raise	With the patient supine, the involved lower extremity is passively flexed to 30° with the knee in full extension	Reproduces pain in the buttock, posterior thigh, and posterior calf in conditions with S1 radicular pain
Reverse straight leg raise	With the patient prone, the involved lower extremity is passively extended, the knee flexed	Reproduces pain in the buttock and anterior thigh in conditions with high lumbar (e.g., L3 and L4) radicular pain
Crossed straight leg raise	With the patient supine, the contralateral lower extremity is passively flexed to 30° with the knee in full extension	Reproduces pain in the ipsilateral buttock, posterior thigh, and posterior calf in conditions with S1 radicular pain
Sitting root	With the patient sitting, the involved lower extremity is passively flexed with the knee extended	Reproduces pain in the buttock, posterior thigh, and posterior calf in conditions with S1 radicular pain
Lasegue's test	With the patient supine, the involved lower extremity is passively flexed to 90°	Reproduces pain in the buttock, posterior thigh, and posterior calf in conditions with S1 radicular pain

(Continued)

Table 12-2—Cont'd
Spinal Physical Examination Maneuvers

Maneuver	Technique	Result
Bragard's maneuver	With the patient supine, the involved lower extremity is passively flexed to 30°, with dorsiflexion of the foot	Reproduces pain in the buttock, posterior thigh, and posterior calf in conditions with S1 radicular pain
Gaenslen's maneuver	Position the patient supine with the affected side flush with the edge of the examination table. The hip and knee on the unaffected side are flexed, and the patient clasps the flexed knee to the chest. The examiner then applies pressure against the clasped knee, extends the lower extremity on the ipsilateral side, and brings it under the surface of the examination table	Reproduces pain in patients with sacroiliac joint syndrome
Sacroiliac joint compression	With the patient side lying, apply compression to the joint	Reproduces pain in patients with sacroiliac joint syndrome
Pressure at the sacral sulcus	With the patient in a prone position, apply pressure on the posterosuperior iliac spine (PSIS) (dimple)	Reproduces pain in patients with sacroiliac joint syndrome
Patrick's test/ FABER test	With the patient supine, the knee and hip are flexed. The hip is abducted and externally rotated	Reproduces pain in patients with sacroiliac joint syndrome, facet joint arthropathy (pain is reproduced in the low back), and degenerative joint disease of the hip (pain is reproduced in the groin)
Yeoman's test	With the patient prone, the hip is extended and the ilium is externally rotated	Reproduces pain in patients with sacroiliac joint syndrome
Iliac gapping test	Distraction to the anterior sacroiliac ligaments can be performed by applying pressure to the anterosuperior iliac spine	Reproduces pain in patients with sacroiliac joint syndrome

Deep Tendon Reflexes

Examination of the deep tendon reflexes is helpful in the diagnosis of radiculopathies, especially if asymmetrical reflexes are present (Table 12-3). Deep tendon reflexes may be diminished secondary to multiple neurological conditions or as a result of age. On the other hand, deep tendon reflexes may remain unaffected in radiculopathies or may even be hyperactive in radiculopathies accompanied by upper motor neuron lesions.

Manual Muscle Testing

Manual muscle testing is performed on the four extremities to determine whether a myotomic weakness is present. To detect myotomic weakness, two different muscles supplied by the same nerve root and two different peripheral nerves usually are tested. For example, to examine the L5 nerve root for muscle weakness, the extensor hallucis longus (L5, deep

Table 12-3
Deep Tendon Reflexes

Deep Tendon Reflex	Nerve Root Affected
Biceps	C6
Triceps	C7
Quadriceps	L4
Medial hamstring (not commonly elicited)	L5
Gastrocsoleus	S1

peroneal nerve) and the gluteus medius and minimus (L5, superior gluteal nerve) are tested. This testing rules out different neurological conditions that cause weakness, such as myopathies, peripheral nerve injuries, and plexopathies.

Spinal Range of Motion

Range of motion usually is restricted in patients with spinal pain because of degenerative spinal conditions and muscle guarding around the painful structure.

Imaging Studies

Imaging studies are essential to confirm a suspected diagnosis. Also, imaging must be done before spinal intervention procedures are performed. With the advances in imaging technology, a high number of false positive findings may be encountered. Imaging of the spine solely identifies anatomical changes but not biochemical or physiological changes that cause pain. It is important to correlate the imaging findings with the clinical picture. As an example, anatomical changes, which are visualized through various radiologic/imaging studies can be attributable to the aging process. These changes, however, may not cause symptoms. Ordering unnecessary imaging studies without a clear management plan is not beneficial. Sorting out the positive findings is really the clinician's task. When the imaging studies are properly correlated with the clinical picture and other investigations, the accuracy of the diagnosis, and therefore management, is optimized.

Clinical Point

Always correlate the findings from diagnostic imaging with the clinical findings.

Radiographic Imaging

Traditionally, radiographic imaging is the first step in the evaluation of painful spinal disorders. Although x-ray films cannot be used to evaluate soft tissues, such as the intervertebral discs, nerves, or spinal cord, it is useful for screening for fractures, bone changes, and anatomical deformities. Radiographic studies can be used to evaluate the alignment of the spine and the integrity and architecture of the radiopaque structures. Dynamic x-ray images, such as flexion and extension views, can be used to evaluate spinal instability.

Plain x-ray film anteroposterior, oblique, and lateral views constitute a routine examination. These views provide information about intervertebral disc heights, spondylotic changes, foraminal size variability, deformities, and bony alignment. X-ray films can be useful for identifying malignancy and destructive, metabolic, and rheumatological diseases. The usefulness of ordering x-ray films for acute low back pain is the subject of debate in the literature. Because the pain from this condition improves in a short time, radiographic results usually are not significant and do not affect management. X-ray films should be requested in atypical presentations. Deyo and Diehl[36] suggested criteria for ordering x-ray films to evaluate painful conditions of the lumbar spine. The purpose is mainly to exclude other significant conditions that can manifest as low back pain. These criteria and their rationales are summarized in Table 12-4.

Common Spinal Pathology X-ray Series

- Anteroposterior view
- Oblique view
- Lateral view

Computed Tomography

Computed tomography (CT) scans use two x-ray beams focused on a particular plane of an object. Multiple images are taken, and composite axial images are created using a computer and a rotating x-ray beam. With advances in digital reformatting of the axial images, coronal and sagittal images can be obtained.

A CT scan of the spine provides superior quality imaging of the bone structures. With a CT scan, the clinician can identify subtle fractures that are not identifiable on plain x-ray films. CT scans also provide information about destructive bone pathologies (e.g., infection and malignancy) and on

Table 12-4
Criteria for Use of X-Ray Imaging in Acute Low Back Pain

Criteria	Rationale
Age >50 years	Higher risk of osteoporotic fractures
Significant trauma	Risk of fractures
Neurological deficit	Sign of radiculopathy
Unexplained weight loss	Occult spinal lesion (e.g., malignancy)
Suspicion of ankylosing spondylitis	Spine and sacroiliac joint x-ray films are diagnostic for this condition
History of alcohol or drug abuse	Risk of infection (e.g., osteomyelitis)
History of cancer	Possible spinal metastasis
Corticosteroid use	Osteoporotic fractures
Fever	Possible osteomyelitis
Pain that persists longer than 1 month	Pain is becoming chronic, and further management is recommended
Litigation	To further establish the cause of pain

Data from Deyo RA, Diehl AK: Lumbar spine films in primary care: current use and effects of selective ordering criteria, *J Gen Intern Med* 1:20-25, 1986.

bony union after surgery. Using myelography in conjunction with CT scans enhances imaging for painful spinal disorders. Myelography involves injection of a contrast material into the spinal canal, after which the CT scan is done. (Before the use of CT scans, myelography was performed with plain x-ray films). CT scan myelography provides information about the status of the spinal canal in addition to the spinal bony elements. CT scans and CT myelograms are important in the postoperative workup of painful spinal conditions involving implanted ferromagnetic hardware and in patients unable to have magnetic resonance imaging (MRI) because of implanted devices.

Bone Scan

Bone scanning (also called *bone scintigraphy*) allows the clinician to assess both the anatomy and the physiological activity of tissues. It is an effective screening modality for evaluating systemic pathologies because it covers the whole body. Before and as part of the bone scan, the patient is given an intravenous injection of nuclear tracers that emit small amounts of γ-gamma radiation proportional to the uptake from a specific tissue. Imaging of the radiation produced in tissues allows evaluation of the location of tissue metabolic pathologies. Technetium-99m is used in the evaluation of bone pathologies, and gallium-67 is used in the evaluation of infections. Healthy bones are in a constant state of normal turnover of bone breakdown (osteoclast activity) and bone rebuilding (osteoblast activity). An increased concentration of the technetium-99 tracer suggests increased bone turnover, which can occur in pathologies such as osteoblastic malignant lesions and acute fractures. Lack of radioactive tracer activity indicates cessation of bone activity (cold defect), which can occur with osteonecrosis. Imaging of the radiotracer traditionally is performed in uniplanar anteroposterior fashion. Single photon emission computed tomography (SPECT) now allows tomographic images to be obtained, which improves the sensitivity and specificity of this modality.

Bone scanning is particularly useful for evaluating for occult lesions and suspected infections and as a screening tool for metastases. Because most metastatic spinal lesions are osteoblastic in origin, bone scans detect high bone turnover activity with these lesions. A minority of malignancies involving the spine (e.g., multiple myeloma) may involve osteoclastic activity; in these cases, a bone scan result is negative. If a bone scan result is positive, further imaging of the involved area or areas is done using other modalities, such as CT scanning and MRI studies, which provide anatomical details.

Magnetic Resonance Imaging

MRI is the most recently introduced imaging modality. It was first used in the late 1970s and had gained popularity by the mid-1980s. MRI has become the imaging modality of choice for evaluating painful spinal conditions. It provides a detailed anatomical picture that surpasses the results of other modalities, allowing the clinician to better visualize and evaluate structures such as the nerve roots, spinal cord, paraspinal area, and soft tissues (e.g., intervertebral discs). MRI is sensitive to bone marrow abnormalities found in malignancy, infection, and disc degeneration. With the use of intravenous contrast (gadolinium), MRI provides optimum information on spinal cord lesions, demyelination, infections, and tumors. In the evaluation of postoperative spinal pain recurrence, comparison of the MRI images before and after intravenous administration of gadolinium contrast helps differentiate new disc herniations, recurrence, and postoperative scarring.

MRI technology does not involve the use of ionizing radiation. Instead, it uses magnetic fields and pulsed radiofrequency through which computer-generated sagittal, axial, and coronal images are produced. An external magnet polarizes the hydrogen protons in water molecules, and a specific radiofrequency is pulsed into the body. Images are generated according to the tissues' mobile intrinsic hydrogen ions.

Two frequency spin sequences are used for MRI imaging: T_1-weighted imaging (the longitudinal relaxation time) and T_2-weighted imaging (the transverse relaxation time). On T_1-weighted images, fat-rich tissues have a bright signal. On T_2-weighted images, extracellular free water has a bright signal.

The most common terminology used by clinicians to describe MRI spinal findings are presented in Table 12-5, and findings are shown in Figures 12-4 to 12-11.

Spinal Intervention Procedures

The two main types of spinal intervention procedures are diagnostic interventions and therapeutic interventions.

Diagnostic Intervention Procedures

The purpose of diagnostic spinal interventions is to establish and confirm a suspected diagnosis. In many cases the physical examination, imaging techniques, and electrodiagnostic studies fail to provide an accurate assessment of spinal pathologies. This often is due to multiple-level imaging findings or a lack of imaging or electrodiagnostic evidence of a painful spinal disorder. Through the use of local anesthetics, diagnostic interventions attempt either to "block" the painful structure and eliminate or reduce the pain or to provoke pain to allow an accurate assessment of the location of the pathology based on the patient's response.

Pharmacological Intervention Procedures

Local Steroid Injections

Therapeutic interventions are widely used to treat painful spinal conditions. These can include local steroid injections or newly introduced devices and procedures, such as radiofrequency and percutaneous disc decompression. Administration of a local steroid injection in or around the painful structure is considered an efficient way to use steroids in small amounts without systemic side effects.

Steroids are a potent anti-inflammatory medication. They reduce inflammation around the intervertebral discs, spinal nerves, and facet joints. At the cellular level, steroids inhibit the action of phospholipase A2, preventing the formation of arachidonic acid and inflammatory mediators. They also act as membrane stabilizers, blocking the conduction of nociceptive C fibers that carry pain signals. Steroids diminish the sensitization of the dorsal horn cells by reducing prostaglandins. After the inflammation has been reduced, edema around the nerve roots subsides and microcirculation is improved, reducing nerve ischemia. The steroids most often used in spinal interventions are listed in Table 12-6.

Interlaminar and Caudal Epidural Injections

Interlaminar epidural injections are the traditional and most frequently used spinal therapeutic intervention in the management of axial discogenic pain and radicular pain. Dogliotti[39] first introduced epidural injections in 1933. The injections were first used in the management of lumbosacral pain in 1952.[40] Currently, the use of interlaminar and caudal epidural injections versus transforaminal

Table 12-5
Common Magnetic Resonance Imaging Terminology and Descriptions

Term	Description
Disc dissecation	Reduction of the bright nuclear signal on the sagittal T_2-weighted images; this finding signifies disc degeneration and reduction of the water content of the nucleus
Disc bulge	Circumferential, broad-based extension of the annulus beyond the vertebral end plate
Disc herniation	General term used to describe the displacement of the nucleus pulposus beyond the disc itself
Focal disc protrusion	More specific term describing disc displacement. The nuclear material protrudes into the annulus without disrupting its outer wall; this results in a change in the contour of the annulus (see Figures 12-4 to 12-10)
Disc extrusion	Nuclear material protrudes through the outer wall of the annulus. The protruded material can remain contained by the posterior longitudinal ligament (subligamentous extrusion) or may extend beyond it (transligamentous extrusion)
Sequestered disc	Nuclear material is detached from the disc and migrates in the spinal canal cranially or caudally
High intensity zone	An area of high intensity on T_2-weighted images in the annulus;[37] it occurs secondary to an area of vascularized granulation tissue in the outer region of the annulus
Foraminal stenosis	Narrowing of the neural foramen; this commonly occurs secondary to a lateral disc herniation, bone spurs, or spondylolisthesis
Central stenosis	Narrowing of the central canal; this commonly occurs secondary to a combination of disc herniation and/or ligamentum hypertrophy, facet joint hypertrophy, and spondylolisthesis
Myelomalacia	T_2-weighted signal changes in the spinal cord commonly present in severe central stenosis
End plate changes (Modic changes[38])	Changes in the end plates associated with degenerative disc disease at the level of involvement, first described by Modic et al.[38] Type 1 changes decrease signal intensity on T_1-weighted images and increase signal intensity on T_2-weighted images. Type 2 changes increase signal intensity on T_1-weighted images and isointense or slightly increase signal intensity on T_2-weighted images Type 3 changes show a decreased signal intensity on both T_1- and T_2-weighted images. These changes in signal intensity appear to reflect a spectrum of vertebral body marrow changes associated with degenerative disc disease

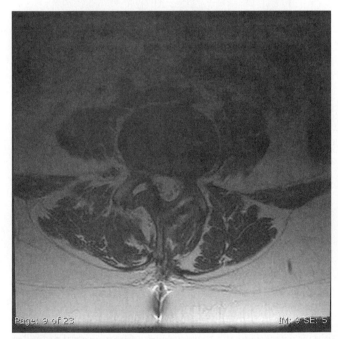

Figure 12-4
Axial T_2-weighted image demonstrating fluid in the right L4-5 facet joint after left L4 laminectomy and facetectomy, indicating stress on the right L4-5 facet joint with possible pain.

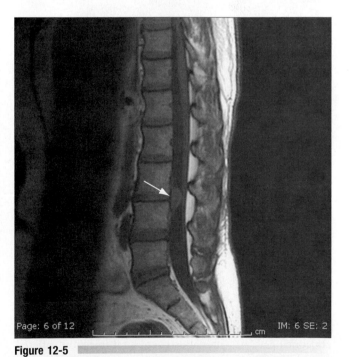

Figure 12-5
Sagittal T_1-weighted image with a large focal protrusion at the L3-4 disc level.

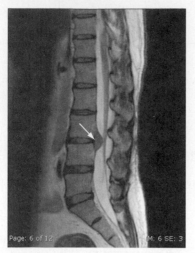

Figure 12-6

Sagittal T_2-weighted image with a large focal protrusion at the L3-4 disc level.

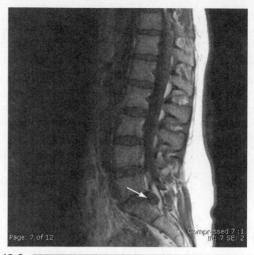

Figure 12-8

Sagittal T_1-weighted image with a large focal protrusion at the L5-S1 disc level.

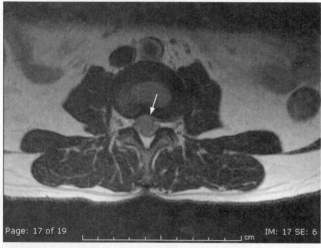

Figure 12-7

Axial T_2-weighted image with a large focal protrusion at the L3-4 disc level.

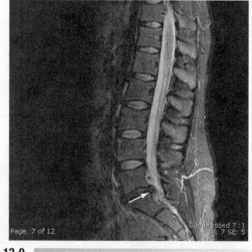

Figure 12-9

Sagittal T_2-weighted image with a large focal protrusion at the L5-S1 disc level.

epidural injections is the subject of debate. Interlaminar and caudal epidural injections are considered nontarget specific compared to transforaminal injections. Steroids are injected into the posterior epidural space but do not reach the anterior space because of the presence of ligaments. In a randomized, double blind trial, Carette et al.[41] administered up to three interlaminar epidural injections of methylprednisolone acetate or isotonic saline to 158 patients with sciatica caused by a herniated nucleus pulposus. No significant differences in outcomes were seen in the short term or the long term (1 year). These researchers concluded that interlaminar epidural injections offered no significant functional benefit, nor did they reduce the need for surgery. The major flaw in this study was that fluoroscopic guidance was not used. Needle positioning was not confirmed either with fluoroscopy or by adding local anesthetic, and transient sensory and motor deficits were not monitored after the epidural injection.

Koes et al.[42] reviewed data from 12 randomized studies and reported that the efficacy of interlaminar epidural steroid injections was not established. The benefits of epidural steroid injections, if any, were of short duration only. Watts and Silagy[43] reviewed 11 randomized studies involving a total of 907 patients and reported no long-term adverse outcomes. They also provided quantitative evidence from meta-analysis that epidural administration of corticosteroids is effective in the management of lumbosacral radicular pain. In a retrospective study of 75 patients, Manchikanti et al.[44] compared pain relief after blind interlaminar epidural injections, caudal epidural injections, and transforaminal

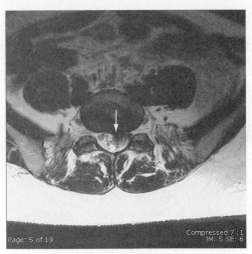

Figure 12-10
Axial T$_2$-weighted image showing a large, left focal protrusion at the L5-S1 disc level compressing the left S1 nerve.

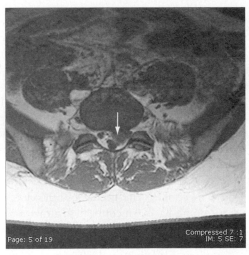

Figure 12-11
Axial T$_1$-weighted image showing a large, left focal protrusion at the L5-S1 disc level compressing the left S1 nerve.

epidural injections. The response was most favorable with transforaminal injections, followed by caudal injections, which surpassed the outcome for blind interlaminar injections.

Indications for Interlaminar and Caudal Epidural Injections

- Overall, studies have shown better outcomes for interlaminar and caudal epidural injections in acute rather than chronic pain, with a longer duration of improvement for radicular pain.
- Interlaminar epidural injections are declining in popularity among interventionalists, whereas transforaminal epidural injections are growing in popularity because of their better outcomes.

Interlaminar epidural injections are performed blindly or with fluoroscopic guidance. In a prospective study that included 316 patients undergoing blind epidural injections, needle positions were evaluated using fluoroscopy.[45] Renfrew et al.[45] reported that, even in experienced hands, blind placement of the injection needle was optimal in only 60% of cases. They recommended fluoroscopic control and contrast administration to ensure correct needle placement and to prevent inadvertent venous injections.

Technique for Interlaminar Epidural Injections. With fluoroscopic guidance, the level of the injection can be accurately assessed and the epidural location can be accurately confirmed using contrast. This reduces the patient's discomfort. Using contrast helps reduce the incidence of intravascular injections; such an injection can be readily identified because the contrast has a quick runoff (i.e., fast flow of contrast under fluoroscopy when the medium is injected into a blood vessel). The use of fluoroscopy and contrast is highly recommended in postoperative patients because it readily identifies the surgical level and confirms needle positioning.

The patient is placed in the prone position on the fluoroscopy table. A pillow is placed under the abdomen to open up the interlaminar space. Conscious sedation can be used but is not recommended; avoiding its use provides extra protection from accidental neural trauma. Light sedation is suggested if the patient is very anxious or has a history of vasovagal events. The blood pressure, pulse, and pulse oxymetry are monitored. The skin is prepped with iodine and draped with sterile drapes. The interlaminar space is properly identified under fluoroscopy by adjusting the end plates and aligning the spinous processes. A midline interspinous or slightly paraspinal entry point is identified. Using a 25 gauge, 4-cm (1½-inch) needle, the clinician injects 0.5 cc of lidocaine 1% subcutaneously, forming a skin wheal. This injection is used to numb the skin, and it also provides the clinician with a needle introduction site.

For the intralaminar injection, 17 to 22 gauge Tuohy needles are used. These are special needles with curved tips designed to reduce the incidence of dural punctures. In most cases 9-cm (3½-inch) needles are used, but 13-cm (5-inch) needles occasionally are needed for obese patients. Pencil point tip (Whitacre and Sprotte), sharp tip (Quincke), and blunt tip needles are also used.

The needle is introduced through the skin and advanced into the midline of the interlaminar space. The needle stylet is removed, and a loss of resistance syringe is applied. A "loss of resistance" syringe is a special syringe made of plastic or glass. The clinician introduces the needle, under fluoroscopic guidance, while applying continuous pressure on the syringe plunger. Once the needle passes through the thick ligamentum flavum, the clinician feels a sense of give and encounters a loss of resistance on the syringe plunger. Aspiration is performed to ensure that there is no leakage of cerebrospinal fluid. Contrast is injected to confirm the needle's position.

Table 12-6

Common Medications Used for Spinal Intervention Procedures

	Hydrocortisone	Methylprednisolone (Depo-Medrol)	Triamcinolone Acetonide (Kenalog)	Betamethasone Sodium Phosphate and Acetate (Celestone, Soluspan)	Dexamethasone Sodium Phosphate (Decadron Phosphate)
Relative anti-inflammatory potency	1	5*	5*	25*	25*
pH	5-7	7-8	4.5-6.5	6.8-7.2	7-8.5
Onset	Fast	Slow	Moderate	Fast	Fast
Duration of action	Short	Intermediate	Intermediate	Long	Long
Concentration (mg/cc)	50	40-80	20	6	4 mg/cc
Relative mineralocorticoid activity	2+	0	0	0	0

* Relative to hydrocortisone as 1.

When the epidural flow is confirmed, steroids and local anesthetics are injected. The needle is then removed. If the vital signs are stable, the patient is transferred by stretcher or wheelchair to the waiting area for monitoring for about 15 minutes. As soon as the lower extremities regain their full strength, the patient is discharged.

Vasovagal Events (Vasovagal Attack)

- Lightheadedness (dizziness)
- Paleness
- Sweating
- Nausea
- Decreased blood pressure
- Decreased heart rate
- Loss of consciousness

The cervical spine is a narrower space; however, the same technique is used. Cervical interlaminar epidural injections are performed at the C6-7 or C7-T1 level because of the relative increase in spinal canal diameter at those levels. Performing the injections at these levels is relatively safer, because the wider central canal reduces the chances of spinal cord injury and provides a better space for introducing catheters. A needle and catheter technique frequently is used to perform cervical interlaminar epidural injections. An epidural catheter is inserted through an epidural needle placed at the C6-7 or the C7-T1 level. The epidural needle is introduced with the loss of resistance technique. Once the positioning is confirmed with fluoroscopy, a 20 gauge catheter is introduced and driven cephalad in the epidural space near the level of the pathology. Contrast is used to confirm the catheter's presence in the epidural space before medications are injected. This technique has the advantage of introducing the medication near the pathology while accessing the epidural space in the lower cervical spine.

Caudal epidural steroid injections are performed blindly or with fluoroscopic guidance. In the blind technique, the patient is placed in the prone position, and the sacral hiatus is palpated. The skin is prepped and draped in the usual sterile manner. A spinal needle is introduced at 45 degrees. A pop is felt as the needle passes through the sacrococcygeal ligament. The angle of the needle is reduced, and the needle is advanced rostrally. The loss of resistance technique is used to confirm the needle's position. Once the epidural positioning has been confirmed, a mixture of steroids and local anesthetics is injected. With the fluoroscopically guided technique, the sacral hiatus is identified, and the needle's position is confirmed with contrast.

Transforaminal Epidural Injections

Transforaminal epidural injections are administered only under fluoroscopic guidance. This injection aims for the disc and spinal nerve interface. The needle is introduced into a triangular space within the anterosuperior third of the neural foramen; this space, known as the "safe triangle" (Figure 12-12), is bounded by the pedicle superiorly, the exiting nerve inferomedially, and the lateral margin of the neural foramen laterally. The needle is lodged at the 6 o'clock position, just inferior to the pedicle. If the needle is introduced farther medially, so that the safe triangle is violated, a dural puncture may result. Once the needle is in position, the medication can be efficiently injected into the lateral epidural space or around the emerging nerve root depending on the needle position and the bevel (slanted) orientation.

This approach is commonly used in the treatment of radicular pain,[12] and it also is used in the management of

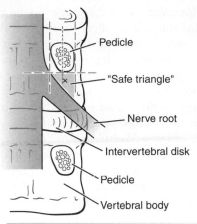

Pedicle

"Safe triangle"

Nerve root

Intervertebral disk

Pedicle

Vertebral body

Figure 12-12
The safe triangle.

axial discogenic pain. In experienced hands, the transforaminal technique is safe and produces a good outcome. Transforaminal epidural steroid injection is gaining popularity over the interlaminar approach because it is more effective at administering the medication at the spinal nerve/disc interface in the lateral epidural space rather than in the dorsal epidural space, which is separated from the lateral epidural space by the ligamentum flavum. Fluoroscopic guidance is essential for this procedure, and administration of steroids at the level of the pathology is crucial to effectiveness.

Transforaminal epidural injections have both diagnostic and therapeutic value. If the pathology is unclear or if multiple pathologies are present, administration of local anesthetic (without a steroid) has diagnostic value if pain is relieved immediately after the injection is given. For therapeutic purposes, steroids are injected with the goal of pain relief 2 or 3 days after the injection. The effectiveness of therapeutic transforaminal epidural injections has been the subject of a number of studies. In a prospective study, Lutz and Wisneski[14] evaluated the outcomes of therapeutic transforaminal epidural steroid injections in 69 patients for a mean period of 80 weeks. They found that 75% of their patients reported improvement of pain intensity of at least 50% and near return to functional activities after 1.8 injections.

In a prospectively randomized study, Riew et al.[46] evaluated 55 patients with lumbar radicular pain with radiographic confirmation of nerve root compression. All of their patients had requested operative intervention and were considered surgical candidates. Instead the patients were randomized and underwent a selective nerve root injection with either bupivacaine alone or bupivacaine with betamethasone. The treating physicians and the patients were blinded to the medication. Twenty-nine patients did not have surgery during a follow-up period of 13 to 28 months. Of the 27 patients who had received bupivacaine alone, nine did not have surgery. Of the 28 patients who had received bupivacaine and betamethasone, 20 decided not to have surgery.

A study by Vad et al.[47] prospectively included 50 patients with lumbar radicular pain that had lasted longer than 6 weeks. All of the patients had MRI evidence of a herniated nucleus pulposus (HNP) with less than 50% narrowing of the neural foramen, along with radicular pain corresponding to the MRI positive level of pathology. The patients were randomized into two groups. The treatment group received fluoroscopically guided transforaminal epidural injections, and the control group received trigger point injections. Forty-eight patients completed the study, and the average follow-up was 16 months. Outcome measures were the Roland Morris Questionnaire, a visual analogue scale, and the finger to floor test. An 84% improvement was seen in the study group, and only a 24% improvement in the control group.

In a prospective study, Botwin et al.[48] included 34 patients with unilateral radicular pain, caused by degenerative spinal stenosis, who were not responding to conservative management. Their patients received an average of 1.9 fluoroscopically guided transforaminal epidural injections on the symptomatic side. A visual analogue scale score, the Roland 5-point pain scale, standing and walking tolerance, and a patient satisfaction scale were assessed 2 months and 12 months after the injections. The results showed that 75% of the patients reported a pain score reduction of greater than 50% after the injection therapy; also, 64% had improved walking tolerance and 57% had improved standing tolerance at 12 months.

Slipman et al.[12] retrospectively evaluated 20 patients who had had cervical radicular pain for longer than 5 months. Their patients received an average of 2.2 cervical transforaminal epidural injections in addition to physical therapy. The patients were followed for 21 months. Their pain scores, medication use, work status, and satisfaction were assessed. Sixty percent of the patients reported excellent or good outcomes, and 30% underwent surgery.

Huston et al.[13] prospectively studied the side effects and complications of transforaminal epidural injections. An analysis of 350 consecutive cervical and lumbar transforaminal injections identified no instance in which dural punctures occurred. Lutz and Wisneski[14] found no epidural punctures or other major complications in 50 patients who received lumbar transforaminal epidural injections. Botwin et al.[15] reviewed complications in 322 transforaminal lumbar epidural injections done on 207 patients. They reported a complete absence of post dural puncture headache (PDHD). The most common complication found in their study was headache, which occurred in 3.1% of patients. These headaches were transient and resolved after 24 hours. These patients' epidurograms were reviewed, and no intrathecal pattern was noted.

Spinal cord injury has been reported after lumbosacral nerve root block with steroid injections.[49] This is postulated to occur secondary to an injury or to injection of particulate steroids in patients with an aberrant artery of Adamkiewicz. Another possibility is occlusion of the anterior spinal artery, with resultant spinal cord infarction, after inadvertent injection into a feeder artery in the neural foramen. This has occurred only recently, because Celestone, the medication of choice, is not consistently available. Clinicians are using Depo-Medrol and Kenalog preparations as a substitute, and these preparations form large particulate granules, which can occlude the anterior spinal artery unless a meticulous technique is followed.

Technique for Cervical Transforaminal Epidural Injections. The patient is placed in the supine position on the fluoroscopy table. A bolster is placed under the contralateral shoulder. The blood pressure, pulse, and pulse oxymetry are monitored. The fluoroscopy beam is rotated to visualize the neural foramen in a perpendicular plane to the radiographic imager. Once the neural foramen has been properly visualized, a 25 gauge needle is introduced through the skin. The needle is advanced until it abuts the superior articular process of the corresponding neural foramen. The needle then is slightly advanced into the foramen. Contrast (0.3 cc of Omnipaque 300) is used to confirm the needle's position. When contrast clearly outlines the exiting nerve root, 2 cc of Celestone (6 mg) and 0.5 cc of lidocaine 1% are given in therapeutic injections (Figure 12-13) If Celestone is not available, Depo-Medrol is the preferred substitute. For diagnostic puroposes only, 0.8 cc of lidocaine 2% is given without steroids (diagnostic injection).

Technique for Thoracic and Lumbar Transforaminal Epidural Injections. The patient is placed in the prone position on the fluoroscopy table. The blood pressure, pulse, and pulse oxymetry are monitored. The fluoroscopy beam is rotated to visualize the neural foramen in an oblique plane with the superior articular process dissecting the corresponding pedicle. Once the neural foramen has been properly visualized, a skin wheal is made with

0.5 cc of lidocaine 1%. A 22 gauge needle is introduced through the skin and advanced to the 6 o'clock position under the pedicle (the safe triangle) under fluoroscopic guidance. Needle positioning is confirmed using the anteroposterior plane. The needle should not extend medial to the pedicle on the anteroposterior view. Contrast (0.3 cc of Omnipaque 300) is used to confirm the needle's position. When the contrast clearly outlines the exiting nerve root, 1.6 cc of Depo-Medrol (40 mg) (or 2 cc of Celestone [6 mg] in thoracic injections) and 1 cc of lidocaine 1% are given as therapeutic injections (Figures 12-14 and 12-15). For diagnostic puroposes only, 0.8 cc of lidocaine 2% is given without steroids (diagnostic injection).

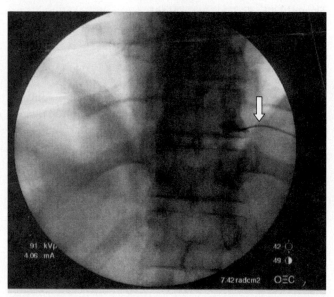

Figure 12-14
Right T10 transforaminal epidural injection.

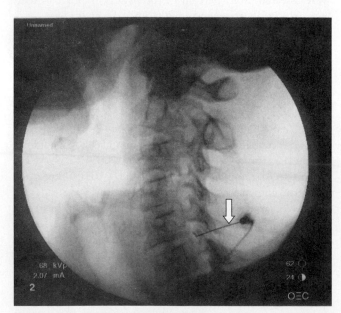

Figure 12-13
Left C6 transforaminal epidural injection.

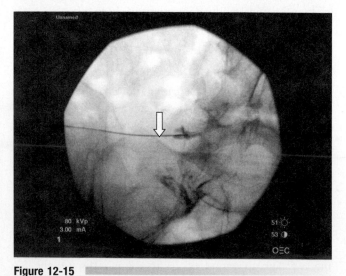

Figure 12-15
Left L5 transforaminal epidural injection. Note the presence of left S1 flow (an S1 transforaminal injection had been given just before the L5 injection).

Guiding Principles for Transforaminal Epidural Injections

- The needle must be carefully positioned in the safe triangle.
- The needle's position must be confirmed radiographically in the anteroposterior plane.
- For a cervical transforaminal injection, oblique planes, rather than lateral planes, should be used to perform the injection. The depth of the needle cannot be noted if lateral planes are used.
- Live fluoroscopy should be used while contrast material is injected.
- If possible, Celestone should be used for cervical and thoracic injections (Celestone has less particulate substance than Depo-Medrol or Kenalog, which are suspected of causing vascular clogging).
- Cervical and thoracic transforaminal injections should be administered only by a well-trained physician experienced in performing these procedures.
- With thoracic transforaminal injections, the risk of pneumothorax arises if the pleura is punctured. The interventionalist should always keep the needle medial to the costovertebral junction.

While performing the transforaminal epidural injections, the clinician must take special precautions to prevent vascular injections and spinal cord injuries.

Facet Joint Injections

Neither the clinical examination nor imaging studies can confirm a diagnosis of facet-mediated pain. The gold standard for this diagnosis is the use of a local anesthetic to block a particularly painful joint.[21,24,50-52] Barnsley et al.[53] evaluated the effect of intra-articular cervical facet joint steroid injections in 41 patients with chronic neck pain. The patients were carefully selected by means of differential diagnostic cervical facet joint block with a long-acting and a short-acting anesthetic. Under double blind conditions, patients received intra-articular injections of either 1 cc of bupivacaine (20 patients) or 1 cc of betamethasone (21 patients). Patient follow-up was conducted either in the office or by telephone until the patient reported a return of 50% of the pain. The median time to a return of 50% of pain was 3 days in the steroid group and 3.5 days in the local anesthetic group. Only 20% of the patients had substantial relief after 1 month. The authors concluded that the improvement was due either to a placebo effect or secondary to facet joint distention. This study had some flaws; the sample number was small, and all the patients included had traumatic injury with whiplash.

Lilius et al.[54] evaluated 109 patients with chronic low back pain who did not respond to conservative management. Their patients were separated into three groups: the first received intra-articular steroid and a local anesthetic; the second received saline; and the third received pericapsular steroid and a local anesthetic. The authors reported improvement of pain in all three groups. The major flaw of this study was that the patients were selected without undergoing diagnostic injections to identify the level of therapeutic injections.

In a prospective study, Carette et al.[55] compared the effect of intra-articular saline with that of intra-articular methylprednisolone in 101 patients after positive lidocaine joint injection. At 6 months, 46% of the methylprednisolone group and 15% of the saline group reported marked pain relief.

In a prospective study, Lynch and Taylor[56] evaluated 50 patients. Of these, 23 received extra-articular steroid injections and 27 received intra-articular steroid injections without a local anesthetic. Nine of the 27 patients who had received intra-articular injections had total improvement, whereas none of the control group (those who had received extra-articular injections) experienced total improvement. Only two members of the intra-articular group had no improvement.

Technique for Intra-articular Facet Joint Injections. These injections are performed only under live fluoroscopic visualization. For cervical facet joint injections, the patient is placed in the lateral position on the fluoroscopy table. A bolster is placed beneath the patient's head with the ipsilateral side bent 5° to 15° for better visualization of the upper joints. For C1-2 injections, the patient is positioned prone with the bolster placed beneath the forehead and the neck in slight extension of 5° to 10°. For lumbar facet joint injections, the patient is placed prone with or without a bolster under the ipsilateral side. The blood pressure, pulse, and pulse oxymetry are monitored. The skin is prepped and draped in the usual sterile manner. The target ipsilateral joint is properly identified in a plane perpendicular to the radiographic imager. A 25 gauge, 4-cm (1½-inch) needle (for cervical injections) or a 22 gauge 9-cm (3½-inch) spinal needle (for lumbar injections) are used. The needle is advanced to the midportion of the superior articular process (for level C1-2, the needle is introduced through the lateral third of the joint). After the depth has been checked, the needle is advanced to pierce the joint capsule (Figure 12-16). About 0.15 cc of Omnipaque 300, a water-soluble contrast agent, is injected into the joint for proper identification. After a positive arthrogram has been identified, 0.8 cc of Xylocaine 2% is given as a diagnostic injection. A greater than 80% improvement in pain is considered a positive diagnostic injection. For therapeutic injections, 0.8 cc of Depo-Medrol (40 mg) (or another type of steroid) and 0.2 cc of lidocaine 1% are injected.

Medial branch blocks instead of intra-articular injections are primarily performed for the diagnosis of facet joint syndrome.[57] Technically, they are easier to perform than the

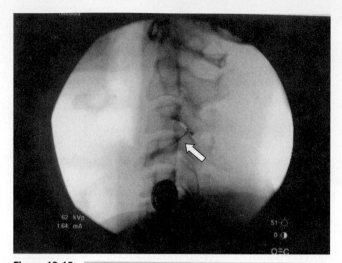

Figure 12-16
Left C3-4 intra-articular facet joint injection.

intra-articular facet joint injections. The spinal needle is positioned at the junction of the superior articular process and the transverse process under fluoroscopic guidance (Figure 12-17).

Facet Joint Radiofrequency Ablation

From a spinal intervention perspective, radiofrequency ablation is considered the ultimate management of facet joint mediated pain. This procedure results in ablation of the medial branch nerves that provide sensory innervations to one or more facet joints. In a randomized, double blind trial, Lord et al.[24] included 24 patients with chronic neck

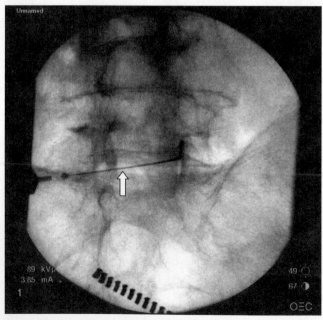

Figure 12-17
Right L5-S1 intra-articular facet joint injection.

pain with a median duration of pain of 34 months. All the patients had developed pain after a motor vehicle accident. The radiofrequency procedure was compared to an identical procedure in which the machine was not turned on. The patients were split into two groups of 12 receiving each treatment. The radiofrequency level was selected using double blind, placebo-controlled facet blocks. Follow-up consisted of clinic visits and phone interviews until the patient's pain had returned to the 50% level. The median time for pain return was 263 days in the active treatment group and 8 days in the control group. At 27 weeks, seven patients in the active group and one patient in the control group were pain free. The study had a good design and good methodology; however, the sample size was small.

In a prospective study, Dreyfuss et al.[58] included 15 patients with chronic low back pain who reacted positively to a double local anesthetic comparative block (with lidocaine and bupivacaine). Patients underwent lumbar facet joint radiofrequency therapy and were followed for 12 months. To determine the outcome of the study, the investigators evaluated a number of factors: the patients' use of prescription analgesic medications; the results of the McGill Pain Questionnaire and Short Form SF-36; the North American Spine Society treatment expectations; the patient's ability to perform isometric push and pull, dynamic floor to waist lifts, and above the shoulder lifting tasks; and the results of needle electromyography of the L2 to L5 bands of the multifidus muscles done before and 8 weeks after the procedure. Sixty percent of patients had at least a 90% pain reduction, and 87% of the patients had a 60% pain reduction for 12 months.

McDonald et al.[59] followed 28 patients for 5 years. All the patients underwent radiofrequency treatment of the cervical spine after undergoing placebo-controlled blocks. The median pain relief time after the first procedure was 219 days.

Technique for Radiofrequency Ablation of the Facet Joints. Radiofrequency ablation is performed only under live fluoroscopic visualization. The blood pressure, pulse, and pulse oxymetry are monitored. For cervical facet joint radiofrequency ablation, the patient is placed in the lateral position on the fluoroscopy table. A bolster is placed beneath the patient's head with the ipsilateral side bent 5° to 15° to allow better visualization of the upper joints. For treatment of a lumbar facet joint, the patient is placed in the prone position. The skin is prepped and draped in the usual sterile manner. A grounding pad is applied to the patient's shoulder (or any other area of dry skin) and connected to the radiofrequency generator.

For the cervical spine, the target facet joint is properly visualized in a plane perpendicular to the radiographic imager. A 22 gauge, 4-cm (1½-inch), specially insulated needle is introduced and advanced under fluoroscopic guidance in a ventral and medial direction until it abuts the superior articular process, transverse process, and pedicle. The C3 medial branch (third occipital nerve) needs to be lesioned in two or three locations along the C2-3 facet, because it is larger.

For the lumbar spine, the fluoroscopy beam is rotated 10° to 20° to visualize the ipsilateral superior articular process and the transverse process clearly. Then 0.5 cc of lidocaine 1% is injected subcutaneously. A 22 gauge, specially insulated spinal needle is introduced under direct fluoroscopic visualization. The needle is advanced until it abuts the junction of the base of the superior articular process, the pedicle, and the transverse process. The needle then is slightly "walked off" over the transverse process; this places the needle close to the medial branch at that level.

Once the needle is in the proper position, sensory testing is performed at 50 Hz with a voltage of 0-1 V. The patient is asked whether sensory symptoms ranging from pressure, tingling, burning, to pain are experienced. The symptoms must be localized in the paraspinal area and not in the extremities. If sensory symptoms are not elicited or felt in the extremities, the needle's position is changed. Once sensory testing has been confirmed, motor testing is performed by switching the frequency to 2 Hz with a voltage of 1-10 V. The clinician's hand is placed over the immediate ipsilateral paraspinal area to check for rhythmic muscle contractions. When contractions are identified, the voltage is doubled and the clinician's hand is placed over the limb muscles supplied by the nerve root corresponding to the medial branch level. Neither the clinician nor the patient should feel any rhythmic contractions in the limb muscles. If contractions in the limb muscles are identified, the needle's position is changed. Sensory testing and motor testing confirm that the radiofrequency needle is positioned close to the medial branch and away from the corresponding nerve root.

Once correct positioning of the needle has been confirmed, 0.5 cc of lidocaine 2% is injected into the cervical levels and 3 cc of lidocaine 1% is injected into the lumbar spine. Radiofrequency lesioning is then performed at 80°C (176°F) for 90 seconds. The radiofrequency denervation of each facet joint implies lesioning of the medial branch at the joint level and the medial branch of the level cephalad to that joint.

Radiofrequency ablation is a safe procedure if performed according to the technique just described. The most common complication is the sensation of pain, which can last 7 to 10 days. Pain rarely lasts longer than 2 weeks[60] because of the denervation process of the ablated medial branches.

Sacroiliac Joint Injections

Injections into the SI joint are either diagnostic or therapeutic for SI joint syndrome. No physical examination test or imaging study can be used to confirm this diagnosis.[35,61] Diagnostic injections are used to further assess the pain emanating from the joint. If the patient has a positive response to the diagnostic injection, a therapeutic injection is administered.

Technique for Intra-articular Sacroiliac Joint Injections. The patient is placed in the prone position on the fluoroscopy table. The skin is prepped and draped in the usual sterile manner. The blood pressure, pulse, and pulse oxymetry are monitored. The fluoroscopy beam is slightly rotated in an oblique position. The most caudal part of the joint is visualized with the ventral and the dorsal aspects superimposed. At the needle entry point, a skin wheal is made using 0.5 cc of lidocaine 1%. Under direct fluoroscopic visualization, a 22 gauge, 9-cm (3½-inch) needle is introduced into the most caudal aspect of the SI joint. After the needle's positioning in the joint has been confirmed, 0.3 cc of contrast (Omnipaque 300) is injected. Intra-articular contrast should be properly visualized. For diagnostic injections, 1 cc of lidocaine 2% is used; for therapeutic injections, 1.6 cc of Depo-Medrol (40 mg) and 0.5 cc of lidocaine 2% are used.

Discograms
Diagnostic Discograms

In 1970 Henry Crock first described **internal disc disruption syndrome (IDDS)** after conducting a retrospective analysis of patients who continued to experience leg and back pain despite multiple surgical procedures. He postulated that IDDS was caused by alterations in the internal structure and metabolic function of one or more discs, the alterations having developed after significant trauma.[62] Subsequent studies have established the morphology of the disrupted disc to be a degenerated nucleus pulposus with radial fissures extending to the periphery of the annulus fibrosus.[63] Patients with IDDS usually present with axial back pain that is dull or aching and difficult to localize and that often produces somatically referred symptoms.

Provocative discography is considered the best available test for diagnosing IDDS.[64] A discogram is considered only when the option of spinal fusion is entertained, whether for failure of conservative measures to control pain or for the management of spinal instability. A discogram confirms the disc level causing pain. However, discograms are plagued by a high false positive rate, and even experienced physicians should perform the procedure meticulously. A patient undergoing a discogram should not be sedated and should be blinded to the disc level assessed. Sedation can cloud the patient's sensation of pain. It is important for the patient to be completely conscious so that the pain provoked during the test can be accurately described.

Technique for Diagnostic Lumbar Discogram

The patient starts the test in the side lying position with a roll under the L4-5 area. The blood pressure, pulse, and pulse oxymetry are monitored. The fluoroscopy beam is rotated to visualize the intervertebral discs with parallel end plates and dissected by the superior articular process.

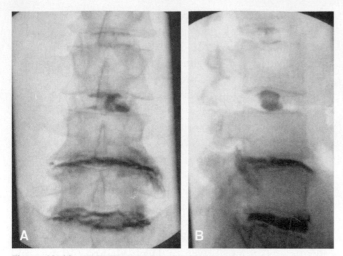

Figure 12-18

Fluoroscopic anteroposterior (**A**) and lateral (**B**) views of intradiscal contrast after a diagnostic lumbar discogram at L2-3, L3-4, L4-5, and L5-S1. The L4-5 and L5-S1 discs are degenerated, but only the L5-S1 level provoked concordant pain; therefore, the L5-S1 level is the positive level.

To visualize the L5-S1 disc, the fluoroscopy beam should be tilted caudally to avoid the ipsilateral iliac crest. Using a double needle technique (an 18 gauge outer discography needle and a 22 gauge inner discography needle), the clinician places the needles into the disc using a posterolateral approach. After needles placement, the patient's position is changed to prone. Omnipaque 300 is used for disc injection, and needle placement is assessed using fluoroscopic imaging (Figure 12-18). The patient is blinded to the intervertebral disc injected. The pain response and its distribution are recorded after each disc injection (P0, no pain on injection; P1, partial concordant pain; P2, discordant pain; and P3, concordant pain with same intensity and distribution). A discographic injection is considered positive if the pain response is P3 at the injected level. Negative levels are considered control levels in each discographic study. The pain response encompasses the skin, the underlying soft tissue, and the viscera located in these areas.

Immediately after discography, a CT scan is performed. Discs that appear lobular or cotton ball shaped (grade 0, 1, or 2 on the Modified Dallas Discogram Scale)[65] are classified as normal; discs that have an irregular discogram pattern with extravasation of dye to or through the outer annulus (grade 3, 4, or 5 on the Modified Dallas Discogram Scale) are classified as abnormal.

Percutaneous Discectomy

Patients with radicular pain who fail to improve with conservative management, including spinal nerve root blocks, are candidates for percutaneous discectomy, an evolving spinal procedure. This procedure aims to achieve disc decompression without the side effects of conventional surgical procedures. Regardless of the technique used, percutaneous disc decompression is based on the principle that a small reduction of volume in a closed hydraulic space, such as an intact disc, results in a disproportionately large drop in pressure. Once the intradiscal pressure declines, the disc is believed to downregulate inflammatory mediators and decrease in size, and a healing process is believed to commence, thereby alleviating the chemical, mechanical, and neural genesis of discogenic pain.[66]

Percutaneous discectomy was first introduced in 1964 with the use of intradiscal chymopapain injections (chemonucleolysis). However, chymopapain was reported to be associated with severe anaphylactic reactions and transverse myelitis, and its use was discontinued.[67]

Hijikata[68] introduced instrumented percutaneous disc decompression in 1975. Although his procedure was reported to be effective, it did not become widely accepted. Among the reasons cited were the potential complications, including nerve root and/or vascular injury caused by the large canula (5-8 mm in diameter), repeated entrance into the disc space with an increased risk of infection, inability to relieve foraminal or lateral recess stenosis, lack of applicability among patients who had previously undergone surgery, difficulty performing the procedure on obese patients, and inaccessibility of the L5-S1 disc.

In 1985 Maroon and Onik introduced the automated lumbar discectomy device.[69] The device was criticized for its low success rate and for reports of major cauda equina injury. Laser discectomy became popular, but its use subsequently declined because of postprocedural complications, such as moderate to severe intraoperative pain secondary to the thermal effect of the laser, postoperative low back pain and spasm, bowel necrosis resulting from inadvertent perforation of the anterior annulus, nerve root injury, and inability to visualize the tip of the laser beam under fluoroscopy.[70] Most recently, the technologically advanced devices Nucleoplasty[71] and Decompressor[72] were introduced. Reports suggest that these devices are effective, especially in the management of small disc protrusions with radicular pain, and that they cause minimal and transient side effects and complications. Randomized studies to validate their use have yet to be performed.

Technique for Lumbar Percutaneous Discectomy

The patient starts the procedure in the side-lying position with a roll under the L4-5 area. The blood pressure, pulse, and pulse oxymetry are monitored. The fluoroscopy beam is rotated to visualize the intervertebral discs with parallel end plates and dissected by the superior articular process. To visualize the L5-S1 disc, the beam should be tilted caudally to avoid the ipsilateral iliac crest. Conscious sedation is used. A 17 gauge, 15-cm (6-inch) spinal needle is introduced into the disc using a posterolateral extrapedicular approach. The needle is positioned at the junction of the annulus and the nucleus. After the needle placement, the patient's position is changed to prone. The discectomy device's catheter is placed into the spinal needle. Under real-time imaging, the tip of the catheter is withdrawn simultaneously with the introducer needle until it is positioned approximately 1 mm distal to the proximal annular-nuclear interface. The catheter then is advanced slowly until it reaches the distal nuclear-annular interface. The process of decompression involves advancing and withdrawing the catheter to form channels in the disc. A minimum of six channels is created, at the 12, 2, 4, 6, 8, and 10 o'clock positions. Additional channels, up to 12, are created if resistance to catheter advancement is perceived. Postoperatively, patients are allowed unlimited walking, standing, and sitting. They are instructed not to perform any lifting, bending, or stooping. Return to sedentary or light work is permitted at 3 to 4 days after the procedure. A lumbar stabilization program is started 2 weeks after the procedure.

Intradiscal Electrothermoplasty

Intradiscal electrothermoplasty (IDET) was introduced in 1997 for the management of discogenic axial pain. The procedure consists of the insertion of a flexible catheter in a circumferential manner into the annulus of a painful disc. Heating the annulus via the catheter is thought to coagulate the nerve fibers in the annulus and inflammatory products, stiffen the collagen fibers, and heal disc tears.[60,73] IDET gained popularity among clinicians shortly after its introduction. It is used in the management of discogenic pain proved by discography. IDET is seen as a last step before lumbar fusion surgery is considered. It is performed primarily in the lumbar spine and seldom in the thoracic spine.

Technique for Intradiscal Electrothermoplasty

The patient starts the procedure in the side-lying position with a roll under the L4-5 area. The blood pressure, pulse, and pulse oxymetry are monitored. The fluoroscopy beam is rotated to visualize the intervertebral discs with parallel end plates and dissected by the superior articular process. To visualize the L5-S1 disc, the beam should be tilted caudally to avoid the ipsilateral iliac crest. Conscious sedation is used. A 17 gauge, 15-cm (6-inch) needle is introduced until it contacts the annulus fibrosis. After the needle placement, the patient's position is changed to prone. A flexible electrode is introduced through the needle and navigated through the posterior annulus. The catheter is heated for 16 minutes at 90°C (194°F). After the procedure, the patient wears a lumbar corset for 6 weeks.

Complications of Intradiscal Procedures

When good techniques are used, these interventional procedures are minimally invasive and have few complications or side effects. The side effects are transient and include temporary worsening of radicular or axial pain. Discitis is a possible complication, although the incidence is extremely low. Collis and Gardner[74] reported on 2187 disc injections and mentioned only one intervertebral disc infection. Wiley et al.[75] reported a review of the literature, which showed only 30 cases of discitis in approximately 5000 disc injections, an incidence of 0.6% per disc. Fraser et al.[76] reviewed 432 cases and found an overall infection rate of 2.3% of patients, or 1.3% per disc. The study breaks down the incidence of infection based on different techniques. The incidence of infection fell to 0.7% when a double needle technique was used. Aprill[77] examined 2000 patients who had undergone discography involving a single needle technique and reported only one case of acute discitis in that group.

Percutaneous Vertebroplasty

Percutaneous vertebroplasty (PV) was first introduced in France in 1984 for the management of aggressive vertebral hemangiomas.[78] The procedure later was used in the management of painful vertebral compression fractures and painful vertebral malignancies. The procedure involves the injection of polymethylmethacrylate (PMMA; also called *bone cement*) into the vertebral body. PV is an outpatient procedure performed with the patient under conscious sedation. Sterile preparation is applied. The procedure is performed in the thoracic and lumbar spine using a transpedicular (posterior) approach. A 17 gauge needle is introduced into the vertebral body through the pedicles, and the needle is positioned in the junction between the posterior and middle thirds of the vertebral body. Once the needle's position has been confirmed, PMMA is injected. This process is performed either unilaterally or bilaterally.

Complications

Complications of PV are rare, and the use of good technique can obviate them. The most severe complication is injury to the spinal cord, the nerve roots, or the venous plexuses if the needle breaches the medial pedicle; this necessitates immediate surgical decompression. Pedicle fracture can occur, which is not destabilizing to the spine but may be painful for many weeks. Extravasation of bone cement into neural structures and blood vessels can occur, although the occurrence of this can be minimized by mixing the cement with the contrast and injecting them under live fluoroscopy.

Kyphoplasty

Kyphoplasty is a recently developed procedure for the management of compression fractures. A balloon is placed through a needle into the vertebral body. The balloon is inflated to reduce the fracture, and PMMA is injected under low pressure. The supporters of this procedure believe that the restoration of height of the vertebral body improves the biomechanics of the spine and may reduce kyphosis. The injection of PMMA under low pressure is also believed to reduce extravasation into surrounding structures.

Summary

Nonsurgical interventional procedures for the spine are becoming a prominent management tool for painful spinal disorders. Physicians and surgeons currently consider using these procedures more frequently than recommending surgical interventions. These procedures, when performed by experienced physicians, have good outcomes and minimal complications. With advances in technology, improved techniques and the development of more effective equipment are expected. Interventions should always be followed up with an active spinal rehabilitation program after the patient's symptoms improve. Nonsurgical techniques, combined with a rehabilitation program, can restore function and minimize the recurrence of back pain.

References

To enhance this text and add value for the reader, all references have been incorporated into a CD-ROM that is provided with this text. The reader can view the reference source and access it online whenever possible. There are a total of 78 references for this chapter.

CHAPTER 13

Spinal Pathology, Conditions, and Deformities: Surgical Intervention

C. Dain Allred and Glenn R. Rechtine

Introduction

Successful surgical management of spinal pathology can be simplified into two basic concepts: decompression and stabilization. The neural elements, including the spinal cord and nerve roots, must be freed from impingement to halt the progression of neurological deficit and potentially to allow improvement in function. Segmental instability must also be addressed, because this leads to pain and deformity and may result in neurological impairment. This chapter focuses primarily on degenerative derangements of the spine; however, similar principles of decompression and stabilization hold true for spinal pathology caused by trauma, neoplasms, infection, and other etiologies.

Critical Questions Regarding Surgical Success

- Which neurological structure is compromised (spinal cord, nerve roots, or both)?
- What is the source of compression (e.g., disc herniation, osteophyte, fracture fragment, tumor)?
- Does the compressive force arise from the anterior side, posterior side, or both?
- How many levels are involved?
- What is the spinal alignment?
- Are there levels of segmental instability?
- What are the relevant medical co-morbidities?

Patient selection is perhaps more important than the technical aspects of surgery for achieving a successful surgical outcome in the treatment of spinal disorders. When surgery is indicated, careful planning of the operation is vital for success; this planning is based on a knowledge of the pathological process and its influence on local anatomy and neurological function. Armed with the answers to critical questions, the surgeon can select an operation that will adequately address the pathology, alleviate symptoms, and restore function.

Cervical Disc Disease

Degenerative cervical disc disease comprises a number of derangements of the cervical spine, ranging from isolated, single-level disc herniation to multilevel spondylosis with osteophyte formation. The clinical evaluation of patients with cervical disc disease requires interpretation of a detailed history, a meticulous examination, and appropriate diagnostic testing. Proper diagnosis and differentiation of patients with nerve root disorders (radiculopathy), spinal cord compression (myelopathy), or axial neck pain give the clinician insight into the natural history of the process and direct the treatment plan.

Differential Diagnosis of Cervical Disc Disease

- Radiculopathy (nerve root)
- Myelopathy (spinal cord)
- Axial neck pain

Cervical spondylotic radiculopathy usually presents as upper extremity pain associated with dysesthesias or paresthesias in a dermatomal pattern. Symptoms stem from impingement of a single or multiple nerve roots as a result of the degenerative changes of the bony and soft tissue anatomy. The natural history of cervical radiculopathy is favorable. Radiculopathy appears to be a distinct disorder, because progression from radiculopathy to myelopathy is uncommon. Most patients' acute symptoms improve with nonoperative management as the inflammatory cycle initiated by nerve root compression resolves. The short-term success of medical management is generally accepted; however, over a longer period, radiculopathy commonly recurs. Gore et al.[1] reported that 50% of patients with cervical radiculopathy who were treated conservatively had persistent symptoms at 15-year follow-up. In their long-term observations, Lees and Turner[2] reported that 30% of patients complained of intermittent symptoms, whereas 25% experienced persistent radiculopathy. On plain x-ray films, separating normal, age-related degenerative changes from those causing symptoms often is difficult. In asymptomatic adults over 50 years old, the prevalence of significant radiographic degenerative changes mirrors age; that is, in a cohort of 60-year-olds, approximately 60% will have radiographic spondylosis.

Surgery for radiculopathy is indicated for patients who have demonstrated symptoms of sufficient duration and magnitude despite conservative management. Generally, patients considered for surgery are those with at least 3 months of persistent or recurrent arm pain or neurological deficits that interfere with personal or professional function and those for whom nonsurgical treatment has failed. A correlation of clinical findings with an identifiable lesion on neuroradiography also portends more consistent relief of symptoms after surgery.

Indications for Surgery for Radiculopathy

- Persistent or recurrent arm pain of more than 3 months' duration
- Neurological deficits that interfere with function
- Failure of conservative treatments

Upper motor neuron symptoms, including hyper-reflexia, fine motor dysfunction, and gait disturbances, are the typical manifestations of cervical spondylotic myelopathy. The natural history of myelopathy is less favorable, with a tendency for acute episodes of neurological decline separated by periods of relative stability of symptoms. Clarke and Robinson[3] first reported on the natural history of myelopathy. They found that in more than 100 patients, motor symptoms worsened over time, and none of the patients returned to a normal neurological status. Lees and Turner[2] reported similar findings for long-term observations. Nurick[4] classified patients into six grades based on their disability with ambulation. His observations demonstrated long periods of no disease progression after early deterioration. Surgical intervention can be recommended when moderate to severe symptoms significantly affect a patient's quality of life or ability to work;

such symptoms include unsteady gait, hand dysfunction, or neurogenic bowel or bladder. Surgery also is indicated when a patient has a clinical history of disease progression, and in milder cases when significant stenosis is seen on imaging studies.

Indications for Surgery for Myelopathy

- Moderate to severe symptoms that affect the patient's quality of life or ability to work
- Unsteady gait
- Hand dysfunction
- Neurogenic bowel or bladder
- Stenosis
- Progressive disease

Axial neck pain is pain that is localized to the cervical area and does not radiate into the upper extremities. It can manifest as unilateral or bilateral pain, headaches, or stiffness. The most common cause of axial neck pain is cervical strain, commonly referred to as whiplash or whiplash-associated disorders (WADs). Treatment for whiplash is universally nonoperative, and in most cases symptoms resolve within 6 to 8 weeks. Patients with cervical degenerative disease associated with axial pain are more challenging to manage. Surgical outcomes have been unpredictable, and success has been limited when the sole indication for operative intervention is neck pain.[5-7] However, more recent studies have found that surgery has yielded beneficial results in patients with severe, persistent neck pain in whom the disease was limited to one or two levels with sparing of the remaining discs. Garvey et al.[8] reported 82% good or excellent results at greater than 4-year follow-up and concluded that single- or two-level cervical fusion could provide more reliable outcomes. Likewise, Palit et al.[9] demonstrated a 79% satisfaction rate among patients who underwent one- to three-level fusions. Despite these more promising reports, the surgeon should exercise considerable restraint in recommending operative care for axial neck pain, and the patient must understand the relative unpredictability of surgery in the relief of symptoms.

Surgical Treatment of Cervical Radiculopathy

The surgical options for treating cervical radiculopathy include anterior cervical discectomy and fusion (ACDF), anterior corpectomy and fusion (ACF), posterior laminotomy with foraminotomy, and laminectomy or laminoplasty with or without fusion. The procedures most commonly performed for cervical radiculopathy resulting from soft disc herniations are ACDF and foraminotomy; the other procedures (ACF, laminectomy, and laminoplasty) are reserved for more advanced ankylosis and multilevel disease (these are discussed in more detail in the section on the surgical management of myelopathy). Robinson and Smith[10] first described a technique for ACDF in 1955. This procedure has the advantages of (1) halting further osteophyte formation, (2) leading to regression and remodeling of existing osteophytes after solid fusion, and (3) distracting the disc space, which reduces buckling of the ligamentum flavum and enlarges the neuroforamen.[11]

The Smith-Robinson technique uses a horseshoe-shaped, tricortical iliac crest bone graft (Figure 13-1). The graft height should be 2 mm more than the pre-existing disc space, with a minimum height of 5 mm. Overdistraction can occur if an attempt is made to enlarge the disc space by more than 4 mm; this may result in overcompression, graft collapse, and pseudarthrosis. Various other graft configurations have been described, including the dowel-shaped Cloward graft, the iliac crest strut graft reported by Bailey and Badgley, and the keystone graft described by Simmons (Figure 13-2).[12-14] In addition to these techniques, which use autogenous bone graft, success has been reported with the use of allograft bone, carbon fiber composite cages, titanium-threaded cages, polymethylmethacrylate, coral, and ceramics. However, these have not been shown to be superior to autografting.[11] Osteoinductive agents, such as recombinant bone morphogenic proteins, currently are under investigation for use in fusions in the cervical spine.

The anterior cervical spine may be approached from the right or left side. After the skin and platysma have been incised, dissection is carried down to the spine, following the natural fascial planes. The sternocleidomastoid and carotid sheath are retracted laterally, and the trachea, esophagus, and thyroid are moved medially. Along with the risk posed to these large structures, a risk of injury to the recurrent laryngeal nerve exists. The disc space is identified, and the annulus is incised. The disc contents and end plate cartilage are removed to the uncovertebral joints on either side and to the posterior longitudinal ligament (PLL)

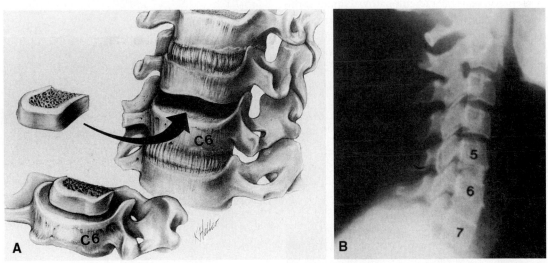

Figure 13-1

A, Schematic showing a Smith-Robinson graft (horseshoe-shaped tricortical iliac crest) placed in the disc space after excision of disc material. **B,** Lateral x-ray film showing ACDF at C5-6 and C6-7 using the Smith-Robinson technique. (From Herkowitz HN, Garfin SR, Balderson RA et al, editors: *The spine,* ed 4, p 499, Philadelphia, 1999, WB Saunders.)

Figure 13-2

Schematic showing some of the various graft configurations for ACDF. **A,** Cloward dowel graft. **B,** Bailey and Badgley iliac strut. **C,** Simmons keystone graft. (From Herkowitz HN, Garfin SR, Balderson RA et al, editors: *The spine,* ed 4, p 499, Philadelphia, 1999, WB Saunders.)

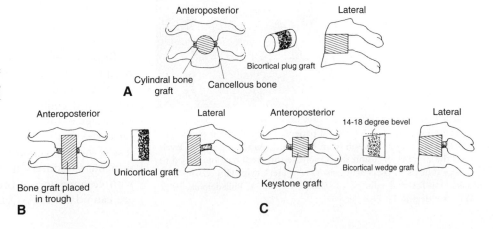

posteriorly. If sequestered disc material is behind the PLL or if a rent is noted in the PLL, the ligament is removed and the fragment is identified and excised; otherwise, the PLL may be left intact. The end plates are prepared to expose bleeding subchondral bone, and the contoured graft is placed into the disc space.

Controversy continues about the need for instrumentation in the surgical management of cervical disc disease. The purported advantages of internal fixation are to provide immediate stability, increase the fusion rate, prevent loss of graft fixation and position, improve postoperative rehabilitation, and reduce the requirement for a cervical orthosis.[15] Considerable debate exists about the efficacy of anterior cervical plating for single-level fusions. As the procedure is performed at an increasing number of levels, more compelling data support the use of rigid internal fixation because of the increased likelihood of bone graft nonunion (Figure 13-3).

Posterior approaches can also be used effectively in the surgical treatment of cervical radiculopathy. Laminotomy with foraminotomy is used primarily for unilateral radiculopathy at one or more levels. This technique is particularly useful for disc herniations or osteophytes that occur in

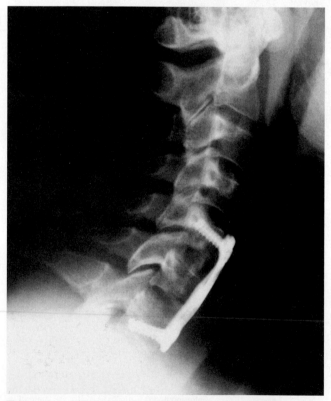

Figure 13-3

Lateral x-ray film of a 48-year-old patient who underwent two-level ACDF with internal fixation from C5 to C7. As the number of levels (and the number of fusion sites) increases, internal fixation is used to reduce the risk of pseudarthrosis. (From Herkowitz HN, Garfin SR, Balderson RA et al, editors: *The spine,* ed 4, p 534, Philadelphia, 1999, WB Saunders.)

relatively lateral positions. An incision is made posteriorly between the spinous processes at the affected level or levels, and dissection is carried down to expose the laminae on the symptomatic side. A keyhole-shaped laminotomy is performed using a combination of rongeurs, a high speed burr, and angled curets (Figure 13-4). The nerve root can then be exposed, and a probe is used to ensure adequate decompression. If a soft disc herniation is present laterally, the nerve root can be retracted gently and the disc fragment excised. At least 50% and preferably as much as 75% of the facet joint surfaces should be preserved to prevent iatrogenic segmental instability.[16]

Surgical Options for Cervical Radiculopathy

- Anterior cervical discectomy and fusion (ACDF)
- Anterior corpectomy and fusion (ACF)
- Posterior laminectomy with foraminotomy
- Laminectomy or laminoplasty with or without fusion

Surgical Treatment of Cervical Myelopathy

The goal of surgery in the treatment of cervical spondylotic myelopathy is to halt the neurological progression of the disease and to reduce pain. Although neurological improvement occurs in some cases, it cannot be reliably predicted, nor should it be the expected outcome for the patient or the clinician. Because neurological improvement cannot be ensured, when possible surgical intervention should occur before the deficits progress to the level of disability. The choice of surgical technique and approach is based on the location of the neural compression, the number of involved levels, the presence of instability, the alignment in the sagittal plane, and the surgeon's familiarity and comfort level.

Surgical Considerations for Cervical Myelopathy

- Location of neural compression
- Number of levels involved
- Presence of instability
- Sagittal plane alignment
- Surgeon's experience

Because cervical spondylosis typically results in cord compression from anterior structures, the anterior approach allows for direct access to the pathological anatomy and decompression of the neural elements. Another advantage of the anterior approach is that it allows for better correction of sagittal plane deformity in patients with loss of normal cervical lordosis, a deformity that is more difficult to address from a posterior approach. Patients with compression of the cord primarily at the disc levels are candidates for ACDF using the techniques described

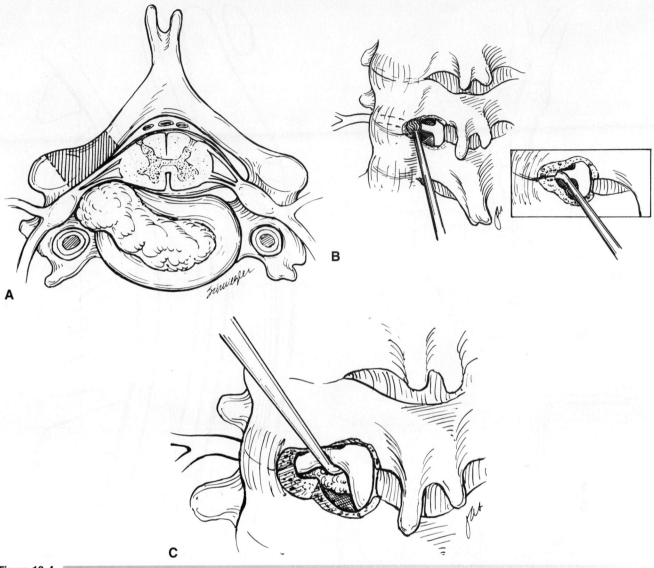

Figure 13-4
A, Posterolateral disc herniation causing nerve root compression. **B,** Laminotomy is performed; a portion
of the laminae superiorly and inferiorly is removed and the nerve root is identified. **C,** After foraminotomy,
the nerve root is retracted, revealing the herniated disc, which is excised. (From Herkowitz HN, Garfin
SR, Balderson RA et al, editors: *The spine,* ed 4, p 512-513, Philadelphia, 1999, WB Saunders.)

previously. ACDF can be used successfully in single-level
or multilevel disease; however, most surgeons do not
advocate its use for more than three levels because of the
increased risk of pseudarthrosis.[17] Posterior stabilization
sometimes is added to improve rates of successful fusion
when multiple levels are involved. As mentioned previously, iliac crest autograft is the gold standard, and the
use of internal fixation becomes more important in two-
and three-level procedures.

When myelopathy is caused by osteophytes, disc herniation, or ossification of the posterior longitudinal ligament
(OPLL) that extends above or below the disc space (behind
the vertebral bodies), corpectomy is indicated for satisfactory
decompression of the spinal cord. The term *corpectomy*
implies removal of the central portion of the vertebral body
and the discs above and below, as well as decompression of
the joints of Luschka. The anterior approach for anterior corpectomy and fusion (ACF) is the same as for ACDF; that is,
following the natural fascial planes between the trachea,
esophagus, and thyroid medially and the sternocleidomastoid and carotid sheath laterally to expose the anterior cervical spine. The appropriate discs are incised and removed back
to the PLL. A rongeur is used to remove the bulk of the central portion of the vertebral body (Figure 13-5). After this
initial trough is made, a high-speed burr is used to remove
the remaining vertebral body back to the posterior cortex.
Small angled curets are then used to remove the posterior
cortex from the dura. The cervical spine is stabilized after

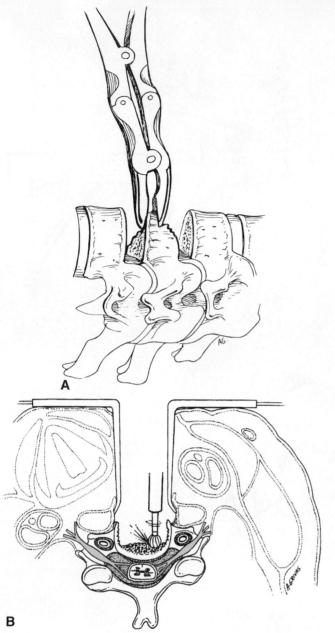

Figure 13-5

A, After removal of the disc above and below, a Leksell rongeur is used to remove the anterior two thirds of the vertebral body. **B,** A high-speed burr is used to remove the remaining bone back to the posterior cortex. The residual cortex is then removed with a small curet. (From Winter RB, Denis F, Lonstein JW, Smith M, editors: *Atlas of spine surgery,* p 63, Philadelphia, 1995, WB Saunders.)

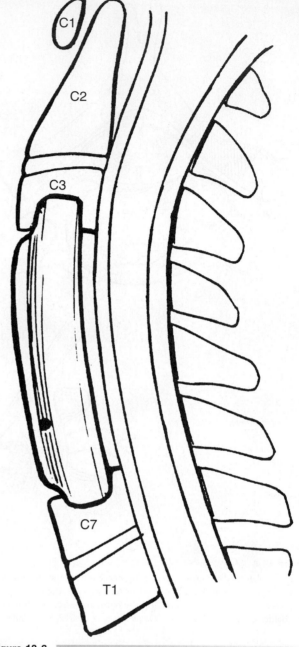

Figure 13-6

Schematic showing corpectomies of C4-6 with placement of a strut graft from C3 to C7. Note that the vertebral bodies have been notched to secure the graft in position. (From Winter RB, Denis F, Lonstein JW, Smith M, editors: *Atlas of spine surgery,* p 69, Philadelphia, 1995, WB Saunders.)

corpectomy with strut grafts. Ideally, the iliac crest is used for fusion of up to two vertebral bodies; its curve precludes its use in longer fusions. For more than two levels, strut allograft is biomechanically sound.[18] Figure 13-6 shows the use of a fibular strut graft for a C3-7 fusion following corpectomies. Internal fixation in the form of anterior cervical plating often is indicated to provide additional rigidity, reduce graft dislodgement, and possibly reduce the rate of pseudarthrosis (Figure 13-7). Postoperatively, a rigid cervical orthosis is often used. After prolonged surgery, the patient may remain intubated overnight to reduce the risk of respiratory complications.

Figure 13-7

Postoperative AP (**A**) and lateral (**B**) x-ray films of a 58-year-old patient who underwent anterior corpectomy and fusion from C4 to C7 for cervical myelopathy. Internal fixation was used to provide added stability. (From Herkowitz HN, Garfin SR, Balderson RA et al, editors: *The spine,* ed 4, p 535 Philadelphia, 1999, WB Saunders.)

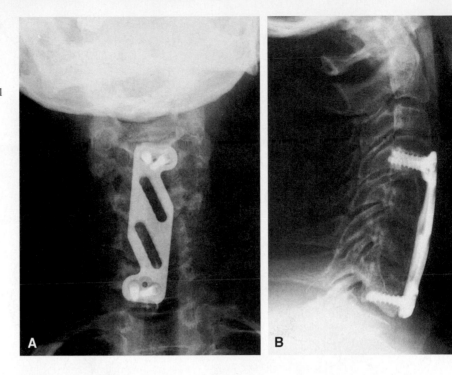

Posterior surgery for the management of cervical myelopathy is indicated in patients with dorsal spinal cord compression, diffuse canal stenosis, multilevel spondylosis, and OPLL. Posterior surgery may be preferable to long anterior exposures for diffuse disease, because posterior approaches are less technically demanding and do not endanger structures such as the trachea, esophagus, and recurrent laryngeal nerve. It must be remembered that for posterior decompression of the spinal cord to be effective, the cord must move posteriorly (dorsally) in the thecal sac. For this to occur, a lordotic alignment of the cervical spine is necessary; kyphosis in the sagittal plane is a relative contraindication to posterior surgery, because the spinal cord is less likely to move posteriorly when it is "draped over" the kyphotic vertebral bodies. Laminectomy with or without fusion and laminoplasty are the principle posterior procedures used to treat myelopathy.

Isolated cervical laminectomy currently has narrow indications. Laminectomy alone can increase instability and lead to postoperative kyphosis, neurological deterioration, and progression of OPLL. For these reasons, laminectomy without posterior stabilization probably should be reserved for patients with short segment posterior compressive lesions and a normal cervical lordosis. With more diffuse disease, it should be combined with instrumentation and fusion. The procedure is performed through a posterior midline incision. The paraspinal muscles are dissected from the spinous processes and laminae bilaterally. A high-speed burr is then used to create two troughs at the lateral aspects of the laminae down to the inner cortex (Figure 13-8, *A*). A Kerrison rongeur is used to complete the trough, through the inner table and ligamentum flavum. The spinous processes and lamina can then be removed as a block, held together by the ligamentum flavum. Figure 13-8, *B* shows a laminectomy of C3-7 with the dura decompressed. The facet joints lateral to the troughs are left intact to the extent possible while still allowing adequate decompression. Partial facetectomy can have a significant effect on spinal stability.

Posterior cervical instrumentation and fusion are often indicated after posterior laminectomy, for failed anterior fusion, and for segmental instability. Traditionally, wiring techniques have been used to stabilize the posterior cervical spine. Figure 13-9 shows a commonly used triple wiring technique, which also secures two corticocancellous strips of bone graft. Most wiring techniques require the spinous processes as points of fixation; however, after laminectomy, these have been removed. Screw fixation into the lateral masses can also be used for stabilization; these can be plate and screw constructs or rod and screw constructs (Figure 13-10).

Combined anterior and posterior approaches are necessary in some patients. This circumferential approach most often is indicated for patients with a combination of severe sagittal plane kyphosis and multilevel stenosis, postlaminectomy kyphosis, or severe osteoporosis. In these challenging cases, the anterior procedure (multilevel corpectomy with strut graft) is directed at restoring sagittal alignment and decompressing the spinal cord. The posterior procedure (lateral mass screws with plate or rod fixation) typically is used to enhance stabilization, minimize anterior graft complications, and reduce pseudarthrosis rates. These can be done as one procedure or as staged procedures on different days.

Because of the high incidence of spinal cord compression secondary to OPLL in Japan, Japanese surgeons have

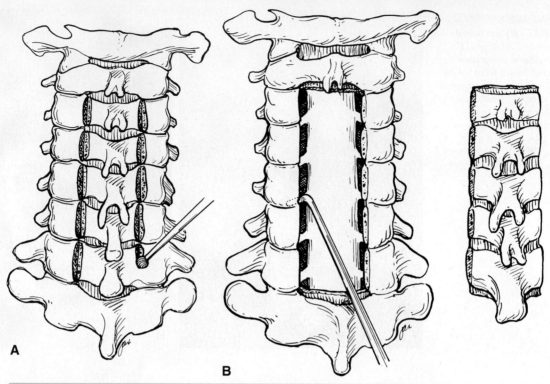

Figure 13-8

Technique for cervical laminectomy. **A,** Troughs are created bilaterally in the lamina using a high-speed burr. **B,** The troughs are completed, allowing for en bloc resection of the spinous processes, laminae, and ligamentum flavum. A blunt probe is used to assess the decompression of the nerve roots. (From Herkowitz HN, Garfin SR, Balderson RA et al, editors: *The spine,* ed 4, p 529-530, Philadelphia, 1999, WB Saunders.)

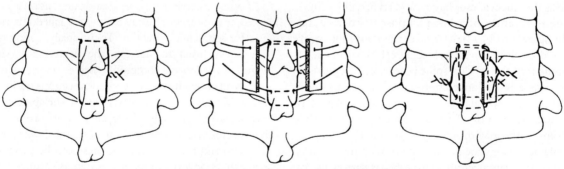

Figure 13-9

Triple wiring technique in the posterior cervical spine. This serves as a tension band as well as securing two corticocancellous strip grafts in position bilaterally. (From Benzel EC, editor: *Spine surgery: techniques, complication avoidance, and management,* ed 2, p 398, Philadelphia, 2005, Elsevier.)

been very innovative in developing decompressive procedures. Laminoplasty was designed to reduce postoperative instability while maintaining spinal motion. Although various laminoplasty techniques have been described, the common goal of each is to expand the area of the spinal canal (effecting decompression) while preserving the posterior bony and ligamentous structures. Retaining the posterior elements allows segmental muscle reattachment, promoting stability and allowing motion.

The two most common laminoplasty techniques are the open door technique, in which the posterior arch is opened on one side with the contralateral side acting as a hinge, and the French door technique, in which the lamina is opened in the midline with bilateral hinges.[19,20]

The exposure for laminoplasty is a posterior midline approach, dissecting the paraspinal musculature from the posterior elements. Care is taken to preserve the interspinous ligaments and facet joint capsules. A high-speed burr

Figure 13-10

AP (**A**) and lateral (**B**) x-ray films showing lateral mass plating and fusion from C3 to C7 after laminectomy for severe multilevel myelopathy. (From Herkowitz HN, Garfin SR, Balderson RA et al, editors: *The spine,* ed 4, p 539, Philadelphia, 1999, WB Saunders.)

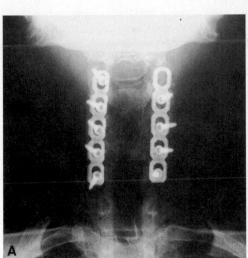
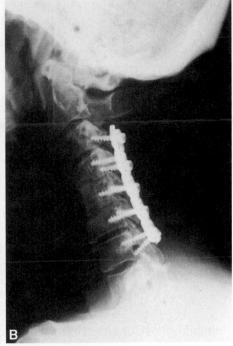

generally is used to create lateral troughs in the lamina bilaterally. The trough can then be completed and opened on one side and hinged on the other (open door technique) (Figure 13-11, *A*). A midline osteotomy can also be performed; the lamina is opened centrally, hinging on the bilateral troughs (French door technique) (Figure 13-11, *B*). Various methods of holding the laminoplasty open have also been detailed, including wiring, sutures, small plates, and interposition bone grafts.

Surgical Treatment of Axial Neck Pain

Operative treatment for axial neck pain has narrow indications and should be used when all nonoperative options have been exhausted. Surgery may be indicated for a patient who continues to have unrelenting neck pain despite conservative treatment and has one- or two-level cervical degenerative disease. ACDF is the primary procedure used to treat axial neck pain. Anterior fusion eliminates the diseased disc (thought to

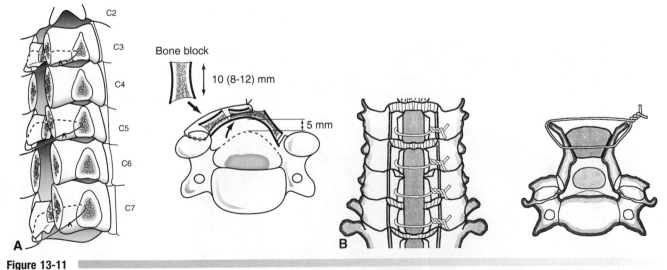

Figure 13-11

Two common techniques for vertebroplasty. **A,** Open door technique. **B,** French door technique. These procedures allow for preservation of motion and maintain the posterior ligamentous structures while decompressing the spinal canal. (**A** redrawn from Itoh T, Tsuji H: Technical improvements and results of laminoplasty for compressive myelopathy in the cervical spine, *Spine* 10:729-736, 1985; **B** from Herkowitz HN, Garfin SR, Balderson RA et al, editors: *The spine,* ed 4, p 556-557, Philadelphia, 1999, WB Saunders.)

Table 13-1

Rehabilitation Considerations After Surgery on the Cervical Spine

Expected Hospital Course	Outpatient Course	Red Flags
Length of stay: 0-3 days Ambulation and upper extremity range of motion (ROM) Bracing: May or may not be used (surgeon's preference, 2-24 weeks)	Aerobic conditioning, upper extremity stretching/strengthening Active cervical spine ROM when brace is removed No passive ROM for 3 months (at affected levels) May shower when wound is healed For fusions: No heavy lifting/exercise for 3 months	Change in neurological examination findings or symptoms Worsening pain Difficulty swallowing Erythema/fever/wound drainage

be the major pain generator) and stops motion of the uncovertebral joints and facet joints, which may also play a role in causing neck pain. A posterior approach may also be helpful in patients with failed anterior surgery or when posterior decompression is indicated. The anterior approach generally is preferred, because it does not involve extensive paraspinal muscle stripping and the disc is removed in its entirety.

Rehabilitation Considerations

Little data in the literature provide evidence on ways to optimize postoperative rehabilitation. The surgeon's preference and local opinion generally influence the rehabilitation process, lending anecdotal guidance to such things as the use of bracing, activity limitations. The authors' guidelines are outlined in Table 13-1; however, there is a wide range of variability among surgeons.

Thoracic Disc Disease

Thoracic disc herniation is a relatively unusual diagnosis among patients who seek care for spinal problems. Because the presenting symptoms can be quite varied, this uncommon diagnosis often goes unrecognized. However, with the improvement in magnetic resonance imaging (MRI) and other advanced imaging techniques, patients are being diagnosed earlier and with greater accuracy. Figures 13-12, A and 13-12, B show spinal cord impingement caused by

soft and hard disc herniations, respectively. Disc herniations in the thoracic spine affect mostly middle-aged individuals; nearly 80% are seen in the 4th through 6th decades, with 33% occurring in those in their forties.[21] Surgery for thoracic disc disease is estimated to account for 0.15% to 1.8% of all discectomies performed.[22,23] No clearcut syndrome has been described for this condition, because the presentation varies considerably. The most common initial symptom is pain (in 57% of patients), followed by sensory complaints and, least commonly, motor and bladder disturbances.[21] Three fourths of disc herniations in the thoracic spine occur between T8 and L1, with T11-12 being the most affected level (26%);[21] this is thought to be related to the increased stress on the spine at the thoracolumbar junction.

Patients without myelopathy can be treated conservatively with narcotic pain medications, anti-inflammatory drugs, physical therapy, activity modification, and occasionally bracing. In general, surgery is regarded as the treatment of choice for symptomatic patients with myelopathy to prevent the sequelae of cord compression. Indications for operative intervention for herniated thoracic discs include progressive myelopathy, lower extremity weakness, and unremitting pain after conservative treatment.

Surgical Treatment

When surgery is indicated, the approach taken to remove the diseased disc is determined by its nature and location,

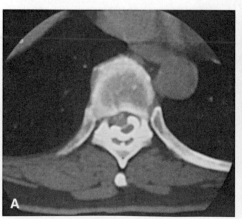 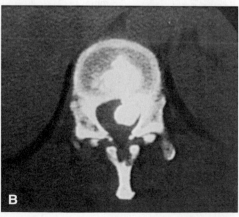

Figure 13-12

Thoracic disc herniations. **A,** CT scan after myelography showing a centrolateral "soft" disc herniation. **B,** CT scan showing a "hard," or calcified, centrolateral disc herniation. (From Herkowitz HN, Garfin SR, Balderson RA et al, editors: *The spine,* ed 4, Philadelphia, 1999, WB Saunders.)

the level of the pathology, and the surgeon's experience. Historically, thoracic myelopathy was treated with a direct posterior laminectomy and disc excision. This approach has been abandoned because of its unacceptably high rate of neurological deterioration, which results from manipulation of the spinal cord to access the disc for excision.[24] The widely accepted techniques for thoracic discectomy are the transthoracic approach, costotransversectomy, the transpedicular (posterolateral) approach, and video-assisted thoracoscopy (VATS).

The transthoracic approach gives the widest exposure to the disc space (especially for central and intradural herniations), accessibility of multiple levels, and the ability to place bone graft; however, with these advantages comes the morbidity of a thoracotomy.[22] A left-sided approach usually is preferred to avoid the inferior vena cava and the liver in the lower thoracic spine. With the patient in the

lateral decubitus position, a standard thoracotomy is performed, and the chest cavity is entered one or two levels above the level of interest. Mobilization of the parietal pleura and segmental vessels and nerves is then performed. Partial or complete discectomy can be undertaken anteriorly without manipulation of the spinal cord (Figure 13-13). Fusion is indicated when stability is compromised by the decompression, as in the case of complete discectomy with partial corpectomy. A chest tube is placed at the end of the surgery.

For posterolateral and lateral disc herniations, the costotransversectomy approach may be used. This approach has the advantages of avoiding entry into the pulmonary cavity and providing access to all thoracic levels, but it requires disruption of the paraspinal musculature and more extensive bone resection. The patient is positioned

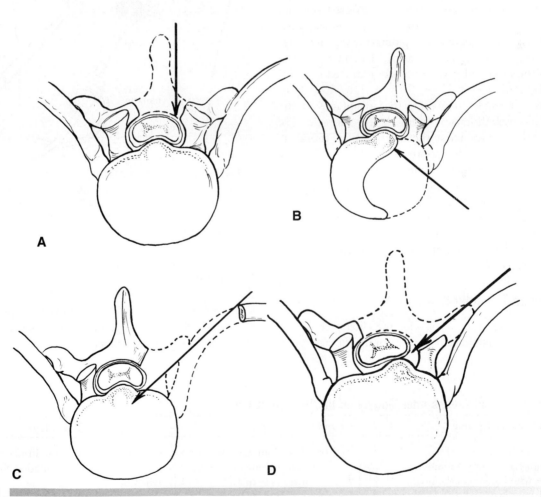

Figure 13-13

A, Decompression of thoracic disc herniations from a standard laminectomy approach requires manipulation of the spinal cord and results in a high rate of neurological injury. **B,** A transthoracic approach allows the most direct access to the disc without encountering the spinal cord.
C, Decompression using a costotransversectomy approach allows safe excision of the disc posteriorly.
D, For posterolateral and foraminal disc herniations, a transpedicular approach can give access to the lesion. (From Herkowitz HN, Garfin SR, Balderson RA et al, editors: *The spine,* ed 4, p 590-592, Philadelphia, 1999, WB Saunders.)

prone, and a paramedian incision is made. The paraspinal muscles are retracted medially or split transversely. The posterior medial portion of the rib is resected, and the pleura is mobilized and retracted anteriorly. The transverse process and pedicle on the affected side are excised, providing access to the lateral aspect of the disc. The disc fragment is removed, often along with a posterolateral portion of the adjacent vertebral bodies. Disc herniations that do not cross the midline can be effectively decompressed with this technique without manipulation of the spinal cord, minimizing neurological complications.

A transpedicular (or posterolateral) approach to the thoracic spine is useful only for posterolateral or foraminal herniations. This approach gives only limited exposure of the disc, but it avoids thoracotomy, it does not necessitate rib resection, and it requires less extensive dissection. With the patient prone, a midline exposure is performed. The lamina, facet joint, and pedicle on the affected side are removed. The lateral portion of the involved disc can then be excised with small curets and pituitary rongeurs. Segmental stability may be compromised, depending on the amount of the facet and pedicle that are removed to facilitate visualization.

VATS may be able to provide the advantages of the anterior (or transthoracic) approach to thoracic disc pathology while minimizing the morbidity of thoracotomy (Figure 13-14). This approach is more technically demanding and has a steep learning curve for the surgeon and staff; incomplete decompression and failure to resolve symptoms can result from inadequate visualization or unreliable excision of disc material. Limited data are available on the effectiveness of VATS, because this technique is evolving; however, preliminary series in the literature appear promising.[25]

Rehabilitation Considerations

Little information is available in the literature about postoperative rehabilitation after surgery of the thoracic spine.

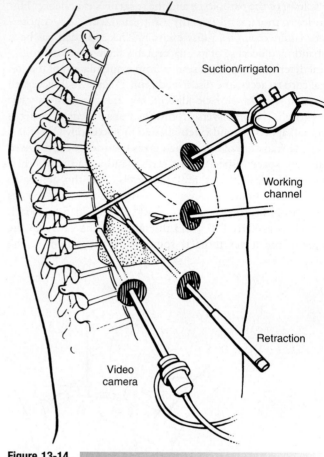

Figure 13-14

Diagram of the typical portals and instruments used in video-assisted thoracoscopy for decompression of a T8-9 herniated disc. (From Herkowitz HN, Garfin SR, Balderson RA et al, editors: *The spine,* ed 4, p 606, Philadelphia, 1999, WB Saunders.)

Many surgeons routinely use rigid orthoses, whereas others feel that the inherent stability of the thoracic spine, combined with modern instrumentation (for more extensive procedures), is sufficient to forego bracing. Table 13-2 presents the authors' preferred guidelines for rehabilitation.

Table 13-2
Rehabilitation Considerations After Surgery on the Thoracic Spine

Expected Hospital Course	Outpatient Course	Red Flags
Length of stay: 3-7 days Bed rest until chest tube is removed Ambulation when able to be out of bed Bracing: May or may not be used after chest tube is removed (surgeon's preference, 2-24 weeks)	Aerobic conditioning, upper extremity/lower extremity stretching/strengthening Active spinal range of motion (ROM) when brace is removed No passive ROM for 3 months (at affected levels) May shower when wound is healed Brace off for shower, activities of daily living No heavy lifting/exercise for 3 months	Change in neurological examination findings or symptoms Worsening pain Shortness of breath Erythema/fever/wound drainage

Lumbar Disc Disease

An estimated 80% of the population experiences low back pain at some time in their lives, resulting in one of the most common causes of disability among people living in industrialized nations.[26] In most patients, low back pain is self-limiting and requires no treatment; however, 7% to 14% have symptoms that persist longer than 2 weeks, and 1% to 2% eventually undergo surgery of the lumbar spine.[27] The most common disorders of lumbar discs can be divided into syndromes that cause predominantly back pain and those in which the primary complaint is leg pain (sciatica).

Statistics for Lumbar Disc Disease

- 80% of the population will experience low back pain
- 7% to 14% will have symptoms longer than 2 weeks
- 1% to 2% will undergo surgery

Discogenic pain syndromes of the lumbar spine present with low back pain as the chief symptom. Some associated buttock or sporadic leg pain also may be reported. As the name implies, the lumbar intervertebral discs are thought to be the principal pain generators and are the focus of diagnosis and treatment. These syndromes can be classified into three categories: internal disc disruption (IDD), degenerative disc disease (DDD), and segmental instability. IDD usually follows trauma and is marked by damage to the internal structure and metabolic function of the intervertebral disc. X-ray films generally are normal. DDD, on the other hand, is atraumatic, with a gradual onset of symptoms that usually manifest in middle-aged individuals.[28] Radiographic findings include disc space narrowing, osteophyte formation, and end plate sclerosis. Segmental instability describes excessive motion, either translational or rotational, of the spinal segments; this manifests as spondylolisthesis, lateral listhesis, rotatory subluxation, or scoliosis.

Disc Syndromes

- Internal disc disruption (IDD)
- Degenerative disc disease (DDD)
- Segmental instability

Lumbar disc herniation can cause impingement and inflammation of neural elements, most commonly the nerve roots. This leads to pain that radiates down the leg on the affected side, called *radiculopathy*. Irritation of the posterior primary ramus may result in localized back pain as well. In a healthy disc, the inner nucleus pulposus is contained by the annulus fibrosus. When fissuring or tearing of the inner annulus occurs but the outer portion remains intact, the nucleus can bulge or protrude posteriorly, causing root impingement. As further fissuring occurs, the nucleus can push through and exit the annulus, causing extrusion of the disc material. When an extruded fragment becomes detached from the remaining nucleus pulposus, it is said to be sequestered (Figure 13-15).

Nonoperative treatment of symptomatic lumbar disc disease most often results in a return to normal activity. Conservative treatment plans commonly consist of several modalities, including drug therapies and the use of a wide variety of physical therapy interventions, such as exercise, traction, and counterirritation techniques to manage pain (i.e., electrical nerve stimulation, acupuncture, biofeedback), as well as bracing and manipulation. Epidural and selective nerve root injections may also be helpful and are discussed fully in Chapter 12.

Surgery is indicated urgently for patients presenting with cauda equina syndrome or progressive motor deficit. In the absence of these findings, surgery generally is indicated only after conservative measures have failed. The major goal of surgery for these patients is pain relief. The most predictable results can be expected when the history, physical examination, and radiographic findings are consistent. Abnormal findings on MRI are not by themselves an indication for surgery.

Surgical Procedures for Lumbar Disc Disease

- Discectomy
- Posterior interbody fusion
- Anterior interbody fusion
- Artificial disc replacement

Discectomy

Surgery is indicated for patients with unilateral radiculopathic leg pain, for whom imaging studies confirm a correlating lumbar disc herniation, if nonoperative management fails after a trial of 6 to 8 weeks or if the patient has a severe or worsening motor deficit.[29,30] Conventional discectomy is performed with the patient positioned prone on a frame or in the kneeling position; this allows the abdomen to hang free, preventing pressure on the vena cava, which reduces intraoperative bleeding. The proper spinal level is identified, and a midline incision is made. Subperiosteal dissection is performed, exposing the spinous process and lamina. When proper exposure of the posterior elements is obtained, laminotomy (or laminectomy) of the affected side is carried out with the appropriate rongeurs and curets. Care must be taken not to remove too much of the facet, because this may result in iatrogenic instability. The ligamentum flavum is excised to expose the dura. The nerve root is inspected and retracted to reveal the underlying disc herniation (Figure 13-16). The posterior longitudinal ligament and posterior annulus are incised, and pituitary

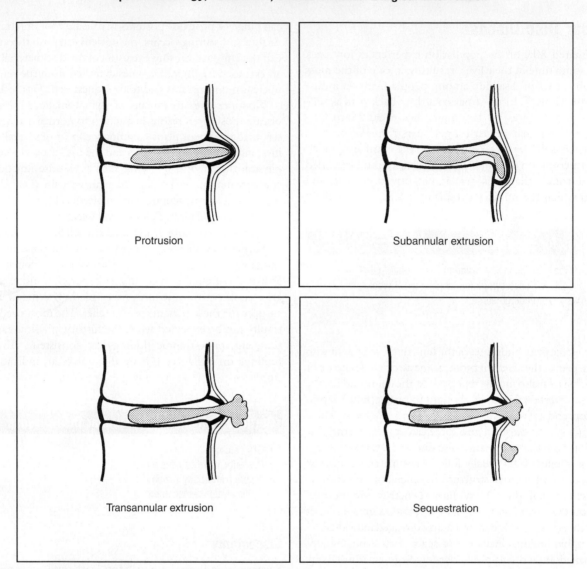

Figure 13-15

Classification of disc herniations. (From Herkowitz HN, Garfin SR, Balderson RA et al, editors: *The spine,* ed 4, p 706, Philadelphia, 1999, WB Saunders.)

rongeurs are used to remove the herniation in a piecemeal fashion. A blunt probe can then be inserted to ensure that a sufficient amount of disc material has been removed for adequate decompression of the nerve root. After meticulous hemostasis is achieved, the wound is closed in layers.

Alternative forms of discectomy have been described, with the goal of reducing the size of the incision and limiting dissection, and thereby minimizing postoperative morbidity, reducing the potential for scar formation, and allowing for quicker mobilization and rehabilitation. Two of the more common alternate techniques are microdiscectomy and arthroscopically assisted microdiscectomy.

Using the operating microscope or loupes with a headlamp coaxial to the line of sight allows the surgeon to obtain illumination and visualization of deep spinal structures through a small incision. With this advantage, microdiscectomy can be performed through incisions 2 to 3 cm

(1 to 1.2 inches) long. The surgical technique is similar to that for conventional discectomy, in which dissection of the paraspinals, laminotomy, and removal of the ligamentum flavum are required to allow visualization of the pathological disc and decompression of the nerve root. This operation can be safely performed as an outpatient procedure.[31] However, its role is somewhat controversial, because several reports show similar results for microdiscectomy and conventional discectomy.[32,33]

Arthroscopic assisted microdiscectomy (AMD) uses a percutaneous, posterolateral approach to the lumbar disc. The potential advantages of this technique are as follows: it does not require muscle stripping, bone resection, or retraction of inflamed nerve roots; it allows irrigation and dilution of inflammatory mediators; and it minimizes epidural bleeding and subsequent scar formation.[34] For AMD, the patient is positioned prone on a radiolucent

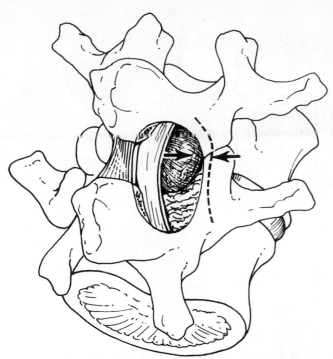

Figure 13-16

Technique for lumbar discectomy. Parts of the superior and inferior laminae and ligamentum flavum are removed to expose the nerve root and underlying disc herniation *(left arrow)*. The disc fragment is excised, and a blunt probe is used to ensure adequate decompression. Excessive bone removal (past dotted line) can cause iatrogenic instability. (From Benzel EC, editor: *Spine surgery: techniques, complication avoidance, and management,* ed 2, Philadelphia, 2005, Elsevier.)

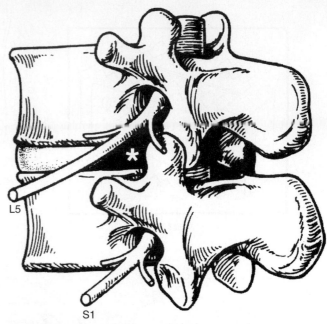

Figure 13-17

The triangular working zone used for arthroscopically assisted microdiscectomy. The zone is bordered anteriorly by the spinal nerve from the level above, posteriorly by the articular process of the lower vertebral level, inferiorly by the end plate of the lower vertebral body, and medially by the dura. (From Herkowitz HN, Garfin SR, Balderson RA et al, editors: *The spine,* ed 4, Philadelphia, 1999, WB Saunders.)

table, and standard sterile skin preparation and draping are followed. Under fluoroscopic guidance, a needle is inserted approximately 10 cm (4 inches) from the midline and directed toward the triangular working zone and into the disc (Figure 13-17).[34] A guide wire is placed through the needle, and the needle is removed. An obturator and canula are then advanced over the guide wire, providing access for the arthroscope and instruments. This approach allows for manual removal of the disc fragments causing nerve root compression, as well as annular fenestration, which reduces intradiscal pressure and creates a "path of least resistance" away from the nerve root for any future herniations. Success rates of 70% to 90% have been reported for AMD, with minimal complications.[35,36]

Posterior Lumbar Interbody Fusion

Numerous authors have reported on the success of posterior lumbar interbody fusion (PLIF) techniques in the treatment of lumbar degenerative disease, spondylolisthesis, and discogenic back pain. PLIF allows for decompression of the neural elements, distraction and realignment of the disc space, and stabilization of the painful motion segment. Some debate exists as to the surgical indications for PLIF

(or a modification, transforaminal lumbar interbody fusion [TLIF]); however, most would agree that only patients who still have persistent, disabling pain after an aggressive, prolonged nonoperative therapy program should be recommended for the operation. Provocative discography has also been recommended as a diagnostic tool to confirm that a particular disc space is the focus of pain generation.[37]

Patients undergoing PLIF surgery are positioned prone with the abdomen free, usually on a Jackson spinal table, which allows for easy access of fluoroscopy. A longitudinal midline incision is made, and subperiosteal dissection is carried down to expose the posterior elements of the lumbar spine. A portion of the lamina and the superior and inferior facets is removed to allow access to the spinal canal. Further decompression may be performed as necessary. The neural elements may then be retracted to expose the lateral aspect of the disc. The disc space is entered, and the disc material is removed bilaterally. Intradiscal shavers of different widths are used to excise the remaining disc material and prepare the end plates for fusion. Structural grafts are then placed in the interspace to restore alignment and allow for fusion (Figure 13-18). Multiple techniques and graft choices have been described, including autograft bone, allograft bone, and metal and carbon fiber cages filled with cancellous bone, and all of these choices come in a number of shapes and configurations. Although most variations of the PLIF technique involve grafting of the interspace and the use of implants, the need for posterior segmental instrumentation

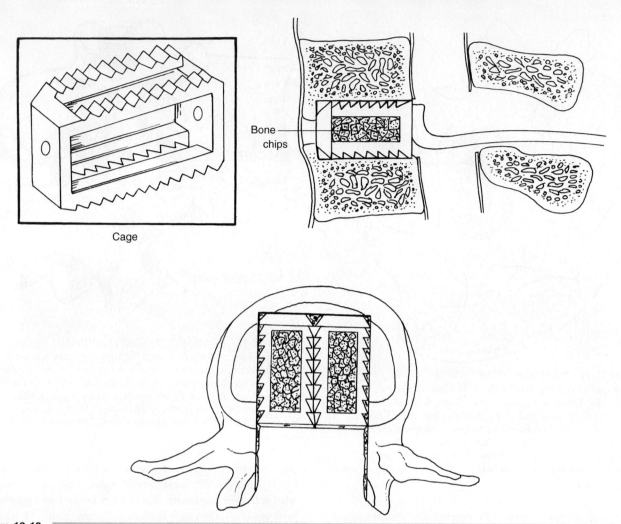

Figure 13-18

Posterior lumbar interbody fusion. The diagram shows the interbody positioning of two carbon fiber cages packed with cancellous bone graft. The cauda equina (not shown) is retracted to each side as the cage is impacted into the disc space. (From Benzel EC, editor: *Spine surgery: techniques, complication avoidance, and management,* ed 2, p 460, Philadelphia, 2005, Elsevier.)

and the addition of posterolateral fusion are the subject of debate. PLIF may be performed as a stand-alone procedure, or pedicle screw fixation with or without intertransverse fusion can be added (Figure 13-19). All methods have been reported successful.[38-40]

Anterior Lumbar Interbody Fusion

Anterior lumbar interbody fusion (ALIF) has become an increasingly popular surgical option because it allows reconstruction of the anterior column, improves sagittal alignment (i.e., restores lumbar lordosis), stabilizes the painful motion segment, enlarges the neuroforamina through distraction of the disc space, and avoids paraspinal muscle damage and scarring. The primary indication for ALIF is chronic low back pain, generally caused by degenerative disc disease, degenerative spondylolisthesis, or failed posterior surgery. As with other surgical techniques for the treatment of

degenerative lumbar conditions, ALIF is indicated when disabling symptoms have persisted for a prolonged period and when conservative management options have been exhausted. It is used primarily in the treatment of L4-5 and L5-S1, but it also may be used at more rostral levels. Neural compression is a relative contraindication for ALIF; decompression of the canal and neuroforamen is most safely and effectively carried out dorsally.

ALIF is performed with the patient supine on a radiolucent table. An anterior retroperitoneal approach is used, usually from the left side. An abdominal or vascular surgeon commonly performs the procedure in conjunction with the spinal surgeon. A paramedian incision is made low on the abdomen, the rectus sheath is incised, and the muscle is retracted. The retroperitoneal space is entered, and the peritoneum is mobilized and retracted to expose the lower lumbar spine. The iliac vessels are retracted to allow access to the disc space or spaces that are to be fused. The anterior

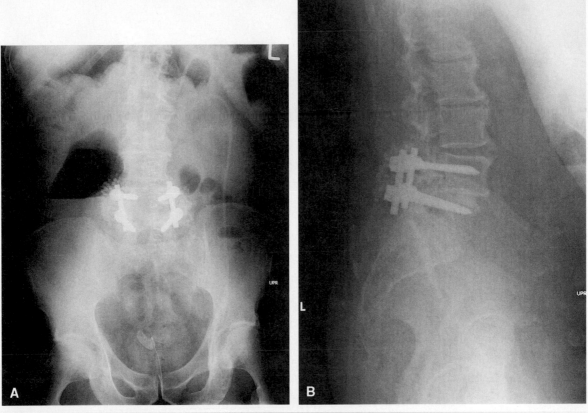

Figure 13-19

AP (**A**) and lateral (**B**) x-ray films showing an instrumented PLIF of L4-5. (From Benzel EC, editor: *Spine surgery: techniques, complication avoidance, and management,* ed 2, Philadelphia, 2005, Elsevier.)

longitudinal ligament and anterior annulus are excised, along with the remainder of the disc material. The subchondral bone of the end plates is prepared, and a graft slightly larger than the disc space is inserted to achieve the desired level of sagittal correction and distraction of the foramina. The choice of graft varies and, as with PLIF, successful outcomes and fusion have been achieved using tricortical autograft, shaped allograft, and cages. Hemostasis is achieved, followed by a standard closure. A nasogastric tube is used postoperatively until bowel function returns. Retrograde ejaculation is a recognized complication that may develop after ALIF; it most often occurs after L5-S1 fusion and is a result of injury to the autonomic nerves overlying that interspace.

Lumbar Artificial Disc Replacement

The U.S. Food and Drug Administration (FDA) recently approved the use of lumbar artificial disc replacement for the treatment of symptomatic lumbar disc disease. The artificial disc is an alternative to fusion procedures. The proposed advantage of disc replacement is the ability to restore pain-free motion of the intervertebral segment and to protect adjacent segments from increased loading and failure. The current indications for disc replacement are quite limited; only about 5% of patients considered for surgical intervention meet the criteria.[41] Candidates for lumbar arthroplasty are patients 18 to 60 years old in whom nonoperative treatment for at least 6 months has failed, who have single-level degenerative disc disease confirmed by MRI and discography, and who have no previous lumbar fusion, no instability, and no extruded disc material.[42] Proper patient selection has been advocated as the most important parameter for a successful clinical outcome.[43]

The only implant currently approved in the United States is the SB-Charité disc prosthesis. Three others currently in trials are the ProDisc II, Maverick, and FlexiCore. The SB-Charité prosthesis consists of cast cobalt-chromium-molybdenum (Co-Cr-Mo) alloy end plates that engage the bone with small spikes and an ultra high molecular weight polyethylene insert with a less constrained, mobile bearing design (Figure 13-20). Short-term follow-up of these implants has demonstrated a relatively high success rate and has shown results equivalent to or slightly better than the ALIF control group (stand-alone BAK cages with autograft).[42] The approach for implantation is similar to that for ALIF, a left anterior retroperitoneal exposure of the lower lumbar spine. The disc is excised, and the end plates are prepared. The prosthetic end plates are sized and implanted, followed by a polyethylene spacer of the

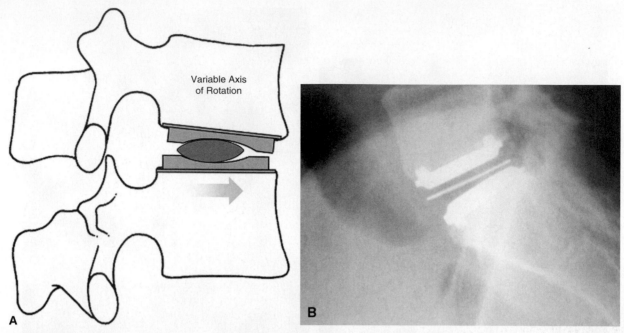

Figure 13-20

A, Schematic of SB-Charité artificial disc prosthesis. The mobile bearing design of this device accommodates the dynamic changes in the spine's axis of rotation. **B,** Lateral x-ray film showing the SB-Charité device at the L5-S1 disc space of a 39-year-old woman. (From Benzel EC, editor: *Spine surgery: techniques, complication avoidance, and management,* ed 2, pp 1647, 1650, Philadelphia, 2005, Elsevier.)

appropriate height to restore lordotic alignment of the segment. Long-term survival data are limited, as are reports of successful methods for revision or salvage when implant failure occurs.

Rehabilitation Considerations

Spinal surgeons vary widely in the use of postoperative bracing and activity restrictions after surgery on the lumbar spine, partly because of a lack of evidence-based literature. In a series of 50 open discectomies, Carragee et al.[44] urged patients to return to full activities as soon as possible, with no restrictions at all. They found that this resulted in a

quicker return to work and no increase in complications. This study is helpful for patients undergoing simple discectomy, but it should not be extrapolated to those undergoing fusion procedures. The authors' suggested guidelines for rehabilitation can be found in Table 13-3.

Lumbar Spinal Stenosis and Spondylolisthesis

The term *lumbar spinal stenosis* describes a complex set of symptoms, physical findings, and radiographic abnormalities caused by narrowing of the spinal canal. The etiologies of spinal stenosis are degenerative, congenital, traumatic,

Table 13-3
Rehabilitation Considerations After Surgery on the Lumbar Spine

Expected Hospital Course	Outpatient Course	Red Flags
Length of stay: 0-3 days for discectomy, laminectomy; 3-7 days for instrumented fusions Nasogastric tube (for anterior approach) Ambulation and upper extremity/lower extremity range of motion (ROM) Bracing: May or may not be used (surgeon's preference, 2-24 weeks)	Aerobic conditioning, upper extremity/lower extremity stretching/strengthening Active spine ROM/strengthening No passive ROM for 3 months (at affected levels) May shower when wound is healed Brace off for shower, activities of daily living No heavy lifting/exercise for 3 months	Change in neurological examination findings or symptoms Worsening pain Bowel/bladder changes Erythema/fever/wound drainage

and iatrogenic in nature, as well as a few others. The most common form of spinal stenosis is degenerative and usually occurs in the 6th and 7th decades.[45] The degenerative changes result in hypertrophy of the facet joints, capsule, and ligamentum flavum; in addition, disc degeneration leads to posterior bulging and loss of height, which add to both central and foraminal narrowing.

As would be expected in most degenerative disorders, the symptoms of lumbar stenosis can have an insidious onset. Initially they may include a low back ache that worsens with activity and is relieved by rest. As the stenosis progresses, symptoms of neurogenic claudication can begin to interfere with daily activities. These symptoms are classically described as vague cramping, aching, or burning pains in the back, buttocks, and legs that are exacerbated by standing or walking and relieved by sitting, squatting, or flexing the lumbar spine.[46] Spinal stenosis must be differentiated from vascular claudication, a somewhat similar but distinct symptom complex caused by peripheral vascular disease.

Lumbar spondylolisthesis can be classified into five groups according to the underlying abnormality:[47] congenital (dysplastic), isthmic (spondylolytic), degenerative, traumatic, and pathological. The most common form is isthmic spondylolisthesis, which is associated with a defect in the pars interarticularis; this form can be found in 5% to 7% of adults in the United States.[48] Many of these individuals are asymptomatic. Back pain and hamstring tightness are the most common presenting complaints, and few progress to high grade slips. The degenerative form, caused by intersegmental instability resulting from long-standing degenerative changes of the disc and facet joints (usually at L4-5), can cause or contribute to spinal stenosis and symptoms of neurogenic claudication.

Conservative management is the mainstay of treatment for most patients with spinal stenosis or degenerative spondylolisthesis. Pharmacological treatment (i.e., nonsteroidal anti-inflammatory drugs [NSAIDs], antidepressants, pain relievers, and muscle relaxants), injections, manipulation, bracing, exercise, traction, physical therapy, and other modalities (e.g., heat/cold applications, ultrasound) all have been reported to be helpful. Because the natural history of this disorder suggests that few patients will have short-term deterioration, a thorough trial of these nonoperative measures is suggested before surgery is considered.[49] Patients with moderate symptoms may be treated conservatively for 2 to 3 years.

Surgical Procedures for Lumbar Spinal Stenosis and Spondylolisthesis

- Laminectomy
- Posterolateral fusion

Lumbar Laminectomy

Decompressive laminectomy for spinal stenosis of the lumbar spine is indicated in patients with intractable pain recalcitrant to nonoperative treatment and those with neurological deficits that significantly impair their lifestyle and ability to function. Because of the potential destabilizing effects of lumbar decompression, laminectomy without stabilization is reserved for patients with no significant deformity or instability. Laminectomy is a safe, effective procedure; it may have a success rate in the range of 85% to 90% for eliminating neurogenic claudication.[50,51]

Laminectomy is performed with the patient positioned prone on a spine frame or in the kneeling position with the abdomen hanging free. A midline incision is made over the lumbar spine, and dissection proceeds down to expose the spinous processes and laminae bilaterally. The proper level or levels are identified radiographically, and the spinous processes are removed. The decompression is divided into three stages. In the first stage, the central canal is decompressed by means of removal of the laminae and ligamentum flavum (Figure 13-21). A number of methods can be used for this, including use of a high speed burr, Kerrison rongeurs, or osteotomes, depending on the surgeon's familiarity and experience. In the second stage, hypertrophied tissue is removed from the lateral recesses. A Kerrison rongeur is used to excise the medial aspect of the inferior and superior facets, along with excess ligamentum flavum, out to the level of the pedicle. In the third stage, each individual neuroforamen is decompressed. The nerve roots are identified, and a blunt probe is used to palpate the foramen. The bone spurs and soft tissue are removed until the probe can be passed freely into the foramen. Care must be taken to preserve the integrity of the pars interarticularis as well as that of the facets. The wound is closed in layers, and a suction drain is commonly used.

Minimally invasive and microsurgical techniques have also been developed for lumbar decompression. Little difference is apparent in the long-term outcomes of these procedures compared with the standard approach.[52,53] These techniques use the advantages of coaxial light and stereopsis, which the operating microscope provides, to perform the decompression through smaller incisions and with less morbid dissections. This may lead to less pain, shorter hospital stays, and quicker rehabilitation.[31] Preservation of the spinous processes, along with the interspinous and supraspinous ligaments, may also minimize the risk of iatrogenic instability.

Posterolateral Fusion

Dorsolateral arthrodesis of the lumbar spine may be used to treat many disorders that result in deformity and instability. This procedure is widely recommended for many patients in whom trauma, tumor, or infection have rendered the spine unable to support physiological loading.[54] It also is

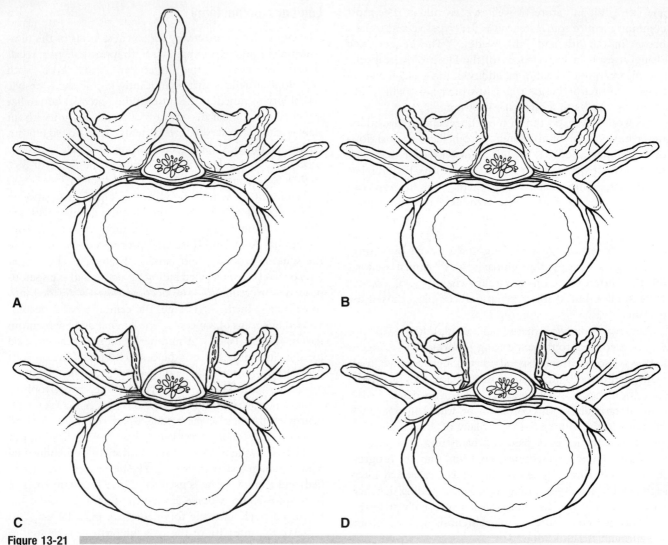

Figure 13-21

Lumbar laminectomy technique. **A,** Depiction of an axial view of the lumbar spine with typical hypertrophic degenerative changes. **B,** First stage: The spinous processes, midline laminae, and ligamentum flavum are removed to expose the dura. **C,** Second stage: Decompression of the lateral gutters is performed, with removal of the remaining laminae and the medial aspect of the superior facets. **D,** Third stage: Decompression of the neuroforamina is performed. (From Herkowitz HN, Garfin SR, Balderson RA et al, editors: *The spine,* ed 4, Philadelphia, 1999, WB Saunders.)

indicated for instability secondary to previous surgery or isthmic spondylolisthesis. Its use in degenerative disorders, however, is the subject of considerable debate. No benefit has been shown to adding arthrodesis to routine discectomy or after laminectomy in the stable lumbar spine.[55] Controversy exists over the need for fusion in degenerative spondylolisthesis when decompression is performed for associated spinal stenosis. Recent data suggest that more successful outcomes result when posterolateral arthrodesis is added to the decompressive operation when degenerative instability is present.[56,57]

Indications for the addition of internal fixation, namely segmental pedicle screw instrumentation, to posterolateral fusions are also debated. In patients with degenerative spondylolisthesis and spinal stenosis, segmental internal fixation has been shown to improve fusion rates, but this did not lead to improved clinical outcomes.[58] Instrumentation may help correct deformity, stabilize the spine, enhance arthrodesis rates, minimize the number of segments that need to be fused, and reduce rehabilitation time and brace wear. Instrumentation often is indicated in the treatment of fractures, when structural support is compromised by tumor or infection, for failed in situ fusion, or in cases of high grade translational motion.

Patients undergoing posterolateral fusion are positioned kneeling on an Andrews table or prone on a radiolucent Jackson frame (especially for instrumented cases). Most often, a midline approach and subperiosteal dissection are

Figure 13-22

Postoperative lateral (**A**) and AP (**B**) views of a 31-year-old man who underwent pedicle screw instrumentation and posterolateral fusion for a grade II spondylolisthesis at L4-5. (From Benzel EC, editor: *Spine surgery: techniques, complication avoidance, and management,* ed 2, p 818, Philadelphia, 2005, Elsevier.)

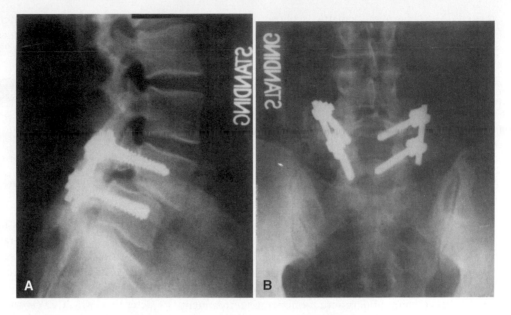

done to expose the posterior elements. Exposure is continued out to the tips of the lateral processes. Decompression is then performed as needed. Decortication of the dorsal aspect of the transverse processes and the lateral aspect of the superior facets and pars interarticularis, as well as removal of the facet joint capsule and cartilage, prepares the spine bed for fusion. Instrumentation (if used) is then implanted, using screws that pass through the pedicles into the vertebral bodies interconnected with rods (Figure 13-22). The gutters overlying the lateral process are filled with bone graft (Figure 13-23), and the wound is closed in layers over a suction drain.

Complications of posterolateral fusion may include hemorrhage, infection, and neurological injury in the perioperative period. Later, pseudarthrosis, hardware failure, or recurrent symptoms may lead to failures of treatment.

Rehabilitation Considerations

The authors' postoperative guidelines for laminectomy and dorsolateral fusion are the same as for procedures treating lumbar disc disease (see Table 13-3). When the wound produces no drainage, early showering may be allowed. Carragee and Vittum[59] reported no increase in wound complications after posterior surgery when patients were allowed to shower 2 to 5 days after surgery, compared to a historic cohort by the same surgeon who kept the wound dry for 10 to 14 days.

Spinal Deformities

Spinal deformity generally is categorized as frontal plane deformity (scoliosis) or sagittal plane deformity (kyphosis).

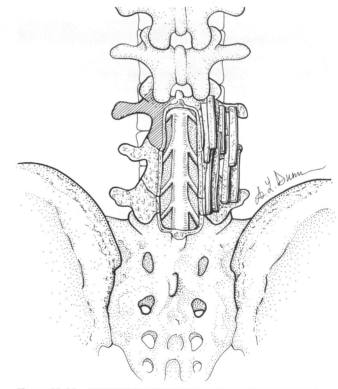

Figure 13-23

Diagram of a posterolateral fusion after lumbar laminectomy. Bone graft is shown in the lateral gutters; the fusion bed includes the transverse processes, the facet joints, and the pars interarticularis. (From Benzel EC, editor: *Spine surgery: techniques, complication avoidance, and management,* ed 2, Philadelphia, 2005, Elsevier.)

However, scoliosis most often includes a rotational or torsional malalignment and sagittal plane disturbance. In children and adolescents, scoliosis is broadly classified as idiopathic, congenital, neuromuscular, or syndrome related. Most cases of pediatric scoliosis are idiopathic. Kyphosis may be related to congenital abnormalities, neuromuscular disorders, trauma, infectious or neoplastic processes, or metabolic disorders, but Scheuermann's disease is the diagnosis in most cases.

The magnitude and progression (or risk for progression) of the curve are the major indications for surgical treatment of scoliosis.

In adolescent idiopathic scoliosis (AIS), the risk for curve progression is largely a factor of growth remaining and the magnitude of the present curve. In a growing child, bracing usually is indicated when the curve reaches 25° to 30°, with an upper limit of approximately 45°, beyond which curves are less amenable to bracing. Most data have shown that bracing halts curve progression, but correction cannot be anticipated. The indications for surgical correction in AIS are a growing child who presents with a curve of 40° to 45°, progression of a curve to 40° in a child undergoing nonoperative treatment, and a curve greater than 50° to 60° in a skeletally mature adolescent.[60]

Scoliosis Treatment

- Bracing: Curve 25° to 45°
- Surgery: Growing child with a curve of 40° to 45°
  Curve that progresses to 40° in a child undergoing bracing
  Curve greater than 50° to 60° in a skeletally mature adolescent

The normal range for thoracic kyphosis in the adolescent is generally considered to be 20° to 40°. Patients with Scheuermann's disease often have kyphosis greater than 45°, with associated end plate irregularities, Schmorl's nodes, and vertebral wedging on x-ray films. Deformity is the most common presenting complaint, and pain is another common symptom. Bracing for Scheuermann's disease has led to improvement in vertebral wedging and kyphotic angle but was less effective in patients with greater than 75° of initial kyphosis.[61] Surgical intervention may be indicated for rigid kyphosis greater than 75° and for those who have unrelenting pain despite conservative treatment.[62]

Deformity in adults presents a diagnostic as well as a therapeutic challenge for the clinician. Adult deformity most often can be divided into cases in which a curve was present before maturity; cases in which the curve developed de novo as a result of metabolic bone disease or degeneration; and cases in which degenerative changes are superimposed on pre-existing scoliosis. Nonoperative management is directed at treatment of symptoms, usually pain. Operative intervention is indicated to treat persistent, disabling pain that is refractory to conservative treatment, to correct

and stabilize progressive deformity, to restore coronal and sagittal balance, and to decompress neural elements associated with spinal stenosis.[63]

Surgical Procedures for Spinal Deformities

- Posterior arthrodesis
- Anterior arthrodesis

Posterior Arthrodesis

Preoperative planning for surgical correction of thoracic and lumbar deformities is important. Standing posteroanterior (PA) and lateral x-ray films of the entire spine are used to gauge the magnitude of the deformity and spinal balance. Bending films are also commonly used to assess the flexibility of the curve. This information is used to determine which levels to include in the fusion and how much correction of deformity can be expected.

Posterior reconstructive surgery is performed with the patient prone on a radiolucent spine frame. A long midline incision is made, and subperiosteal dissection is carried deep to expose the spinous processes, laminae, and lateral processes of the levels to be included in the fusion. Intraoperative x-ray films or fluoroscopy is used to positively identify the correct levels. The spinous processes generally are removed, the facet joint cartilage and capsule are excised, and decortication of the lateral processes and facet joints is performed to prepare the bed for later bone grafting.

Modern segmental instrumentation systems allow for multiple points of fixation along the spine. This enhances the procedure by adding stability to the construct, allowing for correction of deformity, improving fusion rates, and preserving normal sagittal plane alignment. Flat-back syndrome was common after nonsegmental Harrington rod fixation. Segmental fixation can be achieved using a number of techniques or combinations of techniques, including sublaminar wires or cables, hooks, and pedicle screws (Figures 13-24 to 13-26). These are affixed to rods, which are bent to accommodate the normal anatomy while providing correction of the existing deformity.

In adults, deformities associated with degenerative changes present added difficulty. These curves are stiff and cannot be passively corrected. Circumferential interbody techniques may be used to aid correction of the deformity and increase the fusion area. Osteotomies sometimes are needed in more severe cases to restore spinal alignment and balance (Figure 13-27). Decompressive surgery also is often required to relieve impingement of the cord or nerve roots.

After instrumentation, the posterolateral gutters are packed with autogenous cancellous bone graft. The wound

Figure 13-24

Preoperative x-ray films showing 56° curves in a 13-year-old girl with idiopathic adolescent scoliosis. She was treated with posterior fusion using the Harri-Luque technique (i.e., segmental fixation was obtained with sublaminar wires). The curves were corrected to 29 and 28°. (From Herkowitz HN, Garfin SR, Balderson RA et al, editors: *The spine,* ed 4, p 361, Philadelphia, 1999, WB Saunders.)

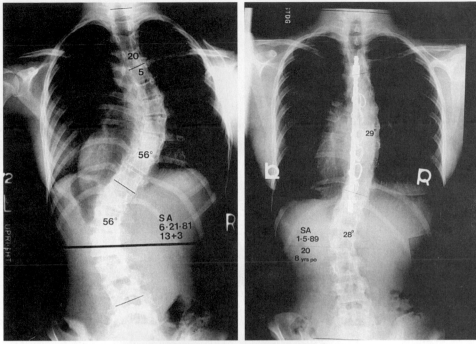

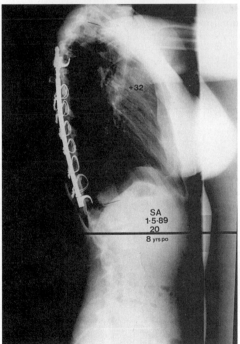

is closed in layers. The rigidity of modern instrumentation reduces the need for postoperative bracing or casting. Patients may be mobilized early and light activity advanced as pain permits.

Anterior Arthrodesis

For some thoracic and thoracolumbar curves, anterior instrumentation and fusion are preferred. The anterior approach has several potential advantages.[64] The crankshaft phenomenon, which may occur with continued growth after posterior arthrodesis, is essentially eliminated by ventral fusion. The hardware is anterior to the axis of rotation, making anterior fusion kyphogenic; this is helpful in AIS when hypokyphosis of the thoracic spine is present (although this can be a problem in the lumbar and thoracolumbar regions, where kyphosis is detrimental, or in the treatment of kyphotic deformities). In addition,

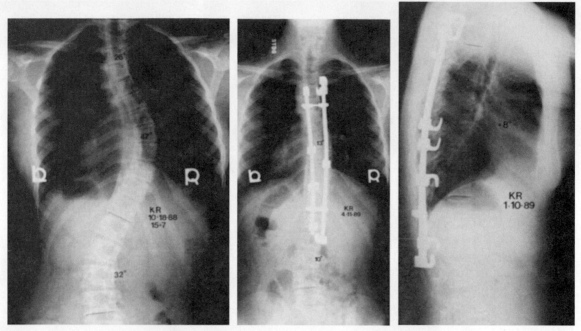

Figure 13-25

A 14-year-old with a 47° right thoracic curve. The condition was treated with posterior fusion from T4 to L1 using C-D instrumentation (hooks and rod construct). (From Herkowitz HN, Garfin SR, Balderson RA et al, editors: *The spine,* ed 4, p 364, Philadelphia, 1999, WB Saunders.)

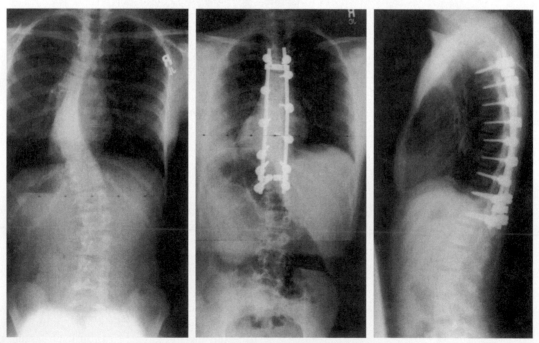

Figure 13-26

X-ray films of a 12-year-old girl with a left thoracic curve associated with a complex cervicothoracic syrinx. The syrinx was treated, and the patient underwent T4-12 posterior fusion with pedicle screw fixation. Postoperative x-rays show near complete correction of the curve. (From Benzel EC, editor: *Spine surgery: techniques, complication avoidance, and management,* ed 2, pp 846-847, Philadelphia, 2005, Elsevier.)

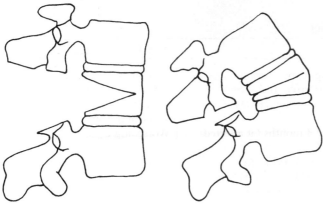

Figure 13-27

With adults with more severe sagittal deformities, an osteotomy can improve the surgical correction of alignment and balance. The diagram shows a pedicle subtraction closing wedge osteotomy used to restore lordosis. (From Van Royen BJ, De Gast A: Lumbar osteotomy for correction of thoracolumbar kyphotic deformity in ankylosing spondylitis: a structured review of three methods of treatment, *Ann Rheum Dis* 58:399-406, 1999.)

anterior instrumentation in thoracolumbar curves allows correction while preserving additional lumbar motion segments.

The patient is placed in the lateral decubitus position, and the spine is approached from the side of the curve's convexity. Depending on the levels to be included, a thoracotomy, retroperitoneal approach, or combination of the two with detachment of the diaphragm is needed for adequate exposure. Thorascopic techniques have also been described, which have the potential to reduce the morbidity of the open exposures. The segmental vessels are ligated, and the psoas muscle is mobilized. The discs are excised, and the end plates are removed to expose bleeding surfaces for fusion. Screws are placed in the lateral aspect of the vertebral body and are measured to achieve bicortical fixation. A rod is placed into the screw heads, and correction is performed, converting scoliosis to lordosis (Figure 13-28). The disc spaces are packed with cancellous bone graft (usually from the rib, harvested during the exposure); vertebral compression

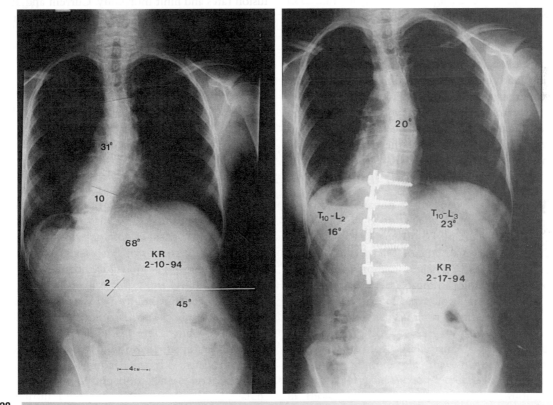

Figure 13-28

Adolescent girl with a progressive, 68° thoracolumbar curve that was treated with anterior instrumentation and fusion from T10 to L2. A standing postoperative x-ray film shows correction of the primary curve to 23°, with preservation of most of the lumbar segments. (From Herkowitz HN, Garfin SR, Balderson RA et al, editors: *The spine*, ed 4, pp 367-368, Philadelphia, 1999, WB Saunders.)

Box 14-1 Synopsis of the Assessment of the Pelvic Girdle

Patient History

Observation

Posture
- Between the pelvic girdle and thorax, pelvic girdle and legs
- Within the pelvic girdle (between the innominates and sacrum)

Gait

Examination

Active movements
- Pelvic girdle associated with movements of the trunk and hip joints
- Intrapelvic movements
- Hip and lumbar spine

Passive movements
- Joint play tests for sacroiliac joint mobility
- Stress tests for pain provocation for the sacroiliac joints and pubic symphysis

Resisted tests

Special tests
- Neurological mobility and conduction
- Palpation
- Diagnostic imaging

Modified from Magee DJ: *Orthopedic physical assessment,* ed 5, St Louis, 2007, Saunders.

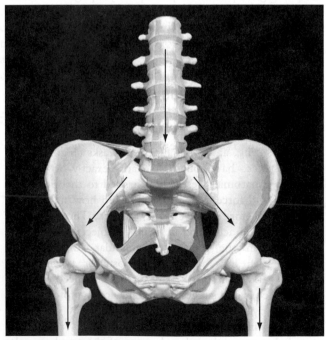

Figure 14-1

An understanding of how loads are effectively transferred through the pelvic girdle forms the basis of all subsequent assessment tests. (Courtesy Primal Pictures Ltd., London, UK.)

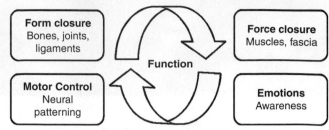

Figure 14-2

The integrated model of function has four components: form closure (considers the role of the bones, joints, and ligaments), force closure (considers the forces produced by myofascial action), motor control (the specific timing and modulation of muscle action and inaction during loading), and emotions.

the pelvic girdle have been developed[23-26] and treatment protocols proposed.[27-35] Both clinically and scientifically, the impact of chronic pain and emotional states on motor control has become evident, and clinical outcomes are now known to be influenced significantly by the patient's thoughts and beliefs.[36-44]

The integrated approach to the treatment of pelvic girdle pain has evolved from this collective body of research. This approach has four components (Figure 14-2), three that are physical (form closure, force closure, and motor control) and one that is psychological (emotions). This model proposes that joint mechanics can be influenced by multiple factors (articular, neuromuscular, and emotional) and that management of pain and dysfunction requires attention to all of them.

Stability is required for the effective transfer of loads through the pelvic girdle; this in turn requires optimum functioning of three systems: the passive system, the active system, and the control system (Figure 14-3).[45] Collectively these three systems produce approximation of the joint surfaces,[4,5] the amplitude of which is variable and difficult to quantify because it depends on an individual's structure and the forces needing control. The European guidelines on the diagnosis and treatment of pelvic girdle pain included a definition of joint stability.[1]

Clinical Point: Definition of Pelvic Joint Stability

The European guidelines on the diagnosis and treatment of pelvic girdle pain described joint stability as "the effective accommodation of the joints to each specific load demand through an adequately tailored joint compression, as a function of gravity, coordinated muscle and ligament forces, to produce effective joint reaction forces under changing conditions. Optimal stability is achieved when the balance between performance (the level of stability) and effort is optimized to economize the use of energy. Nonoptimal joint stability implicates altered laxity/stiffness values, leading to increased joint translations, resulting in a new joint position and/or exaggerated/reduced joint compression, with a disturbed performance/effort ratio."[1]

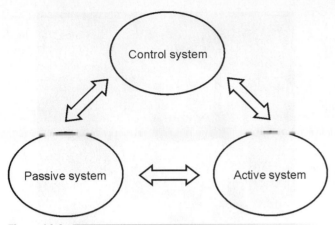

Figure 14-3

Panjabi's model for stability requires optimum functioning of three systems: the passive system, the active system, and the control system. (Modified from Panjabi MM: The stabilizing system of the spine. I. Function, dysfunction, adaptation, and enhancement, *J Spinal Disord* 5:383-389, 1992.)

According to this definition, analysis of pelvic girdle function requires tests for joint compression (mobility) and motion control (stability) during functional tasks (one leg standing and active straight leg raise). Joint mobility can be affected by factors intrinsic to the joint (e.g., the capsule and ligaments) or extrinsic to the joint (e.g., over-activation/underactivation of muscles that compress the joint). Motion control of the joints requires the timely activation of various muscle groups (i.e., neuromuscular function) such that the co-activation pattern occurs at minimal cost to the musculoskeletal system. Analysis of neuromuscular function requires tests both for motor control (i.e., timing of muscle activation) and muscular capacity (i.e., strength and endurance), because both are required for intrapelvic and regional control (i.e., control between the thorax and pelvis and the pelvis and legs), and maintenance of whole body equilibrium during functional tasks.

Effective management of pelvic girdle pain should include techniques to reduce joint compression where necessary (e.g., joint mobilization, muscle release techniques), exercises to control joint motion where and when necessary (e.g., motor control and muscle capacity training), and patient education to foster an understanding of both the mechanical and emotional components of the patient's experience.

Form Closure: Joint Mobility and Stability

New research has helped clarify the reasons that tests for mobility and stability of the sacroiliac (SI) joint have not shown reliability or validity. This new evidence requires clinicians not only to re-examine the tests commonly used in clinical practice and how the results have been interpreted, but also the research methodology that sought to validate or negate them.

For many decades the SI joint was thought to be immobile because of its anatomy. Researchers now know that mobility of the SI joint is not only possible[23,46-48] but also essential for shock absorption during weight-bearing activities and that this mobility is maintained throughout life.[49] The amount of motion is small (both for angular and translatoric motion) and varies from individual to individual.[46-48] Using Doppler imaging to view the transmission of a vibration impulse across the SI joint, Buyruk et al.[50-52] and Damen et al.[53-55] established that the SI joint has a high degree of individual variance with respect to its stiffness. Within the same subject, asymptomatic individuals had similar values for the left and right SI joint, whereas individuals with unilateral posterior pelvic girdle pain had different stiffness values for the left and right sides. In other words, asymmetry of stiffness between the left and right SI joint correlated with the symptomatic individual. In keeping with this research, the emphasis of manual motion testing should focus less on *how much* the SI joint is moving (amplitude) and more on the symmetry or asymmetry of the motion palpated.

The one leg standing, or stork, test (also known as the *Gillet test*) is commonly used to analyze the active range of motion of the SI joint. Hungerford et al.[23] established that, during this test, the non-weight-bearing innominate rotates posteriorly relative to the sacrum during ipsilateral hip flexion (Figure 14-4). The motion is compared bilaterally, and often a diagnosis of hypermobility or hypomobility of the SI joint is assigned. Before the work of Hungerford et al.,[23] Jacob and Kissling[46] and Sturesson et al.[48] independently investigated the amplitude of SI joint motion during the stork test. In the study by Jacob and Kissling, healthy, asymptomatic subjects were tested, whereas in the study by Sturesson et al., subjects with posterior pelvic girdle pain and suspected SI joint instability were investigated. The two studies found similar amplitudes of motion in their subjects. This suggests that this *active* mobility test cannot be used to determine the amplitude of *passive* mobility of the SI joint. The subjects in the study by Sturesson et al. did not demonstrate increased *active* amplitude of SI joint motion, perhaps because the joints were overly compressed by the activation of certain lumbopelvic muscles. Unstable joints often are associated with hypertonicity of the regional muscles, which occurs in an attempt to provide more functional stability during active movements. Therefore, current research supports the use of the stork test to determine whether the compression forces are symmetrical or asymmetrical between the left and right sides of the pelvic girdle; however, clinicians must keep in mind that this test does not differentiate the cause of any asymmetry noted. Further tests of passive mobility and stability of the SI joint are required to implicate or exonerate this joint.

Another challenge for clinicians who strive to be evidence based in their practice is that the one leg standing test has not yet shown intertester reliability for determining

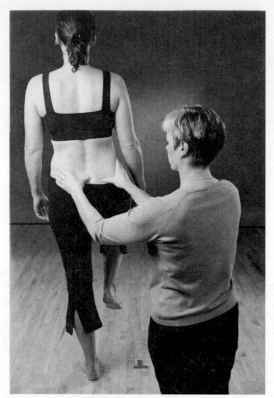

Figure 14-4
One leg standing test (stork, or Gillet, test). The individual transfers weight through one leg and flexes the contralateral hip joint to approximately 90°. When analyzing mobility, the examiner palpates the innominate and sacrum on the non-weight-bearing side. The innominate should rotate posteriorly relative to the sacrum,[23] and the motion should be symmetrical bilaterally. (Reproduced with permission from Diane G. Lee Physiotherapist Corporation and Linda-Joy Lee Physiotherapist Corporation.)

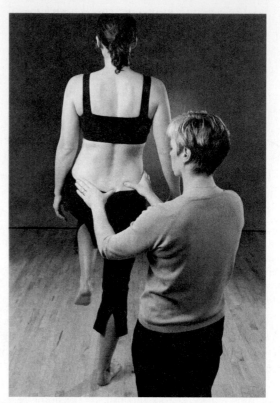

Figure 14-5
One leg standing test (stork test). The individual transfers weight through one leg and flexes the contralateral hip joint to approximately 90°. When analyzing stability, the examiner palpates the innominate and sacrum on the weight-bearing side. The innominate should remain posteriorly rotated relative to the sacrum. In patients with failed load transfer through the pelvic girdle, the innominate rotates anteriorly. Further tests are required to differentiate the cause of the functional instability. (Reproduced with permission from Diane G. Lee Physiotherapist Corporation and Linda-Joy Lee Physiotherapist Corporation.)

how much (amplitude) the SI joint is moving in either symptomatic or asymptomatic subjects.[56-62] However, the literature is marked by considerable discrepancy in the methods used, the subjects tested, the standardization of the technique, the skill of the tester, and the statistical analysis used. In other words, many clinicians doubt the quality of the research regarding this test.[23,63] New studies are underway to retest the reliability of the one leg standing test for motion analysis of the SI joint, and these studies are giving consideration to standardization of technique (i.e., the skill of the testers, how the motion is palpated) and the interpretation of the findings. The focus is on noting the pattern of motion and the symmetry or asymmetry, as opposed to simply judging the amplitude of motion.

The work of Hungerford et al.[23] has suggested another role for the stork test. These researchers noted that in healthy subjects, the innominate *on the weight-bearing side* remained posteriorly rotated relative to the sacrum during loading (the SI joint remained close packed) (Figure 14-5), whereas in subjects with posterior pelvic girdle pain and failed load transfer, the innominate rotated anteriorly

(unlocked). Hungerford recently completed an intertester reliability study for this part of the one leg standing test and was able to demonstrate a 97% confidence interval when the pattern of innominate motion was compared during the weight transference portion of the test.[64]

The passive tests for SI joint mobility and stability (joint play movements) are described in volume 1 of this series, *Orthopedic Physical Assessment.* The research of Buyruk et al.,[50-52] Damen et al.,[53,54] and Hungerford et al.[23] suggests that clinicians should re-examine how the findings of these tests are interpreted. Instead of assigning a diagnosis of normal, hypermobile, or hypomobile to the tested SI joint, the clinician should arrive at a judgment with respect to the quality and symmetry of resistance between the right and left SI joints. Because the muscular system is known to increase compression across the SI joint,[65,66] resistance during passive gliding of the joint can be due either to extrinsic causes (i.e., muscular) or intrinsic causes (i.e., capsule, ligaments).

When the SI joint is unilaterally truly stiff because of fibrosis of the capsule, the amplitude of motion is asymmetrical and reduced on the stiff side. In addition, the resistance to motion is increased. When the SI joint is unilaterally resistant to movement because of overactivation of certain lumbopelvic muscles, the amplitude of motion is also asymmetrical and reduced on the compressed side. However, in addition to an increase in the resistance to motion (i.e., muscular end feel), trigger points are palpable in the overactive, hypertonic muscles.

When the SI joint is unilaterally loose as a result of laxity of its capsule and ligaments, the amplitude of motion is asymmetrically increased and the resistance to motion decreased (i.e., soft end feel). This presentation also is seen with underactivation of the deep stabilizing muscle system, and differentiation requires retesting of the joint glide in a position that should tighten the capsule and ligaments (i.e., the close-packed position). For the SI joint, this position is nutation of the sacrum (posterior rotation of the innominate) (Figure 14-6). No glide should be felt in the anteroposterior plane between the innominate and the sacrum when the joint is held in the close-packed position (Figure 14-7). A SI joint that is loose because of laxity of the capsule or ligaments *does not* stiffen when joint glide

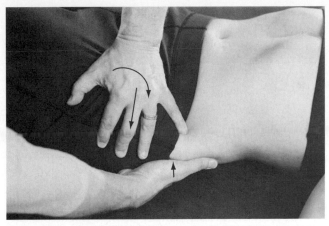

Figure 14-7

To test the integrity of the capsule and ligaments of the sacroiliac (SI) joint (form closure), the sacrum is nutated with the fingers of the dorsal hand *(arrow on the hand palpating the sacrum)* while the ventral hand simultaneously posteriorly rotates the innominate *(curved arrow)*. The SI joint is held in this close-packed position, and the anteroposterior glide *(vertical arrow on the hand palpating the innominate)* is repeated. No palpable motion of the SI joint should be present if the capsule and ligaments are intact and capable of effectively stabilizing the joint. (Reproduced with permission from Diane G. Lee Physiotherapist Corporation and Linda-Joy Lee Physiotherapist Corporation.)

is tested in the close-packed position, whereas a SI joint that is loose secondary to underactivation of the stabilizing muscle system *does* stiffen with the joint glide test.

Force Closure/Motor Control

Function would be significantly compromised if joints were stable only in the close-packed position. Stability for load transfer is required throughout the entire range of motion and is provided by the active system, directed by the control system, when the joint is not in the close-packed position. Optimum force closure of the pelvic girdle requires application of just the right amount of force at just the right time. This in turn requires a certain capacity (i.e., strength and endurance) of the muscular system, as well as a finely tuned motor control system that can predict the timing of the load and prepare the system appropriately. The amount of compression needed depends on the individual's form closure and the loading conditions (e.g., speed, duration, magnitude, predictability and threat value). Therefore, multiple optimum strategies are possible, some for low loading and/or predictable non-threatening tasks and others for high loading and/or unpredictable or threatening tasks.[67] The compression, or force closure, is produced by an integrated action and reaction between the muscle systems, their fascial and ligamentous connections, and gravity. The timing, pattern, and amplitude of the muscular contractions depend on an appropriate efferent response from both the central and peripheral nervous

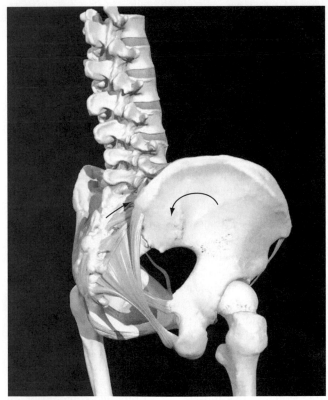

Figure 14-6

Nutation of the sacrum, or posterior rotation of the innominate, tightens the greatest number of ligaments of the sacroiliac joint and is the close-packed position, the most effective position for transferring high loads.[9] (Courtesy Primal Pictures Ltd., London, UK.)

systems, which in turn rely on appropriate afferent input from the joints, ligaments, fascia, and muscles. It is indeed a complex system, often difficult to study; yet, returning to the definition of joint stability (i.e., the ability to transfer loads with the least amount of effort that controls motion of the joints), one that is not difficult to assess or treat.

A healthy, integrated neuromyofascial system ensures that loads are transferred effectively through the joints while mobility is maintained, continence is preserved, and respiration is supported. Nonoptimum strategies result in loss of motion control (i.e., excessive shearing or translation), which often is associated with giving way (Figure 14-8) and/or excessive bracing (rigidity) of the hips (Figure 14-9), low back, and/or rib cage (Figure 14-10). These strategies often produce an excessive increase in intra-abdominal pressure,[68] which can compromise urinary or fecal continence or both. In addition, a nonoptimum respiratory pattern, rate, and rhythm can develop. Patients with failed load transfer through the pelvic girdle often present with inappropriate force closure, in that certain muscles become overactive while others remain inactive, delayed, or asymmetrical in their recruitment.[17] The possibility of these alterations in motor control must be considered during the assessment, because if they are present, the

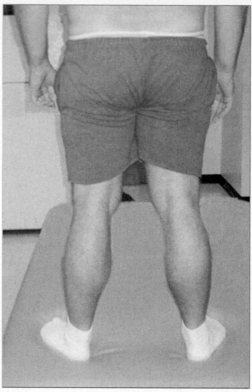

Figure 14-9

This individual is not conscious of the muscle activity in his buttocks, even though he uses excessive bracing through the inferior aspect of the pelvic girdle and hip joints as a strategy to compensate for nonoptimum stabilization of the pelvic girdle. This posture is called butt-gripping, for obvious reasons. (Reproduced with permission from Diane G. Lee Physiotherapist Corporation and Linda-Joy Lee Physiotherapist Corporation.)

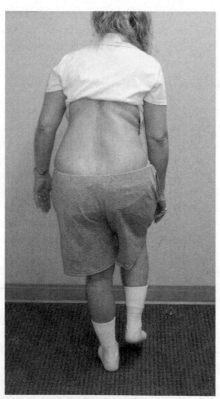

Figure 14-8

This individual shows marked loss of motion control through the left side of the pelvic girdle during one leg standing. (Reproduced with permission from Diane G. Lee Physiotherapist Corporation and Linda-Joy Lee Physiotherapist Corporation.)

system is not prepared for the loads that reach it, and repetitive strain of the passive soft tissues can result. Recent evidence on the role of the transversus abdominis, the deep fibers of the lumbar multifidus, and the pelvic floor muscles suggests that these components may be particularly significant.

Although the transversus abdominis (TrA) does not cross the SI joint directly, it can affect the stiffness of the pelvis through its direct anterior attachments to the ilium, as well as its attachments to the middle layer and the deep lamina of the posterior layer of the thoracodorsal fascia.[3,69] Richardson et al.[65] suggested that contraction of the TrA produces a force that acts on the ilia perpendicular to the sagittal plane (i.e., approximates the ilia anteriorly) (Figure 14-11, *A*). They also proposed that the "mechanical action of a pelvic belt in front of the abdominal wall at the level of the transversus abdominis corresponds with the action of this muscle." Theoretically, compression of the anterior aspect of the pelvic girdle (i.e., compressing the anterior superior iliac spines [ASISs] toward one another) (Figure 14-11, *B*) simulates the force produced by contraction of this muscle.

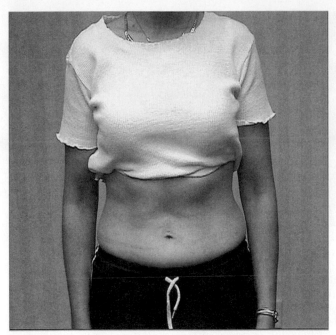

Figure 14-10
This individual is not aware of the excessive bracing of her lower rib cage; this is another compensatory strategy for nonoptimum stabilization of the low back and pelvic girdle. Note the telltale vertical lines down the anterolateral wall of the abdomen, a sure sign of overactivation of the oblique abdominals. This posture, called *chest-gripping*, can severely limit optimum respiration. (Reproduced with permission from Diane G. Lee Physiotherapist Corporation and Linda-Joy Lee Physiotherapist Corporation.)

In studies of patients with chronic low back pain, a timing delay of TrA was found in which the TrA failed to anticipate the initiation of arm and/or leg motion.[13,19,70,71] This delayed activation of the TrA could imply that the thoraco-dorsal fascia is not sufficiently pretensed (and therefore the pelvis is not optimally compressed) in preparation for external loading, leaving it potentially vulnerable to the loss of intrinsic stability during functional tasks. Other studies have shown altered activation in the TrA in subjects with long-standing groin pain,[19] low back pain,[70] and neck pain.[14]

Hides et al,[72,73] and Danneels et al,[74] have studied the response of the multifidus (deep, superficial, and lateral fibers) in patients with low back and pelvic girdle pain. They note that the deep fibers of the multifidus (dMF) become inhibited and reduced in size in these individuals. It is hypothesized that the normal "pump up" effect of the dMF on the thoracodorsal fascia (Figure 14-12, *A*), and therefore its ability to compress the pelvis, is lost when the size or function of this muscle is impaired.

Using the Doppler imaging system, Richardson et al.[65] noted that when the subject was asked to "hollow" the lower abdomen (resulting in co-contraction of the TrA and the dMF), the stiffness of the SI joint increased. These researchers stated that "under gravitational load, it is the transversely oriented muscles that must act to compress the sacrum between the ilia and maintain stability of the SI joint." Although the multifidus is not oriented transversely, both it and several other muscles (i.e., the erector

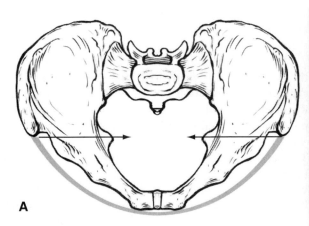

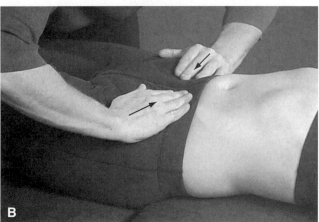

Figure 14-11
A, Contraction of the transversus abdominis bilaterally creates a force that approximates the ilia anteriorly *(arrows)*, providing the anterior abdominal fascia is not overly stretched. **B,** During tests of load transfer in the supine position (active straight leg raise test), the force of the transversus abdominis and the anterior abdominal fascia can be simulated by applying a bilateral compression force to the anterolateral aspect of the ilia such that the anterior superior iliac spines (ASISs) are approximated and the sacroiliac joints are compressed anteriorly. (Reproduced with permission from Diane G. Lee Physiotherapist Corporation and Linda-Joy Lee Physiotherapist Corporation.)

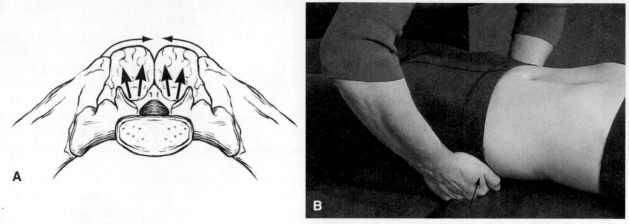

Figure 14-12
A, When the deep fibers of the sacral multifidus contract, they broaden (swell) within the confines of the posterior aspect of the sacrum, the medial walls of the innominates, and the roof of the thoracodorsal fascia. Much like air in a balloon, this swelling creates tension of the relatively inextensible roof (thoracodorsal fascia), which subsequently provides a posterior approximation force between the posterior superior iliac spines (PSISs) bilaterally. **B,** During tests of load transfer in the supine position (active straight leg raise test), the force of the deep fibers of the multifidus and the posterior thoracodorsal fascia can be simulated by applying a bilateral compression force to the posterolateral aspect of the ilia such that the PSISs are approximated and the sacroiliac joints are compressed posteriorly (only one arrow can be seen on this figure). (Reproduced with permission from Diane G. Lee Physiotherapist Corporation and Linda-Joy Lee Physiotherapist Corporation.)

spinae, gluteus maximus, latissimus dorsi, and internal oblique) can generate tension in the thoracodorsal fascia and thus impart compression to the posterior pelvis.[2,64] Theoretically, compression of the posterior aspect of the pelvic girdle (compressing the posterior superior iliac spines [PSISs] toward one another) could simulate the force produced by contraction of the multifidus (Figure 14-12, *B*).

The muscles of the pelvic floor play a critical role in the maintenance of urinary and fecal continence,[10,75-80] and recently attention has been directed to their role in the stabilization of the joints of the pelvic girdle.[18,28,29,81,82] The research suggests that motor control (i.e., the sequencing and timing of muscular activation) is an essential element of the ability to effectively force close the urethra, stabilize the bladder, and control motion of the SI joint during loading tasks.

It also is recognized that, although individual muscles are important for regional stabilization and mobility, an understanding of how they connect and function together is crucial. A muscle contraction produces a force that spreads beyond the origin and insertion of the active muscle. This force is transmitted to other muscles, tendons, fasciae, ligaments, capsules, and bones that lie both in series and in parallel to the active muscle. In this manner, forces are produced quite distant from the origin of the initial muscle contraction. These integrated muscle systems produce a continuum of force (also known as an *integrated muscle sling*[8]) that assists in the transfer of load. A muscle may participate in more than one sling, and the slings may overlap and interconnect, depending on the task being

demanded. The hypothesis is that the slings have no beginning or end, but rather connect to assist in the transference of forces. The slings may all be part of one interconnected myofascial system, and different loading situations may require the activation of selective parts of the whole sling. Specific muscle dysfunction (i.e., inappropriate timing, insufficient strength, and/or lack of endurance) can be identified and addressed within any sling to ensure that all components of stability (segmental, regional, and postural equilibrium[67]) are maintained while adequate mobility between the pelvic girdle, thorax, and hips is ensured for the task at hand.

The active straight leg raise (ASLR) test demonstrates the patient's ability to transfer load through the pelvis in the supine lying position and has been validated for reliability, sensitivity, and specificity for pelvic girdle pain after pregnancy.[24-26] It also can be used to identify nonoptimum stabilization strategies for load transfer through the pelvis. The supine patient is asked to lift the extended leg 20 cm (about 8 inches) and to note any difference in effort between the left and right leg (i.e., does one leg seem heavier or harder to lift). The strategy used to stabilize the lumbopelvic region during this task is observed, and the effort is scored on a scale of 0 to 5. The pelvis then is compressed passively (anterior, posterior, and oblique[29,63]), and the ASLR test is repeated; any change in strategy and/or effort is noted (see Figures 14-11, *B* and 14-12, *B*).

Subsequently, the patient's ability to voluntarily contract the TrA, the dMF, and the pelvic floor is assessed, and the results are co-related to the findings of the ASLR test.

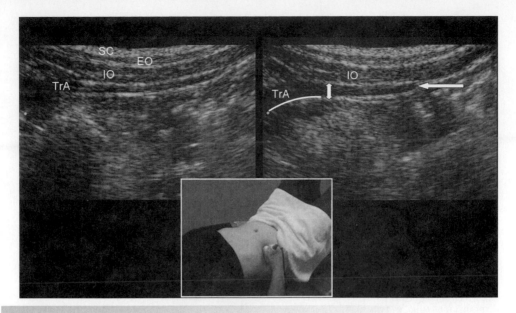

Figure 14-13

Ultrasound imaging of the anterolateral abdominal wall to assess the real-time activation of the lateral abdominal muscles in response to verbal cues and commands (e.g., the patient is asked to contract the muscles around the urethra, lift the vagina/testicles, lift the leg, or do a curl up). A transverse approach is used to generate a resting image *(inset)* of the three layers of abdominal muscles *(dark layers)* and the fascia *(white lines)* that separates them. The deepest, thinnest muscle is transversus abdominis (TrA); superficial to this is the internal oblique (IO), and above that is the external oblique (EO) and subcutaneous tissue (SC). The image on the left is the abdominal wall at rest; the image on the right shows an isolated contraction of the TrA. When an isolated TrA contraction occurs in response to a cue, characteristic features are seen. Specifically, there is an observable lateral slide of the anterior medial fascia of the TrA under the IO *(medial arrow)*, a relative increase in width and corseting (curving) of the TrA around the lateral aspect of the abdominal wall without an associated increase in width or corseting of the IO. (Reproduced with permission from Diane G. Lee Physiotherapist Corporation and Linda-Joy Lee Physiotherapist Corporation.)

To assess the ability of the left and right TrA to co-contract in response to a pelvic floor cue, the clinician palpates the abdomen just medial to the ASISs bilaterally at a sufficient depth to monitor the activity of the TrAs and asks the patient to gently squeeze the muscles around the urethra or to lift the vagina/testicles. When a bilateral contraction of the TrAs is achieved in isolation from the internal oblique, a deep tensioning is felt symmetrically and the lower abdomen hollows (moves inward).[33,34,83,84]

The dMF is palpated bilaterally close to the spinous process or the median sacral crest. In a healthy system, a cue to contract the pelvic floor should result in co-contraction of the dMF (clinical experience[29,63]). When a bilateral contraction of the dMF is achieved, the muscle can be felt to swell symmetrically beneath the fingers.[33,34] The examiner should not detect any evidence of substitution from the more superficial multisegmental fibers of the multifidus, which produces extension of the lumbar spine and a phasic bulge of the substituting muscle. The TrA should co-activate with the dMF; both muscles can be palpated unilaterally to assess co-contraction during a verbal cue to contract the pelvic floor (clinical experience[29,63]). The activation patterns of the deep muscle system can also be assessed using rehabilitative ultrasound imaging[29,33,85] (Figures 14-13 to 14-15).

When the force closure mechanism is effective, co-contraction of these deep muscles should compress the joints of the lumbar spine[86] and the SI joints,[65] thereby increasing stiffness. To test the ability of the active force closure mechanism to control motion of the SI joint sufficiently, the examiner first should ask the patient to co-contract the deep muscles. The joint play tests are repeated with the joint in a neutral position (i.e., hook lying) while the patient maintains this gentle co-contraction. Joint stiffness should increase, and no translation should occur even though the joint is in a neutral (i.e., loose-packed) position. This means that an adequate amount of compression has occurred and that the force closure mechanism is effective for the amount of load applied.

Emotions, Pain, and Motor Control

Emotional states play a significant role in human function and are often reflected in the musculoskeletal system.[42,87] In addition to their functional complaints, many patients with pain present with symptoms similar to those seen in

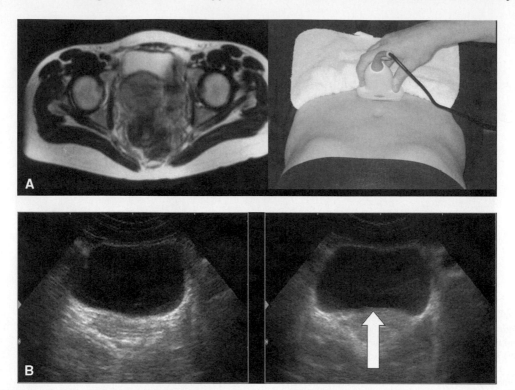

Figure 14-14

A, Ultrasound imaging with a suprapubic transverse abdominal probe *(right)* can be used to demonstrate the response of the muscles of the pelvic floor and their impact on the bladder. For example, the patient can be asked to contract the muscles around the urethra, lift the vagina/testicles, lift the leg, or do a curl up, and the impact of these commands on the bladder is imaged. The magnetic resonance imaging (MRI) scan *(left)* depicts the midline structures beneath the probe; the bright white structure is a moderately full bladder. **B,** The left ultrasound image is a suprapubic transverse abdominal view of a moderately full bladder with the pelvic floor muscles at rest. The right ultrasound image depicts the impact of optimum contraction of the pelvic floor muscles *(arrow)* on the bladder, as evidenced by a central and symmetrical indentation. (Reproduced with permission from Diane G. Lee Physiotherapist Corporation and Linda-Joy Lee Physiotherapist Corporation.)

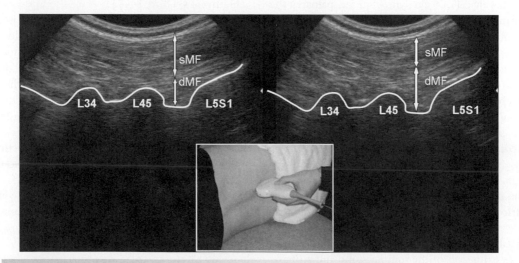

Figure 14-15

Ultrasound imaging of the lumbar multifidus with a sagittal probe placed just lateral to the spinous processes of the lumbosacral junction *(inset)*. The left ultrasound (RUI) image is a resting image of the deep multifidus (dMF) and the superficial multifidus (sMF) in relation to the articular processes of L3-4, L4-5, and L5-S1. The right image shows an isolated contraction of the deep fibers of the multifidus, seen as an increase in girth and preferential activity in the deeper aspects of the muscle. Assessment of an optimum contraction should be correlated with the findings on palpation. (Reproduced with permission from Diane G. Lee Physiotherapist Corporation and Linda-Joy Lee Physiotherapist Corporation.)

individuals who have experienced traumatic events.[88] Negative emotional states, such as fear, anxiety, and insecurity, can express themselves in maladaptive defensive or aggressive postures, which lead to altered muscle activity and further strain on the musculoskeletal system.

Clinically, it appears that if individuals do not have the coping mechanisms necessary to confront the symptoms, they learn to avoid activities that result in pain.[43] This avoidance can persist because of their fear of reinjury or an underlying belief that they are unable to perform because of their condition (i.e., fear-avoidance). The muscles of the region can reflect this fear and can become hypertonic, thereby increasing force closure, which subsequently results in excessive compression of the pelvic girdle. This can perpetuate pain and may be a factor in peripheral and/or central sensitization of the nervous system,[36,42,87,89] which in turn can create substantial barriers to rehabilitation.

It is important to understand the patient's emotional state and belief systems, because the resultant detrimental motor patterns often can be changed only by affecting the emotional state. Sometimes the answer can be as simple as restoring hope through education[36,40-42] and awareness of the underlying mechanical problem and providing a clear, understandable diagnosis and a logical course of action. Other times, professional cognitive behavioral therapy is required to retrain more positive thought patterns.

Management of Pelvic Girdle Pain and Impairment

Treatment for the impaired pelvic girdle must be prescriptive, because every individual has a unique clinical presentation. Ultimately, the goal is to teach the patient a healthier way to live and move, such that sustained compression and/or tensile forces on any one structure are avoided. The clinician uses manual skills to facilitate this process; however, the primary role is to educate and coach the patient through the recovery process, because only the patient can make the changes necessary for optimum function. Rarely is only one dysfunction present (e.g., one stiff joint or one poorly controlled joint); more commonly, multiple problems coexist, so that the most effective treatment consists of a combination of techniques and exercises that are patient specific (Figures 14-16 and 14-17).

In the first instance (i.e., existence of one dysfunction), the clinician may decide to use manual techniques and exercises that decompress the joints (increase mobility) and follow this with an exercise plan that re-establishes an optimum stabilization strategy. In the second instance (i.e., existence of multiple problems), the clinician may decide to start a program that emphasizes retraining of the stability muscle system and then add decompression techniques and exercises (increase mobility) later as

necessary. The most common scenario is one in which a combination of decompression and stabilization is required. In this case, the clinician uses techniques to decompress specific areas while concurrently prescribing exercises and/or support (e.g., belting or taping) for increased stability in other areas.

Pelvic Treatment Principles to Help Guide the Clinician

The first step in the treatment of pelvic disorders is to analyze the findings from the assessment. The clinician should determine whether the condition appears to involve:
- Primarily too much compression from stiff, fibrosed joints or hypertonicity of the global muscle system
- Primarily poor control of loose joints (loss of capsular/ligamentous integrity) or underactivation of the deep stabilizing muscle system (local system)
- A combination of too much compression and too little control in different areas of the lumbopelvic-hip complex

Assessment Findings That Indicate Excessive Compression

- Reduced movement on active mobility tests
- Decreased neutral zone on passive joint play tests
- Active straight leg raise (ASLR) test result that does not change or that worsens with compression
- Palpable hypertonicity in specific muscles that often is accompanied by nonoptimum patterns of muscle recruitment during movement or in response to verbal cueing

Assessment Findings That Indicate Poor Motion Control

- Increased neutral zone and soft end feel on passive joint play tests
- Active straight leg raise (ASLR) test result that improves with compression
- Nonoptimum pattern of muscle recruitment in response to verbal cueing
- Loss of joint position during functional load transfer tests (e.g., anterior rotation of the innominate during the one leg standing test)

Treatment Principles

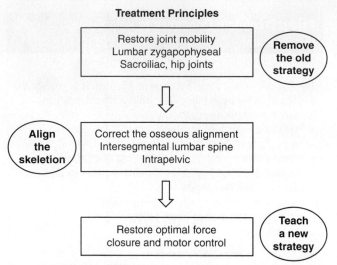

Figure 14-16

For most patients with lumbopelvic pain, the treatment plan includes techniques and exercises for decompression or mobilization of some regions and stabilization of other regions. The goal is to teach the patient a new way to live in the body, such that old habits that have led to pain and dysfunction are abandoned. (Modified from Lee LJ, Lee DG: Treating the lumbopelvic-hip dysfunction. In Lee DG: *The pelvic girdle,* ed 3, Edinburgh, 2004, Elsevier; and Lee DG, Lee LJ: An integrated approach to the assessment and treatment of the lumbopelvic-hip region, DVD, 2004. www.dianelee.ca)

Treatment Principles if Decompression Is Necessary

- Restore zygapophyseal, sacroiliac, and/or hip joint mobility
- Correct the osseous alignment within and between the lumbar spine, pelvic girdle, and femur
- Restore optimum force closure and motion control of the joints through training of the deep stabilizing muscle system
- Retrain the integration of the deep stabilizing muscle system with the superficial regional muscle systems with exercises and tasks that include functional movements (rehearse activities of daily living and work- or sport-specific movement patterns)
Also see Figures 14-16 and 14-17

Treatment Principles if More Control Is Necessary

- Correct the osseous alignment within and between the lumbar spine, pelvic girdle, and femur
- Restore optimum force closure and motion control of the joints through training of the deep stabilizing muscle system
- Provide an external support (if necessary) to augment the training being taught (sacroiliac [SI] belt, taping)
- Restore articular mobility and stability to extrinsic joints (knee, foot, thorax), because dysfunction in these areas can contribute to compensatory patterns that put excessive stress on the joints of the pelvis

Treatment Principles

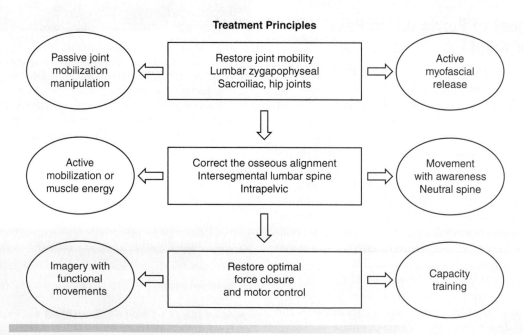

Figure 14-17

A treatment approach that follows the integrated model of function is multimodal; the clinician must be skilled in techniques of manual therapy (mobilization, manipulation, myofascial release) and alignment (muscle energy, re-educating movements with awareness for restoring neutral joint position). The clinician also must be able to provide instruction in exercises for motor control (timing and sequencing of muscle activation and relaxation) and muscle capacity (strength and endurance). (Modified from Lee LJ, Lee DG: Treating the lumbopelvic-hip dysfunction. In Lee DG: *The pelvic girdle,* ed 3, Edinburgh, 2004, Elsevier; and Lee DG, Lee LJ: An integrated approach to the assessment and treatment of the lumbopelvic-hip region, DVD, 2004. www.dianelee.ca)

Principles for Reducing Articular Compression

Excessive compression of the SI joint can be due to intrinsic factors, such as inflammatory pathology (e.g., ankylosing spondylitis), or to fibrosis of the capsule secondary to trauma. The joint also can be compressed by factors extrinsic to the joint, namely, overactivation of certain lumbopelvic and thoracopelvic muscles, specifically the external rotators of the hip, the pelvic floor muscles,[82] the oblique abdominals, the latissimus dorsi and gluteus maximus,[66] and the superficial fibers of the lumbosacral multifidus. In both types of compression (articular and muscular), the resistance to movement of the SI joint is increased; however, the clinical management is quite different (Figure 14-18).

For joint compression caused by fibrosis, specific passive articular mobilization techniques are the most effective treatment. Although the technique is graded according to the irritability of the articular tissues, long-standing fibrosis generally requires a sustained, grade 4+ passive mobilization (Figure 14-19).[29]

For joint compression caused by overactivation of muscles, many neuromuscular techniques can reduce the hypertonicity, including the following:

1. Functional or craniosacral techniques
2. Muscle energy techniques[90]
3. Trigger point techniques[91]
4. Dry needling[92]
5. Release with awareness (Figure 14-20)
6. Surface electromyography (EMG) or rehabilitative ultrasound imaging to foster "relaxation" of the targeted muscle[29,33]
7. Manual therapy techniques (i.e., joint mobilization, manipulation)[28,29]
8. Exercise and retraining of optimum postural and movement strategies[28,29,31,93]

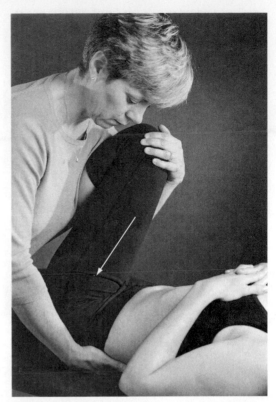

Figure 14-19
When the sacroiliac joint is sprained, the innominate rotates anteriorly to accommodate the swelling, and this is the position in which the joint tends to stiffen. The goal of the specific articular mobilization technique is to mobilize the joint into posterior rotation. To perform this technique, position the patient supine, with the hips and knees flexed. Then, with the long and ring fingers of one hand, palpate the sacral sulcus just medial to the posterosuperior iliac spine (PSIS). Next, support the patient's flexed hip and knee against your shoulder and arm. Flex the femur until you perceive the motion barrier for posterior rotation of the innominate. If you encounter a muscle barrier of either the hip or the sacroiliac (SI) joint, apply a gentle muscle energy technique by having the patient push gently into your shoulder. Resist the force (thus activating the hamstrings to release the anterior hip flexors) and facilitate a centering of the femoral head. Engage the motion barrier for the hip joint by maintaining this flexed position and adducting and internally rotating the femur. From this position, distraction of the SI joint is achieved by applying a dorsolateral force along the length of the femur (*arrow*). The SI joint can be felt to distract posteriorly. The degree of force applied is dictated by the joint and myofascial reaction. (Reproduced with permission from Diane G. Lee Physiotherapist Corporation and Linda-Joy Lee Physiotherapist Corporation.)

Treating the Compressed/Stiff Joint

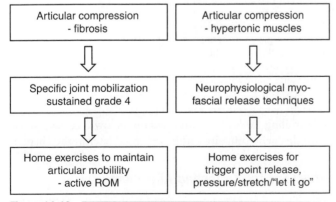

Figure 14-18
Treatment techniques and exercises vary, depending on the cause of the excessive articular compression. For a stiff, fibrotic joint, the most effective technique is a specific, passive articular mobilization sustained at grade 4 for up to 3 minutes. For a myofascially compressed joint, numerous techniques are effective, and all target the neurophysiology of the impaired, overactive muscles.

When a force is applied to the SI joint sufficient to stretch or tear the articular ligaments, such as in a hard fall on the buttocks or a lifting/twisting injury, the muscles respond to prevent dislocation and further trauma to the joint. The resulting spasm may fix the joint in an abnormal resting position, and marked asymmetry of the pelvic girdle (i.e., innominate and/or sacrum) may be present. This is an unstable joint under excessive compression, and the pelvic girdle is malaligned in a nonphysiological position (i.e., joint fixation). In this case, treatment that focuses on exercise without first addressing the fixation of the joint tends

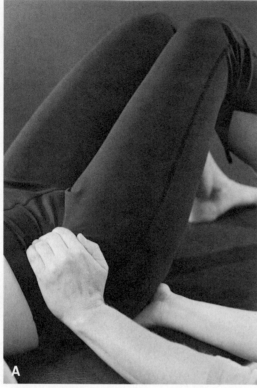

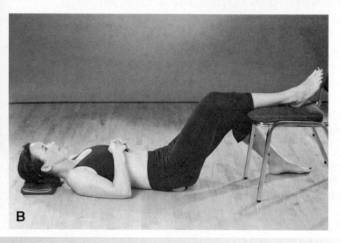

Figure 14-20

If the sacroiliac joint is stiff secondary to overactivation of the posterior wall of the pelvis (ischiococcygeus), the following technique and home exercise can be used to decompress the joint.[28,29,96] **A,** Position the patient supine with the hips and knees comfortably flexed. With your cranial hand, palpate the iliac crest. With your caudal hand, palpate the muscle (or muscles) in the posterior pelvic wall that is overactive (look for a tender trigger point somewhere along a line from the inferior lateral angle of the sacrum to the ischium along the medial aspect of the inferior arcuate band of the sacrotuberous ligament). Very gently, apply a lateral pressure to the ilium and a medial pressure to the ischium (adduct the innominate); that is, approximate the origin and insertion of the muscle. Monitor the muscle response; do not force the innominate or evoke a reflex muscle contraction, merely provide a proprioceptive cue to the nervous system as to the direction of release for which you are looking. Then, rotate the innominate anteriorly, posteriorly, internally, or externally, or a combination of these, to find the position that gives the greatest relaxation in the muscle you are monitoring. Hold this combined position for up to 90 seconds and wait for a softening sensation in the muscle. Give the patient verbal cues and images (release with awareness) to let the 'sitz bones' widen, to let your fingers sink into the hypertonic muscle, simply put – to let go. After you release the muscle, recheck the joint play test to see whether the technique has been successful at restoring the SI joint's mobility; you should feel an increase in the neutral zone of motion, and the tenderness in the muscle should be much reduced. **B,** Home exercise: The patient lies on the floor with the affected leg supported on a footstool or chair. A small ball is placed posteriorly on the tender trigger point. The patient then relaxes the posterior buttock (lets the ball sink into the muscles of the buttock) and thinks about allowing the sitz bones to move apart (open the posterior pelvic floor and wall). (Reproduced with permission from Diane G. Lee Physiotherapist Corporation and Linda-Joy Lee Physiotherapist Corporation.)

to be ineffective and commonly increases symptoms. Conversely, if treatment includes only manual therapy (i.e., mobilization, manipulation, or muscle energy techniques), relief tends to be temporary, and dependence on the health care practitioner to provide the manual correction is common. This impairment requires a multimodal therapeutic approach that includes manual therapy to decompress and align the pelvic girdle (specific articular manipulation technique) (Figure 14-21) followed by exercises and patient education to restore optimum motor control, strength, and endurance for functional tasks (see Principles for

Controlling Articular Compression below). A case study with this pelvic impairment is presented later in the chapter.

Principles for Correcting Alignment

Loads are transferred more effectively through joints that are properly aligned, so that the compression and tension forces induced are shared among all structures. Malalignment (Figure 14-22) can create excessive stress on individual structures (i.e., tension or compression) and ultimately leads to tissue breakdown, resulting in inflammation and pain.

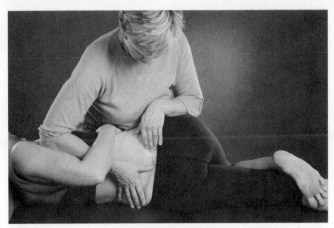

Figure 14-21
A manipulation technique is used to decompress a shear fixation of the sacroiliac (SI) joint. The clinician distracts the posterior aspect of the SI joint with a focused, high velocity, low amplitude thrust while simultaneously maintaining a "locked" L5-S1 joint. This is not a technique that can be learned from a book, and clinicians who want to become manipulative practitioners should pursue a certified program to ensure patients' safety and their own competence. In all cases, it is essential that the clinician be able to recognize those patients who require a manipulative technique so that an appropriate referral can be made. (Reproduced with permission from Diane G. Lee Physiotherapist Corporation and Linda-Joy Lee Physiotherapist Corporation.)

A common observation is that if motor control and stabilization exercises are prescribed when malalignment is present, the resultant muscle contractions are asymmetrical and suboptimal (e.g., a unilateral TrA contraction occurs instead of a bilateral contraction). Therefore, techniques that correct alignment are necessary in most treatment plans. Nonphysiological malalignment of the pelvic girdle suggests the presence of a shear lesion and requires a manipulative technique for correction. Physiological malalignment arising from muscle imbalance (e.g., anterior innominate, posterior innominate, forward/backward sacral torsion) can be addressed with several manual therapy techniques, including the following:

1. Active mobilization and alignment techniques (muscle energy techniques)[90,94]
2. Movement with awareness exercises (finding the neutral spine position and restoring the optimum pelvic base; that is, postural re-education) (Figure 14-23).[28,29,93,95,96]

These techniques should be followed by an exercise program and patient education to restore motor control, strength, and endurance if optimum alignment is to be maintained (see the following section).

Principles for Controlling Articular Compression

Inadequate or inappropriate motor control results in poor control of the SI joint during movement and loading.[17] The patient often complains of sensations of giving way

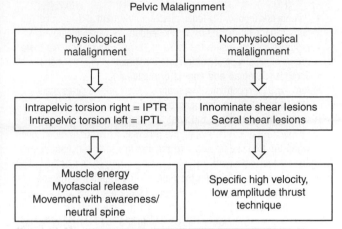

Pelvic Malalignment

Figure 14-22
Treatment techniques for a malaligned pelvic girdle vary, depending on the cause of the distortion. Physiological malalignment occurs secondary to muscle imbalance, and the posture of the pelvis can be corrected in many ways. An intrapelvic torsion (IPT) is a physiological malalignment. An IPT right consists of a left anteriorly rotated innominate, a right posteriorly rotated innominate, and a right sacral rotation. An IPT left consists of a right anteriorly rotated innominate, a left posteriorly rotated innominate, and a left sacral rotation. Techniques that restore optimum tension, tone, or balance in the muscles of the lower extremity, pelvis, and trunk and also restore a neutral pelvic position include muscle energy techniques, release with awareness techniques, strain/counterstrain techniques, movement with awareness exercises, and neutral spine exercises. Nonphysiological malalignment occurs secondary to an intra-articular shear lesion of either the innominate or the sacrum. These lesions (also known as *innominate upslips*, *downslips*, or *anterior/posterior sacral subluxations/fixations*) require a specific, high velocity, low amplitude thrust technique to restore a neutral pelvic position, followed by an exercise program for restoring force closure and motor control of the pelvic girdle.

or a lack of trust when loading through the involved extremity (see Figure 14-8). Treatment for this impairment requires the restoration of both motor control and muscle capacity (strength and endurance) with specific exercises that initially train an optimum recruitment strategy for control of the pelvic girdle, followed by exercises that challenge stability during functional tasks. A sacroiliac belt or tape can be used temporarily to augment force closure during this stage of rehabilitation (Figure 14-24).[28,29,49,97,98]

Important General Principles for the Progression of Exercise Programs[28,33,34,93]

- *Connect first;* that is, as the starting point for each exercise, teach the patient to perform a precontraction of the deep local stabilizers.
- Initially the patient may need to relax the local stabilizer co-contraction after each repetition of movement; however, the goal is to encourage a maintained local muscle co-contraction for several repetitions of movement, as long as substitution strategies are not observed. The number of repetitions possible with one local muscle activation increases as control improves.

- Palpate and monitor the local muscle recruitment and control of the joint position during the exercises, especially when adding a new progression. Make sure the muscles do not turn off and that there are no signs of loss of control into the direction of hypermobility.
- Focus on low load and control of movement.
- Aim for high repetitions (endurance). Start with only as many repetitions as the patient can perform with an effective local system co-contraction and control of the movement (sometimes as low as 3 to 5 repetitions) and progress to 15 to 20 repetitions when the exercise is easy and requires minimal concentration to control the movement.
- Use manual cues to help the patient attain neutral spine and isolate the local stabilizers. Provide tactile feedback and assist control at the levels where segmental hypermobility or multisegmental collapse occurs during the exercise movements.
- Avoid fast, ballistic movements.
- Progress from stable to unstable surfaces to increase proprioceptive input and challenge.

- Check for excessive global muscle activity by monitoring the breathing pattern (lateral costal and abdominal expansion should continue) and by monitoring for bracing or rigidity.
- Incorporate local muscle co-contraction into daily functional activities as early and as often as possible; break down functional tasks into component movements and use separate components as an exercise.
- Focus on co-contraction and control of position instead of strengthening of a single muscle.
- Include exercises that address rotational control to restore full function.
- If high load and high speed activities are required for work or sport, add these at the end stages of rehabilitation and make sure that low load, slow speed control is present for the same movement pattern first. High speed, high load activities should be only one part of the patient's exercise program; low load exercises should be continued concurrently to ensure continued functioning of the local system.

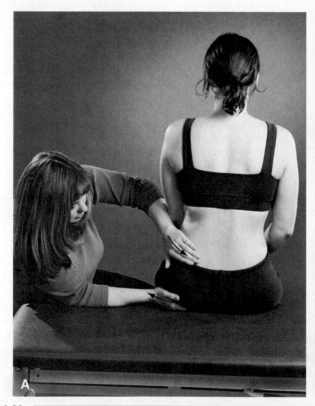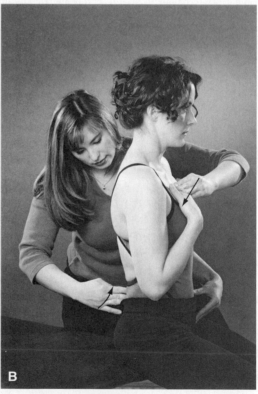

Figure 14-23

A, Setting the optimum pelvic base. Restoration of a neutral spine position begins with setting the optimum base of the pelvis. In this figure, the clinician facilitates abduction of the left innominate and reseats the left femoral head, steps that are commonly needed for a unilateral butt-gripper. The patient is taught to do this by using the hand to passively pull the ischium lateral (and often posterior). The goal is to have the patient sit with the weight central between the two ischia and midway between the pubic symphysis and the coccyx. **B,** Once the pelvic girdle has been set into neutral, the clinician can use manual and verbal cues to align the thorax and lumbar spine (regionally and segmentally) over the pelvic girdle.[28,29,93,96] (Reproduced with permission from Diane G. Lee Physiotherapist Corporation and Linda-Joy Lee Physiotherapist Corporation.)

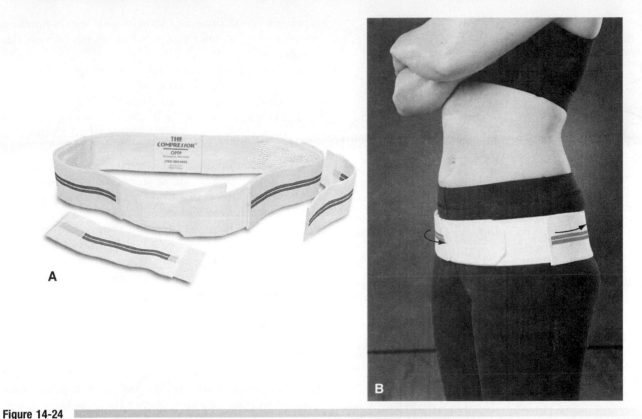

Figure 14-24

A, The COM-PRESSOR™, a belt designed for the pelvic girdle, allows specification of both the amount and location of compression support. Four elastic straps are provided with the belt such that two can be overlapped for more compression. The location of application of the compression straps is determined by the results of the active straight leg raise test and by which type of compression (anterior, posterior, or oblique) provides the best response (least effort required) for lifting the leg in the supine position. **B,** In this figure the straps are applied to the left posterior pelvic girdle and the right anterior pelvic girdle, simulating the forces of the left deep multifidus and the right transversus abdominis. Many other belts on the market are also effective for generally compressing the pelvic girdle, but the advantage of this model is the specificity of the compression. Further research is required to establish the need for this specificity. (**A,** From Orthopaedic Physical Therapy Products; **B,** Reproduced with permission from Diane G. Lee Physiotherapist Corporation and Linda-Joy Lee Physiotherapist Corporation.)

Recent research has increased our understanding of muscle and joint function and consequently changed the way exercises for back pain and dysfunction are prescribed.[13-15,21,30,32-35,39,67,71-73,86,99-102] New concepts of how joints are stabilized and how load is transferred through the body highlight the importance of proprioception, automatic muscle activity, and motor control for regaining optimum movement after injury. This body of evidence makes it clear that successful rehabilitation of back and pelvic girdle pain and dysfunction requires different exercises from those used to condition and train healthy, pain-free individuals (Figure 14-25).

The treatment plan should prescribe exercises as part of a multimodal approach. If exercise is prescribed before joint and neuromeningeal mobility is restored (i.e., before articular compression and neuromeningeal tension are reduced), the patient's pain and dysfunction often worsen.

This may lead some to conclude that certain exercises are "bad" or unsuccessful in treating back pain, when in fact the problem may be merely *inappropriately timed exercise intervention.* In addition, the *type* of exercise prescribed is of utmost importance. For lumbopelvic pain, the evidence supports correction of deficits in motor control before focusing on the strength and power of individual muscles (i.e., core training before core strengthening). One randomized, controlled trial on a subgroup of patients with pelvic girdle pain (after pregnancy) showed efficacy with this approach to exercise intervention.[35] In this trial, considerable attention was paid to *how* the exercises were performed, and each patient's program was specific to her needs.

Patients who go through a routine of exercises without awareness often have limited success in retraining motor patterns; in fact, they may even get worse with exercise if poor patterns and control are reinforced, because this may

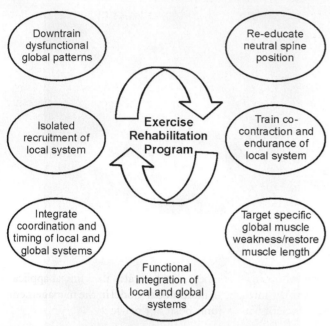

Figure 14-25

Insufficient compression of the sacroiliac joint and/or pubic symphysis during loading may be due to poor motor control (inappropriate force closure secondary to an alteration in the timing/recruitment pattern of muscles) or to insufficient muscle capacity (strength/endurance), or to a combination of these two factors. To restore optimum force closure and motor control for the pelvic girdle, the clinician first must address any hypertonicity in the global muscles (see Figure 14-18) and then restore neutral alignment of the pelvic girdle and low back (see Figure 14-22). This is followed by specific exercises that address any motor control deficits in the deep stabilizing muscle system (local muscles). Images and cues are used to facilitate the activation of these muscles; cues are then combined to restore co-activation of the muscles. This is followed by exercises that integrate both the local and global muscle systems with functional tasks, such as squats, sit to stand, lunges, and so forth. (Modified from Lee LJ, Lee DG: Treating the lumbopelvic-hip dysfunction. In Lee DG: *The pelvic girdle*, ed 3, Edinburgh, 2004, Elsevier; and Lee DG, Lee LJ: An integrated approach to the assessment and treatment of the lumbopelvic-hip region, DVD, 2004. www.dianelee.ca)

result in irritation of joint structures and exacerbation of symptoms. Often the problem is not *which* exercise was prescribed but *how* the exercise was performed.

Exercises for motor control are aimed at retraining strategies of muscular patterning so that load transfer is optimized through all joints of the kinetic chain. Optimum load transfer occurs when there is precise modulation of force, coordination, and timing of specific muscle contractions, ensuring control of each joint (i.e., segmental control), orientation of the spine (i.e., spinal curvatures, thorax on pelvic girdle, pelvis in relation to the lower extremity), and control of postural equilibrium with respect to the environment.[67] The result is stability with mobility, characterized by stability without rigidity of posture, without episodes of collapse, and with fluidity of movement.

Optimum coordination of the myofascial system produces optimum stabilization strategies. Patients who achieve this are able to:

1. Find and maintain control of neutral spinal alignment both in the lumbopelvic region and in relationship to the thorax and hip (see Figure 14-23)
2. Consciously recruit and maintain a tonic, isolated contraction of the deep stabilizers of the lumbopelvis to ensure segmental control and then to maintain this contraction during loading (Figure 14-26)
3. Move into and out of a neutral spine (i.e., flex, extend, laterally bend, and rotate) without segmental or regional collapse
4. Maintain all of the above in coordination with the thorax and the extremities in functional, work-specific, and sport-specific postures and movements

Further information on the specific exercises that address each component of this type of program is provided by Lee and Lee[28,29] and Richardson et al.[33,34] The purpose of this chapter is not to describe these exercises in detail, but rather to outline the key principles of an integrated, multimodal treatment program for the pelvic girdle. After reading this section, clinicians are encouraged to reconsider how they prescribe exercises for patients with pelvic girdle pain and whether their current practices are in keeping with current research. Specifically, cues, images, and facilitation techniques are needed to address deficits in the functioning of the deep stabilizing muscle system.

The process of restoring optimum recruitment of the deep stabilizing muscles and ensuring their appropriate activity during functional progressions can be enhanced by the use of rehabilitative ultrasound imaging (RUI),[85,103,104] which can serve not only in the diagnosis[19,70] but also as a biofeedback tool.[28,29,34,105]

Subsequently, exercises that are patient specific according to the person's functional work and recreation demands need to be integrated into the program. For most patients with pelvic girdle pain, this requires education and exercises that address optimum sitting posture (see Figure 14-23), getting into and out of a chair or car, optimum techniques for squatting (getting objects off the floor) (Figure 14-27), and climbing stairs.

Proprioceptive challenges, such as exercises on a gym ball, rocker board, or SitFit, are added to facilitate the automatic recruitment of the stability system and also to prepare the patient for unanticipated changes in the base of support, which are common in daily life. The clinician should monitor the stability of the SI joint (watch for anterior rotation of the innominate) during the introduction of all new exercises (Figure 14-28) to make sure that the patient is ready for any new load challenge. The deep stabilizing muscle system must be checked often to ensure that optimum recruitment co-contraction is being carried forward into the higher levels of task demands.

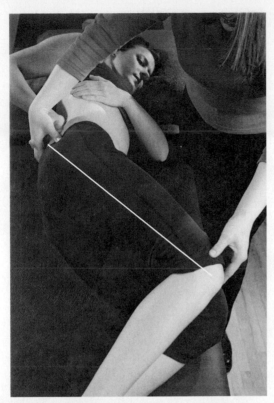

Figure 14-26

Images and cues (verbal and tactile) of lines, guy wires, and connections have been found clinically to facilitate contraction of the deep local muscle system. Briefly, images that create the idea of the spine being "suspended" are effective for facilitating contraction of the deep multifidus (dMF). The patient is instructed to imagine that the spine or sacrum is a central pole that needs to be suspended by equal tension in suspension or guy wires on both sides. If unilateral loss of activity in dMF is present, motion control often is lost during loading, and the pelvis or spine collapses, buckles, or gives way on that side. The image of energy coming up vertically along the wires to support the spine and sacrum helps create the sense of suspension. The dMF is palpated at the dysfunctional level; this is the point where the guy wire attaches. The inferior attachment of the wire can vary; the image ultimately chosen is the one that produces the best response in the dMF. The timing of the tactile pressure from the clinician's hands creates the image and provides feedback as to how quickly the muscle should contract. The fingers should sink into the dMF and provide a cranial pressure to encourage a lifted or suspended feeling. The inferior attachment of the wire can be just medial to the anterosuperior iliac spine (ASIS), superior to the pubic bone, or on the pelvic floor; the sequence of tactile feedback is from the anterior palpation point first, then up into the dMF palpation point. Ideally, a slow development of firmness in the muscle will be felt as a deep swelling and indentation of the pads of the palpating fingers. A fast contraction indicates activation of the superficial multifidus (sMF) and/or the lumbar erector spinae; in this case, the fingers are quickly pushed off the body. A fast generation of superficial tension can also be palpated if the thoracic erector spinae are contracting. The common tendon of the erector spinae muscle overlies the lumbar multifidus, and activity in the muscle changes tension in the tendon, especially in individuals in whom this muscle is well developed. No pelvic or spinal motion should be observed, and no activity in the global abdominal muscles or the hip musculature. A co-contraction of the transversus abdominis (TrA) is acceptable and desired. In this figure the clinician cues the patient to imagine a guy wire that connects the distal end of the knee through the pelvic girdle to the location of the deficient multifidus *(line)* and then to connect along this wire. No movement of the lumbar spine, pelvic girdle, or hip should be felt during the connection phase; however, a slow swelling of the deficient multifidus in response to this cue should be felt. The patient is then instructed to maintain this connection and to slowly lift the top knee 5 cm (2 inches) (clamshell). This lift is held initially for 3 to 5 seconds to build capacity (strength and endurance) of both the local muscle system (dMF and TrA) and the global muscle system (gluteus medius). The connection to the local system (i.e., the image) is maintained until the leg is lowered. This task is repeated up to 10 times, building up to 10-second holds for each repetition. The lifted leg should feel light, and no rotation of the lumbar spine should occur; all articular motion should be at the hip joint. (Reproduced with permission from Diane G. Lee Physiotherapist Corporation and Linda-Joy Lee Physiotherapist Corporation.)

Principles for Integrating the Emotional Component

The patient's emotional state can maintain a detrimental motor pattern and prevent a successful outcome. The clinician can help relieve patients' anxiety about their current physical status and the future by explaining the possible causal factors[36,39-42] and by helping them to understand the physiology of pain. Restoring hope by providing a patient-specific treatment plan often is motivational and helps build trust. When positive changes in function occur, the treatment plan is reinforced, and this builds commitment. Ultimately, it is critical to teach people to accept responsibility for their health through education and motivation.

Case Report

The following case report demonstrates the clinical application of the integrated, multimodal model in the management of a patient with chronic posterior pelvic girdle pain.

Patient History

Ms. K is a physiotherapist with an extensive athletic history (18 years of dance training, competitive beach volleyball, and recreational mountain biking). Over the past 4 years, she has had multiple falls on her left posterior buttock. Her primary complaint was unilateral left low back and left posterior pelvic girdle pain (left L5-S1 and left SI joint) with intermittent referral into the left L5 dermatome. The initial onset of pain occurred after she fell on her left buttock while playing competitive beach volleyball. After this, she experienced difficulty with activities that vertically loaded the left side of her pelvis (especially jumping or pushing off from the left leg). She did not seek any specific treatment, and her pain resolved over time. Two years later, she was hiking downhill and fell very hard on the inferior aspect of her left buttock. The low back and pelvic girdle

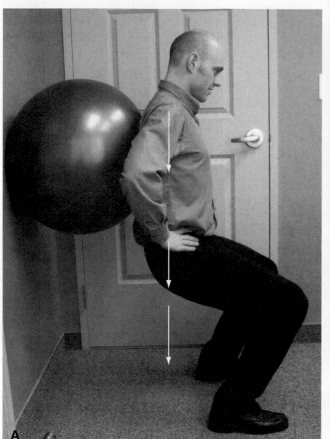 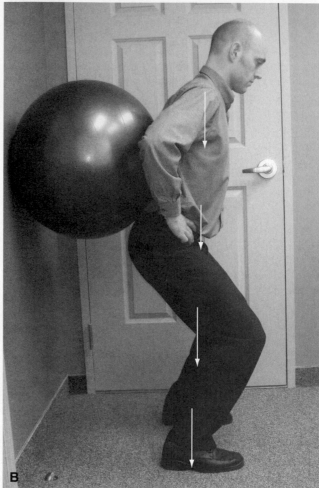

Figure 14-27

A, This is a nonoptimum strategy for squatting, yet it is frequently seen in the gymnasium. Note how the center of gravity is well behind the feet *(arrows),* and the pelvic girdle is in a position of posterior tilt. **B,** This is a much better strategy for a functional squat. As the patient releases the hips and knees into flexion, the pelvic girdle tilts anteriorly over the femurs, carrying the trunk with it so that the line of gravity is optimally situated through the pedal base *(arrows).* This strategy facilitates loading in lumbopelvic neutral. (Reproduced with permission from Diane G. Lee Physiotherapist Corporation and Linda-Joy Lee Physiotherapist Corporation.)

pain recurred and was referred distally into the left L5 dermatome. After this fall, she also noticed immediate difficulty with any weight bearing through the left leg. She reported that something was definitely wrong in her pelvic girdle and that her left side felt suddenly shorter. She sought two treatments from an osteopathic practitioner (the left SI joint was manipulated), and she did her own "core stabilization" exercises (details are unknown). One year later, she fell off her bike and landed hard once again on the posterolateral aspect of her left buttock. Her symptoms remained unresolved after this last fall.

At the time she sought treatment, her pain was aggravated by running (worst), sitting, and sustained forward bending activities. She could still cross-country ski, and she trained three to four times a week to keep her pain

under control. This training included 1.5 hours of cardiovascular exercise (i.e., treadmill, stepper, cross-country machine), gym ball core stability training (mostly muscle capacity–type exercises), and light weights. She complained of some sleep disturbance, specifically, waking to change position frequently during the night. She noted that she could not sleep prone or in any position that posteriorly rotated the left innominate.

Observation

Posture

In standing, Ms. K's pelvic girdle was rotated to the left in the transverse plane. With respect to the intrapelvic position, the left innominate appeared to be translated ventrally

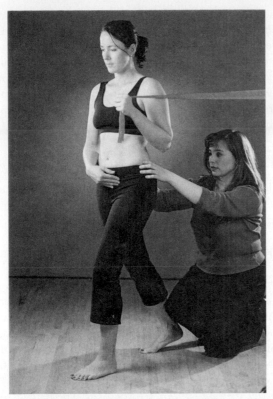

Figure 14-28
Forward lunge with rotation resistance (exercise band). The clinician monitors the left sacroiliac joint to make sure the patient retains intrapelvic motion control (no unlocking) during the exercise. The patient monitors the lower abdomen to make sure that optimum contraction of the deep anterior local muscle system is maintained. (Reproduced with permission from Diane G. Lee Physiotherapist Corporation and Linda-Joy Lee Physiotherapist Corporation.)

and superiorly compared to the right. This is a nonphysiological alignment for the pelvic girdle and suggests the presence of a joint fixation or shear lesion.

Examination

Active Movements

Pelvic Girdle Movements Associated With Trunk Movements: Load Transfer Tests. Ms. K used a lumbar strategy to forward bend (Figure 14-29), backward bend, and lateral bend (i.e., minimal pelvic tilt was associated with any trunk movements), and the intrapelvic malalignment noted in standing did not worsen or improve.

Intrapelvic Movements: One Leg Stand Test. During left hip flexion and unilateral right leg standing, no palpable motion could be felt between the left innominate and the left side of the sacrum. Marked hiking of the left side of the entire pelvic girdle (i.e., left lateral bending of the thoracolumbar spine) occurred as she attempted to raise her knee toward her chest (Figure 14-30). During right hip flexion and unilateral left leg standing, the right

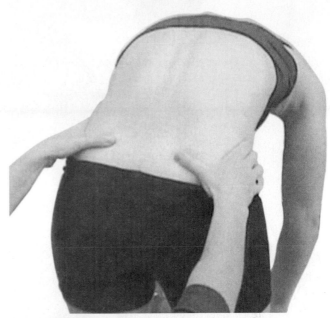

Figure 14-29
Forward bending test in standing. Note the lack of anterior pelvic tilt, the excessive flexion of the thoracolumbar spine, and the "twist" in the pelvic girdle. (Reproduced with permission from Diane G. Lee Physiotherapist Corporation and Linda-Joy Lee Physiotherapist Corporation.)

innominate rotated posteriorly relative to the sacrum. Thus the motion was asymmetrical between the left and right sides of the pelvic girdle. Further tests of passive joint mobility were required to determine the cause (articular versus neuromyofascial) of the increased compression and resultant decreased active movement through the left SI joint.

Active Straight Leg Raise Test. Ms. K had marked difficulty lifting either leg while in the supine position; however, she sensed that the left leg lift was harder than the right (Figure 14-31), and she used a marked abdominal bracing/breath holding strategy to perform this usually low load task. When manual compression was applied to her pelvis, the patient noted the effort required to lift the left leg *increased*. Regardless of where compression was applied, no decrease was reported by the patient in the effort required to lift either leg. This suggests that the pelvic girdle was already under excessive compression and that techniques for decompression were required initially.

Passive Tests (Form Closure Tests of Joint Mobility and Stability)

No motion of the left SI joint could be palpated in either the anteroposterior or craniocaudal plane. The right SI joint was mobile in both the anteroposterior and craniocaudal planes. The malalignment of the left innominate relative to the sacrum, noted in the standing position, persisted in the sitting, supine, and prone positions. This suggested that the left SI joint was fixated and that the first technique of choice was a distractive manipulation aimed at reducing the joint compression and correcting the malalignment (see Figure 14-21). Further tests of force closure/motor control would be irrelevant until the joint compression had been reduced.

Treatment: First Session

The left SI joint was manipulated with a distractive manipulation (grade 5) technique. Immediately after the manipulation, the following was noted:

Active Movements

1. *One leg standing (stork) test:* The left innominate now was able to rotate posteriorly relative to the sacrum, and the motion was more symmetrical compared to the right side (Figure 14-32). The patient had marked difficulty standing on the left leg, and unlocking of the SI joint occurred during the transference of weight to the left leg (the innominate rotated anteriorly).
2. *Active straight leg raise (ASLR) test:* The patient found it much easier to lift her left leg (Figure 14-33), and even less effort was required when compression was applied bilaterally to the posterior aspect of the pelvic girdle.

Passive Movements

1. *Form closure tests of mobility and stability:* Asymmetry was noted between the left and right SI joints. The left SI joint was looser than the right in the anteroposterior plane when the test was done with the joint in a neutral

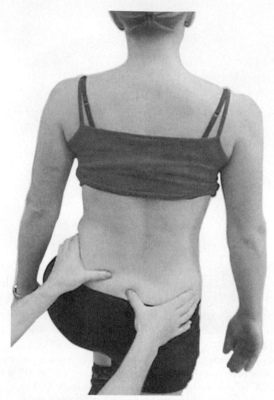

Figure 14-30
Ms. K, one leg standing test. No palpable motion is present between the left innominate and the sacrum during flexion of the left hip, and marked hiking of the entire pelvic girdle (associated with excessive left lateral bending of the thoracolumbar spine) is required for Ms. K to achieve 90° of flexion at the hip joint. This suggests that something was overly compressing the left side of the pelvic girdle. Further tests were required to differentiate the cause. (Reproduced with permission from Diane G. Lee Physiotherapist Corporation and Linda-Joy Lee Physiotherapist Corporation.)

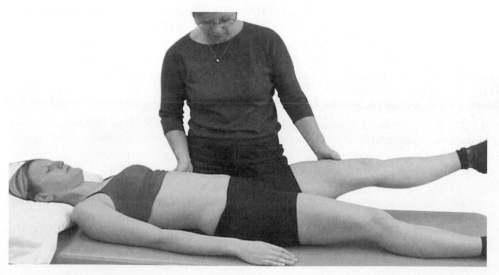

Figure 14-31
Ms. K, active straight leg raise test. Note the excessive effort in Ms. K's face as she attempts to lift the left leg. Compression of the pelvic girdle made lifting the left leg more difficult, which also suggests that the pelvic girdle is already under excessive compression. (Reproduced with permission from Diane G. Lee Physiotherapist Corporation and Linda-Joy Lee Physiotherapist Corporation.)

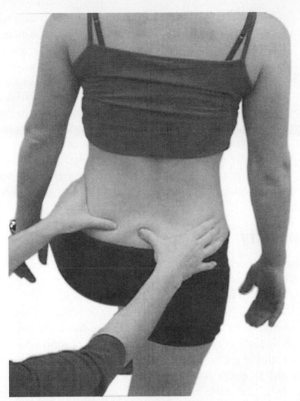

Figure 14-32
Ms. K, one leg standing test immediately after decompression of the left sacroiliac joint with a high velocity, low amplitude thrust technique. The innominate now can rotate posteriorly relative to the sacrum, and much less compensatory thoracolumbar left lateral bending is present as she flexes her left hip to 90°. (Reproduced with permission from Diane G. Lee Physiotherapist Corporation and Linda-Joy Lee Physiotherapist Corporation.)

Figure 14-33
Ms. K, active straight leg raise test immediately after decompression of the left sacroiliac joint. Ms. K now can effortlessly lift her left leg off the table (note the reduced effort in her face and even a smile of surprise!), and the effort was reduced further when compression was applied bilaterally to the posterior aspect of the pelvic girdle. (Reproduced with permission from Diane G. Lee Physiotherapist Corporation and Linda-Joy Lee Physiotherapist Corporation.)

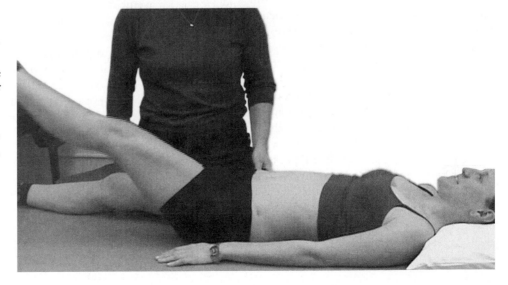

position. When the joint was close packed (i.e., the sacrum nutated and the innominate posteriorly rotated), the patient's pain was provoked (the capsule and ligaments stretched); however, the joint glide was reduced. This suggested that although the soft tissue had been stretched and some static stability from the passive elements had been compromised, the anatomical integrity of the capsule and ligaments was intact. Time would tell whether sufficient soft tissue integrity remained to afford stability to the left SI joint as treatment of the muscle system progressed.

Force Closure/Motor Control Tests

1. *Response of the deep stabilizing muscles to a verbal cue (i.e., "Contract the pelvic floor."):* A proper symmetrical response was elicited from the TrA (isolated from the internal oblique); no response was elicited from the left dMF at the level of the left SI joint. These findings suggest the presence of a motor control deficit (and likely a muscle capacity deficit) of the deep fibers of the left lumbosacral multifidus. The patient was given a sacroiliac belt (the COM-PRESSOR; see Figure 14-24, *A*) with a compression strap applied posteriorly on the left side of the pelvic girdle. This supported force closure posteriorly and simulated the function of the left dMF.

The goal of treatment over the next 3 weeks was to retrain the left dMF to co-contract with the TrA and the pelvic floor muscles and then to integrate this co-contraction into functional tasks, especially those involving weight transference through the left leg. As the force closure mechanism and the associated motor control improved, it was hoped that the motion control impairment of the left SI joint would be corrected and the recurrent fixation of the left SI joint (as well as the patient's pain) would resolve.

Treatment: Second Through Fourth Treatments, First 2 Weeks

Ms. K was taught to isolate the dMF using imagery (see Figure 14-26 for details of this technique). Once she could isolate a contraction of the left dMF at the level of the left SI joint, she was taught to combine this contraction with contraction of the TrA and pelvic floor muscles and to maintain this co-contraction for 10 seconds as she breathed normally. Subsequently, loads were added to the pelvic girdle through the lower extremity in both the supine and side lying positions to further challenge the capacity of the co-contraction (strength and endurance). These exercise progressions included supine bent knee fallouts, alternating single heel slides, and single leg lift and side lying leg loading tasks. All leg loading was done with preactivation of the deep muscle system.

Response to Treatment and Subsequent Progression

By the third week of treatment, Ms. K was experiencing less pain and more functional stability in that she could transfer weight through the left leg without the sense of giving way. She was still wearing the COM-PRESSOR belt intermittently. Her functional load transfer tests revealed that she was able to maintain a stable position of the left SI joint (i.e., posterior rotation of the innominate) during the left one leg standing test. However, she still needed to "think about" the precontraction of the deep stabilizing system (especially the left dMF). In other words, the timing of muscle activation was still not fully integrated and automatic. Her active straight leg raise test was still easier when compression was applied to the posterior aspect of the pelvic girdle. Passive joint play testing showed that asymmetry of motion still existed between the left and right SI joints (the left side was more mobile); however, no palpable joint glide was detected when the joint was in the close-packed position (i.e., the form closure mechanism was intact). These findings suggested that the patient needed more "bulk" and resting tone in the left dMF. She was encouraged to continue with the exercises previously prescribed. In addition, she was ready to begin further exercises that increased vertical loading through the pelvic girdle.

Ms. K's exercise program was progressed to include wall squats, split squats (stride stance position), and lunges. She was taught to monitor the position of the left innominate under vertical loading (i.e., to feel for any unlocking of the left SI joint). This ensured that if unlocking occurred, she stopped the exercise, corrected her technique (i.e., she focused on preactivation of the local system), and tried again. If she was unable to perform the exercise without the left SI joint unlocking, that session of exercise was over. She was encouraged to use a biomechanical analysis of when to stop, as opposed to waiting for the onset of pain or discomfort.

Once Ms. K could perform three sets of the previously mentioned exercises with ease (5 weeks into treatment), further proprioceptive challenges were added by introducing balance board work. At 6 weeks after the initial assessment, she was discharged from treatment with a home maintenance program of exercises. Two years later, she was able to function at a higher level of sport (including running, which she had not been able to do before) and was able to work without any exacerbation of her low back or pelvic girdle pain. She was taught that she likely would still require intermittent focus on her local system exercises, especially during tasks requiring high loads, to prevent recurrences.

Summary

It long has been recognized that physical factors affect joint motion. The integrated, multimodal approach to the management of pelvic girdle pain suggests that joint mechanics are influenced by multiple factors, some of which are intrinsic to the joint and others that are produced by muscle action, which in turn is influenced by the emotional state. More studies are required to identify subgroups of patients with pelvic girdle pain according to specific impairments, because these patients do not all have the same impairments. Clinicians need to develop more diagnostic tests relevant to motion and load transfer for both the SI joint and the pubic symphysis and then to test them for reliability, sensitivity, and specificity for pelvic girdle pain. Only then will clinicians have the ability to develop more rigorously designed studies to test the efficacy of treatment programs specific to each subgroup of impairment that leads to pelvic girdle pain. Until then, the best evidence-based treatment involves a multimodal approach that considers the biomechanical, neuromuscular, and emotional needs of the patient with pelvic girdle pain.

This chapter has briefly outlined the principles for management of the articular (form closure) and muscular (force closure and motor control) factors that affect the functioning of the SI joint and consequently the ability of the pelvic girdle to transfer load. Effective management of pelvic girdle pain and dysfunction requires attention to all four components of the integrated model: form closure, force closure, motor control, and emotions, with the ultimate goal of guiding patients to a healthier way to live in their bodies.

References

To enhance this text and add value for the reader, all references have been incorporated into a CD-ROM that is provided with this text. The reader can view the reference source and access it online whenever possible. There are a total of 105 references for this chapter.

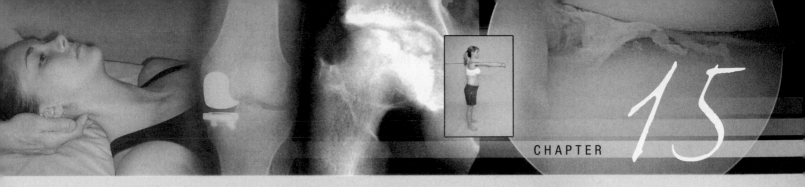

CHAPTER 15

Hip Pathologies: Diagnosis and Intervention

Timothy L. Fagerson

Introduction

This chapter explores adult hip pathologies, their diagnosis, and appropriate interventions. Most hip conditions are discussed, except for pediatric conditions and hip joint arthroplasty, which are covered elsewhere in this text (Chapters 24 and 26). Clinicians need a good working knowledge of hip pathologies so that they can select, perform, and interpret the appropriate tests for the diagnostic process and then decide what interventions need to be included to treat the patient's condition most effectively.

Adult hip pathologies can be divided into six subcategories based on the type of disorder (Table 15-1). It also can be helpful to think of hip disorders in relation to age, because their prevalence rate often is age dependent (Table 15-2).

Another useful approach is to classify a condition based on the need for diagnostic imaging or laboratory tests to confirm the diagnosis and initiate appropriate medical or surgical management. The following diagnostic classification system can be applied not only to hip pathologies but also to all clinical problems:[1]

1. Diagnoses that can be made on the basis of the history and physical examination alone (e.g., sprains, strains, muscles imbalances, nerve entrapments). Rehabilitation should be initiated as appropriate.
2. Diagnoses that tentatively can be made on the basis of the history and physical examination, but further diagnostic imaging and laboratory studies are necessary to confirm the diagnosis (e.g., osteoarthritis, rheumatoid arthritis, herniated disc). Rehabilitation can be initiated to assist symptom management and maintain maximum function while a definitive diagnosis is pursued.

3. Red flag diagnoses (e.g., fracture, dislocation, osteonecrosis, infection, metastatic disease). These conditions require definitive medical or surgical intervention. Rehabilitation should follow when appropriate.

When possible, a diagnosis should be the lowest common denominator driving a clinical presentation. Table 15-3 presents a summary of musculoskeletal diagnoses for rehabilitation management.[2]

When one of these lowest common denominators cannot be identified or associated with an anatomical structure and pathology (i.e., if a tissue level or pathoanatomical diagnosis cannot be made), one of the next levels of rehabilitation diagnosis should be used; for example, component impairment (i.e., the tissue at fault) or functional limitation (see Figure 19-9 in volume 2 of this series, *Scientific Foundations and Principles of Practice in Musculoskeletal Rehabilitation*).[3]

The primary reason a patient seeks outpatient clinical care is pain. The exact location of hip-mediated pain varies. Khan and Woolson[4] reported that of patients presenting for total hip replacement, 73% had groin pain (Table 15-4). Other common locations were the lateral hip (trochanter) and buttocks (gluteals).[4] Hip pain from osteoarthritis (OA) can also refer to the anterior knee and to the low back. Sometimes these are the only symptoms produced by hip OA. Although groin pain often is associated with hip pathology, the groin is not the only place that symptoms originating from the hip are felt; nor is the groin region immune to pain referral from sources other than the hip. In contrast to the findings of Khan and Woolson,[4] a study by Wroblewski[5] rated the groin area as the fourth most common site of pain in patients with OA of the hip, behind the greater trochanter, the anterior thigh, and the

Table 15-1
Types of Hip Disorders

Type of Disorder	Examples
Soft tissue disorders	Bursitis Tendonitis/tendinosis Muscle strain Osteitis pubis Hip pointer Snapping hip syndrome Sports hernia Contracture Hip capsule contracture
Joint disorders	Osteoarthritis Femoroacetabular impingement Labral tears Loose bodies
Osseous disorders	Osteonecrosis Osteoporosis Heterotopic ossification Transient osteoporosis Osteoid osteoma Symptomatic herniation pit Brodie's abscess
Fractures and dislocations	Hip fracture Femoral head fracture Acetabular fracture Stress fracture Traumatic dislocation
Nerve entrapment syndromes (commonly described types)	Piriformis syndrome Meralgia paraesthetica Hamstring syndrome Superior gluteal nerve entrapment
Pediatric disorders (not covered in this chapter)	Developmental dysplasia of the hip (DDH) Congenital coxa vara Acute transient synovitis Legg-Calvé-Perthes (LCP) disease Slipped capital femoral epiphysis (SCFE) Avulsion fracture

Table 15-2
Hip Disorders Related to Age

Disorder	Age
Developmental dysplasia of the hip	Newborn/infancy
Congenital coxa vara	1-3 years
Acute transient synovitis	2-10 years
Legg-Calvé-Perthes disease	2-10 years
Slipped femoral capital epiphysis	10-16 years
Avulsed ASIS, AIIS, lesser trochanter	12-16 years
Osteoid osteoma (femoral neck)	5-30 years
Malignancy	Any age
Rheumatoid arthritis	Any age (20-40 years)
Stress fractures	14-25 years
Avascular necrosis	20-40 years
Paget's disease	40 years +
Osteoarthritis	45 years +
Hip fracture	65 years +

Modified from Fagerson TL, editor: *The hip handbook,* p 40, Boston, 1998, Butterworth-Heinemann.
ASIS, Anterosuperior iliac spine; *AIIS,* anteroinferior iliac spine.

Table 15-3
Manual Therapy Diagnoses

Principal Diagnosis	Type of Problem
Pain	Mechanical Chemical
Misalignment	Structural Functional
Hypomobility	Contracture Adhesion Restriction
Hypermobility	Instability Tissue insufficiency
Weakness	Motor control Muscle imbalance Tissue weakness

Modified from Dyrek DA: Assessment and treatment planning strategies for musculoskeletal deficits. In Sullivan SD, Schmitz T J, editors: *Physical rehabilitation: assessment and treatment,* ed 3, pp. 61-82, Philadelphia, 1994, FA Davis.

knee. Hip OA can also cause medial buttock, shin, and low back pain.[5] In addition to pain referred from the hip, the buttock, lateral hip, and groin are common sites of pain referred from the lumbar spine and sacroiliac joints.[6,7]

Differentiating Hip Disease from Lumbar Disease by Physical Examination

Because the lumbar spine can refer symptoms to the hip region (and to a lesser extent vice versa), the clinician should always rule out involvement of the lumbar spine when a hip problem is suspected. The examination, therefore, may be extensive, involving the hip, lumbar spine, and pelvis. Brown et al.[8] identified a limp, groin pain, and limited hip medial rotation as signs that significantly predicted a hip problem rather than a lumbar problem.[8] Clinically, Cyriax's screening tests for a noncapsular pattern of the hip and a positive "sign of the buttock" have been identified as predictors for further workup.[9] With a capsular pattern of the hip, the pattern of hypomobility is one where medial rotation, and abduction and flexion are the most limited motions.[10] Extension and

Table 15-4

Location and Frequency of Hip Pain in Patients with Intra-articular Hip Pathology

Location	Frequency (%)
Groin only	43
Trochanter only	18
Gluteal only	6
Groin/trochanter	12
Groin/gluteal	16
All locations	3
No hip pain	3
Groin only or groin with other locations	73

Modified from Khan NQ, Woolson ST: Referral patterns of hip pain in patients undergoing total hip replacement, *Orthopedics* 21:123-126, 1998.

lateral rotation may also be limited, and adduction is the least limited in a true capsular pattern.

Cyriax[10] described the sign of the buttock as a means of differentiating a major lesion of the buttock (e.g., infection, tumor, fracture) from a minor lesion (e.g., bursitis, tendonitis, arthritis). Major lesions obviously are red flags indicating the need for further workup. For the sign of the buttock test, hip flexion is performed in the supine position, first with knee flexion and then with knee extension. Normally, hip flexion combined with knee flexion results in a greater hip flexion range of motion (ROM) than does hip flexion with knee extension, because hamstring muscle tension limits the motion when the knee is in extension. However, if the hip flexion ROM is the same with the knee extended and the knee flexed (i.e., an empty end feel is noted, usually the result of pain), this is a positive sign of the buttock.[9,10]

Signs Predicting a Hip Rather Than a Lumbar Problem[8]

- Limp
- Groin pain
- Limited hip medial rotation
- Capsular pattern of the hip (medial rotation, abduction, flexion)
- Positive "sign of the buttock"

The lumbar spine can refer symptoms into the hip region and lower extremity even when the lumbar spine itself is symptom free. Dermatomes for the lumbar spine are shown in volume 1 of this series, *Orthopedic Physical Assessment*. The L1 dermatome covers the anterior and lateral hip. The L2 dermatome covers the iliac crest (buttock) and medial thigh. The L3 dermatome covers the iliac crest (buttock) and medial thigh and knee. The clunial nerves, which supply the skin over the buttocks from the iliac crest

to the greater trochanter, originate as the lateral branches of the dorsal primary divisions of the upper three lumbar nerves. A disc herniation at L4-5 can cause groin pain via the sinuvertebral nerve.[6]

Restricted hip movement often can be an etiological factor in low back pain. Greater limitation of medial than of lateral rotation of the hip is seen more frequently in patients with low back pain (LBP) than in individuals without LBP.[11] Limited hip extension also has been correlated with an increased incidence of LBP.[12]

Adult Hip Pathologies
Soft Tissue Disorders

Soft tissue disorders are considered first, because the soft tissues are essentially the tissues the rehabilitation clinician can influence the most significantly with intervention. The ability of the living tissues of the body, especially the soft tissues, to adapt and deform to imposed demands makes strong repair and functional remodeling possible with appropriately directed intervention.

Rehabilitation clinicians usually conceptualize their role in health care using some variation of the Nagi disablement model.[3] Although it is often assumed from the Nagi model that impairments result from active pathology, the converse also is true: active pathology can be partly or fully caused by impairments (e.g., abnormal postural alignment and/or muscle imbalances can lead to OA). Obviously, impairments and pathology can each affect the other. Sahrmann[13] defines these differing mechanisms as the *pathokinesiology model* (pathology causing impairments) and the *kinesiopathology model* (impairments causing pathology). Soft tissue problems are dealt with first because they frequently are the primary problem at the hip, and they also are common sequelae to other types of pathology (e.g., OA, hip fracture).

Trochanteric Bursitis

In the region of the greater trochanter, three bursae are consistently present, two major bursae and one minor bursa (Figure 15-1).[14] The subgluteus maximus bursa lies between the greater trochanter and the fibers of the gluteus maximus and tensor fascia lata muscles as they blend into the iliotibial band (ITB). The subgluteus medius bursa lies at the superoposterior tip of the greater trochanter and prevents friction between the gluteus medius muscle and the greater trochanter and also between the gluteus medius and gluteus minimus muscles. The subgluteus minimus bursa is a minor bursa lying between the gluteus minimus attachment and the superoanterior tip of the greater trochanter.

Trochanteric bursitis and gluteal tendonitis are the most common soft tissue disorders affecting the hip.[15] Some have said that trochanteric bursitis should be considered a

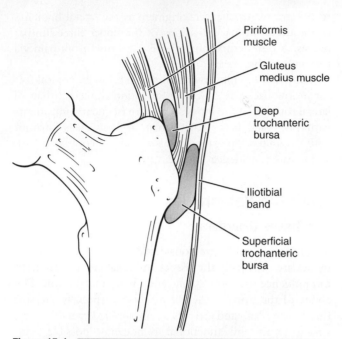

Piriformis muscle

Gluteus medius muscle

Deep trochanteric bursa

Iliotibial band

Superficial trochanteric bursa

Figure 15-1
Schematic diagram of bursae around the greater trochanter.

Box 15-1 Clinical Criteria for Diagnosis of Trochanteric Bursitis

1. *Both* of the following conditions must be present:
   - Aching pain in the lateral aspect of the hip
   - Distinct tenderness around the greater trochanter
2. *One* of the following three conditions must be present:
   - Pain at the extreme of rotation, abduction, or adduction, especially positive Patrick's (FABER) test
   - Pain on forced hip abduction
   - Pseudoradiculopathy (pain extending down the lateral aspect of the thigh)

Modified from Shbeeb MI, Matteson EL: Trochanteric bursitis (greater trochanter pain syndrome), *Mayo Clin Proc* 71:565-569, 1996; data from Ege Rassmusen KJ, Fano N: Trochanteric bursitis: treatment by corticosteroid injection, *Scand J Rheumatol* 14:417-420, 1985.

clinical diagnosis rather than an anatomical diagnosis, because it cannot be distinguished from gluteal tendonitis by signs and symptoms alone. Use of the term *lateral hip pain* has been suggested when an anatomical source cannot be specified.[16] Another alternative name is *greater trochanteric pain syndrome*.[14]

Trochanteric bursitis is more common in arthritic conditions and fibromyalgia and with leg length discrepancy. It also is more common in females than males (2-4:1 ratio), with a peak incidence occurring between 40 and 60 years of age.[14] Trochanteric bursitis, especially in athletes, may result from a fall onto a hard surface or friction of the ITB over the greater trochanter during repetitive flexion/extension motion of the hip, such as occurs in running (similar to ITB friction syndrome at the knee).

Trochanteric bursitis is characterized by an aching pain over the lateral aspect of the hip accompanied by distinct tenderness on palpation around the greater trochanter. A widely accepted diagnostic classification for trochanteric bursitis includes both of these features and one of three other findings (Box 15-1).[17] Symptom relief through peritrochanteric injection of a corticosteroid and an anesthetic is required for more definitive diagnosis of trochanteric bursitis. In a study by Shbeeb et al.,[18] 77% of patients treated for trochanteric bursitis with glucocorticosteroid injection had relief at 1 week after the injection, and 61% had lasting relief at 26 weeks.

Rehabilitation intervention for trochanteric bursitis can include modalities such as ultrasound/phonophoresis, iontophoresis, and nonsteroidal anti-inflammatory drugs (NSAIDs) to alleviate the inflammatory response; however, treatment also should include manual therapy/mobilization techniques and therapeutic exercises to address potential causative factors, such as ITB contracture; flexion contracture; abnormal lumbopelvic alignment, mobility, and stability; and gluteus medius weakness. The patient should be advised to avoid aggravating activities or positions, such as lying on the painful side or excessive walking and running, until the inflammatory process abates. Use of a contralateral cane can prove useful in acute and irritable cases of trochanteric bursitis.

The location of symptoms and the related diagnostic label (i.e., trochanteric bursitis) often can be merely the tip of the iceberg. The actual cause of the inflammation may be a mechanical problem in the region, such as a soft tissue contracture. The most common soft tissue contractures at the hip are flexion contractures, ITB contractures, and abduction contractures.

Gluteus Medius/Gluteus Minimus Tears and Tendinosis

The quadriceps muscle has been described as "the key to the knee"; similarly, the key muscle for hip joint function is the gluteus medius muscle.[3] The gluteus medius is critical for balancing the pelvis in the frontal plane during one leg stance, which accounts for approximately 60% of the gait cycle.[3,19] Janda[20] has described one leg stance as the most common posture for humans because it is the lowest common denominator during locomotion, the primary functional task that humans perform. When the gluteus medius is weak, Trendelenburg's gait pattern or a compensated Trendelenburg's gait pattern is seen (Figure 15-2). During one leg stance, approximately three times the body weight is transmitted through the hip joint, and two thirds of that is generated by the hip abductor mechanism (Figure 15-3). To reduce this load in cases of hip pain or dysfunction, the patient often shows a compensating Trendelenburg's lean over the affected hip; this reduces

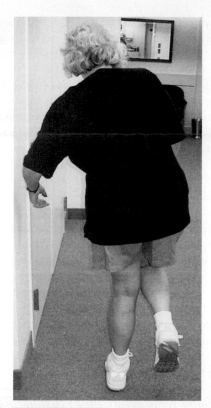

Figure 15-2
Compensated Trendelenburg's lurch over the left hip.

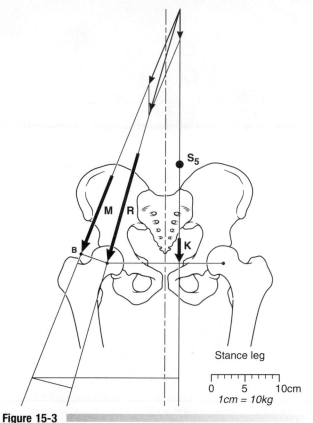

Stance leg

0   5   10cm
1cm = 10kg

Figure 15-3
Forces exerted on the hip when a person stands on one leg. *S5,* center of gravity of the mass of the body acting on the hip (head, trunk, upper limbs, and opposite leg); *K,* force exerted by the partial body mass; *M,* force exerted by the abductor muscles to counterbalance K; *R,* resultant of forces K and M. (Modified from Pauwels F: *Biomechanics of the normal and diseased hip,* New York, 1976, Springer-Verlag.)

the lever arm for body weight and therefore the counterbalancing hip abductor contraction. This counterbalancing effect can stress the lumbar spine, and a cane in the opposite hand is an excellent alternative.[21] The contralateral cane can act as a gait assist to unload the abductors as the patient is progressively rehabilitated. Walking is an excellent endurance and strengthening activity for the hip abductors and is preferred over specific abductor strengthening exercises if the abductors are easily irritated. A cane in the contralateral hand (Figure 15-4) can help create the noncompensatory mechanical environment that assists a weak gluteus medius and gluteus minimus in regaining their strength.

The gluteus medius has been likened to the supraspinatus in the shoulder, and the hip can sustain rotator cuff–like injuries.[22] If the hip "complex" were compared to the glenohumeral "complex," the likenesses would be as follows: the gluteus medius would be comparable to the supraspinatus, the gluteus minimus to the infraspinatus, the piriformis to the teres minor, the iliopsoas to the subscapularis, and the reflected head of the rectus femoris to the long head of the biceps brachii; these, along with the other deep rotators of the hip (i.e., the gemellus superior, obturator externus, gemellus inferior, obturator internus, and quadratus femoris muscles) would be considered the "rotator cuff" of the hip. The tensor fascia lata (TFL) and the gluteus maximus, feeding into either side of the ITB proximally,

act in a fashion similar to the deltoid in the shoulder; they provide a strong, superficial fascial umbrella around the hip. Sahrmann[13] emphasized the importance of enhancing motor control of the one-joint hip muscles (i.e., iliopsoas, gluteals, and deep external rotator muscles), which control the position of the femoral head in the acetabulum, over the two-joint muscles (i.e., rectus femoris, hamstrings, TFL-ITB), which have distal attachments that are at a distance from the hip joint center.

"Rotator Cuff" Muscles of the Hip (with Shoulder Equivalents)

- Gluteus medius (supraspinatus)
- Gluteus minimus (infraspinatus)
- Piriformis (teres minor)
- Iliopsoas (subscapularis)
- Rectus femoris (long head of the biceps)
- Tensor fascia lata (deltoid)
- Gluteus maximus (deltoid)

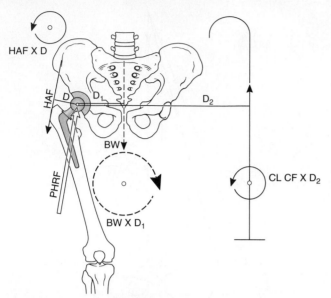

Figure 15-4

The balance of torques acting in the frontal plane about a right prosthetic hip while in single limb support. The diagram depicts a cane used contralateral to the prosthetic hip. Assuming static equilibrium, the sum of the clockwise torque produced by body weight (BW) (*dashed circle*) equals the combined counterclockwise torques produced by hip abductor force (HAF) and the contralateral cane force (CLCF) (*solid circles*). The prosthetic hip reaction force (PHRF) is shown directed toward the right prosthetic hip. The force vectors are not drawn to scale. *D,* Moment arm used by HAF; *D1,* moment arm used by BW, *D2,* moment arm used by CLCF. (Modified from Neumann DA: An electromyographic study of the hip abductor muscles as subjects with a hip prosthesis walked with different methods of using a cane and carrying a load, *Phys Ther* 79:1163-1173, 1999.)

Tendinosis and tears of the gluteus medius and gluteus minimus were a common finding in an magnetic resonance imaging (MRI) study of patients presenting with buttock, lateral hip, or groin pain.[23] Recent work by Khan et al.[24] has shown that most cases of tendinopathy are in fact tendinosis, not tendonitis. The primary problem is collagen degeneration, not inflammation. Because differentiating tendinosis from tendonitis is difficult and because tendinosis is much more common than tendonitis, Khan et al.[24] suggested treating all cases initially as if the problem were collagen degeneration. The differences between overuse tendinosis and overuse tendonitis can be found in Table 15-5. Eccentric strengthening has been shown to be the most effective method of treating tendinosis, probably because eccentric muscle action stimulates mechanoreceptors, which encourage tendon cells to produce collagen. Loading the tendon also improves collagen cross-linking and alignment, resulting in greater tensile strength.[24] As mentioned previously, walking is an excellent eccentric exercise for the gluteus medius, and it should be incorporated into any program. Other approaches (e.g., rest, ice, compression, ultrasound treatment, and anti-inflammatory medication) can and should

be used when appropriate for acute injury. Soft tissue mobilization (e.g., transverse friction, passive stretching) can be helpful in the treatment of a collagen scar and can help improve tissue length.

Twelve musculotendinous structures (the gluteus medius, gluteus minimus, TFL, ITB, gluteus maximus, the six short lateral rotators, and the vastus lateralis muscle) attach to or cross over the greater trochanter, making this region the "Grand Central Station" of the hip. The use of soft tissue mobilization techniques for muscles attaching to the greater trochanter are extremely beneficial for restoring optimum hip joint mechanics. Particularly beneficial is the application of sustained, deep pressure, load and release techniques to various points in the gluteus medius, gluteus minimus, and TFL muscles above the greater trochanter, combined with sustained ipsilateral passive hip abduction performed in the side lying position (Figure 15-5). This technique helps release the abductor mechanism and thereby paradoxically improves hip abduction ROM by allowing the abductors to fold in on themselves; loading the abductors just proximal to the greater trochanter with the hip in abduction also acts as a medioinferior mobilization of the hip capsule and pubofemoral ligament.

Iliotibial Band Contracture and Proximal Iliotibial Band Friction Syndrome

ITB contracture can lead to trochanteric bursitis by increasing compression and friction of the subgluteus maximus bursa between the ITB and the greater trochanter. The classic test for ITB contracture is Ober's test (see volume 1 of this series, *Orthopedic Physical Assessment*). For this test, the patient is in the side lying position with the leg to be tested uppermost. In most cases the hip should be able to adduct so that the knee touches the table without the pelvis moving caudally. To prevent a false negative result, the following are important: (1) the clinician should use one hand to firmly stabilize the patient's pelvis; (2) the hip should be extended to 0°, with the clinician using the other hand to engage the ITB over the greater trochanter; and (3) the hip must not be allowed to flex or to rotate medially as the knee is lowered toward the table (Figure 15-6). To prevent a false positive result, the clinician must ensure that the patient is fully relaxed and allows the leg to be lowered toward the table. Performing the test with the knee flexed 90° takes up slack in the rectus femoris and the anterior fascia lata and is more sensitive to change than performing the test with the knee extended. However, care must be taken to avoid excessive valgus stress to the medial knee when the knee is flexed for the test.

ITB contracture is best treated using a combination of soft tissue mobilization and hold/relax–type stretching in the Ober's test stretch position. In addition, stretching of the rectus femoris and iliopsoas is important, because these muscles are enveloped by the fascia lata. The patient should be taught self-stretching to maintain and improve what is achieved in manual therapy sessions. Foam rollers have

Table 15-5
Implications of a Diagnosis of Tendinosis Compared With a Diagnosis of Tendonitis

Trait	Overuse Tendinosis	Overuse Tendonitis
Prevalence	Common	Rare
Time required for recovery (early presentation)	6-10 weeks	Several days to 2 weeks
Time required for full recovery (chronic presentation)	3-6 months	4-6 weeks
Likelihood of full recovery to sport from chronic symptoms	About 80%	99%
Focus of conservative therapy	Encouragement of collagen-synthesis maturation and strength	Anti-inflammatory modalities and drugs
Role of surgery	Excision of abnormal tissue	Not known
Prognosis for surgery	70% to 85%	95%
Time required to recover from surgery	4-6 months	3-4 weeks

From Khan KM, Cook JL, Taunton JE, Bonar F: Overuse tendinosis, not tendinitis, *Phys Sportsmed* 28:38-48, 2000.

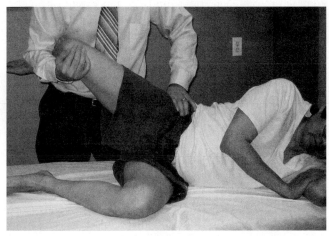

Figure 15-5
Hip abductor soft tissue release technique.

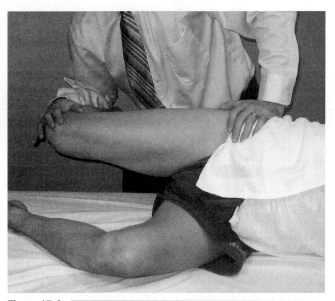

Figure 15-6
Ober's test.

become popular in the personal training arena as a means of self-mobilization of the ITB. Improving the strength and stability of the lumbopelvic region also is important to reduce tension in the ITB. The ITB and hip abductors can tighten in an ineffective attempt to compensate for lack of lumbar control and stability.

Flexion Contracture

Hip flexion contracture is common with hip dysfunction, probably as a result of protective guarding and the positioning of the hip into flexion (the resting position) in response to pain. The likely causes of hip flexion contracture can be one or more of the following: shortening of the iliopsoas muscle, shortening of the rectus femoris muscle, shortening of the tensor fascia lata muscle, or contracture of the anterior hip capsule. Hip flexion contracture can occur in response to osteoarthritis, after injury to the hip region, or as part of a repetitive, flexed posture or movement habit. As a consequence of hip flexion contracture,

loading through the hip joint is shifted to a thinner region of hyaline cartilage in both the femur and the acetabulum, the pelvis is placed in anterior tilt with increased lumbar lordosis, and the hip extensors are placed in a state of constant, low level muscle tension because the line of gravity shifts anterior to the center of mass.[25] Therefore it is important for the clinician to examine for flexion contracture and, if it is reversible, to intervene appropriately.

Causes of Hip Flexion Contracture

- Shortening of the iliopsoas
- Shortening of the rectus femoris
- Shortening of the tensor fascia lata
- Shortening of the anterior hip capsule

The Thomas test assesses for contracture of the iliopsoas muscle. In this test, the hip opposite the affected one is flexed to the point of flattening the lordosis in the lumbar spine, and the involved hip then is extended. If the involved hip stays flexed (i.e., is not able to extend to 0°), this is a positive test result for a flexion contracture (Figure 15-7). For an accurate test result, it is very important to negate the lumbar lordosis. For a more sensitive assessment when comparing with the opposite side and certainly when the maneuver is used for treatment, the clinician should flex the opposite knee fully to the chest. During treatment, a rolled towel can be placed immediately distal to the ischial tuberosity to minimize anterior rotation torque of the innominate during hip extension. If the hip stays abducted during the Thomas test, this is indicative of a tight TFL; if the knee cannot be flexed beyond 90° in the stretch position, this is indicative of shortening of the rectus femoris.

In addition to testing the length of the iliopsoas muscle, it is important that the clinician palpate the iliacus muscle at its origin at the internal superior rim of the iliac crest and palpate the psoas major muscle down to the inguinal ligament to assess for increased density (Figure 15-8).

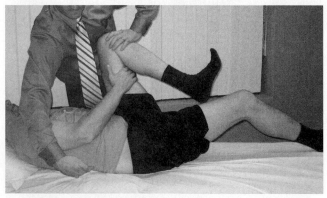

Figure 15-7
Thomas test. With the back flat to the table and the contralateral hip flexed, any flexion indicates a hip flexor contracture.

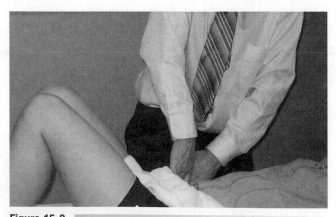

Figure 15-8
Iliacus soft tissue release.

To ensure that palpation of the psoas major muscle occurs, and not loading of some other abdominal structure, the examiner resists active hip flexion by asking the patient to push up with their thigh against the examiners caudal hand while simultaneously, with the cephalad hand, the examiner palpates the psoas major muscle in the abdomen a few inches lateral to the umbilicus. *Because of the abdominal contents, extreme caution should be observed if this soft tissue technique is to be used; the aortic pulse should be identified and then avoided with the soft tissue load, and female patients of childbearing age should be queried about pregnancy.*

Ely's test (prone knee flexion, then added hip extension) can be used to assess for contracture of the rectus femoris muscle; most athletes knees can be flexed to touch the heel to the buttock in prone lying, however, the stretch should be stopped if pain is felt in the knee or lumbar spine. Hip joint capsuloligamentous contracture is distinguished from contracture of the rectus femoris by hip extension in the prone position with the knee extended and also by assessment of the end feel on a posteroanterior glide of the hip. Anterior hip capsule restriction can be treated with a combined hip extension and posteroanterior glide technique with the patient in the prone position.

Iliopsoas Syndrome (Iliopsoas Bursitis and Tendonitis)

Iliopsoas syndrome is defined as anterior hip pain associated with inflammation of the iliopsoas bursa or tendon. This often is the result of repetitive overuse or sudden overload in sports. Iliopsoas bursitis or tendonitis can result from repetitive friction of the iliopsoas myotendon over the anterior femoral head or iliopectineal eminence. Signs and symptoms of this syndrome typically include tenderness in the femoral triangle over the iliopsoas myotendon, decreased hip extension ROM, hip flexion contracture, positive anterior snapping hip, and weakness of hip medial and lateral rotation at 90° hip flexion.[26]

Signs and Symptoms of Iliopsoas Syndrome

- Tenderness in the femoral triangle
- Decreased hip extension
- Hip flexion contracture
- Anterior snapping hip
- Medial and lateral rotation weakness at 90° hip flexion

Johnston et al.[26] described a hip rotation strengthening program for treatment of iliopsoas syndrome. The program consists of medial and lateral rotation strengthening exercises in sitting to the affected leg (Figure 15-9), performed daily for 2 weeks, 3 sets of 20 repetitions on the weaker rotation, 2 sets of 20 repetitions on the stronger rotation.

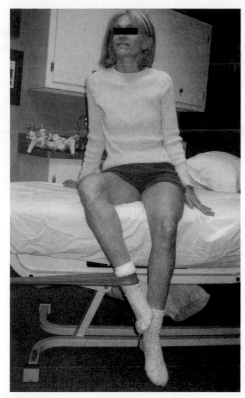

Figure 15-9
Sitting hip internal and external rotation resistance.

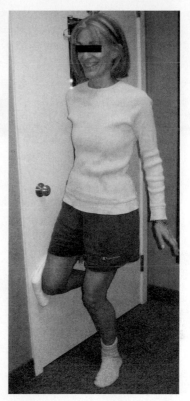

Figure 15-10
One-leg squat with contralateral abduction against a wall.

After 2 weeks the frequency of this exercise is reduced to two to three times a week. At the 2-week point, side-lying abduction/lateral rotation against Thera-Band resistance is introduced (Figure 15-10), with 3 sets of 20 repetitions on the affected side, 2 sets of 20 repetitions on the unin-jured side; this is continued daily for 2 weeks. At the 4-week mark, a one-leg standing minisquat is introduced, keeping the knee tracking over the outside of the foot (Figure 15-11); the regimen is 3 sets of 20 repetitions on the affected side and 2 sets of 20 repetitions on the unin-jured side. At this point, all strength exercises were per-formed two to three times per week. The hip flexors, quadriceps, lateral hip/piriformis, and hamstrings are stretched daily. The patient is instructed to perform twice as many stretches on the affected side as the uninjured side and to repeat the stretches as often as possible during the day. The stretching program continues as long as the pain persists. Gluteal re-education during gait also is incorporated with a conscious, voluntary contraction of the gluteal muscles of both the affected and the uninjured leg during the middle to late portion of the stance phase of the gait cycle. This is performed a maximum of 10 to 15 steps at a time, two or three times per day.[26] The advan-tages of this program are that it is cost-effective and practi-cal for a patient to perform independently at home. Further research is necessary to corroborate the good results seen in the preliminary retrospective case series.[26]

Hip Capsule Contracture

The capsule of the hip joint can develop a contracture simi-lar to adhesive capsulitis in the shoulder (frozen shoulder). The capsular pattern is the typical pattern of contracture of a joint capsule in cases of arthritis. At the hip joint, the most limited movements classically were described by Cyriax as "maximum loss of medial rotation, flexion, abduction and a minimal loss of extension."[10] Extension and lateral rotation can also be limited, and adduction is the least limited motion. In fact, as abduction range decreases, adduction range can be seen to increase in patients with progressing OA of the hip. Kaltenborn[27] described the hip capsular pattern as extension more lim-ited than flexion, medial rotation more limited than lateral rotation, and abduction more limited than adduction. The only difference between the descriptions of Cyriax and Kaltenborn are the contributions of flexion and extension to a capsular pattern; these authors agree that abduction is more limited than adduction and medial rotation more limited than lateral rotation in a true capsular pattern.

The arthrokinematic motions at the hip are anterior glide, posterior glide, medial glide, long axis distraction, lateral distraction, and short axis distraction. (Short axis distraction is a pull in line with the angle of the femoral neck, whereas lateral distraction is a direct lateral pull of the proximal end of the femur.) These accessory motions are used for joint mobilization purposes, primarily to treat

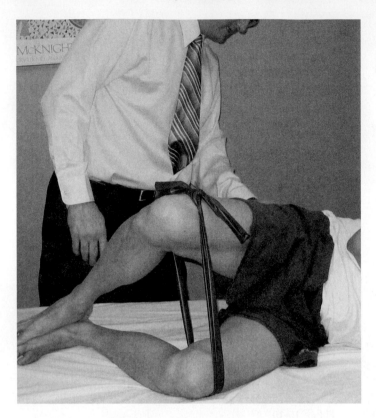

Figure 15-11
Side-lying hip abduction (clam) exercise with Thera-Band. The focus should be on contraction of the posterior gluteus medius muscle and deep external rotators.

a capsuloligamentous restriction. Mulligan[28] described a technique combining arthrokinematic with osteokinematic motions that he called *mobilization with movement* (MWM). Short axis distraction combined with medial or lateral rotation is particularly effective for improving rotation ROM (Figure 15-12).[28] Manual posterior mobilization can be useful for assessing and treating a posterior hip capsule contracture that would limit flexion and medial rotation ranges of motion (Figure 15-13).

End feel is a very important component of joint mobility assessment, both in osteokinematic assessment of the quality of overpressure and in arthrokinematic assessment of the quality of end range tissue resistance.[3] Normal end feels at the hip are soft tissue approximation for flexion and a firm, capsuloligamentous end feel for extension,

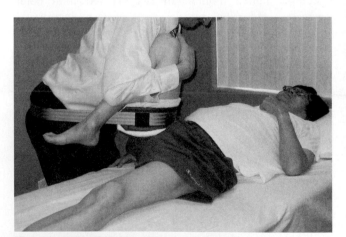

Figure 15-12
Mulligan's mobilization with movement (MWM) technique to increase range of motion of hip internal rotation.

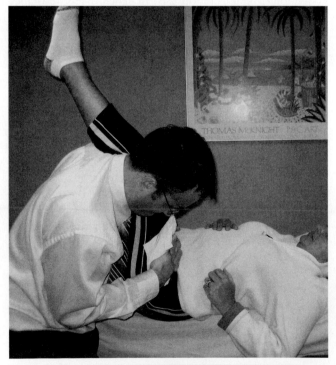

Figure 15-13
Posterior hip mobilization to stretch the posterior capsule of the hip.

medial and lateral rotation, abduction, and adduction. Abnormal end feels common at the hip are a firm capsular end feel before expected end range (e.g., from capsular contracture), an empty end feel from severe pain (e.g., very acute bursitis), and a bony block (eg., from osteophytes in advanced OA).

Proximal Hamstring Strain

Hamstring strains are common, especially in athletes. In American football players, hamstring strains have been reported to be the most common hip region injury and the third most common injury overall, after injuries to the knee and the ankle.[29] In a general sports medicine population, however, hamstring strains are the third most common hip or pelvic injury, after gluteus medius strain/tendonitis and trochanteric bursitis.[15] Two types of hamstring injuries can occur: muscle tears (grades I to III) and tendonitis/tendonosis caused by overuse. Muscle tears tend to occur at the stress risers of the musculotendinous or tenoperiosteal junctions or at the site of scar tissue from a previous injury (an acquired form of stress riser). The most widely accepted theory about the hamstrings' vulnerability to injury is that they are a two-joint muscle functioning to eccentrically control knee extension and hip flexion. The biceps femoris muscle tends to be the most commonly injured component of the hamstrings, perhaps because the nerve supply to the short head of the biceps femoris is from the peroneal division of the sciatic nerve, whereas the long head of the biceps femoris and the other components of the hamstrings have their nerve supply from the tibial division of the sciatic nerve.[29,30] It is proposed that the differing nerve supplies to the biceps femoris result in poor neuro-muscular coordination between the two heads of the muscle and thus a greater susceptibility to injury.

During walking and even jogging, the hamstrings are not fully recruited. It is with sprinting that high eccentric resistance from the hamstrings is required to decelerate the rapid leg swing (both knee extension and hip flexion); therefore, the hamstrings are most vulnerable to injury during sprinting. With running, the hamstrings have three primary functions: eccentric contraction to decelerate the leg swing that starts at approximately 30° flexion; eccentric contraction at foot strike to control and facilitate hip extension; and, eccentric contraction at push-off to assist the gastrocnemius in extending the knee.[30] If gluteus maximus recruitment for propulsive hip extension is insufficient at push-off, the hamstrings may have this additional role.

A hamstring injury also can occur during eccentric control of hip flexion in sports (e.g., lunging for a ball in tennis). This may occur when a player has not sufficiently flexed the knee, causing the hamstrings to strongly contract and lengthen at the same time. An important component of rehabilitation of such hamstring strains is emphasizing to the player the importance of bending the knees for practically everything so that even when a lunging, top heavy

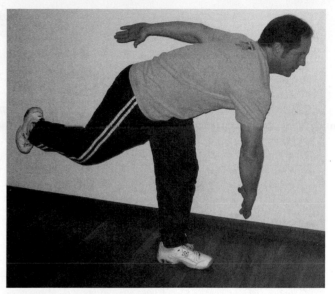

Figure 15-14
Windmill touches for eccentric hamstring contraction.

movement occurs, it does not result in sudden or cumulative tissue overload. Another theory on rehabilitation of this mechanism is to strengthen the hamstrings for this type of function with activities such as single leg stand windmill touches (Figure 15-14). In the controlled rehabilitation environment, this activity is appropriate for the few times this movement might occur in a sport. However, this author discourages lunging with a straight knee and strongly emphasizes lunging in sports over a bent knee to prevent this type of injury; besides, bending the knees is better technique for reaching low in most sports.

Golfers can strain the proximal hamstring of the non-target-side leg from the propulsion required for the drive in the golf swing. The gluteus maximus should contract strongly on the non-target-side leg during the forward swing. Inadequate recruitment from the gluteus maximus may result in overcompensation and strain of the proximal hamstrings.[31]

Rehabilitation of hamstring strains using progressive agility and trunk stabilization exercises (Box 15-2) has been found to be more effective than a program emphasizing isolated hamstring stretching and strengthening.[32] Sherry and Best[32] reported that only one of 13 subjects in the core stabilization group sustained a recurrent injury during the 1-year follow-up, whereas in the static hamstring stretch/progressive hamstring strengthening group, seven of 10 subjects had recurrent hamstring strains. Fredericson et al.[33] also recommended incorporating eccentric hamstring strengthening based on the rationale that it is the only proven treatment for chronic tendinopathies.[24,33]

Strain or overload of the hamstring tissues also may be due to a pelvic alignment fault or malalignment that changes the length/tension relationship of the hamstrings. Athletes with hamstring strains often show an anterior

---

Box 15-2 Progressive Agility and Trunk Stabilization Approach for Treating Hamstring Strains

Phase 1*
1. Low to moderate intensity† sidestepping: 3 × 1 minute.
2. Low to moderate intensity grapevine stepping (lateral stepping with the trail leg going over the lead leg and then under the lead leg), both directions: 3 × 1 minute.
3. Low to moderate intensity steps forward and backward over a tape line while moving sideways: 2 × 1 minute.
4. Single leg stand, progressing from eyes open to eye closed: 4 × 20 seconds.
5. Prone abdominal body bridge (abdominal and hip muscles are used to hold the body in a face down, straight plank position with the elbows and feet as the only points of contact): 4 × 20 seconds.
6. Supine extension bridge (abdominal and hip muscles are used to hold the body in a supine hook lying position with the head, upper back, arms, and feet as the points of contact): 4 × 20 seconds.
7. Side bridge (i.e., side plank) each side: 4 × 20 seconds.
8. Ice in long sitting: 20 minutes.

Phase 2
1. Moderate to high intensity sidestepping: 3 × 1 minute.
2. Moderate to high intensity grapevine stepping: 3 × 1 minute.
3. Moderate to high intensity steps forward and backward while moving sideways: 2 × 1 minute.
4. Single leg stand windmill touches: 4 × 20 seconds of repetitive alternate hand touches.
5. Push-up stabilization with trunk rotation (starting at the top of a full push-up, the patient maintains this position with one hand while rotating the chest toward the side of the other hand as it is lifted to point toward the ceiling; the patient pauses and then returns to the starting position): 2 × 15 repetitions on each side.
6. Fast feet in place (jogging in place with increasing velocity, picking up the feet only a few inches off the ground): 4 × 20 seconds.
7. Proprioceptive neuromuscular facilitation trunk pull-downs using a Thera-Band: 2 × 15 repetitions to the right and left.
8. Symptom-free practice without high speed maneuvers.
9. Ice for 20 minutes if any symptoms of local fatigue or discomfort are present.

Modified from Sherry M, Best T: A comparison of 2 rehabilitation programs in the treatment of acute hamstring strains, *J Orthop Sports Phys Ther* 34:116-125, 2004.
*Progression criteria: The patient is progressed from exercises in phase 1 to exercises in phase 2 when the individual can walk with a normal gait pattern and do a high knee march in place without pain.
†*Low intensity* is a velocity of movement that is less than or near that of normal walking; *moderate intensity* is a velocity of movement greater than normal walking but not as great as sports activity; *high intensity* is a velocity of movement similar to sports activity.

---

innominate tilt on the affected side, and manipulation of the sacroiliac joint can enable these patients to regain muscle function and return to activity more quickly than those treated with more conservative measures.[34] This same response has been identified with runners experiencing anterior or lateral hip pain.[35]

Muscle Strain Management
Management of muscle strains should follow a rational, evidence-based progression based on the extent, mechanism, symptoms, and healing stage of the injury. In the acute, or early, phase, the PRICEM regimen should be followed (*P* for protect, prevent, promote; *R* for relative rest; *I* for ice or cryotherapy; *C* for compression; *E* for elevation; and *M* for modalities, medication, massage, mobilization, and movement). Acute phase management should be used for the first 2 to 5 days and sometimes longer, depending on the extent of the injury. Rehabilitation then progresses through a subacute and a late phase. Return to sport after a muscle strain may take anywhere from a few weeks to many months, depending on the extent of injury.[3]

Acute Injury Treatment Regimen

P	Protect injury, prevent further injury, promote healing
R	Relative rest
I	Ice/cryotherapy
C	Compression
E	Elevation
M	Modalities, medication, massage movement, mobilization

Adductor Muscle Injury
As in other regions of the body, contractile tissue injuries at the hip come in two forms: strain (a muscle tear) and tendonitis (acute) or tendinosis (chronic). Participants in sports such as soccer, hockey, and football are susceptible to adductor muscle pulls ("groin" strain) because of the explosive lateral and rotatory hip movements involved, along with end range abduction stresses. Hyperabduction (overstretching) and forceful abduction of the thigh during adduction (e.g., during a soccer tackle) are the most

common mechanisms of groin injury. Overuse adductor muscle injury also is common with repetitive, high velocity limb movement that usually involves a change in direction (e.g., ice hockey or soccer). Adductor injuries usually are felt in the groin, and any of the adductor muscles can be affected, although the adductor longus is most commonly injured.[36]

Defects in the abdominal musculature (i.e., "sportsman hernia"), osteitis pubis, inguinal hernia, and referred pain from the hip joint or lumbar spine should be ruled out in any assessment of the hip. A general but useful test to differentiate abdominal injury from adductor injury is to have the patient perform a situp or a situp with trunk rotation; an abdominal injury is most likely to be painful with these maneuvers.

In a study comparing active and passive management of adductor strains, Holmich et al.[37] found the active treatment group (i.e., those who performed adductor strengthening, lumbopelvic strengthening and stabilization, and balance work) did much better than the passive treatment group (i.e., those who received transverse friction massage, transcutaneous electrical nerve stimulation, laser therapy, and adductor stretching). These findings support the notion that deficient collagen (quality and quantity) is part of the problem. An active loading program (including eccentric exercise) stimulates collagen synthesis and produces better long-term results than a passive loading program. Box 15-3 outlines an active loading program for adductor strain rehabilitation.

A mechanism of groin pain that deserves further study is the effect of a positional fault on the lumbopelvic region. A case example seen by this author was acute onset left groin pain that occurred during the split-step on a serve and volley in tennis. Immediate pain, tightness, and spasm occurred in the adductor muscles and could not be relieved by an adductor stretch. Because stretching to relieve the adductor spasm did not have any appreciable effect and because the mechanism was not likely to have resulted in an adductor strain (the mechanism was a sudden load in slight lumbopelvic-hip flexion), the author asked the patient to perform a standing lumbar backward bend that immediately and permanently relieved the symptoms. Whether the source of the symptoms was a flexion positional fault in the lumbar spine or pelvis, a lumbar disc bulge that referred the symptoms to the groin, or an iliopsoas spasm, in this case lumbopelvic extension was an effective treatment.

Athletic Pubalgia (Sports Hernia)

Athletic pubalgia is a complex injury of the flexion/adduction apparatus of the hip.[38] When surgery is performed, the findings typically include a laddered appearance of the external oblique aponeurosis; separation of the conjoined tendon of the rectus abdominis from the inguinal ligament; and laxity of the transversalis fascia.[39] The syndrome presents as disabling lower abdominal and groin pain on exertion, typically progressing to involve the adductor longus tendon, as well as the abdomen and groin musculature on the opposite side. Resisted situps or situps with trunk rotation and resisted hip adduction often can reproduce the symptoms.[38] The condition occurs mostly in male elite athletes in ice hockey, soccer, and football who are involved in vigorous training and competition schedules and whose sport involves repetitive hyperextension of the hip along with trunk rotation.[39] Abdominal hyperextension with thigh hyperabduction, with the pivot being the pubic symphysis, has also been reported as a mechanism.[38] Often patients report an initial incident of a hyperextension injury of the hip in which the anterior pelvis or pubic symphysis is the pivot. Both the rectus abdominis and adductor longus tendons insert at the pubic symphysis and are sites of pain in athletic pubalgia.[38]

Meyers et al.[38] hypothesized that the abdominal component of the injury usually is the initial injury in athletic pubalgia and that it allows the pelvis to rotate anteriorly (as evidenced by the fact that in the cadaver, when a portion of the rectus abdominis is cut, the pelvis rotates anteriorly with ease). The anterior tilt of the hemipelvis causes a compartment syndrome in the proximal adductors, because the adductors are now relatively unopposed as a result of injury to the lower abdominals (creating an unbalanced force couple).[38]

Meyers et al.[38] described their pelvic floor (abdominal) repair as a broad surgical reattachment of the inferolateral edge of the rectus abdominis muscle and its fascia to the pubis and anterior ligaments. They also performed an adductor release that involved complete division of all the anterior epimysial fibers of the adductor longus 2-3 cm (1 to 1.2 inches) distal to the insertion on the pubis, as well as multiple longitudinal incisions at the tendinous attachment site on the pubis.[38] Surgical repair for athletic pubalgia boasts a 95% success rate.[38,39] A typical postoperative rehabilitating protocol is outlined in Box 15-4. Athletes usually are able to return to competitive sports by 12 weeks after surgery.

A course of conservative management should be attempted for sports pubalgia before surgery is considered. A key component of conservative rehabilitation is core strengthening, including emphasis on eccentric adductor and oblique abdominal strengthening.[40] A particularly effective form of core strengthening for athletic pubalgia uses diagonal elastic tubing resistance between the upper and lower extremities. Alex McKechnie developed this approach and has had considerable success using it with professional athletes.[41] A key component of this method is to have the patient simultaneously contract the pelvic floor and transversus abdominis and hold a low level contraction while performing activities such as squats, lunges, and sport-specific moves repetitively, with additional core resistance coming from a Thera-Band wrapped around each thigh and held in the contralateral hand (Figures 15-15 and 15-16).

Box 15-3 Postinjury Program for Adductor Strain

Phase I (Acute)
- Rest, ice, compression, and elevation (RICE)
- Nonsteroidal anti-inflammatory drugs (NSAIDs)
- Massage
- Transcutaneous electrical stimulation (TENS)
- Ultrasound
- Submaximum isometric adduction from knees bent to knees straight, progressing to maximum isometric adduction, pain free
- Non-weight-bearing hip progressive resistive exercise (PRE) with weight in antigravity position (all except abduction)
- Pain-free, low load, high repetition exercise
- Upper body and trunk strengthening
- Contralateral lower extremity (LE) strengthening
- Flexibility program for noninvolved muscles
- Bilateral balance board
  Clinical milestone: Concentric adduction against gravity without pain

Phase II (Subacute)
- Bicycling/swimming
- Sumo squats
- Single limb stance
- Concentric adduction with weight against gravity
- Standing with involved foot on sliding board moving in frontal plane
- Adduction in standing position on cable column or with Thera-Band
- Seated adduction machine
- Bilateral adduction on sliding board moving in frontal plane (i.e., bilateral adduction simultaneously)
- Unilateral lunges (sagittal) with reciprocal arm movements
- Multiplane trunk tilting
- Balance board squats with throwbacks
- General flexibility program
  Clinical milestone: Involved lower extremity passive range of motion (PROM) equal to that of the uninvolved side and involved adductor strength at least 75% that of the ipsilateral abductors

Phase III (Sport-Specific Training)
- Phase II exercises with increase in load, intensity, speed, and volume
- Standing resisted stride lengths on cable column to simulate skating
- Sliding board
- On-ice kneeling adductor pull-togethers
- Lunges (in all planes)
- Correction or modification of ice skating technique
  Clinical milestone: Adduction strength 90% to 100% of abduction strength and involved muscle strength equal to that of the contralateral side

Modified from Tyler TF, Nicholas SJ, Campbell RJ, et al: The effectiveness of a preseason exercise program to prevent adductor muscle strain in professional ice hockey players. *Am J Sports Med* 30:680-683, 2002.

Snapping Hip Syndrome

Snapping hip syndrome (coxa saltans) is defined as an audible snap or pop as the hip moves through a range of motion, usually when the flexed hip is extended.[42] It often is painless, but it can become symptomatic in athletic individuals. The syndrome is more common in young athletic females. The cause of the snapping or clicking can be intra-articular or extra-articular (Table 15-6).

Intra-articular snapping or clicking can occur as a result of labral tears, loose bodies, synovial chondromatosis, and osteocartilaginous exostosis. In these cases, it is more commonly a clicking sensation or sound. These problems may not be amenable to conservative treatment and may require arthroscopic intervention. An internal pop, called the *suction phenomenon,* is related to the hip's natural negative pressure environment. It is benign and usually symptom free.[42]

Extra-articular snapping hip syndrome has been categorized into two general subtypes: external and internal snapping hip. Extra-articular snapping hip is most likely caused by the ITB snapping over the greater trochanter (external snapping hip) or the iliopsoas muscle-tendon

Box 15-4 Postoperative Protocol for Surgical Repair of a Sports Hernia

0-4 Weeks Relative rest	
4-6 Weeks No resistive exercises	

0-4 Weeks   Relative rest
4-6 Weeks   No resistive exercises
    Posterior pelvic tilt (5-6 second hold): sets of 10
    Gentle stretching
        5 repetitions, hold 30 seconds each
        Side bending
        Hip flexion
        Quadriceps
        Hamstrings
        Adductors
    Pool exercises
        Walking, forward and backward
        Standing hip abduction/adductio/flexion/extension:
            3 × 10 repetitions
        Partial squats: 30 repetitions
        Heel raises: 3 × 10 repetitions
6 Weeks   Progressive resistance exercises
    Hip flexion/adduction/abduction/extension with
        body weight (add resistance in 1 pound
        [0.45 kg] increments as tolerated)
    UE PREs: Light dumbbells
    Cardiovascular exercise
        20 to 30 minutes in any combination of the
            following:
            Upper Body Ergometer (UBE)
            Stairmaster
            Stationary bike
            Elliptical glider
    Pool exercises
        Running, forward and backward
        Side slides
        Carioca
        Jumping jacks
        Swimming (flutter kick; *no butterfly*)

7 Weeks   Previous exercises, increase weights as tolerated
    Strengthening
        Abdominal crunches
        Bridging
    Jogging: ½ mile (0.8 km)
    Backward jog: 100 yards (91.4 m) × 5 repetitions
8 Weeks   Previous PREs
    Trunk stabilization exercises
        Lunges
        Swiss ball
        Crunches
        Bridging
        Obliques
        Superman
        Trunk extension
        Reverse fly
    Jogging: ½-1 mile (0.8-1.6 km)
    Backward jog: 100 yards (91.4 m) × 5 repetitions
    Agility drills
        Sprinting: 50 yards (45.7 m); avoid sudden starts
            and stops

        Figures-of-eight
        Cariocas
    Plyometrics
        Rope jumping
        Side to side
        Front to back
9 Weeks   Previous exercises
    LE PREs
    Sport-specific drills
        Soccer—*No* shooting or long volleys
10-12 Weeks   Continued increase in exercise with the goal of
    return to play at 12 weeks after surgery

Modified from Meyers W, Ryan J: Drexel University College of Medicine, Department of Surgery, Hahnemann Sports Medicine Center.
UE, Upper extremity; *PREs,* progressive resistance exercises; *LE,* lower extremity.

snapping over the pelvic brim (internal snapping hip).[42] Other reported causes are snapping of the biceps femoris over the edge of the ischial tuberosity, snapping of the gluteus maximus over the greater trochanter as it blends into the ITB, and snapping of the iliopsoas over the anterior femoral head.[42]

The classic test for snapping of the iliopsoas muscle over the anterior pelvic brim or hip is reproduction of the snap as the hip is extended from a position of flexion, abduction, and lateral rotation (the extension test). It is helpful to identify the location of the snap or click by simultaneous palpation during the test. Often firm manual pressure during the extension test can reduce the snapping by preventing the lateral to medial subluxation of the tendon over the pelvic brim.[42] Commonly,

shortening of the iliopsoas muscle and malalignment of the pelvis are associated with snapping of the iliopsoas muscle.

A test for a snapping ITB is flexion of the adducted hip with the knee extended.[43] Ober's test is also likely to show shortening of the ITB (see the section on ITB contracture).

An extra-articular snapping hip often is asymptomatic, but it can result in inflammation of a gluteal tendon or bursa. Treatment with NSAIDs and ice can be helpful in the short term. For long-term benefit, the cause of the snapping must be resolved, or at least its frictional effect must be reduced. This can involve soft tissue mobilization and stretching techniques for myotendinous contractures, correction of muscle imbalances, correction of

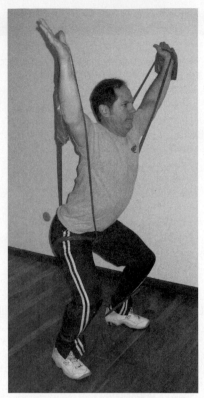

Figure 15-15
McKechnie squat with Thera-Band.

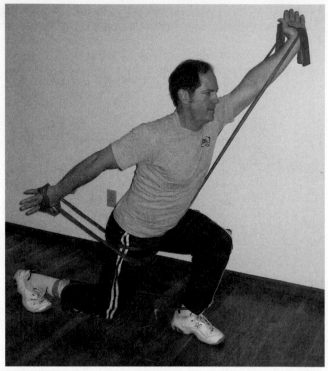

Figure 15-16
McKechnie lunge with Thera-Band.

malalignment of the pelvic girdle, movement pattern adjustments to minimize or abolish the click, and prescription orthotics for patients with pronating feet.

If conservative measures do not resolve symptoms associated with snapping hip syndrome and surgery is required, good results have been reported for surgical release and lengthening techniques for both the iliopsoas and proximal ITB.[42,43]

Joint Disorders

Osteoarthritis

Osteoarthritis is a complex disorder of synovial joints characterized by both deterioration of articular cartilage and new bone formation, resulting in joint pain and dysfunction.[44] Radiographically, the deterioration of articular cartilage presents as joint space narrowing, and new bone formation presents as osteophytes. The hip is one of the more common

Table 15-6
Causes of Snapping Hip

| | Anterior | | |
Intra-articular	Internal	External	Posterior
Loose bodies	Iliopsoas tendon snapping over pelvic brim	Iliotibial band snapping over greater trochanter	Long head of biceps femoris tendon sliding over ischial tuberosity
Synovial chondromatosis	Iliopsoas tendon snapping over femoral head	Gluteus maximus tendon snapping over greater trochanter	
Osteochondral injury	Iliopsoas tendon snapping over bony ridge on lesser trochanter		
Subluxation of the hip	Tendonitis of iliopsoas or rectus femoris		
Labral tears	Anterosuperior labrum most common site		

From Gruen GS, Scioscia TN, Lowenstein JE: The surgical treatment of internal snapping hip, *Am J Sports Med* 30:607-613, 2002.

sites of involvement, and OA of the hip affects approximately 1.5% of the adult population in the United States.[45] Pain from OA of the hip usually is felt in the groin, lateral hip, and/or buttock.[4,5] Women account for 2/3 to 3/4 of adults with OA of the hip and OA in general.[45]

OA can be divided into primary and secondary types. Primary OA occurs without some predisposing mechanical alignment factor. Secondary OA is the end result of another disease 'process. Eighty percent of OA of the hip is secondary in nature.[46] Predisposing factors to secondary OA of the hip are disorders such as osteonecrosis, Legg-Calvé-Perthes disease, developmental dysplasia of the hip, slipped capital femoral epiphysis, congenital coxa vara or coxa valga, and hip fracture.

The primary signs and symptoms of OA are joint pain and stiffness. Radiographically, OA is characterized by joint space narrowing in the weight-bearing region and by osteophyte formation (Figure 15-17). Rheumatoid arthritis (RA), on the other hand, shows uniform joint space narrowing, which progresses to protrusio acetabuli (protrusion of the femoral head through the acetabulum) at the end stage. Routine x-ray views of the hip usually are sufficient to diagnose OA. Routine views for the hip are an anteroposterior (AP) pelvic view (which captures both proximal femurs, the pelvis, and the distal lumbar spine), AP hip view, and lateral hip view (either true lateral or frog lateral).

Routine X-Ray Views for the Hip

- Anteroposterior (AP) pelvis
- AP hip
- Lateral view (either true lateral or frog lateral)

Advanced OA of the hip (i.e., radiographic evidence of OA with persistent severe symptoms or functional loss) can be very effectively treated with total hip arthroplasty (THA), discussed in Chapter 26. Because THA is not without risks and limitations, it is reserved for more advanced cases of OA that have not responded to medical management. A number of nonoperative (medical) approaches can be used to manage OA, including pharmacological and nonpharmacological measures. Nonpharmacological methods include patient education and physical and occupational therapy, which have been described as the foundation of treatment for patients with OA.[47]

Rehabilitation management of OA of the hip should be directed toward maintaining function, relieving symptoms, preventing deformity, and educating the patient in ways to protect the hip joint. Function can be maintained by changing the person to fit the environment or by changing the environment to fit the person. Examples of factors that can be changed in the person are inflammation, joint alignment, range of motion, and muscle length and strength. Changing the environment may involve adaptive equipment, home modifications, and social services.

In published trials of nonmedicinal and noninvasive treatments for hip OA, aerobic-type exercise has shown the greatest benefit.[48] Exercise therapy with the goals of improving muscle function (i.e., endurance, strength, and coordination), range of motion, pain relief, and walking ability has been shown to be effective for OA of the hip.[49] However, in a study by Hoeksma et al.,[50] manual therapy for the hip was shown to be even more effective than exercise therapy in improving pain, stiffness, hip function, and range of motion. The manual therapy these researchers used was stretching of the iliopsoas, quadriceps, tensor fascia lata, sartorius, adductors, and gracilis. The hold time was 8 to 10 seconds for each muscle, repeated 2 times. The stretching was followed by a series of five traction manipulations (long axis traction), as described by Cyriax, starting with the hip in the maximum loose-packed position; with each subsequent manipulation, the hip was placed in a position of more restriction.[50,51]

Acupuncture was found to be helpful for symptom relief in a group of patients with OA who were awaiting total hip replacement.[52] Pain from OA of the hip and knee has also

---

Figure 15-17

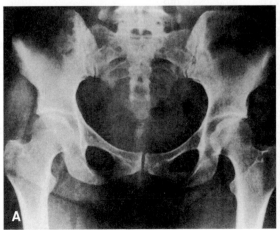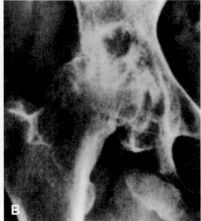

A, Normal hip joints on plain x-ray film, AP view. **B,** Osteoarthritis of the hip joint. Note the superior and lateral joint space narrowing, subchondral sclerosis, superior acetabular bone cyst, medial femoral neck, and lesser trochanteric sclerosis with buttressing. (From Frontera WR, Silver JK: *Essentials of physical medicine and rehabilitation,* Philadelphia, 2002, Hanley & Belfus.)

been shown to diminish when patients wear magnetic bracelets.[53]

The findings of Hoeksma et al.[50] have been corroborated by this author, who has found manual therapy techniques extremely helpful for improving hip function in individuals with OA and other hip conditions. Combinations of manual soft tissue techniques, joint mobilization, and manual stretching are very effective in improving ROM, and muscle length, reducing pain, and improving gait and other functions. A published case study has shown that ROM, strength, function, and gait can be improved and pain reduced in a person with hip OA who follows through with a rehabilitation program that includes manual therapy, therapeutic exercise, and education that addresses the presenting impairments.[54] Often patients with progressive OA may eventually need a hip replacement when walking becomes too painful, but the appropriate rehabilitation intervention can delay the operation and make for a better postoperative outcome. Delaying hip replacement too long, however, especially if function and exercise capability are significantly limited, is not wise, because it can result in worsening cardiovascular health in particular.[55]

The decision on whether to change a joint's range of motion depends on whether that joint's range can be expected to increase and whether the hip currently is functionally limited. The decision as to whether the joint's range can be increased depends primarily on the end feel. If the end feel is a bony block, the joint's range cannot be changed. If the end feel is not a bony block, the joint's range may be changeable. A balance between symptoms, range, and function must be found. Much of the pain from OA arises from the inflammatory process. In most cases, reducing inflammation produces concomitant symptom and functional improvements. A rationale for improving range of motion is that restricted motion could be causing an inflammatory response from abnormal joint surface arthrokinematics. If this hypothesis is not supported by treatment, the approach for improving ROM must be modified or discontinued.

It is important to teach the patient the principles of hip joint protection, especially considering that normal gait causes approximately three times the body's weight to load through the hip during walking (see Figure 15-3). These protection principles can be grouped into body weight reduction, load carrying modification, and assistive device use. For every pound of body weight lost, a 3-pound reduction in load through the hip occurs; therefore body weight reduction is an admirable goal. However, the weight-bearing exercise required to lose body weight can irritate the hip. Pool exercises, swimming, and upper body workouts can be used for weight reduction without exacerbating hip inflammation. Workouts on stationary bikes and rowing machines also are often well tolerated until OA is more advanced.

Hip Joint Protection Principles

- Weight reduction
- Exercise modification
- Load carrying modification
- Use of assistive device

When the patient needs to carry something, it should be as light as possible and should be carried on the back in a knapsack. If a unilateral load is carried, it should be carried on the side of the hip problem. A cane should be used on the side contralateral to the hip problem. Both the contralateral cane and ipsilateral load advice are based on the opposing torque explanation.[56] For example, during one-leg stance on the right leg, the right hip has body weight creating a counterclockwise torque and the hip abductors creating a clockwise torque (see Figure 15-4). Use of a cane in the contralateral (left) hand or holding a weight in the ipsilateral (right) hand also creates a clockwise torque about the right hip, thereby assisting the right hip abductors in clockwise torque generation.

Besides rehabilitation intervention, medication is an important component of nonoperative treatment for OA. The main indication for the use of medication in OA is pain relief.[57] Acetaminophen is recommended for mild to moderate pain because its efficacy is comparable to that of NSAIDs for this level of pain, and it has a more favorable side effect profile, provided the dosage does not exceed 4 g per day. NSAIDs are recommended for moderate to severe hip pain and in cases in which acetaminophen does not provide significant relief or the clinical presentation suggests significant inflammation.[47] Because of the cardiovascular risks associated with the cyclo-oxygenase-2 (COX-2) inhibitors, the nonselective traditional NSAIDs ibuprofen and naproxen are usually recommended as a first line of treatment. However, celecoxib (200 mg daily [qd]) and naproxen (500 mg twice per day [bid]) appear to be safer than other agents with regard to cardiovascular risk.[58] For long-term use of a nonselective NSAID or in individuals with an increased risk of an upper gastrointestinal adverse event, a gastroprotective agent (e.g., misoprostol) is recommended.[47]

Other pharmacological measures for hip OA are intra-articular injection of glucocorticosteroids, intra-articular injection of hyaluran, and opioid analgesics (e.g., Tramadol).[47] Some patients find that glucosamine and/or chondroitin sulphate help take the edge off their symptoms.

Femoroacetabular Impingement

Although femoroacetabular impingement was first recognized as a mechanism for early hip OA in 1965, it was not until recently that increased interest in this condition as a primary etiological factor behind labral tears and OA has been considered.[59] One recent study has documented that acetabular labral tears rarely occur in the absence of bony

Figure 15-18

Plain x-ray film of the pelvis showing a "pistol grip" deformity of both proximal femora. This deformity is so named because the nonspherical femora resemble pistol grips. (From Shetty VD, Villar RN: Hip arthroscopy: current concepts and review of literature, *Br J Sports Med* 41:64-68, 2007.)

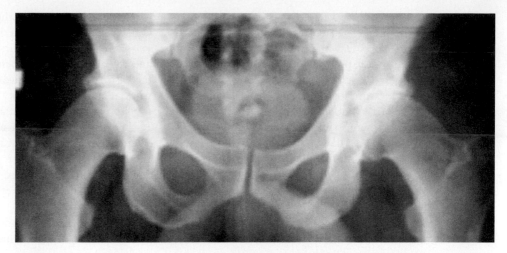

abnormalities.[60] Femoroacetabular impingement has been identified as the most common cause of end stage OA in young men and a common cause in young women.[61] Two mechanisms of impingement have been identified: cam impingement, caused by jamming of an abnormal femoral head (e.g., from pistol grip deformity) into the acetabulum with increasing hip flexion; and pincer impingement, which occurs when the acetabular rim contacts the femoral head-neck junction at end range of flexion, causing a leverage of the opposite side of the femoral head up against the posteroinferior edge of the acetabulum. Pincer impingement is more likely to be seen in patients with retroversion.[62]

Hip (Femoroacetabular) Impingement

- Cam
- Pincer

Symptoms of femoroacetabular impingement typically are seen in athletic, younger middle-aged individuals who experience groin pain with sports activity. The pain initially is intermittent and can be aggravated by increased athletic activity, prolonged walking, and prolonged sitting.[62]

The impingement test is described as hip flexion of the adducted hip with progressively increasing medial rotation; this elicits groin pain with a positive test result.[62] The imaging workup should include a cross-table lateral view, which gives good visualization if either flattening of the normally concave femoral neck (pistol grip deformity) and/or a nonspherical femoral head is present (Figure 15-18); MRI is necessary to evaluate for acetabular version (especially for a retroversion problem). MR arthrography often is necessary to identify labral tears (Figure 15-19).[63]

Conservative treatment involves modification of activity to avoid the impingement positions and NSAIDs to reduce inflammation. To maintain a higher level of function and to prevent early onset of OA, the surgeon and patient

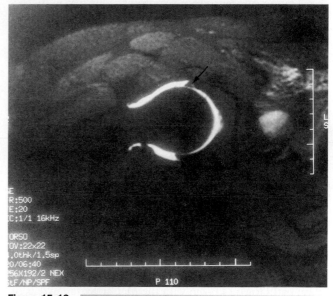

Figure 15-19

Magnetic resonance arthrogram showing an acetabular labral tear. (From DeLee J, Drez D, Miller M: *DeLee and Drez's orthopaedic sports medicine,* ed 2, Philadelphia, 2003, WB Saunders.)

may opt for arthroscopic debridement of the source of impingement through contouring of the femoral head and neck to a more normal anatomy (cheilectomy), or a periacetabular osteotomy may be needed if an acetabular torsion problem is present.[64] During surgery, repair of labral tears and microfracture of any chondral lesions may also be performed.[63]

Labral Tears

With the increasing use of arthroscopy at the hip, labral tears have been found to be more common than previously thought. It is believed that labral tears may precipitate and/or accelerate the process of osteoarthritis. Most labral tears (86%) are in the anterior quadrant of the labrum. Chondral lesions double in the presence of a labral tear, and 40% of patients with a labral tear have severe chondral lesions.[65]

The mechanism for labral tears is associated with either repetitive microtrauma associated with pivoting and twisting movements in sports or with a specific traumatic event. Often the specific traumatic event involves extension and lateral rotation with the femoral head moving anteriorly and overstressing the anterior labrum.[65]

The symptoms of a labral tear usually are mechanical in nature: buckling, catching, painful clicking, and restricted ROM. Several special tests have been described to assess for labral pathology; these tend to be variations of two primary tests:[66,67]

1. The **impingement test** involves medial rotation of the flexed and adducted hip while it is held in at least 90° flexion and at least 15° adduction. If pain is not reproduced with the test performed slowly, a rapid application of the medial rotation at end range can reproduce symptoms. This test is suggestive of a wide range of anterior hip disorders, including anterior labral tear, anterosuperior impingement, and iliopsoas tendonitis.
2. The **apprehension test** consists of lateral rotation of the extended hip. If symptoms are not reproduced, a rapid application of end range lateral rotation can be performed. With a positive test result, this maneuver elicits apprehension or groin pain and suggests anterior hip instability, anterior labral tear, or posteroinferior impingement.

The McCarthy hip extension sign is a further test for labral pathology. In this test, both hips are flexed, and while the uninvolved hip is kept flexed, the involved hip is extended from the flexed position first in lateral rotation and then in medial rotation. Reproduction of the patient's pain is a positive test result. McCarthy considered positive results on three different tests to be the key to predicting labral pathology: (1) pain with the McCarthy hip extension sign; (2) painful impingement with hip flexion, adduction, and lateral rotation; and (3) inguinal pain on a resisted straight leg raise.[68]

McCarthy's Signs Predicting Hip Labral Pathology

- Positive McCarthy hip extension sign
- Painful impingement on hip flexion, adduction, and lateral rotation
- Inguinal pain on resisted straight leg raise

The active and, if necessary, resisted straight leg raise in the early range (test 3 in McCarthy's three-test battery) has been labeled the Stinchfield resisted hip flexion test, and the result is often positive with intra-articular disorders such as labral tears, arthritis, synovitis, occult femoral neck fractures, and prosthetic failure or loosening.[69] It also is positive with iliopsoas tendonitis/bursitis.

Fitzgerald[70] described the following variations to differentiate anterior from posterior labral tears. To test for *anterior* labral tears, the hip first is flexed with lateral rotation and full abduction and then extended with adduction and medial rotation. A positive test result is hip pain with or without an associated click. To test for *posterior* labral tears, the hip is first fully flexed, adducted, and medially rotated. It then is extended with abduction and lateral rotation. Again, a positive test result is pain with or without an associated click.[70] Pain with a resisted straight leg raise (resisted SLR) and pain with forced hip medial rotation combined with axial traction are other tests that can load the anterolateral labrum.[71]

Millis and Kim[67] found that MRI with gadolinium enhancement provides a more sensitive and specific diagnosis of labral tears than was previously possible (although it does not identify all tears present on arthroscopy), and arthroscopy provides a means to resect or stabilize the tear.[72]

The rehabilitation of patients after hip arthroscopy is outlined in Table 15-7. This program follows a gradual rehabilitation progression over the course of several months. Hyperextension past neutral of the hip is avoided for the first 5 weeks after surgery to protect the anterior labrum as are rotational movements of the hip.

The ideas of Sahrmann[13] are worth incorporating into both the nonoperative and postoperative rehabilitation of patients with labral pathology. Sahrmann emphasized the importance of keeping the femoral head well seated in the acetabulum. This requires accurate diagnosis of the movement impairment syndrome, followed by prescription of the appropriate stretches, motor control and strengthening exercises, and patient education. Sahrmann has identified 11 movement impairments at the hip, of which anterior femoral glide is the most common. Anterior femoral glide syndrome can result in injury to the anterior labrum of the hip through a directional susceptibility of the hip into extension (common in runners and dancers) that causes the femoral head to increase pressure against the anterior joint structures, causing irritation and injury. Anterior femoral glide syndrome can also cause impingement of anterior hip structures (e.g., the iliopsoas myotendon and anterior labrum) as a result of inadequate posterior glide of the femoral head during hip flexion. For treatment, the clinician should advise the patient to avoid activities and exercises that load the anterior labrum (e.g., into end range extension and/or lateral rotation) and prescribe exercises and activities that encourage posterior glide of the femoral head (e.g., rocking back and forward in the quadruped position, hinging at the hips, with the back held flat in the neutral spine position), as well as emphasizing control of one joint hip stabilizers (e.g., iliacus, gluteus maximus, and posterior gluteus medius) and de-emphasizing two-joint stabilizers (e.g., hamstrings, rectus femoris).[13]

Table 15-7
Hip Arthroscopy Rehabilitation Guidelines

Range of Motion	Postoperative Week							
	Phase I		Phase II			Phase III		
	1	2	3	4	5	6	7	8
Avoid hyperextension	▓	▓	▓	▓	▓			
Ankle pumps, circles								
Active IR/ER—seated								
Active abd/add								
AA flexion—heel slides								
Seated A/P, lateral weight shift								
Single knee to chest								
Seated trunk flexion								
Hip flexor stretch to neutral						Begin to stretch past neutral		
Pelvic tilts								

Resistance Training	Postoperative Week							
	Phase I		Phase II			Phase III		
	1	2	3	4	5	6	7	8
Isometrics and abdominals (level I)—supine								
Standing isometric abduction	▓	▓						
Bridging	▓	▓						
Unilateral bridging	▓	▓	▓					
Three-way SLR (flex, abd, add)	▓	▓				4-way		
Prone knee flexion	▓							
Seated knee extension								
Nautilus knee extension	▓	▓	▓					
Seated hip flexion	——Pain-free range——							
Abdominal bracing								
PNF pelvic patterns								
Upper body strengthening								
PNF diagonals—(full range) LE patterns	▓	▓	▓	▓	▓			
Stairmaster	▓	▓	▓	▓	▓			
Closed kinetic chain exercises								
Heel raises, ¼ squats								
Lunges, full squat	▓	▓	▓	▓	▓			
Step-ups	▓	▓	▓			Retro		
Multihip machine, operative leg	▓				—Abd, add, flex only—			
Operative leg extension	▓	▓	▓	▓	▓	▓		
Nonoperative leg					—All directions—			

Continued

Table 15-7

Hip Arthroscopy Rehabilitation Guidelines—Cont'd

Balance/Coordination	Postoperative Week							
	Phase I		Phase II			Phase III		
	1	2	3	4	5	6	7	8
Unilateral stance	▓	▓						
Rebounder	▓	▓	▓					
BAPS—bilateral to unilateral	▓							

Conditioning	Postoperative Week							
	Phase I		Phase II			Phase III		
	1	2	3	4	5	6	7	8
Stationary bicycle	▓	▓						
Swimming—flutter kick only	▓	▓						
Running	▓	▓	▓	▓	▓			
Upper body cycle								

Pool Activities (Wounds must be completely healed)	Postoperative Week							
	Phase I		Phase II			Phase III		
	1	2	3	4	5	6	7	8
Deep water walking with float	▓	▓						
Buoyancy-assisted ROM	▓	▓						
Buoyancy-resisted ROM	▓	▓	▓					
Shallow water walking	——————Increase speed. Increase stride length as tolerated.——————							
Plyometrics								

Sport-Specific Activities	Postoperative Week							
	Phase I		Phase II			Phase III		
	1	2	3	4	5	6	7	8
Fitter	▓	▓	▓	▓	▓			
Slide	▓	▓	▓	▓	▓			
Plyometrics	▓	▓	▓	▓	▓			
Cutting drills	▓	▓	▓	▓	▓			
Sport cords	▓	▓	▓	▓	▓			

Modified from Dirocco S, McCarthy JC, Busconi BD, et al.: Rehabilitation after hip arthroscopy. In McCarthy JC, editor: *Early hip disorders: advances in detection and minimally invasive treatment*, p. 180, New York, 2003, Springer-Verlag.

Return to sports depends on full pain-free range of motion, strength 90% of the opposite limb, and completion of a running or jogging program. Grey areas indicate the period in which exercises should not be performed.

IR/ER, internal rotation/external rotation; *abd/add*, abduction/adduction; *AA*, active-assisted; *A/P*, anteroposterior; *SLR*, straight leg raise; *flex*, flexion; *PNF*, proprioceptive neuromuscular facilitation; *LE*, lower extremity; *BAPS*, biomechanical ankle platform system (BAPS) board; *ROM*, range of motion.

Sahrmann's Movement Impairments of the Hip

- Femoral anterior glide syndrome without medial rotation
- Femoral anterior glide syndrome with medial rotation
- Femoral anterior glide syndrome with lateral rotation
- Hip adduction syndrome without medial rotation
- Hip adduction syndrome with medial rotation
- Femoral lateral glide syndrome
- Hip extension with knee extension
- Hip extension with medial rotation
- Femoral hypomobility syndrome with superior glide
- Femoral accessory hypermobility syndrome
- Hip lateral rotation syndrome (shortened piriformis)

From Sahrmann SA: *Diagnosis and treatment of movement impairment syndromes*, pp. 176-191, St Louis, 2002, Mosby.

Loose Bodies

Loose bodies have been more frequently diagnosed at the hip with improved arthroscopic technology and technique—and more easily removed. In fact, treatment of symptomatic loose bodies has been described as the most widely reported and accepted application for arthroscopy of the hip.[73] Loose bodies are classified as ossified or non-ossified. The ossified group is more frequently diagnosed because the ossification can be visualized on plain x-ray films. The primary symptom of loose bodies is anterior inguinal pain with locking episodes. Other signs and symptoms include painful clicking, buckling, giving way, and persistent pain with activity.[73] Loose bodies can damage the articular cartilage of a joint, therefore prompt diagnosis and treatment are essential to prevent progression to OA.

Although arthroscopy has become the ideal method of addressing loose bodies definitively, Cyriax described a technique for repositioning a loose body that may have some temporary benefit in lieu of arthroscopic removal.[10] Cyriax likened his technique for loose body treatment to repositioning a pebble in your shoe; you shake it around until it moves to a pain-free position.[10] Cyriax described loose bodies as presenting with sudden, sharp pain on weight bearing.[10] The technique for "reducing" a loose body in the hip involves applying strong, long axis traction to the hip while it is in 80° flexion and then lowering the hip to 0° flexion while maintaining the traction and applying several small amplitude, high velocity lateral rotation maneuvers. If this method is unsuccessful, the procedure is performed again, but this time small thrusts into medial rotation are used.

Another alternative suggested by Cyriax entails applying traction to the hip at 90° flexion (the knee also is at 90° flexion), passively moving the hip to the extreme of lateral rotation, and then applying a quick, short overpressure.[10] The effect on pain and function should be dramatic if indeed a mobile loose body is the culprit. The clinician should not persist if the treatment is not effective after several attempts, but if

it works, it should be repeated as needed. If conservative treatment does not provide lasting relief, arthroscopy may be necessary.

Osseous Disorders

Osteonecrosis

Osteonecrosis is a multifactorial disease in which osteocyte death occurs in the femoral head via a variety of proposed pathogenic pathways. It has both clinically and radiographically recognizable patterns to aid diagnosis. Osteonecrosis can occur anywhere in the body but is most common in the femoral head.

The two general subtypes of osteonecrosis are traumatic osteonecrosis and nontraumatic osteonecrosis. The traumatic type often occurs secondary to a hip fracture or dislocation, and for this reason, displaced femoral neck fractures are treated by replacement of the femoral head. With a hip dislocation, the risk for osteonecrosis is increased if hip reduction is not performed within 8 hours.[70]

Types of Osteonecrosis

- Traumatic
- Nontraumatic

In the nontraumatic type of osteonecrosis, the symptoms are hip pain (often a fairly abrupt onset of severe pain), decreased hip ROM, and stiffness. These symptoms are not specific to this condition, and no specific physical examination tests exist for osteonecrosis. The examiner therefore needs to rely on the history as the clue to pursue diagnostic imaging that would result in a definitive diagnosis. The male to female ratio for osteonecrosis is 4:1. The most common age range for onset is between the 3rd and 5th decades. Bilateral involvement is seen in more than 50% of cases. Red flags for nontraumatic osteonecrosis include a history of corticosteroid use, alcohol abuse, or sickle cell disease. Clinicians should keep in mind that plain x-ray films are not sensitive to osteonecrosis in the early stages, therefore being alert to any historical red flags is crucial. MRI is both sensitive and specific for diagnosing osteonecrosis (Figure 15-20), and the classic MRI finding is the crescent sign. The crescent sign is seen early on MRI as decreased signal indicative of the necrotic bone; when the crescent sign is observed on plain films at a more advanced stage of the disease process it is from a subchondral fracture between necrotic bone and healthy bone.

Red Flags for Hip Osteonecrosis

- History of corticosteroid use
- Alcohol abuse
- Sickle cell disease

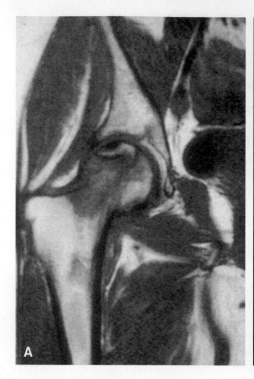
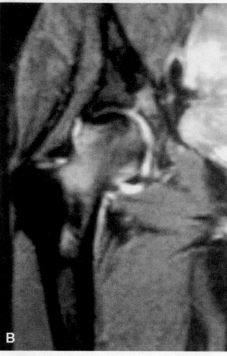

Figure 15-20

Osteonecrosis. Corresponding coronal T₁-weighted (TR/TE, 600/20) **(A)** and fat-suppressed fast T₂-weighted (TR/TE, 4000/70) **(B)** spin-echo magnetic resonance images reveal an area of osteonecrosis in the right femoral head, with associated articular collapse and joint effusion. Note the diffusely distributed abnormalities in the femoral head and neck compatible with marrow edema and the crescent sign on the superior femoral head. (From Resnick D, Kransdorf MJ: *Bone and joint imaging,* ed 3, p 1076, Philadelphia, 2005, WB Saunders.)

Treatment for osteonecrosis covers the gamut of surgical options for treatment of the hip. Mild cases respond well to core decompression, in which a hole is drilled up into the femoral head to release pressure. Moderately severe cases can be treated by osteotomy or vascularized fibular grafts. Severe or late stage cases require hemiarthroplasty or total hip replacement.[75]

It is very important for clinicians to be aware of osteonecrosis, because patients may be seen for hip pain that is mistakenly thought to be of soft tissue origin, when the real source of symptoms is osteonecrosis.[3] The prognosis is much better if the problem is diagnosed in the early stage, when core decompression can be performed.

Osteitis Pubis

Osteitis pubis is the most common inflammatory disorder affecting the pubic symphysis.[76] It generally is a self-limiting inflammation that occurs secondary to overuse, trauma, pelvic surgery, or childbirth. Although it can occur at any age, it is most common in males in their 3rd or 4th decade. Those most at risk are athletes who participate in sports involving repetitive shearing forces at the pubic symphysis and multidirectional deceleration and acceleration forces (e.g., soccer, ice hockey). Long distance runners are also prone to develop osteitis pubis. The gracilis muscle that attaches to the pubic symphysis has been implicated as a component in the etiology, and contracture or weakness (or both) of the gracilis often is seen with osteitis pubis.

A "groin burn" is a common complaint in patients with osteitis pubis. Depending on the irritability of the condition, the pain can be brought on by walking, running, climbing stairs, one leg stance, pivoting, kicking, and even coughing or sneezing. Rest usually relieves the pain. A prolonged, bilateral adductor contraction with the patient squeezing the clinician's fist between the knees can elicit groin pain. Resisted rectus abdominis contraction (situp) can also be painful. Tenderness is present at the superior or inferior pubic ramus (or both), and often both sides can be tender. Other conditions to consider in the differential diagnosis are groin strain, pubic rami stress fracture, hernia, and infectious osteitis pubis (most often occurring after urological or gynecological surgery).[76]

The imaging studies of choice are plain x-ray films and radionuclide bone scans. The x-ray findings, which may be negative in the early stage of osteitis pubis, usually include decreased definition of the cortical bone (irregular cortical margins and patchy sclerosis), and widening of the pubic symphysis may be seen. To assess for pubic symphysis widening, one-leg standing (flamingo) views are recommended. Bone scans usually show unilateral uptake at the pubic symphysis. Imaging helps differentiate osteitis pubis from other causes of groin pain, such as athletic pubalgia.

Treatment should begin with rest from the causative activity (e.g., soccer or running) and avoidance of aggravating activities. NSAIDs and ice can be helpful for the inflammation. If NSAIDs are not helpful, a corticosteroid injection into the site of maximum tenderness can be considered. Prolotherapy injections are also effective in some cases. Once the symptoms have abated, progressive rehabilitation stretching and strengthening of the hip musculature are initiated. Exercise in water can be particularly helpful. Heat-retaining compressive shorts can be helpful for dry land exercise and sport.[77]

Less Common Bone Pathologies

Like osteonecrosis, other bone pathologies can be the source of hip pain but can present with tenderness on palpation and produce positive results on hip tests (e.g., Patrick's test, the flexion/adduction test) and decreased ROM. Often these pathological conditions are not identifiable on plain x-ray films, and MRI may not be thought to be warranted. In addition to red flags in the history, a noncapsular pattern of ROM restriction suggests the need for further diagnostic workup. Examples of such bone pathologies are transient osteoporosis of the hip and symptomatic herniation pit.[78]

Transient Osteoporosis

Transient osteoporosis is a self-limiting, painful osteoporosis, usually of the proximal femur. Its cause is unknown, but the condition is most common in women in the third trimester of pregnancy and in men in their 4th or 5th decade. The onset of pain from transient osteoporosis can be sudden or gradual. Range of motion is often limited because of pain, and weight bearing is painful. X-ray films initially are normal, but by 6 weeks they usually show severe osteopenia with indistinctiveness of subchondral cortical bone.[79] MRI shows a nonspecific, diffuse pattern of bone marrow edema. Because the condition is self-limiting and usually resolves within 6 to 12 months, treatment involves protected weight bearing for pain relief and to prevent insufficiency fractures. The clinician should reassure the patient that this is a self-limiting condition. The patient should be encouraged to use touchdown weight bearing, or "feathering" (less than 10% of body weight), with crutches, and during pregnancy a wheelchair may also be helpful to limit the distance walked (e.g., for physician visits at a hospital). Rehabilitation intervention may be necessary to prevent the secondary effects of limited mobility, particularly a flexion contracture. An aquatic program has been described as an effective mode for ROM, hip strengthening (forward, backward, sidestepping ambulation), and trunk stabilization exercises postpartum.[80]

Symptomatic Herniation Pit

A herniation pit in the femoral neck is a normal variant in 5% of the population. It can become painful, at which time it becomes clinically significant. The pathogenesis of a herniation pit is related to an abrasive effect to the femoral neck from the iliopsoas tendon where it is tightly applied to the medial part of the capsule. The herniation pit can become symptomatic in athletes when rapid and forceful shortening and lengthening of the iliopsoas occurs. The pit also can enlarge and cause a painful cortical fracture.[81] Femoroacetabular impingement has also been implicated as a cause of herniation pits.[62]

Fractures and Dislocation

Hip (Proximal Femur) Fracture

Hip fracture is the orthopedic problem with the highest incidence, cost, and risk.[82] More than 300,000 hip fractures occur each year in the United States, with a 1-year mortality rate of nearly 25%, a life expectancy reduction of 25%, and lifetime health care costs approaching $25 billion.[83] The morbidity rate after fracture is 32% to 80%.[83] One interpretation of this data is that a hip fracture is part of a downward spiral of health. Although partly true, this view ignores evidence that many older adults are able to tolerate and make improvements in physical attributes and function.[84-86]

Approximately 90% of hip fractures result from a simple low energy fall.[87] The most common risk factors for falls (and thus hip fractures) are age, gender, race, institutionalization/hospitalization, medical co-morbidities (cardiac disease, stroke, dementia, prior hip fracture, osteoporosis), hip geometry, medication, bone density and body habitus, diet, smoking, alcohol consumption, fluorinated water, urban versus rural residence, and climate.[88] A fall results from poor balance reactions and decreased strength. The fall results in a hip fracture because the bone is weaker (usually osteoporotic), less soft tissue padding is present for shock absorption in the frail elderly, and older elders tend to fall on the hip because of their slower gait speed (Figure 15-21), whereas younger elders often fall forward onto an outstretched arm, resulting in a Colles' fracture at the wrist (Figure 15-22).[89]

Risk Factors for Falls and Hip Fractures[88]

- Older age
- Female
- Caucasian
- Institutionalization
- Medical co-morbidities
- Poor balance
- Decreased strength
- Hip geometry
- Medication
- Bone density
- Body habitus
- Diet
- Smoking
- Alcohol consumption
- Fluorinated water
- Urban residence
- Climate

Hip fracture is defined as a fracture of the proximal third of the femur. Most hip fractures need to be treated surgically. The type of fixation required depends on the location and degree of displacement of the fracture. Hip fractures are most simply categorized as intracapsular or extracapsular. Femoral neck fracture is the typical intracapsular fracture, and

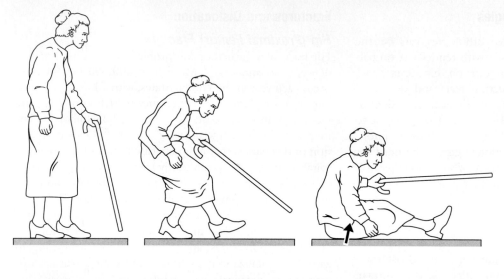

Figure 15-21

A fall that occurs while a person is standing still, walking slowly, or slowly descending a step has little forward momentum. With little forward momentum, the principal point of impact is near the hip. (Modified from Cummings SR, Nevitt MC: A hypothesis: the cause of hip fractures, *J Gerontol* 44: M107-M111, 1989.)

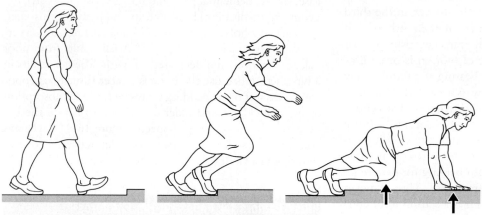

Figure 15-22

A fall that occurs while a person is walking rapidly has enough forward momentum to carry the individual onto the hands or knees instead of the hip. (Modified from Cummings SR, Nevitt MC: A hypothesis: the cause of hip fractures, *J Gerontol* 44: M107-M111, 1989.)

intertrochanteric fracture is the typical extracapsular fracture. A nondisplaced femoral neck fracture can be treated with pins or screws. A displaced femoral neck fracture requires hemiarthroplasty because the blood supply to the femoral head has been disrupted.

The two types of hemiarthroplasty are the unipolar type and the bipolar type. The bipolar implant has a pole of movement within the prosthesis that is designed to reduce wear on the acetabular cartilage. The bipolar endoprosthesis is more expensive than the unipolar design and is used with younger patients (approximately those less than 70 years of age) who might require revision to a total hip replacement during their lifetime usually because of acetabular cartilage degeneration. The original unipolar design (e.g., the Austin-Moore prosthesis) tends to be used on less active and older patients who are unlikely to outlive the hip implant. Recently, total hip arthroplasty has been advocated as the optimum treatment for displaced femoral neck fractures in the elderly. THA is associated with more independent living, it is more cost-effective, and there is a longer interval to reoperation or death than with open reduction and internal fixation (ORIF) and unipolar or bipolar hemiarthroplasty.[90]

For intertrochanteric fractures (stable or unstable), the sliding hip screw, which is available in a variety of designs, is the implant of choice.[87] Unstable intertrochanteric fractures sometimes are treated with an intramedullary device, but no difference in functional outcomes has been seen between it and the sliding hip screw.[87] THA is recommended for treatment of intertrochanteric fractures in patients with RA.[91] Figure 15-23 shows some of the implants commonly used in hip surgery.

Rehabilitation after a hip fracture must be intensive and multidisciplinary, because appropriate rehabilitation efforts can restore many patients to a prefracture functional status.[3] Weight bearing as tolerated (WBAT) for gait has been found to result in improved function for hip fracture patients over partial weight bearing (PWB) restriction, without deleterious effect to the surgical fixation.[92] In the acute care setting, more than one physical therapy visit per day has been shown to be predictive of achievement in basic function and of discharge home from the acute care setting.[82] Binder et al.[85] found that 6 months of extended outpatient rehabilitation, including progressive resistance training, for frail elderly patients with a hip fracture improved the patients' physical function and quality of life and reduced

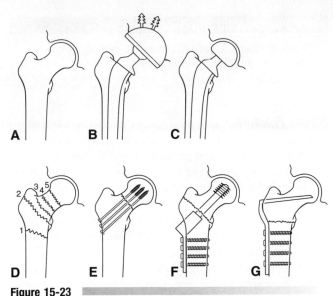

Figure 15-23
Various types of hip reconstructions and implants. **A,** Normal hip joint. **B,** Total hip arthroplasty. **C,** Hemiarthroplasty. **D,** Levels of proximal femoral fractures: *1,* Subtrochanteric; *2,* intertrochanteric; *3,* basicervical; *4,* transcervical (femoral neck); *5,* subcapital. **E,** Multiple screw fixation of a femoral neck fracture. **F,** Screw and plate fixation of an intertrochanteric hip fracture. **G,** Blade plate fixation of a proximal femoral osteotomy. In this drawing, no rotation of the proximal fragment was performed (Modified from Shinar AA: Surgeries of the hip: the approaches and the basics. In Fagerson TL, editor: *The hip handbook,* p. 239, Boston, 1998, Butterworth-Heinemann.)

their disability compared with a low intensity "standard" home exercise program. Mangione et al.[86] found that a sample of frail elderly patients who had ORIF or hemiarthroplasty for a hip fracture could tolerate a moderate to high intensity home exercise program of either resistance training or aerobic exercise with appropriate supervision.

Acetabular Fracture

Acetabular fractures are socket-side hip fractures but are categorized with fractures of the pelvis, unlike fractures of the proximal femur, which are designated as hip fractures. Most acetabular fractures occur as a result of high energy trauma, and they can be displaced or nondisplaced. Displaced acetabular fractures are treated with ORIF to allow earlier ambulatory function and to reduce the risk of post-traumatic arthritis. The ORIF hardware (screws and plates) is placed outside the joint to act as an "internal cast" until the bone heals. The hardware is not routinely removed.[93]

Perhaps more than in most other hip conditions or surgeries, application of a knowledge of in vivo force and pressure data is extremely important in the rehabilitation of surgical or nonsurgical acetabular fractures. Table 15-8 presents an evidence-based loading progression that is particularly useful for rehabilitation of acetabular fractures based on data from in vivo force and pressure measurements at the hip.[21] Most patients with an acetabular fracture begin with touch-down (feathering) weight bearing (TDWB), which, when performed correctly, results in less acetabular contact pressure than even non-weight-bearing (NWB), which can cause joint loading from hip muscle co-contraction. The exercise program should also follow a graduated loading progression that mirrors the healing stages of the fracture and is in synchronization with the physician's prescribed weight-bearing status.

Traumatic Hip Dislocation

Dislocation of the hip is most common after total hip arthroplasty; the incidence ranges from less than 1% to as high as 9%.[74] Dislocation of the hip in nonsurgical instances

Table 15-8

Progression of Activities of Daily Living and Exercise Based on in vivo Force and Pressure Data at the Hip

Low Load	Low Moderate Load	Moderate Load	High Moderate Load	High Load
TDWB gait performed correctly	PWB gait	FWB gait	AROM (standing) *no support*	Getting into and out of low chairs
NWB gait	Chair rise *with technique**	AROM (standing) *with support*	Maximum isometrics	Up and down stairs
PROM	Stairs *with technique*	One-leg stance *(with support)*	One-leg stance *no support*	Accidental stumble
AAROM	AROM (supine and prone) *no resistance*	Hip abduction (side lying) *no external resistance*	Slow jogging	Abductor resistance
Submaximum quad sets	Submaximum gluteal isometrics	Low resistance exercise (supine and prone)		Jumping
Bridging	Bridging			Running
Double leg stance				
Bicycle (no resistance)				

Modified from Fagerson TL: *Home study course: current concepts of orthopaedic physical therapy—hip,* La Crosse, WI, 2001, Orthopaedic Section, American Physical Therapy Association.
* *With technique* refers to the use of a load modifying variable, which a physical therapist can teach a patient. For example, for a chair rise, this could involve use of the armrests, having the affected leg out in front, sitting in a higher chair, or a combination of these. For stairs, *with technique* could involve ascent and descent one leg at a time, use of a banister and a crutch, or both.
TDWB, touch-down weight bearing; *NWB,* non weight bearing; *PROM,* passive range of motion; *AAROM,* active-assisted range of motion; *PWB,* partial weight bearing; *AROM,* active range of motion; *FWB,* full weight bearing.

is very rare; it usually occurs secondary to some form of trauma and often is associated with an acetabular and/or a femoral head fracture. Most traumatic hip dislocations are posterior (85% to 90%), and this usually is related to a mechanism of injury in which the hip is flexed and in some degree of adduction and the knee is flexed while a dislocating force drives the femoral head posteriorly out of the acetabular socket.[94] The classic mechanism is the dashboard injury in motor vehicle accidents, although the use of seat belts is reducing the incidence of this injury. In contact sports (e.g., football, rugby, ice hockey, wrestling), a fall or tackle onto a flexed hip and knee can also drive the femur posteriorly.

Posterior hip dislocations can be recognized based on the mechanism of injury. The patient has considerable posterior thigh and buttock pain, and the leg appears shortened and is held in flexion, adduction, and medial rotation. Prompt recognition and early reduction are essential for a good outcome. Before reduction under anesthesia is attempted, plain x-ray films should be taken to rule out a fracture of the femoral head or acetabulum. Reduction of a dislocated hip should be performed within 6 to 8 hours to reduce the risk of avascular necrosis of the femoral head, which occurs as a later complication in 10% to 15% of patients after posterior hip dislocation. For dislocated hips that are not reduced within 8 hours, the rate of femoral head osteonecrosis increases to 40%. Most traumatic dislocations of the hip are reduced using spinal or general anesthesia. However, before anesthesia is administered, one attempt at reduction can be made with an analgesic for pain and muscle spasm using the Allis or Stimson methods.[74] These methods use hip traction in 90° flexion with firm counterstabilization of the pelvis. The Allis method is performed with the patient in the supine position, whereas in the Stimson method the patient is prone with the hip flexed over the end of the examination table.[74]

A complication of hip dislocation for which the clinician should monitor is sciatic nerve palsy. Sciatic nerve injury occurs in 10% of posterior dislocations, and although it resolves in most cases over time, in some cases permanent footdrop develops. Vascular insufficiency is rare but can occur with anterior or open dislocations.

Fracture-dislocations usually require open reduction because attempts at closed reduction could further displace the fracture and increase the rate of complications. If less than 20% of the posterior margin of the acetabulum is fractured, conservative management is acceptable; however, larger fractures require ORIF.[74]

Once the dislocated hip has been reduced, management may require limited motion with a hip brace and patient education about risk positions. The risk position for posterior dislocation is combined flexion, adduction, and medial rotation. The risk position for anterior dislocation is combined extension and medial rotation. These movements, done rapidly, further increase the risk for redislocation.

Risk Positions for Hip Dislocation
- Posterior: Flexion, adduction, and medial rotation
- Anterior: Extension and lateral rotation

Stress Fracture

Stress fractures in the hip region usually are seen at the femoral neck, pubic rami, and proximal femoral shaft. Although most stress fractures occur in the lower leg and foot, 8.8% of lower extremity stress fractures are reported to occur in the hip and pelvic region.[95]

Stress fractures typically occur as a result of repetitive overuse that exceeds the intrinsic ability of bone to repair itself. Osteoclastic old bone resorption typically exceeds osteoblastic new bone formation by 3 to 4 weeks, and increased stress to the bone during this time (e.g., an increase in running mileage) can result in microfractures, which result in a stress fracture if the increased stress to the bone is continued. Resting and unloading the bone can allow the osteoblastic new bone formation to catch up.[96]

Early detection and appropriate management of stress fractures of the proximal femur are very important, because these fractures have a high rate of complication from nonunion, progression to complete fracture, and osteonecrosis.[97] A study of 23 athletes with femoral neck fractures found that the diagnosis was not confirmed, on average, until 14 weeks after the onset of symptoms, and this delay forced elite athletes to end their careers; this underscores the importance of keeping an open mind to diagnostic possibilities and ordering the necessary imaging earlier rather than later in the course of management.[98] The recommended imaging modalities for diagnosing stress fractures are bone scans or MRI, because stress fractures often can be missed on plain x-ray films.[99] Computed tomography (CT) also can be used.

Risk Factors for Stress Fractures[97]
- Participation in sports involving running and jumping
- Rapid increase in physical training program
- Poor preparticipation physical condition
- Female gender
- Hormonal or menstrual disturbances
- Low bone turnover rate
- Decreased bone density
- Decreased thickness of cortical bone
- Nutritional deficiencies (including dieting)
- Extremes of body size and composition
- Running on irregular or angled surfaces
- Inappropriate footwear
- Inadequate muscle strength
- Poor flexibility
- "Type A" behavior

The classic symptom of a lower extremity stress fracture is progressive, activity-related pain that is relieved by rest. Local tenderness often is present. A single leg hop test usually reproduces symptoms, and percussion of bone distal to the fracture site may reproduce symptoms.[100] A femoral neck stress fracture causes anterior thigh or groin pain (often an ache) that is relieved by rest, although night pain may be present in chronic cases. An antalgic (painful) gait, pain at the extremes of hip rotations (especially medial rotation), and pain with axial compression are common findings.[101] Clinicians should consider referral for further workup for stress fractures if continuous therapeutic ultrasound increases the patient's pain; this has been reported for lower leg stress fractures, and although it is not a sensitive tool for this diagnosis, the occurrence of increased pain with ultrasound used in treatment of suspected soft tissue injury should be a prompt for further workup.[102]

Stress fractures can be defined as fatigue or insufficiency fractures. Fatigue fractures tend to occur in young and middle-aged individuals from repetitive mechanical stress (e.g., distance running or military training). Insufficiency fractures tend to occur in older individuals when the bone is weakened from disease states, such as osteoporosis or osteomalacia. Fullerton and Snowdy[103] defined femoral neck fractures as compression, tension, and displaced fractures. Compression stress fractures tend to occur in the inferomedial femoral neck, and because they tend to be more stable, they can be treated with protected weight bearing and follow-up x-ray films (to ensure that no fracture displacement occurs during the healing process) until the patient is pain free. Tension stress fractures occur on the superolateral femoral neck, and because they are potentially unstable, they should treated with multiple screws or a sliding hip screw. Displaced fractures should be treated with ORIF.[19]

Nerve Syndromes

Theoretically, any nerve in the hip region can be injured. The nerves of the hip can be categorized into three groups of five nerves: five major nerves (the sciatic, femoral, obturator, superior gluteal, and inferior gluteal nerves); five minor nerves (the nerve to the quadratus femoris and inferior gemellus, the pudendal nerve, the posterior femoral cutaneous nerve, nerve to the obturator internus and superior gemellus, and the lateral femoral cutaneous nerve); and five "referring" nerves (the iliohypogastric nerve, the ilioinguinal nerve, the genitofemoral nerve, the cluneal nerves, and the sinuvertebral nerve). Irritation of nerve roots of the lumbar and sacral plexuses can also refer symptoms to the hip and buttock region.

Nerve injuries occur as a result of one of three mechanisms: compression, traction, or ischemia. The three types of nerve injury are neuropraxia, axonotmesis, and neurotmesis (described in greater detail in Chapter 20). Most nerve injuries about the hip have been described as a complication of total hip replacement, in which injury to the sciatic nerve is by far the most common complication. Surgeons also are very aware that the incision must not be extended more than 6 cm (2.4 inches) directly proximal beyond the tip of the greater trochanter, to avoid causing denervation of a branch of the superior gluteal nerve.[104]

In the nonsurgical setting, most nerve injuries at the hip occur as the result of mechanical entrapment, which causes a neuropraxia. Neuropraxia is an intact neural structure with decreased function because of local pressure, which produces ischemia and contusion of the nerve; usually full function is recovered after appropriate management. These nerve entrapments often are related to alignment, contractures, and repetitive or a single excessive overload or overstretch. The two most common nerve entrapments in relation to the hip are sciatic nerve entrapment by the piriformis muscle in the greater sciatic foramen and lateral femoral cutaneous nerve entrapment at the lateral edge of the inguinal ligament. Entrapments of other nerves in the hip region also have been reported in the literature, including the ilioinguinal nerve, femoral nerve, obturator nerve, genitofemoral nerve, lateral cutaneous branches of the subcostal and iliohypogastric nerves, and entrapment of the sciatic nerve at the level of the ischial tuberosity (hamstring syndrome).[21]

Nerve entrapments or injuries are easiest to diagnose when the symptoms include specific neurological features (i.e., motor weakness, sensory changes [numbness or tingling], and reflex change). Nerve entrapments are most difficult to diagnose when the primary symptom is pain, especially buttock pain or groin pain that mimics a muscle strain or tendonitis. Causalgia-like pain or reflex sympathetic dystrophy occasionally complicates recovery after a nerve injury.[104]

The two more common nonsurgical nerve entrapments at the hip are piriformis syndrome and meralgia paresthetica.

Piriformis Syndrome

Piriformis syndrome is a confusing diagnosis, because some practitioners believe that it is overdiagnosed, others that it is underdiagnosed, and some do not believe that it exists![105] Often it is a diagnosis of exclusion, when no other reason for pain in the buttock can be determined. Piriformis syndrome may account for up to 5% of cases of low back, buttock, and leg pain. It most commonly is seen in the 30 to 40 age range, and it often is associated with some form of trauma to the buttock.[106] Buttock tenderness is present over the piriformis muscle (especially in the greater sciatic notch) and surrounding tissues, and referred leg symptoms can arise from sciatic nerve irritation or from trigger points in the muscle itself. Flexion, adduction, internal (medial) rotation (FLADIR) of the hip usually causes buttock pain with piriformis syndrome. Numerous tests for piriformis syndrome have been described in the literature. Basically, they involve either passive stretching or resisted contraction of the piriformis muscle, and a positive test result is reproduction of symptoms in or emanating from the buttock.[3]

The piriformis is the only muscle that passes through the greater sciatic notch, along with six nerves (sciatic nerve, superior gluteal nerve, inferior gluteal nerve, pudendal nerve, posterior femoral cutaneous nerve, and the nerve to the quadratus femoris) and three vessel sets (superior gluteal artery and vein, inferior gluteal artery and vein, and internal pudendal artery and vein). Therefore a problem with the piriformis logically would have magnified effects because of its close anatomical relationship to numerous other neurovascular structures. A change in sacral or innominate alignment can also change the position of or tension in the piriformis in relation to these structures and thus potentially cause buttock and/or referred pain.

Several definitions of piriformis syndrome have been presented in the literature.[106] This author believes that treatment is best guided by an approach in which a diagnosis of piriformis syndrome is complemented by a statement of symptom mechanism and a statement of symptom distribution (e.g., "local buttock pain from fall onto buttock," or, "buttock and posterior leg pain to foot from sciatic irritation by piriformis in greater sciatic notch"). Differentiating piriformis syndrome from other lumbopelvic causes of referred pain into the buttock and posterior leg is important.

Piriformis syndrome is characterized by symptoms in the sciatic nerve distribution. Pain in the buttock alone is not piriformis syndrome; the term *piriformis syndrome* is associated with sciatic nerve irritation by the piriformis muscle. As mentioned, the piriformis muscle is the only muscle that passes through the greater sciatic foramen, which makes it the most likely muscular source of sciatic entrapment.

Likely aggravating factors for piriformis syndrome are walking, stair climbing, and activities involving trunk rotation. Less severe cases of piriformis syndrome can be exacerbated by repetitive or resistive lateral rotation (e.g., from kicking a soccer ball).[3] A positive piriformis test produces buttock pain with possible radiation into the leg. Travell and Simons[107] described the piriformis as "the double devil," because it can refer pain from irritation of the sciatic nerve or irritation of the piriformis trigger points.[107]

Treatment can include gentle, static stretching; ice massage; a vapocoolant spray and stretch technique; ultrasound; and NSAIDs. Techniques to promote balanced and optimal alignment, mobility, and stability of the lumbo-pelvic region are also worth pursuing. A heel insert of up to 0.64 cm (¼ inch) on the nonaffected side may take some tension off the piriformis. Rest from sporting activity for several weeks often is necessary.[3]

Meralgia Paresthetica

Entrapment of the lateral femoral cutaneous nerve of the thigh as it emerges from the pelvis adjacent to the anterior superior ischial spine (ASIS) can result in tingling, numbness, and pain in the nerve's sensory distribution on the anterolateral thigh. This condition is called *meralgia paresthetica*. It can present during pregnancy, in obese individuals, in laborers who carry heavy tool bags around their waists, and from direct trauma near the ASIS during sports. Sensory testing can confirm the diagnosis, and a positive Tinel's sign may be elicited by tapping adjacent to the ASIS and inguinal ligament. The diagnosis should not be made before other hip, lumbar, or intrapelvic pathology has been ruled out. Treatments that can be beneficial include correction of mechanical contributing factors, as well as rest, ultrasound, and NSAIDs if needed. In some cases, injection of an analgesic and a corticosteroid is warranted. In rare cases, when conservative measures have failed, surgical release of the nerve can be performed.[108]

Summary

Applying the information presented in this chapter to live clinical situations requires good clinical judgment. The most logical method for making clinical decisions is the risk-reward ratio: balancing cost (risk) against benefit (reward). The F balance (Figure 15-24) is an expansion of the risk-reward ratio that can be particularly helpful to the clinician in making decisions about a person presenting with hip pathology. In rehabilitation terms, clinicians balance achievement of best possible function against the risk of tissue failure (tissue breakdown or damage). Controlled forces (e.g., movement, mobilization, exercise) are used to improve form (e.g., strength, flexibility, endurance, balance), and both controlled forces and improved form are

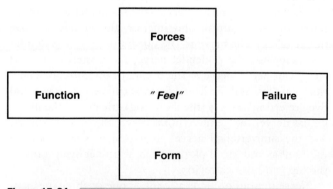

Figure 15-24

The F balance: A model for clinical decision making. (From Fagerson TL, editor: *The hip handbook*, p. 248, Boston, 1998, Butterworth-Heinemann.)

used to optimize function (e.g., transfers, walking, stairs, sports activity). The patient should always be the focus of the rehabilitation process; "feel" at the center of the F-balance refers to the importance of asking "how does the patient feel?" and incorporating his/her goals into the treatment plan.

References

To enhance this text and add value for the reader, all references have been incorporated into a CD-ROM that is provided with this text. The reader can view the reference source and access it online whenever possible. There are a total of 108 references for this chapter.

CHAPTER 16

KNEE: LIGAMENTOUS AND PATELLAR TENDON INJURIES

Michael M. Reinold, Eric M. Berkson, Peter Asnis, James J. Irrgang, Marc R. Safran, and Freddie H. Fu

Introduction

Successful nonsurgical and surgical management of knee ligament and patellar tendon injuries requires knowledge of the functional anatomy and biomechanics of the knee. This understanding forms the basis for the physical examination of the knee and foundation for treatment options. When a patient sustains a knee ligament injury or patellar tendon injury, the clinician must be able to integrate this information to evaluate the knee and to develop an appropriate treatment regimen.

The following chapter presents the scientific background of the principles of treatment of knee ligament and patellar tendon injuries. The functional anatomy and biomechanics of the knee are brought to a clinical level as the physical examination of the ligamentous injuries are presented. Specific ligamentous injuries are then discussed in terms of epidemiology, operative and nonoperative approaches to treatment, and rehabilitation.

Foundation for Surgical and Nonsurgical Management of Ligament and Patellar Tendon Injuries of the Knee

Functional Anatomy and Biomechanics of the Knee

The tibiofemoral joint is the articulation between the distal end of the femur and the tibial plateau. The femoral condyles are convex in the anterior and posterior and the medial and lateral directions. They are separated by the intercondylar notch, which serves as the site of attachment for the anterior and posterior cruciate ligaments. The width of the intercondylar notch may be an important consideration for the risk of injury to the cruciate ligaments and for the development of loss of extension after reconstruction of the anterior cruciate ligament. The transverse anterior to posterior dimension of the lateral femoral condyle is greater than that of the medial femoral condyle (Figure 16-1).[1] As a result, the lateral femoral condyle projects farther anteriorly than the medial femoral condyle, providing a bony buttress to minimize lateral displacement of the patella. The radius of curvature of the femoral condyles decreases from anterior to posterior and is shorter on the medial side than on the lateral side.[2] The anterior to posterior length of the articular surface of the medial femoral condyle is longer than that of the lateral femoral condyle.[1] The longer articular surface of the medial femoral condyle facilitates external rotation of the tibia as the knee approaches terminal extension.

Static (Passive) Restraints of the Knee

- Joint capsule
- Menisci (2)
- Ligaments, primarily:
  - Medial collateral ligament
  - Lateral collateral ligament
  - Anterior cruciate ligament
  - Posterior cruciate ligament
  - Posterior oblique ligament
  - Arcuate popliteus complex (meniscofemoral ligaments; ligaments of Humphrey and Wrisberg)

Dynamic (Active) Restraints of the Knee

- Quadriceps
- Hamstrings
- Gastrocnemius
- Iliotibial band (tensor fascia lata)
- Gracilis
- Sartorius
- Popliteus

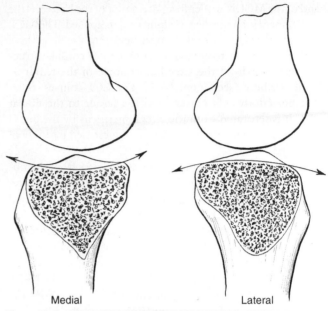

Figure 16-2
The medial tibial plateau is concave anterior to posterior, whereas the lateral tibial plateau is convex anterior to posterior. (From Kapandji IA: *The physiology of the joints: annotated diagrams of the mechanics of the human joints,* Edinburgh, 1970, Churchill Livingstone.)

The medial tibial plateau is concave from anterior to posterior and from medial to lateral. The lateral tibial plateau is convex from anterior to posterior (Figure 16-2). The concavity of the tibial plateaus is increased by the presence of the menisci. The bony configuration of the knee lends little inherent stability. Stability of the knee depends on static and dynamic restraints. The static restraints include the joint capsule, ligaments, and menisci. Dynamic stability is provided by muscles that cross the knee, including the quadriceps, hamstrings, and gastrocnemius.

The ligamentous restraints of the knee include the collateral, cruciate, and capsular ligaments. The medial collateral ligament (MCL) is a broad band that runs from the medial epicondyle of the femur to insert on the tibia two to three finger widths below the medial joint line (Figure 16-3). The MCL, which has been described as a thickening of the medial capsule, is divided into deep and superficial layers. The deep MCL is intimately attached to the medial meniscus and consists of the tibiomeniscal and femoromeniscal ligaments. The superficial band of the MCL runs from the medial epicondyle to insert distal to the tibial plateau. Because the superficial

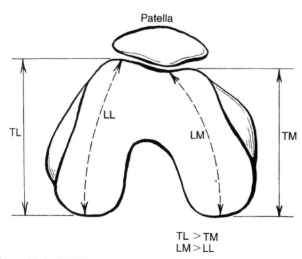

Figure 16-1
The transverse anterior-posterior dimension of the lateral femoral condyle *(TL)* is greater than that of the medial femoral condyle *(TM).* The anterior to posterior length of the articular surface of the medial femoral condyle *(LM)* is longer than the anterior to posterior length of the articular surface of the lateral femoral condyle *(LL).* (From Cailliet R, editor: *Knee pain and disability,* ed 3, Philadelphia, 1992, FA Davis.)

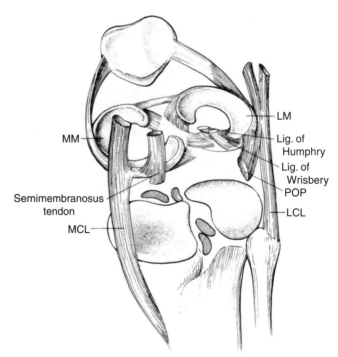

Figure 16-3
Ligamentous structures and menisci at the knee. *MM,* Medial meniscus; *LM,* lateral meniscus; *POP,* popliteus tendon; *MCL,* medial collateral ligament; *LCL,* lateral collateral ligament. (From Girgis FG, Marshall JL, Monngem ARS: The cruciate ligaments of the knee joint: anatomical function and experimental analysis, *Clin Orthop* 106:218, 1975.)

band of the MCL is farther from the center of the knee, it is the first ligament injured when a valgus stress is applied. The MCL courses anteriorly as it runs from the femur to the tibia.

The lateral collateral ligament (LCL) is a cordlike structure that runs from the lateral epicondyle of the femur to the fibular head (see Figure 16-3). The LCL courses somewhat posteriorly as it passes from the femur to the fibular head. It is separated from the lateral meniscus by the popliteus tendon, which partly explains the increased mobility of the lateral meniscus.

The anterior cruciate ligament (ACL) arises from the tibial plateau just anterior and medial to the tibial eminence. From the tibia, the ACL courses superiorly, laterally, and posteriorly to insert on the posterior margin of the medial wall of the lateral femoral condyle (Figure 16-4). The ACL has been described as being composed of two bundles: the anteromedial bundle, which is taut in flexion, and the posterolateral bundle, which is taut in extension (Figure 16-5).

The posterior cruciate ligament (PCL) arises from the posterior margin of the tibia just inferior to the tibial plateau. From the tibia, the PCL courses superiorly, anteriorly, and medially to insert on the lateral wall of the medial femoral condyle (Figure 16-6). The PCL has been described as consisting of two bands: the anterolateral band, which is taut in flexion, and the posteromedial band, which is taut with the knee in extension.

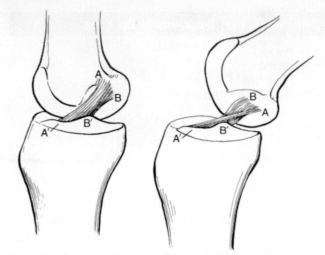

Figure 16-5

The anterior cruciate ligament is composed of two bundles. The anteromedial bundle (A-A′) is taut in flexion. The posterolateral bundle (B-B′) is taut in extension. (From Zachazewski JE, Magee DJ, Quillen WS, editors: *Athletic injuries and rehabilitation,* p 625, Philadelphia, 1996, WB Saunders.)

A synovial fold covers both cruciate ligaments. The ACL and PCL, therefore, are intrarticular but are considered to be extrasynovial. The predominant blood supply of the cruciate ligaments is the middle geniculate artery. Branches of this artery form a plexus within the encompassing synovial

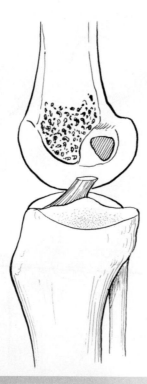

Figure 16-4

The anterior cruciate ligament arises from the tibial plateau anterior and medial to the tibial eminence and courses superiorly, laterally, and posteriorly to insert on the medial wall of the lateral femoral condyle. (From Zachazewski JE, Magee DJ, Quillen WS, editors: *Athletic injuries and rehabilitation,* p 625, Philadelphia, 1996, WB Saunders.)

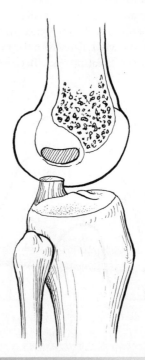

Figure 16-6

The posterior cruciate ligament arises from the posterior margin of the tibial plateau and courses superiorly, medially, and anteriorly to insert on the lateral wall of the medial femoral condyle. (From Zachazewski JE, Magee DJ, Quillen WS, editors: Athletic Injuries and Rehabilitation, p 625, Philadelphia, 1996, WB Saunders.)

sheath.[3] Disruption of this plexus is the source of the hemarthrosis typically seen after ACL injury.

The meniscofemoral ligaments course in a direction similar to that of the PCL. They arise from the posterior horn of the lateral meniscus and course superiorly and medially to insert on the lateral wall of the medial femoral condyle (see Figure 16-3). The ligament of Humphrey lies anterior to the PCL, and the ligament of Wrisberg lies posterior to the PCL. The meniscofemoral ligaments become taut with internal rotation of the tibia.

The posterolateral corner of the knee has a complex anatomy consisting of the biceps femoris, the LCL, and the popliteus complex. Dynamic and static components, including the popliteofibular ligament, the fabellofibular ligament, and the arcuate complex, add to this stability and prevent excessive posterior translation, varus rotation, and posterolateral rotation. The arcuate complex consists of the arcuate ligament, popliteus tendon, LCL, and posterior third of the lateral capsule.[4] The arcuate ligament arises from the fibular head and LCL to course superiorly and medially to insert along the popliteus tendon and lateral condyle of the femur. The popliteofibular ligament may be present in 98% of knees, but the anatomy of the posterolateral corner can vary significantly.[5] The presence of a fabella, a variable sesamoid bone in the tendinous portion of the gastrocnemius muscle, correlates with the presence of a fabellofibular ligament.

The medial and lateral menisci lie between the tibial plateaus and femoral condyles (see Figure 16-3). The menisci improve stability of the knee by increasing the concavity of the tibial plateaus. The menisci also absorb shock and distribute weight bearing over a greater surface area.

The outer third of the menisci is vascularized by the middle genicular artery, and the inner third of the menisci is considered to be avascular. Peripheral tears of the menisci, therefore, have the potential to heal and often are repaired surgically; however, tears in the inner third (the avascular zone) do not heal, and partial meniscectomy often is required. Baratz et al.[6] demonstrated the effects of a partial or total meniscectomy on the articular contact area and stress in the human knee. Total meniscectomy resulted in a concentration of high contact forces on a small area of the tibial plateau. Partial meniscectomy resulted in a smaller increase in contact stress. With a total meniscectomy, the increased tibiofemoral contact forces that result may predispose the patient to long-term degenerative changes. Therefore, partial meniscectomy is preferred to minimize this risk.

During flexion and extension of the knee, the menisci move posteriorly and anteriorly, respectively (Figure 16-7). This movement is a result of the bony geometry of the tibiofemoral joint. Posterior movement of the medial meniscus during flexion also is partly due to the insertion of a portion of the semimembranosus into the posterior horn of the medial meniscus. Similarly, fibers from the popliteus tendon inserting on the posterior horn of the lateral meniscus pull the

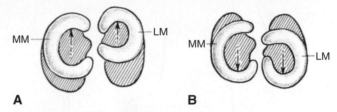

Figure 16-7

The menisci move anteriorly with extension (**A**) and posteriorly with flexion (**B**). The right knee is shown. *MM,* Medial meniscus; *LM,* lateral meniscus. (From Kapandji IA: *The physiology of the joints: annotated diagrams of the mechanics of the human joints,* Edinburgh, 1970, Churchill Livingstone.)

lateral meniscus posteriorly during flexion. Anterior-posterior movement of the lateral meniscus is greater than that of the medial meniscus, which reduces the susceptibility of the lateral meniscus to injury. During rotation of the knee, the menisci move relative to the tibial plateaus. During external rotation of the tibia, the medial meniscus moves posteriorly relative to the medial tibial plateau, whereas the lateral meniscus moves anteriorly relative to the lateral tibial plateau. During internal rotation of the tibia, movement of the menisci relative to the tibial plateaus is reversed.[2]

Flexion and extension of the knee combine rolling and gliding of the joint surfaces to maintain congruency of these surfaces. During flexion of the knee, the femur rolls posteriorly and glides anteriorly. During extension, the femur rolls anteriorly and glides posteriorly. The combined rolling and gliding of the joint surfaces maintains the femoral condyles on the tibial plateaus. Disruption of the normal arthrokinematics of the knee results in increased translation of the joint surfaces, which can lead to progressive degenerative changes of the articular surfaces.

Muller[7] described the ACL and PCL as a four-bar linkage system that maintains the normal arthrokinematics of the knee (Figure 16-8, *A*). Two of the four bars are the ACL and PCL. The remaining two bars are the line connecting the femoral attachments of the ACL and PCL and the line connecting the tibial attachments of the ACL and PCL. The ACL and PCL are inelastic and maintain a constant length as the knee flexes and extends. As a result, the four-bar linkage system controls rolling and gliding of the joint surfaces as the knee moves. During flexion, the femur rolls posteriorly. This increases the distance between the tibial and femoral insertions of the ACL. Because the ACL cannot lengthen, it guides the femoral condyles anteriorly (Figure 16-8, *B*). Conversely, during extension of the knee, the femoral condyles roll anteriorly and the distance between the femoral and tibial insertions of the PCL increases. Because the PCL cannot lengthen, it pulls the femoral condyles posteriorly as the knee extends (Figure 16-8, *C*). Disruption of the ACL or PCL disrupts the four-bar linkage system and results in abnormal translation

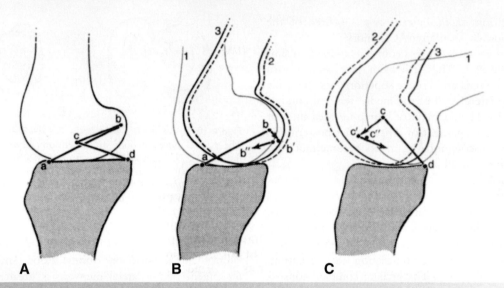

Figure 16-8

Four-bar linkage system. **A,** The four bars consist of the anterior cruciate ligament (ACL) *(line ab);* the posterior cruciate ligament (PCL) *(line cd);* the line connecting the femoral attachments of the ACL and PCL *(line cb);* and the line connecting the tibial attachments of the ACL and PCL *(line ad).* **B,** During flexion, the femur rolls posteriorly; this increases the distance between the tibial and femoral insertions of the ACL. Because the ACL cannot lengthen, it guides the femoral condyles anteriorly. **C,** During extension of the knee, the femoral condyles roll anteriorly and the distance between the femoral and tibial insertions of the PCL increases. Because the PCL cannot lengthen, it pulls the femoral condyles posteriorly as the knee extends. (From Kapandji LA: *The physiology of the joints: annotated diagrams of the mechanics of the human joints,* Edinburgh, 1970, Churchill Livingstone.)

of the femoral condyles. Disruption of the normal arthrokinematics of the knee may lead to repetitive injury of the menisci and joint surfaces and to the development of progressive degenerative changes over time.

Ligamentous Restraints of the Knee

The primary restraint to anterior translation of the tibia is the ACL, which provides approximately 85% of the total restraining force to anterior translation of the tibia.[8,9] The remaining 15% of the restraining ligamentous force to anterior displacement of the tibia is provided by the collateral ligaments, the middle portion of the medial and lateral capsules, and the iliotibial band (Table 16-1).

The primary restraint to posterior displacement of the tibia is the PCL. The PCL provides approximately 85% to 95% of the total restraining force to posterior translation of the tibia.[8] The remaining 5% to 15% of the total ligamentous restraining force to posterior displacement of the tibia is provided by the collateral ligaments, the posterior portion of the medial and lateral capsules, and the popliteus tendon. The ligaments of Humphrey and Wrisberg also provide restraint to posterior translation of the tibia, and their ability to do so increases with internal rotation of the tibia (see Table 16-1).

The primary restraint to valgus rotation is the MCL. The ACL and PCL serve as secondary restraints to valgus rotation. When the knee is in full extension, the posterior

Table 16-1
Primary and Secondary Restraints of the Knee

Tibial Motion	Primary Restraint	Secondary Restraints
Anterior translation	ACL	MCL, LCL; middle third of medial and lateral capsule; iliotibial band
Posterior translation	PCL	MCL, LCL; posterior third of medial and lateral capsule; popliteus tendon; anterior and posterior meniscofemoral ligaments
Valgus rotation	MCL	ACL, PCL; posterior capsule when knee is fully extended
Varus rotation	LCL	ACL, PCL; posterior capsule when knee is fully extended
External rotation	MCL, LCL	
Internal rotation	ACL, PCL	Anterior and posterior meniscofemoral ligaments

From Zachazewski JE, Magee DJ, Quillen WS, editors: *Athletic injuries and rehabilitation,* p 627, Philadelphia, 1996, WB Saunders.
ACL, anterior cruciate ligament; *MCL,* medial collateral ligament; *LCL,* lateral collateral ligament; *PCL,* posterior collateral ligament.

capsule becomes a significant restraint to valgus rotation (see Table 16-1). For varus rotation, the primary restraint is the LCL, and the ACL and PCL serve as secondary ligamentous restraints. The restraining force provided by the ACL and PCL, as well as the posterior capsule, increases when the knee is in full extension (see Table 16-1).

External rotation of the tibia is restrained by the collateral ligaments, whereas internal rotation is restrained by the cruciate ligaments and the ligaments of Humphrey and Wrisberg (see Table 16-1).

The quadriceps and hamstrings serve as dynamic stabilizers of the knee. In doing so, they assist the passive restraints in controlling kinematics of the knee. These muscles work synergistically with the cruciate ligaments to control motion of the knee dynamically. Unopposed contraction of the quadriceps is synergistic to the PCL and antagonistic to the ACL. Conversely, isolated contraction of the hamstrings is synergistic to the ACL and antagonistic to the PCL. It is theorized that activities that promote co-contraction of the hamstrings and quadriceps minimize tibial translation, and activities of this type have been advocated for rehabilitation of knee ligament injuries.[10] Dynamic stabilization of the knee to control abnormal motion depends on muscular strength and endurance, as well as on the development of appropriate neuromuscular control.

Role of Proprioception

Researchers have shown increased interest in the role of proprioception in the prevention and progression of knee injuries.[11-14] Proprioception has been described as a variation in the sense of touch; it includes the senses of joint motion (kinesthesia) and joint position. Proprioception is mediated by sensory receptors in the skin, musculotendinous unit, ligaments, and joint capsule. These sensory receptors transduce mechanical deformation to a neural signal, which modulates conscious and unconscious responses. It has been hypothesized that proprioception is important for providing smooth, coordinated movement and for protecting and dynamically stabilizing the knee.[13,15-17]

Mechanoreceptors in the knee may mediate protective reflexes. Solomonow et al.[13] described an ACL-hamstring reflex arc in anesthetized cats. High loading of the ACL resulted in increased electromyographic (EMG) activity in the hamstrings, with electrical silence in the quadriceps. The increase in hamstring EMG activity was not evident when low to moderate loads were applied to the ACL. It originally was thought that the ACL-hamstring reflex arc protected the ACL during high loading conditions. However, recent studies have shown that this reflex has a relatively long latency in humans; therefore, rather than being a protective reflex, it may be important for updating motor programs.[18]

Other proprioceptive reflexes originating from the joint capsule or musculotendinous unit probably exist. This was demonstrated by Solomonow et al.,[13] who reported increased hamstring EMG activity in a patient with an ACL-deficient knee during maximum slow speed isokinetic testing of the quadriceps. The increased hamstring EMG activity occurred simultaneously with anterior subluxation of the tibia at approximately 40° knee flexion and was associated with a sharp decrease in quadriceps torque and inhibition of quadriceps EMG activity. Because the ACL was ruptured, reflex contraction of the hamstrings could not have been mediated by receptors originating in the ACL. It was proposed that this reflex contraction is mediated by receptors in the joint capsule or hamstring muscles.

Several clinical studies have evaluated proprioception in terms of threshold to detection of passive motion and reproduction of passive joint position. Barrack et al.[11] demonstrated deficits in threshold to detection of passive motion in subjects with a unilateral ACL-deficient knee. Barrett[16] demonstrated high correlations between measurements of proprioception and function ($r = 0.84$) and patient satisfaction ($r = 0.90$) in 45 patients who had undergone ACL reconstruction. Standard knee scores and clinical examination results correlated poorly with the patient's own opinion and the results of functional tests. Lephart et al.[14] studied the threshold to detection of passive movement in patients who had undergone ACL reconstruction. Testing was performed at 15° and 45° flexion. Three trials were performed, moving into flexion and extension. The results indicated that the threshold to detection of passive movement was less sensitive in the reconstructed knee than the noninvolved knee. Also, the threshold to detection of passive motion was more sensitive in both the reconstructed knee and the normal knee at 15° flexion than at 45° flexion. Sensitivity to detection of passive motion was enhanced by the use of a neoprene sleeve, which has implications for bracing after ACL injury and/or reconstruction. Use of a sleeve or compressive wrap or garment may help the patient develop a greater sense of perception of the knee during rehabilitation and progressive activity.

Injury to the knee may result in abnormal sensory feedback and altered neuromuscular control, which may lead to recurrent injury. Proprioceptive training after knee injury and/or surgery should attempt to maximize the use of sensory information mediated by the ligaments, joint capsule, and/or musculotendinous unit to stabilize the joint dynamically. Proprioceptive training requires repetition to develop motor control of abnormal joint motion and may be enhanced with the use of EMG biofeedback. Initially, control of abnormal joint motion requires conscious effort. Through repetitive training, motor control of abnormal movement becomes automatic and occurs subconsciously. It should be noted, however, that the extent to which an individual can develop neuromuscular control of abnormal joint motion to stabilize the knee dynamically currently is unknown. Further research is required to determine the effectiveness of proprioceptive training to stabilize the knee dynamically.

Biomechanics of Exercise

Open kinetic chain (OKC) exercise is exercise in which the distal segment is free to move, resulting in isolated movement at a given joint. At the knee, OKC exercise results in isolated flexion and extension. OKC knee extension is a result of isolated contraction of the quadriceps, and open chain knee flexion occurs as a result of isolated contraction of the hamstrings. Baratta et al.[17] and Draganich et al.[19] demonstrated low levels of co-activation of the quadriceps and hamstrings during open chain knee extension. It is hypothesized that the hamstrings become active during the terminal range of extension to decelerate the knee and act as a synergist to the ACL to minimize anterior tibial translation produced by contraction of the quadriceps. During open chain knee extension, the flexion moment arm increases as the knee is extended from 90° flexion to full extension (0°). This requires increasing quadriceps and patellar tendon tension, which can increase the load on the patellofemoral and tibiofemoral joints.

During closed kinetic chain (CKC) exercises, the distal segment is relatively fixed; therefore movement at one joint results in simultaneous movement of all other joints in the kinetic chain in a predictable manner. The lower extremity functions as a closed kinetic chain when a person squats over the fixed foot, resulting in simultaneous movement of the ankle, knee, and hip. CKC exercise for the lower extremity results in contraction of muscles throughout the lower extremity. During CKC exercises for the lower extremity, the flexion moment arms at the knee and hip increase as the squat is performed, and increased force of contraction of the quadriceps and hamstrings is required to control the knee and hip, respectively.

OKC and CKC exercises have different effects on tibial translation and ligamentous strain and load. During active OKC knee extension, the shear component produced by unopposed contraction of the quadriceps depends on the angle of knee flexion (Figure 16-9). Sawhney et al.[20] investigated the effects of isometric quadriceps contraction on tibial translation in subjects with an intact knee. Tibial translation was measured with the KT1000 Ligament Arthrometer (MEDmetric, San Diego, CA) at 30°, 45°, 60°, and 75° flexion. Open chain isometric quadriceps contraction against 10 pounds (4.5 kg) of resistance applied to the distal aspect of the leg resulted in anterior tibial translation at 30° and 45° flexion. No significant tibial translation occurred at 60° or 75° flexion. It was determined that the quadriceps-neutral Q angle (i.e., the angle at which quadriceps contraction produces no anterior or posterior tibial translation) occurs at 60° to 75° flexion (see Figure 16-9, *A*). OKC knee extension at angles less than the quadriceps-neutral position results in anterior translation of the tibia. This was demonstrated by Grood et al.[9] in intact cadaveric knees. Anterior translation of the tibia during OKC knee extension increased with loading of the quadriceps at angles less than 60° flexion. Sectioning of the ACL increased anterior translation during loaded and unloaded open chain knee extension. Anterior tibial translation produced by the quadriceps at knee flexion angles less than the quadriceps-neutral angle is a result of the anteriorly directed shear component of the patellar tendon force (see Figure 16-9, *B*). OKC knee extension at knee flexion angles greater than the quadriceps-neutral position results in posterior tibial translation. This is the result of a posteriorly directed shear component of the patellar tendon force at these angles of knee flexion (see Figure 16-9, *C*).

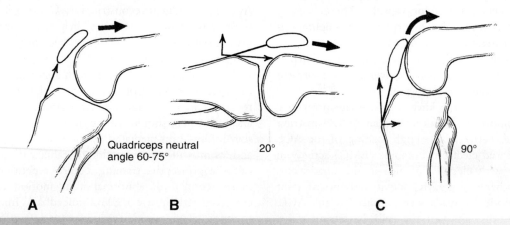

Figure 16-9

During open chain knee extension, tibial translation is a function of the shear force produced by the patellar tendon. **A,** Quadriceps neutral position. The patellar tendon force is perpendicular to the tibial plateaus and results in compression of the joint surfaces without shear. **B,** At flexion angles less than the angle of the quadriceps neutral position, orientation of the patellar tendon produces anterior shear of the tibia. **C,** At angles greater than the angle of the quadriceps neutral position, patellar tendon force causes a posterior shear of the tibia. (From Daniel DM, Stone ML, Barnett P, Sachs R: Use of the quadriceps active test to diagnose posterior cruciate ligament disruption and measure posterior laxity of the knee, *J Bone Joint Surg Am* 70:386-391, 1988.)

OKC knee flexion is produced by isolated contraction of the hamstrings. This has been shown to result in posterior translation of the tibia and was demonstrated by Lutz et al.,[21] who found posterior tibial shear forces during isometric open chain knee flexion at 30°, 60°, and 90° knee flexion. The posterior shear force increased as flexion progressed from 30° to 90° flexion.

Several methods of biomechanical analysis have been used to study rehabilitation of the knee, including cadaveric, EMG, kinematic, kinetic, mathematical modeling, and in vivo strain gauge measurements. These studies are best evaluated by delineating the findings according to the tissue or structure examined, such as the ACL, the PCL, and the patellofemoral joint.

Anterior Cruciate Ligament

Most biomechanical research on rehabilitation of the knee has focused on the ACL. After years of theoretical and anecdotal assumptions, researchers now are better able to scrutinize more closely the efficacy of OKC and CKC exercises. Markolf et al.[22] examined the effect of compressive loads on cadaveric knees to simulate body weight. These authors reported that compressive forces reduce strain on the ACL, compared to OKC exercises, thus providing a protective mechanism. Fleming et al.[23] investigated this theory using in vivo strain gauge measurements in the ACL. This method allows direct measurement of ACL strain during activity. The authors noted that strain on the ACL increased from −2% during non-weight-bearing to 2.1% in a weight-bearing position. Although an increase in ACL strain was observed in a weight-bearing position, it still is unclear whether a 2% strain is detrimental to a healing ACL graft. Clinical experience has shown that early weight bearing does not result in poor functional outcomes in postoperative ACL reconstructions.

CKC exercises have also been theorized to reduce ACL strain by providing co-contraction of the hamstrings and quadriceps. Wilk et al.[24] examined the EMG activity of the quadriceps and hamstrings during the CKC squat and leg press and the OKC knee extension. These authors noted that co-contraction occurred from 30° to 0°, during the ascent phase of the squat, when the body is positioned directly over the knees and feet, but it did not occur at other ranges of motion or during the CKC leg press or OKC knee extension. Therefore, not all CKC exercises produce a co-contraction of the quadriceps and hamstrings. Rather, several factors appear to affect muscle activation during CKC exercises, including the knee flexion angle, body position relative to the knee, and the direction of movement (ascending or descending). Clinically, exercises performed in an upright and weight-bearing position with the knee flexed to approximately 30° (e.g., squats and lateral lunges) may be used during knee rehabilitation to promote co-contraction of the quadriceps and hamstrings.

Wilk et al.[24] also used mathematical modeling to estimate the shear forces at the tibiofemoral joint during the squat,

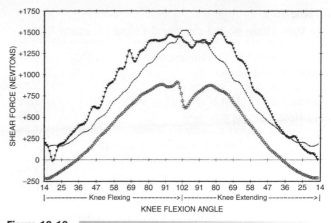

Figure 16-10

Tibiofemoral shear forces observed throughout the range of motion during closed kinetic chair squat *(filled triangles)* and leg press *(small points)* exercises and open kinetic chain knee extension exercises *(open circles)*. (From Wilk KE, Escamilla RF, Fleisig GS et al: A comparison of tibiofemoral joint forces and electromyographic activity during open and closed kinetic chain exercises, *Am J Sports Med* 24:522, 1996.)

leg press, and knee extension exercise (Figure 16-10). The authors reported that a posterior tibiofemoral shear force was observed during the entire range of motion during both the CKC squat and leg press (peak, 1500 newtons [N]), and during deep angles of OKC knee extension from 100° to 40° (peak, 900 N). Anterior tibiofemoral shear force (peak, 250 N), and theoretically ACL strain, was observed during the OKC knee extension exercise from 40° to 10°.

Similar to the results of Wilk et al.,[24] Beynnon et al.,[25] using in vivo strain gauge measurements, found that the greatest amount of ACL strain (2.8%) occurred during 40° to 0° OKC knee extension. This strain was found to increase significantly in a linear fashion with the application of an external 45 Newton boot (3.8%). However, the authors also reported an ACL strain of 3.6% during the CKC squat exercise. In contrast, application of external loading did not significantly increase the amount of strain on the ACL (4%).

Based on the findings of Fleming et al.[23], Wilk et al.,[24] and Beynnon et al.,[25] both OKC and CKC exercises should be performed during rehabilitation of a reconstructed ACL, although the patient often is limited to 90° to 40° during the OKC knee extension when heavy resistance is applied.

The bicycle and stair climbers also are commonly used during ACL rehabilitation. Fleming et al.[26] analyzed six different bicycle riding conditions, manipulating speed and power. These authors found no significant differences among these conditions (minimal mean ACL strain of 1.7%). The greatest amount of strain was observed when the knee reached the greatest amount of extension. Similarly, Fleming et al.[27] analyzed two cadences of stair climbing (80 and 112 steps per minute) and noted a similar 2.7%

Table 16-2
In Vivo Strain on the Anterior Cruciate Ligament

Isometric quadriceps contraction at 15°	4.4%
Squatting with resistance	4.0%
Active knee flexion with resistance	3.8%
Lachman's test (150 N of anterior shear at 30°)	3.7%
Squatting without resistance	3.6%
Active knee flexion without resistance	2.8%
Quadriceps and hamstring co-contraction at 15°	2.7%
Isometric quadriceps contraction at 30°	2.7%
Stair climbing	2.7%
Anterior drawer test (150 N anterior shear at 90°)	1.8%
Stationary bicycle	1.7%
Quadriceps and hamstrings co-contraction at 30°	0.4%
Passive knee range of motion	0.1%
Isometric quadriceps contraction at 60° and 90°	0.0%
Quadriceps and hamstrings co-contraction at 60° and 90°	0.0%
Isometric hamstring contraction at 30°, 60°, and 90°	0.0%

Modified from Fleming BC, Beynnon BD, Renstrom PA et al: The strain behavior of the anterior cruciate ligament during stair climbing: an in vivo study, *Arthroscopy* 15:185-191, 1999.

Table 16-3
Posterior Tibiofemoral Shear Forces

Source	Activity	Knee Angle (Degrees)	Force (× Body Weight)
Kaufman[30]	60°/sec flexion isokinetic	75	1.7
	180°/sec flexion isokinetic	75	1.4
Morrison[28]	Level walking	5	0.4
Morrison[29]	Descending stairs	5	0.6
	Ascending stairs	45	1.7
Smidt[31]	Isometric flexion	45	1.1

strain on the ACL. Again, the greatest strain was observed during terminal knee extension. Therefore, both bicycling and stair climbing are safe exercises to perform that put low strain on the ACL compared to other rehabilitation exercises (Table 16-2). Furthermore, the finding that the greatest amount of strain occurred as the knee moved into terminal knee extension was similar to the results seen by Wilk et al.[24] and Beynnon et al.[25] during OKC and CKC exercises.

Posterior Cruciate Ligament

Historically, rehabilitation after injury to the PCL has had mixed results. Poor functional outcomes have often been attributed to residual laxity after surgical reconstruction. The biomechanics of the tibiofemoral joint during exercise must be understood so that the rehabilitative process does not have deleterious effects on the PCL.

Posterior tibiofemoral shear forces that occur during specific activities, such as level walking,[28] ascending and descending stairs,[29] and resisted knee flexion exercises,[30,31] have been documented.[32] Level walking and descending stairs have a relatively low posterior tibiofemoral shear force, 0.4 × body weight (BW) and 0.6 × BW, respectively (Table 16-3). However, high posterior shear force has been noted during several commonly performed activities of daily living, such as climbing stairs (1.7 × BW at 45° knee flexion)[29,33] and squatting (3.6 × BW at 140° knee flexion), which may have an effect on residual laxity after surgery. Further studies have shown that isometric knee flexion at 45° places a posterior shear force of 1.1 × BW on the tibiofemoral joint.[31]

Tremendous shear forces on both the PCL and the tibiofemoral joint occur during OKC resisted knee flexion. Posterior tibial displacement is attributed to the high EMG activity of the hamstring muscles during resistive knee flexion. Lutz et al.[21] reported a maximum shear force of 1780 N at 90°, 1526 N at 60°, and 939 N at 30° during isometric knee flexion. Kaufman et al.[30] also noted a PCL load of 1.7 × BW at 75° during isokinetic knee flexion exercise. Because PCL stress increases with the knee flexion angle, isolated OKC knee flexion exercises should be avoided for at least 8 weeks after surgery or, in patients who did not undergo surgery, until symptoms subside.

Excessive stress on the PCL has also been observed during deeper angles of OKC knee extension. Several studies have proven that resisted knee extension at 90° flexion causes a posterior tibiofemoral shear and potential stress on the PCL.[13,20,21,24,34] Wilk et al.[24] documented a posterior shear force from 100° to 40° with resisted OKC knee extension. The greatest amount of stress on the PCL was seen at angles of 85° to 95° during knee flexion. Conversely, the lowest amount of posterior shear force occurred from 60° to 0° of resisted knee extension.[24] Kaufman et al.[30] also reported that posterior shear forces are exerted until 50° to 55° knee flexion. Jurist and Otis[34] documented stress on the PCL at 60° flexion during an isometric knee extension exercise when resistance is applied at the proximal tibia. To reduce the excessive posterior shear force on the PCL, OKC resisted knee extension should be performed from 60° to 0°.[32]

The stress applied to the PCL during CKC exercises depends on the knee flexion angle produced during the exercise. Wilk et al.[24,35] reported an increase in posterior shear force as the knee flexion angle increased during CKC exercise. Stuart et al.[36] also documented a linear increase in posterior shear force from 40° to 100° knee flexion during the front squat maneuver. Therefore, to reduce PCL stress during CKC exercises, leg presses and squats should be performed from 0° to 60° knee flexion.[32]

Patellofemoral Joint

The effects of OKC versus CKC exercises on the patellofemoral joint must be considered in a rehabilitation regimen after knee ligament injury and/or surgery. The patellofemoral joint consists of the articulation between the patella and the distal end of the femur. The patella is embedded in the knee extensor mechanism and is the largest sesamoid bone in the body. Proximally, the quadriceps inserts into the patella through the quadriceps tendon. Distally, the patella is connected to the tibia through the patellar tendon. The patella protects the anterior aspect of the knee, increases the effective moment arm of the knee extensor mechanism, and centralizes the divergent forces produced by the quadriceps. The tendency of the patella to sublux laterally (produced by the Q [quadriceps] angle, the vastus lateralis, and the lateral retinacular structures) must be counterbalanced by the oblique fibers of the vastus medialis. Maintaining this balance is crucial to normal function of the knee extensor mechanism.

The patella is a triangular bone with the base directed superiorly and the apex directed inferiorly. The patella is described as having three facets on its posterior aspect. A central ridge that runs from superior to inferior divides the patella into medial and lateral facets. The odd facet lies on the medial border of the patella and engages the femur only during the extreme range of flexion. The posterior margin of the patella is covered by a thick layer of articular cartilage, which is thicker centrally than peripherally. This layer of articular cartilage is thicker than at any other joint in the body, perhaps up to 5 mm thick.[37] It is important for reducing friction and aiding lubrication of the patellofemoral joint.

The stability of the patellofemoral joint depends on static and dynamic restraints. Static restraints consist of the shape of the patellofemoral joint and the medial and lateral patellofemoral ligaments. The lateral femoral condyle projects farther anteriorly than the medial femoral condyle and serves as a buttress to minimize lateral displacement of the patella. Dynamic stability of the patellofemoral joint is provided by the quadriceps. The vastus medialis oblique (VMO) and medial retinaculum provide medial stabilization of the patella. The vastus lateralis, lateral retinaculum, and iliotibial band pull the patella laterally. The Q angle is the angle formed by lines that connect the anterior superior iliac spine (ASIS) to the midpatella and the midpatella to the tibial tubercle. The Q angle results in lateral displacement of the patella when the quadriceps contracts. Lateral displacement of the patella is dynamically resisted by the VMO and medial retinaculum. Weakness of the VMO allows the patella to track laterally. In addition, tightness of the lateral retinaculum and overpull from the vastus lateralis and iliotibial band can result in lateral displacement of the patella.

Prevention and/or treatment of patellofemoral symptoms after knee ligament injury or surgery should seek to maintain or restore the balance of the medial and lateral stabilizers of the patellofemoral joint.

Hungerford and Barry[38] described the patellofemoral contact pattern as the knee moves through a full range of motion (Figure 16-11). The patella initially makes contact with the femur in the trochlear groove at approximately 20° flexion. Initial contact is between the trochlear groove and the inferior pole of the patella. As flexion progresses, the contact area on the patella progresses superiorly, so that by 90° flexion, the entire articular surface of the patella, except for the odd medial facet, has articulated with the femur. As flexion continues beyond 90°, the quadriceps tendon articulates with the trochlear groove and the patella moves into the intercondylar notch area of the femur. At full flexion, the odd medial facet and

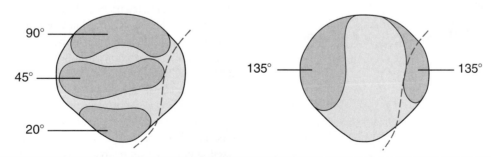

Figure 16-11

Patellofemoral contact pattern. Initial contact between the trochlear groove and the inferior pole of the patella occurs at approximately 20° flexion. As flexion progresses, the area of contact migrates superiorly so that by 90° flexion, the entire articular surface of the patella except for the odd facet has articulated with the trochlear groove. At full flexion, the odd medial facet and lateral facet articulate with the intercondylar notch. (From Magee DJ: Orthopedic Physical Assessment, ed 3, p 729, St. Louis, 2007, Saunders.)

lateral facet of the patella articulate with the intercondylar notch. The odd medial facet articulates with the femur only at the end range of flexion.

A knowledge of the patellofemoral contact pattern is useful for determining the limits of motion when patients with patellofemoral symptoms perform OKC and CKC exercises. *Generally, exercises should be performed in the pain-free and crepitus-free range of motion.* It should also be noted that the patellofemoral contact area increases from 20° to 90° flexion. This increase helps distribute patellofemoral joint reaction forces over a larger area to reduce patellofemoral contact stress per unit of area. (Chapter 18 presents a more detailed discussion of the impact of patellofemoral forces and mechanics during rehabilitation and activity.)

Alterations in the Q angle often are associated with patellofemoral disorders. They may alter the contact areas and thus the amount of joint reaction forces of the patellofemoral joint. Huberti and Hayes[39] examined the in vitro patellofemoral contact pressures at various degrees of knee flexion from 20° to 120°. The maximum contact area occurred at 90° knee flexion, where contact pressure was estimated to be 6.5 × BW. An increase or decrease in the Q angle of 10° resulted in increased maximum contact pressure and a smaller total area of contact throughout the range of motion. Clinicians can use this information in prescribing rehabilitation interventions to ensure that exercises are performed in ranges of motion that place minimal strain on damaged structures.

Patellofemoral joint reaction force is a function of quadriceps and patellar tendon tension and of the angle formed between the quadriceps and patellar tendons (Figure 16-12).

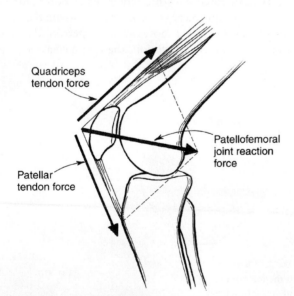

Figure 16-12

Patellofemoral joint reaction force. This is a function of patellar and quadriceps tendon tension and the angle formed between the quadriceps and patellar tendons. This force increases with increasing patellar and quadriceps tendon tension and an increasing angle of knee flexion. (From Zachazewski JE, Magee DJ, Quillen WS, editors: *Athletic injuries and rehabilitation*, p 633, Philadelphia, 1996, WB Saunders.)

This force compresses the patellofemoral joint, with increasing patellar and quadriceps tendon tension and an increasing angle of knee flexion. Patellofemoral joint reaction forces during functional CKC activities were calculated by Reilly and Martens[40] and were found to be 0.5 × BW during level walking, 3.3 × BW on stairs, and 7.8 × BW during a full squat. These results are consistent with activities that increase patellofemoral symptoms.

OKC and CKC exercises produce different effects on patellofemoral joint reaction force and contact stress per unit area. During open chain knee extension, the flexion moment arm for the knee increases as the knee is extended from 90° flexion to full extension (0°), which results in increased quadriceps and patellar tendon tension and increasing patellofemoral joint reaction forces. For CKC exercises, the flexion moment arm of the knee increases as the angle of knee flexion increases. In the case of OKC exercises, the patellofemoral joint reaction forces may be concentrated in a relatively small contact area, resulting in larger contact stresses per unit area; this can create forces that ultimately result in symptoms such as pain and possibly degenerative change. Conversely, for CKC exercises, the flexion moment arm of the knee increases as the knee flexion angle increases. Greater quadriceps and patellar tendon tension is required to counteract the increasing flexion moment arm. By controlling the position of the foot, ankle, knee, and hip in this weight-bearing position, it may be possible to influence the position and "tracking" of the patella, which results in increasing patellofemoral joint reaction force as the knee flexes. This force is distributed over a larger patellofemoral contact area, minimizing the increase in contact stress per unit area.

The effectiveness and safety of OKC and CKC exercises during patellofemoral rehabilitation have been heavily scrutinized in recent years. CKC exercises replicate functional activities, such as ascending and descending stairs, but OKC exercises often are important for isolated muscle strengthening when specific muscle weakness is present.[41]

Steinkamp et al.[42] analyzed patellofemoral joint biomechanics during the leg press and extension exercises in 20 normal subjects. Patellofemoral joint reaction force, stress, and moments were calculated during both exercises. At 0° to 46° knee flexion, the patellofemoral joint reaction force was less during the CKC leg press. Conversely, at 50° to 90° knee flexion, joint reaction forces were lower during the OKC knee extension exercise. Joint reaction forces were minimal at 90° knee flexion during the knee extension exercise. Similar findings have been reported by Escamilla et al.,[43] who studied patellofemoral compressive forces during the OKC knee extension and the CKC leg press and vertical squat. OKC knee extension produced significantly greater forces at angles less than 57° knee flexion, whereas both CKC activities produced significantly greater forces at knee angles greater than 85°. The results of these two studies should influence clinicians' choice of the range of motion in which they have their patients perform OKC and CKC exercises to develop quadriceps strength while protecting the patellofemoral joint.

In analyzing the biomechanics of the OKC knee extension, Grood et al.[9] reported that quadriceps force was greatest near full knee extension and increased with the addition of external loading. The small patellofemoral contact area observed near full extension, as previously discussed, and the increased amount of quadriceps force generated at these angles may make the patellofemoral joint more susceptible to injury. At lower angles of extension (closer to full extension, or 0°), a greater magnitude of quadriceps force is focused onto a more condensed location on the patella. Therefore, if the results of Steinkamp et al.,[42] Escamilla et al.,[43] and Grood et al.[9] are applied, it appears that during OKC knee extension, as the contact area of the patellofemoral joint decreases, the force of quadriceps pull subsequently increases; as a result, a large magnitude of patellofemoral contact stress is applied to a focal point on the patella while it is seated in the trochlear groove, in a position to articulate with the femur. In contrast, during CKC exercises, the quadriceps force increases as the knee continues into flexion. However, the area of patellofemoral contact also increases as the knee flexes, leading to a wider dissipation of contact stress over a larger surface area.

Recently, Witvrouw et al.[44] prospectively studied the efficacy of OKC and CKC exercises during nonoperative patellofemoral rehabilitation. Sixty patients participated in a 5-week exercise program consisting of either OKC or CKC exercises. Subjective pain scores, functional ability, quadriceps and hamstring peak torque, and hamstring, quadriceps, and gastrocnemius flexibility all were recorded before and after rehabilitation and at 3 months after the program ended. Both treatment groups reported a significant decrease in pain, increase in muscle strength, and increase in functional performance at 3 months after intervention.

The studies seem to show that both OKC and CKC exercises can be used to maximize the outcomes for patellofemoral patients if they are performed within a safe range of motion. Exercises prescribed by the clinician should be individualized according to the patient's needs and the clinician's assessment. If CKC exercises are less painful than OKC exercises, then that form of muscular training is encouraged. In addition, for postoperative patients, regions of articular cartilage wear must be considered carefully before an exercise program is designed. Clinicians most often allow open kinetic exercises, such as knee extension at 90° to 40° knee flexion. This range of motion provides the lowest patellofemoral joint reaction forces while providing the greatest amount of patellofemoral contact area. CKC exercises, such as the leg press, vertical squats, lateral step-ups, and wall squats (slides), are performed initially at 0° to 16° and then progressed to 0° to 30°, where patellofemoral joint reaction forces are lower. As the patient's symptoms subside, the ranges of motion performed are progressed to allow greater muscle strengthening in larger ranges. Exercises are progressed based on the patient's subjective reports of symptoms and the clinical assessment of swelling, range of motion, and painful crepitus.

Examination of the Knee

Subjective Assessment and History

A thorough history and physical examination are essential for making the correct diagnosis and determining appropriate treatment. Most injuries about the knee can be diagnosed with a thorough clinical evaluation, which often can eliminate the need for advanced imaging. (A full discussion of the history and physical examination can be found in volume 1 of this series, *Orthopedic Physical Assessment,* Chapter 12.)

The history can help determine the patient's activity level before injury and expectations after recovery. This can help in the planning and timing of treatment and in ensuring that patients have a realistic expectation of the outcome after the injury.

The clinician first must determine whether the injury is of traumatic origin. With traumatic injuries, the patient should be asked about the mechanism of injury and the location of the pain. This information provides a clue as to which anatomic structures are at risk. The examiner should determine whether the foot was planted, whether the injury was a twisting injury, whether the injury resulted from direct contact, and the direction of the forces involved. It is important to determine whether the patient had injured the same knee before and if so, how it was treated. Was the patient able to leave the scene unassisted or was assistance required? This may indicate the severity of the injury. The patient may be able to relate hearing or feeling a pop at the time of injury, which may indicate a cruciate ligament tear or osteochondral fracture. Determining whether any deformity was present that may have been reduced before the patient was evaluated is helpful in diagnosing a patellar or tibiofemoral dislocation or periarticular fracture. Determining the time course of swelling of the knee after injury also is helpful, because an acute effusion or hemarthrosis may differentiate an intra-articular fracture or torn cruciate ligament from a peripheral meniscal tear or patellar dislocation.

The same history is required for a subacute or chronically dysfunctional knee, because the injury may have been initiated by a traumatic event but never treated. The examiner must determine when the symptoms began in relation to a traumatic event. The patient must relate whether the primary complaint is popping or clicking, giving way (instability), locking, pain, or swelling. The relationship between activity and the patient's symptoms can also be helpful in determining the cause of the problem. Pain on takeoff (and, to a lesser extent, landing) in jumping often is due to extensor mechanism problems (patella, patellar tendon, quadriceps tendon), whereas instability on landing suggests ACL insufficiency or quadriceps weakness. A history of popping or clicking frequently is elicited, and these sounds can be caused by a variety of conditions, both pathological and normal.

Instability often is described as giving way, sliding, slipping out of socket, buckling, or the sensation that the knee may give out. Giving way usually indicates intra-articular pathology, including a displaced meniscal tear or cruciate ligament injury, resulting in a loose body or rotary instability. Impending giving way may be due to patellar subluxation or weakness of the extensor mechanism. Most patients with chronic rotatory instability can ambulate and perform activities of daily living without pain or instability. These patients complain of buckling during activities such as running, jumping, pivoting, or cutting. True locking is a mechanical block to full extension with uninhibited flexion, and it usually indicates a displaced meniscal tear. Other causes of locking include loose bodies, joint effusion, hamstring spasm, posterior capsulitis, and sometimes disruption of the quadriceps mechanism.

A history of swelling commonly is obtained after an injury; however, the time from injury to the onset of swelling and the location and amount of swelling should be determined, as well as its response to rest, activity, and medications. The development of a large, acute hemarthrosis within 2 to 6 hours after injury occurs secondary to an ACL rupture approximately 70% of the time,[45] although it also may be due to an intra-articular or osteochondral fracture. Alternatively, an acute hemarthrosis may be due to patellar dislocation; however, because the capsule is torn, the swelling usually is not as large as with a cruciate ligament disruption or fracture. An effusion that develops 1 or more days after injury usually is a hydrarthrosis, which occurs secondary to a meniscal tear, synovitis, or sympathetic effusion. Chronic synovitis and its attendant effusion indicate intra-articular inflammation. It usually is caused by a meniscal tear, advanced chondromalacia patella (patellar dysfunction, or excessive lateral patellar compression syndrome), rotatory instability, or loose bodies. The differential diagnosis must also include pigmented villonodular synovitis, osteochondritis dissecans, inflammatory and/or rheumatological arthritis, and other causes of synovitis.

Physical Examination

A thorough physical examination complements a good history. (We recommend that the reader review Chapter 12 in volume 1 of this series, *Orthopedic Physical Assessment,* for a detailed explanation of how to complete various physical examination techniques associated with examination of the knee.) Clinicians not only must be able to perform a physical examination accurately, they must understand the rationale for using specific examination techniques to diagnose ligamentous instability. This understanding is critical for an accurate, efficient patient examination.

The motion resulting from a clinical test in a relaxed patient depends on the position of the limb at the start of the test, the point of application and direction of the force, and the examiner's ability to detect displacement. Manual

examination of the knee compares the two sides to differentiate normal laxity from pathological instability. In a normal patient, left to right, side-to-side differences usually are negligible, therefore an internal control often exists for most patients. Most knee ligament tests assess for pathological motion by stressing a specific ligament or ligament complex. The motion detected during this examination depends on whether the primary or the secondary restraints have been disrupted (see Table 16-1). When a primary restraint is disrupted, pathological motion occurs, but its extent is limited by the remaining structures, called *secondary restraints*. Disruption of a secondary restraint does not result in pathological motion if the primary restraint is intact; however, disruption of the secondary restraint when the primary restraint is disrupted enhances pathological motion. For all clinical laxity tests, the femur is held steady and the tibial translation or rotation (joint space opening) is measured. A summary of the examination of the knee is presented in Box 16-1.

Specific Tests

Medial Collateral Ligament

Abduction (Valgus Stress) Test. The valgus stress test assesses the integrity of the MCL and medial instability in one plane only. With the patient supine and the leg held in slight external rotation, a gap opens in the medial joint line when a valgus stress is applied across the knee (Figure 16-13). The examiner's hand is placed on the lateral joint line to feel for opening of the medial joint line when valgus stress is applied from the lateral aspect of the knee. The knee is tested first in full extension and again in 20° to 30° knee flexion. It is imperative to examine both knees, because some ligamentous laxity may be normal in some individuals. The severity of injury to the MCL and associated structures can be determined by the amount of medial joint line opening in extension and slight flexion. With the knee in full extension, capsular and other secondary restraints resist valgus stress, even when the MCL is disrupted. Flexion of the knee to approximately 30° relaxes the secondary restraints for primary testing of the MCL.

If increased medial joint line opening is seen in the affected knee at 20° to 30° flexion, the posterior oblique ligament and posteromedial capsule may be injured.

If excessive medial joint opening is seen in full extension, a more severe injury to the secondary structures must be assumed. Medial joint line opening with the knee in full extension indicates injury to the MCL (superficial and deep fibers), posterior oblique ligament, ACL, PCL, posteromedial capsule, medial quadriceps expansion and retinaculum, and semimembranosus. With this more severe injury, the results of one or more rotatory instability tests are also positive.

MCL injuries are graded as first, second, or third degree. A grade I MCL injury is indicated by pain and tenderness

Box 16-1 Physical Examination of the Knee

Standing Position
- Mechanical alignment and symmetry of the lower extremity
- Foot type
- Gait
- Heel-and-toe walking
- "Duck" walk

Sitting Position
- Palpation:
  - Medial joint line
  - Lateral joint line
  - Patellar tendon
  - Tibial tubercle
  - Proximal tibia (pes anserine bursa, Gerdy's tubercle)
- Sulcus-tubercle angle (Q angle at 90°)

Supine Position with Knees Extended
- Palpation:
  - Warmth
  - Swelling
  - Patellar facets
  - Quadriceps tendon
  - Lateral collateral ligament in figure-of-four position
- Active and passive flexion and extension
- Patellofemoral and tibiofemoral crepitus
- Sag sign
- Godfrey's sign
- Quadriceps active test
- Anterior and posterior drawer tests
- Lachman's test
- Varus-valgus stress test
- O'Donoghue-McMurray test
- Medial and lateral pivot shift tests
- Reverse pivot shift test
- External rotation recurvatum test
- Quadriceps atrophy
- Hamstring and calf tightness

Side Lying Position
- Ober's test

Prone Position
- Heel height difference (flexion contracture)
- Apley's compression/distraction test
- External rotation of the tibia at 30° and 90° flexion
- Reverse Lachman's test
- Quadriceps flexibility

From Zachazewski JE, Magee DJ, Quillen WS, editors: *Athletic injuries and rehabilitation*, p 639, Philadelphia, 1996, WB Saunders.

injury or complete disruption of the MCL and associated structures is indicated by a soft end point, and the joint space opens more than 5 mm more than that of the normal knee in 20° flexion and full extension.

Lateral Collateral Ligament

Adduction (Varus Stress) Test. The varus stress test assesses the integrity of the LCL, and thus lateral instability, in one plane. With the patient supine and the leg held in slight external rotation, a gap opens in the lateral joint line when a varus stress is applied to the knee (Figure 16-14). External rotation of the leg uncoils the cruciate ligaments, requiring the collateral ligament to resist this stress. The examiner's hand is held on the medial joint line to feel for opening of the lateral joint line when varus stress is applied from the medial aspect of the knee. The knee is tested first in full extension and again in 30° knee flexion. It is imperative to examine both knees, because some ligamentous laxity may be normal in some individuals.

The severity of injury to the LCL and associated structures can be determined by the amount of lateral joint line opening in extension and slight flexion. With the knee in full extension, capsular and other secondary restraints (e.g., the biceps femoris and popliteus) resist varus stress, even when the LCL is disrupted. Flexion helps relax the secondary restraints for primary testing of the LCL.[46]

If excessive lateral joint line opening is seen in full extension, a more severe injury to the secondary structures must be assumed. Lateral joint space opening with the knee in full extension indicates some degree of injury to the LCL, posterolateral capsule, arcuate-popliteus complex, iliotibial band, biceps femoris tendon, ACL, PCL, and lateral head of the gastrocnemius. With this more severe injury, the results of one or more rotatory instability tests are also positive.

Grading of these injuries is the same as for MCL injuries and is based on the degree of opening of the lateral joint line.

Palpation of the LCL. With the patient supine, the hip is flexed to approximately 70°, abducted maximally, and externally rotated with the knee flexed 70° to 90° so that the ipsilateral foot rests on the patient's contralateral leg (i.e., figure-of-four position). As the knee is allowed to relax passively, the examiner palpates the LCL from the fibular head to the femoral condyle. A firm, taut band (i.e., the LCL) should be easily palpated. If the patient's knee is not relaxed, the examiner may be fooled by the insertion of the biceps femoris. Both knees should be examined to compare the intact LCL with the injured one.

Anterior Cruciate Ligament

Lachman's Test. Outside of the operating room, Lachman's test is the most sensitive clinical test for determining disruption of the ACL, particularly the posterolateral band.[47-49] Lachman's test isolates the ACL, which

along the ligament or at its insertion, and the joint space opening is within 2 mm of the contralateral side, with a firm end point. In a grade II injury, the end point is relatively firm and the joint space opens 3 to 5 mm more than the contralateral side in 20° flexion and less than 2 mm more than the normal knee in full extension. A grade III

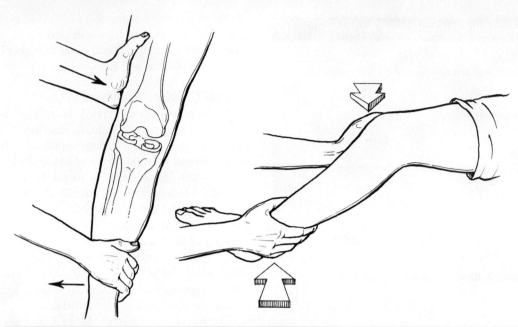

Figure 16-13

Valgus stress test in 30° flexion. A gap opens in the medial joint line when a valgus stress is applied across the knee. At 30° flexion, this test assesses the integrity of the medial collateral ligament. (From Zachazewski JE, Magee DJ, Quillen WS, editors: *Athletic injuries and rehabilitation*, p 640, Philadelphia, 1996, WB Saunders.)

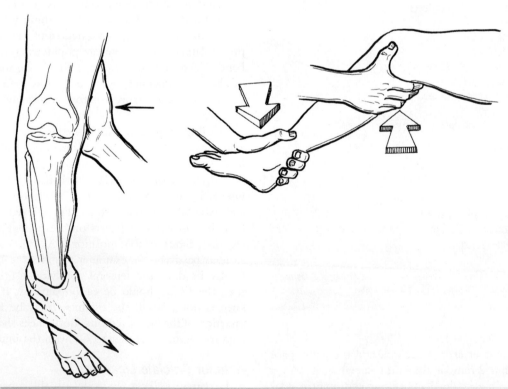

Figure 16-14

Varus stress test in 30° flexion. A gap opens in the lateral joint line when a varus stress is applied to the knee; this indicates injury to the lateral collateral ligament. (From Zachazewski JE, Magee DJ, Quillen WS, editors: *Athletic injuries and rehabilitation*, p 641, Philadelphia, 1996, WB Saunders.)

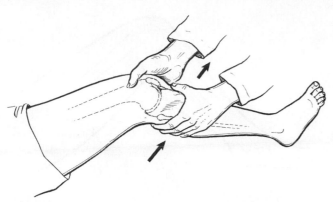

Figure 16-15
Lachman's test. This test is performed with the knee in 20° to 30° flexion. The examiner stabilizes the distal femur with one hand while pulling the proximal tibia anteriorly with the other hand. (From Zachazewski JE, Magee DJ, Quillen WS, editors: *Athletic injuries and rehabilitation,* p 642, Philadelphia, 1996, WB Saunders.)

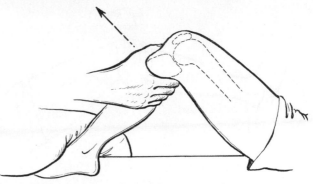

Figure 16-16
Anterior drawer test. This test is performed with the knee in 90° flexion, with the examiner sitting on the patient's foot. The examiner palpates the hamstring tendons to make sure they are relaxed. The thumbs should be placed in the joint line medially and laterally to palpate anterior translation of the tibia during the test. (From Zachazewski JE, Magee DJ, Quillen WS, editors: *Athletic injuries and rehabilitation,* p 642, Philadelphia, 1996, WB Saunders.)

acts as the primary restraining force preventing anterior translation of the tibia relative to the femur. The test is performed by stabilizing the distal femur with one hand while moving the proximal tibia forward with the other hand (Figure 16-15). The leg is held in 20° to 30° flexion, effectively relaxing the secondary constraints of anterior translation. The amount of anterior translation and the quality of the end point indicate potential injury to the ACL.

The grade of laxity is measured in comparison to the normal contralateral knee, not as the degree of absolute translation. Anterior tibial translation is measured in millimeters. The end point is graded as firm (normal), marginal, or soft. If the end point and translation are normal, the Lachman's test result is negative. If the end point is soft and/or if anterior translation is increased, the test result is positive. The degrees of anterior translation can be affected by several other factors. A large effusion or displaced meniscal tear can diminish the degree of translation. Muscular guarding and the position of the foot can also affect the side-to-side difference. With an incompetent PCL, the tibia sags posteriorly at rest, giving a false sense of increased anterior translation. Also, a false negative result on Lachman's test can occur if the ACL scars to the PCL to the roof of the intercondylar notch. A pseudo-endpoint is detected in these cases.

Anterior Drawer Test. This test determines anteroposterior uniplanar instability (Figure 16-16). With the patient supine, the ipsilateral hip is flexed to 45° and the knee is flexed to 90°. In this position, the ACL is nearly parallel to the tibial plateau. The examiner sits on the patient's forefoot to stabilize the leg. The examiner then grasps the back of the proximal tibia with the index fingers and palpates the hamstring muscles to ensure that they are relaxed. The examiner's thumbs are placed on the anterior medial and anterior lateral joint line to palpate anterior translation as the tibia is drawn forward on the femur. A stepoff at the medial tibial plateau should be palpated

to ensure the proper starting position. The knee is tested with the foot in three positions: neutral rotation, external rotation, and then internal rotation. The amount of translation and the end point are compared with those in the contralateral (normal) knee. If excessive anterior translation is evident, the ACL (primarily the anteromedial bundle), posterolateral capsule, posteromedial capsule, deep MCL, iliotibial band, posterior oblique ligament, and arcuatepopliteus complex may be injured.

Truly isolated acute ACL tears often produce only minimally increased anterior translation when the secondary stabilizers of the knee are intact, including the posterior capsule and posteromedial and posterolateral capsular structures. For this reason, the anterior drawer test is not as sensitive as Lachman's test for ACL injury. False negative results also can occur with a displaced ("bucket handle") meniscal tear, hamstring spasm, and hemarthrosis.

Pivot Shift Test. This test is used to test for injury to the ACL and to assess anterolateral rotatory instability of the knee.[50-52] During this test, the tibia subluxes anterolaterally on the femur.[52] This recreates the anterior subluxation-reduction phenomenon that occurs during functional activities when the ACL is torn. During the test, subluxation occurs in extension and reduction occurs between 20° and 40° flexion; as a result, the patient feels the sensation of instability that occurs when the knee buckles (Figure 16-17). The pivot shift result is graded as grade 0 (normal) if no shift is present; grade 1 if there is a smooth glide; and grade 2 if the tibia "jumps" back into the reduced position. A grade 3 pivot is marked by transient locking of the tibia in the subluxed position before reduction.[53]

A positive pivot shift test is pathognomonic for ACL deficiency. Unfortunately, the sensitivity of the test is affected by guarding and muscular splinting. The sensitivity improves dramatically if the test is done with the patient

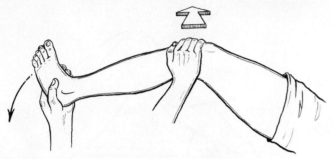

Figure 16-17

Lateral pivot shift test. This test is performed with the patient supine. The examiner places the heel of one hand behind the head of the fibula and the other hand on the foot. Internal rotation and valgus force of the lower leg are produced with the knee in full extension to sublux the lateral tibial plateau anteriorly. The knee then is flexed to 20° to 30°, which results in reduction of the lateral tibial plateau. (From Zachazewski JE, Magee DJ, Quillen WS, editors: *Athletic injuries and rehabilitation,* p 643, Philadelphia, WB Saunders, 1996.)

under anesthesia.[54] Varying the position of the hip (abduction and slight flexion) and external rotation of the tibia can enhance the pivot shift.[50]

The pivot shift test can differentiate partial tears of the ACL from complete injuries. Partial tears produce increased anterior translation, as documented by Lachman's test or instrumented laxity testing, but they produce a negative pivot shift test result under anesthesia. A tear is considered complete if rotational instability is demonstrated by a positive pivot shift test result. For this reason, the pivot shift test can be considered the most important assessment in the evaluation of an ACL injury.

Posterior Cruciate Ligament and Posterolateral Corner

Stepoff Test. This is a sensitive uniplanar test for determining posterior cruciate injury and posterior instability. Normally, the medial tibial plateau protrudes anteriorly 1 cm beyond the medial femoral condyle when the knee is flexed to 90° (Figure 16-18, *A*).[55] This stepoff is lost when there is a posterior sag of the tibia associated with injury to the PCL and other secondary restraints to posterior translation of the tibia (Figure 16-18, *B*). The patient is examined in the supine position with the knee flexed to 90°. The examiner places the hands on either side of the proximal tibia at the joint line and palpates the hamstrings with the fingers to ensure that they are relaxed. The medial tibial plateau, which is easier to palpate than the lateral plateau, is felt in relation to the femoral condyle with the examiner's thumb. A 0.5-cm (¼ inch) difference in the stepoff between the involved and the uninjured knee is considered a grade I laxity; a 1-cm (½ inch) difference, in which the tibia and femoral condyles are flush, is considered a grade II laxity. If the anterior tibia lies posterior to the femoral condyle, indicating a difference of more than 1 cm (½ inch) between the involved and the noninvolved knee, a grade III laxity is present.[56,57]

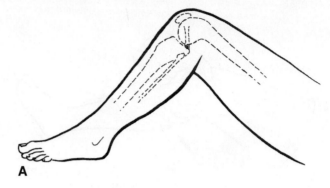

A

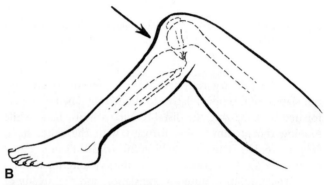

B

Figure 16-18

Stepoff test. **A,** Normal relationship of the tibiofemoral joint. The medial tibial plateau protrudes anteriorly approximately 1 cm (0.5 inch) beyond the medial femoral condyle. **B,** With injury to the posterior cruciate ligament, the stepoff is lost. The medial tibial plateau now lies either in line with or posterior to the medial femoral condyle. (From Zachazewski JE, Magee DJ, Quillen WS, editors: *Athletic injuries and rehabilitation,* p 645, Philadelphia, 1996, WB Saunders.)

Posterior Sag Test. This is a uniplanar, passive test of PCL function and posterior instability. With the patient supine, the hip is flexed to 45°, and the knee is flexed to 90°. The examiner then views the knee from the lateral side; with a PCL-deficient knee, a loss of tibial tubercle prominence will be seen (Figure 16-19). If the PCL is torn, gravitational forces cause the tibia to fall back or sag on the femur. The posterior tibial displacement is more noticeable when the knee is flexed 90° to 110° than when the knee is only slightly flexed. This test is less obvious when significant swelling of the knee is present. The examiner must be aware of tibial tubercle enlargement (as a result of Osgood-Schlatter disease) or tibial plateau osteophytes, which can give a false negative result. Different degrees of posterior sag represent varying degrees of injury to the PCL, arcuate-popliteus complex, posterior oblique ligament, and ACL. The quadriceps active drawer test[58] and Godfrey's sign (Figure 16-20) also can be used to test the PCL.

Posterior Drawer Test. An isolated tear of the PCL leads to increased posterior translation of the tibia that increases with knee flexion. The most accurate means of

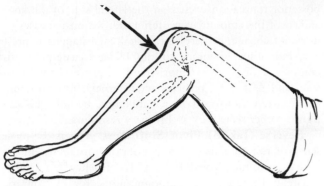

Figure 16-19

Posterior sag test. When a posterior cruciate ligament–deficient knee at 90° flexion is viewed from the side, loss of prominence of the tibial tubercle can be seen. (From Zachazewski JE, Magee DJ, Quillen WS, editors: *Athletic injuries and rehabilitation,* p 645, Philadelphia, 1996, WB Saunders.)

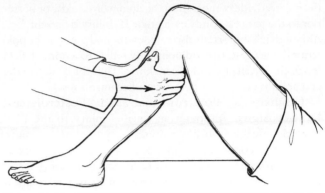

Figure 16-21

Posterior drawer test. The posterior drawer test is performed with the knee in 90° flexion. The examiner palpates the hamstrings posteriorly to make sure they are relaxed. The thumbs are placed in the anterior joint line to palpate posterior translation of the tibia when a posterior force is applied. (From Zachazewski JE, Magee DJ, Quillen WS, editors: *Athletic injuries and rehabilitation,* p 646, Philadelphia, 1996, WB Saunders.)

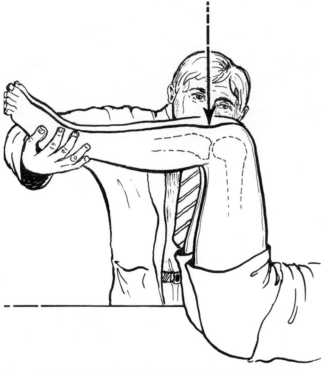

Figure 16-20

Godfrey's test. This posterior sag test is performed with the patient's hips and knees flexed to 90°. Disruption of the posterior cruciate ligament results in loss of prominence of the tibial tubercle. (From Zachazewski JE, Magee DJ, Quillen WS, editors: *Athletic injuries and rehabilitation,* p 645, Philadelphia, 1996, WB Saunders.)

diagnosing this injury is the posterior drawer test with the knee flexed at 90°.[59,60] The examiner's thumbs are placed on the anterior joint line to feel posterior translation as the tibia is drawn backward on the femur. The medial tibial plateau should be palpated as a 1 cm (½ inch) anterior stepoff from the medial femoral condyle to ensure the proper starting position. The knee is tested with the foot

in three positions: neutral position, external rotation, and then internal rotation. The amount of translation and the end point are again compared with those in the contralateral (normal) knee. If excessive posterior translation is evident, the PCL (primarily the anterolateral bundle), arcuate-popliteus complex, posterior oblique ligament, and ACL may be injured (Figure 16-21).

Truly isolated acute PCL tears often produce only minimally increased posterior translation when the secondary restraints of the knee are intact, particularly the posterior capsule and posteromedial and posterolateral structures. Some studies have suggested that the meniscofemoral ligaments are strong and may act as secondary stabilizers to PCL function. A posterior drawer test with the leg in internal rotation is reduced if the posterolateral structures or, as some investigators have suggested, the meniscofemoral ligaments, are intact.[61] Some investigators believe that a posterior drawer cannot occur with an intact arcuate-popliteus complex, although laboratory studies have revealed that a posterior drawer of no greater than 10 mm (½ inch), as compared to the contralateral side, can occur with an isolated PCL injury. False negative results can occur with a displaced bucket handle meniscal tear, hamstring or quadriceps spasm, and hemarthrosis.

Grading of this test also requires comparison of the injured knee with the normal knee. A grade I injury is one in which the injured to noninjured side-to-side difference in posterior translation is less than 5 mm (¼ inch), which usually corresponds to posterior displacement of the tibial plateau to a position that is still anterior to the femoral condyles. A grade II PCL injury results in 5 to 10 mm more posterior tibial displacement on the involved side. This corresponds to posterior translation of the tibial plateau to the level of the femoral condyles. If the tibia can be posteriorly displaced 10 mm (½ inch) or more on the involved side compared to the noninvolved side, or posterior to the femoral condyles, a grade III injury is present.[56,57] Although it is important also to assess the end point of the posterior drawer test, the end point may return to a normal, firm feel in chronically PCL-deficient knees. Thus the quality of the end point is not as sensitive as with Lachman's test.

Hughston's Posteromedial and Posterolateral Drawer Signs. Although an isolated injury to the PCL has little effect on tibial rotational laxity or varus or valgus angulation, concomitant injury to the secondary extra-articular restraints results in some aspects of rotatory instability. Posteromedial and posterolateral drawer tests assess rotatory instability combined with PCL injury and are analogous to the Slocum test for rotatory instability associated with ACL injury.[62] With the patient positioned as for the posterior drawer test, the foot is internally rotated 30°. Posteromedial rotatory instability is present if most of the posterior translation occurs on the medial side of the knee and/or if the amount of posterior translation increases or does not change. Posteromedial rotatory instability is a result of varying degrees of injury to the PCL, posterior oblique ligament, MCL (deep and superficial), semimembranosus muscle, posteromedial capsule, and ACL (posteromedial corner).

Next, the patient's foot is placed in 15° external rotation as the examiner sits on the patient's forefoot. If most of the

posterior translation occurs on the lateral side of the knee and/or if the amount of posterior translation increases or does not change, posterolateral rotatory instability is present, indicating an injury to the PCL, arcuate-popliteus complex, LCL, biceps femoris tendon, posterolateral capsule, and ACL (i.e., posterolateral corner). Over-rotating the foot can lead to a false negative test, because this can tighten other secondary and tertiary restraints.

Reverse (Jakob) Pivot Shift Test. This is the most sensitive test for posterolateral rotatory instability and is analogous to the pivot shift for ACL deficiency.[53,63] Unfortunately, the test is not pathognomonic for PCL injury, because up to 35% of normal knees may have a positive reverse pivot test result.[64] During this test (Figure 16-22), the posterolateral tibial plateau subluxes laterally and posteriorly on the femur. The knee starts in the subluxed position; the clunk associated with the test indicates reduction. The external rotation recurvatum test[62] (Figure 16-23) and the tibial external rotation (dial) test[46] (Figure 16-24) also test for posterolateral rotatory instability.

Posteromedial Pivot Shift Test. A positive result on this test indicates injury to the PCL, MCL, and posterior oblique ligament.[65] All three structures must be injured for a positive test result. The patient is positioned supine, and the knee is flexed to greater than 45° while a varus stress is applied, combined with axial compression and

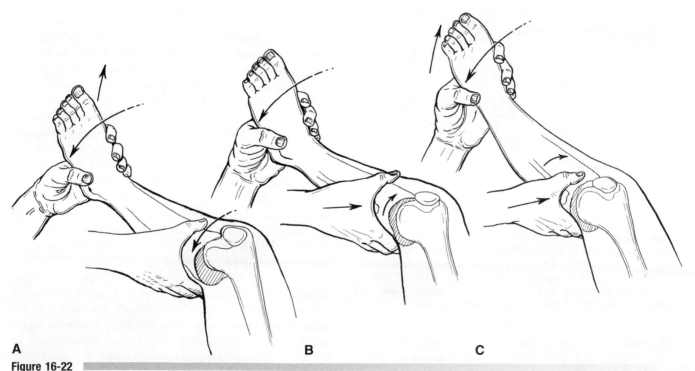

A   **B**   **C**

Figure 16-22
Reverse pivot shift test. **A,** The knee is flexed to 70° to 80°. The examiner uses the proximal hand to externally rotate the lower leg to sublux the lateral tibial plateau posteriorly. **B,** A valgus force is applied as the knee is passively extended. **C,** The lateral tibial plateau reduces as the knee approaches 20° flexion. (From Zachazewski JE, Magee DJ, Quillen WS, editors: *Athletic injuries and rehabilitation*, p 647, Philadelphia, 1996, WB Saunders.)

Figure 16-23

External rotation recurvatum test. To perform this test, the examiner grasps the individual's big toes and lifts the leg, allowing both knees to go into passive hyperextension. The test result is positive if the affected knee hyperextends to a greater degree than the noninvolved knee and appears to be in valgus alignment. Also, the tibial tuberosity is displaced laterally as the lateral tibial plateau subluxes posteriorly. (From Zachazewski JE, Magee DJ, Quillen WS, editors: *Athletic injuries and rehabilitation*, p 648, Philadelphia, 1996, WB Saunders.)

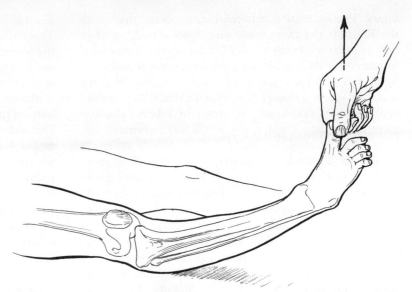

A

B

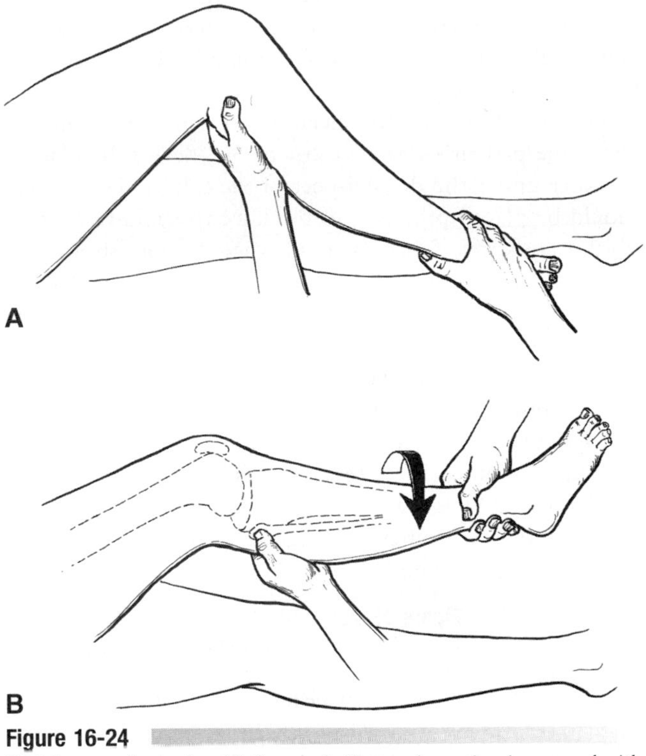

Figure 16-24

Tibial external rotation (dial) test. **A,** External rotation is assessed with the knee at 90° flexion. **B,** External rotation is assessed with the knee at 30° flexion. (From Zachazewski JE, Magee DJ, Quillen WS, editors: *Athletic injuries and rehabilitation*, p 648, Philadelphia, 1996, WB Saunders.)

internal rotation. With a positive test result, this action causes the medial tibial plateau to sublux posterior to the medial femoral condyle. As the knee is brought into extension, the tibia reduces at approximately 20° to 40° knee flexion. Occasionally the femur appears to rotate internally suddenly as the knee is extended.

Instrumented Testing of the Knee

Several knee ligament arthrometers are commercially available for clinical use to quantify laxity of the knee. These include the KT1000 Knee Ligament Arthrometer, mentioned previously, the Acufex Knee Signature System (Acufex Microsurgical, Norwood, MA), the Genucom Knee Analysis System (FaroMedical, Toronto, Canada), and the Stryker Knee Laxity Tester (Stryker Corp., Kalamazoo, MI). Of these, the KT1000 arthrometer appears to be the most widely used.

The reliability and validity of these devices have been widely studied.[66-77] The Acufex and Genucom arthrometers appear to be less reliable than the KT1000.[72,73] The standard deviations of measurements from these devices are higher than the KT1000. Also, the Genucom tends to produce greater differences in displacement between the right and left knees of normal subjects.[75,76] The reliability of the Stryker arthrometer has been questioned by King and Kumar,[71] who reported that more than 20% of normal knees showed more than a 2 mm variation between knees when tested by different examiners on the same day, as well as when tested by the same examiner at a 3-week interval. Boniface et al.[70] reported that the Stryker arthrometer is valid for detecting ACL injury. They reported that 89% of subjects with unilateral ACL injury had an increase of 2 mm or more compared to the uninjured side.

Intratester reliability and intertester reliability for the KT1000 have been reported to be high, both within and between days.[77] Wroble et al.[73] indicated that the 90% confidence limit for right-left difference with the KT1000 was ±1.6 mm when measured at 89 N and ±1.5 mm when measured at 134 N. A confidence interval of this magnitude is within acceptable limits for the clinical diagnosis of ACL injuries. In vitro and in vivo studies have shown the KT1000 to be a valid measure for the detection of ACL injury. The correlation between measurements made with the KT1000 and those made with direct transducer readings in cadaveric knees was 0.97.[66] The mean anterior displacement in ACL-intact cadaveric knees was found to be 5.8 mm, which increased to 12.1 mm when the ACL was sectioned. In vivo studies demonstrated that 92% of normal subjects had a side-to-side difference in anterior displacement of less than 2 mm, whereas 96% with confirmed unilateral disruption of the ACL had a side-to-side difference in anterior displacement greater than 2 mm.[66] Stratford et al.[67] and Highgenboten et al.[68] found that testing with the KT1000 is more sensitive when performed with a 134 N load or with manual maximum force. Highgenboten et al.[68] measured the knees of 68 patients with the KT1000 at 15, 20, and 30 pounds (6.8, 9, and 13.6 kg) of force. They found that more patients demonstrated a side-to-side difference greater than 2 mm between the injured and noninjured legs at 30 pounds (13.6 kg) of force than at 20 pounds (9.1 kg) of force. It should be noted that even at 30 pounds (13.6 kg) of force, approximately 20% of patients with an ACL-deficient knee demonstrated a side-to-side difference less than 2 mm.

Based on this research, the KT1000 appears to be a clinically applicable instrument that can be used to assess anterior laxity in patients with an ACL-deficient knee. The KT1000 measures anterior-posterior movement of the tibia relative to the femur. It has both a patellar and a tibial sensor pad (Figure 16-25). The patellar sensor pad rests on the patella. When the patella is compressed against the femur, the patellar sensor pad indicates the position of the femur. The tibial reference pad rests in the area of the tibial tuberosity and provides a point of reference for the tibia. Relative motion between the patellar and tibial sensor pads indicates anterior and posterior translation of the tibia on the femur. The KT1000 also has a force-sensing handle that can be used to provide an anteriorly directed force of 15, 20, and 30 pounds (6.8, 9, and 13.6 kg), as well as a posteriorly

directed force of 15 and 20 pounds (6.8 and 9.1 kg). Tibiofemoral motion is measured in millimeters as the relative motion between the patellar and the tibial sensor pads and is displayed on a dial that can be zeroed to the neutral starting position.

Before using the KT1000 to assess anterior-posterior laxity of the knee, the clinician must screen for PCL injury. This is done by observing for lack of a stepoff between the medial femoral condyle and the medial tibial plateau. The posterior sag test or the active quadriceps drawer test (or both) also can be done to rule out injury to the PCL. Failure to detect a PCL-deficient knee before testing with the KT1000 may result in a false positive result for anterior laxity. With a PCL-deficient knee, gravity causes the tibia to sublux posteriorly. If this goes undetected, the reference position of the tibia is posterior to the true neutral position of the tibiofemoral joint. Performing a KT1000 test from a starting position at which the tibia is posteriorly subluxed results in a false positive increase in anterior translation. This occurs as the tibia is translated anteriorly from the posterior subluxed position to the neutral position. Failure to detect a PCL injury when performing a KT1000 test invalidates the results.

Once PCL injury has been ruled out, the examiner places the patient's knees in 20° to 30° flexion by placing a bolster under the distal aspect of the thighs. The bolster should be placed proximal to the knee to avoid restricting tibial translation. The angle of knee flexion should be recorded so that it can be repeated for future tests. A footrest is placed under the patient's feet just distal to the lateral malleoli to block external rotation of the leg, which produces relative internal rotation of the tibia in relation to the femur. Accurate placement of the footrest is important to obtain symmetrical tibiofemoral rotation, which is necessary for an accurate test result (Figure 16-26).

The KT1000 is applied to the lower leg so that the arrow on the arthrometer is aligned with the tibiofemoral

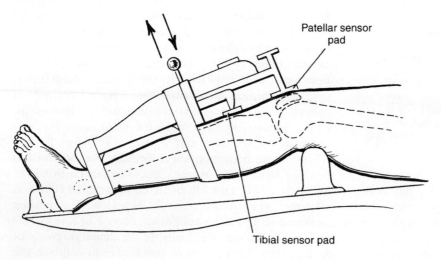

Patellar sensor pad

Tibial sensor pad

Figure 16-25

Use of the KT1000 arthrometer (MEDmetric, San Diego) to quantify tibial translation. Relative movement of the tibiofemoral joint is measured as motion between the patellar and tibial sensor pads. (From Zachazewski JE, Magee DJ, Quillen WS, editors: *Athletic injuries and rehabilitation,* p 650, Philadelphia, 1996, WB Saunders.)

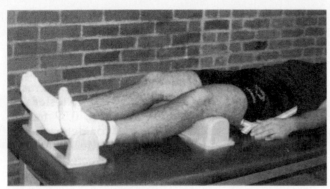

Figure 16-26

Position of the lower extremity for the KT1000 arthrometer test. A bolster is placed under the distal aspect of the thigh to flex the knee to 20°-30°. A foot rest is placed distal to the lateral malleolus to produce symmetrical internal rotation of the tibia on the femur. (From Zachazewski JE, Magee DJ, Quillen WS, editors: *Athletic injuries and rehabilitation,* p 651, Philadelphia, 1996, WB Saunders.)

joint line. The arthrometer also should be slightly rotated on the leg so that compression of the patellar sensor pad against the patella causes the patella to compress directly against the femur without medial or lateral displacement. The height of the patellar reference pad is adjusted so that the needle on the dial faces the 12 o'clock position. Once the arthrometer has been placed accurately, it is secured to the leg with two Velcro straps (Figure 16-27).

The examiner encourages the patient to relax by oscillating the tibiofemoral joint. Several posterior pushes are performed to establish the neutral reference position before

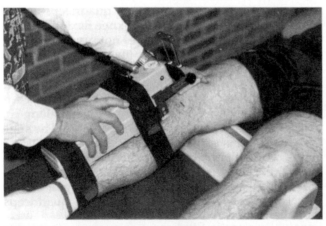

Figure 16-27

Proper alignment of the KT1000 arthrometer on the lower leg. The arrow on the arthrometer is aligned with the medial joint line, and the arthrometer is slightly rotated onto the leg so that compression of the patellar sensor pad directly compresses the patella against the femur without medial or lateral displacement. The height of the patellar sensor pad is adjusted so that the needle faces the 12 o'clock position on the dial. (Med Metric: KT-1000 Knee Ligament Arthrometer, Med Metric, San Diego) (From Zachazewski JE, Magee DJ, Quillen WS, editors: *Athletic injuries and rehabilitation,* p 651, Philadelphia, 1996, WB Saunders.)

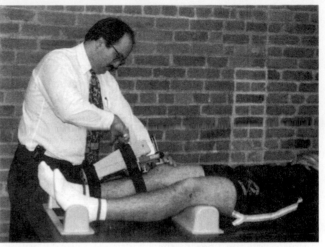

Figure 16-28

Anterior and posterior displacement are measured with the KT1000 arthrometer. (Med Metric, San Diego.) (From Zachazewski JE, Magee DJ, Quillen WS, editors: *Athletic injuries and rehabilitation,* p 651, Philadelphia, 1996, WB Saunders.)

the test is started. Once the neutral starting position of the tibiofemoral joint has been determined, the dial is rotated so that zero lies under the needle; this indicates the reference-neutral position for the test. Once the zero reference position has been set, the test is conducted by performing successive anterior pulls and posterior pushes through the force-sensing handle (Figure 16-28). The amount of anterior displacement is recorded with the application of 15, 20, and 30 pounds (6.8, 9, and 13.6 kg) of force, as indicated by the force-sensing handle. Posterior displacement with the posterior push through the force-sensing handle is measured at 15 and 20 pounds (6.8 and 9.1 kg) of force. After each anterior-posterior cycle, the needle on the dial should return to the zero reference position. Failure to return to the zero reference point may indicate that the patient is not fully relaxed or that the arthrometer has moved from its initial starting position. Care should be taken when performing the test to avoid rotating or moving the arthrometer in a superior or inferior direction. The anterior drawer test is also performed with a maximum manual force, which is applied to the posterior aspect of the proximal calf. The quadriceps active drawer test is performed by having the patient contract the quadriceps with sufficient force just to raise the heel off the table. Both the noninvolved and involved knees are tested.

Side-to-side differences are calculated for each level of force by subtracting translation of the involved side from the noninvolved side. Positive values indicate increased translation on the involved side. A side-to-side difference in anterior or posterior translation less 2 mm is considered normal. A side-to-side difference of 3 mm or more for anterior translation is considered diagnostic for injury to the ACL (Table 16-4).

Table 16-4
Interpretation of Side-to-Side Differences With the KT1000 Arthrometer

Test	Normal (mm)	Equivocal (mm)	Diagnostic (mm)
20 Pound (9.1 kg) anterior drawer	<2	2-2.5	≥3
30 Pound (13.6 kg) anterior drawer	<2	2-2.5	≥3
Maximum manual anterior drawer	<2	2-2.5	≥3

From Zachazewski JE, Magee DJ, Quillen WS, editors: *Athletic injuries and rehabilitation,* p 652, Philadelphia, WB Saunders, 1996.

The procedure for the KT1000 test must be modified if the patient is suspected of having a torn PCL. In patients suspected of having a PCL injury, the test should be performed with the knee in the quadriceps-neutral position. The quadriceps-neutral position is defined as the angle of knee flexion at which contraction of the quadriceps does not result in anterior or posterior translation of the tibia. The quadriceps-neutral position is determined on the noninvolved knee by placing the knee in approximately 70° to 90° flexion. The patient then is instructed to contract the quadriceps by sliding the heel along the table while translation of the tibia is palpated. The angle of knee flexion is adjusted until no tibial translation is felt with isolated contraction of the quadriceps. Once the quadriceps-neutral angle has been determined, it is measured with a standard goniometer. Daniel et al.[58] found that the quadriceps-neutral angle averages 71°.

After the quadriceps-neutral angle is found, the KT1000 arthrometer is placed on the leg so that the arrow on the arthrometer is in line with the tibiofemoral joint line. The arthrometer is held in place with Velcro straps. When the arthrometer is secure and in place, the height of the patellar pad is adjusted so that the needle on the dial is directed toward the 12 o'clock position. The dial is adjusted to set the zero reference position for the knee. Anterior translation and posterior translation of the tibia are measured with 20 pounds (9.1 kg) of force. In addition, the patient is instructed to contract the quadriceps with the KT1000 in place to determine the active quadriceps drawer displacement. Once measurements are completed on the noninvolved knee, the involved knee is placed at the same angle of knee flexion as the quadriceps-neutral angle found on the noninvolved knee. The KT1000 arthrometer is applied to the leg, and anterior translation and posterior translation at 20 pounds (9.1 kg) of force are measured. The active quadriceps drawer is measured by having the patient contract the quadriceps muscle.

The active quadriceps drawer measurements are used to calculate corrected anterior and posterior translation for the noninvolved and involved knees. The corrected posterior drawer is calculated by adding the active quadriceps drawer to the measured posterior drawer. The corrected anterior drawer is calculated by subtracting the active quadriceps drawer from the measured anterior drawer (Figure 16-29). Side-to-side differences for corrected anterior and posterior tibial translation are determined by subtracting the values for the involved knee from those for the noninvolved knee. A positive value indicates more translation on the involved side. A noninvolved to involved difference in corrected posterior translation greater than 3 mm indicates injury to the PCL.

Huber et al.[78] found moderate test-retest reliability within and between novice and experienced testers. This was determined on 22 subjects who had a PCL-deficient knee or had undergone PCL reconstruction. Intraclass correlation coefficients (ICCs) for the novice tester were 0.67 for corrected posterior translation, 0.59 for corrected anterior translation, and 0.7 for determination of the quadriceps-neutral angle. For the experienced tester, ICC values were 0.79 for corrected posterior translation, 0.68 for corrected anterior translation, and 0.74 for determination of the quadriceps-neutral angle. Reliability between testers was 0.63 for corrected posterior translation and 0.64 for corrected anterior translation. Standard of error measurements were used to construct 95% confidence intervals (CIs). For the novice tester, the 95% CI for corrected posterior translation was ±3.0 mm, whereas for the experienced tester it was ±1.2 mm. The 95% CI between testers for corrected posterior translation was 2.0 mm. These results indicate that the KT1000 can be used with moderate reliability to measure anterior and posterior translation in a PCL-deficient knee. Also, the experience of the tester is an important consideration in the interpretation of the test results.

Special Diagnostic Studies

Radiography

Radiographs of the knee should be obtained after any acute trauma. If the trauma was severe and the patient complains of pain when the knee is moved, radiographs should be obtained before the physical examination is started. Fractures must be ruled out before the knee is manipulated, because displacement of the fracture may damage other structures, including neurovascular structures.

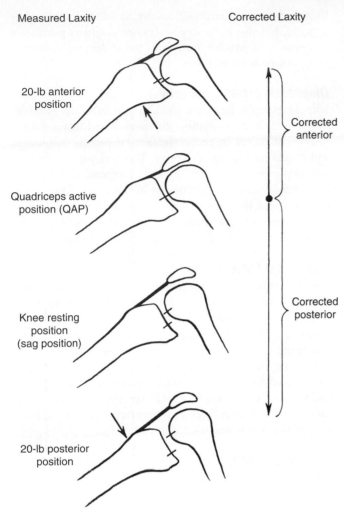

Measured Laxity

20-lb anterior position

Quadriceps active position (QAP)

Knee resting position (sag position)

20-lb posterior position

Corrected Laxity

Corrected anterior

Corrected posterior

Figure 16-29

Use of quadriceps active drawer measurements to calculate corrected anterior and posterior translation in a posterior cruciate ligament–deficient knee. The corrected posterior drawer is calculated by adding the active quadriceps drawer to the measured posterior drawer. The corrected anterior drawer is calculated by subtracting the active quadriceps drawer from the measured anterior drawer. (From Daniel DM, Stone ML, Barnett P, Sachs R: Use of the quadriceps active test to diagnose posterior cruciate ligament disruption and measure posterior laxity of the knee, *J Bone Joint Surg Am* 70:386-391, 1988.)

Our standard radiographic series for the knee includes a flexion weight-bearing anteroposterior (AP) and lateral and skyline views. Because ligaments and menisci are radiolucent, radiography is used for the most part to exclude other causes of knee pain, swelling, deformity, and/or loss of function. Other radiographs obtained in special circumstances that may be beneficial include a long cassette AP weight-bearing view to assess alignment; stress radiographs in cases of suspected ligamentous or physical injury; a cross-table lateral view to look for hemarthrosis with a fat-fluid level, an indication of a fracture; and external and internal rotation views to look for loose bodies or oblique fracture lines.

When viewing standard radiographs of the knee, the examiner should look for any obvious intra-articular or osteochondral fractures, calcifications, joint space narrowing, epiphyseal damage, osteophytes or lipping, loose bodies, tumors, accessory ossification centers, alignment deformity (varus-valgus), patellar alta or baja, asymmetry of the femoral condyles, and dislocations. Secondary signs can be seen on plain radiographs to help diagnose ligamentous or meniscal injury.

Soft tissue swelling as seen on radiographs is helpful when the injured structures are surrounded by fat. An MCL injury may reveal only soft tissue swelling on the medial aspect of the knee. A bloody effusion, often associated with intra-articular ligament damage, is detected as a soft tissue density in the suprapatellar pouch on the lateral view. Fat in the effusion, or lipohemarthrosis, suggests a fracture (osteochondral or intra-articular) and is identified as a fat-fluid level on a cross-table lateral projection. Although fat globules occasionally are seen in many other types of effusions, the accumulation of fat is much greater in cases of trauma.[79] Meniscal tears, although often associated with effusions, do not produce as large an effusion as a cruciate ligament disruption or intra-articular fracture. Furthermore, the timing of the radiograph in relation to the time of injury is important, because cruciate ligament injuries are associated with acute effusions, but meniscal tears usually do not produce a significant effusion for at least 12 hours.

Although extensive fractures about the knee are readily identified by standard radiographs, careful evaluation of the films may be required to detect avulsion injuries at the attachment sites of ligaments. This is particularly true in children, in whom cruciate ligament injuries frequently involve avulsion fractures. An avulsion of the ACL insertion may be seen on the flexion AP radiograph or on the lateral view by identifying the displaced fragment superior and anterior to the tibial spine.[80] Segond's fracture, also known as the lateral capsular sign, is an avulsion fracture of the lateral capsule posterior to Gerdy's tubercle on the proximal lateral tibia.[81] This fracture, seen on AP radiographs, is an indirect sign of ACL injury. The thin fragment of bone is vertically oriented and located proximal and anterior to the fibular head and should not to be confused with a lateral ligamentous injury. Avulsion of the tibial insertion of the PCL may be seen on lateral radiographs in the posterior intercondylar area. A PCL avulsion may be a small flake of bone or a large bony fragment. Lateral ligamentous injury may be identified on an AP or external rotation view as an avulsion of the biceps femoris or LCL insertion from the fibular head. Uncommonly, the MCL or LCL may avulse from the femoral condyle with a bony fragment. These injuries can be identified on AP radiographs.

Chronic knee injuries may also produce abnormal findings on radiographic studies. The lateral notch sign, an expansion of the normal indentation of the lateral condyle by 2 mm or more, has been correlated with an ACL-deficient knee.[82]

A chronic MCL injury may result in calcification at the site of injury. When this occurs at the femoral origin of the MCL, it is called Pelligrini-Stieda disease. Although the natural history of isolated cruciate ligament injuries is debated, most authors agree that if left untreated, the unstable knee develops degenerative osteoarthritic changes. Osteoarthritic change in the cruciate-deficient knee tends to occur first in the medial compartment, but the compartment with meniscal pathology often develops degenerative changes.[83] This is best seen on 45° flexion, weight-bearing, posteroanterior (PA) radiographs.[84] Degenerative changes identified on radiographs in a patient with a history of trivial trauma with signs of possible meniscal pathology may suggest a degenerative meniscal tear.

Stress radiography has been advocated for knee ligament injuries, but it is difficult to carry out after acute trauma.[85] In chronic injury or in the anesthetized patient, these radiographs are more easily obtained and can be valuable. In children with varus or valgus instability, these films can differentiate between ligamentous disruption and a Salter I physeal fracture (fracture through the growth plate without displacement). Stress radiography is particularly popular in Europe to document knee instability in the sagittal and frontal planes;[86-90] however, it is not used as often in the United States.

Arthrography

Traditionally, single contrast and double contrast arthrography served as the gold standard for evaluating the menisci and plica and, to a lesser extent, the cruciate ligaments and articular surfaces.[91-97] However, this method is limited in that it is an uncomfortable, invasive procedure that requires a great deal of expertise to perform and interpret, and it exposes the patient to irradiation. It was more widely used before the advent of arthroscopy and magnetic resonance imaging (MRI). Arthrography has been largely replaced by those two modalities in most centers, but it still may be used in specialized situations to resolve a specific question or when the availability or quality of MRI is limited.

Radionuclide Scintigraphy

Radionuclide scintigraphy uses technetium-99 methylene diphosphonate (MDP) to screen for a variety of abnormalities. In general, the scintigram reflects the relative blood flow to an area and the degree of bone turnover (osteogenesis and osteolysis). The test is sensitive but nonspecific. It provides more information about osseous physiology than structural characteristics. The technique traditionally has been used to evaluate arthritic joints, stress fractures, tumors, osteonecrosis, infection, osteolysis, metabolic or metastatic bone disease, and reflex sympathetic dystrophy.

Increased osseous metabolic activity, as determined by scintigraphy, has also been seen with knee disorders previously considered to involve only soft tissue failure, including symptomatic tears of the ACL.[98-104]

Diagnostic Ultrasonography

Ultrasonography has been used to evaluate various structures of the knee, including the menisci and ligaments.[105] It is most useful in the evaluation of patellar tendonitis and partial patellar tendon tears. This technique is technician dependent, and although it is inexpensive, it has not been popularized for routine use in the evaluation of ligamentous and meniscal injuries. It is used in the United States primarily for evaluating patellar tendonitis and masses about the knee.

Computed Tomography

Ever since the early application of computed tomography (CT) to the musculoskeletal system, this technique has been used to evaluate many disorders of the knee.[106-108] However, CT scanning is best used for bony detail, because soft tissue detail is better with MRI or arthroscopy. Many conflicting descriptions have been reported with respect to the need for and type of intra-articular contrast material and patient positioning in the CT scanner. Therefore clinical use of CT scanning after meniscal and ligamentous injury currently is not widely accepted.

Magnetic Resonance Imaging

MRI is a sensitive, noninvasive, nonionizing radiation means of evaluating the structural integrity of the knee. It is particularly helpful for visualizing soft tissue structures. At first, MRI met some resistance because initial studies were less accurate than double contrast arthrography, and the procedure was time-consuming and expensive.[109-112] Improvements in hardware and software, as well as increasing expertise in the interpretation of these studies, have overcome these problems, and MRI has become the procedure of choice for evaluating acute knee injuries.[113-118] Partial and complete tears of ligaments and menisci, as well as other pathological changes, such as bone bruises and effusions, can be identified with MRI. Evaluation of the knee by MRI is reader dependent, but its accuracy approaches 100% in diagnosing lesions of the PCL, ACL, medial meniscus, and lateral meniscus (diagnosis is least accurate with the lateral meniscus).[113,116,118-121] Some clinicians believe this technique is overused,[122] and in the future its use may be limited by the expense. Nonetheless, MRI can help diagnose injuries when the patient cannot relax for an adequate examination and can provide additional information about concomitant intra-articular knee injuries.

Increased signal intensity in the subchondral bone (bone bruises) has been found in specific patterns. Up to 80% of patients with an ACL injury show increased subchondral signal in the posterior aspect of the lateral tibial plateau and the anterior aspect of the lateral femoral condyle as a result of abnormal impaction of these surfaces secondary to the transient subluxation of the lateral compartment after an ACL injury.[123-125] This pattern is distinctly different from bone bruises seen after patellar dislocation and PCL injury. Bone bruises are less common after isolated PCL injuries.

The authors' current indications for an MRI are as follows:

- An acutely injured knee in which an ACL tear is likely but it is unclear whether the patient has associated meniscal or chondral pathology
- Complete evaluation for preoperative planning for a knee with multiple-ligament injuries
- An unclear diagnosis based on the history, physical examination, and standard radiographs
- A patient who cannot relax or cooperate during the physical examination
- A clinical course not commensurate with the clinical diagnosis
- A high level athlete with an acute injury who needs an immediate, thorough evaluation to determine the extent of injury and the need for surgical or nonoperative treatment
- Evaluation of an occult fracture
- Investigation of the cause of poor range of motion after ligament reconstruction surgery

Other uses of MRI include evaluation for soft tissue masses, tumors, osteonecrosis, osteochondritis dissecans, and extensor mechanism injuries, including tendonitis.

Arthroscopy

Arthroscopy currently is the most commonly performed orthopedic procedure in the United States. It allows for direct visualization of all intra-articular structures, and it can be used to diagnose and surgically treat lesions of the knee. For many acute knee injuries, the best opportunity for complete recovery is with prompt, appropriate surgical treatment. The benefit of arthroscopy, therefore, is that all pathology can be correctly identified and treated as needed. Arthroscopy uses smaller incisions than open surgery, allows better visualization with less morbidity, and can be performed without the use of a tourniquet. Partial tears of the ACL sometimes cannot be differentiated from complete tears, even with an examination under anesthesia. Using arthroscopy, the surgeon can determine whether the ACL is partially or completely torn. Furthermore, if the ligament is partially torn, the extent of injury can be ascertained to guide treatment. Arthroscopy can also be used to evaluate meniscal pathology and determine whether the lesion should be left alone, repaired, or excised. It also has been shown that complete, isolated PCL disruptions may yield a negative posterior drawer sign, even under anesthesia, but these can be diagnosed with arthroscopy.[126]

Although invasive, arthroscopy is a relatively low risk procedure; it has a complication rate of less than 1% and an infection rate of approximately 0.1%.[127,128] Although the risk of anesthesia exists, some authors have found local anesthesia to be effective and safe.[129-133] This is important, because several investigators are evaluating the efficacy of diagnostic and therapeutic office arthroscopy. Nonetheless, diagnostic arthroscopy has been largely replaced by MRI.

Epidemiology, Biomechanics, and Classification of Knee Ligament Injuries
Straight Plane Versus Rotatory Instabilities

The terminology used to classify knee ligament injuries is the source of much confusion. This partly arises from the use of inappropriate terminology to describe and classify movement of the knee. Noyes et al.[134] defined terms that should be used to describe the motion and position of the knee. Motion of the knee is accompanied by rotation and translation of the joint surfaces. *Translation* refers to movement that results when all points of an object move along paths parallel to each other. A fixed point on one surface engages successive points on the opposing surface, much like a tire sliding on an ice patch when the brakes are locked. In the knee, translation of the tibia has three independent components, known as *translational degrees of freedom:* medial-lateral translation, anterior-posterior translation, and proximal-distal translation. Translation of the tibia is commonly reported in millimeters of motion.

Rotation occurs when successive points on a given surface meet successive points on an adjacent surface. The surface appears to be going in circles about an axis of rotation. Rotation of the joint is similar to a tire rolling down a road. In the knee, rotation has three independent degrees of freedom. Flexion and extension rotation occurs in the sagittal plane about an axis located through the femur, which lies in the coronal plane. Abduction and adduction rotation occurs in the coronal plane through an axis in the sagittal plane. Internal and external rotation occurs in the transverse plane around a vertical axis, which is located near the PCL. Rotation of the knee is measured in degrees of motion.

Motion of the knee involves a complex combination of rotation and translation of the joint surfaces. According to the convex-concave rule, flexion of the knee is associated with posterior translation and rotation of the tibia. When the tibia is fixed, flexion of the knee occurs as posterior rotation and anterior translation of the femur. Extension of the knee involves anterior rotation and translation of the tibia. When the tibia is fixed, extension of the knee involves anterior rotation and posterior translation of the femur. This combination of rotation and translation is necessary to keep the femur centered over the tibial plateaus throughout the range of motion. As described earlier, rotation and translation of the joint surfaces during movement of the knee are controlled by the geometry of the joint surfaces, tension in the ligamentous structures, and muscular contraction. Disruption of ligamentous or musculotendinous structures alters the normal arthrokinematics of the knee and may lead to progressive degeneration of the joint surfaces.

The terms *laxity* and *instability* often are used interchangeably. The meaning of these terms must be clarified to improve communication among health care professionals in the evaluation and treatment of knee ligament injuries. The term *laxity* can be used to indicate slackness or lack of tension in a ligament or to describe looseness of a joint. *Laxity* also is used to indicate the amount of joint motion or play that results with the application of forces and moments. Laxity of a joint can be normal or abnormal; therefore the adjective *abnormal* should be used to indicate laxity that is pathological. In addition, *laxity* can refer to either translation or rotation, and this should be clearly specified. For example, *anterior laxity* of the knee can refer either to anterior translation or to rotation of the tibia. If *anterior laxity* is used to describe translation of the tibia, the more precise (and preferable) term is *anterior translation*. The amount of laxity often is recorded as the difference between the involved and noninvolved knees, and this should be clearly indicated. Owing to the ambiguity in the use of the term *laxity,* Noyes et al.[134] recommended that it not be used to describe joint motion or displacement. They recommended that the term be used in a more general sense to indicate slackness or lack of tension in a ligament. When referring to motion of the knee, it is preferable to describe the specific motion as *translation* or *rotation.*

According to Noyes et al.,[135] the term *instability* can be used to describe the symptom of giving way or the physical sign of increased mobility of the joint. To avoid ambiguity, they recommend avoiding use of the term *instability* to indicate an episode of giving way. They prefer to use it to indicate a physical sign that is characterized by an increased or excessive displacement of the tibia resulting from traumatic injury to the stabilizing structures.

Ligamentous injury to the knee results in varying degrees of abnormal laxity or instability, as just described. Hughston et al.[136] classified instability that arises as a result of a knee ligament injury as straight plane or rotatory instability.

A straight plane instability implies injury that allows for equal translation of the medial and lateral tibial plateaus. According to Hughston et al.,[136] straight plane instabilities include posterior, anterior, medial, and lateral instability. Posterior instability occurs with injury to the PCL combined with injury to the arcuate complex and posterior oblique ligament; this results in equal posterior translation of the medial and lateral tibial plateaus when a posterior drawer force is applied. Straight anterior instability occurs with a tear of the ACL and PCL, along with the medial and lateral capsular ligaments. With a straight anterior instability, the two tibial plateaus sublux anteriorly an equal amount when an anterior drawer test is performed. Straight medial instability occurs with a tear of the medial compartment ligaments and the PCL; this results in a positive valgus stress test with the knee in full extension. Straight lateral instability occurs with a tear of the lateral compartment ligaments and the PCL; this results in a positive varus stress test when the knee is in full extension.

Rotatory instabilities involve unequal movement of the medial and lateral tibial plateaus and can include anteromedial, anterolateral, and posterolateral instabilities. Anteromedial rotatory instability occurs when the medial compartment ligaments, including the posterior oblique ligament, are torn. Anteromedial rotatory instability may be accentuated by a tear of the ACL. With anteromedial rotatory instability, a valgus stress test at 30° flexion is positive. In addition, increased anterior translation of the medial tibial plateau is seen when an anterior drawer test is performed with the tibia externally rotated, and the medial pivot shift test may be positive.

Anterolateral rotatory instability occurs with injury to the middle third of the lateral capsular ligaments and is accentuated by a tear of the ACL. With anterolateral instability, an anterior drawer test results in increased anterior translation of the lateral tibial plateau. The lateral pivot shift test also is positive.

Posterolateral rotatory instability implies greater posterior translation of the lateral tibial plateau compared to the medial tibial plateau when a posterior drawer force is applied. Posterolateral instability occurs with a tear of the arcuate complex, which results in a positive varus stress test at 30° flexion. The external rotation recurvatum test also is positive.

Combined rotatory instabilities, such as anteromedial and anterolateral rotatory instability, also can occur.

Butler et al.[8] developed the concept of primary and secondary ligamentous restraints. For each plane of motion of the knee, one ligamentous structure serves as the primary restraint. This structure is responsible for restraining most of the motion in a given direction. For example, the ACL is the primary restraint for anterior translation of the tibia, providing approximately 85% of the restraining force.[8] As the name implies, secondary restraints are structures that take on a secondary role in restraining motion in a particular direction. For example, the secondary restraints for anterior tibial translation are the collateral ligaments, the middle portion of the medial and lateral capsule, and the iliotibial band. These structures are responsible for providing approximately 15% of the total restraining force to anterior translation of the tibia.[8]

The amount of ligament laxity or instability after injury to the ligamentous structures of the knee depends on the extent of injury and the amount of force applied. Injury to the primary restraint that leaves the secondary restraints intact may result in a minimal increase in laxity during manual examination of the knee. However, if both the primary and secondary restraints are injured or stretched, clinical tests for laxity may demonstrate a large increase in motion compared to the noninvolved side. For example, isolated injury to the ACL may result in only a slight increase in anterior tibial translation if the secondary restraints are intact. Over time, with repeated episodes of giving way, the secondary restraints may stretch out, resulting in increased anterior tibial translation. It is important to note that the secondary stabilizers are not as effective as the primary stabilizers in restraining motion in a particular direction. Therefore, over time, the secondary restraints tend to stretch out gradually when the primary restraint has been lost.

Another important consideration for clinicians in performing and interpreting a clinical laxity test is the amount of force applied to the knee. Forces applied during a clinical laxity test are small, ranging from 9.1 to 18.1 kg (20 to 40 pounds). This is much less than the forces involved in in vivo activities, which may exceed 45.4 kg (100 pounds) with strenuous exercise.[8] As a result, clinical laxity tests may not accurately describe the stability of the knee in performing strenuous physical activities. The clinical laxity test may demonstrate only a slight degree of increased laxity. When more strenuous activities are performed, higher loads are placed on the knee, which may result in greater laxity and in complaints of giving way.

Anterior Cruciate Ligament

The ACL is one of the most commonly injured ligaments in the knee. Some studies suggest that the ACL is the most commonly injured ligament in the general population.[137-139] Other investigators, however, believe that of all knee ligament injuries, including those that do not result in pathological motion (grade I and grade II injuries), the MCL is the most commonly injured ligament.[137] The ACL is the primary stabilizer for resisting anterior translation of the tibia on the femur and serves to control hyperextension of the knee. The ACL also serves as a secondary stabilizer to resist internal and external rotation, as well as varus and valgus stress. The ACL can be injured by contact or noncontact mechanisms of injury. Pathomechanics include a valgus force applied to a flexed, laterally rotated knee with the foot planted, or hyperextension, often combined with medial rotation. Less common mechanisms of injury include hyperflexion or a direct valgus force.

Mechanisms of Injury to the Anterior Cruciate Ligament

- Valgus force applied to a flexed, laterally rotated knee with the foot planted
- Hyperextension (often combined with medial rotation)
- Hyperflexion
- Direct valgus force

Daniel et al.[140] reported that the incidence of acute ACL injury among members of a managed health care plan was 31 per 100,000 members annually. Ninety percent of ACL injuries occurred in patients 15 to 45 years of age. Most ACL injuries occur as a result of sports activities, particularly those that place high demands on the knee (e.g., those involving jumping and hard cutting).[141] Skiing may be a particularly high risk activity; the incidence of ACL injury among adult skiers is 1 in 2000.[142]

Mounting evidence indicates that a narrow intercondylar notch may place a patient at greater risk of injury. LaPrade and Burnett[143] reported a higher incidence of acute ACL injuries in individuals with a narrow notch width index. The notch width index is the ratio of the width of the anterior outlet of the intercondylar notch divided by the total condylar width at the level of the popliteal groove. These researchers' prospective study involved 213 athletes at a Division I university, representing 415 ACL-intact knees. Intercondylar notch stenosis was found in 40 knees (i.e., a notch width index less than 0.2), and 375 individuals had a normal notch width index. During the 2-year follow-up period, seven ACL injuries occurred, six in knees with a narrow notch and one in a knee with a normal notch width. Souryal and Freeman[144] demonstrated similar results in 902 high school athletes followed prospectively. The overall rate of ACL injury during the 2-year follow-up was 3%. Athletes who sustained noncontact ACL tears had a statistically smaller notch width index. Of the 14 athletes with noncontact ACL injuries, 10 had a notch width index at least 1 standard deviation (SD) below the mean.

Currently, no data support the premise that poor conditioning or increased physiological laxity places an individual at greater risk of ACL injury; however, women may be at higher risk for this type of injury. Malone[145] reported that women participating in National Collegiate Athletic Association (NCAA) Division I basketball were eight times more likely than their male counterparts to sustain an ACL injury. Further research is needed to identify factors that may place women at higher risk for ACL injury. Females appear to have some unique characteristics that may predispose them to injury, including a wider pelvis, increased genu valgum, altered muscular recruitment patterns, increased laxity, and different biomechanical patterns during athletic participation.[145-148]

Seventy-five percent of ACL ruptures occur in the midsubstance, 20% involve the femoral attachment, and 5% involve the tibial attachment.[149] Associated injuries include meniscal tears in 50% to 70% of acutely injured knees and in up to 90% of chronic, ACL-deficient knees,[45,126,150] chondral injuries in 6% to 20% of ACL-injured knees,[45,126] collateral ligament injuries in 40% to 75% of ACL-injured knees,[150,151] and occasionally capsular injuries and knee dislocations.

The patient often reports an audible crack or pop at the time of initial injury. The patient also notes swelling within the first 2 to 6 hours and inability to continue the activity.

Classification of ACL injuries is based on the extent of the tear and the resulting instability and is largely a clinical diagnosis. Partial tears have increased anterior translation, as documented by Lachman's test or instrumented laxity testing, but they have a negative pivot shift test under anesthesia. If loss of ligament function and rotational instability are demonstrated by a positive pivot shift test, the ACL tear is considered complete. Although this determination often can be made in the clinic or by MRI alone, an examination under anesthesia may be required to establish a definitive diagnosis.

The natural history of an ACL-deficient knee is still unclear. A torn ACL does not heal.[152,153] ACL deficiency leads to rotatory instability in many patients and results in functional disability. This can occur with activities of daily living in some, with sports activities such as running (deceleration), cutting, and jumping in others, and with no functional instability in still another undetermined group. Repetitive episodes of instability may result in meniscal tears, which can result in arthritis. Debate exists as to whether isolated ACL tears, without meniscal pathology, result in degenerative changes within the knee joint.[51,138,140,150,152,154,155] ACL-deficient patients who undergo meniscectomy without ACL reconstruction develop degenerative changes more quickly; this is more apparent in patients with higher activity levels.[156] A direct relationship exists between giving way (instability) and the activity level, but many patients with an ACL-deficient knee can return to sports at a less stressful level of activity. Furthermore, functional instability may also be related to meniscal pathology. As is discussed later in the chapter, meniscal injury directly relates to the level of disability, pain, and swelling and the frequency of reinjury.

Posterior Cruciate Ligament

Although the true incidence of PCL injuries is unknown, they are thought to account for 3% to 40% of all knee injuries.[137,157-159] PCL injury may be more common than realized. PCL injuries are easily missed, because physicians are less familiar with the clinical examination findings. Injuries often go undiagnosed and manifest later as instability or pain.

The PCL is the strongest ligament in the knee,[160] and a significant force is required to rupture it. Most PCL injuries occur as a result of athletic, motor vehicle, or industrial accidents. The mechanism of most athletic PCL injuries is a fall on the flexed knee with the foot and ankle plantar-flexed.[61,161] This imparts a posteriorly directed force on the proximal tibia, which ruptures the taut ligament that is parallel to the force vector, usually resulting in an isolated PCL injury.[162] Similarly, in a motor vehicle accident, the knee is flexed and the tibia is forced posteriorly on impact with the dashboard. Another mechanism of injury to the PCL is a downwardly directed force applied to the thigh

while the knee is hyperflexed, such as when landing from a jump.[55] Hyperflexion of the knee without a direct blow to the tibia can also result in an isolated PCL injury.[163]

Mechanisms of Injury to the Posterior Cruciate Ligament

- Fall on a flexed knee with the ankle plantar flexed
- Dashboard injury
- Downward force to the thigh while the knee is hyperflexed
- Hyperflexion

Other mechanisms can result in injury to the PCL, but these usually also involve injury to other ligaments. Forced hyperextension does not usually result in injury to the PCL.[164] Rather, hyperextension is more likely to lead to injury to the posterior knee capsule, popliteal vessel, or ACL.[157] A posteriorly directed force applied to the antero-medial tibia with the knee in hyperextension may also cause injury to the posterolateral corner[157] and results in lateral and posterolateral instability. Significant varus or valgus stress injures the PCL only after rupture of the appropriate collateral ligament. Therefore, when the PCL is torn, the integrity of the rest of the knee must be carefully evaluated.

Seventy percent of PCL disruptions occur on the tibial side, with or without an associated bony fragment, 15% occur on the femoral side, and 15% involve midsubstance tears.[149] Associated injuries with acute "isolated" PCL tears include chondral defects in 12% and meniscal tears in 27%, which occur more commonly in the lateral compartment.[165] As with chronic ACL tears, the incidence of meniscal and chondral lesions is higher in chronic PCL-deficient knees,[165] although in contrast to acute injuries, these more commonly involve the medial compartment.

The patient often reports an audible crack or pop at the time of the initial injury. The patient also notes mild to moderate swelling within the first 2 to 6 hours; however, unlike with ACL injuries, these individuals may return to activity, and the injury often is thought to be a minor event. Patients frequently complain of an unstable gait, but pain with weight bearing or anterior knee pain is common. Pain in patients with a chronic PCL-deficient knee also may be partly due to degeneration of the medial or patellofemoral compartments.[164] The pain is exacerbated by walking down stairs.

As with the classification of ACL injuries, grading of PCL injuries depends on the extent of the tear and the degree of resulting laxity. A grade I PCL sprain involves microscopic partial tearing of the ligament, which overall remains intact. The ligament fibers are stretched, causing hemorrhage and microscopic disruption of the ligament. Examination of a grade I PCL injury reveals no increased laxity compared to the contralateral knee, and the end point is firm. A grade II sprain is also a partial tear, although the injury results in partial loss of function, as determined by a slight increase in posterior translation during a posterior drawer test; however, a definite end point is noted, and the reverse pivot shift test is negative. This may be a macroscopic or microscopic tear that results in hemorrhage and stretching of the ligament, but the ligament is still in continuity and functions to some degree. A grade III sprain of the PCL is a complete tear of the ligament. Loss of ligament function and joint stability are seen; the posterior drawer test result is 2+ to 3+; and the posterior sag test, Godfrey's sign, the quadriceps active drawer test, and the reverse pivot shift test are positive. Posterior tibial translation is excessive, and the end point is soft.

The natural history of the PCL-deficient knee remains controversial. Some patients experience almost no functional limitation and compete in high level athletics, whereas others are severely limited during activities of daily living.[161,163,166,167] Parolie and Bergfeld[161] suggested that, if adequate quadriceps strength can be obtained, most patients do well with nonoperative treatment. Dejour et al.[168] suggested that patients are symptomatic for the first 12 months, during which time they learn to adapt to the PCL injury. After this time, patients do well, and a high percentage return to sports. They also reported the development of degenerative changes involving the medial and anterior compartment in chronic PCL-deficient knees,[168] but this finding has not been reported by others.[61,161,166]

More recently, these positive results of nonoperative treatments have been challenged. Clancy et al.[61] reported degenerative changes in the medial compartment in 90% of patients at the 4-year follow-up. Dandy and Pusey[169] followed patients for an average of 7.2 years. Seventy percent had pain while walking, and 55% had patellofemoral symptoms. No correlation was seen between ligament laxity and functional results. Keller et al.[167] reported on a series of 40 patients at the 6-year follow-up. The longer the interval between injury and follow-up, the lower the knee score. The presence of radiographic degenerative changes directly correlated with lower knee scores despite excellent muscular strength.

Similarly, with long-term follow-up (15 years), Dejour et al.[168] found progressive deterioration of results. Eighty-nine percent of patients with isolated PCL injuries had pain, and 79% of knees had degenerative changes. These researchers described the natural history of PCL deficiency as having three phases: functional adaptation, functional tolerance, and osteoarthritic deterioration.

Laboratory studies confirm that PCL deficiency results in increased medial compartment and patellofemoral contact pressures that can result in arthritis of the knee.[170] Whether surgical reconstruction can alter the development of long-term degenerative changes is unclear. Furthermore, in some patients the PCL apparently may heal, although in a lengthened position.[171] This may explain the variable results of long-term studies of the PCL-deficient knee.

Medial Collateral Ligament

As noted earlier, the MCL is the most commonly injured ligament in the knee.[137] However, the incidence of grade III injuries to the MCL may be lower than the incidence of high grade ACL tears.[137] The MCL is injured by a valgus stress to the knee that exceeds the strength of the MCL. This most commonly occurs from a blow to the lateral aspect of the knee during a sports event. Uncommonly, a noncontact valgus injury to the knee, such as occurs in skiing, can produce an isolated tear of the MCL.

Mechanism of Injury to the Medial Collateral Ligament

• Valgus stress to a weight-bearing knee

MCL injuries most commonly involve the femoral insertion site, which accounts for approximately 65% of all MCL sprains. Approximately 25% of MCL sprains involve the tibial insertion. The remaining 10% of MCL injuries involve a deep portion of the MCL at the level of the joint line.[149] Associated tears of the medial meniscus occur in 2% to 4% of grade I and grade II MCL sprains, but medial meniscal tears generally do not occur with grade III MCL sprains.[172-174] This is most likely because compression of the medial compartment is required to tear the medial meniscus, whereas injury to the MCL requires tension that unloads the medial compartment.

The diagnosis of an MCL injury can be made from the history and physical examination alone and usually does not require MRI or arthroscopy. However, if the physical examination is difficult to perform or if damage to other intra-articular structures is suspected, an MRI can be helpful for determining the full extent of the injury. The patient often recalls being hit by another athlete while the foot was planted, feeling the impact on the lateral aspect of the knee and pain on the medial aspect of the knee. In rare cases patients may note a pop at the time of injury, but they more commonly state that they felt a tearing or pulling on the medial aspect of the knee. Swelling occurs quickly at the site of injury, and ecchymosis may develop 1 to 3 days after injury. With a grade I or II sprain, the patient may be able to continue to play, but with a grade III sprain, the patient usually cannot continue to participate in sports. These patients usually walk with a limp and with the knee partially flexed, because extension stretches the ligament and causes further pain. The patient may not have an effusion if the injury is isolated to the MCL.

Classification of MCL sprains depends on the extent of the tear and the degree of laxity that results. A grade I sprain involves microscopic tearing of the ligament, which overall remains intact. The ligament fibers are stretched, causing hemorrhage and microscopic disruption of the ligament. Examination of the MCL by the aforementioned tests reveals no increase in laxity compared to the contralateral knee, and the end point is firm. However, tenderness is present along the ligament. A grade II sprain of the MCL is also a partial tear, but the injury results in partial loss of function, as determined by a slight degree of increased joint opening (3 to 5 mm) on a valgus stress test with the knee in 30° flexion; a definite end point is noted. In full extension, the knee joint opens less than 2 mm more than the contralateral knee. A grade II sprain may represent macroscopic or microscopic tearing, resulting in hemorrhage and stretching of the ligament, but the ligament is still in continuity and functions to some degree. An acute grade II MCL injury is tender to palpation, and the patient notes pain with stress testing. A grade III sprain is a complete tear of the ligament. Loss of ligament function occurs, and a joint space opening of more than 5 mm compared to the noninvolved knee is seen on a valgus stress test in 30° flexion; an opening of more than 3 mm compared to the noninvolved knee occurs in full extension. Also, no definite end point is noted with stress testing. Significant joint opening in full extension indicates medial capsular injury and possibly injury to the cruciate ligaments. The severity of tenderness does not correlate with the extent of injury. A grade III sprain usually hurts less than a grade II or grade I injury.

The natural history of isolated MCL tears is a process of healing, regardless of the degree of injury.[173-179] Patients with proximal injuries involving the femoral insertion tend to have a higher incidence of stiffness. Also, proximal MCL injuries heal with less residual laxity compared to injuries involving the tibial side.

Lateral Collateral Ligament

Isolated injuries to the LCL of the knee are uncommon. In fact, they tend to be the least common injury to the knee, causing only 2% of all knee injuries that result in pathological motion (grade III injuries).[137] The injury usually is the result of a direct varus stress to the knee, generally with the foot planted and the knee in extension.[127] Injury to the LCL tends to occur as a result of nonsports, high energy activities,[127,137] because a direct blow to the medial aspect of the knee is an unusual occurrence in sports. Varus stress to the knee may also occur during the stance phase of gait, with sudden imbalance and a shift of the center of gravity away from the side of injury resulting in tension on the lateral structures. This mechanism does not require an external force to the knee. Another cause of a varus stress to the knee is a sideswipe injury, in which one knee has a valgus stress and the other a varus stress. The varus injury often has a rotational component.

Mechanism of Injury to the Lateral Collateral Ligament

• Varus stress to a weight-bearing, extended knee

Straight varus injuries result in LCL disruptions. These tend to be tears from the fibular head, with or without avulsion in 75% of cases, from the femoral side in 20%, and midsubstance tears in 5%.[149] Associated peroneal nerve injuries are common (up to 24%), because the nerve is tethered as it courses around the fibular head.[127] These nerve palsies have a poor prognosis for complete recovery.[180]

Patients with injury to the LCL may hear or feel a pop in the knee and have lateral knee pain. An intra-articular effusion may represent a capsular injury or an associated meniscal or chondral lesion. Because the LCL is extra-articular, isolated LCL lesions do not commonly result in an effusion of the knee.

Often LCL injuries occur in association with injury to other ligaments in the knee. A severe varus stress results in an LCL disruption, followed by disruption of the posterolateral capsule and PCL. The posterolateral corner should be assessed with stress tests for increased varus rotation and external rotation at 30° and 90° and compared to the opposite knee.[181]

Classification of LCL sprains depends on the extent of the tear and the resulting degree of laxity. A grade I sprain involves microscopic partial tearing of the ligament, but the ligament overall remains intact. The ligament fibers are stretched, causing hemorrhage and microscopic disruption within the ligament. Varus stress testing reveals no increase in laxity compared to the contralateral knee, and the end point is firm; however, tenderness is present along the ligament. A grade II sprain is also a partial tear, but the injury results in partial loss of function, as determined by a slight increase in joint opening with varus stress testing (3-5 mm) compared to the noninvolved knee with the knee in 30° flexion; however, a definite end point is noted. In full extension, the knee joint opens less than 2 mm more than the contralateral knee. A grade II LCL sprain may represent macroscopic or microscopic tearing, resulting in hemorrhage and stretching of the ligament, but the ligament is still in continuity and functions to some degree. A grade II acutely injured LCL is tender to palpation, and the patient notes pain with stress testing. A grade III sprain is a complete tear of the ligament. Loss of ligament function occurs, and a joint space opening of more than 5 mm compared to the noninvolved knee is seen with varus stress testing in 30° flexion; an opening of 3 mm or more than the noninvolved knee is seen in full extension. In addition, no definite end point is noted with varus stress testing. Palpation of the ligament in the figure-of-four position reveals absence of tension in the ligament proximal to the fibular head.

The natural history of the untreated, complete LCL disruption has yet to be determined. Only a few studies with limited subjects have involved isolated LCL injuries. DeLee et al.[127] suggested that severe, straight lateral instability with more than 10 mm of joint opening compared to the contralateral knee usually implies that the ACL or the PCL (or both) has been injured. From the few studies that have been reported, truly isolated LCL injuries appear to do well with nonoperative treatment.[127,176,179]

Dislocations and Multiple-Ligament Knee Injuries

Knee dislocations and other, less severe multiple-ligament injuries account for approximately 20% of all grade III ligament injuries of the knee.[137] This diverse group of injuries has a variable severity and co-morbidity. Other than combined ACL-MCL injuries, combined ligament injuries account for fewer than 2% of all knee ligament injuries.[137] Frequent combinations of two-ligament injuries include the ACL-MCL (most common), PCL-MCL, PCL-LCL, ACL-LCL, and ACL-PCL.

To dislocate the knee, at least three ligaments must be torn.[182] In most knee dislocations, both cruciate ligaments and one collateral ligament are torn. Fractures occasionally are associated with knee dislocations, but these fracture-dislocations are considered a different entity from a dislocated knee and involve injury only to the ligaments.

A person may dislocate the knee by simply stepping in a hole and hyperextending the knee (low energy). Dislocations also can result from a high energy blow to the knee, such as can occur in a motor vehicle accident. Athletes have sustained low energy knee dislocations during collisions in baseball, rugby, football, and soccer.

Neurovascular injury is uncommon with knee injuries that involve only two ligaments. However, an LCL injury combined with a cruciate ligament injury can result in enough lateral joint opening to produce injury to the peroneal nerve.

Although the knee can dislocate in any direction, the most common directions are anterior and posterior.[183,184] Knee dislocations may involve damage to multiple structures within the knee, including the cruciate and collateral ligaments, capsular structures, menisci, articular surface, tendons, and neurovascular structures. The nerves and blood vessels in the popliteal space of the knee are easily stretched and torn during dislocation of the knee, and neurovascular injury must be ruled out in all cases. Associated injuries include vascular damage in 20% to 40% of knee dislocations and nerve damage in 20% to 30%. Some knee dislocation case series reports had an amputation rate of the involved extremity of up to 49%.[183,185,186] Posterior knee dislocations are associated with the highest incidence of popliteal artery injury,[183] and posterolateral rotatory dislocations have the highest incidence of nerve injury.[187] Some

evidence suggests that low velocity knee dislocations may uncommonly result in neurovascular injury.[188] On the other hand, ultra-low velocity knee dislocations in morbidly obese individuals have a very high rate of vascular injury.[189]

Evaluation of vascular status should include palpation of pulses and comparison of the ankle-brachial index (ABI). This test involves taking the blood pressure at the ankle and on the arm at rest and is repeated at both sites after 5 minutes of treadmill walking. It is used to predict the severity of peripheral arterial disease (PAD). If pulses are asymmetrical, or if an abnormal ABI is obtained, an arteriogram is required. Recent evidence suggests that serial vascular examinations may replace the arteriogram if ankle-brachial indices are normal.[190]

Osteochondral and meniscal injuries are rare, particularly with low velocity knee dislocations. This is most likely because a distraction force is required to dislocate the knee, whereas osteochondral and meniscal injuries are caused by compressive forces.[188]

The patient with a multiple-ligament injury frequently gives a history of severe injury to the knee, although, as noted earlier, the mechanism may be trivial. The patient often hears a pop. Swelling occurs within the first few hours, but it is not always large because of the associated capsular injury and extravasation of the hemarthrosis. The patient may note deformity of the knee if the knee dislocated and remains unreduced. The patient complains of instability and inability to continue with sports and activities of daily living.

Tibiofemoral dislocations are classified by the direction in which the tibia translates in relation to the femur. As mentioned, the knee can dislocate in any direction. For example, if the tibia lies anterior to the femur, the injury is an anterior dislocation. Posterior, medial, and lateral dislocations of the knee also can occur. Rotatory dislocations occur when the knee dislocates in more than one direction; these include anteromedial, anterolateral, posteromedial, and posterolateral dislocations. Unfortunately, knee dislocations can reduce spontaneously; therefore this classification scheme is not useful. Furthermore, the amount of tibial displacement that occurs at the time of injury cannot be estimated from physical or radiographic findings. It therefore is helpful to describe the dislocated knee by the ligamentous structures that have been disrupted.

The natural history of knee dislocations and multiple-ligament injuries is unknown. This is due to the uncommon nature of these injuries and to the many types of dislocations and mechanisms of injury (low velocity versus high velocity) that can occur. However, vascular injury associated with knee dislocation, if left untreated or if not repaired within 8 hours of the time of injury, results in an 86% amputation rate. If surgery to correct vascular injury is completed within 6 to 8 hours, the amputation rate is only 11%.[188] Associated nerve injuries have a poor prognosis for recovery, regardless of the treatment.[191,192]

The development of instability, loss of motion, and arthritis is unclear with nonoperative treatment. The level of function of patients with multiple-ligament injuries is worse than those with an isolated knee ligament injury. Knee dislocations treated with immobilization and aggressive rehabilitation have surprisingly good results with regard to stability, absence of pain, and the range of knee flexion up to 90°.[193] The incidence of arthritis after multiple-ligament injuries has yet to be determined, but increased instability would be expected to result in a greater degree of arthritic change.

Treatment of Knee Ligament Injuries

Guidelines for Progression of Rehabilitation

Progression of the rehabilitation program after knee ligament injury and/or surgery should proceed in a logical sequence. Generally, the phases of this progression overlap. For example, muscle function may be addressed before full range of motion and flexibility have been restored. Progression of the patient through the sequence must be individualized and depends on the nature of the injury and/or surgery, principles of tissue healing, individual signs and symptoms, and the response to treatment. Adequate time must be allowed for tissue healing and remodeling. During rehabilitation, care must be taken to avoid overaggressive treatment, which is indicated by a prolonged increase in pain after treatment and/or regression in the patient's progress.

Determinants of Rehabilitation Progression

- Nature of injury
- Nature of surgery
- Tissue healing principles
- Tissue healing timelines
- Patient's signs and symptoms
- Patient's response to treatment

The initial phase of the rehabilitation program should promote tissue healing and reduce pain and swelling. During this period, treatments such as cold and compression may be beneficial for decreasing pain and swelling. A balance must be achieved between mobility and immobility. The healing tissues must not be overloaded. Overaggressive treatment during this period can disrupt the healing process, but prolonged immobilization can also have adverse effects. Prolonged immobilization is associated with decreased bone mass, changes in the articular cartilage, synovial adhesions, and decreased strength and increased stiffness of ligaments and the joint capsule, which lead to joint contracture and loss of motion. Disuse results in atrophy and diminished oxidative capacity of muscle. Immobilization appears to affect slow muscle fibers more than fast muscle fibers.[194,195]

The time required for soft tissue healing varies. The response of soft tissue to injury is acute inflammation, which typically lasts several days or until the noxious stimulus has been neutralized. During this period, applications of cold and compression may be used to limit and control acute inflammation. Inflammation is followed by fibroplasia, which involves the proliferation of fibroblasts and the formation of collagen fibers and ground substance. Fibroplasia usually lasts for several weeks and results in the formation of granulation tissue, which is fragile, vascularized connective tissue. During this period, protected motion is encouraged, because it stimulates collagen formation and alignment. Excessive loading of the healing tissue should be avoided, because it may disrupt the healing tissue and reinitiate the inflammatory process. Over time, granulation tissue matures and remodels and can withstand greater loads. This process is gradual and depends on the stresses imposed on the tissue; stresses should be gradually and progressively increased to allow the tissues to adapt to the functional demands placed on them.

Rehabilitation of the knee should ensure that full motion symmetrical to the uninvolved knee is restored. Loss of motion after knee ligament injury and/or surgery adversely affects function. Loss of extension affects gait and results in patellofemoral symptoms. Loss of flexion interferes with activities such as stair climbing, squatting, and running. In the early phases of rehabilitation, passive, active-assisted, and active range of motion exercises can be used to increase and/or maintain motion of the knee. In the latter stages of rehabilitation, active and passive stretching can be used to restore motion. Stretching should be sustained and should use low force to maximize creep and relaxation of connective tissue to produce permanent elongation. Application of heat before and during the stretch and maintaining the stretch during cooling may also help produce permanent elongation.[196] Neurophysiological stretching techniques, such as contract/relax or contract/relax/contract, can help restore motion if the limitation is due to muscular tightness.

Mobilization of the patella also may be helpful in restoring motion. Inferior glide of the patella is necessary for flexion, and superior glide is necessary for normal functioning of the extensor mechanism. Decreased superior mobility of the patella interferes with the ability of the quadriceps to pull through the knee extensor mechanism and results in the development of a knee extensor lag. Medial glide and lateral tilt of the patella are necessary to stretch the lateral retinacular structures. The force used during patellar mobilization must be appropriate for the degree of inflammation present. Overly aggressive patellar mobilization aggravates pain and swelling, which can contribute to loss of motion. Mobilization of the tibiofemoral joint is rarely necessary but can help restore motion if the limitation of motion is due to hypomobility of the tibiofemoral joint.

Rehabilitation after knee ligament injury and/or surgery must restore function of the muscles that cross the knee as well as the muscles that influence segments proximal and distal to the knee. After acute knee injury or in the immediate postoperative period, the emphasis should be on regaining motor control. Often acute pain and swelling result in inhibition of the quadriceps, and a knee extensor lag develops. During this period, quadricep sets, straight leg raises (SLRs), co-contraction in weight bearing (CKC) and isometric hamstring exercises can be performed. Facilitation techniques such as vibration and tapping, as well as biofeedback and electrical stimulation, may be helpful in regaining motor control. Generally, gaining quadriceps control is more difficult than gaining control of the hamstrings.

Resistive exercises are initiated when the individual has regained full active motion of the knee. Initially, resistive exercises should be performed with light resistance and high repetitions to improve muscle endurance. This minimizes stress on healing structures about the knee and improves the aerobic capacity of slow twitch muscle fibers. OKC exercises can be used to provide isolated exercise for the hamstrings and quadriceps. Precautions must be taken to avoid overloading healing tissues and to prevent the development of patellofemoral symptoms. CKC exercises can be used to improve muscle function in functional patterns while minimizing patellofemoral stress. CKC exercises are progressed as tolerated and may include wall slides, minisquats, step-ups, and leg presses. Cycling is an excellent exercise for developing endurance of the lower extremity musculature while minimizing stress on the patellofemoral and tibiofemoral joints. The use of toe clips and pedaling with one leg can help increase hamstring activity. Other forms of endurance exercise for the lower extremities include step machines, cross-country ski machines, and swimming.

In the later phases of rehabilitation, resistive exercises can be progressed to high resistance, low repetition exercises to develop muscle strength and power. High resistance, low repetition OKC exercises are used to improve isolated muscle strength, but care must be taken to avoid overloading the patellofemoral joint, as described earlier in this chapter. High resistance, low repetition CKC exercises can be used to improve strength in functional patterns with less risk of patellofemoral symptoms; however, patellofemoral mechanisms should always be considered with the rehabilitation of any knee injury.

Exercises should incorporate both the concentric and eccentric phases of contraction. Concentric muscle function is necessary to accelerate the body, whereas eccentric muscle function is necessary to decelerate the body. During a concentric contraction, the muscle shortens as it contracts, whereas during an eccentric contraction, the muscle elongates as it contracts. The force-velocity relationship is different for concentric and eccentric contractions. During a concentric contraction, muscle force decreases as the speed of shortening increases. During an eccentric contraction, muscle force increases as the speed of lengthening increases. Eccentric contractions produce higher levels of force as a result of lengthening of the series elastic component and facilitation of the stretch reflex. To ensure full restoration of function, rehabilitation should include concentric and eccentric exercises. Failure to incorporate eccentric exercise into the rehabilitation program results in the development of muscle soreness and an increased risk of reinjury with return to activity.

For athletes who require power to perform their sport, plyometric exercises should be incorporated into the final stages of the rehabilitation program. Plyometric exercises develop power and speed and incorporate lengthening of the muscle immediately before a powerful concentric contraction. These exercises include depth drops and jumps from heights of 15.2 to 45.7 cm (6 to 18 inches), bounding, hopping, and ricochets. The plyometric program must be carefully planned and implemented to avoid injury.

Once the strength and endurance of the lower extremity musculature have been established, neuromuscular control must be developed to enhance dynamic stability of the knee. This requires learning how to recruit muscles with the proper force, timing, and sequence to prevent abnormal joint motion. Initially it requires conscious effort, often with the help of biofeedback. Through practice and repetition, control of abnormal joint motion becomes automatic and occurs subconsciously.

Proprioceptive neuromuscular facilitation techniques, such as rhythmic stabilization and timing for emphasis, may be helpful for developing dynamic stability. A variety of functional activities can also be used to develop dynamic control of abnormal joint motion. These activities generally are progressed from slow to fast speed, from low to high force, and from controlled to uncontrolled activities. The emphasis should be on establishing proper movement patterns to enhance dynamic stability of the joint. EMG biofeedback may be used to ensure that muscles are being recruited in the proper sequence to maintain joint stability. Activities for enhancing dynamic stability progress from walking, jogging-running, acceleration-deceleration, sprinting, jumping, cutting, pivoting, and twisting. Research is needed to determine the effectiveness of these techniques.

Anterior Cruciate Ligament Injuries

Treatment of ACL injuries must be individualized. It depends on the extent of pathology and the level of disability experienced by the patient during sports and activities of daily living. Therefore, decisions regarding the treatment of the ACL-deficient knee must be made in collaboration with the patient, physician, physical therapist, and athletic trainer. The type of treatment depends on many factors, including age, activity level, occupation, desire to continue sports, amount of functional instability, presence of associated injuries and arthritic changes, and amount of laxity. The patient's willingness to modify activity to a level compatible with functional stability is the most important factor governing treatment options.

Most studies of the natural history of conservative treatment of ACL injuries have shown poor results in young patients. Persistent instability is common. Noyes et al.[197] reported a 65% incidence of giving way during activity, which was associated with persistent pain and disability for several days thereafter. Hawkins et al.[198] reported that 86% of patients in his case series had similar findings. Furthermore, the ability to return to strenuous activity is limited without reconstruction; only 14% to 22% of patients in this younger age group return to the same level as their previous activity.[197-199]

In older patients, who accept limitations on their activities, results generally are better. Ciccotti et al.[200] evaluated a series of patients 40 to 60 years old who were treated conservatively for ACL tears. Ninety-seven percent had a grade 2 or grade 3 on Lachman's test, and 83% had a positive result on the pivot shift test; the overall satisfaction rate was 83%.

Even so, without treatment, ACL insufficiency predisposes the patient to injury of other knee structures. The risk for additional lesions of the menisci and cartilage increases with time.[152,199,201-204] Progressive degeneration of the knee has been cited, especially when associated with meniscal tears.[199,205] Osteoarthritic changes have been noted to occur with ACL insufficiency in 21% to 100% of patients.

Factors associated with a good outcome for nonoperative treatment include intact collateral ligaments, absence of meniscal injury and/or arthritis, and participation in low demand sports that do not require running, jumping, or cutting. A factor that militates against a surgical approach is a minimal increase in tibial translation with laxity testing.

Surgical reconstruction of the ACL-deficient knee should be considered if instability of a knee prevents the patient from participating in sports and other activities. It also should be considered if associated collateral ligament damage or meniscal injury is present or if a large increase in anterior tibial translation is seen with laxity testing. Surgery should be considered in most patients who have high expectations and plan to compete in sports that place high demands on the knee.

Partial tears of the ACL involving more than 50% of the ligament are more likely to progress to complete tears if treated nonsurgically.[134] In general, however, there is little correlation between the percentage of the tear and the clinical outcome.[134] Also, the extent of tearing may be difficult to quantify accurately. For this reason, the distinction between a partially torn ACL and a complete tear usually is a clinical one. A positive result on the pivot shift test, regardless of whether the patient is awake or under anesthesia, defines functional instability and an incompetent ACL.

ACL tears in skeletally immature individuals are more common than previously suspected. Initially these patients usually are treated nonoperatively. If functional instability persists after rehabilitation, consideration must be given to reconstruction of the ACL. Skeletal immaturity is no longer an absolute contraindication to ACL reconstruction, but the patient must be followed closely to ensure that growth has not been arrested.

Nonoperative Treatment

Nonoperative treatment after injury to the ACL generally has fallen out of favor, because advances in surgical and rehabilitative techniques have improved outcomes and reduced morbidity. Nonetheless, conservative treatment of ACL injuries may be indicated for more sedentary individuals who have an isolated injury without damage to other structures and who are willing to modify their lifestyle to avoid activities that cause pain, swelling, and/or episodes of instability. Nonoperative treatment of ACL injuries does not mean that the injury is ignored. Treatment should actively involve the patient and includes exercise, functional training, bracing, and patient education.

Treatment after acute injury to the ACL should focus on resolving inflammation, restoring range of motion, regaining muscle control, and protecting the knee from further injury. Cold and compression can be used to decrease pain and swelling. Range of motion exercises should be performed to restore motion, which should improve as pain and swelling subside. Failure to regain motion, particularly extension, may indicate a torn meniscus, and further diagnostic studies and/or surgery may be indicated. Isometric exercises for the quadriceps and hamstrings should be initiated to regain motor control and minimize atrophy. Assistive devices should be used for ambulation while the knee is still actively inflamed. The use of assistive devices can be discontinued once the patient has regained full extension without a quadriceps lag and can walk normally, without gait deviations.

More aggressive rehabilitation can begin once inflammation has resolved and full range of motion has been restored. The emphasis at this time should be on improving the strength and endurance of the muscles that cross the knee. Particular emphasis should be placed on the muscles that pull the tibia posteriorly (i.e., the hamstrings and gastrocnemius). The normal quadriceps to hamstring ratio at a slow contractile velocity is approximately 3:2. It has been suggested that rehabilitation of an ACL-deficient knee should strive to develop a hamstring-dominant knee so that the quadriceps to hamstring ratio approaches 1:1. This seems to be a logical goal for rehabilitation of ACL injuries, but it should not be achieved at the expense of quadriceps weakness.

OKC and CKC exercises can be used to improve strength and endurance. OKC exercises can be used to provide isolated exercise for the hamstrings and quadriceps. Precautions must be taken to prevent the development of patellofemoral symptoms with OKC knee extension. Standing and seated calf raises can be used to develop the gastrocnemius and soleus, respectively. CKC exercises can be used to develop strength and endurance of the muscles of the lower extremity in functional patterns while minimizing patellofemoral stress. CKC exercises are progressed as tolerated.

Once the strength and endurance of the lower extremity muscles have been established, neuromuscular control must be developed to enhance dynamic stability of the knee. Emphasis should be placed on learning to recruit the posterior muscles to minimize anterior subluxation of the tibia. The patient should be taught to "set" the hamstrings and gastrocnemius before foot strike.

Sherrington[206] proposed co-activation of the antagonist during contraction of the agonist. Baratta et al.[17] and Draganich et al.[19] demonstrated co-activation of the hamstrings during resisted OKC knee extension. Antagonist-agonist co-activation probably originates from the motor cortex in the phenomenon known as *direct common drive*.[207] Activation of the muscle spindle can also facilitate contraction of the antagonist.[13] As the knee extends, muscle spindles lying within the hamstrings are activated and facilitate contraction. Training the hamstrings to stabilize the knee dynamically should capitalize on the phenomenon of co-activation.

A functional brace may be helpful as the patient returns to activity. Exactly how knee braces work is unclear, but many patients report improved function with the use of a knee brace. Whether functional braces provide a physical restraint to abnormal joint motion is doubtful. Several studies[208-210] have indicated that knee braces may restrain tibial translation at low force levels but are ineffective at controlling abnormal joint motion at functional force levels. It has been proposed that knee braces function by improving proprioception. Lephart et al.[14] reported enhanced awareness of joint movement sense with the application of a neoprene sleeve. Application of a knee brace may stimulate cutaneous receptors and enhance proprioception. In addition, knee braces may enhance conscious or subconscious awareness of the injury, helping the individual to protect oneself from further injury.

Another important component of nonoperative management of ACL injuries is modification of the patient's lifestyle to avoid activities associated with pain, swelling, and episodes of instability. Repeated episodes of instability cause further injury to the joint, including stretching of secondary restraints and injury to the menisci and joint surfaces. Recurrent pain and swelling with activity indicate additional damage to the joint. Activities that are not tolerated by the joint should be eliminated to prevent irreversible degenerative changes. Activities that place high stress on the ACL-deficient knee include those that involve jumping, landing, cutting, pivoting, and rapid acceleration or deceleration on the involved extremity. Nonoperative management is likely to fail patients who are unwilling or unable to modify their lifestyle to avoid activities associated with increased pain, swelling, and instability; therefore these individuals should consider surgical reconstruction.

Surgical Treatment

Surgical treatment of a torn ACL includes direct repair, repair with augmentation, and reconstruction with autografts or allografts. Results of direct repair have been poor.[151,211,212] A few investigators, however, have been encouraged by repair with augmentation.[213,214] From a historical perspective, reconstructions using synthetic ligaments led to early failure and the development of wear particle debris that leads to reactive synovitis.[215-217]

Reconstruction has been successful and remains the treatment of choice.[215-217] Reconstruction with augmentation does not appear to improve the results compared to reconstruction alone.[218-220] In addition, the use of a ligament augmentation device may result in stress yielding of the graft, which may delay remodeling.

The timing of surgery after acute injury is an important consideration in minimizing the risk of postoperative loss of motion. Most authors recommend delaying surgery until inflammation has subsided and range of motion and muscle function have been restored.[221,222] A decreased incidence of loss of motion and a faster return of quadriceps strength were noted when surgery was delayed 3 to 4 weeks after acute ACL injury.[221,223,224]

Currently, ACL reconstruction is most commonly performed using an arthroscopically assisted technique with the goal of recreating the normal anatomy of the ACL. An arthroscope is inserted into the knee through two or three small portals. A tibial tunnel is drilled with an intra-articular exit point at the posterior half of the native ACL insertion. A second tunnel is drilled in the femur at the origin of the native ACL. Position of the femoral tunnel is often dictated by the tibial tunnel position as the tibial tunnel is used to drill the femur. An anatomical and isometric reconstruction of the ACL is performed by positioning a graft within these tunnels.

Multiple surgical variables contribute to the success of the operation. Tunnel placement, graft type, graft fixation, tension, rotation, and notch preparation affect the biomechanics of the reconstruction. Graft fixation can be performed by multiple techniques. If a patellar tendon graft is used, fixation usually is achieved with interference screws (Figure 16-30). Soft tissue grafts (e.g., hamstring, tibialis) can be fixed with an EndoButton, spiked washers, or a special interference screw. An adequate "notchplasty" must be performed to allow enough space for the graft so that the knee can extend fully without impingement. This should

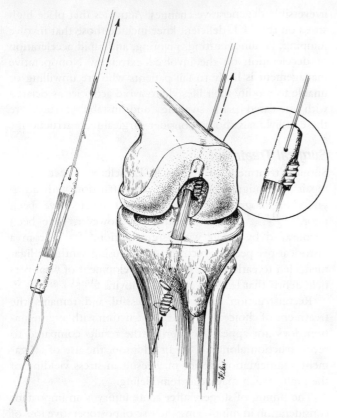

Figure 16-30
Anterior cruciate ligament reconstruction using a bone–patellar tendon–bone graft. Interference screw fixation is used to fix the graft within the tunnels. (From Zachazewski JE, Magee DJ, Quillen WS, editors: *Athletic injuries and rehabilitation,* p 665, Philadelphia, 1996, WB Saunders.)

be determined intraoperatively, and the notch should be enlarged if the graft impinges in the intercondylar area.

ACL reconstruction techniques have evolved with advances in the biomechanical evaluation of the knee. Computer-assisted surgery, high resolution MRI, and evaluation of in vivo three-dimensional kinematics recently have provided new insights into functional evaluations of ACL reconstructions. These analyses have led to an increased emphasis on optimization of graft placement. Several surgeons have proposed that the two functional bundles of the ACL, the anteromedial bundle and the posteromedial bundle, be reconstructed individually.[225-227] The clinical importance of this technique has yet to be determined.

Multiple types of grafts have been used to reconstruct the ACL. Currently the most common sources of autograft tissue (i.e., tissue from the same individual) are the bone–patellar tendon–bone (BPTB)[61,228,229] and hamstring tendons,[230-232] but other graft sources have been used with success.[233,234] The use of allograft tissue (i.e., tissue from another human being) for reconstruction has become more prominent, especially in older individuals, as a result of advances in disease screening techniques, increased tissue

availability, and ease of use in surgery.[235-237] Differences in graft tissue strength, stiffness, and graft fixation strength lead to differences in surgical technique and postoperative rehabilitation.

The ultimate load to failure of various tissues has been reported by several investigators (Table 16-5). The quadrupled hamstring tendon graft is approximately 91% stronger than the native ACL and 39% stronger than the patellar tendon. The patellar tendon graft is approximately 37% stronger than the native ACL. Although three of the four potential grafts listed in Table 16-5 are stronger than native ACL, graft fixation strength must be factored into the equation when a rehabilitation program is developed.

Empirically, the healing of bone to bone in the osseous tunnel would seem to occur more quickly than the healing of tendon to bone. However, this has not been proved scientifically. Furthermore, with delayed healing of tendon to bone, aggressive rehabilitation or activities may appear to cause the graft to stretch out. Also, the theoretical advantage of a larger, stronger allograft allowing for more aggressive rehabilitation remains unproven.

Recently, Brand et al.[242] reported biomechanical data on various graft fixation techniques for ACL reconstruction. These authors reported that the tibial fixation strength for a patellar BPTB graft was highest with a 9-mm interference screw (load to failure, 678-758 N).[243] The femoral fixation of the BPTB graft was optimal with a metal interference screw (640 N).[244,245] Fixation strengths also were reported for soft tissue grafts. Hamstring graft tibial fixation was greatest with a washer plate (9.5 N),[246] and with an Endo-Button with #5 suture on the femoral side.[247,248] Noyes et al.[249] have estimated the strength required for activities of daily living to be 454 N, based on the failure strength of the ACL.

The authors' clinical approach to designing a rehabilitation program based on ACL graft selection is to be less aggressive initially with soft tissue grafts, such as the quadrupled hamstring grafts.[250] This approach is based on the premise that soft tissue to bone healing takes approximately 12 weeks, whereas bone to bone healing occurs in approximately 8 weeks in most cases. With our current operative technique, patients generally return to sports within 6 to 9 months.

Postoperative Management for Reconstruction of the Anterior Cruciate Ligament

Rehabilitation after ACL reconstruction must consider initial graft strength, fixation, and healing and maturation of the graft. Initial graft strength depends on the quantity and quality of the material used and has been investigated by Noyes et al.[249] The central and medial thirds of the patellar tendon were found to be 186% and 159% of the strength of the native ACL, respectively. Weaker graft materials include the semitendinosus (70%), gracilis (49%), distal iliotibial track (44%), and fascia lata (36%). The use of

Table 16-5

Ultimate Load to Failure and Stiffness of Various Graft Selections

Graft Selection	Ultimate Strength to Failure (Newtons)	Stiffness (Newton-Meters)
Native anterior cruciate ligament (Woo et al.[238])	2160	240
Patellar tendon (Race and Amis[239])	2977	455
Quadrupled hamstring (Hamner et al.[240])	4140	807
Quadriceps tendon (Staubli et al.[241])	2353	326

stronger graft materials with solid fixation, such as that provided by an interference screw, allows more aggressive rehabilitation in the immediate postoperative period.

Graft strength is strongest at the time of reconstruction. Over time, the graft undergoes necrosis and remodeling. Healing and maturation of autogenous BPTB grafts in the animal model[251-254] and in humans[251,255] have been described, as have healing and maturation of allograft BPTB grafts in animal models[255-259] and humans.[254] Initially, the graft is avascular. By 6 weeks, the graft is enveloped in a synovial sheath. Revascularization begins 8-10 weeks after surgery and is nearly complete by 16 weeks. Histologically, the graft shows signs of avascular necrosis 6 weeks after reconstruction. The graft is invaded by mesenchymal cells 8 to 10 weeks after reconstruction. These cells proliferate and form collagen by postoperative week 16. One year after reconstruction, the graft takes on the appearance of a ligament, with dense, oriented collagen bundles. Graft strength decreases during the period of necrosis and then increases as the graft remodels and matures.

Although the graft takes on the appearance of a normal ligament, it does not function the same as the native ACL. Evidence suggests that at 6 months after surgery, allografts demonstrate a greater decrease in their structural properties from the time of implantation, a slower rate of biological incorporation, and prolonged presence of an inflammatory response compared to autografts.[259] Although clinical results have not demonstrated a significant difference between allograft and autograft reconstruction, rehabilitation after allograft reconstruction may need to be less aggressive than that following autograft reconstruction. In spite of the research that has been done, little is known about the graft's ability to withstand loads and strain during healing and maturation. Therefore it is difficult to base rehabilitation after ACL reconstruction strictly on the time required for healing and maturation of the graft.

Postoperative rehabilitation after ACL reconstruction must minimize the adverse effects of immobility without overloading healing tissues. As discussed earlier, basic data are lacking on the strain and loads that the graft can withstand during healing and maturation. In addition, studies on strain and loads imposed on the graft during exercise and activity are incomplete. For these reasons, current trends in rehabilitation after ACL reconstruction are based on clinical experience.

Rehabilitation after ACL reconstruction has undergone significant changes over the last decade. In the 1970s and early 1980s, rehabilitation after ACL reconstruction was conservative. Paulos et al.[260] described a five-phase program that imposed time restraints thought to be necessary for graft healing and controlled forces that may have been deleterious to the healing process. In this program, range of motion was limited to 30° to 60° in a cast brace, and the patient was non-weight-bearing on crutches for 6 weeks. Toe touch weight bearing was initiated in week 7. The patient was allowed gradually to begin partial weight bearing on crutches at 12 weeks and was allowed to be in full weight bearing without assistive devices by week 16. Resisted exercises consisted of hamstring and limited arc quadriceps exercise using light resistance and high repetitions. No mention was made of CKC exercises. Full return to activity was delayed for 9 to 12 months.

An interest has developed in accelerated rehabilitation after ACL reconstruction, which initially was popularized by Shelbourne and Nitz.[261] The essential features of their program included early emphasis on restoration of full knee extension symmetrical to the noninvolved side, immediate full weight bearing, use of CKC exercises to improve lower extremity muscle function, and return to full sports participation in 4 to 6 months. These researchers compared the results in a group of patients who underwent an accelerated rehabilitation program with those in a group that underwent a more traditional rehabilitation program, which included immobilization in 10° flexion, delayed weight bearing, reliance on OKC exercises to improve quadriceps and hamstring function, and delayed return to full activity. The study found that the accelerated rehabilitation program resulted in an earlier and more complete return of full extension and an earlier return to final flexion without any adverse effect on the stability of the knee, as indicated by side-to-side differences in knee laxity scores. In addition, isokinetic testing of the quadriceps revealed a higher mean percentage of involved to noninvolved scores from 4 to 10 months postoperatively. However, these differences in isokinetic scores were eliminated 1 year after surgery. No differences were seen in the patients' subjective assessment of their knee function. A second surgical procedure to recover loss of extension was required less often in patients who underwent the accelerated program. Based on these results, the use of an accelerated rehabilitation program after ACL reconstruction was recommended because it resulted in earlier restoration of motion, strength, and function without compromising stability of the knee.

Loss of motion has been described as the most common complication after ACL reconstruction.[222,262-266] Sachs et al.[265] reported a 24% incidence of a knee flexion contraction greater than 5° after ACL reconstruction; this was positively correlated with quadriceps weakness and patellofemoral pain. Harner et al.[222] reported an 11% incidence of loss of motion, which they defined as a knee flexion contracture of 10° or more and/or knee flexion less than 125°. All patients with loss of motion experienced loss of extension, and two thirds also had loss of flexion. Factors significantly related to the development of loss of motion included reconstruction within 4 weeks of the initial injury, concomitant knee ligament surgery involving the medial capsule, and gender (male). Patients with loss of motion tended to have had an autograft rather than an allograft and to be older, but these trends did not reach statistical significance. Also, patients who developed loss of motion used a postoperative brace that limited full extension more often than did patients who had normal motion after surgery. Loss of extension after ACL reconstruction leads to an abnormal gait, quadriceps weakness, and/or patellofemoral pain. Preoperative, intraoperative, and postoperative recommendations to minimize the risk of loss of motion were provided.

The goal for postoperative management after ACL reconstruction is to provide a stable knee that allows return to the highest level of function while minimizing the risk for loss of motion. To reduce the risk of loss of motion, postoperative management after ACL reconstruction should emphasize control of inflammation, restoration of full extension symmetrical to the noninvolved knee, early range of motion and quadriceps exercises, and restoration of normal gait.

The authors currently use two rehabilitation programs for patients with an isolated ACL reconstruction.[250] An accelerated rehabilitation approach is used for young, athletic patients, and a slower program is used for older patients whose needs are more recreational. The main difference between the two programs is the rate of progression through the various phases of rehabilitation and the period of time required for rehabilitation before running and sports can be resumed.

The authors' accelerated rehabilitation program is organized into six phases. Certain criteria must be met before the patient can progress to the next phase. ACL rehabilitation begins preoperatively, immediately after the injury occurs. The goals during this phase are to reduce pain, inflammation, and swelling, restore normal range of motion (ROM), and prevent muscle atrophy. Emphasis is placed on achieving full passive knee extension to minimize postoperative complications and arthrofibrosis.[261]

Another critical aspect of the rehabilitation program is re-establishing voluntary muscle activation of the quadriceps muscle. After damage to the ACL, a protective mechanism of quadriceps reflex inhibition and hamstring facilitation has been observed.[267,268] The patient therefore is instructed to recruit as much quadriceps firing as possible. This is facilitated through the use of electrical muscle stimulators or biofeedback units to achieve greater quadriceps muscle activation.

Patient education is another valuable component of preoperative rehabilitation. The surgical procedure and the postoperative rehabilitation program are explained to the patient as part of the mental preparation. During this phase, an appropriate date of surgery is determined. Some authors have suggested that delaying the timing of surgical intervention enhances results.[221,224] Based on clinical experience, we believe that surgery should be delayed until knee motion and effusion are normalized. Effective preoperative rehabilitation followed by an accelerated postoperative program appears to achieve the best results with minimal complications.

ACL Rehabilitation Goals: Phase 0 (Preoperative Phase)

- Explain the surgical procedure
- Explain the course of postoperative rehabilitation
- Determine the date of surgery

Postoperative ACL rehabilitation begins on the first day after surgery. The goals of phase I, the immediate postoperative phase, are to reduce pain and swelling, regain full passive knee extension, re-establish quadriceps control, and restore patellar mobility and independent ambulation. A commercial cold wrap is applied to the knee while the patient is in the recovery room to reduce pain and swelling. Quadriceps muscle contractions and full passive knee exercises are emphasized to prevent the development of arthrofibrosis on the first post operative day. A postoperative hinged knee brace is worn and locked at 0° knee extension during ambulation. Weight bearing is permitted as tolerated with the assistance of two crutches.

ACL Rehabilitation Goals: Phase I (Immediate Postoperative Phase)—Week 1

- Reduce pain
- Reduce swelling
- Regain full passive knee extension
- Re-establish quadriceps control
- Restore patellar mobility
- Restore independent ambulation

These primary goals continue through the first week of postoperative rehabilitation. To reduce pain and swelling, the patient wears the continuous cold unit as much as possible. The rehabilitation specialist and the patient perform patellar mobilizations to prevent the negative effects of immobilization. In addition, the patient's knee flexion ROM is gradually increased. By postoperative day 5, the patient should have 90° of knee flexion; by day 7, the person should have at least 100° of knee flexion. CKC functional training also begins during the first week with exercises that include minisquats (0° to 40°), balance drills, and proprioceptive training activities.

Phase II, the early rehabilitation phase, includes weeks 2 to 4. The goals during this phase include maintaining full passive knee extension, gradually increasing knee flexion, and restoring proprioception. Restoration of full passive knee extension should be emphasized early in the postoperative program. Some patients may show hyperextension of the tibiofemoral joint. Whether full hyperextension should be restored is the subject of debate. Some authors have reported that restoring full hyperextension does not affect ligament stability.[269] It is suggested that, in the clinic, the patient regain only 5° to 7° of hyperextension through stretching techniques; the remaining hyperextension may be achieved through functional activities. The authors believe that this allows the patient to gain a greater degree of neuromuscular control rather than clinically stretching to excessive motion.

ACL Rehabilitation Goals: Phase II—Weeks 2-4

- Maintain full passive knee extension
- Increase knee flexion
- Restore proprioception
- Restore muscle strength and endurance
- Achieve full weight bearing
- Begin gait training
- Begin functional exercises

Knee flexion is increased gradually during the early rehabilitative phase. The rate of progression is based on the patient's unique response to surgery. If substantial effusion is present, range of motion is advanced at a slower rate, allowing adequate time for the swelling to subside. Also, the rate of knee flexion motion is adjusted based on the patient's ligamentous end feel. A firm end feel indicates an aggressive rate of progress, and stretching is appropriate. Conversely, when a patient has a capsular, or soft, end feel, a slower rate of progression is suggested.

Muscle training is progressed with OKC and CKC exercises during this phase. Electrical muscle stimulation is applied to the quadriceps muscle during therapeutic exercise to facilitate active quadriceps contraction and to prevent muscle inhibition from pain and swelling.[270,271] Other exercises to enhance proprioception and weight distribution also are initiated. A critical goal during week 2 is to train the

patient to assume full weight bearing on the involved leg. A force platform often is used to assess the exact percentage of body weight used by the involved limb and to provide biofeedback training. OKC exercises initiated at this time include hip abduction and adduction and knee extension in a restricted ROM (90° to 40°). This restricted range has been shown to reduce strain on the healing ACL graft.[24]

In weeks 3 to 4, functional exercise drills to strengthen the lower extremity are incorporated. Such activities include lateral step-ups, front step-downs, lateral lunges, and lateral cone step-overs. The patient rides a stationary bike to stimulate ROM. Lastly, as the incision heals, a pool program is begun to facilitate proper gait training and to provide a safe environment for initiation of more advanced drills.[272]

Phase III, the intermediate phase, usually begins by week 4 and continues through week 10. Progression is based on the accomplishment of the specific goals of previous phases; therefore, the actual time frame varies from patient to patient. The goals in phase III are to establish full normal ROM while improving muscular strength, proprioception, and neuromuscular control. The strengthening program is progressed in weight, repetitions, and sets. CKC exercises are advanced to include the leg press (100° to 0°) and wall squats (0° to 70°). Proprioception and functional exercises are advanced to enhance dynamic joint stability; such drills include squatting on an unstable platform and lateral lunges with a resistance cord attached to the patient's waist. Ball tosses are incorporated into the proprioception exercises as the patient tolerates, to remove the patient's conscious awareness of joint position. Aquatic therapy is used during this phase to allow the patient to begin early running and agility drills in the pool. The buoyancy of the water assists the patient by reducing the percentage of body weight, and thus the loads, applied to the lower extremity.

ACL Rehabilitation Goals: Phase III (Intermediate Phase)—Weeks 4-10

- Establish normal range of motion
- Re-establish neuromuscular control
- Improve strength and endurance
- Improve proprioception

Phase IV, the advanced activity phase usually is initiated at week 10 and progresses until week 16. The patient must have met specific criteria to begin this phase. The patient must pass a clinical examination that shows full active ROM and satisfactory isokinetic strength. The muscle performance characteristics of an ACL-reconstructed knee have been documented by Wilk et al.[273] At 10 to 12 weeks, the patient usually demonstrates a 30% deficit in the bilateral peak torque comparison of the quadriceps muscle group and a 0% to 10% deficit of the hamstring muscle group. Once these predetermined criteria have been met, advanced, sport-specific drills can be started.

> ### ACL Rehabilitation Goals: Phase IV (Advanced Activity)—Weeks 10-16
>
> - Begin aggressive strengthening
> - Introduce neuromuscular control drills
> - Initiate advanced activity-specific drills

During the advanced activity phase, emphasis is placed on aggressive strengthening exercises, neuromuscular control drills, and sport-specific training activities. Strengthening exercises are progressed to high weight, low repetition sets for muscle hypertrophy. Plyometric drills are used to enhance dynamic joint stability and neuromuscular control; such exercises include the plyometric leg press and double leg box jumps. Perturbation training also is used to enhance neuromuscular control. The patient is trained to perform these exercises with a knee flexion angle of 15° to 30° to enhance EMG activity of the quadriceps.[24,35,274] In addition, a flat-ground running program is initiated, including agility drills such as backward running, side shuffles, and cariocas. The patient's return to sport-specific drills progresses through a series of transitional drills designed to challenge the neuromuscular system. Pool running is performed before flat-ground running. Backward running and lateral running are performed before forward running. Plyometrics are performed before running and cutting drills to train the lower extremity to dissipate ground reaction forces. These progressions ensure that the patient has ample time to develop the neuromuscular control and dynamic stabilization needed to perform these drills.

Phase V the return to activity phase, typically begins at postoperative week 16. Further isokinetic tests[275,276] and hop tests[276-278] are performed to determine whether the patient can return to sports and work activities. Functional motor patterns are progressed through plyometric and agility drills to accelerate sport- or activity-specific training activities. Once the patient has demonstrated normal movement patterns and the specific criteria have been satisfied, the individual may begin practice activities. The patient is monitored closely until the individual participates in full competition. Normal return to sports activities occurs at about 6 months for the accelerated patient and 6 to 9 months for general orthopedic patients.

> ### ACL Rehabilitation Goals: Phase V (Return to Activity)—Weeks 16+
>
> - Assess for functional motor patterns
> - Ensure normal movement patterns
> - Begin sport practices

Posterior Cruciate Ligament Injuries

Nonoperative Management

PCL injuries occur less frequently than ACL injuries. Isolated injury to the PCL does not produce the same degree of functional instability and disability seen with injury to the ACL. Many patients with an isolated PCL injury can return to their previous level of function with minimal symptoms. The level of function and patient satisfaction appear to be related to the ability of the quadriceps to stabilize the knee dynamically. Parolie and Bergfeld[161] reported the long-term results of 25 patients with PCL injuries who were managed without surgery. All patients who returned to their previous level of function and were satisfied with their results had isokinetic quadriceps torque values on the involved side greater than 100% of those on the noninvolved side. Conversely, patients who were not satisfied with their knees had isokinetic torque values on the involved side that were less than 100% of those on the noninvolved side. The level of function after PCL injury does not appear to be related to the degree of instability.[161,169] It should be noted, however, that long-term follow-up of PCL injuries reveals the development of progressive pain and degeneration of the patellofemoral joint and medial compartment of the tibiofemoral joint.[168] This likely is due to altered arthrokinematics in the PCL-deficient knee.

Treatment after acute injury to the PCL is similar to the management of acute ACL injuries. It should focus on resolving inflammation, restoring ROM, and regaining motor control of the knee. Cold and compression are used to reduce pain and swelling. ROM exercises are performed to restore motion, which should improve as pain and swelling subside. Isometric exercises for the quadriceps, including quadriceps sets and SLRs are used to minimize quadriceps atrophy. Hamstring exercises are avoided at this time, because they contribute to increased posterior laxity. Also, the hamstrings do not appear to be as susceptible as the quadriceps to disuse atrophy. Assistive devices are used for ambulation while the knee is still actively inflamed. The use of assistive devices is discontinued when the patient has regained full extension without a quadriceps lag and can walk normally, without gait deviations.

More aggressive rehabilitation can begin once inflammation has resolved and full ROM has been restored. The emphasis at this time is on improving the endurance and strength of the quadriceps muscles. OKC knee extension exercises should be modified if the patient complains of pain or crepitus. CKC exercises are initiated and progressed as tolerated to improve the endurance and strength of the muscles of the lower extremity in functional patterns.

OKC knee flexion exercises should be avoided, because they contribute to increased posterior tibial translation. For patients with a PCL-deficient knee, the hamstrings are strengthened by performing open chain hip extension with the knee near terminal extension, which minimizes posterior tibial translation at the knee caused by the hamstrings. During CKC exercises, the hamstrings function to counteract the flexion moment arm at the hip. Their effect (i.e., producing posterior tibial translation of the knee) is offset by simultaneous activity of the quadriceps. Proprioceptive training for the PCL-deficient knee should emphasize recruitment of the quadriceps to control posterior translation of the tibia dynamically. The patient is progressed from walking to jogging-running, acceleration-deceleration, sprinting, jumping, cutting, pivoting, and twisting as tolerated.

Generally, patients with a PCL-deficient knee do not complain of instability during physical activity, and a functional brace usually is not necessary. If a patient with a PCL-deficient knee does require a functional knee brace, one that is specifically designed for a PCL-deficient knee should be chosen. Most functional knee braces are designed for an ACL-deficient knee and do not benefit a patient with a PCL-deficient knee. Many patients with a PCL-deficient knee complain of patellofemoral symptoms, and these individuals may benefit from the use of a neoprene patellar sleeve.

Because of the tendency for progressive deterioration of the anterior and medial compartments of the knee, patients with a PCL-deficient knee should be educated to avoid activities that cause pain and swelling. Repetitive activities that involve high loading of the patellofemoral and tibiofemoral joints may accelerate this degenerative process and should be avoided.

Surgical Management

Clinicians must take into account a number of important variables when deciding how best to manage a PCL injury. These include the type of injury; whether associated structures have been damaged; the patient's symptoms, activity level, goals, and expectations; and the acuity or chronicity of the injury. The goal of treatment is to restore the stability and normal kinematics of the knee and to allow the patient to return to the preinjury level of activity. The best way to achieve this is still the subject of debate.

For interstitial tears of the PCL, the decision to perform surgery is based on the degree of resulting functional instability and injuries to associated ligamentous structures. Surgical reconstruction is recommended for isolated PCL disruptions that result in greater than 10 mm of increased posterior tibial translation compared to the noninvolved side or when injury to the PCL is accompanied by injury to other ligamentous structures. Acute repair of a PCL avulsed from the bone or avulsed with bone may be possible with a single screw or suture technique. Most series have shown that acute reconstructions do better than chronic cases, because the potential for stretching out of secondary restraints increases with time.

It is important to note that a posterior drawer greater than 15 mm indicates combined injury to the PCL and posterolateral structures.[46] An occult injury to the posterolateral corner shoulder be evaluated and concomitantly treated.

PCL tears can be reconstructed using an open or an arthroscopic technique. The authors prefer to perform PCL reconstruction using an arthroscopically assisted technique; although it is technically more demanding, it is believed to reduce operative morbidity and to hold promise for improved clinical results. As with reconstruction of the ACL, PCL reconstruction has been performed using a variety of graft materials, including patellar and Achilles tendon allografts, patellar tendon, fascia lata, medial head of the gastrocnemius, semitendinosus-gracilis, and meniscus autografts, and synthetic replacements. Procedures in which the medial head of the gastrocnemius,[55,279-283] the semitendinosus-gracilis,[280,281] the iliotibial band,[282] the meniscus,[283,284] Gore-Tex synthetic ligament,[285] and primary unaugmented repair[286-288] were used all have failed to produce consistent, objective results.

One technique for PCL reconstruction consists of reproducing the anterolateral bundle of the ligament, because this is the largest and strongest band and it functions primarily with the knee in flexion. The procedure is performed by drilling the tibial tunnel so that it reproduces the distolateral portion of the tibial insertion site and drilling the femoral tunnel so that it reproduces the anterior portion of the femoral insertion site. An Achilles tendon allograft is passed through the femoral and tibial tunnels. The authors prefer to use an Achilles tendon allograft because of its length and strength, availability, lack of morbidity to the patient, and ease of passage; one end of the graft is without a bony block and can easily be passed through the acute angle required to go from the femoral to the tibial tunnel. The femoral side, which includes the Achilles bone plug, is fixed with an interference screw, and the tibial side is fixed to the tibia with a screw and soft tissue spiked washer (Figure 16-31).

Although this type of reconstruction may reduce posterior tibial translation at the time of surgery, increased laxity often is noted clinically postoperatively. Recent anatomical and biomechanical studies have shown that the two bundles of the PCL have different roles in the normal arthrokinematics of the knee. The anterolateral bundle becomes taut in flexion, and the posteromedial bundle becomes taut in extension. For this reason, a double bundle technique recently has been advocated for reconstruction of the PCL. This procedure, which uses two separate grafts to restore both the anterolateral and posteromedial bundles of the PCL, requires two femoral tunnels and one common tibial tunnel. During reconstruction, the anterolateral bundle is tensioned in flexion, and the posteromedial bundle is tensioned in extension. Harner et al.[289] recently reported that double bundle reconstruction more closely restores the normal tibial translation and biomechanics of the knee than the single bundle technique. Several authors have described the double bundle procedure in detail.[33,239,289,290] Nonetheless, the advantages of the double bundle technique have not been confirmed in the

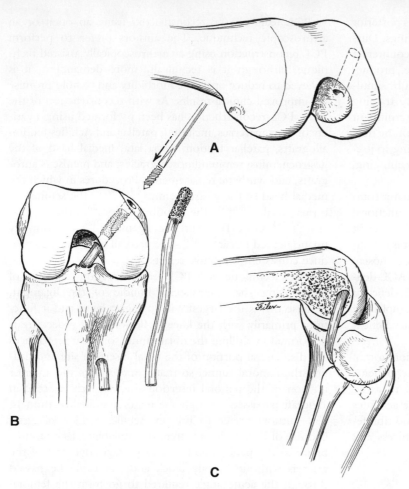

Figure 16-31
Posterior cruciate ligament (PCL) reconstruction.
A, PCL reconstruction is performed with an Achilles
tendon allograft passed through the femoral and tibial
tunnels. **B,** The femoral side is fixed with an interference
screw. **C,** The tibial side is fixed with a soft tissue spiked
washer and screw. (From Zachazewski JE, Magee DJ,
Quillen WS, editors: *Athletic injuries and rehabilitation,*
p 670, Philadelphia, 1996, WB Saunders.)

literature, and much debate still exists over the best technique for PCL reconstruction.

Postoperative Management for Reconstruction of the Posterior Cruciate Ligament

Little is known about the healing and maturation of PCL
grafts. Bosch et al.[291] studied PCL graft fixation in sheep
using a free patellar tendon graft and demonstrated good
bone to bone incorporation at 6 weeks. In their study, postoperative management consisted of immediate partial weight
bearing and range of motion beginning 2 weeks after surgery.
Clancy et al.[253] demonstrated revascularization of free patellar tendon grafts 8 weeks after surgery in rhesus monkeys. As
yet, no studies on graft fixation and incorporation after PCL
reconstruction have been done in humans.

The rehabilitation program after PCL reconstruction has
evolved dramatically over the past several years as a result of
advances in researchers' understanding of the anatomy and
biomechanics of the knee and in surgical techniques.

The goals of rehabilitation include restoring full range of
knee motion, preventing wear of the articular cartilage, gradually increasing the stress applied to the healing PCL graft,
and improving dynamic stabilization of the musculature about
the knee joint. Rehabilitation of PCL injuries focuses on
regaining quadriceps strength and control. In fact, earlier
quadriceps contraction in the gait cycle can increase dynamic
stability in the knee enough to overcome the instability from
an incompetent PCL.[292] Rehabilitation therefore focuses on
regaining or exceeding normal quadriceps strength.[293]

Overall Goals in PCL Rehabilitation

- Restore full range of motion
- Prevent excess articular cartilage wear
- Gradually increase stress to posterior crucial ligament
- Improve dynamic stabilization
- Regain quadriceps strength
- Minimize posterior tibial translation

It is important to minimize posterior tibial translation
during rehabilitation.[294] This is accomplished by protecting
against gravity-induced posterior sag and by avoiding OKC
hamstring exercises. CKC exercises, such as the squat, produce less tibiofemoral shear force. OKC quadriceps extension
exercises at 70° to 0° are used because of the anterior pull of
the patellar tendon on the tibia.

The authors' current program consists of five phases designed to progress the patient gradually to full, unrestricted activities by 6 to 7 months after surgery. The protocol gradually normalizes hemarthrosis, ROM, and strength while preventing degeneration of the articular cartilage at the patellofemoral and tibiofemoral joints.

Immediately after surgery, the knee is wrapped with a compression dressing and continuous cryotherapy (Polar Care, Breg Vista, CA) is applied. The patient uses a drop-lock knee brace that is locked into extension. Ambulation initially involves two crutches and approximately 50% weight bearing. The brace may be unlocked into flexion when the patient sits or performs exercises. Full passive knee extension should be restored soon after surgery to prevent the development of arthrofibrosis within the joint. Range of motion and patellar mobilizations, particularly superior patellar glides, are performed four to five times throughout the day to help restore full knee extension. Knee motion should be progressed gradually to 90° by the end of week 1. Exercises are also performed, including quadriceps setting; isometric knee extension at 0°, 20°, 40°, and 60° of knee extension; and straight leg raises into flexion, abduction, and adduction. Electrical muscle stimulation is applied in conjunction with these exercises to facilitate a quadriceps contraction.[270,295,296] Isolated hamstring exercises are contraindicated for the first 8 weeks because of the large posterior shear force generated with hamstring contraction. Cryotherapy commonly is used for 15 minutes before and after treatment to control pain and edema.

PCL Rehabilitation Goals: Phase I—Weeks 0-1

- Reduce swelling
- Protect the knee in a brace (locked in extension except when exercising)
- Obtain 90° flexion by the end of week 1
- Obtain 50% weight bearing
- Regain full passive knee extension
- Maintain patellar mobility

Range of motion and weight bearing are progressed gradually during weeks 2 to 6. Motion increases from 0° to 90° during week 1; 0° to 105° by week 2; 0° to 115° by week 4; and up to 125° by the end of weeks 5 to 6. Weight bearing is progressed gradually to full weight bearing by week 3. At 14 days the patient begins to ambulate with one crutch, which is discontinued at day 21.

Quadriceps strengthening activities are progressed to include OKC knee extension from 60° to 0° and the CKC leg press from 60° to 0° during week 2. Minisquats are also performed from 0° to 45°. Because the loss of proprioception after PCL injury is well documented,[297] the authors begin proprioceptive drills, such as minisquats on an unstable platform (Biodex Stability System, Biodex, Shirley, NY), soon after surgery. Neuromuscular control drills that train muscular co-activation for dynamic stabilization are also incorporated at this time. Particular drills initiated by week 4 are lateral step-overs performed over cones and lateral lunges. Perturbation training is initiated at this time and is emphasized throughout the program. The stationary bicycle may be used for quadriceps strengthening, motion stimulation, and cardiovascular training when range of motion permits. Also at this time, an aquatic therapy program consisting of pool walking and lower extremity exercise is added. Swimming is permitted between week 6 and week 7, with the precaution of kicking with a straight leg only. All CKC exercises are progressed by weeks 6 to 8 to include lateral step-ups, front step-downs, stair climbing machines, and advanced proprioceptive and neuromuscular control drills. At 8 weeks, resisted hamstring contractions are initiated from 0° to 60° with light resistance. Pool running begins at week 12 to prepare the patient for dry land running and agility drills, including lateral, backward, and forward movements.

PCL Rehabilitation Goals: Phase II—Weeks 2-12

- Progress quadriceps strengthening activities
- Proprioceptive drills
- Reinforce neuromuscular control
- Initiation of pertubation training

The light activity phase begins around 3 to 4 months. Emphasis is placed on advancing strengthening drills, continuing neuromuscular control drills, and beginning sport- or activity-specific training drills. Plyometric exercises are used to enhance dynamic joint stabilization and neuromuscular control. The rapid dynamic loading of the musculature during plyometric drills helps train the stretch-shortening cycle of the musculature. Plyometric drills are progressed from the leg press machine to flat-ground to box jumps to single-leg jumps. Agility drills and sport- or activity-specific training drills may be incorporated at this time for the patient. If satisfactory results are seen on the clinical examination, the return to sport phase is initiated and a running program on dry land begins at 4 to 5 months and gradually progresses in intensity for 4 to 6 weeks.

PCL Rehabilitation Goals: Phase III (Light Activity Phase) —Weeks 13-20

- Emphasize strengthening, neuromuscular control training
- Begin sport- or activity-specific training drills
- Begin plyometric training

PCL Rehabilitation Goals: Phase IV (Return to Sport) —Weeks 21+

- Begin running on dry land
- Gradual progression of training intensity

The authors periodically assess the knee laxity of patients with a reconstructed PCL throughout the program. A KT2000 arthrometer (MEDmetric, San Diego, CA) is used to assess the anteroposterior laxity of the knee joint at 2, 4, 6, 8, and 12 weeks and at 4, 6, 12, and 24 months after surgery. The test is performed at the quadriceps-neutral angle to ensure that anteroposterior laxity is measured accurately. Serial assessment of knee laxity is useful to the rehabilitation specialist for evaluating the integrity of the graft. The rehabilitation program is assessed on the basis of the results of the arthrometric testing and then is adjusted accordingly.

In the authors' experience, patients typically can return to noncontact sports at 5.5 to 6 months after surgery and to contact sports at 6 to 7 months. The authors tend to be more cautious with skiers because of the highly dynamic nature of the sport; they generally permit skiing at 8 to 9 months after surgery.

Medial Collateral Ligament Injuries

The philosophy for managing isolated MCL injuries has changed as a result of basic scientific and clinical studies. In the past, many of these injuries were treated with surgical repair followed by immobilization for 6 weeks. Studies in rabbits by Anderson et al.[76] and Weiss et al.[298] demonstrated that isolated MCL injuries heal when the ACL is intact. Similar findings were noted in clinical studies that demonstrated no difference in stability or function between patients with isolated MCL injuries who were treated nonoperatively and those who had surgery.[154,174,177,299] Isolated MCL tears heal well without surgery, regardless of the degree of injury or the patient's age or activity level.[173-179] Usually some residual valgus laxity can be elicited on physical examination after a grade II or grade III injury, because the ligament may heal in a lengthened state, but this has little effect on knee function. Patients with combined MCL-ACL injuries, however, may require reconstruction of the ACL with or without repair of the MCL to restore stability and function to the knee. Reconstruction of the ACL alone for patients with a combined ACL-MCL injury may restore enough stability to the knee to allow the MCL to heal.

Acute treatment of isolated MCL injuries depends on the stability of the joint. Grade I and grade II MCL sprains that are stable with valgus stress testing are treated symptomatically without the use of a rehabilitation brace. Patients with isolated grade III MCL injuries who are unstable with valgus stress testing and who have a soft end point are treated with a hinged rehabilitation brace for 4 to 6 weeks. The brace typically is set to permit 0° to 90° of motion. The brace controls valgus stresses, allowing the ligament to heal while permitting limited motion of the knee.

Treatment of acute MCL injuries should include the use of cold and compression to control pain and swelling. Early range of motion in the pain-free range is encouraged to facilitate healing and prevent the development of a stiff knee. Transverse friction massage and pulsed ultrasound to the ligament may be beneficial to stimulate healing and orientation of the ligament fibers and to prevent the formation of adhesions. Isometric exercises for the quadriceps and hamstrings are initiated to minimize disuse atrophy. Assistive devices are used for ambulation until the patient demonstrates full extension of the knee without an extensor lag and can walk normally, without gait deviations.

Once inflammation has resolved and ROM has improved, the patient can begin OKC and CKC exercises to increase the endurance and strength of the quadriceps and hamstring muscles. Exercises are progressed as tolerated, with care taken to prevent the development of patellofemoral symptoms. As strength and endurance improve, the patient progresses through functional activities to enhance dynamic stability of the knee and to prepare for return to activity. Patients returning to contact sports may use a functional knee brace to reduce the risk of reinjury. For MCL injuries, the brace should have good medial and lateral stays to control varus-valgus rotation.

Lateral Collateral Ligament Injuries

The treatment of acute, isolated LCL injuries depends on the stability of the joint. Grade I and grade II LCL sprains that are stable with varus stress testing are treated symptomatically without the use of a rehabilitation brace. Patients with isolated grade III LCL injuries who are unstable with varus stress testing and who have a soft end point are treated with a hinged rehabilitation brace for 4 to 6 weeks. The brace usually is set to permit 0° to 90° of motion. The brace controls varus stresses, allowing the ligament to heal while permitting limited motion of the knee.

Treatment of acute LCL injuries is similar to that for MCL injuries. Cold and compression are used to control pain and swelling. Early range of motion in the pain-free range is encouraged to facilitate healing and to prevent the development of a stiff knee. Isometric exercises for the quadriceps and hamstrings are initiated to minimize disuse atrophy. Assistive devices are used for ambulation until the patient demonstrates full extension of the knee without an extensor lag and can walk normally, without gait deviations. Once inflammation has resolved and ROM has improved, the patient can begin OKC and CKC exercises to increase the endurance and strength of the quadriceps and hamstring muscles. As strength and endurance improve, the patient is progressed through functional activities to enhance the dynamic stability of the knee and to prepare for return to activity. Patients returning to contact sports may use a functional brace with good medial and lateral support to reduce the risk of reinjury.

Surgery for isolated grade III LCL injuries is recommended for patients with chronic varus instability that affects their daily function and for patients who want to continue sports activities. Surgery also is recommended for injuries involving a bony avulsion that is displaced more than 3 mm. Reports on the results of LCL reconstruction are lacking. Reconstruction for acute or chronic LCL injuries usually is reserved for knee injuries involving multiple ligaments (see the following section).

The authors' technique for reconstruction of a chronically LCL-deficient knee depends on the acuity and severity of the injury. With an acute LCL tear, the ligament sometimes can be reattached to its insertion with suture anchors, or a primary repair of the ligament can be performed. Often, however, the ligament is torn through its midsubstance and cannot hold sutures for repair. In these cases, as well as in the chronically LCL-deficient knee, the authors use an Achilles tendon allograft for reconstruction of the LCL. The bone plug of the Achilles tendon graft is placed in the fibular head and is fixed with an interference screw. The soft tissue end of the graft is fixed to the anatomical insertion of the LCL on the femoral epicondyle with suture anchors. Care must be taken to avoid putting excessive stress on the graft as the knee is taken through a range of motion. Nonisometric placement of the graft can lead to stretching or tearing. The LCL remnants are sutured to the graft to provide added healing potential and possibly proprioceptive function.[300]

After LCL reconstruction, patients are placed in a postoperative brace for 4 to 6 weeks to minimize varus stress. During this period, limited ROM exercises from 0° to 90° are performed. During the first postoperative week, isometric quadriceps and hamstrings exercises are initiated. A partial weight-bearing gait is used for 4 to 6 weeks after surgery to minimize stress on the graft. The authors have found that early, full weight bearing, particularly in the knee that demonstrates a varus thrust, leads to increased varus laxity. After 6 weeks, the patient is progressed to weight bearing as tolerated. Assistive devices are discontinued once the patient has full knee extension without a quadriceps lag and is able to demonstrate a normal gait pattern.

The rehabilitation brace generally is discontinued at 6 weeks after surgery. At this time, emphasis is placed on regaining full range of motion and on developing muscle function for the lower extremity using OKC and CKC knee exercises. Proprioceptive activities are initiated to regain neuromuscular control of the knee. Gradual sports-specific functional progression allows a return to sports within 6 to 9 months. A functional brace that provides varus stability is recommended for return to sports.

Multiple-Ligament Knee Injuries

Treatment of multiple-ligament injuries of the knee includes a wide spectrum of pathology and requires evaluation of many factors. A knee dislocation can be limb threatening and is associated with a high incidence of neurological and vascular injuries. Immediate surgical intervention is necessary if the multiple-ligament injuries are associated with vascular injury or a compartment syndrome. A grossly unstable knee can be stabilized with an external fixator while these acute issues are addressed.

Knee dislocations can be low or high energy injuries. Low velocity injuries often are athletic injuries and have a better prognosis because fewer vascular injuries are involved. High velocity injuries have a higher incidence of other organ system injuries and neurovascular compromise. However, ultra-low velocity injuries in patients with a body mass index (BMI) of 40 or higher may have a very high rate of vascular injury.[189]

Many knee dislocations reduce spontaneously. If three or more ligaments of the knee are injured, a knee dislocation should be suspected and appropriate neurovascular examinations should be performed.

Based on the work of Taylor et al.[193] on nonoperative versus operative treatment of knee dislocations, it is reasonable to conclude that nonoperative management could result in a functional knee, depending on the patient's demands. However, most authors support open surgical techniques to restore stability and attempt to improve functional outcome.[184,221,301-303] Also, surgical management of a knee with a multiple-ligament injury may prevent or delay the onset of arthritis by improving joint stability. Functional deficiency that results from a multiple-ligament knee injury must be evaluated relative to the patient's age, occupation, and recreational interests and the neurovascular status of the affected extremity before a decision is made to treat the condition surgically.

When the authors opt for surgical management of this injury, reconstruction usually is delayed for 3 weeks after injury to allow soft tissue swelling to decrease. "Sealing" of the capsular injury occurs within a week, which permits the use of arthroscopically assisted techniques. Delayed reconstruction can also prevent the risk of arthrofibrosis by allowing time to regain motion after injury.[187] Even so, early repair of the posterolateral corner should be considered before 3 weeks to allow for the possibility of a primary repair of these structures. In this case, the posterolateral corner is repaired in this first stage, and cruciate ligament reconstruction is performed several weeks later, when motion has been regained.

In general, the treatment of each individual ligament injury is similar to that for an isolated injury of that ligament. Knees with an MCL injury are braced for the first 4 to 6 weeks to allow healing preoperatively. Reconstruction of the cruciate ligaments is then performed concomitantly. The authors prefer reconstruction using allograft tissue to reduce surgical time and patient morbidity. Use of allograft tissue also ensures the availability of graft tissue and minimizes difficulty with graft passage. The procedure is performed with arthroscopic assistance for the cruciate ligaments, particularly if the injury involves the ACL, PCL, LCL, and/or posterolateral corner with the ACL, PCL, or MCL avulsed off the tibial or femoral insertions.

Postoperative rehabilitation for acute reconstructions involves early motion and weight bearing with a gradual restoration of knee flexion. Range of motion is progressed from 0° to 65° on day 5, 0° to 75° on day 7, 0° to 90° on day 10, 0° to 100° beginning week 2, 0° to 115° beginning week 6, and 0° to 125° and beyond beginning week 7. Weight bearing is progressed from 50% body weight at day 7, to 75% body weight at day 12, and finally full weight bearing by week 4. A brace is used for the first 7 to 8 weeks. Patients often are fitted for functional knee braces when the postoperative knee brace is discontinued. CKC exercises are initiated during week 3 with weight shifts and minisquats and progressed to include the leg press, aquatic therapy, and bicycle by week 4. Return to functional activities is allowed beginning with a walking program at week 12, progressing to light running by weeks 16 to 20, and more aggressive agility drills by 5 to 6 months.

Treatment of Patellar Tendon Injuries

Patellar Tendinopathy

Patellar tendonitis is one of the most common causes of anterior knee pain in the athletic population. Activities that involve repetitive jumping, such as basketball and volleyball, have a high rate of patellar tendonitis because of the repetitive eccentric contractions of the quadriceps muscle. Theories about the etiology of these injuries vary and include both intrinsic factors (e.g., muscle tightness, strength imbalances) and extrinsic factors (e.g., sport, training frequency), and both likely relate to the pathological development.

The progression of symptoms has been described by Blazina et al.[304] and can be classified into four stages. Stage I tendinopathy typically occurs after a recent change in sports activity or a change in the intensity of the current sports activity. This stage is characterized by pain that is experienced after activity. Symptoms do not typically limit participation at this stage of the pathology. Stage II is characterized by pain at the start of activities that subsides, only to return as the patient begins to fatigue toward the end of

participation. Stage III involves constant symptoms that limit the activity. Stage IV is defined as tendon rupture.

The stages of pathology defined by Blazina et al.[304] correspond well with the stages of tendinopathy defined by Nirschl.[305] He described an acute period of inflammation of the tendon and paratenon sheath surrounding the tendon (stage I). As the chronicity of symptoms continues, the underlying tendon tissue begins to develop tendinosis, whereas the paratenon continues to show an inflammatory response (stage II). Eventually the pathology becomes chronic enough that inflammation subsides and tendinosis of the tendon continues (stage III.) To develop an appropriate treatment program for patellar tendinopathy, it is imperative that the clinician differentially diagnose the appropriate stage of pathology and treat the patient accordingly.

On clinical examination, the patient often is point tender to palpation at the inferior patellar pole at the patellar tendon junction. The patient also may have symptoms in the midportion or distal attachment of the tendon, although these findings are less common. Resisted quadriceps contraction may elicit symptoms, and the patient often has tightness of the quadriceps musculature. Witvrouw et al.[44] prospectively evaluated predictive factors in the development of patellar tendinopathy and reported that the most common factor was the loss of quadriceps soft tissue flexibility. MRI studies often show abnormal signals in the tendon.

As previously mentioned, conservative treatment for patellar tendinopathy must be appropriate for the stage and progression of pathology. For patients in stage I and early stage II tendinopathy with an acute onset of symptoms and pain after activity, treatment aims at reducing the inflammatory response and balancing the strength and flexibility of the lower extremity. Traditional anti-inflammatory treatments are used, including ice, phonophoresis, iontophoresis, and nonsteroidal anti-inflammatory medications. The patient should try to minimize activities that irritate the tendon, but the concept of "rest" should be avoided. Instead, the patient should continue to work on enhancing quadriceps strength, lower extremity muscle balance, and soft tissue flexibility. Abstaining from all activities and relying on rest and ice often cause further loss of strength and flexibility, which can result in a recurrence of symptoms when activities are resumed.

Nonoperative Treatment

The primary goals of rehabilitation are to control the applied loads and create an environment for healing. The initial treatment consists of phonophoresis, iontophoresis, stretching exercises, and light strengthening exercises to stimulate a healing response. High voltage stimulation and cryotherapy may be used after treatment to reduce pain and postexercise inflammation. The patient should be cautioned against excessive running or jumping activities.

Once the patient's symptoms have subsided, an aggressive stretching and strengthening program is initiated, with emphasis on eccentric quadriceps contractions. Several authors encourage the use of eccentric exercise for patellar tendinopathy to increase the amount of force applied to the tendon.[306-308] A gradual progression through plyometric and running activities precedes the return to full activity participation. Because poor mechanics often are a cause of this condition, an analysis of the mechanics of the activity and proper supervision are critical.

The treatment of more chronic stage II and stage III tendinopathies varies greatly from that used for the acute condition. As the chronicity of the pathology progresses, inflammation subsides and tissue degeneration occurs, creating a tendinosis rather than tendonitis. Thus anti-inflammatory treatments are avoided, and a healing environment is encouraged by attempting to stimulate blood flow to the area. Treatment includes moist heat or a warm whirlpool, ultrasound, transverse friction massage, and eccentric strengthening, which places greater stress on the tendon. The patient is encouraged to exercise in an environment that induces mild microtrauma to the area to stimulate a healing response. Patients therefore should experience mild discomfort when performing their workouts. The authors recommend that, during exercise, general orthopedic patients experience pain they rate as 3 to 4 on a 0 to 10 VAS pain scale, and athletes experience pain they rate as 5 to 6.

Anecdotally, one of the authors (Michael M. Reinold) believes that applying electrical stimulation to the tendon to produce a noxious stimulus often is indicated and is highly effective in creating a healing environment. Neuromuscular electrical stimulation (Russian, 2500 Hz, 50 pps) is applied surrounding the area of pathology, and the current is applied at the highest level tolerable to the patient. The stimulation is applied for 10 to 12 minutes, with a 10-second duty cycle immediately before initiation of strengthening exercises. Subjectively, patients report that their symptoms are decreased and that they are able to perform more aggressive exercises during their workout after application of this noxious stimulus. However, currently no evidence or research confirms this self-reported patient opinion.

Surgical Treatment

Surgery generally is performed for chronic tendinosis that has not responded to conservative treatment for 3 to 6 months. The surgery typically involves debridement of degenerative tissue, which creates an inflammatory response and facilitates a healing response. An incision is made over the area of tendinosis, and dissection is carried down to the underlying tendon. The paratenon is preserved, and the patellar tendon is divided longitudinally. Degenerative patellar tendon tissue is debrided, and the patellar tendon is re-approximated with a high tensile strength suture. Several

surgeons advocate additional stimulation of a healing response by drilling adjacent bone with a Kirschner wire (K-wire).

Postoperative rehabilitation focuses on minimizing pain and swelling and gradually restoring strength and range of motion in the knee. Range of motion is initiated immediately to stimulate healing and collagen tissue organization. The patient typically achieves full knee extension immediately, and full knee flexion is restored gradually over the first 4 to 6 weeks. Aggressive quadriceps strengthening is avoided for the first 2 months and then slowly integrated into the program. Strength is progressed gradually, but aggressive OKC knee extension is avoided until at least 3 months after surgery. The patient can begin a gradual running and jumping program at 3 to 4 months. Depending on the extent of pathology and surgical debridement, this progression may be further delayed for up to 6 months.

Patellar Tendon Rupture

Patellar tendon rupture is a disabling injury that results in disruption of the extensor mechanism and inability to actively obtain and maintain knee extension. Ruptures (grade III strains) often occur in sports as a result of a violent contraction of the quadriceps muscle as the foot is planted and the knee moves into flexion, producing an eccentric contraction of the quadriceps. Forces causing rupture of the patellar tendon typically are greater than 17 × BW.[309] In patients under 40 years of age, these forces are highest at the insertion of the tendon and therefore commonly produce tears at the inferior pole of the patella. Ruptures of the patellar tendon may be more prominent with systemic inflammatory disease, diabetes mellitus, or chronic renal failure. In these patients, rupture of the patellar tendon may more likely occur midsubstance than at the osteotendinous junction.

One of the most commonly observed causative factors in patellar tendon rupture is chronic patient complaints of patellar tendinopathy. Kelly et al.[310] reported a correlation between pre-existing patellar tendinosis and patellar tendon rupture. The relatively poor vascularity and chronic degeneration of tissue associated with patellar tendinosis, combined with repetitive microtrauma, eventually may result in full rupture of the tissue.

Patients almost always report an acute incident of rupture and present with pain, swelling, and inability to actively extend the knee. A palpable defect often is noted upon examination. The patient also has a visible antalgic and quadriceps avoidance gait pattern as the hip musculature attempts to substitute for the lack of quadriceps control. Plain film radiographs are commonly taken in the lateral position. A superiorly orientated patella, or patella alta, may indicate a rupture of the tendon. MRI can confirm the diagnosis of a ruptured tendon and can aid the assessment for concomitant pathology.

Surgical Management

The treatment of an acute tear in the patellar tendon depends on the extent of the tear. If the patient is able to perform a straight leg raise without a quadriceps lag (inability to fully extend the knee), nonoperative treatment can be considered. In most cases, however, patellar tendon rupture results in a disruption of the extensor mechanism and should be repaired surgically.

An anterior longitudinal incision permits exposure of both the patellar tendon and the patella. Because most ruptures occur at the tendosseus junction at the inferior pole of the patella, the patellar tendon cannot usually be simply reapproximated. Instead, three longitudinal drill holes are made in the patella. A running locking stitch is placed in the patellar tendon, and sutures are passed from the tendon through the drill holes in the patella and tied over a bony bridge at the proximal aspect of the patella. The paratenon of the patella is repaired, and the patient is placed in a knee immobilizer or cast.

Postoperative Treatment for Patellar Tendon Repair

The rehabilitation program followed after patellar tendon repair is critical to the long-term success of the procedure. Rehabilitation must protect the healing tendon while gradually returning the patient to functional activities. Traditional rehabilitation programs involve approximately 6 to 8 weeks of immobilization and unloading of the lower extremity after surgery. Although this may be appropriate for patients with poor tissue status, a very active person or competitive athlete who wants to return to vigorous activities may risk the development of joint stiffness and arthrofibrosis. The authors prefer a program that gradually progresses range of motion and weight bearing but does not overload the healing tissue; this is believed to minimize the risk of complications such as knee flexion limitations, patella immobility, and patella baja.[311] The specific pace of the rehabilitation program is based on the quality of surrounding tissue and the fixation strengths of the repair. Communication with the surgeon is vital to develop an appropriate postoperative program.

The immediate postoperative goals include reducing pain and swelling, restoring patellar mobility, initiating early, controlled quadriceps muscle contraction, and gradually restoring range of motion. The patient is instructed to use a brace locked in extension for ambulation. Immediate toe touch weight bearing is initiated, progressing to about 25% of body weight by week 2 and 50% of body weight by week 3. The patient typically progresses to weight bearing as tolerated without crutches by 6 weeks. At this time, the patient may unlock the brace during ambulation but is advised to continue wearing the brace for approximately 8 weeks.

The restoration of passive range of motion is one of the most difficult goals to achieve. Full knee extension is encouraged immediately after surgery, although flexion is limited to 30° for the first 5 days and to 45° by the end of week 1. Motion is gradually progressed to 60° by week 2, 75° by week 4, and 90° by week 6. The rate of progression should be carefully monitored, and a continuous passive motion (CPM) machine may be useful at home. Range of motion is gradually progressed to 105° by week 8, 115° by week 10, and at least 125° by week 12.

Restoring Flexion After Patellar Tendon Repair

First 5 days	30°
7 Days	45°
14 Days	60°
28 Days	75°
42 Days	90°
56 Days	105°
70 Days	115°
84 Days	125°

Initial isometric exercises for the quadriceps and other lower extremity muscles are encouraged. These exercises include quadriceps setting and multiangle straight leg raises by the end of week 2. Use of the pool and gentle cycling also may be beneficial for the patient when range of motion permits, typically by 4 to 6 weeks. Gentle CKC exercises, such as weight shifting and minisquats to 30°, are initiated during week 4 and progressed to include the leg press, wall squats, front lunges, and other lower extremity exercises by weeks 10 to 12. Active OKC knee extension is avoided for the first 8 to 12 weeks. Patients who want to begin a running program are allowed to do so after a satisfactory clinical examination. Running typically begins around 5 to 6 months after surgery, with a gradual return to sports activity at 7 to 9 months.

Assessment of Functional Outcome

Over the past decade, outcome-based research on orthopedic problems of the knee has matured. Research that historically focused on the regional impact of disease (e.g., range of motion, strength, and pain) has broadened to include parameters that characterize the impact of a particular condition on a patient's ability to function in daily life and the relationship of the condition to the patient's general health. In this process, specific and standardized outcome tools have been developed that have been validated to produce accurate and reproducible assessments of a patient population.

This change occurred with recognition of populations of patients with residual knee laxity who may be able to perform at their previous level of activity without symptoms and would consider themselves to have a good outcome.

If outcomes were determined on the basis of joint stability, however, these patients would be classified as having a poor outcome. Conversely, patients may have a good outcome in terms of joint stability but a poor outcome in terms of functional limitations and disability for various reasons, such as pain, apprehension, fear of reinjury, and lack of confidence. Accurate assessment of outcomes after knee injury now requires both measures of knee stability, strength, and motion and assessment of patients' perspective on the impact of the injury on their level of function. In this way, patient-based subjective assessments are combined with objective measures to produce a useful gauge of success.

The tools for making these assessments also have matured in the past decade. Various measures of questionnaire validity are expected before an outcome test is used. Test-test reliability (reproducibility), responsiveness (ability to detect clinically important change), and construct validity are usually defined for each outcome tool.

Successful application of these tools to assess functional outcome requires an understanding of the patient population and the research question at hand.[312] An instrument validated for one population may not be the correct tool to measure a different population. The Western Ontario and McMaster Universities (WOMAC) Osteoarthritis Index, for example, was developed and validated to assess osteoarthritis outcomes in a relatively older population.[313] The usefulness of its comparisons in a population of younger patients with knee instability is uncertain.

Knee Stability and Function

Historically, outcome studies related to treatment of knee ligament injuries focused on reporting physical impairment of the knee, including limitations in range of motion, strength, and stability. The relationship between physical impairment of the knee and functional limitations and disability experienced by the patient has been the subject of research.

It has been hypothesized that deficits in range of motion, strength, and stability result in increased levels of functional limitations and disability. Snyder-Mackler et al.[271] demonstrated a significant relationship between isometric quadriceps peak torque and gait abnormalities. Decreased levels of isometric quadriceps peak torque were associated with an increased angle of knee flexion during gait. Wilk et al.[278] demonstrated a positive correlation between isokinetic knee extension peak torque at $180°/$sec and $300°/$sec and a Modified Cincinnati Knee Rating Score. Lephart et al.[14] failed to demonstrate a significant relationship between isokinetic peak torque and torque acceleration energy for the quadriceps and hamstrings at $60°/$sec and $270°/$sec and physical performance tests, including the shuttle run, carioca, and co-contraction semicircular run. Furthermore, no relationship was found between these isokinetic parameters and the Iowa Athletic

Knee Rating Scale. Research is ongoing to clarify the relationship between isometric and isokinetic strength of the quadriceps and hamstrings and functional limitations and disability experienced by patients.

It has been assumed that increased laxity, measured manually or with instruments such as the KT1000, results in greater functional limitations and disability; however, this has not always been found to be the case. Lephart et al.[14] reported a nonsignificant relationship between the Iowa Athletic Knee Rating Scale score and increased anterior translation of the tibia measured with the KT1000. A variety of functional tests have been proposed to assess outcome after knee ligament injury and/or surgery. Tegner et al.[314] studied the one-legged hop, running in a figure-of-eight, running up and down a spiral staircase, and running up and down a slope in 26 individuals with an ACL-deficient knee and 66 uninjured soccer players. The results indicated significant performance deficits in individuals with an ACL-deficient knee compared to the uninjured soccer players.

Barber et al.[315] evaluated the one-legged hop for distance, one-legged vertical jump, one-legged timed hop, shuttle run with no pivot, and shuttle run with pivot to predict lower extremity functional limitations in individuals with an ACL-deficient knee. Significant differences were found for ACL-deficient subjects compared to a normal group of subjects for all tests except the shuttle run with a pivot. The vertical jump and shuttle run tests were not capable of detecting functional limitations in the ACL-deficient subjects. For the one-legged hop tests, 50% of patients performed normally, but all reported episodes of giving way during high force activities, indicating a lack of sensitivity of such tests to identifying functional limitations in these ACL-deficient patients.

Lephart et al.[14] demonstrated a significant relationship between disability as defined by the Iowa Athletic Knee Rating Scale and performance time on the shuttle run, carioca, and semicircular co-contraction test. Also, those who were able to return to preinjury levels of activity demonstrated significantly better times on the functional performance tests than those who were unable to return to their prior level of activity.

Wilk et al.[278] found weak positive correlations between the Modified Cincinnati Knee Rating Score and the one-legged hop for distance, one-legged hop for time, and one-legged crossover test. Their data demonstrate a positive relationship between functional limitations and disability as measured with the Modified Cincinnati Knee Rating Score and the patient's self-rating on a scale of 0 to 100 for the hop index and the vertical jump index. The hop index is defined as the distance hopped on the involved leg divided by the noninvolved leg multiplied by 100. The vertical jump index is calculated similarly.

It appears that functional performance tests may be better predictors of functional limitations and disability than measurements of physical impairment after knee ligament injury. Deficits in functional performance tests probably would result in functional limitations and disability for a patient. Functional performance tests that reproduce the stresses and strains on the knee that occur during activities may be more likely to demonstrate functional limitations and disability. For example, carioca that involves a cross-cutting maneuver reproduces the pivot shift associated with anterolateral instability. This maneuver would be expected to be more stressful than a one-legged hop for distance in an individual with an ACL-deficient knee. Additional research is needed to identify functional performance tests that can accurately predict functional limitations and disability after a knee ligament injury.

Functional limitations and disability experienced by a patient after a knee ligament injury may have multiple causes. Disability may be related to a combination of factors, such as the type and extent of injury, symptoms, and physical impairment and to psychological factors, such as apprehension, lack of confidence, and fear of reinjury. This diversity has led researchers to use a combination of quality of life and disease-specific evaluation tools.

Multiple measures of patient outcomes have been used to measure clinical success. Questionnaires can be used to measure general health status, pain, functional status, or patient satisfaction. Physiological outcomes, utilization measures, or cost measures can also be defined as end points. Assessment tools can be driven by the health care provider or by patients themselves. Objective measures used by the health care provider can include range of motion, strength, endurance, structural measures (radiographs), proprioception, and joint laxity. Subjective measures, derived from patient-driven data, include general health, pain perception, psychometric evaluations, disability predictions, and overall patient satisfaction. Subjective measurements have been found to be valid measurements of outcome, and in many cases were more reliable than the "objective" tests health care providers have relied on for years. The most appropriate set of tools depends on the question to be evaluated and the patient population; usually a combination of these techniques is required.

Some common knee outcome measures include the Short-Form 36 (SF-36), the Modified Lysholm Scale, the Cincinnati Knee Rating Score, the Activities of Daily Living Scale (ADL), the Knee Injury and OA Outcomes Score, the Quality of Life Outcome Measure for Chronic ACL Deficiency (ACL-QoL), and the International Knee Documentation Committee (IKDC) (see volume 1 of this series, *Orthopedic Physical*).

Summary

Successful treatment and rehabilitation of ligamentous and patellar tendon injuries of the knee require a full understanding of the anatomy and biomechanics of the knee. Although imaging techniques continue to advance technologically, the physical examination remains the most important diagnostic tool. Each knee injury must be treated as an individual and unique case; however, application of the principles outlined in this chapter can lead to improved outcomes over time.

References

To enhance this text and add value for the reader, all references have been incorporated into a CD-ROM that is provided with this text. The reader can view the reference source and access it online whenever possible. There are a total of 315 references for this chapter.

Injuries to the Meniscus and Articular Cartilage

David J. Mayman and Thomas J. Gill

Introduction

Injuries to the articular cartilage and the meniscus of the knee are common. They can be caused by work activities and athletic injuries as well as activities of daily living and degeneration. They can occur as isolated injuries or in combination with injury to ligaments and other knee structures. Meniscal tears and chondral injuries can cause significant clinical symptoms of pain, swelling, loss of motion, and locking, often requiring surgical intervention. Arthroscopic treatment of meniscal tears has become one of the most common procedures in the United States.[1]

To evaluate and treat these injuries, the clinician must have an understanding of the anatomy, histology, and function of the meniscus and articular cartilage. This chapter reviews the anatomy and histology of both the articular cartilage and the meniscal cartilage and the signs and symptoms of injuries to these structures; diagnostic studies and treatment alternatives are then discussed.

Meniscus

Anatomy

The meniscus was first described by Bland-Sutton[2] in 1897 as "the functionless remnants of intra-articular leg muscles." Since that time, the meniscal anatomy has been studied extensively. From a gross anatomical perspective, the menisci are two fibrocartilaginous structures that have strong bony attachments to the anterior and posterior tibial plateau.

In the C-shaped medial meniscus, the anteroposterior dimension of the posterior horn is larger than the anteroposterior dimension of the anterior horn. Some variation is seen in the bony attachments of the medial meniscus. Berlet and Fowler[3] have described four types of anterior horn meniscal attachments, three of which attached to bone. The type four variant had no firm bony attachment, but this type was found in only one of 34 specimens. A similar attachment was described by Nelson and LaPrade;[4] 14% of their specimens had no direct bony attachment of the anterior horn. The remainder of the medial meniscus is attached to the knee joint capsule. The capsular attachment of the meniscus to the tibia is called the *coronary ligament*. The posterior bony attachment consistently lies anterior to the tibial insertion of the posterior cruciate ligament. Johnson et al.[5] studied the surface area of the meniscal bony attachments and found that the anterior horn of the medial meniscus has the largest footprint (61.4 mm^2), and the posterior horn of the lateral meniscus has the smallest (28.5 mm^2) (Figure 17-1).

The lateral meniscus, which is more semicircular in shape, also has anterior and posterior bony attachments. The lateral meniscus covers a larger area of the tibial articular surface than the medial meniscus. A lateral disc-shaped or discoid meniscus that covers the entire tibial articular surface has been reported in 3.5% to 5% of cases.[6] Discoid menisci are the result of a developmental anomaly and may have a familial pattern; they are rarely found medially, are generally thicker than normal, and lack normal posterior attachments. The bony attachment sites of the normally shaped lateral meniscus, the anterior and posterior horns, are much closer together in the lateral meniscus than in the medial meniscus. The anterior horn attaches just adjacent to the anterior cruciate ligament (ACL). The bony attachment site of the posterior horn is located behind the tibial spines and anterior to the insertion site of the medial

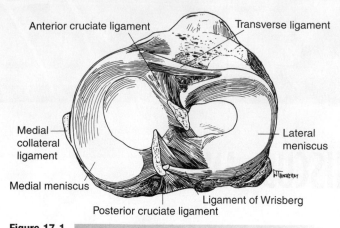

Figure 17-1

Anatomy of the menisci. (From Warren R, Arnoczky SP, Wickiewicz TL: Anatomy of the knee. In Nicholas JA, Hershamn EB, eds: *The lower extremity and spine in sports medicine*, p 687, St. Louis, 1986, Mosby.)

meniscus. The Wrisberg variant of the discoid meniscus lacks a posterior bony attachment, which leaves the posterior meniscofemoral ligament of Wrisberg as the only posterior stabilizing structure; this often allows excess motion and posterior horn instability. The anterior meniscofemoral ligament of Humphry runs from the posterior horn of the lateral meniscus to the posterior cruciate ligament and femur. In the posterolateral corner of the knee, the popliteus tendon lies between the knee joint capsule and the lateral meniscus. This region is called the *popliteal hiatus.* Attachments also are found between the tibia and meniscus through the capsule, but these are not as well developed as on the medial side. Because of the differences in the attachment to the tibia, the lateral meniscus has more mobility through knee joint motion (Figure 17-2). Thompson et al.[7] have demonstrated 11.2 mm of posterior excursion of the lateral meniscus during knee joint flexion, compared to 5.2 mm of excursion of the medial meniscus.

Blood Supply

The entire meniscus is vascular at the time of birth. By 9 months of age, the inner one third has become avascular. The vascularity of the meniscus decreases until approximately age 10, at which time it reaches its adult condition. Ten percent to 25% of the lateral meniscus is vascular, and 10% to 30% of the medial meniscus is vascular (Figures 17-3 and 17-4).[8]

The vascular supply of the menisci is the superior and inferior branches of the medial and lateral genicular arteries. These vessels form a perimeniscal capillary plexus. The region of the popliteal hiatus is a relatively avascular zone of the lateral meniscus. Cell nutrition to the inner 70% to 90% of the menisci comes from diffusion or mechanical pumping.[9]

Innervation

The menisci are innervated by myelinated and unmyelinated nerve fibers. Neural elements are most abundant in the outer portion of the meniscus. The anterior and posterior horns of the meniscus are innervated with mechanoreceptors that may play a role in proprioceptive feedback in the knee.[10]

Function

The menisci are critical structures in the knee. They take load from the femur and distribute it over the entire articular surface of the tibial plateau. The menisci transmit at least 50% to 70% of the load when the knee is in extension. Load transmission increases to 85% at 90° flexion.[11] Radin et al.[12] showed that removal of the medial meniscus results in a 50% to 70% decrease in femoral condyle surface contact area and an increase in joint reactive forces of 100%. Total lateral meniscectomy leads to a 40% to 50% decrease in contact area and an increase in contact stresses of 200% to 300%.[12-14] In addition to being increased, stresses within the joint are distributed

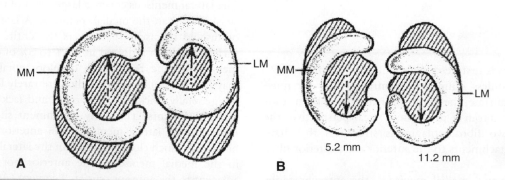

Figure 17-2

The menisci move anteriorly with extension (**A**) and posteriorly with flexion (**B**). The right knee is shown. *MM,* Medial meniscus; *LM,* lateral meniscus. (Modified from Kapandji IA: *The physiology of the joints: annotated diagrams of the mechanics of the human joints,* Edinburgh, 1970, Churchill Livingstone.)

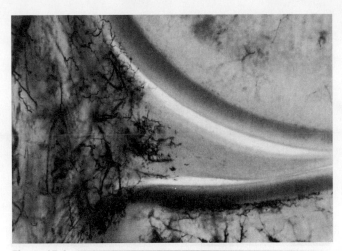

Figure 17-3

Blood supply of the meniscus. Staining studies demonstrate vascular network within the meniscus that is critical for potential for healing. (From Arnoczky SP, Warren RF: Microvasculature of the human meniscus, *Am J Sports Med* 10:90, 1982.)

Shoemaker and Markolf[18] demonstrated that the posterior horn of the medial meniscus is the most important structure in the knee for resisting an anterior tibial force applied to an ACL-deficient knee.

The inner two thirds of the menisci are important for shock absorption and for increasing joint contact surface area, and therefore for reducing contact stresses. The peripheral ring of the menisci is important for load transmission, shock absorption, and knee stability.

Functions of the Menisci

- Load sharing
- Reducing joint contact stresses (by increasing contact surface area)
- Shock absorption
- Passive joint stabilization
- Limiting extremes of flexion and extension
- Proprioception

unevenly, resulting in increased compressive and shear forces across the joint.

The meniscus plays an important role in shock absorption.[15] Compression studies using bovine menisci have demonstrated that articular cartilage is approximately twice as stiff as meniscal fibrocartilage.

The menisci also can play a large role in joint stability.[16] Medial meniscectomy in a knee with an intact ACL does not affect knee stability; however, medial meniscectomy in an ACL-deficient knee results in an increase in anterior tibial translation of up to 58% at 90° flexion. Allen et al.[17] showed that the resultant force in the medial meniscus of an ACL-deficient knee increased 52% in full extension and 197% at 60° flexion under a 134 newton (N) load.

Epidemiology

The mean annual incidence of meniscal tears is 60 to 70 per 100,000,[19,20] and the ratio of males to females varies from 2.5:1 to 4:1. Approximately one third of all meniscal tears are associated with a tear in the ACL.[21] The peak incidence of meniscal tears associated with ACL injury occurs at 21 to 30 years of age in males and at 11 to 20 years of age in females. A traumatic cause is more likely in younger patients, whereas older patients are more likely to have degenerative meniscal tears.

Patients with an acute ACL injury are more likely to have a lateral meniscal tear than a medial meniscal tear.[22] Patients with chronic ACL-deficient knees, on the other hand, are more likely to develop a medial meniscal tear; the role of the medial

Figure 17-4

Schematic of meniscus demonstrating three zones with varying degrees of vascularity and potential for healing. (From Insall JN, Scott WN: *Surgery of the knee,* ed 3, p 476, New York, 2001, Churchill Livingstone.)

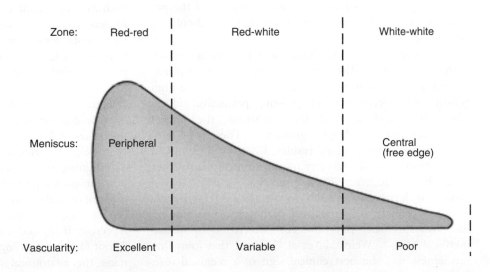

meniscus as an anteroposterior joint stabilizer in ACL-deficient knees is thought to be the reason for this phenomenon.

Diagnosis of Meniscal Tears

Meniscal tears can be diagnosed through a combination of a careful history, a thorough physical examination, and the appropriate diagnostic tests.

History

Younger patients usually have a history of a weight-bearing, twisting, or hyperflexion injury. These patients usually present with acute joint line pain and swelling. Loss of extension with a mechanical block (locking) suggests a displaced bucket handle tear and usually requires acute surgical treatment.

Patients may complain of catching, popping, or locking. These symptoms occur with meniscal tears, but they also may be symptoms of chondral injury or patellofemoral chondrosis. Degenerative tears of the meniscus usually occur in patients over 40 years of age. These tears frequently present with a traumatic history of swelling and joint line pain, and they often are associated with some degree of chondral damage.

Physical Examination

Whenever the clinician suspects meniscal pathology, a complete physical examination of the low back and lower extremity must be performed.

Examination of the knee should begin with inspection of the skin and surrounding tissues. Quadriceps atrophy should be assessed. The knee should be examined for evidence of an effusion. Range of motion should be assessed and compared to the opposite side. The ligamentous structures should be tested. The joint should be palpated to assess for joint line tenderness, tenderness at ligamentous insertion points, and tenderness in the region of the pes anserine bursa. The patellofemoral region also should be palpated.

Numerous special tests have been used to assess for meniscal pathology. Taken in isolation, the various physical examination tests for meniscal tears do not have high sensitivities, specificities, or positive predictive values. These tests include joint line palpation, the flexion McMurray test, and Apley's grind test. These tests have been shown to have mixed results. Evans et al.[23] looked at the flexion McMurray test to determine intraobserver reliability and accuracy. They found that a medially based "thud" with rotation and flexion was the only McMurray sign to correlate with meniscal pathology. This finding had 98% specificity but only 15% sensitivity for medial meniscal tears.[23] Weinstabl et al.[24] found that joint line tenderness was the best clinical sign of a meniscal tear, with a sensitivity of 74% and a 50% positive predictive

value. The presence of an ACL injury makes joint line tenderness less helpful. Shelbourne et al.[25] showed an accuracy of 54.9% for medial meniscal tears and 53.2% for lateral meniscal tears. Terry et al.[26] examined the accuracy of a thorough history, physical examination, and plain radiographs to predict meniscal pathology preoperatively. The overall clinical evaluation had a sensitivity of 95%, a specificity of 72%, and a positive predictive value of 85% for tears of the medial meniscus; it had a sensitivity of 88%, a specificity of 92%, and a positive predictive value of 58% for tears of the lateral meniscus. All tears were confirmed arthroscopically.[26]

Diagnosis of Meniscal Pathology

- History of twisting while weight bearing
- History of hyperflexion of the knee
- Joint line tenderness
- Minimal to moderate synovial swelling
- Pain or forced flexion
- Limited extension with spring block end feel
- Magnetic resonance imaging
- High level of suspicion

Diagnostic Studies

Several types of imaging studies can be used as an adjunct to the history and physical examination. Radiographs, arthrography, magnetic resonance imaging (MRI), and arthroscopy have all been used to help define meniscal pathology.

Radiography

Plain radiographic films should be obtained in the evaluation of all knee pathology. A standard knee series should include a posteroanterior/anteroposterior (PA/AP) weight-bearing view in 30° flexion, a true lateral view, and a tangential image, such as a Merchant or skyline view (Figure 17-5). These images will not confirm the diagnosis of a meniscal tear, but they are still important. Plain radiographic films can be used to assess the knee for joint space narrowing, osteophyte formation, subchondral cysts, and subchondral sclerosis, all findings of osteoarthritis of the knee. Early degenerative changes are better seen on PA/AP views in 30° flexion, because degenerative changes usually are more severe on the posterior femoral condyles than on the distal femur.[27,28] Non-weight-bearing radiographic films are not useful for determining joint space narrowing. The tangential view is best for assessing the patellofemoral joint, which can be a cause of medial or lateral knee pain. Plain radiographic films can also help determine whether any other bony pathology is present. If any question arises about lower limb alignment, 3-foot (1.0 m) standing films should be obtained to determine the anatomical and mechanical axis of the lower extremity.

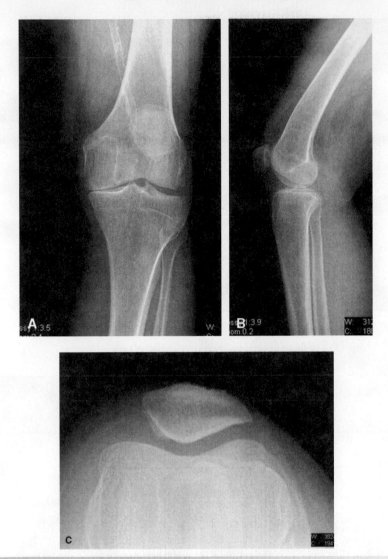

Figure 17-5
Standard radiographic views. **A,** AP weight-bearing view of the knee showing medial joint space loss.
B, Lateral radiograph of the knee. **C,** Tangential view of the patellofemoral joint.

Standard Knee Radiographic Films

- PA/AP weight-bearing view in 30° flexion
- Lateral view
- Merchant or skyline view

Magnetic Resonance Imaging

MRI has proven to be a great advance in the diagnosis of knee pathology, but the scans must be read in the context of the patient's history and the physical examination findings. Some of the advantages of MRI are (1) it allows the clinician to see the ligamentous and cartilaginous structures in the knee; (2) it does not require the use of ionizing radiation; and (3) it is noninvasive. Disadvantages of MRI include (1) a relatively high cost; (2) the amount of time required to obtain the scan; and (3) the tight space in which the patient must lie unless an open magnet machine is used. Normal menisci appear as low signal intensity on all image sequences.

Based on its MRI appearance, the meniscus tear/injury can be categorized according to a four grade system (Figure 17-6). Grade 0 represents a normal meniscus. Grade I and grade II show some degree of intrameniscal signal, but the signal does not abut the free edge of the meniscus. With grade III menisci, the intrameniscal signal exits through the articular surface of the meniscus. The grade III pattern is consistent with a meniscal tear.[29]

MRI is a powerful tool in the diagnosis of meniscal pathology. Several studies have shown meniscal tears on MRI scans of asymptomatic patients. Boden et al.[30] studied 74 asymptomatic patients. Sixty-three were under age 45, and eight of these (13%) were found to have meniscal tears.

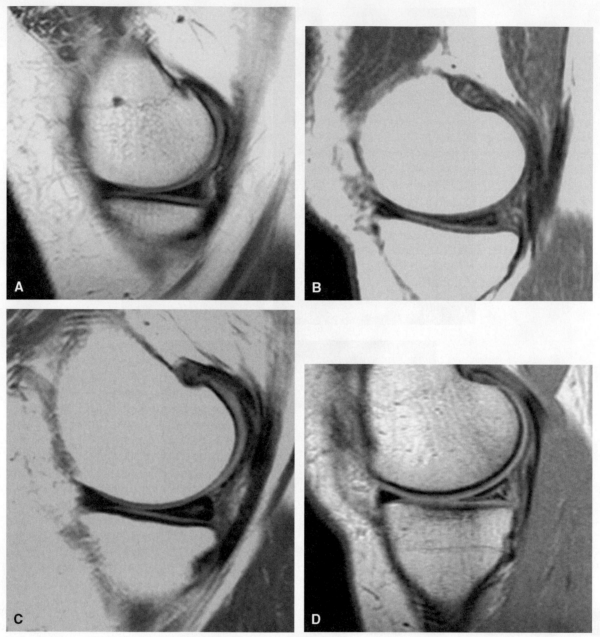

Figure 17-6

Categorization of menisci according to magnetic resonance imaging (MRI) results. **A,** Grade 0: Normal meniscus. **B,** Grade I: Mild intrameniscal signal. **C,** Grade II: Intrameniscal signal. **D,** Grade III: Complex tear of the medial meniscus.

Eleven patients were over age 45, and four (36%) had positive findings on MRI.[30] LaPrade et al.[31] found MRI scans to be positive in 5.6% of knees in asymptomatic patients 18 to 39 years of age who had normal physical examination findings.[31]

Arthroscopy

Arthroscopy is the gold standard for the diagnosis of meniscal tears. Arthroscopic examination allows direct visualization of the tibial and femoral articular surfaces of the meniscus and the meniscocapsular junction. It also allows visualization of the lateral meniscus at the popliteal hiatus and probing to determine whether hypermobility is present.

Classification of Meniscal Tears

Meniscal tears can be classified as oblique, vertical longitudinal, radial (or transverse), horizontal cleavage, or complex (Figure 17-7). Several authors have evaluated the incidence of these tear patterns. Metcalf et al.[32] determined

Figure 17-7
Types of meniscal tears.

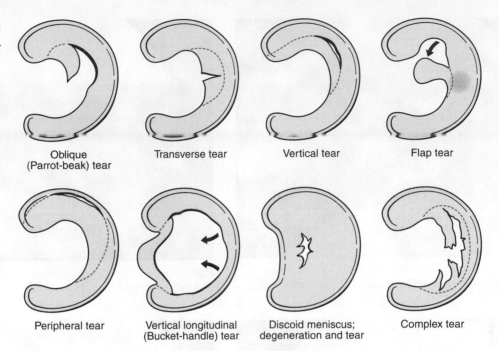

Oblique (Parrot-beak) tear   Transverse tear   Vertical tear   Flap tear

Peripheral tear   Vertical longitudinal (Bucket-handle) tear   Discoid meniscus; degeneration and tear   Complex tear

that 81% of tears were oblique or vertical longitudinal. As patients get older, the incidence of complex tears increases. Most meniscal pathology is found in the posterior horns.

Oblique tears are most commonly found at the junction of the posterior and middle thirds of the meniscus. These tears are commonly called "flap" or "parrot beak" tears (Figure 17-8).

Vertical longitudinal tears, also called "bucket handle" tears, occur most often in young patients. These tears are commonly associated with ACL tears. Binfield et al.[33] showed a 9% incidence of bucket handle tears of the medial

meniscus in ACL-deficient knees. Bucket handle tears occur more often in the medial meniscus, probably because of its more rigid attachments and susceptibility to shear forces. The study by Binfield et al.[33] evaluated knees that, on average, had suffered an ACL injury 23.3 months earlier. This interval is sufficient from the time or original injury for knee instability to generate medial meniscal tears. Vertical longitudinal tears occur most often in the posterior horn of the meniscus and can involve the entire meniscus (Figure 17-9).

Bucket handle tears are unstable and, if large enough, can dislocate into the intracondylar region, causing a

Figure 17-8
Arthroscopic view of an oblique (parrot beak) tear of the meniscus. Symptoms likely result from the flap getting caught in the joint and pulling on the meniscocapsular junction. This also could lead to propagation of the tear.

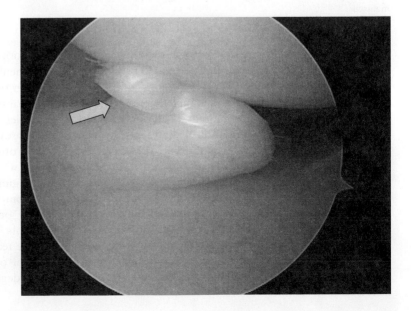

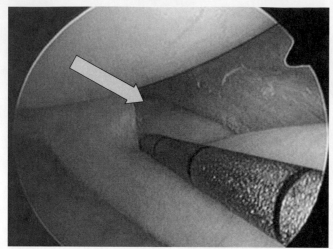

Figure 17-9
Arthroscopic view of a bucket handle tear of the meniscus.

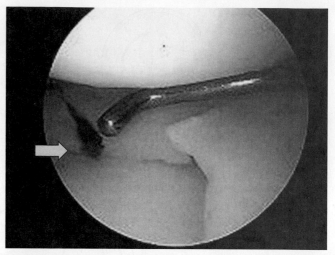

Figure 17-11
Arthroscopic view of a radial meniscal tear.

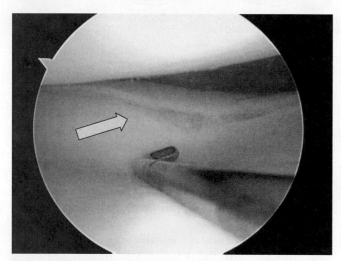

Figure 17-10
Arthroscopic view of an incomplete vertical longitudinal tear of the meniscus.

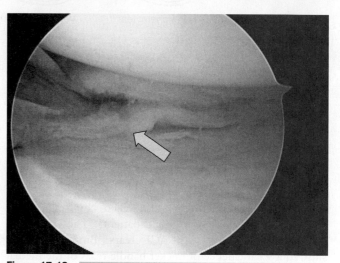

Figure 17-12
Arthroscopic view of a horizontal cleavage tear.

mechanical block to extension (locking). Incomplete vertical longitudinal tears can occur on the femoral or tibial surface of the meniscus (Figure 17-10).

The clinical significance of incomplete bucket handle tears is questionable. Fitzgibbons and Shelbourne[34] found that incomplete vertical longitudinal tears of the lateral meniscus that had been found at the time of ACL reconstruction remained asymptomatic after ACL reconstruction if they were stable at the time of surgery.

Radial, or transverse, tears of the meniscus usually are located at the junction of the posterior and middle thirds of the meniscus. Complete radial tears disrupt the circumferential fibers of the meniscus (Figure 17-11). Jones et al.[35] showed that a complete radial tear completely disrupts the function of the meniscus, leading to significantly increased joint contact stresses.

Horizontal cleavage tears start near the inner margin of the meniscus and extend toward the capsule. Shear forces within the meniscus during load transmission likely cause a separation of the horizontally oriented collagen fiber bundles. The incidence of horizontal cleavage tears increases with age (Figure 17-12). Parameniscal cysts are most often associated with these tears. These cysts often form when horizontal cleavage tears reach the parameniscal region.[36]

Complex tears of the meniscus, often called *degenerative tears,* occur in multiple planes (Figure 17-13). Most patients with complex tears are over 40 years of age. These tears most often occur at the posterior horn of the medial or lateral meniscus and are commonly associated with degenerative changes in the articular cartilage of the knee.

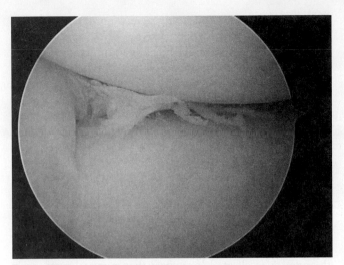

Figure 17-13
Arthroscopic view of a complex meniscal tear. Note the shredding of the meniscus.

Treatment of Meniscal Tears

Indications for Surgical Treatment

Not all meniscal tears require surgical intervention. Before deciding on surgery for meniscal pathology, the clinician must exclude other causes of knee pain, such as degenerative chondral changes. For surgery to be considered, symptoms of meniscal injury should limit activities of daily living, work, or sports. Some meniscal tears heal spontaneously; therefore a trial of conservative management, with activity modification and rehabilitation, should be attempted before surgical intervention. Henning et al.[37] showed that some tears heal spontaneously or remain asymptomatic, including short vertical tears (less than 10 mm), stable vertical longitudinal tears, partial thickness tears (less than 50% of meniscal depth) on the tibial or femoral surfaces, and small radial tears (less than 3 mm).

Indications for Meniscal Surgery

- Symptoms limit activities of daily living, work, or sports
- Conservative treatment has not improved symptoms

If the meniscal injury is associated with an ACL injury, the timing of surgery usually is dictated by the acute rehabilitation after the ACL injury. Factors such as swelling and range of motion dictate the timing of ACL reconstruction. Meniscal pathology usually can be addressed at the time of ACL reconstruction. If a displaced bucket handle meniscal tear is limiting recovery of extension after an ACL injury, the meniscal tear should be dealt with on an urgent basis to allow the patient to regain full extension before proceeding with ACL reconstruction.

Surgical Intervention

Surgeons should develop a standard approach to knee arthroscopy. A diagnostic arthroscopy of the entire knee should be performed as the initial portion of all knee arthroscopies. This diagnostic arthroscopy can be performed in a number of ways, but each surgeon should choose one routine and stick to it to avoid missing pathology. The final decision as to whether the meniscal tear should be repaired or excised should be made after the diagnostic arthroscopy. Most meniscal tears are not amenable to repair. These tears usually require partial meniscectomy to relieve the patient's pain and mechanical symptoms. When a partial meniscectomy is performed, as much of the functioning meniscus as possible is left, to maximize the function of the remaining meniscus and minimize the effect on joint biomechanics.

Indications for meniscal repair can be divided into patient factors and meniscal factors. Patient factors include the chronicity of symptoms, the patient's ability to tolerate the longer rehabilitation required after repair, and the risk of failure of the repair. The patient's age also should be factored into the equation, because younger patients are likely to have a greater chance of progression to arthritis after meniscectomy. Meniscal factors that are favorable for repair include a complete vertical tear longer than 10 mm, a tear within the peripheral 10% to 30% or within 3 to 4 mm of the meniscocapsular junction (red-red zone), an unstable tear that can be displaced by probing, a tear without secondary degeneration or deformity, and tears in stable knees or associated with concomitant ligamentous reconstruction.[30] If both patient and meniscal factors indicate that the tear is amenable to surgical repair, then repair should be performed.

As previously mentioned, some meniscal tears heal spontaneously or remain asymptomatic. If one of these tears is seen at the time of diagnostic arthroscopy and the knee is stable or is undergoing ACL reconstruction, the meniscus can be left alone, or trephination (surgical excision of a circular piece of tissue) and rasping can be performed without surgical stabilization.[37] Weiss et al.[38] reviewed 52 patients with stable vertical longitudinal meniscal tears (less than 3 mm of displacement with probing) and performed repeat arthroscopy. Complete healing was noted in 65% of these patients. Only six patients required further treatment, and four of those had suffered a new traumatic event.[38]

Meniscal Resection

Total meniscectomy used to be a very common procedure. Fairbank[39] first described the damaging effects of total meniscectomy in 1948. As long-term results became available, the progression to osteoarthritis was noted; consequently, total meniscectomy has become a very uncommon procedure.[40,41] With arthroscopic techniques, partial meniscectomy has become feasible (Figure 17-14).

When meniscal repair is not indicated, surgeons now perform a partial meniscectomy. Metcalf et al.[32] established

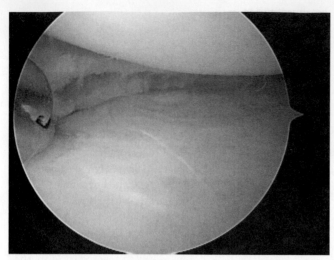

Figure 17-14
Artshroscopic view of a partial meniscectomy.

guidelines for meniscal resection. All mobile fragments of the meniscus that can be pulled past the inner margin of the meniscus into the center of the joint should be resected. The remaining meniscal rim should be smoothed to remove any sudden changes in contour that may lead to further tearing. A perfectly smooth rim is not necessary. A probe should be used to gain information about the stability or mobility of the remaining meniscus. The meniscocapsular junction and the meniscal rim should be retained, if at all possible, to preserve the load transmission properties of the meniscus. Motorized and manual instruments should be used. Manual instruments are more accurate, and motorized shavers can remove loose debris and smooth frayed edges.

Partial Meniscectomy

Studies on the short-term outcome of partial meniscectomy have shown 80% to 90% good results at less than 2-year follow-up.[42] A number of long-term follow-up studies have shown progression of arthritis radiographically after partial meniscectomy. Fauno and Nielsen[43] found that with 8 years of follow-up, radiographic changes occurred in 53% of knees that had undergone partial meniscectomy, compared to 27% of untreated, contralateral knees. Schimmer et al.[44] found good or excellent results in 91.7% of partial meniscectomies at 4 years, but this dropped to 78.1% at 12 years. Articular cartilage damage associated with the meniscal tear had the greatest impact on the long-term outcome. Sixty-two percent of patients who had articular cartilage damage at the time of the index operation had a good or excellent result at final follow-up. In patients with no articular cartilage damage, 94.8% had good or excellent results.[44]

Postoperative Rehabilitation. Rehabilitation after partial meniscectomy usually is uneventful. Postoperatively, rehabilitation focuses on pain control, joint mobilization and range of motion (ROM), gait training, minimization of effusion, regaining full strength, and a progressive return to preinjury or preoperative activity. These goals can be achieved either in a formal rehabilitation setting or with home treatment. Icing and elevation can help minimize pain and effusion in the knee. ROM exercises can be started immediately after surgery. Patients may bear weight as tolerated. Quadriceps strengthening exercises can begin immediately after surgery. Patients should avoid twisting and repetitive impact activities for 4 to 6 weeks after surgery.

Meniscal Cysts

As mentioned, meniscal cysts occur most often with horizontal cleavage tears. These cysts usually can be decompressed at the time of partial meniscectomy from within the joint. Metcalf et al.[32] showed that meniscal cysts rarely recur if the meniscal pathology is dealt with appropriately. The results of arthroscopic decompression of cysts range from 90% to 100% without recurrence. If the cyst is not easily identified from within the joint, a needle can be passed percutaneously through the cyst into the joint and the location of the cyst identified arthroscopically. The cyst then can usually be decompressed by probing or shaving from within the joint.[45,46] If the cyst cannot be decompressed arthroscopically, an open cyst excision should be performed.

Meniscal Repair

Some meniscal tears can heal without fixation. As previously mentioned, meniscal tears that can be left to heal without fixation include vertical longitudinal tears less than 10 mm long, incomplete tears, and stable tears that move less than 3 mm with probing.[34] In such cases, the surgeon can attempt to enhance the healing response with abrasion of the synovial surfaces and meniscal trephination.[47] Synovial abrasion causes a vascular pannus that migrates into the tear and helps produce a healing response. Meniscal trephination is a variation of creating vascular access channels. Horizontally oriented holes are made using a spinal needle through the peripheral vascularized region of the meniscus. Fox et al.[48] showed a 90% success rate in healing incomplete tears with trephination.

When a meniscal tear is found to be amenable to repair and the patient understands the risks of meniscal repair and the rehabilitation required (described later in this chapter), a series of steps must taken to maximize the chances of success of the repair. First, the meniscal bed must be prepared. Loose edges of the tear should be debrided. The torn meniscal edges should be abraded with a rasp or shaver. Rasping of the synovial fringe is also helpful in creating a synovial pannus that can creep into the tear and aid the healing response. Tears that extend into the avascular zone have a lower healing rate. Some think that this can be improved somewhat with trephination.

Open Repair Techniques. Open meniscal repair was first reported by Annandale[49] in 1885. Meniscal repair did not become widely used until it was popularized by DeHaven[50] and Wirth.[51] Open meniscal repair currently is most useful with multiple-ligament injuries in which the collateral ligament injuries may require open repair or tibial plateau fractures require open reduction and internal fixation. With open repair, the meniscus can be sutured directly. The success rate for open meniscal repair is high in multiple-ligament injuries, likely because of the peripheral nature of the tears and the acuteness of the injury and the ensuing hemarthrosis. Rockborn and Gillquist[52] reported a 71% success rate in a 13-year follow-up of patients with open meniscal repairs. Some surgeons still advocate open meniscal repair, suggesting that meniscal preparation and suturing are more readily achieved with an open approach and that the incisions do not need to be much larger than with inside-out arthroscopic repairs.

Arthroscopic Repair. Arthroscopy allows evaluation and treatment of meniscal tears that are not possible with open techniques. Three basic suturing techniques have been used with arthroscopic procedures: the inside-out technique, the outside-in technique, and the all-inside technique. Arthroscopic repairs also can be performed using bioabsorbable implants and suture anchors.

Inside-Out Technique. The inside-out technique was first popularized by Henning et al.[37] in the early 1980s. This technique uses double-armed sutures with long needles, which are positioned through arthroscopically directed cannulas. Skin incisions are then made between the two needles. Soft tissues are dissected down to the capsule, with care taken that no neurovascular structures are trapped between the sutures, and the sutures are then tied, reducing the meniscus. A significant advantage of this technique is that it allows accurate suture placement in the meniscus. The main disadvantage of this technique is the risk to neurovascular structures and the need for incisions between the sutures.

When this technique is performed on the medial side of the knee, branches of the saphenous nerve are most commonly injured.[53] Injuries to the saphenous nerve can cause localized numbness or a painful neuroma. The standard medial incision is a vertical incision approximately 3 cm (1.2 inches) long that starts just above the joint line and runs distally. The incision is made with the knee in 90° flexion. The infrapatellar branch of the saphenous nerve runs approximately 1 cm (0.5 inch) proximal to the joint line. The saphenous nerve usually lies below the subcutaneous fat on the deep fascia covering the sartorius muscle. Keeping the knee in 90° flexion allows the sartorius and saphenous nerve to fall posteriorly. Once the subcutaneous tissue has been bluntly dissected down to the sartorius fascia, the fascia is opened in the direction of its fibers and a plane is dissected down to the knee joint capsule. A retractor can then be placed in this plane, protecting the saphenous nerve. The needles can be visualized as they pass through the capsule.

On the lateral side of the knee, the peroneal nerve is most at risk. The popliteal artery and tibial nerve are at risk as the sutures move more posteriorly. The lateral capsule should be exposed before needles are inserted from within the knee joint. An incision is made on the lateral side of the knee just posterior to the fibular collateral ligament. Again, dissection is performed with the knee in 90° flexion. The peroneal nerve is protected by finding the interval between the biceps femoris and the iliotibial band and retracting the biceps and peroneal nerve posteriorly. The lateral gastrocnemius muscle is found and its fascia is divided in the direction of its fibers. Fibers of the lateral head of the gastrocnemius are dissected off of the posterior capsule. A retractor then can be placed posteriorly in the knee to protect the neurovascular structures. Once this dissection has been performed, needles can be safely passed from inside the knee and retrieved as they exit the capsule, without risk of neurovascular injury.

After the appropriate exposure and neurovascular protection have been obtained, attention can be returned to the meniscal pathology. The meniscal bed is prepared (Figure 17-15), and sutures then can be passed through the meniscus, exiting the knee joint capsule. The sutures should be passed in a vertical mattress pattern for maximum strength; ideally, they should be placed at 2 to 3 mm intervals (Figure 17-16).[54]

Outside-In Technique. The outside-in technique was developed as an attempt to avoid the neurovascular complications that can occur with the inside-out technique. The outside-in technique uses a spinal needle passed percutaneously through the subcutaneous tissue, through the meniscal tear, into the knee joint. A suture then is passed into the joint through the needle and brought out through the anterior portal. A knot is tied in the free end of the suture,

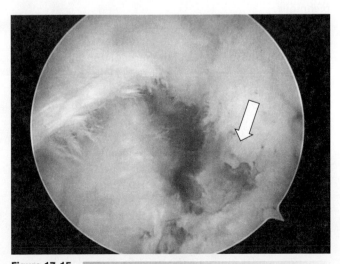

Figure 17-15
Arthroscopic view of a bleeding edge in the red zone of the meniscus.

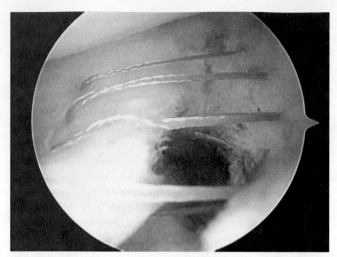

Figure 17-16
Arthroscopic view of vertical mattress sutures in place, ready to be tightened and tied.

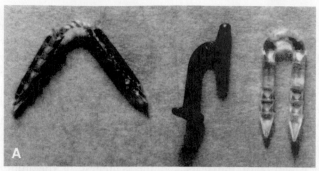

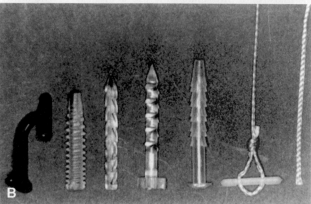

Figure 17-17
Meniscal repair devices. **A,** SDsorb Staple, Mitek Meniscal Repair System, Biomet Staple. **B,** Meniscal repair devices *(left to right):* Miteck Meniscal Repair System, Clearfix Screw, Arthrex Dart, Bionx Meniscus Arrow, Linvatec Biostinger, Smith & Nephew FasT-Fix, and 2-0 Ethibond suture. (From Farng E, Sherman O: Meniscal repair devices: a clinical and biomechanical literature review, *Arthroscopy* 20[3]:273-286, 2004.)

and the suture is pulled back into the joint, reducing the meniscal tear. Adjacent sutures are tied to each other outside the capsule.[55] A small incision is made between the two sutures, the soft tissues are cleared between the sutures down to the capsule (with care taken that no neurovascular structures are caught between the sutures), and the sutures are then tied as in the inside-out technique.

Modifications of the original outside-in technique have emerged. In one such modification, a needle is placed percutaneously, as previously described, to pass the first suture into the knee, followed by a parallel needle with a wire suture retrieval loop. The first suture is passed through the loop and pulled out of the knee joint through the second needle, leaving one intact suture that can be tied outside the capsule. This essentially leaves the patient with the same final configuration of sutures as an inside-out technique.

The outside-in technique is most useful for tears in the anterior or middle third of the meniscus. To perform this technique for posterior tears, the surgeon must use an open approach to allow safe passage of the needles into the knee joint.

All-Inside Technique. The all-inside suture repair is useful for tears of the posterior portion of the medial or lateral meniscus. A posteromedial or posterolateral working portal and a 70° arthroscope are required. Visualization is obtained with the 70° scope, and a curved, cannulated suture passing device is used to pass the sutures through the posterior portal. Arthroscopic knot tying techniques are used to tie the sutures within the knee joint.

Meniscal Repair Devices. A number of devices have been developed to allow meniscal repair without the risk of neurovascular injury or the need for secondary incisions (Figure 17-17).

Barber et al.[56] reported on the BioStinger (Linvatec, Largo, FL). Their study showed a 91% success rate with the device, compared to a 100% success rate for the vertical mattress inside-out suturing technique. Haas et al.[57] reported a 91% success rate for the FasT-Fix (Smith & Nephew, Memphis, TN) when the meniscal tear is associated with an ACL reconstruction and an 80% success rate for isolated meniscal repairs. The Meniscal Arrow (Linvatec) has similar success rates. Meniscal repair devices raise several concerns. Most have been shown to be biomechanically inferior to vertical mattress sutures,[58] and all of these devices can be associated with femoral chondral damage. Gliatis et al.[59] reported on chondral injury caused by migration of a Mitek RapidLoc meniscal repair implant; this report was associated with a successful meniscal repair.

Results of Meniscal Repair. Meniscal repairs have been evaluated using second look arthroscopy, double contrast arthrography, MRI, and clinical examination with the absence of symptoms referable to meniscal pathology. To evaluate the success rates for meniscal repair found in the literature, readers must take into account the definition of successful repair. Success rates are higher for patients who undergo ACL reconstruction at the time of meniscal repair than for patients who have isolated meniscal repairs. When meniscal repair success rates are evaluated, patients who had concomitant ACL reconstruction must be grouped separately and the length of follow-up must be critically evaluated. Studies have been published on the short-term results of meniscal repair, but success rates decline if patients are followed for longer than 2 years. Albrecht-Olsen et al[60] reviewed 27 patients at a median 3-year follow-up, using a clinical examination to determine success. They showed a 63% success rate, and all knees were stable. Buseck and Noyes[61] reviewed 66 repairs associated with ACL reconstruction. All patients underwent second look arthroscopy. Eighty percent were completely healed, 14% were partially healed, and 6% failed. Ninety-eight percent of tears in the outer one third healed. Cannon and Vittori[62] looked at stable knees and knees that underwent ACL reconstruction at the time of meniscal repair. Of the stable knees, 50% healed, whereas 90% of the knees that underwent concomitant ACL reconstruction healed. Healing was confirmed with arthroscopy or an arthrogram.

Rubman et al.[63] evaluated 198 meniscal tears that extended into the avascular (white) zone. Clinical examination showed that 80% of these patients had no symptoms referable to meniscal pathology. Second look arthroscopy was performed in the 20% who had symptoms. Of the 39 knees that underwent second look arthroscopy, only two tears were healed. Thirteen tears were partially healed, and 24 had failed. In the entire group, 91 repairs were evaluated arthroscopically. Of these menisci, 25% were healed,

38% were partially healed, and 36% failed. Seventy-three percent of the patients with unhealed menisci had symptoms referable to the tibiofemoral joint.

Indicators of Successful Meniscal Repairs

- Repairs are done at the same time as ACL reconstruction
- Lateral meniscal repairs are more successful than medial meniscal repairs
- Tear is in the peripheral one third of the meniscus
- A functioning meniscus is present

Postoperative Rehabilitation. Rehabilitation after meniscal repair depends on whether ACL reconstruction was performed at the same time. Although many protocols exist, the principles of rehabilitation include an initial period of non-weight-bearing and limitation of flexion. Standard meniscal repair guidelines are presented in Table 17-1.

If ACL reconstruction is performed concomitantly with the meniscal repair, more aggressive ROM exercises should be performed. Flexion should be limited to 90° for the first 4 to 6 weeks. Arnoczky et al.[64] showed that the meniscus is subject only to small amounts of motion and stress between 15° and 60° flexion. After 6 weeks, more aggressive closed kinetic chain activities can be started. Return to pivoting sports should not be allowed before 6 months.

Complications of Meniscal Repair. The most common complication of meniscal repair is failure of healing

Table 17-1
Rehabilitation Protocol After Meniscal Repair

	Weeks 1-2	Weeks 3-4	Weeks 5-6	Weeks 7-8	Weeks 9-16	Weeks 17-20	Weeks 21-24
Brace	Immobilized	Immobilized	No brace	No brace	No brace	No brace	No brace
Weight bearing	NWB	PWB	WB as tolerated	WB as tolerated	WB as tolerated	WB as tolerated	WB as tolerated
Range of motion	0°-90°	0°-90°	0°-120°	Full ROM	Full ROM	Full ROM	Full ROM
Exercises	Isometric Quad Exercises • Quadsets • SLR	Isometric Quad Exercises • Quad sets • SLR	Begin closed chain exercises	Closed chain exercises Hamstrings Stationary bike	Closed chain exercises Hamstrings Stationary bike Stair climber	Running, straight	Cutting
Manual therapy	Patellar mobilization	Patellar and joint mobilization Passive ROM to 90°	Patellar and joint mobilization Passive ROM to 120°	Patellar and joint mobilization			

NWB, Non-weight-bearing; *PWB,* partial weight bearing; *WB,* weight bearing; *ROM,* range of motion.

and the need for subsequent partial meniscectomy. Other complications specifically associated with meniscal repair include injury to the saphenous nerve or vein, injury to the peroneal or tibial nerve, and injury to the popliteal artery or vein. Loss of motion after repair also can be associated with meniscal repairs.[53,65,66] Deep vein thrombosis, pain, infection, and hemarthrosis can occur but are not seen at a higher rate than with partial meniscectomy. Shelbourne and Johnson[67] reported a 25% incidence of stiffness when ACL reconstruction is performed at the same time as repair of a locked bucket handle meniscal tear. Meniscal repair performed at the same time as ACL reconstruction does appear to be a risk factor for postoperative stiffness; however, meniscal healing rates are higher when meniscal repair and ACL reconstruction are performed at the same time.

Complications of Meniscal Surgery

- Nerve injury (saphenous, peroneal, tibial)
- Vascular injury (saphenous, popliteal)
- Loss of range of motion (stiffness)
- Deep vein thrombosis
- Pain
- Infection
- Hemarthrosis

Meniscal Transplantation

Transplantation of the meniscus was first described by Milachowski et al.[68] in 1989. The experience with human meniscal transplantation was preceded by clinical studies in animals and cadavers. Cadaveric models have shown decreased contact pressures and increased contact surface areas after meniscal transplantation. Both the anterior and posterior horns of the meniscus must be securely attached in their anatomical positions to gain these biomechanical advantages. When both anterior and posterior attachments are released, the decrease in contact stresses is completely lost. If one attachment site is lost, some biomechanical benefit is obtained, but it is significantly reduced.[69]

Arnoczky et al.[70] transplanted cryopreserved medial meniscal allografts in 14 dogs. These menisci healed to the capsule by fibrovascular scar. At 3 months they maintained a normal gross appearance. Histological studies showed that the transplanted menisci maintained a normal cellular distribution. Jackson et al.[71] used a goat model to compare autograft to fresh allograft and cryopreserved allograft. At 6 months, the implanted menisci appeared very similar histologically to the controls. A slight decrease was seen in the cellularity in the central portions of the menisci. Peripheral vascularity was almost normal. The water content of the meniscus was increased and the proteoglycan content was decreased compared to controls. In another study, Fabriciani et al.[72] demonstrated little difference between cryopreserved and deep-frozen meniscal transplants. Their study showed

nearly complete remodeling at 6 and 12 months. Debeer et al.[73] showed that 95% of the deoxyribonucleic acid (DNA) in a human transplanted meniscus was identical to that of the recipient at 1 year, which indicated that the host had repopulated the meniscal cells.

Indications for Meniscal Transplantation. The ideal patient for meniscal transplantation is one who previously has undergone complete or near complete meniscectomy and has joint line pain, early chondral damage, a stable knee, and normal lower limb alignment. Meniscal transplantation can be considered at the same time as ACL reconstruction in an ACL-deficient knee. If axial malalignment is present, tibial or femoral osteotomy should be considered to correct it. Meniscal transplantation is contraindicated in patients with advanced chondral changes.[74] At this point, no evidence supports meniscal transplantation in asymptomatic patients who have undergone complete or near complete meniscectomy. As longer term results become available, the indications may expand to cover asymptomatic young patients with complete meniscectomies.

Indications for Meniscal Transplantation

- Previous complete or near complete meniscectomy
- Joint line pain
- Early chondral damage
- Stable knee
- Normal lower limb alignment

Graft Sizing. Graft sizing is extremely important. To obtain the beneficial biomechanical effects of meniscal transplantation, the transplanted meniscus should vary less than 5% from the original meniscus. Various studies have used computed tomography (CT) scans, MRI, and plain radiography for meniscal allograft sizing. A study by Shaffer et al.[74] showed that MRI was accurate to within 5 mm of width and length measurements in 84% of cases, compared to 79% of cases measured with plain radiographs. Most tissue banks use plain radiographs for allograft sizing.[75]

Surgical Technique. The insertion of meniscal allografts has been described using an open technique with collateral ligament detachment, an open technique without collateral ligament detachment, and an arthroscopically assisted technique. The results of meniscal transplantation seem to depend on patient selection, graft sizing, and secure graft fixation more than surgical technique. As described previously, to increase the contact surface area and reduce contact stresses, the surgeon must securely fix the anterior and posterior horns. Soft tissue fixation, fixation with bone plugs, and fixation with a bony bridge inserted into a trough in the tibial plateau have been described as techniques for secure anterior and posterior horn fixation (Figure 17-18).

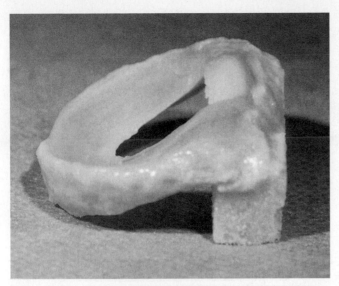

Figure 17-18
Meniscal allograft with bony attachments. (From Insall JN, Scott WN: *Surgery of the knee*, ed 3, p 552, New York, 2001, Churchill Livingstone.)

Results. The results of meniscal transplantation vary significantly with patient selection. Noyes[76] reported on a series of 96 meniscal allografts. MRI and arthroscopic evaluations were used in this study to determine graft success rates. Twenty-two percent healed, 34% partially healed, and 44% failed. When these results were broken down, normal knees had a 70% healing rate, with the other 30% partially healed, whereas knees with severe arthrosis had a 50% failure rate and 50% partial healing. Cameron and Saha[77] reported on 67 meniscal allografts with 87% good or excellent results using a modified Lysholm rating score. These authors performed 34 tibial osteotomies and suggested in their conclusions that limb alignment was important to their success rates. Other studies have shown that meniscal transplantation performed with appropriately sized grafts with secure fixation in patients with normal alignment and only early chondral changes can predictably reduce pain and increase knee function.[75]

Postoperative Rehabilitation. Rehabilitation protocols vary among surgeons who perform meniscal allograft transplantation. In general, rehabilitation protocols are similar to those for meniscal repair. Patients are kept non-weight-bearing or partial weight bearing for the first 4 to 6 weeks. Range of motion is allowed but is limited to 90° flexion for the first 4 to 6 weeks. Muscle strengthening is progressed gradually with closed chain quadriceps and hamstring exercises. Pivoting activities are restricted for the first 6 months.

Summary

The treatment of meniscal pathology is a continually changing field. The art and science of meniscal repairs have advanced tremendously. The future holds potential for meniscal allograft transplantation and for the development of meniscal replacements.

Articular Cartilage Lesions

The treatment of full thickness articular cartilage lesions in the knee is a field that is quickly evolving. Untreated articular cartilage lesions have little or no potential to heal. However, some studies show that a large number of patients will have isolated chondral defects and remain asymptomatic without treatment. Messner and Maletius[78] reviewed a series of 28 patients with isolated chondral lesions; 22 had either good or excellent clinical results without treatment 14 years after diagnosis. Most of these 22 patients had abnormal radiographic findings suggesting progressive degenerative changes. Although these data suggest that isolated chondral defects may predispose patients to the development of further degenerative changes in the knee, long-term prospective data have not been obtained that link isolated chondral defects to progressive degenerative arthritis of the knee that compromises a patient's level of function.

History

The clinical presentation of a full thickness chondral defect can vary. Some patients complain of loose body–type symptoms with locking, catching, and clicking. Other patients complain of crepitus with intermittent mechanical symptoms, and a third group presents with pain as the only symptom. The clinician should obtain a careful history to determine whether the symptoms are indeed coming from within the knee joint and, if so, whether they are coming from the medial, lateral, or patellofemoral compartment.

Physical Examination

A thorough physical examination should be performed for all patients suspected of having chondral defects of the knee. The clinician should begin the examination by watching the patient stand and walk, noting limb length and alignment and observing any gait abnormalities, such as valgus or varus thrust during the stance phase of gait. A low back examination also should be done, and a complete distal neurological and vascular examination should be performed. Examination of the hip is critical in any patient presenting with knee symptoms. A systematic examination of both knees should be performed. Thigh circumference and range of motion should be compared between the two sides. Pain experienced by the patient during range of motion should be noted. The knee should be examined for an effusion.

Knee stability should be examined, including testing of the anterior and posterior cruciate ligaments, the tibial (medial) collateral ligament, the fibular (lateral) collateral ligament, and the posterolateral (popliteus) corner. The knee should be palpated for any local tenderness. The extensor mechanism should be examined for continuity, and the alignment of the extensor mechanism (Q angle) should be measured. The mechanics of the patellofemoral articulation should be examined, and the clinician should observe for a J sign (i.e., deviation of the patella cephalically and laterally in the pattern of an upside-down J), lateral tilt of the patella, lateral retinacular tightness, and patellofemoral crepitation.

Diagnostic Imaging

Diagnostic imaging should begin with plain radiographic films. A standing PA flexion view should be included in the standard knee series. A tangential view of the patellofemoral joint (e.g., Merchant view) should also be included. These plain radiographic films can show joint space narrowing, osteochondral defects, and patellofemoral tilt or subluxation. However, isolated chondral defects often cannot be seen on plain radiographic films.

The imaging study of choice for chondral defects is MRI because of its excellent sensitivity and specificity for this type of lesion. Bredella et al.[79] reported on 130 patients undergoing knee arthroscopy for suspected internal derangement. Of 86 arthroscopically proven abnormalities, 81 were detected with MRI. MRI done with a T_2-weighted, fast spin-echo sequence with fat saturation had a sensitivity of 94% and a specificity of 99% compared to arthroscopy (Figures 17-19 and 17-20).

Nonoperative Management

The goal of nonoperative management of chondral lesions is to minimize symptoms and allow maximum activity. Maintenance of range of motion, muscle strengthening, and a variety of therapeutic modalities to reduce pain and

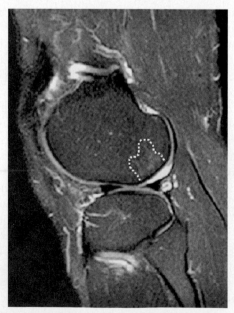

Figure 17-19

T_2-weighted MRI scan of a chondral defect (outlined by *white dotted line*) of the posterior condyle.

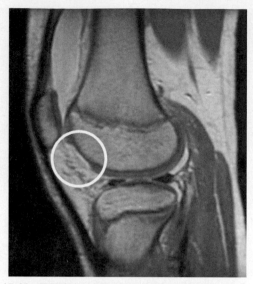

Figure 17-20

T_1-weighted MRI scan of a trochlear chondral defect *(circled).*

inflammation all can minimize symptoms. Orthotics, bracing, and gait training can minimize the stresses on the affected region of the joint. Weight loss in overweight patients can dramatically improve symptoms by reducing patellofemoral and tibiofemoral contact stresses.

Surgical Management

The ultimate goal of surgical treatment is restoration of the microarchitecture of the articular cartilage, which allows complete restoration of the biomechanical and physiological function of the knee. A number of techniques for cartilage repair and regeneration have been developed. The following sections present a detailed look at each of these modalities and review the basic science, surgical techniques, and rehabilitation principles and results.

Abrasion Arthroplasty

The idea of doing something to eburnated bone to cause a reparative tissue response was first proposed by Pridie[80] in 1959. He recommended joint debridement, removal of osteophytes, retention of the patella, shaving of fissured articular cartilage, and drilling of eburnated bone. He described fibrous, reparative-type tissue filling and covering 0.5 cm (0.25 inch) cortical drill holes through the femoral condyle. Most of his poor results involved patients in whom he also performed a patellectomy. Akeson et al.[81] attempted to confirm Pridie's findings in laboratory animals. They removed the articular cartilage and subchondral bone of dog femoral heads. At 1-year follow-up, they concluded that excessive loading destroyed the initial reparative tissue. These results also showed that the proteoglycan concentrations in the reparative tissue were less than half that of normal articular cartilage. Mitchell and Shepard[82] studied rabbit knee joints. They found that after multiple small holes were drilled into the subchondral bone, reparative tissue was stimulated to cover large areas of articular surfaces. The reparative tissue grew out from the drill holes and then spread over the exposed bone. This tissue began to fibrillate and break down within 1 year.[82] These two studies were the first to demonstrate that a fibrocartilaginous repair tissue could be stimulated to form on large areas of articular surface. However, these studies also showed that this reparative tissue did not have the proteoglycan concentration of articular cartilage and that it started to break down quickly with excessive loading.

Abrasion arthroplasty using motorized instrumentation was introduced by Johnson[83] in 1981. Whether the abrasion should be intracortical or cancellous bone should be exposed is the subject of debate. Hjertquist and Lemperg[84] reported that cartilage tissue of mature appearance forms only if the debridement is superficial enough to maintain a cortex.

Surgical Technique. The procedure introduced by Johnson in 1981 is essentially an extension of that described by Pridie. Along with debridement of the joint, a superficial layer of subchondral bone (1 to 3 mm deep) is removed to expose interosseous vessels. This theoretically results in a hemorrhagic exudate that forms a fibrin clot and allows fibrous repair tissue to form over the area of exposed bone.

Rehabilitation. Regeneration of articular cartilage benefits from motion and from limiting the compressive force on the articular cartilage from weight bearing. Patient adherence to a program of motion with limited or no weight bearing is critical. To assist with this, the use of continuous passive motion (CPM) often is considered. Weight bearing often is restricted for up to 12 weeks, with daily CPM, especially in the early postoperative period. Active and passive range of motion are encouraged throughout the postoperative course until weight bearing and strength training can begin.

Results. Eight knees were biopsied in Johnson's original series.[83] Of those eight biopsy specimens, only one showed any type II collagen typical of hyaline cartilage. All other biopsy specimens showed a combination of type I and type III collagen. Bert and Maschka[85] reviewed a series of 59 patients who underwent abrasion arthroplasty with a minimum 5-year follow-up. Of the 59 patients, 15 had conversion to total knee arthroplasty. Biopsies were performed on any remaining fibrous tissue. The fibrous tissue was stained with safranin O to look for proteoglycan. The fibrous surface did not stain, indicating the lack of proteoglycan.

Microfracture

Microfracture can be performed on the patellar, tibial, or femoral articular surface. The general indication for microfracture is a full thickness chondral defect in either a weight-bearing region or a region of contact between the femur and patella. Microfracture can also be performed after debridement of unstable chondral flaps. Contraindications to microfracture include axial malalignment, partial thickness chondral defects, and a patient who is unable or unwilling to comply with a strict postoperative rehabilitation protocol, including minimal weight bearing. Joint space narrowing, chronic lesions, and inability to use a CPM machine may affect the outcome but are not strict contraindications.

Surgical Technique. Microfracture can be performed arthroscopically with a combination of shavers, curets, and picks. The technique has been described by Steadman et al.[86] Three portals are made, allowing use of an inflow canula, the arthroscope, and the working instruments. A diagnostic arthroscopy is performed, and the full thickness chondral defect is identified. Any other work that needs to be performed in the knee is completed before the microfracture procedure is begun. The chondral defect is then inspected, and all cartilage remnants are debrided (Figure 17-21).

The articular cartilage surrounding the defect is inspected and any loose, delaminated cartilage is removed. A perpendicular edge of healthy cartilage is obtained circumferentially around the lesion. The calcified cartilage layer is removed, which care taken not to debride through the subchondral plate.

An arthroscopic awl with the appropriate angle then is used to create perforations in the subchondral plate that are perpendicular to the surface. The awl allows the surgeon to make holes (microfractures) in the subchondral bone with control and without any worry of heat necrosis (Figure 17-22). Attention first is given to the periphery of the lesion. Holes are made at 3 to 4 mm intervals around the periphery and are approximately 3-4 mm deep. Once the holes have been made around the periphery, the remaining surface of the lesion is addressed. Holes should be spaced as close together as possible without fracturing

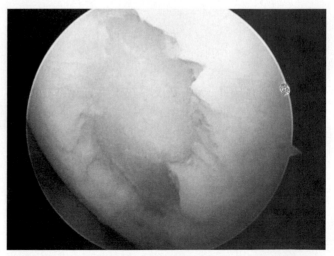

Figure 17-21
Arthroscopic view of a chondral defect debrided to subchondral bone. The calcified cartilage layer has been removed.

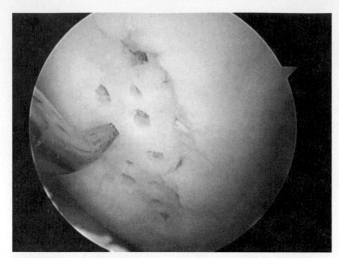

Figure 17-22

Arthroscopic view of a microfracture technique. Multiple pick holes are spaced 3-4 mm apart.

the subchondral bone between two holes (approximately 3 to 4 mm). After the holes have been made, a shaver is used to remove all bony debris. The pump pressure then is turned down to enable the surgeon to visualize fat droplets and blood exiting from all holes (Figure 17-23).

Any holes that do not show bleeding should be checked and possibly made deeper to allow bleeding. After the surgeon has made sure that all holes have been made appropriately, the knee is irrigated, instruments are removed, and the joint is evacuated of fluid. Incisions are closed, and a sterile dressing is applied. The key to this procedure is to establish a clot of pluripotent marrow cells that can then differentiate into stable cartilage under the right conditions.

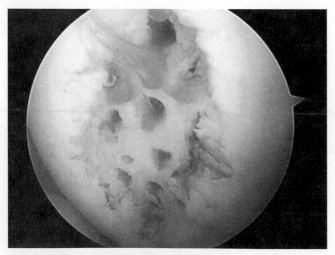

Figure 17-23

Arthroscopic view of a microfracture after reduction of pump pressure shows bleeding from all holes.

Clinical Point

A strict rehabilitation program is essential after microfracture treatment of chondral lesions of the knee.

Rehabilitation. Microfracture creates an environment in which pluripotent marrow cells can be stimulated to produce cartilage. However, the rehabilitation program ultimately determines the success of the procedure. To design an appropriate rehabilitation program after microfracture, the clinician must think about the region that was affected and the kinematics of the knee. The ideal rehabilitation program encourages motion but limits weight bearing and shear stresses on the affected region. For these reasons, the rehabilitation protocol is very different for weight-bearing femoral condyle lesions than it is for patellar or trochlear lesions. All patients are put in a CPM machine postoperatively, and the patient is asked to use the CPM machine up to 10 hours per day.[87] The rate of motion usually is 1 cycle per minute. The CPM is started in a comfortable range and increased as tolerated. Patients with femoral condyle lesions are kept on toe touch weight bearing with crutches for 6 to 8 weeks. At 8 weeks, the patient can progress to weight bearing as tolerated and can begin a more vigorous program of active motion. Strength training with weights or machines should be avoided for 16 weeks. Return to sports that involve cutting, pivoting, and jumping can be allowed at 4 to 6 months.

Patients who have patellar or trochlear lesions are allowed to bear weight as tolerated immediately after surgery; however, the knee must be protected from loaded motion where the defect is engaged. At the time of arthroscopy, the knee joint can be taken through a range of motion to see specifically where the lesion is in contact with the opposing articular surface. In general, a patient with a trochlear or patellar microfracture can be put in a hinged knee brace with the brace set to move from full extension to 20° flexion. The knee should be taken out of the brace for CPM but should be braced at all other times to avoid shear forces across the lesion. The brace can be discontinued at 8 weeks. A recent study by Gill et al.[88] suggested that the period of restricted weight bearing should be increased to 12 weeks. This study evaluated the healing process in cynomolgus macaques. Histological analysis was performed 6 and 12 weeks after microfracture. At 6 weeks, limited chondral repair and ongoing resorption of subchondral bone were seen. By 12 weeks, the cartilage defects were completely filled and showed more mature cartilage and bone repair. Further studies in humans are needed to determine whether this additional length of time makes a clinically significant difference in the long-term outcome.

Results. Steadman et al.[89] looked at a series of 75 knees in 72 patients who underwent microfracture for full thickness traumatic chondral defects. Follow-up was 7 to 17 years. Their three inclusion criteria were (1) a traumatic full thickness chondral defect, (2) no meniscal or ligamentous injury, and (3) patient age under 45 years. Significant improvements were found according to the Lysholm and Tegner knee rating scales. At 7 years after surgery, 80% of patients stated that they were better than before surgery. Some patients took up to 2 years to obtain maximum improvement. Knutsen et al.[90] performed a randomized clinical trial comparing microfracture and autologous chondrocyte implantation (ACI) for isolated chondral defects. Eighty patients were enrolled in the study. Microfracture was performed on 40 patients, and ACI was performed on the other 40. An independent observer performed the follow-up data collection at 12 and 24 months. Both groups showed improvement. According to the Short Form-36 (SF-36) outcome measurement tool, the microfracture group had a significantly greater improvement. Biopsy specimens were obtained from 84% of patients at 2 years. Histological evaluation of repair tissues showed no significant differences between the two groups. Interestingly, no association was found between the histological specimens and the clinical outcome, according to the Lysholm scale, the SF-36, and a visual analog scale.

Mosaicplasty

Autologous osteochondral grafting has shown great promise in that it is a means to transplant bone and hyaline cartilage to a region of a chondral or osteochondral defect. Lane et al.[91] showed that the hyaline cartilage remains viable 12 weeks after transfer. However, two problems were encountered with single plug osteochondral transfers: donor site morbidity and surface incongruity at the recipient site. Mosaicplasty was developed in an attempt to minimize these problems. Mosaicplasty involves the transfer of multiple small osteochondral plugs to a region of chondral or osteochondral defects. The use of multiple small grafts allows for maintenance of donor site integrity and contouring of the new surface.

Surgical Technique. Autologous osteochondral mosaicplasty involves harvesting and transferring small, cylindrical osteochondral grafts (2.7 to 8.5 mm in diameter) from the periphery of the femoral condyles at the level of the patellofemoral joint (Figure 17-24). The cylindrical grafts are then transplanted to prepared recipient sites in the region of the chondral or osteochondral defect.

Combination of different graft sizes allows for coverage of approximately 80% of the lesion. The areas between the osteochondral cylinders are filled with fibrocartilage. At the time of the procedure, a diagnostic arthroscopy is performed. The chondral or osteochondral defect is identified and inspected. All loose cartilage fragments are debrided back to stable, normal articular

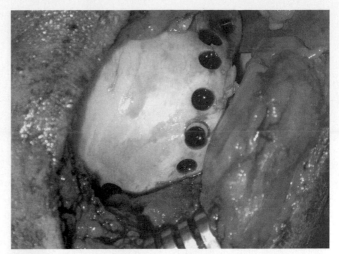

Figure 17-24

View of a graft donor site on the periphery of the lateral femoral condyle.

cartilage. The defect then is sized to determine the number and sizes of grafts needed. If the defect can be accessed adequately arthroscopically, the procedure can be performed arthroscopically. A miniarthrotomy may be required. The grafts can be obtained from either the medial or lateral peripheral margins of the femoral condyles at the level of the patellofemoral joint. The appropriate-sized tube chisel is introduced perpendicular to the donor site, and the harvester is driven into the donor site. For chondral defects, a 15-mm graft is taken. For osteochondral defects, a 25-mm graft is obtained. The chisel is twisted to break the cancellous bone, and the graft is removed. All grafts are harvested with a similar technique (Figure 17-25).

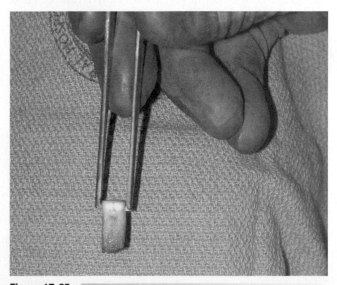

Figure 17-25

Single osteochondral plug.

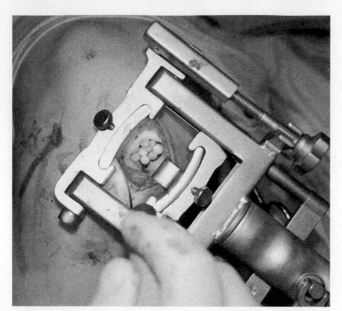

Figure 17-26
Defect filled with multiple osteochondral plugs. (From Insall JN, Scott WN: *Surgery of the knee*, ed 3, p 358, New York, 2001, Churchill Livingstone.)

Attention is then turned to the recipient site. Recipient tunnels are created with drill bits and then an appropriately sized dilator. The grafts are inserted with an adjustable plunger device. It is extremely important to ensure that a smooth surface is created, without prominent or sunken grafts (Figure 17-26).

After all grafts have been put in place, the knee is irrigated and all wounds are closed. Some surgeons place a drain in the knee to try to prevent large postoperative hematomas.

Rehabilitation. Rehabilitation after osteochondral autograft transplantation focuses on early return of range of motion and protected weight bearing. ROM exercises can be initiated immediately after surgery. Patients are kept to toe touch weight bearing for 6 weeks to allow healing of the bony portion of the graft. Patients are allowed to progress to weight bearing as tolerated after 6 weeks and can return to sports activity as soon as they have regained adequate range of motion and strength.

Results. The results of multiple osteochondral autograft transplantation have been promising. Chow et al.[92] reported on 33 patients with 2 to 5 years follow-up. Eighty-seven percent of patients reported their knee as being normal or nearly normal using the International Knee Documentation Committee (IKDC) assessment. Jakob et al.[93] reported on 52 patients with 2 to 5 year follow-up. Ninety-two percent of patients had improvement in knee function at the final follow-up. Hangody et al.[94] reviewed 831 patients undergoing mosaicplasty. Good to excellent results were obtained in 92% of patients with femoral condylar defects, 87% of patients with tibial defects,

and 79% of patients with patellar or trochlear defects. Three percent of patients reported donor site morbidity, and 4% reported painful postoperative hemarthroses. In contrast to the findings of these studies, Bentley et al.[95] reported that only 69% of patients had good or excellent clinical results as assessed by the modified Cincinnati and Stanmore scores. Painful postoperative hemarthroses continue to be a significant complication after mosaicplasty. Feczko et al.[96] used a German Shepherd model and tested donor site plugs. They found that compressed collagen minimized blood loss from the donor sites while still allowing gradual substitution with bone and formation of a fibrocartilage cap at the articular surface.

Autologous Chondrocyte Transplantation

Chesterman and Smith[97] first successfully isolated and grew chondrocytes in culture in 1965. They took epiphyseal chondrocytes from rabbits, grew them in culture, and then implanted them into articular defects in the tibia. They did not show any significant repair. In 1982, Grande et al.[98] began growing articular chondrocytes in culture and then transplanting them into a patellar defect covered with a periosteal flap. These initial results were presented in 1984 and showed 80% filling of the defect with hyaline-like cartilage. In 1987, the first autologous chondrocyte transplantation was performed in the human knee in Sweden. Brittberg et al.[99] reported on the results of the first 23 procedures. Fourteen of 16 patients with femoral lesions had good or excellent results, whereas only two of 7 patients with patellar lesions had good or excellent results.

Surgical Technique. Autologous chondrocyte transplantation requires two operative procedures. The first procedure is a diagnostic arthroscopy and harvesting of chondrocytes. The cultured chondrocytes are implanted during the second procedure. A diagnostic arthroscopy is performed, and the chondral defect is assessed. The defect is not debrided. Any meniscal lesions should be dealt with during the first procedure. Once it has been decided that the patient could benefit from autologous chondrocyte transplantation, cartilage is harvested, typically from the upper medial or upper lateral condyle of the femur. Cartilage most often is taken from the upper medial condyle of the femur at the level of the patellofemoral joint. Three to four slices of cartilage, 3 to 4 mm by 10 mm, should be harvested down to subchondral bone. Two hundred to 300 mg of articular cartilage is required for enzymatic digestion and cell culturing. After harvesting of the cartilage, the knee is irrigated, all arthroscopic instruments are removed, and wounds are closed.

The second procedure involves harvesting of a periosteal flap and implantation of the cultured chondrocytes. A small peripatellar incision is performed to expose the chondral defect. The area of the defect is debrided, with cut vertical edges creating an abrupt transition from healthy cartilage to defect. The excised area is debrided down to subchondral bone without causing bleeding. If bleeding occurs from the subchondral bone, it must be stopped before implantation of the chondrocytes. A separate incision is made to harvest the periosteal flap, which usually is obtained from the upper medial tibia. The periosteal flap is sutured into the healthy cartilage surrounding the defect. The cambium layer of the flap must face the subchondral bone of the defect. Sutures are placed at 5- to 6-mm intervals, and intervals between the sutures are sealed off with fibrin glue. An opening is left in the periosteal patch for injection of the chondrocytes. After injection of the cells, closure of the periosteal patch is completed with sutures and fibrin glue (Figures 17-27 to 17-29).

Rehabilitation. Rehabilitation after autologous chondrocyte transplantation can be broken down into range of motion, CPM, weight bearing, strengthening, and functional training. Patients can begin working on range of motion immediately after surgery. Trochlear groove patients should not work on active extension for the first 4 weeks, because as active extension increases patellofemoral contact stresses. CPM should be used as much as possible for the first 6 weeks. Most patients should be non-weight-bearing for at least the first 2 weeks. Patients then can progress to partial weight bearing. All patients should be in a hinged knee brace that is locked in extension for ambulation. Femoral condyle patients can progress to weight bearing as tolerated at 6 weeks. Trochlear patients can progress to weight bearing as tolerated as soon as they are comfortable as long as they are in the knee brace locked in extension. This keeps the patella out of the trochlear groove and protects the repair. Strengthening can begin

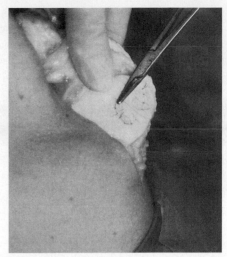

Figure 17-28
Completion of the periosteal patch. (From Insall JN, Scott WN: *Surgery of the knee*, ed 3, p 349, New York, 2001, Churchill Livingstone.)

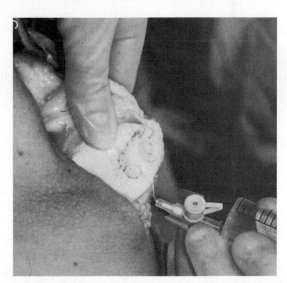

Figure 17-29
Injection of chondrocytes beneath the periosteal patch. (From Insall JN, Scott WN: *Surgery of the knee*, ed 3, p 349, New York, 2001, Churchill Livingstone.)

Clinical Point

It is imperative that the surgeon inform the rehabilitation team of the range of motion to prevent loading, as determined from intraoperative viewing of the lesion during knee range of motion. This allows optimum rehabilitation and protection of the repair.

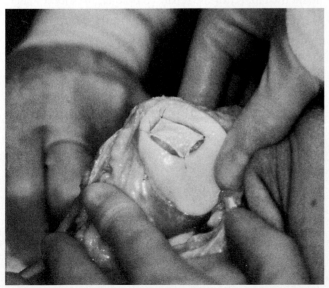

Figure 17-27
Periosteal patch being sewn into place. (From Insall JN, Scott WN: *Surgery of the knee*, ed 3, p 349, New York, 2001, Churchill Livingstone.)

in the first 2 weeks with isometric quadriceps sets and straight leg raises. Closed chain activities can be started at 6 weeks. Positions that stress the region of chondrocyte implantation should be avoided. For anterior femoral condyle lesions, loading in full extension should be avoided. For posterior femoral condyle lesions, loading in flexion should be avoided. For trochlear lesions, deep squats should be avoided. Functional training can begin between weeks 8 and 12.

Positions to Avoid with Autologous Chondrocyte Transplantation

- Anterior femoral condyle lesions—avoid full extension
- Posterior femoral condyle lesions—avoid loaded flexion
- Trochlear lesions—avoid deep squats

Low impact activities, such as cycling, roller blading, and skating, can be started 9 to 12 months after surgery. Repetitive impact loading, such as jogging and aerobics, can be started at 13 to 15 months, and high level sporting activities can be started 16 to 18 months after surgery.

Results. The results of autologous chondrocyte transplantation have been quite promising. Peterson et al.[100] reported on 101 patients treated with ACI with 2 to 9 year follow-up. Ninety-two percent of patients with isolated femoral lesions had good or excellent results. Sixty-five percent of patients with patellar defects had good to excellent results. Second look arthroscopy was performed in 53 patients. Of these, 26 had a hypertrophic response of the periosteum or graft. Seven of these 26 were symptomatic. The incidence of graft failure was 7%. Peterson et al.[101] followed a group of 61 patients treated for isolated femoral or patellar defects for 5 to 11 years to determine the durability of the repair tissue. At 2 years, 50 of 61 patients had good to excellent results. At 5 to 11 year follow-up, 51 of 61 patients had good to excellent results.

Several studies have been performed to evaluate the outcome of ACI compared to the outcomes with microfracture and mosaicplasty. Knutsen et al.[90] compared ACI to microfracture in a randomized trial. Eighty patients with a single chondral defect in the femoral condyle were randomized to ACI or microfracture. Independent observers performed follow-up examinations at 12 and 24 months. Second look arthroscopy was performed at 2 years. Histological evaluation was performed by a pathologist and a clinical scientist, both of whom were blinded to each patient's treatment. Both groups showed improvement at 2 years, but the microfracture group had slightly better improvement as measured by the SF-36.

Biopsy specimens were obtained from 84% of patients. No histological difference was seen between the two groups. Horas et al.[102] compared ACI to osteochondral cylinder transplantation. Forty patients with isolated femoral defects were randomized to ACI or osteochondral cylinder transplantation. Using Lysholm scores, recovery from ACI was slower than recovery from osteochondral cylinder transplantation. After 2 years, clinical results were equal between the two groups. Histomorphological examination of the ACI patients showed a stable resurfacing of the defect in all patients. The tissue consisted mainly of fibrocartilage, with localized areas of hyaline-like regenerative cartilage close to the subchondral bone. Examination of biopsies from the osteochondral cylinder transplantation showed remaining gaps between the graft and intact articular cartilage, but no histological difference was seen between the osteochondral transplants and the surrounding original cartilage.

Numerous studies have shown that autologous chondrocyte transplantation provides good to excellent results in 80% to 90% of patients with isolated chondral defects of the femoral condyles. Results are less predictable for patellar or trochlear defects. Autologous chondrocyte transplantation is one option in the treatment of chondral defects in the knee.

Summary

The treatment of chondral injuries has become an increasingly popular field. As outlined in this chapter, a number of different options are available to today's orthopedic surgeon. The different techniques have varying advantages and disadvantages. The rehabilitation team needs to understand the biology of the repair technique, the biomechanics of the knee, and how the location of the chondral defect affects the biomechanics in order to develop the best rehabilitation program and offer the best rehabilitation advice to each patient.

References

To enhance this text and add value for the reader, all references have been incorporated into a CD-ROM that is provided with this text. The reader can view the reference source and access it online whenever possible. There are a total of 102 references for this chapter.

CHAPTER 18

PATELLOFEMORAL JOINT

Christopher M. Powers, Richard B. Souza, and John P. Fulkerson

Introduction

Disorders of the patellofemoral joint are among the most perplexing and clinically challenging conditions encountered in musculoskeletal practice. Patellofemoral pain (PFP) is one of the most common disorders of the knee, affecting as many as 22% of the general population reporting symptoms.[1] Patellofemoral-related problems are prevalent in a wide range of individuals, but the highest incidence is seen in physically active people, such as runners, tennis players, and military recruits.[2-6] In general, the incidence of patellofemoral-related problems is higher in females (2:1); however, among athletes, the incidence is higher in males (4:1).[1]

Despite the high incidence of PFP in the general population, the pathophysiology of this disorder is sometimes elusive. This is supported by the fact that no clear consensus exists on how PFP should be treated. For example, a myriad of conservative procedures have been advocated (e.g., bracing, taping, foot orthotics, strengthening, stretching),[1,7-14] and numerous surgical techniques have been described.[15-21] Initially, nonoperative care is preferred, but surgical intervention is considered if conservative care fails.[22] Although nonoperative care appears to be successful in the short term,[7,23] the long-term results are less compelling.[14,24,25] A systematic review of 20 randomized, controlled trials evaluating various forms of conservative interventions for PFP revealed that only eight reported a positive outcome.[26] From a surgical standpoint, the success rates for patellofemoral-related procedures are considered equivocally poor compared to other orthopedic operations.[22]

The difficulty involved in treating PFP reflects the complexity of the patellofemoral joint and the multifactorial nature of the disorder. To treat this condition effectively, the clinician must clearly identify the primary cause or causes of the pain. The purpose of this chapter is to provide the reader with an understanding of the relevant anatomy, kinesiology, and biomechanics of the patellofemoral joint and to review current theories related to the etiology of PFP, evaluation methods, and treatment strategies.

Functional Anatomy

The patellofemoral joint consists of the articulation of the patella and the trochlear surface of the femur. It is an integral part of the knee extensor mechanism, and as such it plays a key role in normal knee function and lower extremity biomechanics. The ability of the patellofemoral joint to improve the mechanical efficiency of the extensor mechanism and to accept and redirect forces depends on a host of factors, including the joint's osseous structure and contributions from various soft tissues, such as the quadriceps musculature, quadriceps tendon, patellar tendon, and retinaculum. Clinicians must have an understanding of the anatomical structure of this joint to appreciate both normal and pathological function.

Osseous Structure

Patella

Contained within the quadriceps tendon, the patella has the distinction of being the largest sesamoid bone in the body.[1] The patella consists primarily of cancellous bone covered by thin, compact lamina; its axial length is approximately 4 to 4.5 cm (1.6 to 1.8 inches), and it is approximately 5 to 5.5 cm (2 to 2.2 inches) wide. The thickness of the patella varies considerably, attaining a maximum height of 2 to 2.5 cm (0.77 to 1 inch) at its central portion.[27]

The articular surface of the patella is divided into the medial and lateral facets by a vertical ridge (median ridge) that roughly bisects the patella (Figure 18-1).[28] The lateral facet often is slightly larger than the medial facet.[29] The medial facet is subdivided by a less prominent vertical ridge that separates the medial facet proper and the smaller, odd facet (see Figure 18-1). The articulating surfaces of the

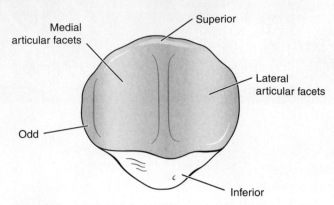

Figure 18-1
Articular facets of the patella.

patella are covered with aneural hyaline cartilage, the thickest cartilage in the body.[30] Maximum cartilage thickness is found at the central portion of the patella (approximately 4-5 mm) and decreases from the median ridge to the medial and lateral borders.

Trochlear Surface of the Femur

The femoral condyles form the trochlear groove that provides the articulating surface of the femur. Similar to the articular surface of the patella, the trochlear surface is divided into medial and lateral facets, the lateral facet being larger and extending more proximally and anteriorly than its medial counterpart (Figure 18-2). This orientation of the lateral femoral condyle provides a bony buttress that helps provide lateral patellar stability.[31] The trochlear groove is shallower proximally than distally, indicating that bony stability is compromised as the patella moves superiorly during terminal knee extension. The cartilage covering the trochlear surface of the femur is much thinner than that covering the patella (i.e., 2 to 3 mm).[30]

Soft Tissue Structures

Synovium

The synovial lining of the patellofemoral joint, which is essentially the synovium of the anterior portion of the knee, has three components: the suprapatellar synovium, the peripatellar synovium, and the infrapatellar synovium. These

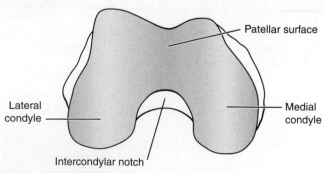

Figure 18-2
Inferior aspect of the distal end of the femur.

three portions blend imperceptibly with each other, allowing free communication with the knee joint proper.[32] The peripatellar synovium creates a small synovial fold or fringe less than 1 cm (0.5 inch) wide that surrounds the patella; this generally is regarded as the true synovium of the patellofemoral joint.[30] Inflammation or scarring of this synovial fold (i.e., plica) can produce symptoms similar to those of cartilage degeneration, and this type of inflammation or scarring is commonly associated with chondromalacia.[33]

Portions of the Synovial Lining of the Patellofemoral Joint

- Suprapatellar synovium (pouch)
- Peripatellar synovium (plica)
- Infrapatellar synovium

Fat Pads

Three fat pads occupy the anterior knee: the quadriceps fat pad, the prefemoral fat pad, and the infrapatellar fat pad (Figure 18-3).[34] The infrapatellar fat pad, or Hoffa's fat pad, is the largest fat pad in the region and has been studied extensively because of its proposed role in various pathologies.[34-38] It is a voluminous structure located just inferior to the infrapatellar pole.[35] It extends inferiorly to the deep infrapatellar bursa at the insertion of the patellar ligament into the tibial tuberosity. Hoffa's fat pad attaches to several structures, including the intercondylar notch via the ligamentum mucosum, the patellar tendon, the inferior pole of the patella, and the anterior horns of the menisci.[34]

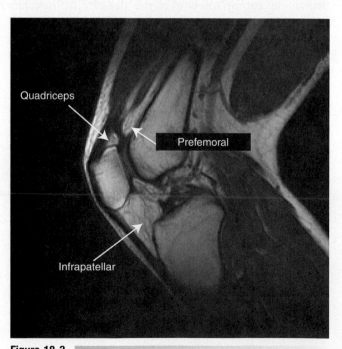

Figure 18-3
Sagittal MRI scan of the knee showing the fat pads that occupy the anterior aspect of the knee.

The quadriceps fat pad, also known as the *anterior suprapatellar fat pad*, lies superior to the suprapatellar pole between the distal quadriceps tendon anteriorly and the suprapatellar recess posteriorly.[39] Just deep (posterior) to the suprapatellar recess and the suprapatellar bursa is the prefemoral fat pad, which is anterior to the femoral shaft and superior trochlear groove.[40]

Fat Pads of the Patellofemoral Joint

- Infrapatellar (Hoffa's) fat pad
- Quadriceps (anterior suprapatellar) fat pad
- Prefemoral fat pad

The fat pads of the knee house neurovascular projections. The infrapatellar fat pad is highly vascularized and highly innervated. Terminal extensions of the inferior genicular arteries anastomose in the infrapatellar fat pad, richly supplying it and its synovial coverings.[37] Substance P immunoreactive pain fibers are widespread and equally distributed throughout the fat pad, retinaculum, and synovium.[38]

Several functions have been proposed for the fat pads, including secretion of synovial fluid, occupation of dead space, and joint stability. Current research concludes that the infrapatellar fat pad appears to play a role in biomechanical support and neurovascular supply to the adjacent structures.[34]

Functions of Fat Pads

- Synovial fluid secretion
- Occupiers of dead space
- Joint stability
- Neurovascular supply

Soft Tissue Stabilizers

Because the patellofemoral joint lacks a tightly closed capsule, external assistance is required to achieve patellar stability within the trochlear groove; this assistance is provided by soft tissue stabilizers. In general, the soft tissue stabilizers of the patellofemoral joint can be described as passive stabilizers or active stabilizers.

Passive Stabilizers

Passive stabilizing structures include the patellar tendon inferiorly and the medial and lateral retinaculum (Figure 18-4). The patellar tendon functions to transmit the forces generated by quadriceps contraction to the tibia. This structure typically is oriented slightly lateral with respect to the long axis of the tibia, thereby creating a slight lateral pull on the patella.[30]

Passive Patellar Stabilizers

- Patellar tendon
- Medial retinaculum
- Lateral retinaculum

A normal patellar retinaculum consists of layered, fibrous connective tissue that traverses the medial and lateral margins of the patella with attachments to the femur, tibia, patella, and patellar ligament.[41] The superficial fibers of the retinaculum originate from the vastus lateralis and vastus medialis fascia, linking the quadriceps to the patella (Figure 18-5).[30,41] This linkage is responsible for the dynamic influence of the quadriceps on the patellofemoral joint during active knee motion.

The lateral retinaculum is composed of two distinct portions, a thinner superficial layer and a thicker deep layer. The deep layer is further divided into three fibrous components: the epicondylopatellar band (or lateral

Figure 18-4
Active and passive soft tissue stabilizers of the patella. (Redrawn from Fulkerson JP, Hungerford DS: *Disorders of the patellofemoral joint,* ed 2, Baltimore, 1990, Williams & Wilkins.)

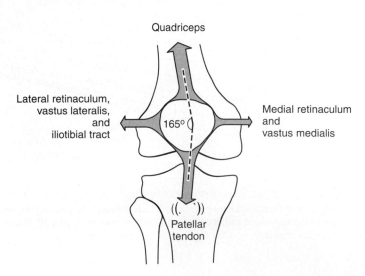

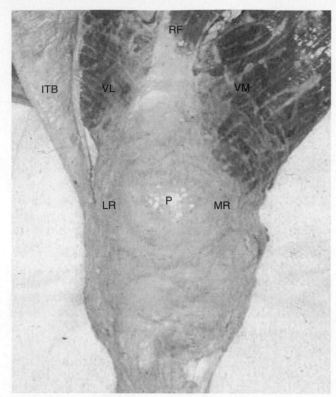

Figure 18-5

Cadaveric dissection showing interdigitation of the quadriceps musculature and iliotibial band with the peripatellar retinaculum. *VM,* Vastus medialis; *RF,* rectus femoris; *P,* patella; *VL,* vastus lateralis; *ITB,* iliotibial band; *LR,* lateral retinaculum; *MR,* medial retinaculum.

patellofemoral ligament), the deep transverse retinaculum, and the patellotibial band (Figure 18-6). These structures connect the patella to the iliotibial band (ITB) and help prevent medial patellar excursion.[42] Because most of the lateral retinaculum originates from the ITB, this structure is drawn posteriorly with knee flexion, placing a lateral force on the patella.[43]

The medial retinaculum forms a tough, fibrous layer that helps to limit lateral patellar excursion. The lateral retinaculum usually is thicker than the medial retinaculum and generally is accepted as providing stronger lateral support.[44]

The specific role of the peripatellar retinaculum as a frontal plane stabilizer of the patellofemoral joint has been well established.[45-48] However, because of its unique orientation, the peripatellar retinaculum plays a complementary load-sharing role with respect to the patellar ligament by resisting tensile forces created by the extensor mechanism.[45,49] Similar to the patellar ligament, the patellar retinaculum provides distal inferior support for the patella through the medial and lateral meniscopatellar ligaments, which connect the patella to the tibia.[46]

The lateral retinaculum contains small nerve endings, which suggests that this structure can be a source of symptoms.[30] In addition, Sanchis-Alfonso et al.[50] reported on the widespread presence of substance P in this area. Fulkerson et al.[51] found that nerve injury in the lateral retinaculum can be a source of pain and may be related to chronic tightness.

Active Stabilizers

Active stabilizers of the patella consist of the four heads of the quadriceps femoris muscle (the vastus lateralis, vastus medialis, vastus intermedius, and rectus femoris), which

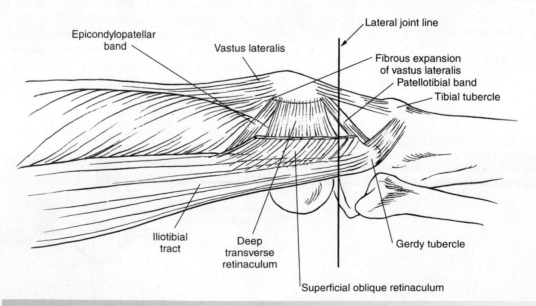

Figure 18-6

Anatomy of the lateral extensor mechanism and retinaculum showing the orientation of the elements that make up the superficial and deep layers. (Redrawn from Fulkerson JP, Gossling HR: Anatomy of the knee joint lateral retinaculum, *Clin Orthop* 153:183-188, 1990.)

Active Patellar Stabilizers

- Vastus lateralis
- Vastus intermedius
- Vastus medialis
- Rectus femoris

fuse distally to form the quadriceps tendon. These muscles, which can be identified at their insertion into the patella, provide dynamic control of the patellofemoral joint.

The rectus femoris (RF) inserts into the anterior portion of the superior aspect of the patella, with the superficial fibers continuing over the superior aspect of the patella and ending in the patellar tendon. The vastus intermedius (VI) inserts posteriorly into the base of the patella but anterior to the joint capsule. Both the vastus lateralis (VL) and vastus medialis (VM) insert into their respective sides of the patella and reinforce the medial and lateral retinaculum.[52,53]

The lower fibers of the VM insert more distally on the patella and at a greater angle from the vertical compared to the VL. In a detailed anatomical analysis, Lieb and Perry[54] determined the angle of insertion of the various heads of the quadriceps muscle with respect to the vertical axis. The fiber alignment in the frontal plane was as follows: VL, 12° to 15° laterally; RF, 7° to 10° medially; and VM, upper fibers, 15° to 18° medially, lower fibers, 50° to 55° medially (Figure 18-7). The fibers of the VI were found to lie parallel to the shaft of the femur.

The distinct and abrupt change in the fiber orientation between the superior and inferior portions of the vastus medialis led Lieb and Perry[54] to consider each of these portions as a separate entity in their mechanical study. The lower fibers were designated the *vastus medialis oblique (VMO)* and the upper fibers the *vastus medialis longus (VML)*. The fiber orientation of the VMO makes this structure particularly effective in providing medial patellar stability.[54]

As a result of the posterior origin of the vasti (linea aspera), any quadriceps muscle contraction (regardless of knee flexion angle) results in compressive forces acting on the patellofemoral joint. Even when the knee is fully extended, substantial joint compression can occur. The posterior angulation of the vastus medialis and vastus lateralis fibers has been reported as approximately 55° from the vertical.[55]

In summary, the bony confines of the trochlea combined with the passive and active soft tissue stabilizers define the limit of patellar excursion and contribute significantly to stability of the patellofemoral joint. The balance between medial and lateral stability is essential for maintaining appropriate alignment of the extensor mechanism and normal biomechanics of the patellofemoral joint.

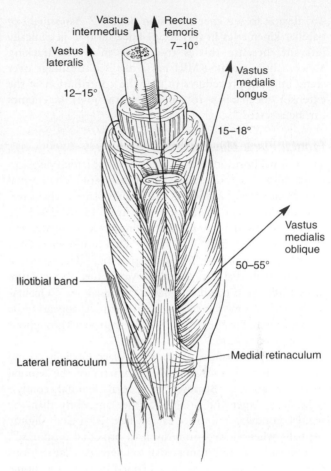

Figure 18-7

Components of the quadriceps-femoris complex. Note the angle of insertion of the various components of the complex. The orientation of the muscle fibers dictates the line of action and the pull on the patella. (Modified from McConnell J, Fulkerson J: The knee: patellofemoral and soft tissue injuries. In Zachazewski JE, Magee DJ, Quillen WS, editors: *Athletic injuries and rehabilitation*, p 697, Philadelphia, 1996, WB Saunders.)

Kinesiology

The complexity of the patellofemoral lies in its dynamic characteristics. Therefore clinicians must understand the normal patellofemoral joint motions before they can determine whether abnormal joint motion is present.

Normal Patellar Kinematics

Inability to visualize the relationship between the patella and the trochlear groove makes clinical assessment of patellar tracking an imprecise task. Also, identifying abnormal patellar motion is difficult if "normal" patellar tracking has not been clearly defined. Kinematic magnetic resonance imaging (KMRI) has been used to quantify patellar movement during resisted knee extension from

45° flexion to full knee extension (0°).[56,57] Assessment of patellar kinematics in this arc of knee motion is clinically relevant, because this is the range in which tracking abnormalities occur. KMRI has a distinct advantage over static imaging procedures in that the contribution of the extensor mechanism to patellofemoral joint kinematics can be assessed.[57]

Frontal Plane Movements

The normal position of the patella is slight lateral displacement throughout knee flexion and extension. The normal pattern of patellar motion in the frontal plane is characterized by slight medial displacement from 45° to 15° knee flexion, followed by slight lateral displacement at the end range of extension (15° to 0°).[58] This motion has been described previously as the C-curve pattern.[59] The estimated amount of medial and lateral movement is about 3 mm in each direction based on quantitative analysis.[58] Qualitatively, with this movement pattern, the patella appears to be evenly centered in the femoral trochlear groove throughout this range of motion.[58]

The tendency of the patella to displace medially during knee extension is related to the geometry of the femoral trochlear groove. Because the lateral femoral condyle typically is larger and projects farther anteriorly than the medial condyle, the trochlear surface is angled slightly medially when viewed from distal to proximal positions.[60] In addition, the shift from medial to lateral patellar motions starting at 18° flexion can be explained by the screw home mechanism of the knee. During terminal extension of the non-weight-bearing knee, the tibia rotates laterally as a result of the unequal curvature between the femoral condyles.[61] As was demonstrated by van Kampen and Huiskes,[60] patellar motion is highly influenced by rotation of the tibia, and lateral rotation induces a lateral patellar displacement.

Transverse Plane Movements

During knee extension from 45° to 0°, the patella tilts medially (5° to 7°) from a laterally tilted position of 10°.[58] As with medial and lateral patellar displacement, this motion pattern appears to be related to the geometry of the femoral trochlear groove.[58] Again, from a qualitative consideration, this movement pattern gives the patella the appearance of being evenly centered in the femoral trochlear groove throughout this range of motion.[58] The fact that the patella typically is lateral to the midline and laterally tilted throughout knee extension suggests that patellar malalignment is more a problem of degree rather than position.

Sagittal Plane Movements

The motions of the patella in the sagittal plane consist of flexion and extension. *Flexion* is defined as the motion in which the inferior pole of the patella moves posteriorly, whereas *extension* is defined as the motion in which the inferior pole moves anteriorly. Flexion of the patella occurs in conjunction with knee flexion; however, the magnitude of patellar flexion is about 20° less than that of knee flexion.[60] For example, when the knee is flexed to 60°, the patella typically is flexed to 40°. Similarly, as the knee extends, the patella also extends from the flexed position.[60]

Patellofemoral Joint Contact Area

During knee flexion, the patella moves from the superior (shallower) portion of the trochlear groove to the inferior (deeper) portion.[58] As such, the articulating surface of the patella on the femur varies throughout the range of knee motion. Movement from full extension to 90° flexion results in a band of contact that moves from the inferior to the superior pole of the patella (Figure 18-8).[62] Normally, the odd facet makes no contact during this range. Between 90° and 135°, the patella rotates laterally with

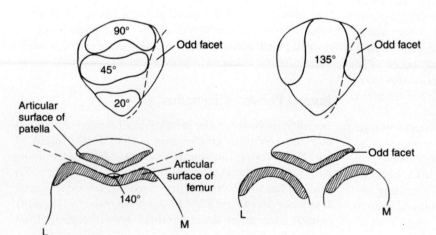

Figure 18-8

Contact area patterns on the patella as a function of the knee flexion angle. In general, contact area increases with increasing knee flexion. *L,* Lateral; *M,* medial. (From McConnell J, Fulkerson J: The knee: patellofemoral and soft tissue injuries. In Zachazewski JE, Magee DJ, Quillen WS, editors: *Athletic injuries and rehabilitation,* p 694, Philadelphia, 1996, WB Saunders.)

the ridge between the medial and odd facets, making contact with the medial condyle. At 135°, the odd facet and the lateral portion of the lateral facet make contact, as does the quadriceps tendon (see Figure 18-8).[62]

Because the patella enters the deeper portion of the trochlear groove during knee flexion, the area of contact between the patella and the trochlear groove increases. In fact, the patellofemoral contact area has been reported to increase threefold, from 0.8 cm² (0.12 in²) at 0° to a maximum of 2.4 cm² (0.4 in²) at 60°.[55] This increase in contact area with increased knee flexion functionally serves to distribute joint forces over a greater surface area, thereby minimizing joint stress.

Frontal Plane Influences

Fulkerson and Hungerford[30] described the natural tendency of the patella to track laterally as the "law of valgus." This tendency is a result of the valgus orientation of the lower extremity. As the quadriceps muscle follows the longitudinal axis of the femur, the quadriceps angle (Q angle) is formed, creating a lateral force vector that acts on the patella (Figure 18-9). This predisposes the patella to lateral tracking forces with quadriceps muscle tension.[63]

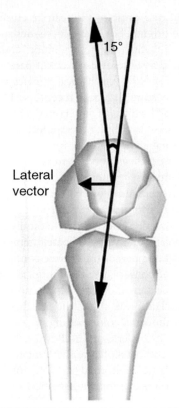

15°

Lateral
vector

Figure 18-9

The orientation of the quadriceps force vector and patellar ligament force vectors creates a lateral force acting on the patella. (From Powers CM: The influence of altered lower-extremity kinematics on patellofemoral joint dysfunction: a theoretical perspective, *J Orthop Sports Phys Ther* 33:639-646, 2003.)

Clinically, the Q angle is measured as the angle formed by the intersection of a line drawn from the anterosuperior iliac spine (ASIS) to the midpoint of the patella and a proximal extension of a line drawn from the tibial tubercle to the midpoint of the patella.[64] The Q angle is greater in women than in men because women have a wider pelvis; the average Q angle is 15° to 18° in women and approximately 12° in men.[31] This variation between the genders may partly explain the higher incidence of PFP in females, because a larger Q angle creates a larger valgus vector and therefore a potentially greater predisposition to lateral tracking.[65]

Joint Biomechanics

The patellofemoral joint is susceptible to the largest loads in the body.[66] Because abnormal forces and stresses are thought to be a primary factor in the origin of patellofemoral pain, it is important that clinicians understand the normal biomechanics of this joint.

Function of the Patella

The primary function of the patella is to facilitate knee extension.[61] This mechanical attribute has been described in detail and has been shown to increase the functional lever arm of the extensor mechanism.[67] Documentation of strength losses in subjects who have undergone patellectomy supports this concept. Fletcher et al.[68] reported a 49% reduction in the torque output of the extensor mechanism after patellectomy.

Functions of the Patella

- Improve the efficiency of the last 30° of extension
- Guide the quadriceps (patellar) tendon
- Reduce friction in the quadriceps mechanism
- Facilitate transmission of quadriceps forces
- Control (through the quadriceps) capsular tension in the knee
- Act as a bony shield
- Improve the esthetic appearance of the knee

The quadriceps muscle lever arm varies throughout the knee range of motion, with reported maximum values ranging from 4.9 cm (1.9 inches) at 30° flexion[69] to 7.8 cm (3.1 inches) at 15° flexion.[70] The effectiveness of the patella diminishes with full flexion because the patella sinks into the trochlear groove, reducing the anterior displacement of the quadriceps tendon. The extensor lever arm is only slightly reduced with full extension (4.4 cm [1.7 inches]).[69]

Apart from improving the moment arm of the quadriceps muscle, the patella provides protection for the articular cartilage of the trochlea and prevents excessive friction between the quadriceps tendon and the femoral condyles, permitting the patellofemoral joint to tolerate high compressive loads. The patella also acts as a guide for the converging heads of the quadriceps muscle, facilitating transmission of the muscular forces to the patellar tendon.[67]

Patellofemoral Joint Reaction Force

Because the quadriceps is the only muscle to cross the patellofemoral joint, the patellofemoral joint reaction force (PFJRF) is determined quasi-statically by the force and moment balance of the quadriceps force vector and the patellar ligament force vector.[71] Early biomechanical descriptions of the patellofemoral joint characterized this articulation as a frictionless pulley where the patellar ligament force (F_{PL}) was assumed to be equal to the force applied by quadriceps tendon (F_Q).[72,73] However, subsequent experimental studies and mathematical representations of the patellofemoral joint suggested that the patella also acts as a lever, thereby creating a force differential between the quadriceps tendon and the patellar ligament.[71,74] This force differential is thought to occur as a result of the varying geometry and shape of the distal femur and patella, as well as the changing point of contact between the patella and femur as the knee flexes and extends.

The PFJRF is the measurement of compression of the patella against the femur, and it depends on the angle of knee flexion, as well as muscle tension.[75] The resultant of the quadriceps muscle force vector and the patellar tendon force vector is equal and opposite to the PFJRF, which evokes compressive stresses on the patellofemoral articular cartilage (Figure 18-10).[76] Previous investigations have

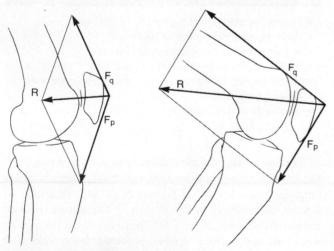

Figure 18-10

The patellofemoral joint reaction force increases as a function of quadriceps force and knee angle. F_q, Force of the quadriceps tendon; F_p, force of the patellar tendon; R, patellofemoral joint reaction force. (From McConnell J, Fulkerson J: The knee: patellofemoral and soft tissue injuries. In Zachazewski JE, Magee DJ, Quillen WS, editors: *Athletic injuries and rehabilitation,* p 700, Philadelphia, 1996, WB Saunders.)

indicated that the PFJRF for level walking is approximately 1 times body weight; it is 3.8 times body weight during stair ascent and descent[77-79] and can be as high as 7 to 11 times body weight during running.[80]

Patellofemoral Joint Stress

From a mechanical standpoint, patellofemoral joint stress (or pressure) is defined as the PFJRF divided by the patellofemoral joint contact area. A high patellofemoral joint reaction force is not necessarily harmful to the patellofemoral joint, because this force can be offset by a large contact area. However, a high joint reaction force combined with a small contact area may be detrimental.

Numerous studies have been done to measure stresses directly from cadaveric knees using pressure-sensitive film. In addition, patellofemoral joint stress has been estimated in vivo by dividing the estimated PFJRF by the patellofemoral joint contact area obtained from the literature or MRI. Heino-Brechter and Powers[78] reported that peak patellofemoral joint stress can vary from 2 megapascals (MPa) for level walking to 6 MPa for stair ambulation.

Pathomechanics

As mentioned, the cause of PFP can be elusive, and it may have multiple origins. For example, tissues such as the subchondral bone, synovium, retinaculum, and fat pad have been implicated as potential sources of patellofemoral joint symptoms.[81] Excessive mechanical stresses in these tissues are believed to stimulate pain receptors. Dye[81] proposed that differential loading of innervated tissue and the loss of tissue homeostasis may be responsible for the genesis of patellofemoral symptoms. In turn, restoration of tissue homeostasis (i.e., alleviation of stress in irritated tissue) is thought to reduce symptoms.

Heino-Brechter and Powers[78] provided evidence supporting the concept of differential loading as a factor in the development of pain. They found that individuals with PFP experience greater amounts of patellofemoral joint stress during walking compared to pain-free controls. Because the primary goal of conservative and surgical management of PFP is to reduce pain and improve function, it is important that the clinician understand the mechanisms that may contribute to abnormal joint loading.

As outlined by Fredericson and Powers,[82] factors that contribute to excessive patellofemoral stress can be broken down into three categories: abnormal patellofemoral joint mechanics; abnormal lower extremity kinematics, and overuse.

Abnormal Patellofemoral Joint Mechanics

The significance of a malaligned patella is related to the fact that, when the patella is not situated firmly in the trochlear groove, contact between the patellar and trochlear surfaces is diminished. For example, a laterally displaced or laterally tilted patella can cause increased lateral facet stress. Two of the more common patellofemoral joint conditions are excessive lateral pressure syndrome and patellar subluxation.

Excessive Lateral Pressure Syndrome

Ficat et al.[83] first described in detail the concept of excessive lateral pressure as a causative factor in patellofemoral articular cartilage pathology. These authors characterized excessive lateral pressure syndrome (ELPS) as a tilt or compression syndrome in which a laterally tilted patella increases the compression between the lateral facet and the lateral femoral condyle (Figure 18-11). This patellar posture also unloads the medial facet.

Tilting of the patella can be isolated, or it can be associated with lateral patellar subluxation.[84-86] Chronic lateral tilt is determined radiologically and has been shown to have a deleterious effect on the articular cartilage. Increased density of the subchondral bone underlying the lateral facet, combined with decreased density of the medial facet subchondral bone, is a sign of the pressure differences seen in this syndrome.[30]

Lateral facet overload and deficient medial facet contact can lead to articular cartilage degeneration at both sites. Abnormal articular cartilage loading of the lateral facet may cross the threshold of cartilage resistance, leading to failure.[30] The primary area of lateral facet degeneration corresponds to the areas of contact in the 40° to 80° knee flexion range.[87]

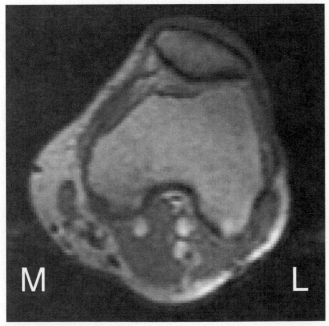

Figure 18-11
Axial MRI of the patellofemoral joint showing excessive lateral tilting of the patella, resulting in increased pressure between the lateral facet and the lateral femoral condyle. *M,* Medial; *L,* lateral.

The mechanism of medial facet articular cartilage damage in ELPS appears to be different from lateral facet degeneration, because this area is susceptible to deficient contact. This form of degeneration likely can be attributed to impaired nutrition, because diminished joint compression results in decreased flow of synovial fluid.[88] Seedholm et al.[87] have stated that areas of relative contact deficiency develop mild degenerative changes and are most probably asymptomatic. When combined with the shearing of the medial facet associated with lateral patellar subluxation, more extensive medial facet degeneration may occur.[30]

Etiology of Excessive Lateral Pressure Syndrome. The natural history of ELPS has been described as congenital tilting of the patella followed by adaptive shortening of the lateral retinaculum. Congenital anomalies cited as possible causes of ELPS include genu varum, femoral anteversion, and dysplasia of the hip.[30] The significance of a tight lateral retinaculum is the increased posterolateral pull on this structure with knee flexion. This, in turn, accentuates lateral facet compression. Insall[89] stated that adaptive shortening of the lateral retinaculum was more likely the result of habitual lateral patellar tracking, in which the VM became stretched and the VL contracted.

Disruption of the medial stabilizers (the VM and the medial retinaculum) also has been implicated as a possible cause of ELPS.[88] Ahmed et al.[90] conducted a mechanical study to measure the static pressure distribution on the retropatellar surface. The results from 24 cadaveric specimens showed that a release of VMO tension created a pressure shift that was transferred almost entirely to the lateral facet of the patella. In addition, the change in the orientation of the pressure zone suggested a considerable frontal plane rotation of the patella relative to the femur.

Some evidence supports both theories, that the shortened retinaculum and the insufficient dynamic medial stabilizers contribute to ELPS. Fulkerson et al.[91] demonstrated the effectiveness of surgical release of the lateral retinaculum in reducing lateral patellar tilt. Based on preoperative and postoperative computed tomography (CT) evaluation, these authors reported a mean tilt improvement of 6° at 10° knee flexion and 15° at 20° knee flexion. These improvements brought the tilt angles of these subjects well within the normal range as demonstrated in the control group.

Douchette and Goble[92] demonstrated the importance of quadriceps muscle weakness and tightness of the lateral structures as contributors to ELPS. They found a decrease in patellar tilt in patients who participated in an 8-week program of quadriceps muscle strengthening and ITB stretching. In addition, 84% of the previously symptomatic patients were pain free after this program.

Patellar Subluxation

Patellar subluxation is abnormal medial or lateral movement of the patella. Abnormal patellar tracking, such that transient medial or lateral displacement occurs during flexion and extension, has been documented as a cause of articular cartilage damage and pain.[93,94] Subluxation of the patella is differentiated from patellar instability or dislocation in that the patella stays in the trochlear groove rather than leaving it (dislocation).

In general, subluxation typically involves increased lateral displacement of the patella;[30] however, medial displacement also can occur.[95] This excessive motion results in a feeling of instability and discomfort.[96] Fulkerson and Hungerford[30] described three types of subluxation: minor recurrent subluxation, major recurrent subluxation, and permanent lateral subluxation. In minor recurrent subluxation, the patella deviates little from its normal course; this type of subluxation is not associated with clinically apparent relocation. In major recurrent subluxation, the patella comes across the lateral trochlear facet and returns to the trochlear groove with an audible snap. Permanent lateral subluxation is a stable lateral displacement in which there was no centering of the patella.

Etiology of Lateral Patellar Subluxation. As mentioned previously, both static and dynamic structures provide resistance to the inherent lateral tracking forces. Disruption of the normal equilibrium of forces may lead to patellar malalignment and associated pathology of the patellofemoral joint. To understand the etiology of a patient's PFP and to formulate an effective treatment program, the clinician must understand the specific mechanism or mechanisms involved in each patient.

Bony Abnormalities. Anatomical variations of the patella or distal femur (or both) can contribute to potential recurrent subluxation.[29,97] Patellar or trochlear dysplasia compromises the inherent stability afforded by the bony structure, making the patella more susceptible to laterally directed forces. Wiberg[29] proposed a system for classifying patella shapes based on axial view radiographs:

- *Type I:* Both facets are slightly concave and symmetrical, and the medial and lateral facets are equal in size (Figure 18-12).
- *Type II:* The medial facet is distinctly smaller than the lateral facet. The lateral facet is concave, whereas the

medial facet is more flat (see Figure 18-12). Wiberg found this to be the most common patellar shape.
- *Type III:* The medial facet is slightly convex and considerably smaller, with marked lateral facet predominance (see Figure 18-12). Wiberg considered this shape a frank dysplastic form.

Apart from the shape of the patella, its position with respect to the trochlear groove can be a potential causative factor in lateral subluxation. Patella alta, as described by Insall,[63] is evident when the resting position of the patella is above the femoral groove (Figure 18-13). The high-riding patella does not sink adequately into the trochlear groove with knee flexion and therefore is prone to lateral displacement.[98] In addition, individuals with patella alta are predisposed to elevated joint stresses, because the contact area is minimal, particularly when the knee is extended.[98] Patella alta is detected with lateral radiographs, and a positive sign is a patellar tendon that is 20% longer than the patella. The excessive length of the patellar tendon is thought to be the primary cause of this condition.[99]

Another bony etiological factor in patellar subluxation is femoral trochlear dysplasia. The trochlear groove of the femur, especially the larger anterior protrusion of the lateral femoral condyle, provides significant bony stability for the patella.[100] The normal trochlear facet (sulcus) angle was established by Brattstrom[101] using a sophisticated radiological technique. Evaluation of 100 normal knees showed that the values for the two genders were similar, with a mean angle of 143° for males and 142° for females. Higher sulcus angles represented a shallower trochlear groove and were associated with recurrent patellar subluxation.[101,102] According to Hvid et al.,[103] a sulcus angle greater than 150° indicates trochlear dysplasia. Using dynamic MRI techniques, Powers[85] reported a strong correlation ($r = 0.76$) between lateral patellar displacement and the depth of the trochlear groove at 0° knee flexion. This suggests that trochlear dysplasia is one of the more important etiological factors contributing to recurrent patellar subluxation.

Abnormal Skeletal Alignment. Abnormal skeletal alignments have been shown to have a profound effect on the magnitude of the Q angle and the subsequent laterally directed component of the quadriceps muscle force.[94,104] Huberti and Hayes[104] documented the deleterious effects of an increased Q angle by measuring patellofemoral contact pressures in 12 fresh cadaver specimens. These authors found that a 10° increase in the Q angle resulted in a 45% increase in peak contact pressure at 20° knee flexion. In half of these specimens, the area of patellar contact shifted laterally, and the peak pressures were evident on the medial portion of the lateral facet.

An increased Q angle often is present with rotational malalignments of the femur and tibia. Such abnormalities include excessive femoral anteversion, lateral tibial torsion and/or lateral displacement of the tibial tubercle, and genu valgum.[1,10,94]

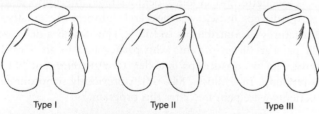

Type I   Type II   Type III

Figure 18-12
Classification of patellar shapes based on axial view radiographs. (From McConnell J, Fulkerson J: The knee: patellofemoral and soft tissue injuries. In Zachazewski JE, Magee DJ, Quillen WS, editors: *Athletic injuries and rehabilitation*, p 694, Philadelphia, 1996, WB Saunders.)

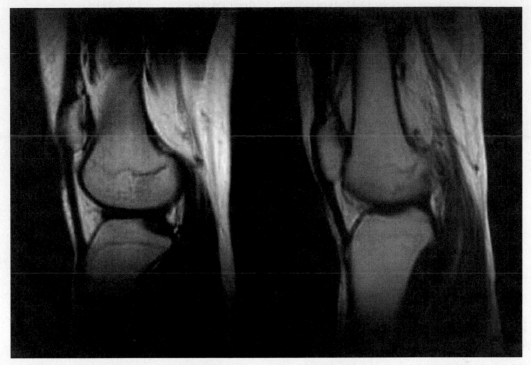

Figure 18-13
Sagittal MRI of the knee obtained at 0° showing patella alta *(left)* and the normal vertical position of the patella *(right)*.

• *Excessive femoral anteversion.* In the transverse plane, the neck of the femur forms an angle of about 15° with the transverse axis of the femoral condyles (Figure 18-14). This places the femoral head anterior to the femoral

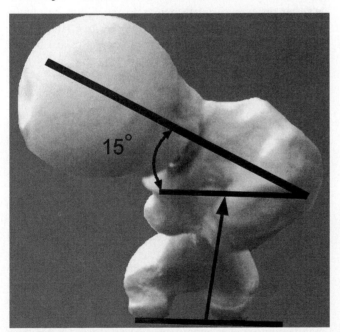

Figure 18-14
Femoral anteversion is measured by comparing the femoral neck and posterior condylar axes in the transverse plane. Normal anteversion is approximately 15°.

condyles. An increase in this angle, or *excessive femoral anteversion,* is associated with medial femoral rotation (Figure 18-15).[31,105-108] Excessive femoral anteversion and subsequent medial femoral rotation cause the trochlear surface of the femur to be placed medially with respect to the tibial tubercle, functionally increasing the Q angle.[10] Clinically, this is manifested by a toed-in gait and the appearance of "squinting patellae."[1,105] Lateral tibial torsion can compensate for this deformity by straightening out the long axis of the leg; however, this also displaces the tibial tubercle more laterally, resulting in an even larger Q angle.[65] Fulkerson and Hungerford[30] have stated that isolated excessive femoral anteversion rarely results in patellar problems; however, femoral anteversion combined with compensatory tibial torsion increases the risk of lateral patellar displacement.

• *Lateral tibial torsion and/or lateral displacement of the tibial tubercle.* A laterally displaced tibial tuberosity with respect to the midline of the tibia and the ASIS acts to increase the Q angle.[10] This anatomical variation typically is the result of increased lateral tibial torsion.[30] Lateral tibial torsion in subjects with PFP has not been clearly delineated and documented, which raises questions as to its clinical importance.

Trillat et al.[21] and Hauser[17] discussed the importance of the laterally displaced tibial tuberosity as a contributing factor in patellar malalignment. These authors described surgical procedures to correct this deformity,

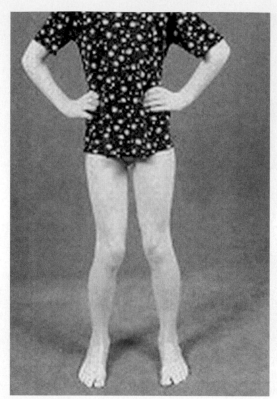

Figure 18-15
Excessive femoral anteversion is associated with increased femoral internal rotation. Note that this posture increases the quadriceps angle (Q angle).

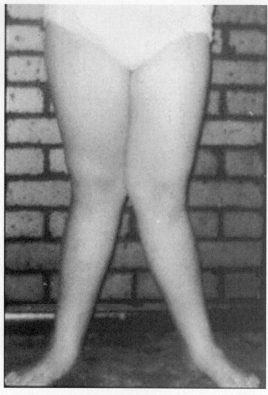

Figure 18-16
Increased angulation of the femur and tibia in the frontal plane is described as genu valgum. Note that this posture increases the Q angle.

involving transfer of the tibial tuberosity medially to reduce the valgus forces created by an excessive Q angle. Hehne[44] studied the effects of this surgery in cadaver specimens and reported that medial transfer of the tibial tuberosity resulted in a significant decrease in the total patellar contact area, especially the contact area of the lateral facet. This reduction in contact area caused a 25% increase in the average patellofemoral joint stress both medially and laterally, leading the authors to dispute the effectiveness of this procedure.

• *Genu valgum.* Increased valgus angulation of the femur and tibia in the frontal plane is called *genu valgum* and is thought to be the result of a tight ITB or excessive femoral anteversion.[31] Genu valgum also is postulated to increase the valgus force vector of the quadriceps muscle (Figure 18-16);[10,109] however, this bony orientation is not consistently present in patients with PFP.

Soft Tissue Influences. Both contractile and noncontractile soft tissue structures can contribute to the lateral forces acting on the patella. Although these effects may be present in conjunction with the abnormalities already described, their potential influence on lateral patellar tracking must be assessed if an effective treatment is to be formulated.

Passive Structures. As mentioned previously, the lateral retinaculum has been implicated as a cause of ELPS and is capable of exerting a lateral force on the patella, potentially contributing to subluxation. Because the lateral retinaculum has an extensive attachment to the ITB, contraction of the tensor fascia lata may exert a dynamic lateral force through this connection.[100] In some cases this attachment has been found to be excessive, causing recurrent dislocation of the patella.[110] Puniello[43] demonstrated a strong relationship between ITB tightness and decreased passive medial patellar glide in a group of 17 subjects with patellofemoral dysfunction. Hughston and Deese[111] found a high incidence (50%) of medial patellar subluxation after lateral retinacular release, which indicates that this structure also plays a role in pulling the patella laterally. These studies support the concept that a functional anatomical relationship exists between the patella and the passive lateral structures of the knee.

Dynamic Structures. A force imbalance between the VM and the VL is widely accepted as a principal cause of patellar subluxation.[31,52,112-114] As such, clinical emphasis has been placed on the dynamic factors associated with patellar instability (i.e., VM weakness). The VM has been identified as the primary structure capable of counteracting the VL in maintaining patellar alignment. VM insufficiency has been associated with muscle atrophy,[100,115] hypoplasia,[100] inhibition caused by pain and effusion,[116,117] and impaired motor control.[118]

According to Fox,[100] hypoplasia of the extensor mechanism is found to a varying degree in 40% of the population. This hypoplasia manifests as incomplete development of the VM, because it is the last of the quadriceps muscle to develop phylogenetically.[100] The effect of an underdeveloped VM is a patellar alignment that is influenced by an overpowering VL; more specifically, the patella is situated more laterally and proximally. The more hypoplastic the VM, the more lateral the position of the patella. In addition, the superior and lateral pull of the patella can cause the development of patella alta. This hypoplasia also has been theorized to influence the development of the tibia, because the unchecked pull of the VL can result in lateral tibial rotation, lateral placement of the tibial tubercle, and genu recurvatum.[100]

Fox[100] theorized that the VM is the weakest muscle phylogenetically and therefore the first component of the quadriceps muscle to atrophy after injury or disuse. Fox considered the potential muscular imbalance between the medial and lateral dynamic stabilizers as a result of this atrophy or weakness to be the major predisposing factor for "hypermobile patella syndromes." Atrophy of the VM was observed by Smillie,[119] who stated that the apparent wasting of the vastus medialis was associated with the inability to complete terminal knee extension. To the contrary, Lieb and Perry[54] stated that apparent atrophy of the VM was the result of a thinner fascial covering (half the thickness) compared to the VL, which made atrophy of the VL less perceptible.

Atrophy of the quadriceps muscle group is thought to be caused by reflex inhibition,[116] with the stimulus being pain[120] or effusion.[121] Inhibition is the result of afferent stimuli from receptors in or around the injured knee that prevent activation of the α-motor neurons in the anterior horn of the spinal cord.[122] Spencer et al.[116] reported that infusion of only 20 to 30 mL of saline into the knee joint exceeded the threshold for quadriceps muscle inhibition, in contrast to other authors, who have proposed much larger volumes (e.g., 100 mL).[121] In an attempt to determine whether selective inhibition of the different heads of the quadriceps muscle was possible, Spencer et al.[116] examined Hoffman's reflex in the individual muscles after intra-articular infusion of saline into the knee. Although the VM appeared to be affected more by small amounts of induced effusion, no statistically significant differences were seen. This finding supported previous work that showed that reflex inhibition caused by effusion affects the entire extensor mechanism and does not predispose the patellofemoral joint to an imbalance of dynamic forces.

Bennett and Stauber[118] proposed a neural component of VM insufficiency, hypothesizing that underdevelopment of this muscle may result from a deficiency in motor control. These authors observed an eccentric muscle contraction deficit with isokinetic testing that demonstrated a rapid reversal with training. The quick return to normal eccentric strength combined with a rapid decrease in symptoms led these researchers to conclude that these subjects had an error in the appropriate use of the VM. Exactly how the training of the quadriceps muscle relieved pain was not presented in this study.

It is apparent from the literature that a host of factors has been postulated to contribute to lateral patellar tracking. Although many theories have been presented, further research is necessary to substantiate these claims.

Do patients with PFP have VMO insufficiency? Documenting imbalances between the VM and the VL in patients with PFP has been of primary interest to the practicing clinician, because conservative treatment of this disorder typically focuses on restoring normal function of the dynamic stabilizers.[9,10] This functional imbalance is widely accepted as a cause of PFP.[123] Despite the interest in the function of the quadriceps femoris in patients with PFP, evidence supporting the concept of vasti muscle imbalance as a cause of lateral patellar subluxation is limited.

Because in vivo strength assessment of the individual vastus muscle is not possible, electromyography (EMG) has been used to compare the relative recruitment of these muscles, under the rationale that decreased activity or impaired timing of the VM relative to the VL may indicate compromised medial patellar stability. Many investigators have studied the EMG activity of the dynamic patellar stabilizers in individuals with PFP; however, the results of these studies are equivocal. Some studies have found significant differences in VM and VL activity in patients with PFP,[124-126] whereas others have not.[127-130] Similarly, some authors have reported that the onset of VL activity precedes that of VM activity in persons with PFP;[131,132] however, vasti timing differences have not been reported in all studies.[133] Direct comparisons of these studies are difficult because of differences in experimental technique, methods of quantifying EMG, and the inherent variability associated with such data.

Another reason for the inconsistent results in these investigations may be the inherent variability among patients with PFP. Because the etiology of PFP has been considered a dynamic entity, a deficiency of the medial stabilizers logically should result in lateral displacement of the patella. However, radiological examinations have documented that fewer than 50% of patients with PFP show isolated lateral subluxation.[83,134] This suggests that lateral patellar tracking is not a universal finding in this disorder, and therefore such an inference cannot be generalized to all patients.

Etiology of Medial Patellar Subluxation. Medial subluxation of the patella is less commonly seen than lateral patellar subluxation. The cause of lateral patellar subluxation is related more to anatomical and soft tissue abnormalities, whereas the etiology of medial subluxation is almost always iatrogenic.[95,111] This condition most commonly is caused by excessive medialization of the extensor mechanism in realignment surgery or by lateral retinacular release in which little or no patellar lateralization was done preoperatively.[30]

Abnormal Lower Extremity Kinematics

Researchers recently have recognized that the patellofemoral joint can be influenced by the segmental interactions of the lower extremity.[135] Abnormal motions of the tibia and femur in the transverse and frontal planes can have a substantial effect on patellofemoral joint mechanics and therefore PFP. An understanding of how the lower kinetic chain can influence the patellofemoral joint is important, because interventions to control abnormal lower extremity mechanics are not focused on the area of pain, but rather on the joints proximal and distal to the patellofemoral joint (i.e., the hip and/or foot and ankle). As noted previously, structural deformities can lead to an increase in the Q angle and the lateral forces acting on the patella; however, abnormal motions of the lower extremity also can be contributing factors.[135] Three principal lower limb motions can influence the *dynamic* Q angle: tibial rotation, femoral rotation, and knee valgus.

Tibial Rotation

The Q angle can be influenced distally through motions of the tibia. Lateral rotation of the tibia moves the tibial tuberosity laterally, thereby increasing the Q angle, whereas tibial medial rotation decreases the Q angle by moving the tibial tuberosity medially (Figure 18-17, *A*). In turn, tibial rotation is influenced by subtalar joint motion. Subtalar joint pronation causes medial rotation of the tibia, and supination causes the tibia to rotate laterally. Normal

subtalar joint pronation occurs during the first 30% of the gait cycle, during which the tibia rotates medially 6° to 10°.[136] This motion occurs in response to the medial rotation of the talus as it falls into the space created by the inferior and lateral movement of the anterior portion of the calcaneus.

As a result of this close biomechanical relationship between the rearfoot and the tibia, abnormal pronation has been linked to several lower extremity conditions, including patellofemoral joint dysfunction. Typically, pronation is considered abnormal if the amount of motion is excessive or occurs at the wrong time (i.e., when the foot should be supinating). When excessive pronation is related to various clinical entities, an assumption is made that abnormal pronation results in excessive tibial medial rotation and that this motion places a rotatory strain on soft tissues of the lower extremity. Although this may be the case with respect to the tibiofemoral joint, the same assumption does not hold true for the vertically aligned patellofemoral joint. In fact, excessive tibial medial rotation caused by subtalar joint pronation would actually *decrease* the Q angle and the lateral forces acting on the patella (see Figure 18-17, *A*).

This discrepancy was noted by Tiberio,[137] who described a scenario in which excessive pronation could affect normal patellofemoral joint function. Tiberio postulated that to achieve knee extension in midstance, the tibia must rotate laterally relative to the femur to ensure adequate motion for the screw home mechanism. To compensate for this lack of tibial lateral rotation because of the failure of the foot to resupinate, the femur would have to rotate medially on the tibia such that the tibia was in

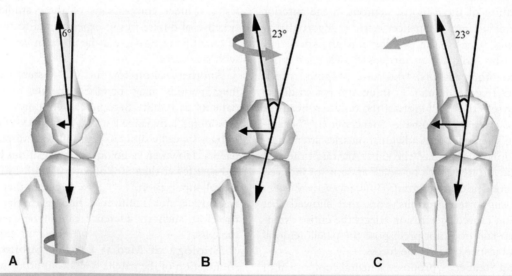

Figure 18-17
Schematic of the influence of femoral and tibial motion on the Q angle. **A,** Tibial internal rotation results in a decrease in the dynamic Q angle. **B,** Femoral internal rotation increases the dynamic Q angle. **C,** Femoral adduction and/or tibial abduction results in knee valgus and an increase in the dynamic Q angle. (From Powers CM: The influence of altered lower-extremity kinematics on patellofemoral joint dysfunction: a theoretical perspective, *J Orthop Sports Phys Ther* 33:639-646, 2003.)

relative lateral rotation. This compensatory medial rotation of the femur would permit the necessary screw home mechanics to allow for knee extension. However, excessive medial rotation of the femur would move the patella medially with respect to the ASIS, thereby increasing the Q angle and the lateral component of the quadriceps muscle vector (Figure 18-17, *B*). This would appear to be a plausible biomechanical means by which pronation could influence the patellofemoral joint; however, to do so, such motion ultimately would have to influence the femur.

An assumption made in the scenario just described is that if excessive pronation is evident in midstance, then excessive medial rotation of the tibia also should be evident. However, a recent study by Reischl et al.[136] reported that the magnitude of foot pronation did not predict the magnitude of tibial or femoral rotation. Also, the magnitude of tibial rotation did not predict the magnitude of femoral rotation, which indicates that excessive rotation of the tibia did not translate into excessive femoral rotation. This is not surprising, considering that the knee has the potential to absorb rotatory forces through its transverse plane motion. It should be noted that all subjects in this study demonstrated pronation and tibial medial rotation during early stance. However, this motion was not a 1:1 ratio. Individual factors, such as the orientation of the subtalar joint axis and the amount of transverse plane motion between the rearfoot and the lower leg, likely influence the degree to which pronation can influence the magnitude of tibial rotation.

Femoral Rotation

The Q angle can be influenced proximally through motions of the femur. As described previously, increased femoral medial rotation results in a larger Q angle, because the patella is moved medially with respect to the ASIS (see Figure 18-17, *B*). Consequently, femoral lateral rotation minimizes the Q angle, because the resultant line of action of the extensor mechanism is more in line with the ASIS.

Apart from increasing the Q angle and the laterally directed forces on the patella, femoral medial rotation can influence patellar alignment and tracking. Because the patella is tethered in the quadriceps tendon, it is not obligated to follow the motions of the femur (i.e., trochlear groove), especially when the quadriceps muscles are contracted. In fact, during weight-bearing activities, medial rotation of the femur can occur independent of patellar motion, thereby bringing the lateral anterior femoral condyle in close approximation to the lateral facet of the patella. Using dynamic MRI methods under weight-bearing conditions (a single-leg partial squat), Powers et al.[138] demonstrated that the primary contributor to lateral patellar tilt in a group of individuals with patellar instability was femoral motion (medial rotation), not patellar motion (Figure 18-18). This finding calls into question the long-held assumption that subluxation is the result of the patella

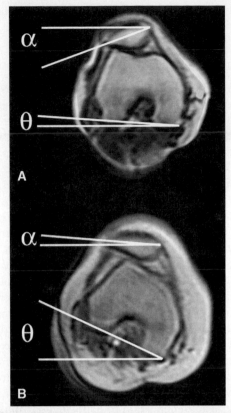

Figure 18-18

Influence of femoral rotation on lateral patellar tilt at 0° knee flexion. During the non-weight-bearing condition **(A)**, lateral patellar tilt was the result of patellar rotation (α) on a relatively horizontal femur (θ). During the weight-bearing condition **(B)**, lateral patellar tilt was a result of internal rotation of the femur (θ) under a relatively horizontal patella (α). (From Powers CM, Ward SR, Fredericson M et al: Patellofemoral kinematics during weight-bearing and non-weight-bearing knee extension in persons with lateral subluxation of the patella: a preliminary study, *J Orthop Sports Phys Ther* 33:677-685, 2003.)

moving on the femur. Although this may be the case during non-weight-bearing activities in which the femur is fixed (i.e., during knee extension in sitting), this study provides evidence that lateral subluxation of the patella during weight-bearing activities may be the result of the femur rotating underneath the patella.

As described previously, excessive medial rotation of the femur during midstance may be a compensatory mechanism to ensure normal knee screw home mechanics in the presence of abnormal pronation and excessive tibial medial rotation. However, motion of the femur also can be influenced proximally. The hip joint offers a great deal of mobility and depends on adequate muscular control for stability. Clinically, weakness of the hip lateral rotators (i.e., gluteus maximus and deep rotators) can result in a "rolling in" of the thigh during early stance and may have a deleterious effect on the patellofemoral joint. In addition, as described previously, excessive femoral anteversion biases the lower extremity into medial rotation and can result in the clinical appearance of "squinting patellae," a toed-in gait, or both.[1,105]

Knee Valgus

Apart from abnormal motions in the transverse plane, excessive frontal plane motions can influence the patellofemoral joint. Most notably, valgus at the knee increases the Q angle, because the patella is displaced medially with respect to the ASIS (Figure 18-17, C). In comparison, a varus position of the knee decreases the Q angle, because the patella is brought more in line with the ASIS.

Knee valgus can be the result of thigh adduction, tibial abduction, or a combination of these two (see Figure 18-17, C). Excessive femoral adduction during dynamic tasks can be the result of weakness of the hip adductors, particularly the gluteus medius. The upper fibers of the gluteus maximus and the tensor fascia lata also assist in abduction at the hip and, if weak, may contribute to excessive thigh adduction.[139] Structural abnormalities of the femur (i.e., excessive anteversion and coxa valga) can reduce the moment arm of the gluteus medius, which may result in a functional weakness. Tibial abduction can be the result of excessive pronation or frontal plane motion at the ankle. However, it should be noted that tibial abduction also could be an accommodation to femoral adduction, because the proximal tibia is obligated to follow the distal femur. Ireland et al.[140] provided evidence supporting the premise that proximal hip weakness may contribute to altered lower extremity motions in individuals with PFP. They reported that these individuals had 26% less hip abductor strength and 36% less hip external rotator strength than pain-free controls.

Overuse

Because only 50% of patients with PFP have tracking abnormalities, other factors must be involved. If patellofemoral joint function and gait mechanics are normal, patellofemoral joint pathology may be related to excessive activity levels, or overuse. For example, the peak PFJRF during weight acceptance has been calculated as 7 to 11 times body weight for healthy runners, a value estimated to be near the physiological limit of involved tissues.[80] Therefore, for a given knee flexion angle, high forces result in elevated patellofemoral joint stress and may be problematic because of the repetitive nature of such activity. This concept is supported by the work of Thomee et al.,[141] who studied 40 women with PFP and concluded that chronic overloading and temporary overuse were the primary causes of symptoms.

Overuse injuries are a function of the magnitude of the applied force and the number of cycles the load is applied. For example, as the load increases, the number of repetitions necessary to cause injury decreases. Conversely, as the load decreases, the number of repetitions necessary to cause injury increases. Activities commonly associated with overuse histories include long distance running and cycling.[142]

Summary

Figure 18-19 summarizes the potential factors that may lead to patellofemoral joint dysfunction and pain. To treat PFP effectively, the clinician must address the root causes of the pain and dysfunction. Therefore the goal of the examination is to identify the likely cause or causes of symptoms so that the most effective interventions can be applied.

Examination

The goal of the examination is to obtain pertinent data to allow the formulation of a hypothesis about the cause of the symptoms. The examination should include both subjective and objective physical components.

Subjective Examination

The subjective examination is essential for making an accurate diagnosis. When taking a patient's history, the clinician should determine what problems are important and what types of examinations may be useful. Key information to obtain includes the patient's current complaints, symptoms, and the mechanism of injury.

Patients typically report pain as diffuse and arising from the anterior aspect of the knee.[140] However, sharp, "stabbing" symptoms can be elicited with provocative testing. Pain often is induced by activity and aggravated with functions that increase patellofemoral compressive forces, such as ascending and descending stairs, inclined walking, squatting, and prolonged sitting.[1,90] The sensation of "giving way" also may be reported and should be differentiated from tibiofemoral joint instability (i.e., ligament tear) or quadriceps muscle inhibition.

Pain along the medial and lateral borders of the patella is a common complaint, and retropatellar and inferior pain often is reported. Patients frequently report crepitus with knee flexion, but this should not by itself cause concern, because asymptomatic patellofemoral crepitus is very common.[143] Painful crepitus may be related to tightness of the deep retinacular tissues, plicae, or patellofemoral joint instability; it is not necessarily suggestive of arthritic changes.

According to Grelsamer and McConnell,[22] the location of symptoms may indicate the specific structures involved and provide direction with respect to a differential diagnosis:

- *Lateral:* Small nerve injury of the lateral retinaculum
- *Medial:* Recurrent stretching of the medial retinaculum/medial patellofemoral ligament

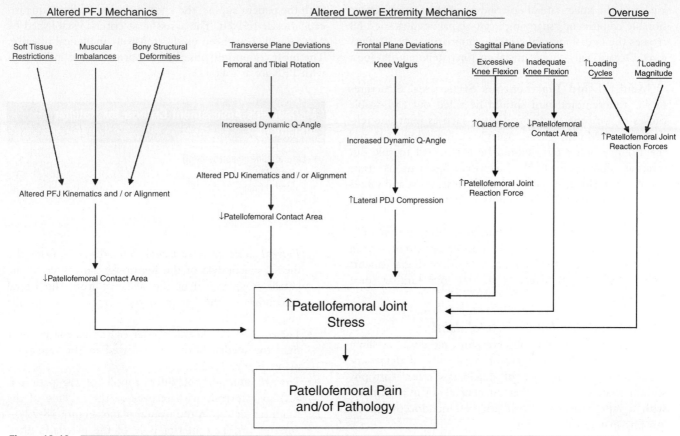

Figure 18-19

Flow diagram of potential mechanisms of patellofemoral pain and/or pathology.

- *Retropatellar:* Articular cartilage damage; stress borne on subchondral bone
- *Superior:* Quadriceps tendonitis/tendinosis
- *Inferior:* Patellar tendonitis/tendinosis; fat pad irritation

Throughout the history process, it is important to ascertain whether the patient's disability is related to pain or instability. Generally speaking, the onset of PFP is insidious and progression is slow. A specific episode or event is not always reported. However, the clinician should pay careful attention to the patient's perceived cause of the injury, making note of changes in lifestyle, activity levels and, with athletes, training habits. A slow onset of symptoms may indicate an underlying biomechanical error or structural faults that manifest themselves over time. A rapid onset of symptoms may be associated with overuse and may or may not have an underlying biomechanical cause.

Histories related to traumatic injury (i.e., direct falls on the patella) or instability related to pain are fairly obvious and self-explanatory. However, biomechanical abnormalities or structural faults may have been present before the injury (e.g., pronation, excessive femoral anteversion), and these factors may be responsible for the perpetuation of symptoms.

Physical Examination

The physical examination should include (1) testing procedures necessary to make a differential diagnosis; (2) evaluation of the patellofemoral joint, including alignment, mobility, and dynamic motion; and (3) assessment of lower extremity alignment and function.

Differential Diagnosis

To diagnose PFP accurately, the clinician must rule out other structures as potential sources of anterior knee pain symptoms.

Patellar Tendonitis/Tendinosis. The symptoms of patellar tendonitis/tendinosis can be very similar to those of PFP, because pain is often induced by activity, especially during high speed eccentric contractions of the quadriceps muscle. A clear distinction can be made between tendonitis/tendinosis and PFP through careful palpation. Local tenderness to the quadriceps tendon (superior to the patella) and patellar tendon (inferior to the patella) indicates tendonitis/tendinosis and should not be confused with retropatellar pain or medial or lateral patellar pain.

Iliotibial Band Friction Syndrome. ITB friction syndrome is characterized by localized pain in the lateral aspect of the knee (lateral epicondyle of the femur). Occasionally crepitus or "snapping" can be palpated as the ITB crosses the lateral femoral condyle (approximately 30° flexion). Occasionally this is mistaken for patellofemoral joint crepitus.

Meniscal and Ligamentous Structures. Structures of the tibiofemoral joint should be ruled out as possible causes of symptoms. Meniscal tests, such as joint line tenderness, McMurray's test, Apley's compression test, and the Bounce home test, should be performed to rule out internal derangement.[144] Likewise, ligamentous tests should be performed (i.e., Lachman's test, varus and valgus stress tests), especially in patients with traumatic histories and/or acute swelling.

Referred Pain. Referred pain from compression and/or irritation of the L3 or L4 nerve roots can manifest itself as vague pain along the lateral border of the thigh. Patients should be carefully screened to rule out lumbar spine pathology.

Evaluation of the Patellofemoral Joint

The examiner should observe for redness, swelling, warmth, dystrophic changes, or obvious joint deformity. In addition, the presence of quadriceps muscle atrophy should be determined (either qualitatively or quantitatively with a tape measure). With athletes, quadriceps muscle atrophy may not be present.

Selective atrophy of the VMO in relation to the rest of the vasti has never been documented in patients with PFP, and evidence suggests that atrophy of the quadriceps muscle affects all of the vasti equally.[145] Because the VMO is the most visible of the vasti (as a result of its superficial fibers and thin retinacular covering), atrophy is more apparent in this muscle. Atrophy of the VL is much more difficult to visualize, because most of its fibers are deep and wrap around to the posterior femur; for this reason, the clinician must be cautious about attributing PFP symptoms solely to VMO atrophy.

Tests for Effusion. Because quadriceps muscle inhibition is associated with slight swelling, general observations about effusion should be made (e.g., joint warmth, redness). Typically, PFP of a nontraumatic nature is associated with only mild effusion. Severe effusion likely indicates a more serious ligamentous injury. Major effusion can be assessed by compressing the patella into the trochlea. A positive ballotable patella sign is seen when the patella quickly "rebounds" or "floats" when compressed into the trochlea.[144]

Minimal joint effusion can be assessed with the knee extended by "milking" fluid from the suprapatellar pouch and the lateral side of the knee into the medial side of the knee. A small bulge medially is a positive sign of mild swelling.[144]

Patellar Alignment. The patella should be assessed for gross alignment abnormalities. Typically this is done

with the patient supine, the knee extended, and the quadriceps muscle relaxed. The assessment criteria established by McConnell[7] have been used extensively in clinical practice. The most commonly observed abnormalities in individuals with PFP are as follows:

McConnell's Assessment Criteria for Patellar Alignment

- Lateral glide (displacement)
- Lateral tilt
- Lateral rotation
- Inferior tilt

- *Lateral glide (displacement).* The distance from the medial epicondyle of the femur to the center of the patella is greater than the distance from the lateral epicondyle of the femur to the center of the patella (Figure 18-20).
- *Lateral tilt.* The lateral border of the patella is lower than the medial border (as viewed in the transverse plane; Figure 18-21).
- *Lateral rotation.* The inferior pole of the patella is rotated externally with respect to the midline of the thigh (as viewed in the frontal plane; Figure 18-22).
- *Inferior tilt.* The inferior pole of the patella is tilted posteriorly compared to the superior pole (sagittal plane; Figure 18-23).

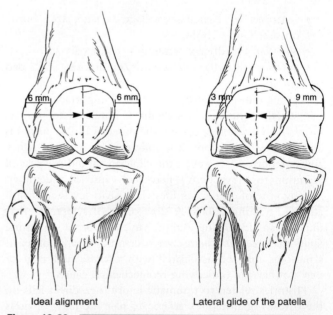

Ideal alignment   Lateral glide of the patella

Figure 18-20

Assessment of the glide component. Ideally the patella should be centered on the superior portion of the femoral articular surface. (From McConnell J, Fulkerson J: The knee: patellofemoral and soft tissue injuries. In Zachazewski JE, Magee DJ, Quillen WS, editors: *Athletic injuries and rehabilitation,* p 711, Philadelphia, 1996, WB Saunders.)

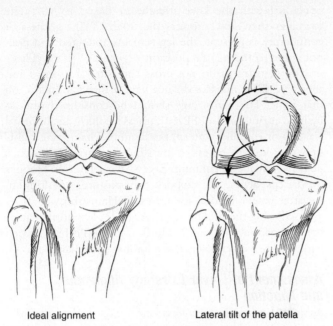

Ideal alignment   Lateral tilt of the patella

Figure 18-21
Assessment of the tilt component. Ideally the patella should be parallel to the frontal plane of the knee. (From McConnell J, Fulkerson J: The knee: patellofemoral and soft tissue injuries. In Zachazewski JE, Magee DJ, Quillen WS, editors: *Athletic injuries and rehabilitation*, p 712, Philadelphia, 1996, WB Saunders.)

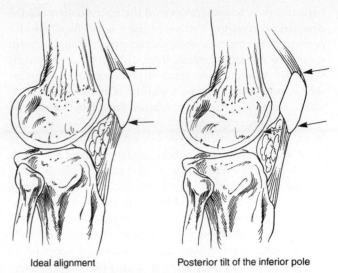

Ideal alignment   Posterior tilt of the inferior pole

Figure 18-23
Assessment of the flexion component. Ideally the superior and inferior poles of the patella should be in line with the long axis of the femur. Excessive inferior tilt of the patella may irritate the infrapatellar fat pad. (From McConnell J, Fulkerson J: The knee: patellofemoral and soft tissue injuries. In Zachazewski JE, Magee DJ, Quillen WS, editors: *Athletic injuries and rehabilitation*, p 712, Philadelphia, 1996, WB Saunders.)

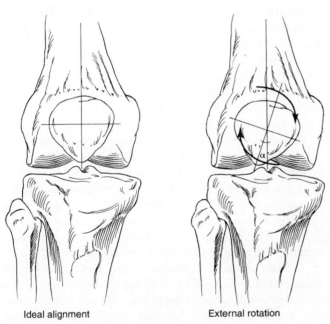

Ideal alignment   External rotation

Figure 18-22
Assessment of the rotation component. Ideally the superior and inferior poles of the patella should be in line with the long axis of the femur. (From McConnell J, Fulkerson J: The knee: patellofemoral and soft tissue injuries. In Zachazewski JE, Magee DJ, Quillen WS, editors: *Athletic injuries and rehabilitation*, p 712, Philadelphia, 1996, WB Saunders.)

Although this classification system is widely used, both the validity and reliability of these techniques in assessing patellar alignment have been challenged.[146,147] Care must be taken in the interpretation of the results of patellar alignment testing, especially because the resting position of the patella tends to be one of slight lateral displacement and lateral tilt. Only obvious abnormalities should be considered relevant.

Passive Patellar Mobility. In addition to static alignment, passive patellar mobility should be evaluated. Because motion of the patella is necessary for normal joint function, assessment of patellar mobility is an important component of the examination. The patella should be able to freely glide superiorly and inferiorly, as well as medially and laterally. Also, the clinician should be able to tilt the patella medially to raise the lateral border. Quite often patellar mobility is restricted after prolonged immobilization or surgery. Tightness of the lateral retinaculum is the most common limiting factor and manifests as decreased medial patellar glide and inability to tilt the patella medially. As the patella moves inferiorly and superiorly and the knee flexes and extends, adequate motion is essential to ensure normal knee motion.

When assessing passive patellar mobility, the clinician also should note excessive translations and/or apprehension to such movements. Excessive lateral translation of the patella may indicate tearing of the medial patellofemoral ligament. Patient apprehension to a lateral glide of the patella suggests recurrent patellar dislocation

Patellar Tracking. Active patellar tracking is best observed with the patient in the sitting position. The patient should be asked to extend the knee slowly while the clinician observes the motion of the patella. As mentioned previously, normal motion is characterized by slight medial motion as the knee extends from 45° to 18°, followed by slight lateral motion in terminal knee extension. Patellar subluxation typically occurs during terminal knee extension, therefore particular attention should be focused on this part of the range. As with static patellar alignment, only large deviations should be considered significant. Clinicians must keep in mind that subtle subluxations are very difficult to pick up, because a large "grey zone" exists between normal and abnormal.

The clinician also should be aware of any painful arc of motion and should note the range in which pain is reproduced. Pain typically is more evident during the last 20°, because greater quadriceps muscle forces are necessary to complete terminal knee extension, and the patellofemoral joint contact area decreases (resulting in elevated patellofemoral joint stress).

As the knee is extending, the examiner should make a qualitative assessment of the state of quadriceps muscle contraction. Does the knee appear to have difficulty completing terminal extension (which suggests quadriceps muscle weakness), or is muscle "quivering" present (suggestive of reflex inhibition)?

Quadriceps Muscle Weakness. General quadriceps muscle weakness or atrophy (or both) is a hallmark of PFP. However, ascertaining whether true weakness is present is difficult, because pain commonly is reproduced with quadriceps muscle contraction and the patient may be hesitant to give a maximum effort, thereby invalidating results.

Tests for Soft Tissue and Muscle Tightness. Tightness of various soft tissues and muscles that cross the knee can have an adverse effect on patellofemoral joint function. In particular, tightness of the rectus femoris, tensor fascia lata/iliotibial band complex, and the hamstrings should be addressed.

Tightness of the rectus femoris can result in excessive patellofemoral joint compression, especially when the knee is flexed and the hip is extended. This posture is particularly evident during the swing phase of the running cycle. The length of the rectus femoris is best assessed using Thomas's test.[148] With the patient supine, both knees are brought to the chest to flatten the lumbar lordosis. The leg being tested then is allowed to extend such that it comes to rest on the table in a neutral position. If the knee cannot flex to 90° with the hip in a neutral position, the rectus femoris is considered tight.

As noted previously, the interdigitation of the ITB and the lateral retinaculum suggests that tightness of this structure may produce a lateral force on the patella, potentially contributing to lateral subluxation and ELPS. Ober's test assesses for tightness of the ITB and tensor fascia lata. For this test, the patient is placed in the side lying position. The examiner passively abducts and extends the patient's

upper leg with the knee straight or flexed to 90°. The examiner then slowly lowers the thigh.[148] If tightness or contracture is present, the leg remains abducted and does not come to the neutral position.

The hamstrings do not cross the patellofemoral joint, therefore these muscles do not have a direct influence on that joint. The hamstrings should be considered only as being contributory to PFP if tightness results in an abnormal walking or running pattern. For example, hamstring tightness may lead to excessive knee flexion during the stance phase of walking or running. Excessive knee flexion requires quadriceps action to support this posture, resulting in elevated patellofemoral joint forces. Hamstring length is assessed using the straight leg raise test.[148] For normal hamstring function, 70° to 80° hip flexion should be achieved with the knee extended and the lumbar spine flattened.

Assessment of Lower Extremity Alignment and Function

As noted previously, recent evidence suggests that patellofemoral pain and dysfunction may be related to abnormal lower extremity mechanics. For this reason, careful assessment of lower extremity alignment and dynamic function is an important aspect of the physical examination.

Standing Posture. The patient should be observed during relaxed standing. The examiner also should observe the alignment of the knee in the sagittal and frontal planes, as well as the transverse plane alignment of the lower extremity.

Sagittal Plane Alignment of the Knee. The knee should be evaluated for hyperextension or excessive knee flexion. Knee hyperextension (genu recurvatum) may result in compression of the inferior pole of the patella into the infrapatellar fat pad. A hyperextended knee also may indicate quadriceps muscle weakness or inhibition, because the patient may rely on the posterior capsule for stability rather than active quadriceps muscle contraction.

Excessive knee flexion (i.e., inability to extend the knee fully) requires greater amounts of quadriceps contraction to maintain this posture. In turn, the quadriceps contraction increases the compressive forces acting on the patellofemoral joint. Excessive knee flexion may be related to loss of terminal knee extension after surgery (particularly anterior cruciate ligament [ACL] reconstruction), hamstring tightness, hip flexion contracture, or a weak calf.[139]

Frontal Plane Alignment of the Knee. Some have suggested that valgus and varus alignment of the knee is related to the structure of the proximal femur. For example, the normal inclination between the femoral neck and the femoral shaft is 125°.[149] A reduction of this angle (i.e., coxa vara) results in a valgus orientation of the knee. An increase in the angle of inclination results in a varus orientation of the knee. Knee valgus tends to increase the Q angle and the lateral forces acting on the patella, whereas knee varus has the opposite effect. However, coxa valga reduces the lever arm of the gluteus medius, thereby reducing the torque-producing capacity of this muscle.[150]

Transverse Plane Alignment of the Lower Extremity. Medial rotation of the femur (medial femoral torsion) results in "squinting patellae," whereas lateral rotation of the femur (lateral femoral torsion) results in the patella pointing outward (i.e., "grasshopper eyes"). (NOTE: Torsion implies actual anatomical rotation of the femur, not the physiological movement of the femur.) Femoral medial rotation may indicate excessive femoral anteversion or femoral torsion, whereas femoral lateral rotation may suggest femoral retroversion or lateral femoral torsion. Careful attention must be paid to whether foot pronation is evident, and whether the entire lower extremity is in a posture of medial rotation or whether the medially rotated position of the femur appears to be an isolated entity.

Dynamic Function. Perhaps one of the most important aspects of the examination is observation of dynamic movement. This should include analysis of level walking, as well as higher demand activities, such as running, ascending and descending stairs, squatting, and jumping. Careful attention should be paid so as to identify movement patterns that increase quadriceps demand and/or increase the dynamic Q angle. Observations also should be made with respect to the speed of ambulation, the force of impact during loading response, and any reproduction of symptoms. Components of the dynamic evaluation should be used to confirm or refute suspected abnormalities based on static testing procedures. Movements should be observed from both the frontal and sagittal views.

Sagittal View. The primary deviations for which the examiner should watch in the sagittal plane are inadequate knee flexion or hyperextension during weight acceptance and excessive knee flexion during stance. Decreased knee flexion during weight acceptance and knee hyperextension during the stance phase may indicate a quadriceps avoidance gait pattern caused by weakness or pain. The functional significance of inadequate knee flexion during weight acceptance is that shock absorption is impaired, and the tibiofemoral joint may be susceptible to excessive impulse loading. In addition, decreased knee flexion reduces the contact area between the patella and femur and therefore may contribute to elevated joint stress.

Excessive knee flexion increases patellofemoral joint reaction forces, because the quadriceps are overly active to support the flexed knee posture. As noted previously, causes of excessive knee flexion include knee flexion contracture, hamstring tightness or spasticity, hip flexion contracture, and weak calf muscles.[139]

Frontal View. In the frontal view, rotation and valgus of the lower extremity are particularly important. An attempt should be made to evaluate for the following abnormalities:

1. Does the patient pronate excessively? If so, does this result in excessive medial rotation of the tibia and femur?
2. Does the patient show excessive medial rotation of the femur? If so, does this medial rotation tend to be present throughout the gait cycle (suggesting a fixed, bony deformity, such as excessive femoral anteversion) or does the patient "collapse" into medial rotation during weight acceptance? The latter is more indicative of poor muscular control or weakness of the hip lateral rotators (Figure 18-24).

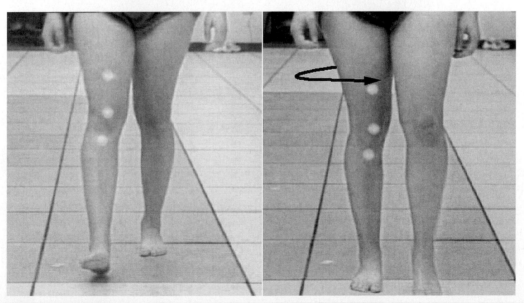

Figure 18-24
Frontal plane observational gait analysis of an individual with patellofemoral pain. Note the collapse into femoral internal rotation in midstance. Markers placed on the distal thigh, patella, and tibial tuberosity aid visualization of segment motions.

3. Does the patient show excessive adduction of the femur and/or a contralateral pelvic drop? This indicates poor muscular control of the hip abductors.

In many instances, frontal and transverse plane abnormalities are not readily evident during walking; therefore higher demand or functional activities specific to the patient need to be assessed. The repetitive step-down test is useful in this respect. The patient stands on a 0.2 m (8-inch) step and then lowers himself or herself with the painful leg and touches the heel to the floor (Figure 18-25). This is repeated 10 times without stopping.

In general, an attempt should be made to determine whether frontal and transverse plane deviations are occurring from the foot upward or from the pelvis downward. If the primary cause of the abnormality is identified, the correct treatment can be applied (i.e., proximal control through the hip versus distal control through the foot).

Additional Tests. Depending on the findings of the assessment of lower extremity alignment and dynamic function, the clinician may require additional information to formulate a hypothesis about the cause of the posture or motion abnormalities. The following tests may be useful:

- *Manual muscle test of the hip lateral rotators and hip extensors.* If excessive dynamic medial rotation and/or adduction of the femur is observed during the dynamic assessment and muscle weakness is suspected, manual muscle testing of the hip abductors, lateral rotators, and extensors is warranted.

- *Assessment of hip range of motion.* Hip range of motion should be evaluated because restricted lateral rotation range of motion can bias a patient into a medial rotation position. Tightness of the hip flexors also can create an medial rotation bias. Hip flexor tightness can be assessed using Thomas's test, as described previously.

- *Craig's test of femoral anteversion.* Excessive femoral anteversion can result in medial rotation of the femur and can have a significant influence on the patellofemoral joint. Craig's test is performed with the patient prone and the knee flexed to 90°. The examiner palpates the posterior aspect of the greater trochanter of the femur, and the hip then is passively rotated medially and laterally until the greater trochanter reaches its most lateral position (Figure 18-26). The degrees of anteversion can be estimated based on the angle of the lower leg with the vertical. Normal femoral anteversion is 15°.

- *Foot evaluation.* If subtalar joint pronation is identified as a potential contributor to faulty lower extremity mechanics, the foot should be examined closely for fixed, bony deformities (i.e., rearfoot varus, forefoot varus), muscle tightness (i.e., gastrocnemius and soleus), and weakness of dynamic stabilizers (i.e., tibialis posterior and peroneals).

Diagnostic Imaging

Different diagnostic imaging procedures have been suggested to further aid the diagnosis and management of patellofemoral pain. However, the wide variability in the

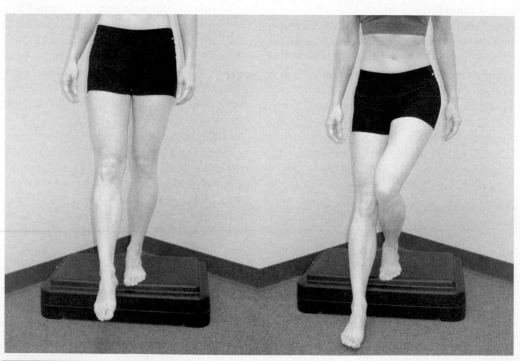

Figure 18-25

Assessment of lower extremity dynamic control. The patient slowly lowers herself with the extremity of interest and touches the heel to the floor without transferring weight to the descending limb. This patient shows medial collapse of the knee (excessive femoral adduction and internal rotation).

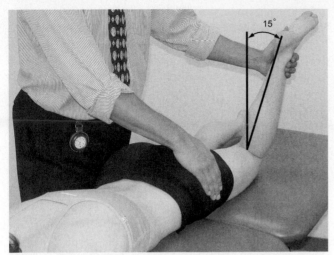

Figure 18-26

Craig's test of femoral anteversion. The examiner palpates the greater trochanter of the femur and rotates the femur internally and externally until the greater trochanter is at its most laterally prominent position. The angle of anteversion is estimated by measuring the angle created by the tibial shaft and a vertical line. Normal femoral anteversion is approximately 15°.

radiographic findings of patients with patellofemoral dysfunction, as well as the difficulty involved in demonstrating radiographic abnormalities consistent with clinical findings, has contributed to confusion in the diagnosis and classification of patients with patellofemoral pain disorders.[85,151,152] Despite this, numerous authors have reported that malposition can be accurately and reliably evaluated radiographically using certain techniques.[85,153-157] One of the main disadvantages of radiographic examination is that the patient's knee usually is x-rayed when it is not weight bearing, with the quadriceps muscle relaxed; therefore the dynamic properties of patellar tracking are not considered.

Overall, few studies have used radiographic measurement of alignment as an evaluation for surgical or conservative treatment. Insall et al.[158] found that, after a proximal surgical realignment of the tibial tubercle, 52 of 57 subjects had congruence angles (i.e., a measure of patellar alignment in the trochlear groove) that were considered normal. Unfortunately, few preoperative measures were available for comparison. Möller et al.[159] investigated patellar alignment in three groups (normal subjects, recurrent subluxers, and those with anterior knee pain) by measuring the congruence angle with and without the quadriceps contracted, before and after 3 months of isometric quadriceps exercises. The congruence angle during a maximum quadriceps contraction became less positive for the recurrent subluxers after the exercise program. It did not change in the other groups. Fulkerson et al.[91] used computed tomography (CT) to assess patellofemoral alignment before and after surgical lateral release. The congruence angle and lateral patellofemoral angle were determined at 0°, 10°, 20°, and

30° preoperatively and postoperatively. The results demonstrated that lateral release significantly reduced abnormal patellar tilting. Reigler[160] had similar results in assessing the outcome of this surgery.

A study by Ingersoll and Knight[161] demonstrated that 3 weeks of biofeedback training to the VMO produced a significant decrease ($p < 0.05$) in the radiographic measurement of the congruence angle, but 3 weeks of general quadriceps strengthening had no effect on the congruence angle.

Roberts[162] investigated the effect of patellofemoral taping on lateral patellar displacement, the lateral patellofemoral angle, and the congruence angle. The subjects were radiographed in the standing position with the knee flexed to 30°. These researchers found that, even though the changes were small, the patellofemoral angle and lateral patellar displacement improved significantly with taping ($p = 0.0003$ and 0.0002, respectively). The changes in the congruence angle were not significant. Bockrath et al.[163] also found no significant change in the congruence angle with taping, but they found that patellar taping significantly reduced perceived pain levels during a 0.2-m (8-inch) stepdown test. They concluded that the reduction in pain was not associated with patellar position changes. McConnell[164] found that when subjects performed maximum isometric contractions between 20° and 70° while a lateral view of the patellofemoral joint was dynamically imaged with video fluoroscopy, a change occurred in the patellofemoral contact point (defined as the midpoint of the contact area) such that when the patella was taped, the contact area was more distal than when the patella was not taped. A corresponding increase in muscle torque was also found when the patella was taped. The reason for this has not yet been established, but pain relief may well account for the improved function.

Basic Radiographic Methods

The anteroposterior (AP) view is used to evaluate the patella for any fracture or bipartite configuration and for gross positional changes, such as dislocation or abnormalities of patellar height. Asymmetry of the femoral condyles may indicate abnormal femoral torsion or femoral neck anteversion.[151] A 30° knee flexion, weight-bearing, posteroanterior (PA) view is most important for evaluating joint space and assessing for evidence of osteoarthritis.

Radiographs for Patellofemoral Pain

- AP view in extension
- AP view in 30° flexion
- Lateral view in full extension
- Lateral view in 30° flexion
- Axial view in 45° flexion
- Tangential view

The lateral view in full extension and at 30° knee flexion is used to determine patellar height and the patella's relationship to the trochlea. At full extension the lateral view should show the distal articular surface of the patella just at the center of the trochlea.[165] Other authors have proposed reliable methods for assessment of patella alta and patella baja.[99,166]

The patellofemoral joint also is visualized on an axial or tangential view. The axial view describes the parallel relationship of the x-ray beam with respect to the axis of the anterior tibia, whereas the tangential view describes the perpendicular relationship of the x-ray beam to the joint surfaces.[154] Both of these methods provide cross sectional information about the relationship of the patella to the trochlear groove.[151] Overall, the most useful axial radiograph is the simple 30° or 45° knee flexion axial view. It is most important to ensure an accurate, reproducible 30° or 45° flexion. A wooden leg holder with pins at the desired flexion angle is helpful. The authors of this chapter recommend obtaining this view, in a standardized fashion, on all patients.

A variety of methods and techniques have been described since the first tangential view was developed by Settegast in 1921. A number of modifications have been proposed, mainly in the variation of the knee flexion angle and the angle of the x-ray beam. For reproducible tangential views, certain requirements must be met. The x-ray beam and x-ray plate must be perpendicular to prevent distortion.[154,167] Views with the knee flexed more than 45° are used[151,154,168] but are much less helpful. The position of potential maximum instability is 0° to 30°, but this position is technically difficult to capture on an axial radiograph.[169,170] For the most reliable and reproducible results, 45° seems to be the preferred position.[156] Some authors contend that tangential projections throughout the range (i.e., 30°, 60°, and 90°) are vital to the assessment of dynamic tracking of the patella.[169,170] However, in the authors' experience, this does not seem worthwhile.

Computed Tomography

CT offers the advantage of a specific, definable plane. In general, CT is best performed using a midpatellar transverse image, including the posterior condyles of the femur. This view enables the clinician to understand the relationship of the articulating midportion of the patella with its reciprocal portion of the trochlea at any degree of knee flexion. Midpatellar transverse images through the posterior condyles with the knee flexed at 0°, 15°, 30°, and 45° provide an excellent depiction of how the patella enters the trochlea during flexion (Figure 18-27). The images may be taken with the quadriceps contracted and with it relaxed. On CT, the patella should be centered in the trochlea by 15° knee flexion.

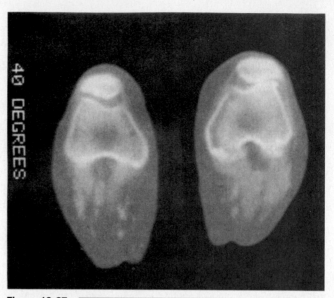

Figure 18-27

CT scan of lateral patellar tilt and displacement with the knee in 40° flexion. Precise midpatellar transverse CT images at 0°, 15°, 30°, and 45° knee flexion give an accurate impression of patellar alignment. (From McConnell J, Fulkerson J: The knee: patellofemoral and soft tissue injuries. In Zachazewski JE, Magee DJ, Quillen WS, editors: *Athletic injuries and rehabilitation,* p 709, Philadelphia, 1996, WB Saunders.)

Magnetic Resonance Imaging

Early magnetic resonance imaging (MRI) had limited value in the evaluation of patients with patellofemoral pain. The use of MRI was prohibitive, based on time and expense and on the quality and usefulness of the information obtained about patellar position and tracking. More recently, however, CT and MRI have been used to image the patellofemoral (PF) joint during active or dynamic flexion and extension activities.[57,134,171,172] Kinematic and conventional modes of MRI of the PF joint offer advantages over CT in that they do not require radiation, and they allow depiction of important passive and active soft issue stabilizers of the PF joint.[57,134,171] It has been suggested that dynamic or kinematic MRI, which allows assessment of the contribution of activated muscles and other soft tissue structures, is more sensitive than static imaging for demonstrating PF alignment and tracking abnormalities.[57,133,169] Statistically significant differences in patellar tracking patterns and imaging parameters (e.g., patellar tilt angle, bisect offset, lateral patellar displacement) between active and passive knee extension have been demonstrated by Brossmann et al.[171] To date, constraints have been encountered in the form of image acquisition time (i.e., 0.5 to 1 images/sec).[57,134,171] The use of echoplanar MRI in the future may dramatically reduce image acquisition time and greatly improve resolution, allowing images of moving or changing structures to be acquired at near real-time rates of 10 to 16 frames/sec.[173]

Bone Scan

A bone scan can reveal whether true intraosseous dysfunction is present and may localize the source of pain. A positive bone scan after knee trauma objectifies the problem. It may even demonstrate whether there is more activity proximally or distally in the patella and may reveal a problem in the trochlea or elsewhere. Dye et al.[174] have been particularly influential in emphasizing the dynamic function of bone in patellofemoral pain and the usefulness of following this with bone (radionuclide) scans.

Conservative (Nonoperative) Treatment

The treatment of PFP should be dictated by objective data obtained through a thorough examination. Treatment decisions also should be based on a solid scientific and biomechanical rationale. Once the examination has been completed, data should be compiled and a hypothesis formulated regarding the cause of the pain. The clinician should attempt to classify patients based on whether the suspected mechanism is a result of local PF joint dysfunction, lower quarter dysfunction, or overuse. Treatment decisions should focus on the identified impairments.

Treatment Classification for Patellofemoral Pain Based on Mechanism

- Local patellofemoral joint dysfunction
- Lower quarter dysfunction
- Overuse

Patellofemoral Joint Dysfunction

Specific treatment strategies for patellar malalignment and/or altered PF joint mechanics should be based on identified causes. As mentioned previously, possible contributing factors are bony and structural abnormalities, tightness of lateral structures, decreased patellar mobility, and quadriceps muscle weakness. From a rehabilitation standpoint, little can be done to correct bony deformities. Although the effects of the Q angle can be minimized through the interventions described below, conditions such as patella alta, trochlear dysplasia, femoral anteversion, and a laterally displaced tibial tuberosity are likely to require surgical intervention.

Tightness of Lateral Structures

If tightness of the lateral retinaculum is found to be contributing to ELPS or lateralization of the patella, treatment interventions should include soft tissue mobilization techniques (e.g., passive stretch, transverse frictions, deep tissue massage) to increase extensibility. Soft tissue techniques in the area of the ITB and its interdigitation with the lateral

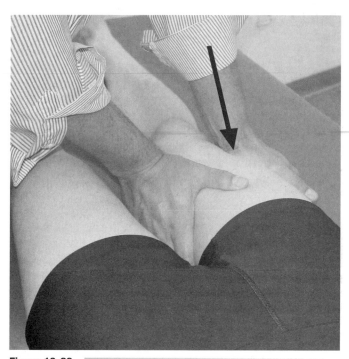

Figure 18-28
Soft tissue techniques in the area of the iliotibial band and its interdigitation with the lateral retinaculum may prove useful for increasing patellar mobility. The arrow indicates the line of force application.

retinaculum may prove useful (Figure 18-28). Because the ITB is a very dense, fibrous tissue, some question whether this structure can be stretched; however, longitudinal deep tissue massage may facilitate the breaking up of adhesions between the ITB and the overlying fascia.

Stretching of the tensor fascia lata also should be considered, because this muscle can influence the tension in the ITB (Figure 18-29). Also, patellar mobilization and patellar taping techniques (discussed in a later section) can be used for passive stretching of the lateral structures. Low level, prolonged passive stretching is preferred so as to take advantage of the creep effect of soft tissue.

Decreased Patellar Mobility

Patellar oscillatory mobilization techniques combined with passive stretching should be performed to improve patellar mobility superiorly and inferiorly, as well as medially and laterally (see Figure 18-29). If the patella lacks normal mobility, forces may be concentrated in localized areas. The most common reasons for reduced patellar mobility are prolonged immobilization, postoperative scarring, and quadriceps tightness.

When oscillatory mobilization techniques are performed, care should be taken to prevent excessive patellofemoral joint compression. To facilitate mobilization of the patella, the knee should be in extension or only slightly flexed (Figure 18-30). If the knee is flexed beyond 20°, the patella becomes seated within the trochlear groove,

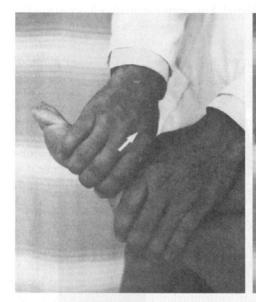
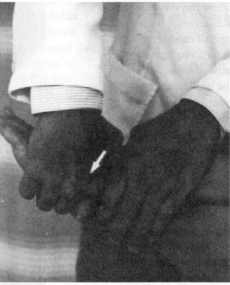

Figure 19-15
Calcaneocuboid mobilization. (From Donatelli RA, Wooden MJ: *Orthopedic physical therapy*, ed 3, p 542, New York, 2001, Churchill Livingstone.)

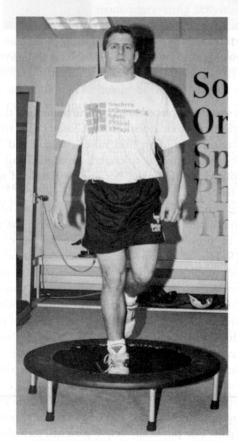

Figure 19-16
Balancing on one foot. (From Shankman GA: *Fundamental orthopedic management for the physical therapist assistant,* St. Louis, 2004, Mosby.)

performed safely and without pain, more ballistic activities can be added, such as jumping and landing from a height.

Patients who suffer mild or moderate ankle sprains often return to activity within a few weeks of injury, even though the clinician knows that the injured ligaments have not had adequate time to heal. This may be the reason recurrence rates are so high. However, conclusive evidence shows that supervised rehabilitation, carried out for at least 4 weeks after an ankle sprain, can reduce the risk of recurrence by more than 50%.[38]

If an ankle sprain does not appear to be improving within the normal time frame, consideration should be given to other pathology, which may require orthopedic referral. Such complications may include syndesmosis involvement, sinus tarsi syndrome, osteochondral fractures of the talus, and peroneal nerve palsy.

Ankle sprains that include tibiofibular syndesmosis damage are referred to as "high" ankle sprains. High ankle sprains must be treated much more conservatively than lateral ankle sprains so that the ligaments stabilizing the syndesmosis can heal; therefore the time frame for return to normal activities is much longer with this type of ankle sprain. These injuries should be immobilized for a minimum of 7 days after injury. If the ankle is not immobilized, the healing ligaments will be stressed repeatedly, because the talus will spread the syndesmosis apart each time the ankle is dorsiflexed. Commonly, the average time of return to high level functional activity after syndesmosis sprain is 6 weeks.[39]

Tarsal Tunnel Syndrome

Tarsal tunnel syndrome is a neuropathy of the tibial nerve where it passes from the leg to the foot at the level of the posterior medial malleolus. The nerve may be injured acutely in conjunction with a fracture of the medial malleolus, or the condition may be an overuse injury. In the latter case, hyperpronation is thought to cause traction to the tibial nerve. Symptoms typically include paresthesia on the medial aspect of the ankle extending into the plantar aspect of the foot and, in severe cases, atrophy of the intrinsic

Figure 19-17

Hopping patterns. (From Norris C: *Sports injuries: diagnosis and management*, ed 3, p 274, Oxford, 2004, Butterworth-Heinemann.)

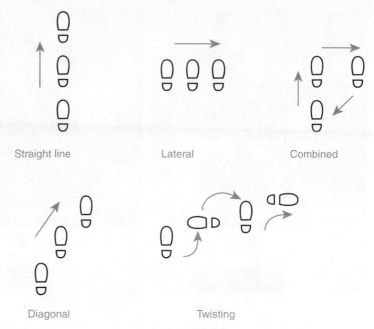

Straight line   Lateral   Combined

Diagonal   Twisting

muscles of the plantar aspect of the foot. Some cases of tarsal tunnel syndrome, including those that are sequelae of tibial fractures, must be treated surgically.

Conservative management of tarsal tunnel syndrome consists of anti-inflammatory medications, rest, ice, and correction of faulty foot mechanics. When hyperpronation is thought to be a contributing factor, the patient should be carefully evaluated for orthotic intervention. Strengthening should include exercises for the intrinsic muscles, especially those on the plantar aspect of the foot. These exercises include towel curls, marble pickups, and walking in sand. A weight-bearing exercise for the plantar intrinsics is the short foot exercise (Figure 19-18).[40] To perform this exercise, the patient keeps the heel and the metatarsal heads on the floor while contracting the muscles of the longitudinal arch in an effort to lift the arch off the floor. This exercise initially can be performed in a bilateral stance and progressed to a single-leg stance with added balance demands.

Plantar Fasciitis

Plantar fasciitis is an overuse injury of the plantar fascia that typically causes symptoms near its calcaneal origin. The plantar fascia normally stabilizes and locks the foot in supination before push-off. The plantar fascia is put under strain by the "windlass mechanism," which occurs during push-off when the metatarsophalangeal joints are hyperextended. It also is stressed by hyperpronation of the foot, as the medial longitudinal arch collapses. The condition is found in both rigid and hypermobile feet. Decreased flexibility in the gastrocnemius-soleus complex commonly is found if the condition is seen in the pes cavus foot. A periosteal reaction at its origin can result in hemorrhage and, ultimately, a heel spur. In many cases heel spurs are asymptomatic, but they are a sign of stress overload to the plantar fascia.

Biomechanical abnormalities of the foot may be significant contributing factors in the development of plantar fasciitis. Overpronation and the resulting stretch and wringing of the plantar fascia during the stance phase can lead to straining of these tissues. If tight posterior muscles limit dorsiflexion, they may force the foot into overpronation to achieve more range in dorsiflexion, which again increases stress on the plantar fascia.

Treatment of plantar fasciitis is aimed at reducing the inflammation and the tension on the plantar fascia, restoring tissue strength and mobility, and controlling any biomechanical abnormality. Inflammation can be controlled

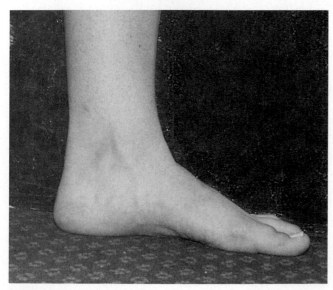

Figure 19-18

Short foot exercise.

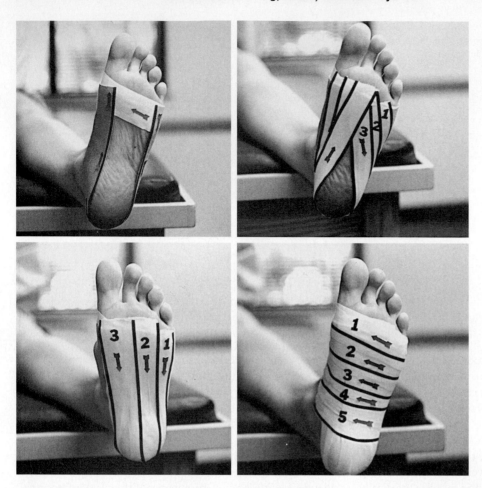

Figure 19-19
Low Dye taping. (From Nawoczenski
DA, Epler ME: *Orthotics in functional
rehabilitation of the lower limb,*
p 163-165, Philadelphia, 1997, WB
Saunders.)

with ice, anti-inflammatory medication and, in recalcitrant
cases, local corticosteroid injection.[41] A combination of
low-Dye arch taping (Figure 19-19) and/or off the shelf
orthotics can help hold the foot in a neutral position and
protect the plantar tissues from constant irritation during
the early stages of rehabilitation.

Gastrocnemius-soleus stretching is important to increase
dorsiflexion and to prevent the foot from going into
increased pronation to compensate for the lack of dorsiflexion in the ankle. Heel lifts, heel cups, low-Dye or modified
arch taping, massage of the plantar fascia, intrinsic foot exercises, and assessment for proper footwear all are important in
the management of plantar fasciitis. Assessment and mobilization of the joints of the ankle and foot also are important.
Of particular interest are the talocalcaneal joint, which often
needs to be mobilized into adduction, and the talonavicular
joint, which needs good translation of the navicular inferiorly on the talus. All other joints of the foot should be
assessed, and mobilization should be performed as needed.

If morning stiffness persists, a night splint to maintain dorsiflexion of the plantar fascia may be useful (Figure 19-20).
With the rare persistent case, surgical consultation is required.
Surgery involves release of the plantar fascia at its origin,
removal of heel spurs, and exploration for nerve entrapment
in scar tissue.

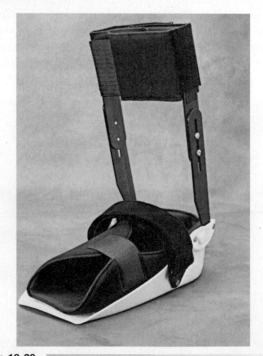

Figure 19-20
Night splint. (From Nawoczenski DA, Epler ME: *Orthotics in
functional rehabilitation of the lower limb,* p 109, Philadelphia, 1997,
WB Saunders.)

In some instances an acute sprain of the medial longitudinal arch may occur distal to the origin of the plantar fascia. The medial longitudinal arch is maintained by its bony arrangement, ligaments, and muscles and by the plantar fascia. The soft tissue may become overloaded during weight bearing, resulting in a sprain, often leading to the navicular bone being forced downward as a result of the weight of the body on the foot. This injury may lead to hyperpronation and lower extremity dysfunction. Clinicians should treat the symptoms and restore proper foot mechanics, which may involve intrinsic foot exercises, proper-fitting footwear, and orthotics.

Midfoot Sprains

Sprains to any of the numerous joints between the distal tarsal bones and the bases of the metatarsal heads can lead to considerable disability. Injuries to the first and second tarsometatarsal joints (Lisfranc's joint) can be particularly problematic. This injury often occurs with landing from a height or a jump, resulting in a sprain of the ligaments stabilizing the tarsometatarsal joints and a diastasis, or widening, of the bases of the first and second metatarsals. In severe cases, there may be accompanying fractures, and some cases may require surgical intervention.

Many cases are treated conservatively. Initial treatment must emphasize protection of the healing tissues. This early treatment often consists of immobilization in a walking boot (see Figure 19-4) for several weeks. After the boot is removed, an orthotic should still be used to provide mechanical stabilization to the midfoot. Rehabilitation should address plantar intrinsic muscle strength and should emphasize the restoration of normal gait mechanics.

Navicular Fractures

Fractures of the navicular bone can be very difficult to diagnose and treat. Injuries include complete fractures, stress fractures and, in skeletally immature patients, traction apophysitis. Fractures and stress fractures of the navicular are notorious for being nonunion fractures.[42] Prolonged immobilization (not modified rest) and bone stimulators often are needed to aid the healing of these fractures. Once the fracture has healed, rehabilitation should emphasize the restoration of ankle and foot ROM, strength, and endurance, as well as normal gait mechanics.

Physically active adolescents, particularly those with excessive foot pronation, can develop traction stress at the insertion of the tibialis posterior into the navicular. Many, in fact, have an accessory navicular bone that develops a traction irritation at the fibrous attachment to the main body of the navicular. This is most commonly seen in patients who participate in sports involving running, jumping, and change of direction. The differential diagnosis must always include a stress fracture, which can be determined by bone and computed tomography (CT) scans. Again, treatment is directed at inflammation and pronation control through the use of orthotics and appropriate shoes for motion control. Resistant cases of symptomatic accessory navicular irritation may require surgical resection with reattachment of the tibialis posterior tendon to the main body of the navicular.

Clinicians must be cautious of pain at the navicular bone in children 4 to 9 years of age. Kohler's disease is an avascular necrosis of the navicular that occurs in children, especially boys. Rest is the most important treatment for Kohler's disease, although a long leg cast sometimes is needed to accomplish this in an active child. This condition typically resolves on its own with no lasting effects.

Metatarsal Fractures

The most common fractures of the metatarsals involve the second or third metatarsal (march fracture) and the shaft of the fifth metatarsal just proximal to the styloid process (Jones's fracture).[43] Metatarsal stress fractures occur most often in the second and third metatarsals and are common in running and jumping sports. Common causative factors, as initially proposed by James et al.,[44] include training errors, changes in exposure to different surfaces, strength/flexibility dysfunction, poor shoes, and biomechanical variants, such as excessive rearfoot and forefoot varus. Crichton et al.[45] noted that the second metatarsal is the most prone to stress fracture because the base of the second metatarsal extends proximally into the distal row of tarsal bones and is held rigid and stable by the bony architecture and ligament support. In addition, if the second metatarsal is longer than the first, as is seen with the Morton-type foot, it theoretically is subject to greater bone stress. Also, in a hypermobile forefoot, the second and third metatarsals are subjected to more stress associated with excessive foot pronation.

These stress fractures do well when treated with modified rest and non-weight-bearing exercise (e.g., cycling, swimming, running in water) to maintain the patient's cardiovascular fitness for 4 to 6 weeks and with a graduated return to running and jumping activities with supportive footwear and orthotics.

A Jones fracture may be an acute fracture that occurs during sudden changes in direction, or it may be an overuse injury. Overuse injuries are especially common in individuals with rigid, pes cavus feet. Like navicular fractures, Jones fractures often result in nonunion and must be treated surgically.[46] Again, as with other overuse foot injuries, appropriate shoes that match the foot type, with adequate stability and shock absorption, are essential for returning the individual to high level functional activity. Attention must also be given to foot control through the use of orthotics. Rehabilitation should emphasize restoration of ankle and foot ROM, strength, and endurance, as well as normal gait mechanics.

Metatarsalgia

Metatarsalgia is a general term for forefoot pain in the area of the lesser metatarsal heads. However, this common term is nondescript and does not identify the specific source of pathology. Two common causes of metatarsalgia are transverse metatarsal arch sprains and Freiberg's infarction.

Transverse Metatarsal Arch Sprain

Transverse metatarsal arch sprains may be due to an acute or chronic mechanism of injury. The plantar ligaments supporting the arch are injured, allowing the adjacent metatarsal heads to excessively plantar flex. This can irritate the metatarsal heads and the subcutaneous tissues on the plantar aspect of the foot. A metatarsal bar made of felt placed just proximal to the metatarsal heads can be used to support the injured structures. Exercises emphasizing strength of the plantar intrinsic muscles should be performed as well.

Freiberg's Infarction

Freiberg's infarction is a painful avascular necrosis of the second or, rarely, the third metatarsal head. It typically is seen in adolescents or young adults who often are involved in running and jumping activities. Early radiographs may be normal, with later development of flattening of the involved metatarsal head. If the condition is caught early, deformity of the metatarsal head, which leads to early degenerative changes, can be prevented. Early treatment consists of exercise modification to eliminate excessive running and jumping plus orthotic foot support with a metatarsal pad or bar to unload the involved metatarsal head. A rocker bar on the shoe may also be required. If pain persists and deformity develops with degenerative osteophytes, surgical consultation is appropriate. Surgical management involves either a cheilectomy (cutting away of bony irregularities on the rim of the affected joint and capsular release) or, with more extensive damage, resection arthroplasty.

Morton's Neuroma

A Morton's neuroma, or interdigital neuritis, is an injury to one of the common digital nerves as it passes between the metatarsal heads. The classic location is between the third and fourth metatarsal heads, where the nerve is thickest, receiving both branches from the medial and lateral plantar nerves. The digital nerves enter the forefoot between the superficial and deep transverse metatarsal ligaments in the interdigital space. Nerve irritation can then occur, with compression between the metatarsal heads when shoes are worn. A fallen transverse metatarsal arch and/or excessive foot pronation can also be a predisposing factor, with more metatarsal shearing forces occurring with the prolonged forefoot abduction.[47]

The patient complains of a burning paresthesia in the forefoot, often localized to the third web space and radiating to the toes. The symptoms are increased with hyperextension of the toes on weight bearing, as in squatting, stair climbing, or running. The symptoms are worse in shoes with a narrow toe box and higher heels. With ongoing nerve irritation and surrounding fibrous reaction or neuroma formation, the pain can become constant. Treatment is aimed at reducing inflammation and unloading the interspace between the bones. Anti-inflammatory medications and modalities (e.g., ice, ultrasound, iontophoresis) can be used in an attempt to provide a local reduction in inflammation. Local corticosteroid injections may be curative, along with an orthotic to prevent excessive pronation and with a metatarsal pad to restore the transverse arch and separate the metatarsal heads.[48] Shoes with low heels and a wide toe box are essential. Failure of conservative management requires surgical excision of the neuroma, which is best done with a dorsal incision.

First Ray Injuries

Injuries to the first ray are particularly problematic because the center of force distribution goes through the first ray during the terminal parts of stance and push off in the gait cycle. Specific injuries include sesamoiditis, hallux valgus, hallux rigidus, and turf toe.

Sesamoiditis

Sesamoiditis involves trauma to the sesamoid bones in the tendons of the flexor hallucis brevis at its attachments to the base of the proximal phalanx of the hallux. This trauma can include a stress fracture, contusion, osteonecrosis, chondromalacia, or osteoarthritis of the sesamoid bones as they slide over and articulate with the head of the first metatarsal. Weight bearing on the toes increases the stress across the sesamoid bones. The patient complains of localized tenderness to the medial (tibial) or lateral (fibular) sesamoid, with localized swelling and pain on weight bearing that increases when the person is on the toes. The diagnosis typically is confirmed with a bone scan.

Treatment is aimed at reducing inflammation and unloading the inflamed sesamoid. Custom-made orthotics with appropriate padding or cutout areas usually are successful. Stress fractures of the sesamoid take 10 to 12 weeks to heal and functional casts, which can be removed for pool exercising, plus daily 8-hour electromagnetic therapy, often can be useful. Ice massage combined with intrinsic foot exercises and calf stretching can be applied to the plantar aspect of the foot and the calf muscles. For persistent pain that is not relieved by conservative means, surgical excision of the sesamoids may be required. The major postoperative concern with removal of the sesamoids is the development of significant hallux valgus, which may be prevented by the prescription of proper footwear and orthotics.

Hallux Valgus

Hallux valgus usually is seen in patients with excessive foot pronation who use narrow footwear. Hallux valgus may occur with widening of the forefoot on weight bearing, resulting in increased laxity of the ligaments of the forefoot, particularly of the first and fifth metatarsal heads.[49] The metatarsal angle increases with hallux valgus from 1° to 2° to approximately 12°, resulting in increased valgus deviation of the great toe toward the second toe. With this altered position, and with pronation and/or compression by footwear, the clinician can see the development of calluses, exostosis, and a bursa thickening (bunion) at the first metatarsal head. Treatment is directed at controlled foot pronation using an orthotic and motion control footwear with adequate forefoot width. The callus can be trimmed, and icing and other modalities (e.g., ultrasound) can be used to treat the bursitis. If not treated adequately, hallux valgus will continue to progress and often must be treated surgically.

Hallux Rigidus

Hallux rigidus, a disabling condition associated with decreased range of motion at the first metatarsophalangeal joint, is accompanied by degenerative changes in the joint. Extension usually is reduced more than flexion, which makes climbing stairs extremely painful. Hallux rigidus is most frequently the result of repeated trauma, but it also can be seen after joint immobilization for a single traumatic episode or infection. The condition progresses, with increasing restriction of joint motion. Radiographic films confirm the hypertrophic degenerative features, such as joint space narrowing, often dorsal osteophytes, transverse joint space widening, and subchondral bone sclerosis. In late stages, as the metatarsophalangeal joint stiffens, hyperextension may be noted at the interphalangeal joint. Treatment is similar to that for turf toe.

Turf Toe

"Turf toe" is a sprain of the first metatarsophalangeal joint that typically occurs when the great toe is forced into hyperextension. It often is associated with sports played on artificial turf when a player catches the foot in a seam, but the condition also is common in those in the performing arts, such as ballet. Treatment is aimed at reducing the inflammation, protection, and restoration of normal range of motion. Anti-inflammatory and analgesic medications and modalities (e.g., ice, ultrasound, iontophoresis) can be used in the early stages after injury. ROM exercises are used early on, with a requirement of at least 10° of extension for walking and stair climbing. ROM exercises can be performed in a cold whirlpool, or contrast baths may be used during the inflammatory stage.

Passive joint mobilizing techniques can be effective for pain relief, starting with accessory (joint play) movements and moving into physiological movement patterns when accessory movements are pain free (Figures 19-21 and 19-22).[50] Sammarco[51] outlined a non-weight-bearing exercise program for rehabilitation of turf toe that involves stretching and strengthening (Table 19-5); this program is also useful for hallux rigidus. The program is combined with taping of the big toe to prevent hyperextension. If normal range of motion cannot be achieved, use of an orthotic with a rocker bar or a stiff-soled shoe with a rocker bar added can allow a pain-free gait. When the individual returns to activity, a properly fitted shoe with a stiffer sole should be used. The shoe can be combined with taping or a stiff insert to prevent hyperextension at the metatarsophalangeal

Figure 19-21

First metatarsophalangeal distraction. (From Donatelli RA, Wooden MJ: *Orthopedic physical therapy,* ed 3, p 543, New York, 2001, Churchill Livingstone.)

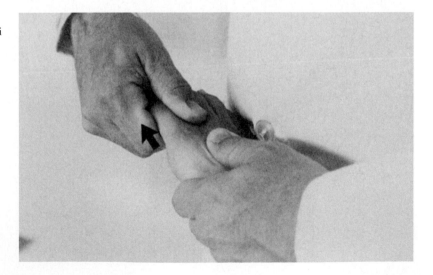

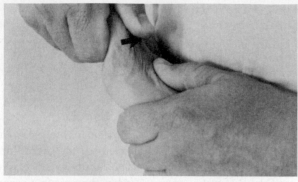

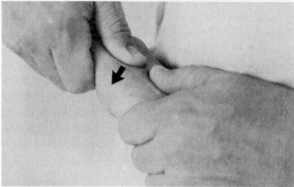

Figure 19-22
First metatarsophalangeal anteroposterior glides. (From Donatelli RA, Wooden MJ: *Orthopedic physical therapy,* ed 3, p 543, New York, 2001, Churchill Livingstone.)

joint. If an orthotic or shoe modification fails to provide relief, surgical consultation is needed. Cheilectomy is the usual procedure, because it improves range of motion without sacrificing joint stability.

Summary

The rehabilitation of patients with foot, ankle, or lower leg injuries must emphasize a return to functional mobility that does not sacrifice the integrity of healing tissue or allow

Table 19-5

Non-Weight-Bearing and Partial-Weight-Bearing Exercises That May Be Initiated When Patients with First Ray Injuries Are Unable to Bear Full Weight

Body Position	Exercise
Long sitting	Open chain toe extension active range of motion (AROM)
	Open chain toe flexion AROM
Seated with foot flat on floor	Open chain toe extension AROM (lift toes off floor while keeping heel on floor)
	Closed chain toe extension AROM (lift heel off ground while keeping toes on floor)
	Closed chain toe flexion AROM (clawing)
	Closed chain circumduction (lift heel off ground and put weight on lateral forefoot; roll from lateral to medial and then lateral again, making a complete circle around the ball of the foot)

Modified from Sammarco JG: How I manage turf toe, *Phys Sports Med* 16:113-118, 1988.

reinforcement of altered neuromuscular patterns. By creating an environment that allows this and by addressing specific functional limitations, such as reduced range of motion and altered gait patterns, mobility and function can be restored safely and effectively.

References

To enhance this text and add value for the reader, all references have been incorporated into a CD-ROM that is provided with this text. The reader can view the reference source and access it online whenever possible. There are a total of 51 references for this chapter.

CHAPTER 20

PERIPHERAL NERVE INJURIES

Caroline Drye Taylor, Robert J. Nee, and James E. Zachazewski

Introduction

Peripheral nerve injuries occur infrequently compared to the multitude of other injuries with which the physician, physical therapist, or athletic trainer must contend. Because they are infrequent, they may be overlooked in the process of differential diagnosis. The authors' purpose in writing this chapter is to alert clinicians to a class of injuries that, although infrequent, can have potentially devastating functional implications.

Scant literature is available documenting the incidence of peripheral nerve injuries, although some reports exist in the athletic injury and trauma literature. Krivickas and Wilbourn[1] reviewed more than 200 cases and found that 86% of peripheral nerve injuries in athletics occurred in the upper extremity. More than one third of those injuries were sustained by individuals playing football, and the most common injury was to the brachial plexus. Takazawa et al.[2] reviewed 9550 injuries treated over a span of 95 years at the clinic of the Japanese Athletic Association. During that period, only 28 cases of peripheral nerve injury were documented. This contrast may be due to the different type of sports or athletic activities in each study. Hirasawa and Sakakida[3] reviewed 18 years of experience with peripheral nerve injuries and reported that only 5.7% (66 of 1167 cases) were associated with athletes. The brachial plexus was involved most often, accounting for 24.2% of injuries (16 of 66). However, this study did not include high contact sports, such as American football.

Noble et al.[4] reported a prevalence of peripheral nerve injuries of 2.8% in a trauma population of 5777. In this study, 83% of the patients were male, and a motor vehicle accident (MVA) was the most common cause of injury (46%). The most frequently injured nerve was the radial nerve in the upper extremity and the common peroneal (fibular) nerve in the lower extremity.

Peripheral nerves may be vulnerable during surgery as a result of prolonged pressure from positioning or retraction of surrounding tissues. One study of iatrogenic nerve injury during abdominal surgery found an incidence of 0.17%.[5] Sciatic nerve injuries were caused by external compression; the mean operating time in those cases was 8.2 hours. Femoral nerves were thought to be injured as a result of prolonged retraction; the mean operating time in those patients was 4.3 hours. Upper and lower extremity injuries have also been reported as a complication of total hip arthroplasty (0.48% and 0.15%, respectively).[6]

Etiology

Injury to a peripheral nerve can occur by means of several mechanisms: stretching, compression (sustained compression or blunt trauma), friction, inflammation, or laceration. The clinical results of stretching or compression of the nerve vary, depending on whether the insult has a rapid onset or is the result of a gradual change. A sudden insult does not allow for any adaptive change in the connective tissue of the nerve and is more likely to cause acute disruption of the nerve's blood supply or connective tissue. Conversely, the nerve can adapt amazingly well to a slow increase in compressive forces, such as that brought on by a growing osteophyte.[7] A classification of peripheral nerve injuries is presented in Table 20-1.[8-11]

Mechanisms of Peripheral Nerve Injury

- Stretching
- Compression
- Friction
- Inflammation
- Laceration

Compression of the nerve can be caused by external sources or by swelling in a rigid compartment, such as the carpal tunnel at the wrist or the anterior compartment of the lower leg.[12] In 1973, Upton and McComas[13]

Table 20-1
Classification of Nerve Injuries[8-11]

Type		Pathological Basis	Possible Causes	Prognosis
Seddon's Classification	*Sunderland's Classification*			
Neuropraxia	Type 1: Focal conduction block Primarily motor function and proprioception are affected Some sensation and sympathetic function may be present	Local myelin injury, primarily larger fibers Axonal continuity No Wallerian degeneration	Electrolyte imbalances, deformation of myelin sheaths, ischemia caused by compression or traction	Recovery occurs within minutes, hours, or days if lesion was due to anoxia or ionic imbalances Mechanical compression or stretch may recover in weeks to months
Axonotmesis	Type 2: Loss of nerve conduction at injury site and distally	Disruption of axonal continuity with wallerian degeneration Connective tissue elements of the nerve remain intact	Compression	Axonal regeneration required for recovery Length of time for regeneration depends on distance of injury from end of nerve Good prognosis
	Type 3: Loss of nerve conduction at injury site and distally	Loss of axonal continuity and endoneurial tubes Perineurium and epineurium are preserved	Compression	Disruption of endoneurial tubes, hemorrhage, and edema produce scarring May have axonal misdirection Poor prognosis May require surgery
	Type 4: Loss of nerve conduction at injury site and distally	Damage to endoneurium and perineurium Epineurium remains intact	Compression	Intraneural scarring and axonal misdirection Poor prognosis Surgery required
Neurotmesis	Type 5: Loss of nerve conduction at injury site and distally	Severance of entire nerve	Compression, traction, laceration	Surgical resection and repair are only means of recovery; full recovery is unlikely Factors that affect extent of recovery include nerve injured, level at which nerve is damaged, extent of injury, time elapsed since injury, and patient's age

Modified from Dumitru D: *Electrodiagnostic medicine,* Philadelphia, 1995, Hanley & Belfus.

theorized that compression at one point along the nerve trunk increased the vulnerability of distal points along the nerve to the effects of compression. They hypothesized that the proximal compression disrupted axonal transport of vital nutrients and possibly the blood supply to the nerve, and they called this type of lesion a *double crush lesion.* They also noted that nerves with some other type of pre-existing physiological disturbance (e.g., diabetic peripheral neuropathy) are more vulnerable to any compressive lesion.

Friction over a nerve trunk can cause inflammation and fibrosis of the nerve's connective tissue elements. Fibrosis of the nerve trunk reduces its extensibility. Loss of

extensibility at one site along the nerve trunk may cause other portions of the nerve to bear increasing tensile loads when the nerve bed is elongated,[14] leading to a mechanical form of a double crush syndrome.[7]

Injury to tissues adjacent to nerve trunks can cause extensive scarring around the nerve trunk, which may impair the nerve's ability to move relative to its interfacing tissue or may compress the nerve if it is enclosed in a rigid space.[7] Laceration injuries can sever the nerve.

Detailed information on the pathology of nerve injuries can be found in volume 2 of this series, *Scientific Foundations and Principles of Practice in Musculoskeletal Rehabilitation,* Chapter 8.

Injuries to the Cervical Nerve Roots and Brachial Plexus

Etiology

Brachial plexus injuries are becoming more common as patients are surviving more severe trauma to the head, chest, spine, and shoulder.[15] The peak incidences of brachial plexus injuries are at birth, from obstetrical trauma, and at 20 to 40 years of age, as a result of motor vehicle accidents or knife or bullet wounds. Up to 10% of all injuries to the peripheral nervous system involve the brachial plexus.[16]

The brachial plexus is vulnerable to injury during surgical procedures, such as median sternotomy for open heart surgery[11,17] and shoulder reconstruction. It also may be compromised by positioning during surgical procedures or during procedures such as axillary arteriography, venous cannulation, and administration of regional anesthetic blocks.[11]

Neoplastic disease also can affect the brachial plexus. Primary brachial plexus tumors are rare; these include schwannomas, neurilemmomas, neurinomas, and neurofibromas. Secondary neoplastic disease of the upper lobe of the lung (Pancoast's or superior sulcus tumors) and breast tissue are more common causes of brachial plexus lesions. Radiation treatment to the breast and lung may further damage the plexus either by direct fibrosis of the nerves or by damage to the vascular tissue and Schwann's cells.[11]

Brachial plexus injuries are the most common nerve injuries in athletics, although they occur infrequently except in American football; the reported incidence in college football players ranges from 15% to 40%.[18,19] To obtain a thorough understanding of the epidemiological factors associated with brachial plexus injuries in football, the clinician must consider the mechanism of injury and the player's position, along with other biomechanical and physical factors.

Because of the incidence of brachial plexus injuries in athletics, many references are made in the chapter to mechanisms of injury, presentation of symptoms, evaluation, and resolution with reference to athletics. The reader should keep in mind that these factors may be very similar to those seen in nonathletic peripheral nerve injuries.

Classically, the following three distinct mechanisms of injury have been described in the literature:

- Head and neck lateral flexion with shoulder depression, causing a traction injury to the brachial plexus (Figure 20-1)[20-27]
- A direct blow to the supraclavicular region in the area of Erb's point, causing direct compression of the brachial plexus at its most superficial point (Figure 20-2)[19-21,24]
- Cervical hyperextension and lateral flexion, causing ipsilateral compression of the nerve roots within the foramina (Figure 20-3)[19,22,28-30] Cumulative trauma from multiple minor compression sprains such as these may lead to

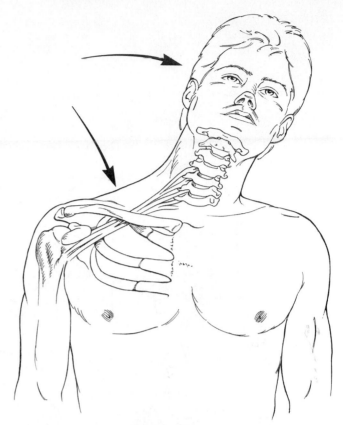

Figure 20-1

The combination of shoulder depression and contralateral cervical side flexion can lead to a traction injury to the brachial plexus; this is commonly referred to as a *burner*. (From Drye C, Zachazewski JE: Peripheral nerve injuries. In Zachazewski JE, Magee DJ, Quillen WS, editors: *Athletic injuries and rehabilitation*, p 442, Philadelphia, 1996, WB Saunders.)

chronic inflammation and secondary narrowing of the foramina where nerve roots exit.[28] A relationship between cervical spinal stenosis and brachial plexus injuries has been demonstrated, with injuries caused by the extension and compression mechanism described earlier.[28]

Clinical Presentation

Brachial plexus injuries in American football usually are the result of tackling or blocking. Therefore, the incidence is highest among defensive players, such as linemen, linebackers, and defensive backs.[31] This injury is commonly referred to as a *burner* or *stinger*. The athlete experiences transient weakness of the shoulder musculature accompanied by upper extremity paresthesia. In the acute syndrome, symptoms usually last several seconds to a few minutes and are followed by complete recovery. Neck pain may or may not be present.[26,32]

The injury usually affects the upper trunks of the plexus (C5 and C6 nerve roots).[21-23,33] Immediately after injury, weakness can be found in the biceps, deltoid, supraspinatus, and infraspinatus muscles. Deep tendon reflexes of the

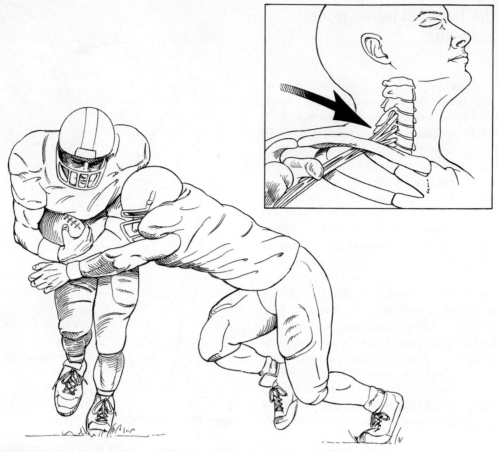

Figure 20-2

A second mechanism for a burner is a direct blow to the base of the neck (Erb's point). This leads to a compression injury to the trunks of the brachial plexus. (From Drye C, Zachazewski JE: Peripheral nerve injuries. In Zachazewski JE, Magee DJ, Quillen WS, editors: *Athletic injuries and rehabilitation,* p 443, Philadelphia, 1996, WB Saunders.)

biceps may also be diminished. Symptoms often can be reproduced by cervical extension and side flexion toward the involved extremity or lateral flexion away from the extremity.[27,32] Any restriction of cervical movement or spinal pain should alert the examiner to the possibility of cervical spine injury. True burners rarely involve restricted cervical mobility.[31] Restriction of shoulder range of motion should alert the clinician to the possibility of a clavicular fracture or acromioclavicular separation.

The injury to the nerve usually is considered a neuropraxic lesion, because it recovers almost immediately.[26,32] A thorough neurological examination can help differentiate spinal cord trauma from injury to the nerve root or plexus (Table 20-2). The patient's neurological status should be monitored closely for several days after the injury to determine the level of recovery accurately. Patients with persistent weakness or sensory loss should be referred to a physician for follow-up evaluation for possible axonotmesis or neurotmesis. Electromyographic (EMG) studies do not differentiate denervation from wallerian degeneration for 10 to 20 days after injury[27]; therefore EMG studies

generally are not performed until a minimum of 2 to 3 weeks after injury. Garrick and Webb[25] suggested that EMG studies be performed 6 weeks after injury. Clinically, Speer and Bassett[24] showed that strength deficits at 72 hours after injury equaled those at 4 weeks after injury.

Acute management mainly involves resting the extremity. If strength and function return completely in 1 to 2 minutes, the athlete can return to play.[32] If any neurological deficits persist after this time, the athlete should not be allowed to continue participation until full strength, range of motion, and sensation are restored in the cervical spine and extremity. Wroble et al.[31] advocate the use of ice, transcutaneous electrical nerve stimulation (TENS), ultrasound, and anti-inflammatory medications if pain and tenderness of the cervical spine and shoulder persist. Neck and shoulder strengthening exercises are prescribed to address any residual weakness.[34]

The athlete returning to play should be advised of the increased risk of reinjury and the likelihood of more severe injury with further trauma. With chronic plexus injuries, the athlete may experience symptoms with subsequent

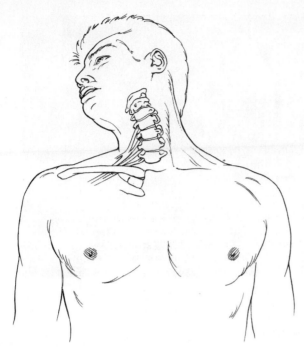

Figure 20-3
A third mechanism of injury in the burner syndrome is cervical extension combined with side flexion to the same side. This leads to compression of the cervical nerve roots in the neural foramina. (From Drye C, Zachazewski JE: Peripheral nerve injuries. In Zachazewski JE, Magee DJ, Quillen WS, editors: *Athletic injuries and rehabilitation,* p 444, Philadelphia, 1996, WB Saunders.)

trauma from a much smaller force. Postural changes (e.g., a dropped shoulder), atrophy of the shoulder muscles, or both may occur.[19] Clearly, more severe neurological losses and the need for longer periods of recuperation indicate that it is less advisable for the athlete to return to play.[31]

Padded neck rolls and shock-absorbing shoulder pads may be of some assistance in preventing recurrent burner injuries in football players.[15,17] However, Garrick and

Webb[25] found most currently used neck rolls to be too small to prevent side flexion injuries. The roll may need to be larger or to have extra padding in strategic locations to prevent excessive motion. An appropriately fitted collar should be worn close to the neck and should restrict cervical extension and side bending (Figure 20-4). Fitted properly, the collar does not restrict cervical rotation. Often the athlete wears the neck roll too low on the shoulder pads in an effort to be able to move the head and neck and see the football more easily; this renders the neck roll ineffective (Figure 20-5). *At no time* should straps running from the shoulder pads to the helmet be used to prevent head and neck movement. Use of straps may predispose the cervical spine to excessive axial loading and resultant fracture or fracture-dislocation by preventing movement of the cervical spine. The U.S. Military Academy has designed augmented shoulder pads that add buffer padding to the neck in an effort to prevent compressive injuries to the plexus (Figure 20-6).[19]

Cervical nerve root avulsion injuries can occur with more severe injuries. Frequently, more than one level avulses at the time of injury; the most common pattern in one study involved the C5-T1 roots.[33] Adjacent roots are always involved if more than one level is avulsed, and associated vascular damage may occur.[15] The patient has complete motor loss in muscles innervated by the affected nerve root levels, and spontaneous recovery does not occur (neurotmesis). Diagnostic findings may include fractures of the transverse processes on cervical radiographs.[34] Rehabilitation consists of maintaining range of motion in the extremity and reconstructive surgery to restore as much function as possible.

Acute Brachial Neuropathy

Acute brachial neuropathy is a rare syndrome characterized by acute or subacute intense shoulder pain, accompanied by weakness and wasting of various muscles of the shoulder

Table 20-2
Neurological Evaluation of Brachial Plexus Injury

Lesion (Root Level)	Motor Findings (Resisted Tests)	Sensory Findings (Light Touch or Pinprick)
C4	Upper trapezius: Shoulder elevation	Top of shoulders
C5	Supraspinatus and deltoid: Shoulder abduction	Lateral upper arm and distal radius
C6	Biceps: Elbow flexion	Lateral forearm, thumb
C7	Triceps: Elbow extension	Index and middle fingertips
C8	Extensor pollicus longus: Extension of distal phalanx of thumb	Fourth and fifth fingers and hypothenar eminence
T1	Intrinsics of the hand: Abduction/adduction of fingers	Medial forearm
Suspected spinal cord lesions	Diffuse motor loss, bilateral weakness, lower extremity motor loss	Diffuse paresthesia and numbness, bilateral sensory loss (nondermatomal)

From Drye C, Zachazewski JE: Peripheral nerve injuries. In Zachazewski JE, Magee DJ, Quillen WS, editors: *Athletic injuries and rehabilitation,* p 444, Philadelphia, 1996, WB Saunders.

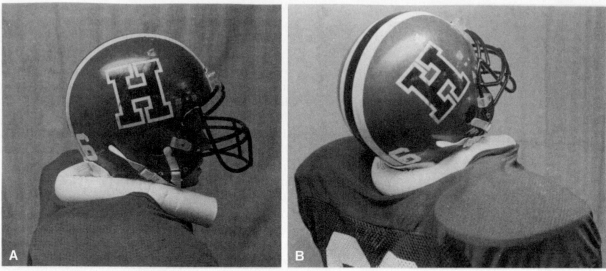

Figure 20-4

Neck rolls often are used to prevent excessive lateral flexion of the cervical spine during tackling in American football. **A,** Proper placement of the neck roll, close to the helmet and cervical spine. **B,** Appropriate restriction of motion of the head and cervical spine. (From Drye C, Zachazewski JE: Peripheral nerve injuries. In Zachazewski JE, Magee DJ, Quillen WS, editors: *Athletic injuries and rehabilitation*, p 445, Philadelphia, 1996, WB Saunders.)

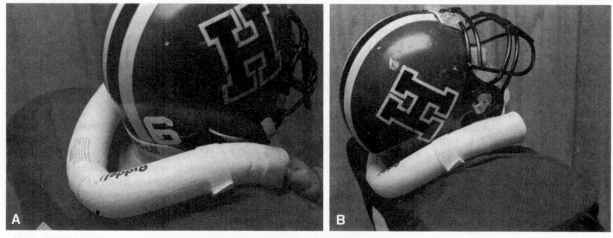

Figure 20-5

The position of padding also determines the effective protection of the spine. **A,** Improper placement of the neck roll, too far from the helmet and cervical spine. **B,** Ineffective restriction of motion of the head and cervical spine. (From Drye C, Zachazewski JE: Peripheral nerve injuries. In Zachazewski JE, Magee DJ, Quillen WS, editors: *Athletic injuries and rehabilitation*, p 445, Philadelphia, 1996, WB Saunders.)

and proximal arm. It should be considered a possible diagnosis if the patient has no clear trauma or history of overuse. The incidence is higher in males than females, and patients in their 30s or 70s are affected more frequently.[35] The disorder has no clear pattern of motor nerve or brachial plexus involvement. Denervation may be limited to one muscle supplied by a peripheral nerve (e.g., normal infraspinatus muscle with denervation of the supraspinatus muscle). Sensory loss usually is limited. Most reported cases occur in the dominant upper extremity.[32,36] The cause of acute brachial neuropathy is unknown.

Management in the acute phase includes rest and analgesics. The patient begins rehabilitation as soon as the pain subsides.[31] The prognosis generally is good, but residual weakness is common for several months or years after diagnosis.

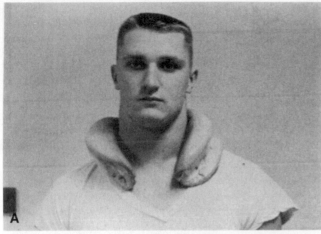

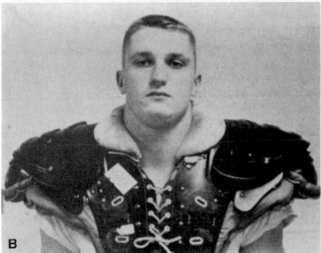

Figure 20-6

A, Orthosis used at the U.S. Military Academy. **B,** Interval pad adds a buffer to the neck opening of football shoulder pads. (From Markey KL, DiBenedetto M, Curl WW: Upper trunk brachial plexopathy: the stinger syndrome, *Am J Sports Med* 21:650-655, 1993.)

Peripheral Nerve Injuries in the Upper Quarter

Nerve Injuries of the Neck and Upper Limb

- Thoracic outlet syndrome
- Spinal accessory nerve
- Long thoracic nerve
- Axillary nerve
- Suprascapular nerve
- Musculocutaneous nerve
- Radial nerve
- Ulnar nerve
- Median nerve
- Combined lesions

Thoracic Outlet Syndrome

Thoracic outlet syndrome (TOS) is a controversial diagnosis consisting of neural and/or vascular compression in the thoracic outlet (Figure 20-7). TOS has a variety of clinical manifestations, depending on the site of compression and the neurovascular structures involved. Vascular symptoms are less common than neurogenic symptoms. The most common neurogenic signs arise from compression of the lower trunk of the brachial plexus, leading to symptoms such as pain and paresthesias of the medial arm and hand, upper extremity fatigue, and muscle atrophy.

TOS may occur in patients with excessive shoulder girdle depression[37] or overly developed trapezius and neck musculature and in work requiring repetitive overhead use of the upper extremity or prolonged wear of heavy body armor for combat soldiers. Swimmers may develop symptoms as a result of hypertrophy of the pectoralis minor muscle. Tennis and baseball players may develop symptoms owing either to greater muscular development of the dominant arm or increased scapular depression as a result of failure to maintain adequate scapular stabilization with repetitive motions.[25,38] Prolonged keyboard use and reaching for a computer mouse can also provoke symptoms. Patients may complain of upper extremity numbness, weakness, and difficulty gripping objects because of intrinsic muscle weakness in the hands.

Because the exact diagnosis of TOS is difficult to confirm, symptoms in the upper extremity should always be evaluated carefully to differentiate true TOS from shoulder instabilities, cervical radiculopathies, and other peripheral nerve injuries. Treatment is directed at restoring posture and muscle balance of the upper trunk and shoulder girdle, restoring diaphragmatic breathing patterns to reduce recruitment of the scalene muscles, and reducing sensitivity to neurodynamic tests in the upper extremity. Modification of technique or avoidance of some activities may be necessary to prevent recurrence of symptoms.[16,39]

Spinal Accessory Nerve Injury

The spinal accessory nerve innervates the sternocleidomastoid muscle and the trapezius. It is vulnerable to injury from blunt trauma (e.g., a blow from a hockey stick or any other mechanism of direct trauma) or a traction injury.[34] Injury can result in paralysis and atrophy of the trapezius muscle. Weakness usually develops soon after the injury and is accompanied by a persistent ache about the shoulder girdle.[40,41] If the nerve does not recover, scapular stabilizing procedures or transfer of the levator scapulae can be performed surgically. However, the prognosis for full return to athletics or other types of vigorous physical activity is usually poor.[40]

Long Thoracic Nerve Injury (Backpacker's Palsy)

The long thoracic nerve originates from the C5-C7 nerve roots and innervates the serratus anterior muscle, which is

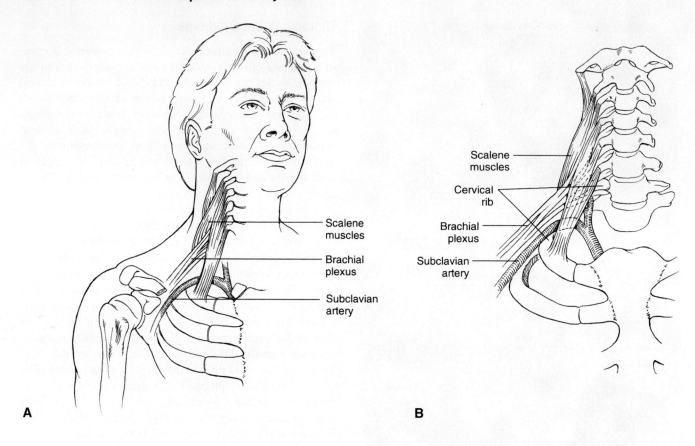

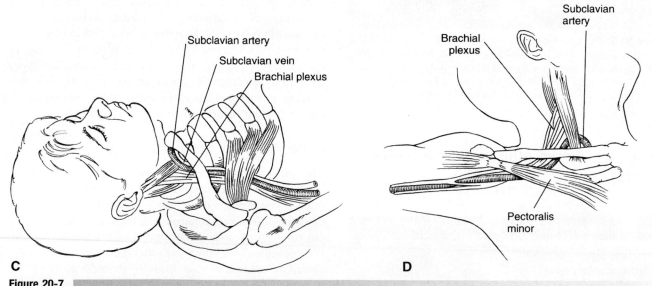

Figure 20-7

Sites of compression in thoracic outlet syndrome (TOS). **A,** Scalenus anterior syndrome. **B,** A cervical rib or a fibrous band can obstruct the neurovascular bundle. **C,** Compression can occur between the clavicle and first rib. **D,** Hyperabduction compresses the neurovascular bundle under the pectoralis minor tendon. (From Drye C, Zachazewski JE: Peripheral nerve injuries. In Zachazewski JE, Magee DJ, Quillen WS, editors: *Athletic injuries and rehabilitation,* p 447, Philadelphia, 1996, WB Saunders.)

essential for scapular stabilization and protraction. The nerve is vulnerable to blunt trauma as it passes from the brachial plexus across the base of the neck and, more distally, where it lies against the chest wall. It may be entrapped in the scalenus medius or as it runs between the clavicle and second rib.[42] It is commonly injured by traction or compression from the strap of a backpack. Traction injury occurs with combined head flexion, rotation, and lateral flexion away from the injured side and shoulder flexion.[43] Paralysis of the serratus anterior has also been reported as an overuse injury in sports such as archery, basketball, bowling, cycling, golf, rope skipping, weight lifting, and tennis.[40] White and Witten[44] reported one incidence of a stretch injury to the long thoracic nerve in a male ballet dancer from aggressive warm-up stretches. The presenting complaint usually is difficulty elevating the arm and winging of the scapula, often accompanied by aching or burning around the shoulder or scapula.[40]

The prognosis is good if the injury is the result of overuse. The injury is treated with rest and exercise to maintain range of motion. Closed injuries have a more guarded prognosis; if the injury was caused by compression, the prognosis depends on how long the compression has been applied. Taping of the scapula can be used to optimize scapular positioning during activities of daily living (ADLs) and exercise.[45] If strength and endurance do not fully recover with conservative management over 24 months, the scapula may have to be stabilized surgically.[40]

Long thoracic nerve injury and thoracic outlet symptoms can be prevented in children who carry backpacks to school. The American Physical Therapy Association suggests that children carry no more than 15% of their body weight. The backpack should fit properly, and both straps should be used. Hip belts and compressive straps help lessen the strain on the upper body.[46]

Axillary Nerve Injury

The axillary nerve is formed from fibers of the C5 and C6 nerve roots. It arises from the posterior cord of the brachial plexus and innervates the deltoid and teres minor muscles. It also provides sensory innervation for a small area of skin over the lateral deltoid. The most common mechanism of injury is an acute anterior shoulder dislocation or its reduction.[38,39] Other mechanisms of injury include blunt trauma to the shoulder, compression by a hematoma, irritation by osteophytes of the glenoid margin, and compression from muscular hypertrophy as the nerve passes through the quadrilateral space.[40,47] Trauma also may occur during many surgical procedures on the shoulder.[40,48]

If EMG findings show incomplete denervation, the prognosis for recovery generally is good, but a long rest from the provoking activity may be necessary.[47] Fortunately, the supraspinatus and infraspinatus muscles can compensate for some of the loss of abduction and external rotation after axillary nerve injury.[40]

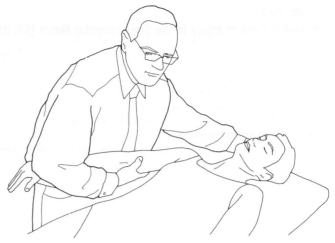

Figure 20-8
Neurodynamic test of the axillary nerve. The test combines internal rotation of the arm, shoulder girdle depression, and lateral flexion of the cervical spine away from the upper extremity. (From Butler D: *The sensitive nervous system*, p 339, Adelaide, 2000, Noigroup Publications.)

Butler[49] proposed a test of the sensitivity of the nerve to mechanical loading based on the geography of the nerve relative to the axes of the shoulder joint (Figure 20-8). This test has not been studied to determine whether it provokes symptoms in the distribution of the axillary nerve.

Suprascapular Nerve Injury

The suprascapular nerve innervates the supraspinatus and infraspinatus and provides sensory branches to the posterior glenohumeral joint and the acromioclavicular joint. The five potential sites of trauma along the nerve are outlined in Table 20-3.[40,50]

The mechanism of injury may be direct trauma, such as a fall on the shoulder or acute dislocation, or traction and friction to the nerve as it passes through the suprascapular notch. Rapid stretching of the accompanying artery may contribute to ischemic injury of the nerve.[50] Laceration of the nerve during distal clavicle resection has also been reported.[51] Volleyball players, swimmers, and other athletes who perform repetitive overhead motions are vulnerable to this injury. It has frequently been reported in baseball players, especially pitchers,[40,50,52] owing to the extreme angular velocities and torque forces acting on the shoulder during the phases of pitching or throwing.[50,53] Clinically, injury has also been seen from prolonged bed rest in left side-lying during a difficult pregnancy with twins. Injury to the nerve in the spinoglenoid notch leads to denervation of the infraspinatus alone.

The onset of symptoms often is insidious, beginning with a vague shoulder ache and weakness without paresthesia or numbness.[40,50] Visible atrophy and EMG changes may be present without noticeable impairment, even in

rest, ice, and muscle stretching and strengthening.[9,27,64] In true radial tunnel syndrome, the most effective treatment usually is surgical decompression of the nerve.[9,64]

Differential diagnosis of lesions to this nerve also must include the possibility of cervical radiculopathy. Gunn and Milbrandt[65] examined the cervical spines of individuals with a history of tennis elbow who had failed to respond to treatment directed at the elbow. All 42 patients in their study had EMG findings "consistent with early radiculopathy or neuropathy of the affected myotomes," and all had increased resistance to passive motion of the C5 and C6 apophyseal joints. Treatment was directed to the cervical spine and included spinal mobilization, traction, various treatment modalities, and isometric exercises. This treatment produced good or satisfactory relief of symptoms in 86% of the patients in an average of 5.25 weeks.

Other authors have explored the relationship between lateral epicondylalgia and cervical dysfunction. A recent retrospective study of patients with lateral epicondylalgia found that adding treatment of the cervical spine to local interventions at the elbow produced successful outcomes in fewer visits (mean, 5.6; standard deviation [SD], 1.7) compared to management directed only at the elbow (mean, 9.7; SD, 2.4).[66] Although this retrospective design does not establish a cause and effect relationship between the cervical spine treatment and successful outcomes in fewer visits, a pilot randomized clinical trial demonstrated that combined cervical manual therapy and local elbow treatment led to greater improvements in self-reported disability and pain at the 6-month follow-up for patients with lateral epicondylalgia compared to local elbow treatment only.[67] The small sample size in this pilot study ($n = 10$) means that the results should be interpreted cautiously, and further randomized studies with larger sample sizes are warranted to explore the role of manual therapy to the cervical spine in influencing longer term outcomes in patients with lateral epicondylalgia.[67]

It also is important to realize that the relationship between lateral epicondylalgia and cervical dysfunction may not be consistent across demographical groups. A prospective study by Waugh et al.[68] revealed that the association between lateral epicondylalgia and cervical joint findings is most likely to be present in women working in repetitive jobs and least likely to occur in men employed in nonrepetitive jobs in whom the onset of lateral elbow symptoms was due to a sports-related injury.

The positive response to treatment of the cervical spine in the aforementioned studies does not necessarily indicate that all the symptoms came from a cervical lesion. It is more likely that treatment directed to the cervical spine removed one component of a double crush lesion involving both the cervical spine and the radial nerve at the elbow. It may also be that manual therapy treatment of the cervical spine stimulated endogenous descending pain inhibitory systems that result in reduced lateral elbow pain.[62] The interplay of proximal and distal components of nerve irritation, as well

as the local effects on the nerve of joint and muscle inflammation, may help explain why the differential diagnosis and treatment of lateral epicondylalgia often are difficult.

Butler[7,49] described this complex interplay between cervical joints and muscle tightness, elbow joint and soft tissue signs, and neural tension tests and neurological findings in the management of a patient with lateral elbow pain. He devised a test known as the **upper limb neurodynamic test 2 (ULNT 2) with a radial nerve bias,** in which mechanical tension is applied to the radial nerve throughout its course. (Some texts refer to this as the upper limb tension test 3 [ULTT 3].[69]) This test consists of a combination of shoulder depression, elbow extension, medial rotation of the extremity, pronation of the forearm, wrist flexion, thumb and finger flexion, and ulnar deviation of the hand (Figure 20-11). If symptoms have not been provoked by this point in the test, shoulder abduction is performed. Cervical lateral flexion away from the extremity also increases the mechanical load on the brachial plexus,[70] further sensitizing the test. The final forearm position in this test (pronation, wrist flexion and ulnar deviation, and thumb flexion) is a position that is commonly used to test flexibility of the common extensor muscles. Pain from muscle stretching in this position can be differentiated from pain from neural structures by the addition of shoulder abduction or cervical lateral flexion. Both of these maneuvers increase mechanical load through the nerve tract without increasing tension in the extensor muscles.

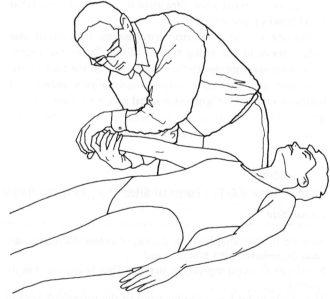

Figure 20-11

The upper limb neurodynamic test 2 (ULNT 2) with a radial nerve bias. The test combines shoulder depression, elbow extension, medial rotation of the whole arm, and wrist and finger flexion. The test is further sensitized with the addition of shoulder depression and abduction and contralateral side flexion of the cervical spine. Symptoms are monitored at each position of the test. (From Butler D: *The sensitive nervous system,* p 329, Adelaide, 2000, Noigroup Publications.)

Yaxley and Jull[71,72] studied the ULNT 2 with a radial nerve bias in 20 subjects with unilateral tennis elbow. Both upper extremities of their subjects had symptoms in the radial forearm, but the symptoms were reported as more intense in the symptomatic arms.[72] They observed a statistically significant difference in available range of shoulder abduction in the symptomatic arms of their subjects (12.45° less than the asymptomatic side). They recommended routine inclusion of this test as a part of the differential diagnosis of lateral epicondylalgia. Further support for this recommendation was provided by a recent prospective case series in which 41% of subjects with lateral epicondylalgia (34 of 83) had their symptoms reproduced during application of the radial bias neurodynamic test.[68]

Ulnar Nerve Injury

The ulnar nerve arises from the medial cord of the brachial plexus. It is most vulnerable to injury at two sites, the cubital tunnel at the elbow and in or near Guyon's canal at the wrist.[61,73,74] The four major etiological factors for injury of the nerve at the elbow are presented in Table 20-5.

Most cases of **cubital tunnel syndrome** have an insidious onset of medial elbow pain radiating down the medial forearm and numbness and tingling in the ulnar aspect of the forearm and hand. Symptoms are aggravated by continued use.[73] Symptoms can occur in computer users working in excessive elbow flexion, violinists or violists practicing for long periods of time and laborers who perform repeated elbow flexion/extension on the job. Injury also is common in athletes who perform repeated throwing motions.[73,74] A normal rise in pressure occurs in the nerve in the cubital tunnel as the elbow is flexed in combination with wrist extension and shoulder abduction, which is the upper extremity position at the beginning stage of throwing.[75] Wright et al.[76] reported that the nerve requires 2 cm (1 inch) of

unimpeded movement at the elbow and can experience strain values that diminish the circulation to the nerve. Entrapment or inflammation of the nerve lessens the nerve's ability to tolerate movement or changes in intraneural pressure.

Various tests for lesions along the path of the ulnar nerve have been described in the literature. Buehler and Thayer[77] suggested using the elbow flexion test as a clinical test for cubital tunnel syndrome (Figure 20-12). A positive response to the test consists of reproduction of paresthesias along the ulnar border of the forearm and hand. Butler's upper limb neurodynamic test with an ulnar nerve bias (ULNT 3) (Figure 20-13) is similar but increases the tensile stress on

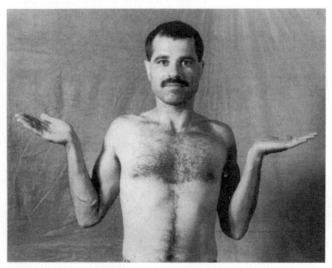

Figure 20-12

The elbow flexion test for ulnar nerve irritation in the cubital tunnel.[77] A positive response is the production of paresthesias along the ulnar border of the forearm and hand. (From Drye C, Zachazewski JE: Peripheral nerve injuries. In Zachazewski JE, Magee DJ, Quillen WS, editors: *Athletic injuries and rehabilitation*, p 451, Philadelphia, 1996, WB Saunders.)

Table 20-5
Ulnar Nerve (C7-T1): Cubital Tunnel Lesions[73,74,76]

Cause/Site	Signs and Symptoms
Traction injuries caused by increased valgus forces: • Prior fracture or injury to the growth plate • Disruption of the medial collateral ligament (MCL) Entrapment under: • Thickened arcuate ligament • Hypertrophic medial triceps, anconeus, or ulnar flexor muscle of the wrist • Postoperative scar or bony callous formation Irregularities in the ulnar groove caused by osteophytes may prevent sliding of the ulnar nerve Subluxation or dislocation of the nerve over the medial epicondyle (usually as a result of laxity of soft tissue restraints) leads to a friction fibrosis	Medial elbow pain radiating to the medial forearm Numbness and tingling in the ulnar aspect of the forearm and hand

Modified from Drye C, Zachazewski JE: Peripheral nerve injuries. In Zachazewski JE, Magee DJ, Quillen WS, editors: *Athletic injuries and rehabilitation*, p 450, Philadelphia, 1996, WB Saunders.

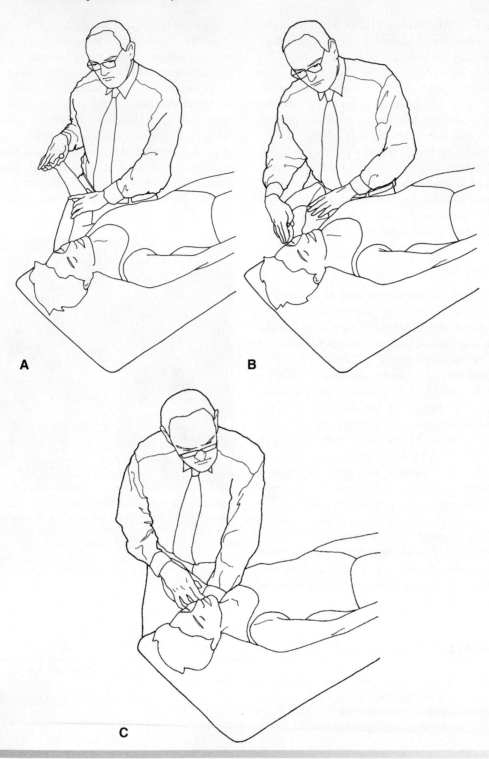

Figure 20-13

The upper limb neurodynamic test 3 (ULNT 3[49]) was designed to place tensile stress on the ulnar nerve. The test consists of (**A**) wrist and finger extension and forearm pronation, (**B**) elbow flexion and lateral rotation of the arm, and (**C**) shoulder abduction and shoulder girdle depression. Contralateral lateral flexion of the cervical spine further sensitizes the test. (From Butler D: *The sensitive nervous system*, p 334, Adelaide, 2000, Noigroup Publications.)

the brachial plexus and proximal portion of the ulnar nerve by adding shoulder girdle depression, glenohumeral abduction, and external rotation[49] (this test has been described elsewhere as the ULTT[37,78] or ULTT 4[69]). Although the test originally was described with the forearm in supination, pronation of the forearm often makes the test more provocative of symptoms. Cervical lateral flexion away from the extremity being tested can also be added.

Responses to Butler's ULNT 3 have been studied in normal patients[78,79] and in symptomatic patients.[78] In most normal subjects, symptoms of tingling or stretching occurred in the medial forearm and hand. Subjects also frequently reported a sensation of stretching or pressure at the medial elbow. Several arms tested in normal subjects had no symptomatic response to the test. In the 18 subjects with a variety of upper extremity or cervical spine symptoms, all subjects had some response to the test. They had more frequent reports of medial upper arm pain (44% versus 18% in healthy subjects) and occasional symptoms in the contralateral extremity.

Twenty-five percent of the subjects tested in the patient group had an onset of symptoms before the addition of shoulder abduction, something that never occurred in healthy subjects. When the range of shoulder abduction at the onset of symptoms in the remaining symptomatic arms was compared with that in healthy subjects, the difference was not statistically significant. Clinically, this seems to indicate that provocation of symptoms in the early stages of the ULNT 3 or with the elbow flexion test is a better measure of the presence of abnormality than the degree of abduction available before the onset of symptoms in the ULNT 3.

Treatment for cubital tunnel syndrome consists initially of rest, ice, and anti-inflammatory medications. The patient should also be examined for any problems in the cervical spine or shoulder that may be contributing to the symptoms. Altering the mechanics of throwing may help minimize stress on the elbow in the athlete. Computer keyboard height should be adjusted to place the elbow in less than 90° flexion during prolonged computer use. A soft splint worn at night can help symptoms by preventing prolonged elbow flexion during sleep.

If conservative treatment fails, surgical treatment should be considered. Surgical options include (1) transposition of the ulnar nerve to the anterior surface of the elbow joint and (2) removal of the medial epicondyle.[61,73,74] Rettig and Ebben[80] retrospectively reviewed the cases of 20 athletes who underwent anterior subcutaneous transfer of the ulnar nerve. The average length of time between surgery and return to sports was 12.6 weeks (range, 6 to 43 weeks), and 19 of 20 athletes returned to their preinjury level of athletic activity.

Compression of the ulnar nerve at the wrist can cause sensory disturbances and motor weakness in the intrinsic muscles of the hand.[61,81] It is a common problem for cyclists.[34,81,82] Fernald[82] studied the incidence of overuse injuries in elite cyclists and found that 21% had sensory

changes in the upper extremities. The abnormality may result from acute or chronic compression of the nerve in Guyon's canal as a result of prolonged weight bearing on the hands or a fall. It also can be caused by traction on the nerve produced by the extended wrist position on the handlebars.[36,81] Normally cyclists bear approximately 45% of their weight on the upper extremities[82]; therefore the combination of compression and vibration from the road increases the likelihood of neurogenic symptoms.

Strategies to prevent irritation to the nerve at the wrist include changing the position of the hands frequently while riding, using padded gloves and handlebars, and adjusting the overall "fit" of the bike to reduce weight bearing on the hands.[81,82]

Digital nerves in the hand are vulnerable to compression and friction injuries. Bowlers are susceptible to compression of the ulnar digital nerve to the thumb, caused by direct pressure from the hole in the bowling ball.[83] Rettig[83] reported a case of digital neuritis in a cheerleader from repetitive clapping.

Median Nerve Injury

The median nerve arises from the medial and lateral cords of the brachial plexus. Three common compression syndromes affect this nerve: pronator syndrome, interosseous syndrome, and carpal tunnel syndrome. Sites of compression in **pronator syndrome** are presented in Table 20-6.[9]

Table 20-6

Median Nerve (C5-T1): Sites of Compression in Pronator Syndrome[9]

Cause/Site	Signs and Symptoms
Swelling from trauma can compress the nerve in the fibro-osseous tunnel created by the ligament of Struthers as it passes between the supracondylar process and the medial epicondyle	Pain with resisted forearm pronation
Abnormal thickness of the bicipital aponeurosis can compress the nerve during resisted elbow flexion	Pain is aggravated by resisted elbow flexion
A fibrous band in the superficial head of the pronator teres muscle may compress the nerve where it passes between the superficial and deep heads	Pain is aggravated by resisted forearm pronation and flexion
The nerve can be compressed under the fibrous arch on the proximal margin of the superficial flexor muscles of the fingers	Pain with resisted flexion of the superficial tendon of the third finger

Modified from Drye C, Zachazewski JE: Peripheral nerve injuries. In Zachazewski JE, Magee DJ, Quillen WS, editors: *Athletic injuries and rehabilitation,* p 452, Philadelphia, 1996, WB Saunders.

Table 20-7
Differential Diagnostic Characteristics of Carpal Tunnel, Pronator, and Anterior Interosseous Nerve Syndromes

	Paresthesia	Nocturnal Symptoms	Muscle Weakness/ Atrophy	Tinel's Test	Phalen's Test	Direct Compression	Electrodiagnostic Tests
Carpal tunnel syndrome (CTS)	Lateral 3½ digits	Yes	Abductor pollicus brevis, opponens pollicis, flexor pollicis brevis	Positive at carpal tunnel	Positive	Positive at carpal tunnel	Diagnostic
Pronator syndrome (PS)	Lateral 3½ digits	No	Not a traditional sign but may involve abductor pollicis brevis, opponens pollicis, flexor pollicis brevis, flexor pollicis longus, flexor digitorum profundus of index and long fingers, pronator quadratus, flexor carpi radialis	Positive at pronator teres <50%	Negative	Positive at pronator teres, negative at carpal tunnel	Rarely diagnostic
Anterior interosseous nerve syndrome (AINS)	None	No	Flexor pollicis longus, flexor digitorum profundus of index and long fingers, pronator quadratus	Negative	Negative	Negative	Diagnostic

From Lee MJ, LaStayo PC: Pronator syndrome and other nerve compressions that mimic carpal tunnel syndrome, *J Orthop Sports Phys Ther* 34:601-609, 2004.

Differential diagnostic characteristics of these syndromes are outlined in Table 20-7.[84]

Anterior interosseous syndrome occurs when the nerve is compressed by a fibrous band of the superficial flexor muscle of the fingers or by anomalous tendons of the forearm. The nerve also is vulnerable to injury from a forearm fracture or corrective surgery.[85] Weakness is confined to the long flexor muscle of the thumb, the deep flexor muscle of the second and third fingers, and the pronator quadratus muscle.[61] Anterior interosseous syndrome is rare compared with carpal tunnel syndrome and pronator syndrome (less than 2%[84,86]).

Carpal tunnel syndrome (CTS) is by far the most common form of compression of the median nerve (88.2% of median nerve injuries[84,86]). Many activities are considered risk factors, including weight bearing on the hands,[36,81] repetitive gripping, throwing, or wrist flexion and extension, and the use of vibrating tools. Other physical characteristics linked to a higher incidence of CTS include female gender, age, race, obesity, pregnancy, diabetes, thyroid disease, and connective tissue disorders.[87] It also can occur after trauma.[83] Splinting in a neutral wrist position may be necessary to facilitate rest. Compliance with the use of splints has been linked to the fit and comfort of the splint and to the ability to continue to work while wearing it.[88] Other adjunct procedures include icing, steroid or lidocaine injection, and resection of the transverse retinacular ligament.[81,83]

Differential diagnosis of median nerve compression syndromes includes ruling out cervical radiculopathies. As with radial and ulnar nerve abnormality, the possibility of a mechanical or physiological double crush lesion must always be considered. Murray-Leslie and Wright[89] found a positive correlation between the incidence of carpal tunnel syndrome and a decrease in the size of the anteroposterior measurements of the cervical spinal canal at C5 and C6 and a decrease in cervical disc height when subjects were compared with age-matched controls.

The authors' clinical experience has been that symptoms may be present in the median nerve distribution that appear to be due to adverse mechanics along the course of the nerve, frequently in the absence of EMG abnormalities. A similar observation led Elvey[70] to develop what is currently considered the first upper limb neurodynamic test (ULNT 1) (Figure 20-14). His cadaveric studies demonstrated that the C5-C7 nerve roots moved laterally during shoulder

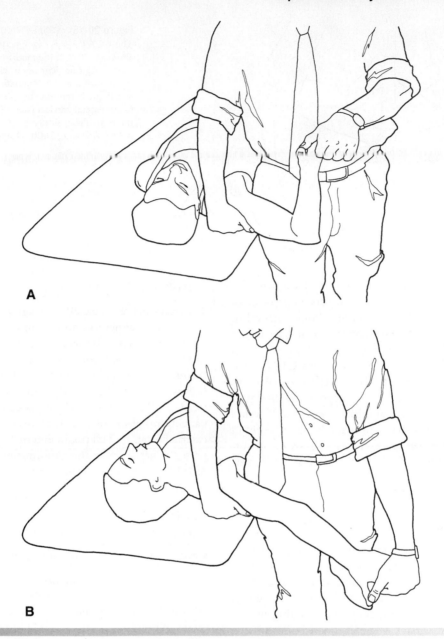

Figure 20-14

The upper limb neurodynamic test 1 (ULNT 1) places tensile stress on the brachial plexus and median nerve throughout its course. The test consists sequentially of **(A)** shoulder abduction, wrist and finger extension, and forearm supination followed by **(B)** shoulder lateral rotation, elbow extension, and contralateral cervical lateral flexion. (From Butler D: *The sensitive nervous system,* p 317, Adelaide, 2000, Noigroup Publications.)

abduction if the shoulder was prevented from elevating. Elbow extension and wrist extension increased the tension on these structures and on the brachial plexus and median nerve. Other studies have confirmed the motion of the median nerve with shoulder abduction, elbow extension, and wrist extension.[14] The response to the end position of the test in asymptomatic subjects is a deep, sometimes painful stretch over the anterior shoulder, elbow, and lateral forearm.[90] It also provokes a mild to moderate amount of tingling in the thumb and first two fingers.

Butler's variation on the ULNT 1 also stresses the median nerve. It uses the same components of motion as Elvey's test but in a different order.[49] Butler developed the ULNT 2 (Figure 20-15) to replicate more closely the functional movements that reproduced patients' symptoms. The final position of the test is similar to the backswing of a forehand shot in tennis. The response to this test in normal subjects is similar to that seen in the ULNT 1.[91,92]

All the upper limb neurodynamic tests described are helpful for determining whether abnormal neurobiomechanics

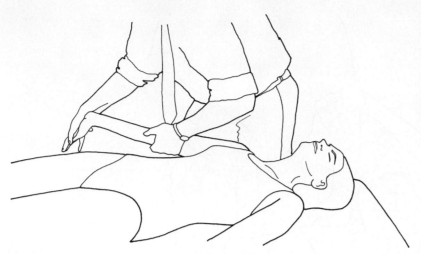

Figure 20-15
The ULNT 2 was developed by Butler[7,49] as an alternative test of the median nerve tract. It consists of shoulder girdle depression, elbow extension, lateral rotation of the arm, supination of the forearm, wrist and finger extension, and shoulder abduction. Contralateral cervical lateral flexion further sensitizes the test. (From Butler D: *The sensitive nervous system*, p 326, Adelaide, 2000, Noigroup Publications.)

are contributing to persistent symptoms. Treatment can then focus on mobilization or release/decompression of the neural tissues involved. Nerve gliding (sometimes called nerve flossing) has been shown to be an effective technique or home exercise for patients with CTS. Seradge et al.[93] used nerve and tendon gliding exercises as part of a CTS prevention program in a meat packing plant. They reported a 45% decrease in the incidence of CTS in response to their program.[93,94] Lee and LaStayo[84] and Rozmaryn et al.[95] found that patients with CTS who performed a home program of nerve gliding exercises had a lower rate of subsequent surgery for CTS (43% versus 71.2% in those who did not perform exercises).

Combined Lesions

Injury to the radial, median, and ulnar nerves can occur as a result of compression in the axilla or upper arm from the misuse of crutches during rehabilitation of lower extremity injuries.[9,61] The median and ulnar nerves are always vulnerable at the wrist during activities requiring weight bearing on extended wrists.[36] The likelihood of combined lesions increases with the magnitude of trauma to the extremity.

Peripheral Nerve Injuries in the Lower Quarter

Nerve Injuries of the Lumbar Spine and Lower Limb

- Sciatic nerve
- Tibial nerve
- Peroneal (fibular) nerve
- Femoral nerve
- Obturator nerve

Sciatic Nerve Injury

The sciatic nerve (Table 20-8) is formed by the fibular (peroneal) and tibial nerves and contains contributions from the L4-S3 nerve roots. The nerve can be irritated as it passes under or through the piriformis muscle in the buttocks.[96] Pain may be due to spasm or scarring of the muscle from straining or overuse.[61] Clinically, pain may radiate down the posterior leg (sciatica). Tenderness is located over the muscle belly. The patient complains of pain with resisted hip abduction and external rotation. Full passive internal rotation can also compress the nerve under the piriformis muscle. The pain is not usually associated with neurological loss.[61]

Table 20-8
Sciatic Nerve (L4-S3): Areas of Entrapment or Irritation

Cause/Site	Signs and Symptoms
Compression as nerve runs under or through the piriformis in the buttocks	Tenderness over the piriformis muscle belly; pain with resisted hip abduction and external rotation; pain with full passive internal rotation or hip adduction in hip flexion
Entrapment in the fibers of the origin of the hamstrings the ischial tuberosity In association with hamstring tear	Pain from ischial tuberosity to posterior thigh; neurological and straight leg raise tests are negative; symptoms provoked by stretching, sitting, and running Differentiation: • Hamstring tear alone: Pain with palpation of muscle, with or without bruising; slump test negative • Sciatic nerve or nerve root involved; slump test positive (see Figure 20-16)

Modified from Drye C, Zachazewski JE: Peripheral nerve injuries. In Zachazewski JE, Magee DJ, Quillen WS, editors: *Athletic injuries and rehabilitation*, p 454, Philadelphia, 1996, WB Saunders.

Hamstring syndrome results from entrapment of the sciatic nerve by tight tendinous bands near the lateral origin of the hamstrings at the ischial tuberosity.[96] It often is found in sprinters and hurdlers. Pain is felt at the ischial tuberosity and may radiate down the posterior thigh. Symptoms are aggravated by sitting, stretching, or running. The results of neurological and straight leg raise tests usually are negative. Surgical release of the tendinous bands usually is successful in relieving symptoms.[96]

Pain from a torn hamstring muscle must be differentiated from irritation of the lumbar nerve roots and the sciatic nerve. The slump sitting test helps to differentiate pain arising from neural or muscular structures (Figure 20-16). The test combines full neck and trunk flexion, knee

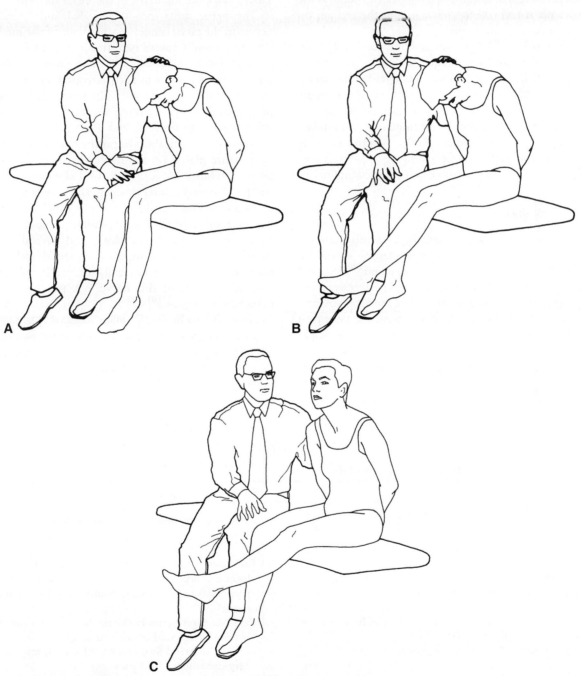

Figure 20-16

The slump test is designed to stress the neural structures in the spinal canal and along the course of the sciatic nerve. The test consists of trunk flexion, neck flexion **(A)**, knee extension **(B)**, and, as needed, dorsiflexion of the ankle and hip flexion, adduction, or internal rotation. If knee extension increases or symptoms decrease when the neck flexion component is released **(C)**, the test is considered positive. (From Butler D: *The sensitive nervous system,* p 292, Adelaide, 2000, Noigroup Publications.)

extension, ankle dorsiflexion, and hip flexion in a sitting position.[7,97] It places tensile stress on the neural tissues throughout the spinal canal and the sciatic nerve. Pain from a stretch on the neural tissue can be differentiated from muscular pain from the hamstrings if the leg is maintained in the same degree of knee extension that reproduces the muscle pain and the head and neck are extended. If the pain is decreased, neural structures are implicated, because the muscle length has not been changed, and the tension on the neural tissues has decreased.[98]

Kornberg and Lew[99] demonstrated that use of the slump sitting test as a treatment technique facilitates faster return to play in Australian football players with grade I hamstring tears, indicating that in some cases motion of the sciatic nerve must be impaired as it passes through the muscle either before the tear or from the inflammation and exudate surrounding the nerve after injury. Butler[7,49] advocates early but gentle motion of the muscle and nerve to prevent scarring and adhesion formation between the muscle and nerve.

Tibial Nerve Injury

The tibial nerve (Table 20-9) usually descends vertically through the popliteal space, where it may be vulnerable to compression by a Baker's cyst.[57,61] Ekelund[100] reported one case of a female athlete who presented with entrapment of the nerve in the proximal portion of the medial gastrocnemius muscle. Her main complaint was posterior knee pain with training. She had tenderness over the nerve on palpation. Surgical release relieved her symptoms completely.

Entrapment of the tibial nerve in the tarsal tunnel (**tarsal tunnel syndrome**) usually occurs as a result of an alteration in the size or shape of the tunnel owing to fracture,

dislocation, trauma, lipoma, tendon sheath cyst, or direct pressure. It also can occur from acute or chronic eversion.[61,101,102] The classic symptoms include pain at the medial malleolus radiating to the sole of the foot, the heel, and sometimes the calf; paresthesia; worsening of the symptoms at night, with walking or running, or with dorsiflexion; and weakness of toe flexion. Pain is reproduced with Tinel's test over the nerve in the tarsal tunnel.[101]

The nerve splits into the medial and lateral plantar nerves in the tarsal tunnel. Entrapment of the medial plantar nerve usually causes paresthesia or pain in the medial three and one half toes.[101,102] The medial plantar nerve can also be entrapped in a hypertrophic or fibrous abductor muscle of the great toe.[61] The repetitive nature of running combined with altered mechanics of the foot and ankle places the nerve at risk for stretch injuries in the tarsal tunnel. Ironically, symptoms may also be provoked by pressure placed on the medial arch by new arch supports.[38] Johnson et al.[103] reported similar problems in a competitive weight lifter owing to the large weight-bearing loads on the foot.

Entrapment of the lateral plantar nerve causes similar symptoms in the lateral foot and lateral two toes. Branches of this nerve supply the medial heel and calcaneus and the long plantar ligament. Irritation of the calcaneal branch of this nerve is a potential source of persistent heel pain.[101,102]

According to Butler,[7,49] many cases of "plantar fasciitis" may be neurogenic in origin. An important part of the differential diagnosis of neurogenic and fascial pain is the use of tests to detect increased mechanical sensitivity of the nerves. To differentiate the cause of pain, the foot and ankle are positioned in a pain-provoking position for

Table 20-9
Tibial Nerve (L4-S3): Sites of Entrapment or Irritation

Cause/Site	Signs and Symptoms
Popliteal space: • Compression by Baker's cyst • Entrapment in proximal portion of medial gastrocnemius	Posterior knee pain, possibly radiating to calf
Tarsal tunnel: • Space-occupying lesion (e.g., osteophyte, ganglion) • Eversion strain (acute or repetitive)	Pain from medial malleolus to the heel, sole of the foot, and occasionally to the calf; worse at night or with walking or running; positive Tinel's test at tarsal tunnel
Medial plantar nerve distal to tarsal tunnel or in hypertrophic abductor muscle of the thumb	Pain and paresthesias in the medial 3½ toes with weight bearing under load or with running
Lateral plantar nerve distal to tarsal tunnel	Pain in the lateral foot and lateral 2 toes; may cause persistent medial heel pain
Interdigital neuromas: • Compression from callus formation under the metatarsal heads • Stretching of nerve under the deep transverse tarsal ligament	Pain and paresthesias at the metatarsal heads that may radiate proximally or to toes

Modified from Drye C, Zachazewski JE: Peripheral nerve injuries. In Zachazewski JE, Magee DJ, Quillen WS, editors: *Athletic injuries and rehabilitation,* p 455, Philadelphia, 1996, WB Saunders.

Figure 20-17

Maximum toe extension and dorsiflexion place tensile stress on the plantar fascia. The position shown is maintained while the lower extremity is raised in a straight leg raise. If symptoms increase with the addition of the straight leg raise, neural structures are implicated, because the tension on the plantar fascia has not changed. (From Butler D: *The sensitive nervous system*, p 280, Adelaide, 2000, Noigroup Publications.)

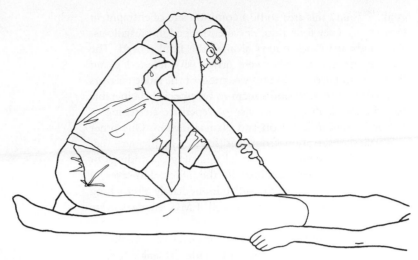

plantar fasciitis (dorsiflexion of the foot and toes), and movement of a proximal part of the limb is superimposed, increasing the tension on the tibial nerve and its branches (Figure 20-17). The plantar fascia is not stressed further by a straight leg raise. Therefore, if symptoms increase in response to the test, they are likely to have at least a partial neurogenic origin.[7]

Interdigital neuromas most often occur in runners and dancers because of the repetitive dorsiflexion of the metatarsophalangeal joints. The nerve is stretched under the deep transverse metatarsal ligament. Compression also can occur as a result of increased pressure on the nerve from callus formation under the metatarsal heads. Pain and paresthesia are felt at the metatarsal heads and may radiate proximally or to the toes.[102] Treatment usually consists of rest, modification of footwear, corticosteroid injection, or surgical excision of the neuroma. Mobilization of the intermetatarsal joints may help alter the mechanical interface among the nerve, the metatarsal heads, and the transverse ligament.[7]

Common Peroneal (Fibular) Nerve Injury

The peroneal or fibular nerve (Table 20-10) is formed from fibers from the L4-S2 nerve roots. It diverges from the sciatic nerve in the upper part of the popliteal space. Nobel[104] described two patients who developed a hematoma of the nerve just distal to the bifurcation from the sciatic nerve after an inversion sprain of the ankle or fracture of the lower leg. He hypothesized that the blood vessels supplying the nerve were ruptured by abrupt longitudinal traction on the nerve. Evacuation of the hematoma relieved the patients' discomfort completely.

This nerve is vulnerable to compression injuries from a direct blow, a lower leg cast, or sustained pressure at the point where the nerve passes around the head of the fibula (e.g., a race car driver leaning his leg against a car door).[27] McMahon and Craig[105] reported common peroneal (fibular) nerve injury after a severe varus force caused disruption of the anterior cruciate ligament (ACL), lateral collateral ligament (LCL), iliotibial band, and biceps tendon. Leach

Table 20-10
Common Peroneal (Fibular) Nerve (L4-S2): Areas of Entrapment or Irritation

Cause/Site	Signs and Symptoms
Traction injury at bifurcation from sciatic nerve	Acute onset of severe lateral leg pain from hematoma formation within the nerve after ankle fracture or inversion sprain
Fibular head: Compression from a blow or entrapment	Pain and/or paresthesias of the lateral leg and foot; electromyogram (EMG) may not be positive in entrapment unless symptoms have been provoked by increased activity
Dorsolateral ankle after a sprain	Lateral foot and ankle pain/paresthesias; possible EMG findings; positive straight leg raise test with plantar flexion/inversion of foot and ankle
Dorsolateral ankle: Superficial or deep fibular nerve compressed by fascial bands, swelling, or ill-fitting boots or shoes	Pain and/or paresthesias in the dorsolateral foot and ankle; symptoms provoked with palpation of the nerve at the site of the lesion; positive straight leg raise test with plantar flexion/inversion of foot and ankle

Modified from Drye C, Zachazewski JE: Peripheral nerve injuries. In Zachazewski JE, Magee DJ, Quillen WS, editors: *Athletic injuries and rehabilitation*, p 457, Philadelphia, 1996, WB Saunders.

et al.[106] found this area to be a common site of entrapment in runners. They found the nerve entrapped in musculofascial bands at various points around the fibular head. The main symptoms reported were progressive lateral leg and foot pain and paresthesia and weakness of the ankle evertors and toe extensors. Runners seem to be especially vulnerable to irritation at this site because of repetitive stretching of the nerve during inversion and plantar flexion. One other important observation from this study was the fact that many of the patients had normal neurological findings or EMG studies when examined in the office. However, if the patients returned to the office immediately after a long run, the neurological findings and EMG changes were much more pronounced.

Common peroneal (fibular) nerve injury should also be considered a probable sequela of grade III ankle sprains or fractures. Grade III sprains involve disruption of the lateral ligaments, the deltoid ligament, and the distal anterior talofibular ligament. Nitz et al.[107] found a high incidence of common peroneal (fibular) and tibial nerve injuries in patients with this type of sprain. Thirty-one of 36 patients (86%) had evidence of common peroneal (fibular) nerve injuries, and 30 of 36 (83%) had tibial nerve injuries; 19 patients in this group also had sensory losses. Of 30 patients with grade II sprains (tearing of lateral ligaments and deltoid ligaments), five had common peroneal (fibular) nerve injuries and three had tibial nerve injuries.

Further evidence of possible neural involvement in ankle inversions sprains was provided by Pahor and Toppenberg.[108] These authors explored responses to the slump test with the foot held in plantar flexion and inversion in 18 subjects who had a history of single or multiple ankle inversion injuries (severity not reported), at least 6 months before neurodynamic testing. Subjects experienced greater reductions in knee extension mobility and more widespread symptoms in the distribution of the common peroneal (fibular) nerve on the involved extremities. Releasing cervical flexion reduced symptoms provoked in the slump test position, confirming a neurogenic contribution to the test response and evidence of increased mechanosensitivity in the common peroneal (fibular) branch of the sciatic tract.

The superficial peroneal (fibular) nerve can be entrapped as it exits from the deep fascia in the lower leg to cross the dorsolateral ankle.[102] Entrapment of this nerve causes numbness or tingling over the dorsum of the foot. The deep peroneal (fibular) nerve can be injured as it crosses the dorsum of the ankle under the extensor retinaculum, where it is vulnerable to compression from ill-fitting boots or shoes or from swelling or osteophytes after a fracture. It also is vulnerable at this site to traction from repetitive ankle sprains.[27] Both sites of injury are more common in runners.[102]

A modification of the straight leg raise test can be used to differentiate neurogenic causes from ligament or joint causes of persistent dorsolateral foot and ankle pain.[7] The

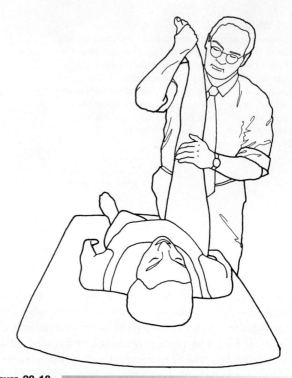

Figure 20-18

The source of lateral ankle pain (i.e., differentiation between a ligament sprain vs. nerve irritation) can be differentiated with the following test. The ankle is placed in the pain-provoking position of inversion and plantar flexion. A straight leg raise is then performed, increasing tensile stresses on the fibular nerve but not on the ankle joint and ligaments. Hip adduction and internal rotation place further tension on the lumbosacral nerve roots and fibular nerve. (From Butler D: *The sensitive nervous system*, p 281, Adelaide, 2000, Noigroup Publications.)

test is similar to the test described earlier for plantar foot pain. In this case, the foot and ankle are held in the pain-provoking position of inversion and plantar flexion, and the entire lower extremity is raised into a straight leg raise (Figure 20-18). Symptoms caused by abnormality along the common peroneal (fibular) nerve tract increase with this test. Symptoms caused by joint and/or ligament abnormality do not change.

Femoral Nerve Injury

The femoral nerve is formed from the posterior branches of the L2-L4 nerve roots.[57] Different mechanisms can cause injury to the nerve. Compression may occur in the iliac compartment as a result of a hematoma, and this possibility should be considered in any patient who is on anticoagulant therapy or who has hemophilia[61] or a history of trauma to the iliacus. Giuliani et al.[109] reported a case of a healthy 14-year-old who developed a hematoma and femoral nerve injury after minor trauma during gymnastics (Figure 20-19). The nerve is vulnerable to compression as it passes under the inguinal ligament in athletes or workers who must squat

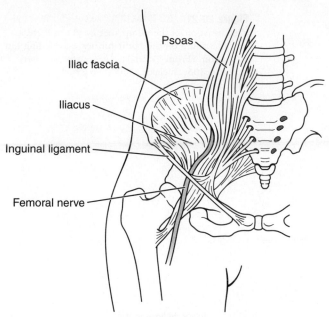

Figure 20-19

Compression of the femoral nerve by an iliacus hematoma. The ballooned right iliacus muscle compresses the femoral nerve against the psoas muscle. (Redrawn from Giuliani G, Poppi M, Acciarri N, Forti A: CT scan and surgical treatment of traumatic iliacus hematoma with femoral neuropathy: case report, *J Trauma* 30:230, 1990.)

for long periods or wear protective clothing that compresses this area. It also may be vulnerable to injury during gynecological or hip surgery.[61]

Sammarco and Stephens[110] described one case of femoral nerve palsy in a modern dancer. The apparent mechanism of injury was traction from dance positions that required simultaneous hip extension and knee flexion. This position is similar to that used in the prone knee bend test for tension on the femoral nerve and L3-L4 nerve roots (Figure 20-20).[3]

Figure 20-20

Prone knee bending is a common test for tension on the femoral nerve and L3 and L4 nerve roots. (From Butler D: *The sensitive nervous system*, p 302, Adelaide, 2000, Noigroup Publications.)

Obturator Nerve Injury

The obturator nerve is derived from the anterior divisions of the lumbar plexus (L2-L4). It emerges from the medial border of the psoas near the brim of the pelvis and passes through the obturator foramen to the medial side of the thigh.[57] Injury can occur from pelvic tumors, obturator hernias, or pelvic and proximal femoral fractures.[57] The nerve supplies the great adductor and external obturator muscles, as well as part of the sensory innervation for the hip joint and medial thigh.

Butler[7] suggested that entrapment of the obturator nerve may contribute to complaints of persistent groin pain in an athlete with an adductor muscle strain. He suggested modifying the slump sitting test to examine for mechanosensitivity of the obturator nerve by positioning the patient in a sitting position with the leg abducted to the point where groin symptoms are felt. If subsequent alteration of trunk or neck flexion or side flexion alters the groin pain, the disorder may have a neurogenic component. Another neurodynamic test used to evaluate the obturator nerve is the slump knee bend test with the involved leg in abduction (Figure 20-21).[49]

Sensory Nerve Injury

The sensory branches of lower extremity peripheral nerves are vulnerable to entrapment or friction at many points in the lower quarter. Symptoms may include paresthesias, areas of numbness, or pain. A patient in one author's practice had compression of the sensory nerves as they passed over the iliac crest to the buttocks after a fall onto the back and buttocks. Palpation of the nerves reproduced the specific sensory complaints that the patient reported.

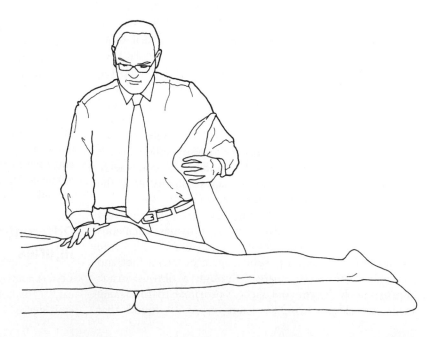

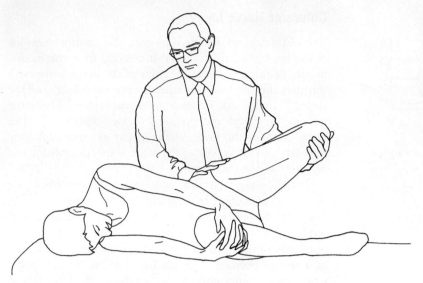

Figure 20-21
This variation of the slump knee bend test increases tensile loading on the obturator nerve by adding hip abduction. (From Butler D: *The sensitive nervous system,* p 306, Adelaide, 2000, Noigroup Publications.)

Meralgia paresthetica is a condition caused by irritation of the lateral cutaneous nerve of the thigh, which provides sensation over the anterolateral portion of the thigh.[57] The nerve is formed from the L3 and L4 nerve roots. It is vulnerable to compression or kinking as it passes from the pelvis through the fascia to the thigh or as it passes under the inguinal ligament. It may be compromised by pressure from protective equipment (e.g., a tight belt used to carry tools), from weight belts that are worn too tight, or by direct trauma.[111] This nerve injury is more common in diabetic, pregnant, and obese patients.[57,61] It also is associated with degeneration of the symphysis pubis in patients over 40 years of age, possibly as a result of increased tension on the ilioinguinal ligament.[112]

The sartorial nerve is a cutaneous branch of the obturator nerve and provides sensation to the medial knee joint.[57,113] It is vulnerable to injury from valgus stresses at the knee and during surgical procedures on the medial knee.[113]

The saphenous branch of the femoral nerve can be entrapped in the adductor canal of the medial thigh (Figure 20-22). The patient may complain of medial knee pain or paresthesias in the medial lower leg. Compression increases during strong muscular contraction, as during squats or knee extension exercises.[38] Pendergrass and Moore[114] reported a case of saphenous nerve injury from a direct blow to the thigh by a heavy truck tire. Release of the resulting fibrotic scar was necessary to resolve the patient's symptoms. Butler[7] has devised a modified femoral nerve stretch test to test for adverse mechanosensitivity along the saphenous portion of the femoral nerve (Figure 20-23).

The sural nerve, derived from branches of the tibial and common peroneal (fibular) nerves, provides cutaneous innervation to the lateral lower leg and foot;[57] this nerve should be considered a possible source of lateral foot and calf pain. The nerve emerges through a fibrous arcade approximately 16 cm (6.3 inches) proximal to the lateral malleolus (Figure 20-24). Fabre et al.[115] found that

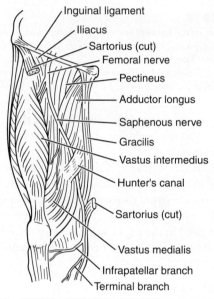

Inguinal ligament
Iliacus
Sartorius (cut)
Femoral nerve
Pectineus
Adductor longus
Saphenous nerve
Gracilis
Vastus intermedius
Hunter's canal
Sartorius (cut)
Vastus medialis
Infrapatellar branch
Terminal branch

Figure 20-22
The saphenous nerve is vulnerable to entrapment in the adductor canal of the thigh.

entrapment at this site was the source of chronic calf pain in 10 runners who failed to respond to conservative treatment. The sural nerve can be palpated laterally in the foot and proximal to the malleolus.[7] Like the fibular nerve, it is vulnerable to injury from repetitive inversion sprains of the ankle or compression from ill-fitting shoes.[7,102]

Differential Diagnosis of Peripheral Nerve Injuries

Leffert's advice, "When in doubt, do a history and physical,"[116] is critical in the differential diagnosis of peripheral nerve injuries. The subjective examination must

Figure 20-23

Tension can be placed on the saphenous nerve by placing the lower extremity in hip extension, external rotation, knee extension, and hip abduction. (From Butler D: *The sensitive nervous system*, p 306, Adelaide, 2000, Noigroup Publications.)

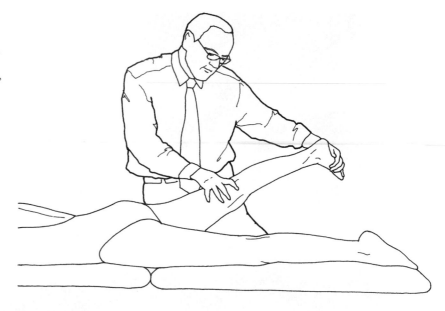

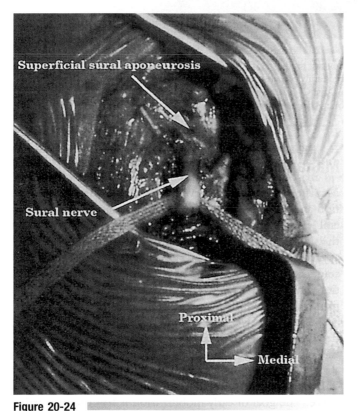

Figure 20-24

The sural nerve can become entrapped in the superficial sural aponeurosis and the fibrous band where the nerve passes through it. (From Fabre T, Montero C, Gaujard E et al: Chronic calf pain in athletes due to sural nerve entrapment, *Am J Sports Med* 28:680, 2000.)

delineate the specific type of symptoms and the area where they are occurring. Paresthesia or sensory losses should be mapped to determine whether the symptoms are in a dermatomal or peripheral nerve distribution.[3]

The precipitating injury or predisposing factors from overtraining or biomechanical abnormalities should give clues as to which nerves might have been injured. A nerve injury should always be suspected if the athlete experiences sensory changes in addition to weakness and/or pain.

Important components of objective testing include reflex, strength, and sensory testing; Tinel's test over the nerve trunks; and palpation along the course of the nerve (Figure 20-25).[7,49] EMG is an important component of the evaluation of peripheral nerve injuries. As mentioned earlier, the timing of the examination is crucial. Abnormalities in the sensory nerve action potentials (SNAPs) and combined motor action potentials (CMAPs) are not evident for 7 to 10 days after injury. Fibrillations caused by denervation of muscles are not evident for 3 to 5 weeks,[34,116] which makes distinguishing between an axonotmesis and a neurotmesis difficult in the first few days and weeks after an injury. According to Wilbourn,[34] EMG examination is most useful when performed between 3 weeks and 3 to 6 months after injury.

In addition to neural conductivity tests, several tests have been described that check for mechanical sensitivity along nerve trunks. These are useful for identifying the pathomechanics of neural structures and their contribution to symptoms. Butler[7,49] and Shacklock[117] detail the applications and variations of these tests in their texts on mobilization of the nervous system. The tests are thought to be clinically significant when a difference exists in any of the following variables when the symptomatic side is compared with the asymptomatic side: available range of motion, resistance to motion as perceived by the clinician, symptom reproduction, or deviation from the established symptomatic responses in normals. The tests are considered particularly relevant if

Correct diagnosis and definitive treatment are important in patients with navicular stress fractures, because delay in diagnosis can result in prolonged disability. Navicular stress fractures treated with rest and a gradual return to activity have a high incidence of delayed union and nonunion.[113] The recommended treatment for navicular stress fractures is immobilization in a non-weight-bearing cast for at least 6 weeks.[113,230] Even complete navicular stress fractures have been shown to heal with this regimen. After 6 weeks, the patient's cast is removed and healing is assessed by palpation on the N spot. Radiographs or bone scans should not be used to monitor progress of the fracture, because imaging signs of healing lag well behind clinical healing. A 6-week rehabilitation program consisting of joint mobilization, muscle strengthening, and gradual return to activity can begin when the patient has no pain on palpation of the N spot.[113,230]

Fifth Metatarsal

Stress fractures of the metatarsals most often occur in the second and third metatarsals. A less common yet important variant is a diaphyseal stress fracture of the fifth metatarsal. This type of stress fracture occurs in the proximal 1.5 cm (0.6 inch) of the diaphysis and sometimes is mistaken for a Jones fracture.[231-233] The term *Jones fracture* should be reserved for an acute fracture of the fifth metatarsal, at the level of the articular facet between the fourth and fifth metatarsals, that does not extend distally.[234] Diaphyseal stress fractures of the fifth metatarsal commonly present with localized pain and tenderness near the base of the metatarsal, and dorsal swelling is seen in this area. Diagnosis is important, because these fractures have a high potential for delayed union, nonunion, and refracture.[231,235]

The treatment of fifth metatarsal diaphyseal stress fractures depends on their classification. Torg et al.[236] described three subtypes of diaphyseal stress fractures: type I is the acute or early form; type II is characterized by delayed union, and type III involves nonunion. A type I stress fracture is an early stress fracture with periosteal reaction that represents healing of an incomplete fracture. Radiography confirms the fracture and shows no medullary sclerosis. This subtype has a good prognosis with immobilization in a nonwalking, short leg cast for 6 weeks,[198,232] after which healing is assessed clinically and radiographically. Patients can then gradually resume activity. An alternative management option is to use intramedullary screw fixation; however, the time to union using this technique is identical to that with conservative management.[237]

Type II and type III stress fractures frequently present as an apparent acute fracture, but when questioned, the patient describes a variable history of pain at the fracture site with activity. Radiography shows a fracture line and, depending on the duration of symptoms, may show medullary sclerosis

or established nonunion with complete intramedullary obliteration. These subtypes may heal with prolonged cast immobilization (3 to 6 months); however, surgical treatment produces more rapid and predictable healing.[238] Intramedullary screw fixation is advocated for type II and type III diaphyseal stress fractures, and bone grafting is variably used for type III stress fractures.[232,237,238] Patients typically return to activity 6 weeks (screw fixation) or 12 weeks (bone grafting) after surgery.[198,219]

Great Toe Sesamoid

The sesamoids of the great toe are embedded in the flexor hallucis brevis and receive fibrous insertions from abductor and adductor brevis muscles. They function to increase the mechanical advantage of the flexor hallucis brevis, assist with weight bearing under the first metatarsal, and elevate the metatarsal head off the ground. As such, they are exposed to repetitive loads and are prone to stress fracture in weight-bearing individuals, especially athletes. Stress fractures most often occur in the tibial sesamoid, because it receives most of the weight transmitted by the first metatarsal.[239]

Sesamoid stress fractures typically present as forefoot pain during loading that increases with dorsiflexion of the great toe and decreases with rest. Palpation is used to determine the presence of localized sesamoid pain. Because these symptoms also are consistent with sesamoiditis, the diagnosis often is delayed. Similarly, the diagnosis can be influenced by the presence of a bipartite or multipartite sesamoid, which frequently is present in normal, asymptomatic individuals.[240] Any delay in the diagnosis of sesamoid stress fractures can be problematic, because prolonged morbidity and progression to nonunion are relatively common. The initial management of sesamoid stress fractures is conservative, with non-weight-bearing for 4 weeks. Given the important functional role of the sesamoids, surgical removal should be considered only if conservative management fails.

Summary

Repetitive stress injuries to bone present along a pathology continuum ranging from stress reactions to complete bone fractures. For this reason, signs and symptoms often vary, depending upon the stage in which a patient presents. Similarly, recovery times also vary. Typically, the earlier an individual is diagnosed, the better and quicker is the response to management. Therefore a certain level of suspicion needs to be maintained at all times in appropriately presenting patients. The diagnosis typically is made clinically by a history consistent with an overuse injury and is confirmed radiographically. In confirmed cases of a repetitive stress injury to bone, management is determined by the risk for healing complications. Low risk stress injures represent relatively straightforward management problems and typically respond to relative rest from the aggravating activity and removal or modification of risk factors. High risk stress fractures, on the other hand, are prone to complication and require specific management.

References

To enhance this text and add value for the reader, all references have been incorporated into a CD-ROM that is provided with this text. The reader can view the reference source and access it online whenever possible. There are a total of 240 references for this chapter.

development of work-related MSDs than men, although this is highly industry dependent.[3,8-10] Advanced age may increase the impact of other risk factors on the severity of MSDs,[3,7,9] and obesity has been shown to predict the onset of MSDs.[11,12]

Work-related MSDs, therefore, have multifactorial causes, and the interaction between physical and nonphysical and workplace and nonworkplace risk factors is complex. This complexity contributes to the persistent controversy surrounding governmental regulation of these disorders. Consequently, private industry in the United States addresses these disorders on a voluntary basis, using industry-specific guidelines provided by the Occupational Safety and Health Administration (OSHA) (www.osha.gov).

Clinical Point

When treating patients with work-related MSDs, health care providers must bear in mind the complexity of causal factors and attempt to identify and address all of them in a comprehensive, holistic approach that emphasizes patient education.

U.S. Department of Labor Survey of Health Statistics

According to the most recent Bureau of Labor Statistics survey, work-related MSDs accounted for 435,180 (33%) lost workday injuries and illnesses in U.S. industry in 2003.[1] Repetitive motion (e.g., grasping tools, scanning groceries, and typing) was one of the most common events or exposures leading to work-related MSDs, and it accounted for the longest absences from work by exposure type (median of 22 lost days). The three occupational groups with the most work-related MSDs were (1) nursing aides, orderlies, and attendants (33,710 cases), (2) laborers and material movers (33,090 cases), and (3) truck drivers (20,580 cases). The first two groups involve jobs requiring heavy and repetitive lifting, whereas truck driving requires prolonged sitting with exposure to whole body vibration.

Work-related MSDs continue to cause substantial worker discomfort, disability, and loss of productivity. Among the remaining top 15 occupations reporting work-related MSDs were stock clerks and order fillers (repetitive moderate lifting and grasping), construction laborers (lifting and use of hand tools, some with vibration), and cashiers (repetitive light to moderate lifting and grasping). The service industries (e.g., health care) accounted for 71% of all MSDs, and goods-producing industries (e.g., manufacturing) accounted for the remaining 29%. Carpal tunnel syndrome was among the major disabling injuries and illnesses in 2003, and it had the highest median of lost workdays (32). Injuries to the wrist had a median of 17 lost workdays. These patterns of lost-workday injuries and illnesses show the impact of upper limb MSDs in the U.S. workforce.

Scope of Workplace Musculoskeletal Disorders in U.S. Industry

- One in three lost-workday injuries and illnesses is a work-related musculoskeletal disorder
- Work-related MSDs caused by repetitive motion had a median of 22 lost workdays
- Carpal tunnel syndrome has the highest number of lost workdays, a median of 32 days
- Wrist injuries have a median of 17 lost workdays

Epidemiological Evidence of Work-Related Repetitive Overuse Injuries of the Hand and Wrist

Two comprehensive reviews of the literature concerning work-related MSDs have been completed since 1997. A review undertaken by the National Institute for Occupational Safety and Health (NIOSH) included more than 600 epidemiological studies, dating from the 1970s to the mid-1990s, concerning work-related MSDs of the neck, upper extremity, and low back.[2] In this review, the framework for evaluating epidemiological evidence for a causal relationship between workplace risk factors and work-related MSDs included an evaluation of strength of association within studies, consistency across reviewed studies, temporality between exposure and work-related MSD outcome, evidence of an exposure-response relationship, and coherence of evidence. Based on this framework, evidence for a relationship between workplace risk factors and the development of work-related MSDs was classified into one of four categories: strong evidence of work-relatedness, evidence of work-relatedness, insufficient evidence of work-relatedness, and evidence of no effect of work factors.

The National Research Council (NRC) and the Institute of Medicine conducted a second, more exclusive review of the work-related MSD literature.[3] The NRC review included studies from the late 1970s to the late 1990s that examined tissue pathophysiology; mechanical, organizational, and psychosocial risk factors; and clinical interventions for work-related MSDs of the upper extremity and low back. For epidemiological studies of the upper extremity, the panel reviewed 42 studies of physical risk factors and 28 studies of psychosocial risk factors. These studies were selected from a larger candidate list of studies based on selection criteria that would allow the reporting or calculation of relative risk or attributable fraction, two epidemiological quantities used to estimate the effect of an exposure on the development of a health outcome.

For the purpose of this discussion, the findings of these two major reviews concerning the epidemiology of the most prevalent work-related hand and wrist disorders are summarized; those disorders are carpal tunnel syndrome and disorders of musculotendinous tissues.

Carpal Tunnel Syndrome

The NIOSH review reported strong evidence for a relationship between exposure to combinations of force and repetition or force and posture and the development of carpal tunnel syndrome (CTS). Evidence of a relationship between cumulative exposure to force, repetition, or hand/wrist vibration and CTS also was seen. The evidence was insufficient to determine the role of awkward postures alone in the development of CTS.

The NRC review included 15 studies of upper limb peripheral nerve disorders. Three studies reported an increased risk of CTS with exposure to high force alone.[4,13,14] Four studies reported an increased risk of sensory disturbances or CTS with exposure to vibration alone.[15-18] Four studies reported an increased risk of CTS with exposure to high repetition alone.[4,13,19,20] One study reported decreased nerve conduction velocity of the median nerve with exposure to a combination of repetitive motion and awkward posture.[21] One study reported an increased risk of CTS with exposure to cold temperatures.[19] Four studies reported an increased risk of CTS with exposure to various combinations of force, repetition, vibration, and cold temperatures.[4,13,19,20]

Musculotendinous Disorders

The NIOSH review reported that strong evidence existed that combinations of force and repetition were associated with the development of hand/wrist tendonitis. Evidence of a relationship between exposure to force, repetition, or awkward postures alone and hand/wrist tendonitis also was seen.

The NRC review included nine studies concerning musculotendinous disorders of the hand and wrist associated with exposure to physical risk factors. Five studies reported an increased risk of musculotendinous disorders with exposure to force alone.[4,22-27] Two studies found an association between exposure to vibration alone and musculotendinous disorders.[15,16] Two studies found an association between musculotendinous disorders and exposure to repetition alone[20] or to a combination of force and repetition.[4] Thirteen studies reported a positive association between psychosocial risk factors ·(e.g., job stress, job satisfaction, work demands) and hand and wrist discomfort or disorders.[4,28-39]

The overall conclusions of the NIOSH and NRC reviews, therefore, were essentially the same: evidence supports associations between workplace physical risk factors and hand and wrist work-related MSDs. The NRC study further examined the importance of psychosocial factors as contributors to the risk of hand and wrist MSD development. Both the NIOSH and NRC reviews identified gaps in the literature in the hope of guiding future research. In subsequent years, investigators began to address some of these issues, and a review of epidemiological studies from 1998 to 2003 concerning CTS and hand/wrist disorders recently was published.[40] Table 22-1 presents a more recent update of the epidemiological literature concerning CTS and hand/wrist musculotendinous disorders.

Epidemiological studies, many of them longitudinal rather than cross sectional, continue to support a causal relationship between prolonged exposure to highly repetitive and/or forceful hand-intensive tasks, vibration, psychosocial stress at work, and the development of CTS or other MSDs related to hand/wrist activities.[11,12,41-45] In addition, a past history of CTS or hand/wrist pain or discomfort increases an individual's risk of developing a new MSD related to upper limb activity or of exacerbating the existing activity-related MSD.[11,12,43,44]

Hours of computer mouse and keyboard use, as well as a history of computer use, are associated with an increased prevalence and incidence of upper limb discomfort and MSDs; however, controversy still exists in the literature concerning the magnitude and severity of computer-related MSDs.[44-48] MSDs related to upper limb activity have a higher prevalence and incidence in women,[45,48] and one author has shown that motherhood exacerbates this gender relationship by providing fewer opportunities for working mothers to relax and exercise outside of work.[49] Several investigators found an increased risk for work-related upper limb MSDs with increasing age and with a body mass index (BMI) near the borderline for obesity.[11,12,41,43]

The studies summarized in this chapter and those summarized in earlier reviews of the epidemiological literature support the contribution of physical and psychosocial risk factors at work to the development of upper limb MSDs. Studies also verify the multifactorial nature of these disorders and the role of nonworkplace risk factors and individual predisposing characteristics in their development. Clinicians need to be aware of all the factors that may have a bearing on the proper treatment of patients with work-related MSDs.

Management of Work-Related Musculoskeletal Disorders

Workplace Management

OSHA currently is developing industry-specific and task-specific ergonomic guidelines for voluntary use by U.S. employers.[50] Thus far, guidelines have been established for meatpacking plants,[51] nursing homes,[52] retail grocery stores[53] and poultry processing.[54] All of these guidelines embrace the same basic program components, which are set forth in the OSHA guidelines for nursing homes:

1. *Management support:* Clearly developed program goals, clearly identified program responsibilities for participants, adequate provision of resources, and oversight to ensure the success of the program.
2. *Employee involvement:* Early employee reporting of problems; also, employees provide insight (suggestions and evaluation) into work design issues and

Table 22-1
Summary of Recent Epidemiological Studies on Work-Related Carpal Tunnel Syndrome and Other Musculoskeletal Disorders of the Hand and Wrist

Authors (Country)	Sample	Study Design	Findings	Conclusions
Alexopoulos et al.[41] (Greece)	430 Dentists	Cross sectional survey of physical and psychosocial workload and complaints of musculoskeletal symptoms	Strenuous shoulder movements, use of vibrating tools, strenuous back postures, repetitive shoulder/hand movements, high perceived exertion, high need for recovery, and moderate perceived general health were associated with increased risk for hand/wrist complaints. Strenuous shoulder/hand movements were associated with increased risk of chronicity and absenteeism. Chronicity increased with age.	Physical load among dentists places them at risk for MSDs. Psychosocial factors, such as perceived health status and perceived exertion, are associated with more severe complaints and absenteeism.
Bovenzi et al.[42] (Italy)	159 Forestry workers and 146 manual laborer controls	Cross sectional, control group design to determine prevalence of vibration-induced white finger, CTS, and soft tissue disorders	Forestry workers showed increased prevalence of peripheral sensorineural disturbances, soft tissue disorders of the upper limbs, and CTS compared to controls. Increased vibration exposure, through the use of chain saws, and increased years of tool use among forestry workers were associated with peripheral neuropathies.	Exposure of forestry workers to a combination of risk factors (segmental vibration, forcefulness, and awkward postures) is associated with the occurrence of peripheral neuropathies and soft tissue disorders of the upper limb.
Gell et al.[43] (United States)	432 Industrial and clerical workers with no history of carpal tunnel syndrome	Longitudinal study over 5.4 years to develop a predictive model for work-related CTS	Average incidence rate of CTS was 1.2% per year. Multiple regression indicated that workers with baseline numbness, tingling, burning and/or pain in the fingers were 5.2 times more likely to develop CTS. For each 0.1 msec increase in median-ulnar peak latency, the relative risk for developing CTS increased 29%. Risk of CTS tended to risk with increased BMI and high risk hand threshold limit values established by the ACGIH.	Incidence rate in this population was higher than in the general population. This study corroborated findings from earlier cross sectional studies; the findings indicated that workers may be predictors of future CTS and that these workers therefore are logical targets for preventive intervention.

Study	Population	Purpose	Results	Comments
Hamilton et al.[46] (United States)	111 Female college students (72 respondents)	Cross sectional study to determine prevalence of computer-related musculoskeletal complaints and their association with hours of use, laptop use, and job strain	Eighty-one percent of respondents reported computer-related musculoskeletal complaints. None of the factors examined were statistically associated with those complaints. Although not statistically significant, 90% of respondents using a laptop computer reported musculoskeletal complaints.	Most students reported computer-related musculoskeletal discomfort. Future studies should include more diverse student populations.
Jensen[44] (Denmark)	2576 Employees who use computers	Longitudinal study to determine risk factors for musculoskeletal symptoms in the neck and hand/wrist	Hand/wrist symptoms were predicted by previous symptoms at baseline and low influence at work for both men and women and by sensorial demands for women only. Almost continual or continual computer use was associated with increased hand/wrist symptoms.	Early intervention for reported hand/wrist symptoms can reduce persistent or recurrent symptoms. Psychosocial issues at work contribute to hand/wrist symptoms. Limiting computer use to less than 0.75 of the workday can help prevent hand/wrist symptoms.
Kryger et al.[45] (Denmark)	6943 Participants from public and private workplaces	Longitudinal study to determine prevalence and incidence of forearm pain, signs of tenderness and nerve entrapment, and association with computer work, physical workplace factors, and psychosocial factors	The 1-year incidence of self-reported forearm pain was 1.3%. Increased risk of new forearm pain was associated with more than 30 hours/week of mouse use and more than 15 hours/week of keyboard use. High job demands and time pressure at baseline increased the risk of new forearm pain. Women had a twofold increased risk of developing forearm pain.	Intensive mouse use and keyboard use were the main risk factors for forearm pain, but the overall incidence was low; therefore these activities cannot be considered severe occupational hazards.
Larsson et al.[134] (Denmark)	6943 Participants from public and private workplaces	Longitudinal study to determine relationship between computer work and elbow and wrist/hand pain, conditions, and disorders (only wrist/hand findings reported in this table)	The duration of mouse use and the duration of keyboard use were significantly associated with wrist/hand pain, and keyboard exposure showed a threshold effect with 12-month wrist/hand pain at 1-year follow-up. Clinical diagnoses on physical examination were not associated with mouse or keyboard exposure.	Self-reported, low force exposures of mouse and keyboard time predicted wrist/hand pain but were not predictors of clinical conditions on physical examination.

(Continued)

factors, which initiate migration of endothelial cells and the growth of new capillaries into the wound site.[74]

Lymphocytes are a third line of leukocytes. They are agranular and are divided into two main subsets, T cells (thymus derived) and B cells (plasma or memory cells that are not thymus dependent). T cells typically arrive 5 days after injury and peak by day 7.[65] They are long-lived cells (months to years) that typically are not seen during acute inflammation; rather, they are more prominent in chronic conditions.[75] T lymphocytes mediate the delayed immune response (cell mediated) by regulating B-lymphocyte and macrophage phagocytic functions.[63] In contrast, B lymphocytes are short-lived and do not play a role in cell-mediated immunity. Instead, they transform into antibody-producing plasma or memory B cells, and through the release of various cytokines (e.g., interferon gamma [IF-γ], IL-2, and TGF-β), they enhance macrophage function.[65] Lymphocytes are not required for the initiation of wound healing, but they are essential for normal repair because they secrete lymphokines, including TGF-β, TNF-α, and fibroblast-activating factor (FAF), all of which induce the proliferation of fibroblasts. However, high concentrations of these lymphokines, particularly TNF-α, are cytotoxic to fibroblasts and other cells.[65,76] Long-term continuation of an acute inflammatory response (i.e., chronic inflammation) can lead to cytotoxicity or fibrosis, and the latter is associated with excessive stimulation of fibroblast proliferation and collagen production.[59,77]

Repair Phase of Wound Healing Versus Chronic Inflammation and Fibrosis

Healing and Repair. The process of wound healing is an effort to restore normal tissue function and architecture after injury. Essentially, three primary outcomes are possible with tissue injury: (1) complete resolution with total restoration of normal tissue structure; (2) repair with scar formation of varying degrees, depending on the level of injury; and (3) chronic inflammation. *Complete restoration* is the regeneration or recreation of the tissue to a state in which it may even be in a better form or condition than before the injury. *Repair* is the process of mending tissue after decay or damage. The mended area may not be complete but may consist of a collagenous scar that fills the damaged tissue region. Substantial tissue injury may also occur in tissues with little capacity for regeneration (e.g., skeletal muscle and nerve) or after prolonged edema. The edematous tissue, injury site, or tissue gap then fills with exudate, immune cells, and fibroblasts before converting to fibrotic connective tissue,[60,78-80] which is later remodeled, albeit slowly.[81] In the case of tendons, a fibrotic scar also fills the tissue gap.[60,79] However, with tendons, although remodeling of the scar area occurs, the tendon never returns to normal structural or biomechanical properties, even after long periods of recovery.[79]

> ### Phases of Wound Healing
>
> **Repair Phase**
> - Infiltration of immune cells to clear debris
> - Fibroplasia (increased fibroblast proliferation and matrix production)
> - Angiogenesis (increased migration and proliferation of endothelial cells)
>   - Increase in capillary beds in wound site
> - Re-epithelialization of skin or mucous membrane
> - Scar formation
>
> **Remodeling Phase**
> - Remodeling and maturation of tissue toward normal, preinjury structure
>   - Collagen conversion: Type III (first to be deposited) to type I
>   - Realignment of fibroblasts in wound

The repair phase begins once the wound site has been cleared of debris, a process that occurs during the acute inflammatory phase of wound healing. The repair phase consists of a proliferation/fibroplasia phase and a remodeling/maturation phase (Figure 22-2).[60] The proliferative phase is characterized by the migration into the injury site of fibroblasts, which proliferate to fill in the wound site. This phase is also called the *granulation tissue formation phase*, because microscopically the wound site appears to be filled with many small immune cells and proliferating fibroblasts. The primary function of fibroblasts is to produce new intracellular and extracellular matrix, such as collagen type III.

The remodeling/maturation phase of repair and healing is characterized by collagen conversion, wound contraction, and scar formation.[59] Collagen type III gradually converts to collagen type I, the collagen becomes cross-linked, and fibroblasts realign along the axis of force through the tissue.[59,60] Unfortunately, some tissues, such as tendons, rarely recover fully to their original structure and strength.

Chronic Inflammation and Fibrosis. Instead of resolving, an acute inflammatory response may be prolonged chronically. Chronic inflammation (sometimes referred to as chronicity) can be considered an interruption of the normal healing progression and can last for months or years. It is associated with certain conditions that prolong the inflammatory response because of chronic exposure to the initiating stimulus or because of a smoldering subacute inflammation or infection. Chronic inflammation is characterized by the prolonged presence of large numbers of macrophages in and around tissues, which contribute to secondary tissue damage through their prolonged phagocytic activity and release of cytotoxic free radicals. Chronic production of inflammatory mediators, such as cytokines,

Figure 22-2
Wound healing response in tendons. (From Lin TW, Cardenas L, Soslowsky LJ: Biomechanics of tendon injury and repair, *J Biomech* 37.866, 2004.)

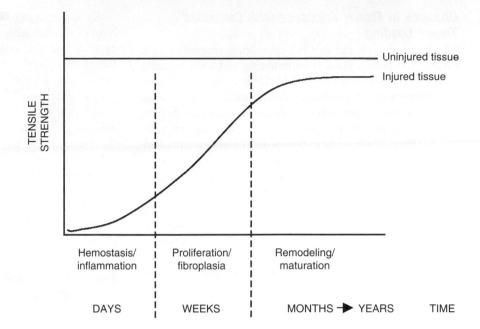

by the macrophages and by cells that are either injured, irritated, or apoptotic can perpetuate the inflammatory cycle, because these molecules are chemotactic for additional immune cells. Cytokines are also fibrogenic mediators, as are connective tissue growth factor (CTGF) and TGF-β. Overproduction or chronic production of fibrogenic mediators can lead to excessive activation of fibroblasts and excessive matrix deposition in and around the wound site, a process called *fibrosis*. Studies now support the hypothesis that chronic inflammation generally precedes fibrosis.[82,83] These same inflammatory and fibrogenic mediators can enter the bloodstream, circulate, and stimulate systemic inflammatory effects, widespread secondary tissue damage, and widespread fibrosis in healthy tissues.[40,77,84]

Chronic Inflammation

- Perpetuation of inflammatory response
  - Continued presence and activity of macrophages in wound site
  - Continued production of inflammatory mediators by cells in wound site
- Fibrosis
- Either or both of these two components may become widespread or systemic

Factors That Affect Wound Healing

Many diverse factors affect wound healing, including ischemia, scar formation, malnutrition, infection, and stress. Circulating cytokines (discussed previously) can induce bone formation, degradation of cartilage and other connective

tissues, and recruitment of leukocytes into widespread tissues areas. Invading neutrophils and macrophages lead to secondary tissue damage through phagocytosis, free radical damage, and tissue and protein catabolism. These cells often invade not only the injury site but also nearby healthy tissue and degrade that tissue as well. The overall health of the tissues and of the individual are also key factors in the end success of wound healing.[6]

Other factors in the success of wound healing are neurogenic in origin and arise from a family of biochemical mediators known as *neuropeptides*. Neuropeptides are secreted by autonomic efferent, nociceptive afferent fibers and perivascular terminals of noradrenergic and cholinergic fibers. They have been shown to play a role in all phases of the healing response. Table 22-2 summarizes the primary effects of several of these neuropeptides during wound healing.

Table 22-2

Neuropeptides Involved in Wound Healing

Neuropeptide	Role in Wound Healing
Substance P	Upregulates endothelial cell receptors that promote leukocyte adhesion and migration; chemotactic for neutrophils and macrophages[101-103]
Catecholamines	Impair T-lymphocyte production and neutrophil phagocytic activity[65]
Glucocorticoids	Impair T-lymphocyte production and neutrophil phagocytic activity[65]

Changes in Tissue Tolerance with Continued Tissue Loading

The authors' work and that of others lends credence to the theory that overexertion is an initiating and a propagating injury stimulus in work-related MSDs and overuse injuries. The authors have speculated that the mechanisms leading to tissue repair are prevented by the continued cycle of tissue trauma in repetitive motion injury.[84,85] Although cumulative loading of viscoelastic tissues in the short term may increase the likelihood that applied loads will result in tissue injury, it is nonetheless an overexertion event that initiates a cyclical and perhaps persistent inflammatory response. Phagocytic cell infiltration, an increase in the number of free radicals, and induction of inflammatory cytokines by persistent injury and inflammation can lead to tissue degeneration, such as tissue necrosis, pathological tissue reorganization, and subsequent biomechanical failure. Repeated bouts of injury, inflammation, and fibrosis eventually contribute to decreasing tissue tolerance over time, such that lower levels of exertion lead to tissue damage, which further reduces tissue tolerance and functional performance. Thus a vicious cycle of injury leading to long-term functional disability is established. Figure 22-3 presents a schematic of this dose-dependent decline in tissue tolerance.

Such decreasing tissue tolerance may explain why analyses of human tissue, such as the flexor tendon synovium in CTS and the extensor carpi radialis brevis tendon in lateral epicondylitis, do not reveal acute inflammatory indicators but instead show tissue degeneration, fibrosis, and/or necrosis.[74,86-89] These patient populations are tested long after the acute inflammation has resolved. The authors agree that designating such soft tissue injuries as noninflammatory informs clinicians of effective treatments for patients seen so late in the process; however, they disagree that the early pathomechanical initiator of these conditions is noninflammatory. The mere presence of fibrotic tissues and anti-inflammatory mediators in the tissues of patients with overuse injuries strongly suggests earlier proinflammatory episodes.

Evidence of Peripheral and Central Neural Changes in the Development of Overuse Injuries

Nerve damage can be caused in numerous ways. Typical modes of injury include compression, overstretching, contusion, and frank tears. Compression and overstretching are the most common types of nerve damage associated with repetitive motion.[78,90-92] However, several other

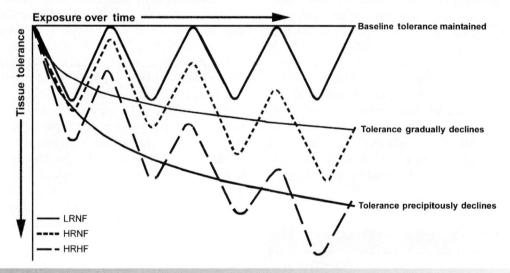

Figure 22-3

Conceptual model of the hypothesized long-term effects of repeated tissue inflammation on tissue tolerance and underlying mechanisms of tissue responses. This model is consistent with the overexertion theory of the development of work-related musculoskeletal disorders. If tissue exposure levels stay below a critical threshold, inflammation resolves (indicated by the episodic fluctuations of tissue tolerance) and adaptive remodeling to the task occurs (indicated by the return to baseline tissue tolerance of the upper low repetition, low force [LRLF] curve between the inflammatory episodes). When tissue exposure exceeds a critical threshold, incomplete healing results (indicated by the lower two curves); exposure-dependent declines in tissue tolerance lead to persistent injury and inflammation followed by tissue disorganization, degeneration, or cell death. Depending on the degree of exertion, this decline in tissue tolerance may be gradual (as in the high repetition, low force [HRLF] group) or precipitous (as in the high repetition, high force [HRHF] group). In addition to the overall decline in tissue tolerance, inflammatory episodes result in transient periods of even lower tissue tolerance, resulting in the fluctuations in tissue tolerance shown. Modification of the tissue exposure level during these transient tissue tolerance episodes may have an important impact on the maximization of tissue tolerance. Furthermore, motor function declines with increasing task demands. (From Barr AE, Barbe MF: Inflammation reduces physiological tissue tolerance in the development of work-related musculoskeletal disorders, *J Electromyogr Kinesiol* 14:83, 2004.)

modes of nerve injury are not exclusive to overuse injuries; these include transection (cutting), crushing mechanisms, immunological causes (creating a chronic autoimmune response in the nerve), chronic constriction injury, and vascular disease. Each of these types of injuries can be a compounding factor in a patient with overuse injuries.

Clinical, Histological, and Biochemical Signs of Nerve Injury

Clinical signs of nerve damage include acute pain, chronic pain, loss of sensation and discrimination, declines in nerve conduction velocity, and motor dysfunction. Examples of motor dysfunction include weakness, atrophy, or paralysis of a muscle. Abnormal sensations, such as hyperalgesia (i.e., hypersensitivity) and mechanical allodynia (i.e., nonnoxious pain), may also develop.

Clinical Signs of Nerve Damage

- Acute pain
- Chronic pain state
- Loss of sensation and discrimination
- Reduced nerve conduction velocity
- Motor dysfunction (weakness, atrophy, or paralysis)

Mechanical disruption of axons and myelin leads to histological signs of nerve damage, such as myelin degradation, Schwann's cell necrosis, and axon degeneration. Macrophage infiltration also occurs as a result of disruption of the blood-nerve barrier or injury-induced chemotaxis, or both. The macrophages then add to the loss of Schwann's cells and axons by phagocytosing even partly injured cells in an effort to debride the injury site and stimulate repair. Each of these histological changes contributes to the decline in nerve conduction by disrupting the flow of current that would occur after loss of the Schwann cell's myelin sheath or by interfering with axoplasmic flow that would occur after disruption of the axons. Nerve compression, edema, and chronic inflammation also lead to the development of fibrotic tissue in extraneural and intraneural tissues,[78,80,91,93-95] which further contributes to nerve compression if the fibrosed area lies within a constrained space, such as the carpal tunnel.

Biochemical signs of peripheral nerve damage include increased production and release of a variety of mediators of pain, inflammation, and vasodilation by Schwann's cells, infiltrating macrophages and mast cells, and the nerve terminal itself. For example, IL-1, TNF-α, and IL-6 are increased after nerve injury and contribute to further inflammation by recruiting macrophages intraneurally. These same cytokines also enhance pain by sensitizing nociceptors through the activation of the neuron or by lowering the threshold for firing in the larger nerve trunk or surrounding tissues. Increased intraneural levels of cytokines also contribute to hyperalgesia and mechanical allodynia.[96-100] Schwann's cells also produce bradykinin, which results in vasodilation, and the nerve terminals produce substance P (SP), vasoactive intestinal peptide (VIP), and calcitonin gene–reactive protein (CGRP), which contribute to immune cell infiltration of intraneural tissues and further sensitization of the nociceptors.[65,101-103]

Peripheral Nerve Trauma Associated with Repetitive Tasks

In work-related MSDs, the primary causes of peripheral nerve trauma are overstretching, increased intracarpal pressure with compression of nerves during flexion or extension or fingertip loading, and overstretching of neuronal tissues during excursion.[90,92,104,105] Experimentally induced nerve compression has been used to determine the pathophysiological effects of compression on nerve tissues (Table 22-3). Such experiments found clear signs of demyelination in a rabbit tibial nerve by 3 weeks after a 2-hour increase of pressure to 200 and 400 mm Hg.[106] In a rat model, demyelination and Schwann's cell death were present in the sciatic nerve by 7 days after an acute increase of pressure to 30 mm Hg.[107]

Animal models of chronic nerve constriction injury using cuff banding or suture ligatures have shown that chronic compression leads to an upregulation of inflammatory cytokines intraneurally, intraneural and extraneural fibrosis (i.e., increases in collagen matrix in and around the nerve), Schwann's cell death, and axonal demyelination and degradation.[80,93,94,96,99,108] These pathological nerve changes lead to loss of electrophysiological function (i.e., decreased nerve conduction).[80,93] Mechanical allodynia and hyperalgesia (discussed later) also were associated with chronic nerve constriction.[96,99,108]

The authors' laboratory has investigated the pathophysiology of repetitive motion injuries of the upper limb caused by voluntary high repetition tasks with or without force.[40,71,78,84,85,91,109-114] The authors have developed an innovative rat model of voluntary repetitive and forceful reaching to answer fundamental questions about the effects of such tasks on musculoskeletal tissues. A force training apparatus was designed in which rats can perform at a range of reach rates and force levels. The apparatus was used to determine the short-term effects (up to 12 weeks) on sensorimotor behavior and the pathophysiological outcomes of forelimb tissues that occurred with (1) a voluntary low force task (less than 15% of maximum grip strength) performed at low frequency reach rates (low repetitions, low force [LRLF], 2 reaches/min) and high frequency reach rates (high repetitions, low force [HRLF]; 8 reaches/min), and (2) a high force task (60% of maximum grip strength) performed at low reach rates (low repetitions, high force [LRHF]) or high reach rates (high repetitions, high force [HRHF]).

Using this model, the authors examined the median nerve for decreased nerve conduction velocity (NCV), a common test used in humans to identify nerve injury. By

Table 22-3
Animal Models of Overuse Injuries and Chronic Nerve Constriction Injury in which Peripheral Nerve Tissues Were Examined

Authors	Model	Tissue and Functional Changes
Chronic Nerve Constriction Injury Animal Models (CCI)		
Mackinnon et al.[80] Mackinnon and Dellon[95]	Rat model Silastic tubing–induced chronic compression of median nerves for 1 to 12 months	Nerve compression, nerve demyelination and degeneration; hypervascularity Intraneural fibrosis; regenerating unmyelinated fibers; ↓ NCV
Mackinnon et al.[93] Mackinnon and Dellon[94]	Primate model Silastic tubing–induced chronic compression of median nerves for 4 to 12 months	↓ Neural tissue in fascicles, demyelination, and ↓ number of myelinated fibers Intraneural fibrosis
Okamoto et al.[108]	Rat model Sutures loosely placed around sciatic nerve for 3 to 45 days	↑ IL-1β and IL-6 (at 7 days), TNF-α (at 14 days), and IL-10 (progressive ↑ to 45 days) ↑ Thermal hyperalgesia and mechanical allodynia days 7 to 14; recovery by 45 days
Schäfers et al.[96]	Rat model Sutures loosely placed around sciatic nerve for 18 days Intraneural application of TNF Ibuprofen and celecoxib therapy	CCI-induced mechanical allodynia and thermal hyperalgesia, a result attenuated by early ibuprofen and celecoxib treatment Mechanical allodynia induced by TNF alone, a result attenuated by ibuprofen treatment
Wagner and Myers[100]	Rat model Sutures loosely placed around sciatic nerve for 3 to 9 days IL-10 therapy (endoneurial application)	CCI-induced thermal hyperalgesia, macrophage influx, and TNF-α expression attenuated by IL-10 therapy
WMSD Animal Model		
Al-Shatti et al.[307] Barr et al.[112]	Rat model Voluntary LRLF reaching and grasping task 1 reach/30 min, 45 mg force 2 hr/day, 3 days/week for 12 weeks	Transient ↑ TNF-α in week 12 No motor changes
Al-Shatti et al.[71] Barbe et al.[110,111] Barr et al.[112,113] Clark et al.[78]	Rat model Voluntary HRLF reaching and grasping task 1 reach/15 min, 45 mg force 2 hr/day, 3 days/week for 8 to 12 weeks	Bilateral ↑ in macrophages in median nerves Transient ↑ IL-1α, IL-1β, TNF-α, and IL-6 in median nerves in weeks 3 to 5; ↑ IL-10 in nerve and muscles in week 5 ↑ Intraneural fibrosis in weeks 10 to 12 ↓ NCV of median nerve ↓ Reach rate and task duration; maladaptive movement patterns (raking) began in week 4, bilateral paw withdrawal response threshold to tactile stimulation, ↓ bilateral grip strength
Clark et al.[91]	Rat model Voluntary HRHF reaching and grasping task 1 reach/15 min, 180 g force, 2 hr/day, 3 days/week for 12 weeks	Bilateral ↑ in macrophages in median nerves ↑ Intraneural fibrosis in weeks 10 to 12 ↓ NCV of median nerve > HRLF ↓ Reach rate and task duration > HRLF Maladaptive movement patterns began in week 4 Hypersensitivity initially, then loss of sensation

HRLF, High repetition, low force; *HRHF*, high repetition, high force; *IL-1*, interleukin-1, a proinflammatory cytokine; *IL-6*, both a proinflammatory and an anti-inflammatory cytokine; *IL-10*, anti-inflammatory cytokine; *LRLF*, low repetition, low force; *NCV*, nerve conduction velocity; *TNF-α*, tumor necrosis factor α; *WMSD*, work-related musculoskeletal disorder.

10 weeks a small but significant decrease (9%) was seen in the NCV,[78] which showed that nerve injury accumulates with continued task performance and leads to a clinically relevant loss of function. The decrease in the NCV was even greater (16%) in rats that performed the HRHF task for 12 weeks, which indicates a positive dose-response relationship between the task exposure level and loss of nerve function.[91] Additional findings were a marked increase in macrophages recruited into the median nerve at the level of the wrist, myelin degradation, and epineural fibrosis after the performance of either the HRLF or the HRHF tasks for 9 to 12 weeks.[78,91] The timing of the fibrosis was associated with the reduction in the conduction velocity of that nerve.[78,91] Finally, significant but transient increases were observed in several cytokines (IL-1α, IL-1β, TNF-α, and IL-6) in the median nerve at the level of the wrist and forearm.[71] The decline in production of these proinflammatory cytokines matched temporally with increased production of an anti-inflammatory cytokine, IL-10, which is known to downmodulate the production of proinflammatory cytokines. These findings and others are summarized in Table 22-3.

Central Nervous System Neuroplasticity Associated with Chronic Pain and Inflammation

Neuroplasticity is a persistent anatomical change that occurs in a neuron as a result of repeated activity across a synapse. It occurs during development, regeneration, or in the mature system. Neuroplasticity can occur at any level of the peripheral and central nervous system, including the spinal cord.

Several mechanisms are possible for neuroplasticity, and two are shown in Figure 22-4. The different mechanisms increase the efficacy of a synapse, unmask or enhance previously ineffective sites, produce changes in neuronal morphology, prune unused neuronal processes, or create electrophysiological changes in the neuron. Peripheral nerve injury results in an increased release of excitatory neurotransmitters and neuropeptides (e.g., SP, glutamate, and CGRP) both peripherally from nociceptor terminals and centrally in a dorsal spinal nerve root or in the dorsal nucleus at the level of the medulla.[115-117] The central release activates postsynaptic receptors for these neurotransmitters, which trigger the release of protein kinases or nitric oxide (NO), or both (see Figure 22-4). The molecules then activate intracellular cascades in the postsynaptic neuron. Chronic or repetitive activation of these cascades results in the upregulation of genes, leading to increased production of neuropeptides, hormones, and enzymes, as well as additional receptors. If additional receptors for neurotransmitters/neuropeptides are inserted into the postsynaptic cell membrane, the postsynaptic neuron's ability to bind these molecules is enhanced, which creates a hyperexcitable neuron. Also, as shown in Figure 22-4, NO is a retrograde messenger that can cross cell membranes to the presynaptic cell. It can increase the release of neurotransmitters from the presynaptic neuron, which can also lead to hyperexcitability of this synapse.

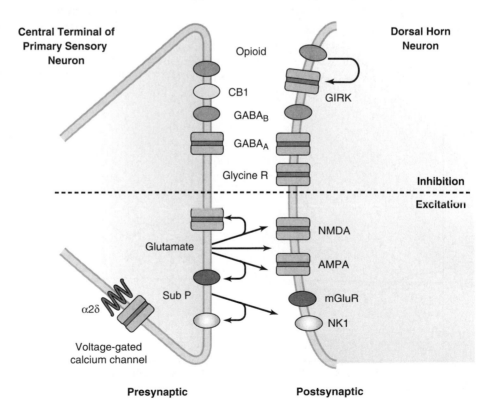

Figure 22-4

Transmission between primary sensory and dorsal horn neurons is subject to presynaptic and postsynaptic excitatory and inhibitory influences. (From Siegel GJ, Albers RW, Brady ST, Price DL: *Basic neurochemistry: molecular, cellular and medical aspects,* ed 7, p 932, Amsterdam, 2006, Elsevier.)

Central Terminal of Primary Sensory Neuron

Dorsal Horn Neuron

Opioid

CB1

GABA$_B$

GABA$_A$

Glycine R

GIRK

Inhibition

Excitation

Glutamate

NMDA

AMPA

Sub P

mGluR

NK1

α2δ

Voltage-gated calcium channel

Presynaptic

Postsynaptic

This hyperexcitability may augment the excitability of the dorsal column–medial lemniscus pathway, or it may lead to abnormal sensations in the peripheral nerve, such as hyperalgesia and mechanical allodynia. Woolf and Salter[118] postulated that these clinical symptoms are due to excessive activation of nociceptors (discussed previously). Chronic pain from chronic peripheral inflammation or the application of irritants to the skin leads to similar central changes. Chronic pain appears to change the efficacy of a synapse by increasing the release of neuromodulators or neurotransmitters from nociceptor terminals or by increasing the number of synaptic vesicles in the nociceptor terminal. Chronic pain also has been shown to alter the enzymatic degradation or reuptake of the neurotransmitter or increase the insertion of receptors into the postsynaptic membrane. Nociceptor hyperexcitability, therefore, may play a role in the pathogenesis of abnormal sensations after peripheral nerve injury. The clinical significance of such neuroplasticity is hyperalgesia, hypersensitivity, and sensory dysfunction.

Abnormal Pain Characteristics

- *Allodynia:* Pain is induced by a normally non-noxious stimulus
- *Hyperalgesia:* A painful stimulus evokes pain of a greater than normal intensity
- *Chronic pain:* Pain of long duration; decreased nociceptor threshold (hyperalgesia)

Hypersensitivity and Spinal Cord Neuroplasticity Associated with Repetitive Tasks

The previously discussed studies prompted the authors to use their model to test sensory function. This was done by observing paw withdrawal in response to palmar stimulation using graded Von Frey monofilaments in the HRHF group. Von Frey monofilaments are calibrated fibers used to test mechanical sensitivity with the application of stimulation to the plantar aspect of the paws. A positive response is defined as immediate withdrawal of the paw from the stimulus and frequently includes licking or shaking of the paw. The authors observed an increase in the paw withdrawal threshold at 12 weeks in the HRHF group,[91] a change indicative of a decrease in sensation (hyposensitivity) (Figure 22-5). The loss of sensation most likely was caused by fibrotic compression of the median nerve and injury or compression-induced demyelination of the neural axons. Interestingly, the hyposensitivity was preceded by a decrease in the withdrawal threshold at 2 to 3 weeks, a change indicative of allodynia or hypersensitivity (see Figure 22-5). Although this decrease was not statistically significant in the eight animals tested, it is noteworthy because of its timing with respect to the onset of the inflammatory response.

The authors also examined the spinal cord for changes in response to peripheral inflammation induced by each of the four task groups. Cervical spinal cord segments were examined using antibodies against SP and two of its receptors, neurokinin-1 (NK-1) and N-methyl-D-aspartase receptor-1 (NMDAr1). An increase was seen in the amount of SP present in the laminae II of the dorsal horns of cervical spinal cord segments, as well as SP receptors, between 4 and 8 weeks of task performance; this increase peaked by 6 weeks in the ipsilateral dorsal horn of cervical cords in the HRLF and the HRHF groups.[109]

Peripheral neuroplasticity also has been observed in conjunction with overuse injuries. Increased innervation and increased levels of neurochemicals (e.g., SP, glutamate, and NMDAr1) have also been observed in tendon attached to the lateral epicondyle of the humerus in patients with chronic tendinopathies, such as chronic

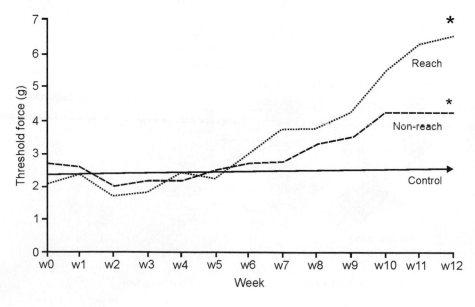

Figure 22-5
Sensory Von Frey outcomes of performing a high repetition, high force (HRHF) task for 12 weeks. Sensory outcomes from the limbs of controls, aged 3 months (n = 15) to 1 year (n = 6), and limbs from experimental rats (reach and nonreach limbs) are depicted (n = 8). The threshold force needed to stimulate a withdrawal of the limb increased dramatically over weeks of task regimen. The sensory threshold of the 1-year-old control rats *(arrow)* did not decline from that of the 3-month-old control rats. Σ:p <0.01.

tennis elbow.[119-123] Using the rat model, the authors found increased levels of SP in flexor forelimb tendons by 3 weeks in the HRHF rats, with additional increases by 12 weeks.[125]

Although, direct correlations need to be made, these human and animal findings suggest that increased neuronal innervation, as well as increased release of neurochemicals from activated nociceptor terminals into peripheral tendon tissues, is linked to painful tendinopathies. Therefore central or peripheral neuroplasticity (or both) may be an underlying cause of some of the motor changes observed in patients with painful tendinopathies.

Evidence of Musculotendinous Injury and Inflammation in the Development of Overuse Injuries

Musculotendinous injuries caused by repetitive and/or forceful tasks are due to repeated overstretching, compression, friction, and ischemia.[90,92,126-128] These insults lead to mechanical injury of membranes and intracellular structures.[81,127,128] The authors hypothesize that these injuries first lead to acute inflammatory responses. If injury and acute inflammation occur repeatedly (as might be the case with a moderate to high demand repetitive task in which the injury cycle overshoots healing), then chronic inflammation, fibrosis, and perhaps even tissue breakdown (disorganization and degeneration) result.

Human Findings

Human studies examining tendons and tendosynovial biopsies from patients with chronic tendinopathies (e.g., epicondylitis, epicondylalgia, tendinosis, and CTS) have found evidence of increased levels of neurochemicals, angiogenesis, inflammatory mediators, fiber and matrix disorganization, and fibrosis (Table 22-4).[86-89,119,121,122,127-130] It should be noted that not all the studies in Table 22-4 found each of these tissue changes. Because only a limited amount of tissue can be collected during a biopsy, the number of questions that can be pursued is limited in a human study. Even so, these studies show that repetitive tasks often lead to fibrotic and degenerative tendon changes and that these changes often are accompanied by localized increases in neurochemicals and their receptors, as well as pain. Furthermore, a study by Hirata et al.[89] showed that the levels of metalloproteinases (MMPs), which are enzymes involved in collagen degradation, correlated with pain severity and that tendon synovial fibrosis increased over time in these patients.

Studies also have been performed on muscle tissue biopsied from patients with long-term chronic overuse syndromes (see Table 22-4). These studies showed evidence of muscle tissue changes, including myopathic changes such as inflammation, muscle fiber necrosis, and cell metabolic changes consistent with injury, denervation, and/or ischemic loss of muscle fibers.[124,131-134]

Serum markers of injury also have been found in patients with overuse injuries. Freeland et al.[129] detected increased serum malondialdehyde, an indicator of cell stress, in patients with CTS. Kuiper et al.[135] found higher levels of biomarkers of collagen degradation and synthesis in a group of student nurses with high numbers of patient handling tasks. Recently, Kuiper et al.[136] examined serum for biomarkers of collagen synthesis and degradation in construction workers involved in heavy manual materials handling. The serum results were compared to those from sedentary workers. Although the levels of collagen synthesis and degradation products were both increased in the workers involved in heavy manual tasks, the overall ratio of the synthesis product to degradation product remained the same as in the sedentary control workers. These results suggested that the tissues had undergone adaptive responses that protected them from unresolved degradation.

A recent pilot study by Carp et al.[137] detected proinflammatory cytokines in the serum of patients treated in an outpatient physical therapy clinic for diagnoses related to severe overuse injuries. The patients were classified into three groups according to symptom severity, as measured by the Upper Body Musculoskeletal Assessment tool (UBMA):[138] mild (UBMA score 51-75; n = 9), moderate (UBMA score 76-100; n = 9), and severe (UBMA score >100; n = 9). A control group was used for comparison; it consisted of unaffected individuals with a UBMA score below 50 (n = 9). The serum results showed significant increases in all proinflammatory cytokines in patients with severe overuse injuries, as well as increases in IL-6 in patients with moderate and mild overuse injuries.[138] Because inclusion in this pilot study required a duration of symptoms no longer than 12 weeks, these findings support the presence of an early inflammatory process in the development of overuse injuries.

One of the challenges involved in studying workers is the difficulty determining the causality between tissue and behavioral responses. Presumably, the initiating injury stimulus is long since past, and the condition of the tissues has been substantially altered from the preinjury state. Whether task-induced injury is followed by inflammation is a point of controversy in the literature, because tissues removed from patients at the time of surgery are collected long after the inflammatory response has resolved. Therefore it is impossible to conclude whether biochemical changes, for example, cause or follow the physiological mechanisms that led to the patient's current clinical presentation.

Animal Studies

A number of animal studies have related exercise loading of tendons to early inflammatory changes (Table 22-5). A study by Nakama et al.[139] found evidence of tendon injury after cyclical loading of the flexor digitorum profundus muscle for 13 weeks at a repetition rate of 2 hours per day, 3 days per week. They observed microscopic

Table 22-4
Selection of Human Studies of Overuse Injuries in which Serum or Musculotendinous Tissues Were Examined

Authors	Description of Patients	Tissue and Functional Changes
Tendon and Tendosynovial Biopsies		
Alfredson et al.[120-122]	ECRB tendon microdialysis, ultrasonography, Doppler, and biopsies of patients with chronic lateral epicondylitis or chronic Achilles tendinosis	↑ Glutamate (mediates pain); ↑ NMDAr1 PGE$_2$ not upregulated in tendon Irregular fiber structure, focal hypoechoic areas Angiogenesis and ↑ innervation of these vessels
Åstrom et al.[130]	Achilles tendon biopsies from 27 patients with chronic Achilles tendonitis	Slight inflammation, bursitis, or fibrosis in five patients Fiber disorganization and activated tenocytes
Campligio et al.[86]	Flexor tendosynovial biopsies from 50 patients with idiopathic CTS	Disorganization and degeneration of collagen fibers Diffuse fibrosis of tendon sheath ↑ Vascularity and arteriosclerosis
Ettema et al.[87]	Subsynovial connective tissue (loose areolar tissue deep to flexor tendons) biopsies from 30 patients with CTS	↑ Fibroblasts, collagen fiber size, and vascular proliferation ↑ Collagen type III fibers; ↑ fibroblasts expressing TGF-β RI
Fenwick et al.[74]	Achilles tendon biopsies from 7 patients with chronic Achilles tendinopathy	Hypercellular, hypervascular; ↑ TGF-β/TGF-β RII Disorganized tendon matrix; ↑ glycosaminoglycan
Freeland et al.[129]	Flexor tendosynovial biopsies and serum examined in 41 patients with CTS	↑ Malondialdehyde in serum and flexor tendosynovium ↑ PGE$_2$ and ↑ IL-6 in flexor tendosynovium (not in serum)
Hirata et al.[88,89]	Flexor tendosynovial biopsies and pain severity testing in 40 patients with CTS; patients divided into symptom duration groups (less than 4 months to longer than 12 months)	Proliferative arteriosclerosis; correlates with symptom duration ↑ MMP-2; correlates with pain severity ↑ Synovial fibrosis with disease progression ↑ PGE$_2$ and VEGF at 4-7 months of symptom duration
Ljung et al.[123]	Flexor tendon biopsies from five patients with tennis elbow (lateral epicondylitis); four patients with medial epicondylalgia	SP and CGRP immunoreactivity in all tendons NK1-R immunoreactivity also in lateral epicondyle tendons

Muscle Biopsies

Study	Subjects	Findings
Kadi et al.[131,308]	Trapezius biopsies from 21 female and 10 male workers with trapezius myalgia, nine male workers without myalgia, and six male controls	Females: ↑ Area and proportion of type I fibers; ↓ capillary: area type I fiber ratio in patients with high pain scores. Males: ↑ Frequency of type II fibers, vascularity, developmental myosin in myalgia group; mitochondrial organization and COX-negative fibers in myalgia group and occupational controls
Larsson et al.[309]	Trapezius biopsies from 17 female workers with trapezius myalgia; Doppler testing of trapezius blood flow	Moth-eaten and ragged red type I muscle fibers worse on pain side; atrophic muscle fibers and fiber splitting. ↓ Blood flow; correlates with pain and ragged red fibers
Larsson et al.[133,134]	Trapezius biopsies from 25 female workers with trapezius myalgia (CM); 25 workers without trapezius myalgia (CC); 21 healthy controls (TC)	↑ Capillary: muscle fiber area in CM; moth-eaten muscle fibers in CM and CC (4%) greater than in TC (2%). Prevalence of ragged red fibers related to working activities and having tender point in trapezius muscle
Ljung et al.[124]	ECRB muscle biopsies from 26 patients with lateral epicondylitis longer than 7 months	Abnormal muscle NADH staining; muscle necrosis. No evidence of muscle inflammation. ↑ Type IIA fibers and muscle fiber regeneration

Serum Samples

Study	Subjects	Findings
Carp et al.[138]	Serum collected from 27 patients diagnosed related to work-related MSDs, nine controls; patients divided into groups based on severity of symptoms	↑ IL-6 in mild and moderate WMSD groups. ↑ IL-6, IL-1α, and TNF-α in severe WMSD group
Kuiper et al.[135]	Serum collected from student nurses with patient-handling activity for 6 months	Higher biomarkers of type I collagen anabolism in exposed group; ↑ with higher exposure levels
Kuiper et al.[136]	Serum collected from male construction workers performing heavy manual materials handling tasks	↑ Type I collagen and ↑ collagen synthesis; no difference in ratio of collagen synthesis to degradation compared to sedentary control workers

CGRP, Calcitonin gene–related peptide; *COX*, cyclo-oxygenase; *CTS*, carpal tunnel syndrome; *ECRB*, extensor carpi radialis brevis; *IL-1*, interleukin 1, a proinflammatory cytokine; *IL-6*, interleukin-6, both a proinflammatory and an anti-inflammatory cytokine; *MMP-2*, matrix metalloproteinase, a collagenase; *MSDs*, musculoskeletal disorders; *NADH*, nicotine-adenine-dinucleotide reductase; *NK-1*, Neurokinin 1, a substance P receptor; *NMDAr1*, N-methyl-ᴅ-aspartase receptor-1 a glutamate receptor; *PGE₂*, prostaglandin E₂; *SP*, substance P; *TGF-β*, transforming growth factor β; *TNF-α*, tumor necrosis factor α, a proinflammatory cytokine; *VEGF*, vascular endothelial growth factor.

Table 22-5

Animal Models of Overuse Injuries in which Serum or Musculotendinous Tissues Were Examined

Authors	Model	Tissue and Functional Changes
Studies Examining Tendons		
Archambault et al.[141]	Rabbit model of Achilles tendinosis Controlled kicking 20 and 75 rep/min, 1 to 2 hr/day, 3 days/week for 6 to 8 weeks	Hypercellularity and ↑ inflammatory cells in tendons; ↑ TNF-α, IL-1 ↑ mRNA of matrix components (e.g., ↑ collagen)
Archambault et al.[142]	Rabbit model of Achilles tendinosis Controlled kicking 75 rep/min, loading of 1.2 Hz, 20 N 2 hr/day, 3 days/week for 11 weeks	No evidence of inflammation ↑ mRNA expression of collagen type III and MMPs
Backman et al.[140]	Rabbit model of Achilles tendinosis Controlled kicking 150 rep/min, 2 hr/session 3 days/week for 5 to 6 weeks	Tendon necrosis, tendon matrix reorganization ↑ Vascularity, ↑ inflammatory cells and edema in paratendon Paratendon fibrosis
Carpenter et al.[143] Soslowsky et al.[144]	Rat model Treadmill running loading of supraspinatus tendon with and without external compression via Achilles tendon allograft 17 m/min on a decline 1 hr/day, 5 sessions/week, up to 16 weeks	Hypercellularity, ↑ tendon cross sectional area Collagen disorganization, rounded tenocytes ↓ Maximum biomechanical stress Tissue changes ↑ with exposure (compression or time)
Messner et al.[145]	Rat model Eccentric loading of Achilles tendon 30 cycles/min 1 hr/day, 3 sessions/week for 7 to 11 weeks	Fibrillation of epitendon ↑ Vascularity of epitendon; ↑ SP and CGRP in epitendon and paratendon Limping gait
Nakama et al.[139]	Rabbit model of medial epicondylitis Cyclical loading of flexor digitorum profundus muscles; tendon examined; 2 hr/day, 3 days/week, for 80 hours total	↑ Microtear area, ↑ tear densities, and ↑ tear size at medial epicondyle attachment site in loaded limbs Regional differences: Outer enthesis > inner enthesis
Topp and Byl[254]	Primate model Repetitive, forceful hand squeezing in owl monkeys 15 squeezes/min, 300 trials/day for 2 to 5 months	Tendon hypercellularity and disorganized collagen in digital flexor tendons of one of three monkeys, attributed to anatomical anomaly No signs of active inflammation in hand tendons
Studies Examining Muscles		
Stauber et al.[127,128]	Rat model Forced lengthening of soleus muscle Slow (10 mm/sec) or fast (25 mm/sec) strain rates 3 sessions/week for 4 to 6 weeks	Hypertrophy, ↑ muscle mass, ↑ myofiber area (adaptation) after slow stretch; ↑ muscle mass, ↓ myofiber area after fast stretch Splitting of myofibers and ↑ type A fibers (regeneration) after fast stretch; collagen struts after slow stretch; clear fibrosis after fast stretch
Stauber et al.[81]	Rat model Forced lengthening (eccentric contractions) of soleus muscle 50 strains/day, 5 sessions/week for 6 weeks Followed by 3 months of cessation of chronic hyperactivity	Hypervascularity ↓ Muscle mass, ↓ myofibers area ↑ Noncontractile tissue, ↑ collagen content Incomplete recovery of tissue changes after 3 months
Studies Examining Muscles, Tendons, and/or Serum		
Barr et al.[112] Fedorczyk et al.[125]	Rat model Voluntary LRLF reaching and grasping task 1 reach/30 min, 45 mg force 2 hr/day, 3 days/week for 12 weeks	No ↑ SP, NMDAr1, or CGRP in epitendon, paratendon, or forelimb muscles No increase in serum IL-1α (only serum examined)

Table 22-5
Animal Models of Overuse Injuries in which Serum or Musculotendinous Tissues Were Examined—Cont'd

Authors	Model	Tissue and Functional Changes
Barbe et al.[111] Barr et al.[112,113] Barr and Barbe[84]	Rat model Voluntary HRLF reaching and grasping task 1 reach/15 min, 45 mg force 2 hr/day, 3 days/week for 8 to 12 weeks	Forearm flexor tendon microfraying Widespread ↑ in macrophages in all muscles, tendons and CTs examined in weeks 3 to 6; ↑COX-2 and IL-1β in cells of muscles, tendons Paratendon fibrosis in weeks 8 to 12 ↑ hsp72 in distal forelimb and palm by week 3 ↑ Serum IL-1α
Fedorczyk et al.[125]	Rat model Voluntary HRHF reaching and grasping task 1 reach/15 min, 180 g force, 2 hr/day, 3 days/week for 12 weeks	↑ SP, NMDAr1, and CGRP in epitendon and paratendon of forelimb muscles
Jarvinen et al.[310]	Rat model Casting for 3 weeks followed by progressively increasing low and high intensity treadmill running, 5 days/week for 7 weeks	Recovery of ↑ tenascin C in myotendinous junction and tendon in dose-dependent manner with treadmill running after casting No de novo synthesis of tenascin C in muscle

CGRP, Calcitonin gene–related peptide; *COX-2*, cyclo-oxygenase 2; *CT*, loose areolar and synovial connective tissue; *IL-1*, interleukin-1; *HRLF*, high repetition, low force; *HRHF*, high repetition, high force; *hsp72*, inducible form of heat shock protein 70/72; *LRLF*, low repetition, low force; *MMPs*, matrix metalloproteinases; *mRNA*, messenger ribonucleic acid; *NMDAr1*, N-methyl-D-aspartase receptor-1, a glutamate receptor; *Rep*, repetitions; *TNF*, tumor necrosis factor; *SP*, substance P.

microtears in the tendons at their epicondylar attachment to the humerus. Backman et al.[140] reported on the use of a controlled kicking model in the rabbit that induced Achilles tendonitis. Inflammatory processes, such as increased vascularity and increased inflammatory cells, were observed in the paratenon, and evidence of necrosis, reorganization, and fibrosis were observed in the tendon by 5 weeks of repetitive kicking.

Archambault et al.[141,142] also found evidence of an inflammatory response and fibrotic responses in the paratenon using this model. They observed increases in proinflammatory cytokines (IL-1 and TNF-α) and increased messenger ribonucleic acid (mRNA) levels of matrix molecules (e.g., collagen type I) by 6 to 8 weeks of task performance. When the kicking protocol was prolonged to 11 weeks, the inflammatory response apparently resolved and remodeling responses occurred (e.g., increased mRNA for collagen type III) in the tendon and paratenon.

Carpenter et al.[143] and Soslowsky et al.[144] developed a rat model of running-induced rotator cuff tendinopathy. Similar to the studies by Backman et al. and Archambault et al., they found evidence of inflammation and fibrosis (hypercellularity and tendon thickening) after 4 weeks of running. These tissue changes persisted through 16 weeks. They also found that biomechanical tissue tolerance decreased in the tendons of experimental animals compared to controls.

Chronic, repetitive contraction of muscles often leads to maladaptive fibrotic repair. Studies by Stauber et al.,[127,128] using a rat model of muscle force-lengthening (eccentric contraction), indicated that repeated muscle strains at fast velocities result in myopathic changes, including muscle fiber splitting, infiltration of macrophages, and fibrosis. These changes are in direct contrast to the compensatory, adaptive responses that occur with repeated slow strains of muscles. Increasing the exposure and duration of repeated forced-lengthening leads to significant decreases in muscle mass and myofiber area and increases in noncontractile tissues (see Table 22-5). In another study, Stauber et al.[81] found that recovery from pathophysiological fibrotic changes is slow, even with complete cessation of the repeated strains for 3 months; this highlights the importance of prevention in the management of such disorders.

In the authors' model of upper extremity overuse injuries in the rat, evidence of musculotendinous damage was found in the forearm flexors of the reach limbs of the rats training under a high rate of repetition with low force (HRLF).[111] Immunohistochemical analyses showed that this tendon disruption was accompanied by an increase in activated exudate macrophages by 6 weeks of task performance. Increases in macrophages in loose connective tissues and at sites of muscle and ligament attachments to bone also were found in these HRLF animals. The increase in the numbers of macrophages rose significantly above those of control animals as early as 3 weeks and peaked at 5 to 6 weeks. Serum levels of IL-1α in these animals increased significantly above control levels in week 8.[111,112] IL-1α did not change significantly with task performance in a low repetition, negligible force (LRNF) group (2 to 4 reaches/min at 15% of maximum grip strength).[112] The authors hypothesized that the net cytokine production in the LRNF group allowed for maintenance of homeostasis through the resolution of an acute inflammatory response. The level of repeated incidents of mechanical injury to the tissues in the HRNF group, on the other hand, led to a net production of IL-1α, indicative of a chronic and systemic inflammatory response to the repetitive task.

Behavioral Changes That Coincide with Tissue Inflammation in Severe Overuse Injuries

The authors have reported on behavioral indicators in the rat model that offer insight into the behavioral consequences of injury and inflammation. The reach rate (RR; reaches/min) is an indicator of the animals' ability to maintain task pace. The reach movement pattern is an indicator of the quality of reaching. The HRLF group showed a significant decline in RR in week 6, which coincided with the peak inflammatory response, and a return toward baseline in week 8.[111,113] The LRLF group did not exhibit any change in RR over 12 weeks.[112] However, the HRHF group underwent a significant decline in RR in weeks 3 to 6 and a significant decrease in sensation, grip strength, and NCV in week 12.[91] All HRLF animals developed progressively degraded

reach movement patterns by 7 weeks of task performance, whereas only 60% to 70% of LRLF animals showed reach movement pattern degradation.[111,112]

Messner et al.[145] reported behavioral changes that develop in their rat model of eccentric loading of the Achilles tendon. Using a repetitive task of 30 cycles/min for 1 hour per day, 3 days per week, for 7 to 11 weeks total, they observed the development of a permanent limping gait that was associated with fibrillation of the epitendon (the outer sheath of the tendon), as well as angiogenic changes and increased expression of neurochemicals in this same tendon region.

These behavioral changes are summarized in Table 22-5, along with the tissue changes observed in the particular study. The findings indicate that functional declines may accompany tissue injury and inflammation. Figure 22-6 shows a timeline that postulates the onset of behavioral changes in relation to the pathological tissue responses.

Role of Proinflammatory Cytokines in "Sickness Behavior"

The psychoneuroimmunological effects of proinflammatory cytokines, specifically IL-1β, TNF-α, and IL-6, have been studied extensively in animal models over the past decade

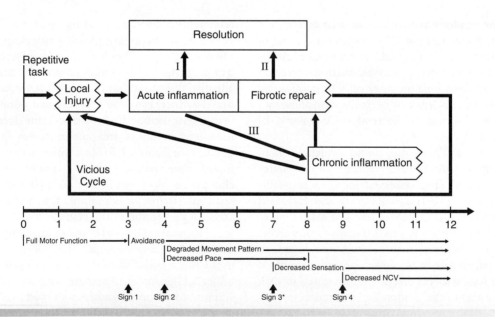

Figure 22-6

Steps in the inflammation-mediated development of work-related musculoskeletal disorders. The vertical zigzagged boundaries indicate uncertainty as to the specific time frame for transitions between progressive steps. The timeline at the bottom of the figure relates these inflammatory events to observations of behavioral indicators in a rat model. At the very bottom of the figure, the physical sign (behavior degradation) that reflects underlying pathophysiology is indicated. The three possible exposure-dependent outcomes in this schematic are indicated as follows: (1) acute inflammation followed by resolution and restoration of normal tissue, as in the LRLF group; (2) acute inflammation followed by fibrotic repair, as in the HRLF group; and (3) acute inflammation followed by chronic systemic inflammation, with or without fibrotic repair, and initiation of a vicious cycle of further injury and inflammation, as in the HRHF group. *LRLF,* Low, repetition, low force; *HRLF,* High repetition, low force; *HRHF,* High repetition, high force. (Modified from Barr AE, Barbe MF: Inflammation reduces physiological tissue tolerance in the development of work-related musculoskeletal disorders, *J Electromyogr Kinesiol* 14:82, 2004.)

for their contribution to a constellation of physiological and behavioral responses known collectively as the *sickness response*. These responses include fever, weakness, listlessness, hyperalgesia, allodynia, decreased social interaction and exploration, somnolence, decreased sexual activity, and decreased food and water intake.[146-149] The sickness response is adaptive in that it results in behavior that minimizes energy expenditure in order to allocate metabolic resources to fighting infection or disease.[146] Furthermore, a sickness response has been shown to be a motivational state with respect to feeding behavior in animals.

"Sickness Responses" Mediated by Proinflammatory Cytokines

- Fever
- Weakness
- Decreased social interaction/exploration
- Somnolence/listlessness/lethargy
- Decreased food and water intake
- Decreased sexual activity
- Hyperalgesia/allodynia

Aubert et al.[150] demonstrated that rats injected with IL-1β reduced the frequency of lever presses to receive a food reward but readily ate food when it was freely presented to them. The interpretation of these results from the motivational standpoint suggests that IL-1β produces an aversion to foraging, which is an energy-intensive activity, rather than to feeding per se. In the authors' model, animals exhibited dose-dependent task avoidance over weeks of task performance.[78,91] The HRLF group declined in duration in week 3, then regained baseline duration by week 6.[78] This avoidance of the task in week 3 matches the onset of inflammatory cytokine production in the median nerves in our model,[71] and the recovery to baseline duration matches temporally the increased production of an anti-inflammatory cytokine, IL-10. The mechanism of action of the proinflammatory cytokines on such behavioral responses has been partly elucidated but is still a subject of intense research. The role of the vagus nerve in facilitating a paracrine signal transduction pathway to the hypothalamic-pituitary-adrenal (HPA) axis has been the most extensively studied in rodent models of bacterial infection.[146] An immediate response to intraperitoneal injection of lipopolysaccharide (LPS), a bacterial endotoxin, is the induction within 60 minutes of IL-1β in the abdominal vagus nerve by glial cells and macrophages.[147] Blocking either the vagus nerve or IL-1β activity reduces sickness behaviors associated with LPS injection. Although these latter findings seem to implicate the vagus nerve in particular, the disease model in this case was most consistent with visceral infection or inflammation. These findings raise the possibility that other peripheral nerves are also capable of facilitating signal transduction between local inflammatory mediators and the HPA axis, inducing a sickness response. Recent studies of bilateral neuropathic pain (i.e., hyperalgesia or allodynia) with a unilateral sciatic nerve lesion strongly suggest that other peripheral nerves are capable of such peripheral-central communication.[151-153]

More recent attention has been given to the possible role of serum circulating proinflammatory cytokines in the etiology of depression and other mood disorders, particularly among cancer patients treated with proinflammatory cytokine therapy.[154] The possibility for patients with chronic inflammatory conditions to succumb to the depressive effects of local and systemic proinflammatory cytokines has implications in the management of severe overuse injuries.

Symptoms of depression and anxiety have been reported in numerous epidemiological and clinical studies of patients with severe overuse injuries.[8,155-157] Bystrom et al[158] reported a lower pressure-pain threshold among women automobile assembly line workers with newly reported work-related forearm and hand symptoms. All of these findings in workers with work-related symptoms may be attributed to the sickness response, which suggests a physiological basis for such symptoms. A more complete understanding of the relationship between repetitive and forceful task demands and induction of the sickness response will help direct effective workplace and clinical management strategies that can reduce the stigmatization often imposed by health care providers on patients who present with such vague and apparently psychological complaints.

Summary

By examining the findings of human and animal studies done on severe overuse injuries, the authors have developed a proposed mechanism of pathophysiological and behavioral changes associated with these injuries.

First, repetitive activity leads to a disruption of cells and tissues (Figure 22-7). This injury activates the acute inflammatory response: infiltration of immune cells into the injury site and increased production of cytokines by these immune cells and by injured cells and tissues. The acute inflammatory response then activates mechanisms of cell proliferation and matrix production related to wound healing. Unfortunately, the continued cycle of tissue trauma by continued performance of the repetitive task halts the process of tissue repair at this point.[84,159] Instead, a chronic inflammatory response (with associated secondary tissue damage) is stimulated, along with an excessive fibrogenic response. This postulated mechanism is supported by the many studies, both human and animal, that have found evidence of tendon tissue thickening and fibrosis, nerve and muscle fibrosis, and tissue disorganization and necrosis. Motor behavior changes related to tissue damage, pain, or both would be clearly apparent at this point as a result of nerve damage, and sensory losses may also be present. Finally, a systemic response is stimulated, apparently by the release of cytokines into the bloodstream from the

CHAPTER 23

MUSCULOSKELETAL DEVELOPMENTAL DISORDERS

Lorrie Ippensen Vreeman, Toby Long, and Zehra H. Habib

Introduction

Numerous musculoskeletal developmental disorders require the expertise of rehabilitation specialists. Many of these disorders, regardless of the pathophysiology, result in complex musculoskeletal and neurological primary and secondary impairments. Ideally, a multidisciplinary team, including the family, coordinates the pediatric patient's plan of care, with the ultimate goal of maximizing the patient's functional potential throughout development. This chapter discusses some of the more common pediatric pathologies.

Arthrogryposis Multiplex Congenita

Definition and Classification

Arthrogryposis multiplex congenita (AMC), a nonprogressive syndrome present at birth, is characterized by severe joint contractures, muscle weakness, and fibrosis.[1] AMC manifests in various forms, including classic arthrogryposis, or amyoplasia (43%),[2,3] contracture syndrome (35%), neuromuscular syndrome (7%), distal arthrogryposis (7%), congenital anomalies (6%), and chromosomal abnormalities (2%). Essentially, two clinical presentations are seen. In one clinical presentation, the lower extremities assume a jackknifed posture (i.e., the hips are flexed and dislocated, the knees are extended), and the patient has clubfeet (Figure 23-1). In the upper extremities, the shoulders are internally (medially) rotated, the elbows are flexed, and the wrists are flexed and ulnarly deviated (Figure 23-2). In the other clinical presentation, the lower extremities assume a frog-leg posture (i.e., the hips are abducted and laterally rotated, the knees are flexed), and the patient has clubfeet. The upper extremities assume the "waiter's tip" posture, with the shoulders medially rotated, the elbows extended, the forearms pronated, and the wrists flexed and ulnarly deviated (Figure 23-3).[2]

Etiology, Epidemiology, and Pathophysiology

The reported incidence of AMC is 1 in 3000 to 4000 live births.[2,4,5] Although AMC is nonprogressive, the long-term sequelae are disabling. The exact etiology of AMC is unknown, but it is probably multifactorial. Reported causes include a maternal fever higher than 37.8°C (100°F), causing hyperthermia in the fetus; prenatal viral infections; vascular compromise between mother and fetus; and a uterine septum.[2,6] The insult occurs during the first trimester of pregnancy and can result from neurogenic, myopathic, or connective tissue disorders.[6] The neuropathic form of AMC involves degeneration of anterior horn cell causing muscle weakness and consequent periarticular soft tissue fibrosis.[7] Failure of muscle function and joint development in the growing fetus leads to stiffness, joint deformation, and intrauterine joint fixation. The chief pathophysiological mechanism is lack of fetal movement;[8] however, decreased amniotic fluid and intrauterine compression are also cited.[2,5]

Diagnosis and Prognosis

No definitive laboratory studies or invasive procedures, such as amniocentesis or chorionic villous sampling, are available to detect AMC. However, detailed level II ultrasound can identify a decrease in fetal movements, which suggests the diagnosis.

In the embryo, muscle formation proceeds normally; however, during fetal development, fibrous fatty tissue replaces muscle. Histologically, weak muscles show fibro-fatty changes. Therefore muscle biopsies and blood tests are done to rule out fatal disorders and to support the diagnosis of AMC. Nerve conduction studies and electromyography (EMG) provide valuable diagnostic information only when the history, examination, and genetic evaluation are unrevealing.[2,9] Children with AMC generally have a positive prognosis. However, family support and the severity

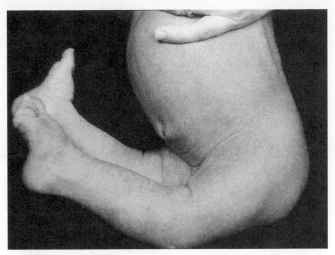

Figure 23-1
Congenital knee dislocation. (From Grosfeld JL, O'Neill J, Coran A, Fonkalsrud E: *Pediatric surgery,* ed 6, vol 2, p 2026, Philadelphia, 2006, Elsevier.)

of the disease, among other factors, influence the prognosis. A study by Sells et al.[10] indicated that by age 5 years, 85% of children with AMC were ambulatory and could perform most of their activities of daily living (ADLs) independently.

Clinical Manifestations and Primary Impairments

The presentation of AMC varies tremendously among infants. Palmer et al.[11] reported that all four extremities are involved in 90% of all cases.[5] Severely affected body parts include the foot (67%), hip (50%), wrist (43%), knee (41%), elbow (30%), and shoulder (4%).[2] Associated clinical

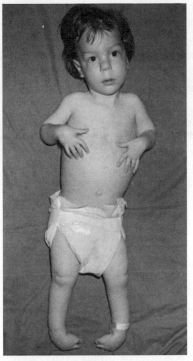

Figure 23-2
This 6-month-old boy has the neurogenic form of arthrogryposis. The marked deformities of the ankles and feet are evident, and the infant has flexion contractures of the wrists, elbows, and knees. (From Swaiman KF, Ashwal S, Ferriero DM: *Pediatric neurology: principles and practice,* ed 4, p 1872, Philadelphia, 2006, Elsevier.)

manifestations include hemangiomas, congenital heart disease, absent or decreased finger creases, facial abnormalities, respiratory problems, and abdominal hernias.[2] Additional congenital changes include low-set ears,

Figure 23-3
A, Infant with arthrogryposis multiplex congenita (AMC) with flexed and dislocated hips, extended knees, clubfeet (equinovarus), internally rotated shoulders, flexed elbows, and flexed and ulnarly deviated wrists.
B, Infant with AMC with abducted and externally rotated hips, flexed knees, clubfeet, internally rotated shoulders, extended elbows, and flexed and ulnarly deviated wrists. (From Donohoe M: Arthrogryposis multiplex congenita. In Campbell SK, Vander Linden DW, Palisano RJ, editors: *Physical therapy for children,* ed 3, p 383, Philadelphia, 2006, WB Saunders.)

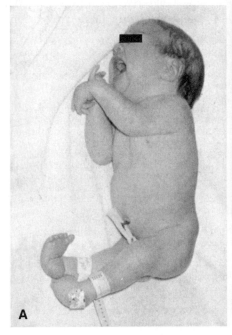

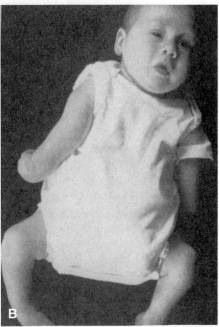

micrognathia, a high-arched palate, and hypoplastic lungs. Speech and intelligence are unaffected.[5]

Primary Impairments in Arthrogryposis Multiplex Congenita

- Severe joint contractures
- Webbing of the joint
- Decreased muscle bulk and weakness
- Impaired integument
- Diminished deep tendon reflexes
- Clubfeet
- Dislocated hips
- Scoliosis

Medical and Surgical Management

Lower Extremity

The most common foot deformity in the newborn period is clubfoot, the most common form of which is taloequinovarus (TEV). Serial manipulation with casting in this period partially corrects the deformity, but recurrence is common.[2,11] Surgical correction of TEV should be deferred until the child demonstrates pull to stand or ambulatory potential.[2,5] The recommended surgical procedures are posteromedial release (i.e., the lateral border of the foot is shortened, and the medial border is lengthened) combined with elongation of the Achilles tendon.[2,5,12,13] After surgery, mandatory use of ankle-foot orthoses (AFOs) is recommended. In severe cases or if the surgery fails, talectomy may be performed.[14]

Hip subluxation or dislocation can be bilateral or unilateral, and its surgical management is an issue of controversy. The basic premise in surgical correction of dislocated hips is that having mobile, painless dislocated hips is more important than having very stiff located ones.[2] However, Asif et al.[15] suggested that open reduction for bilateral dislocated hips in children with AMC is a suitable option that produces satisfactory results. Along with other authors, they recommend surgery at an earlier age for optimum functional outcome.[5] Because high unilateral hip dislocation can lead to severe pelvic obliquity and secondary scoliosis if left untreated, open reduction is essential in these cases.[2,5,16,17]

Knee surgery is reserved for moderate to severe contractures and resistant cases. Posterior capsulotomy and medial and lateral hamstring lengthening are the recommended procedures for young children with a knee flexion deformity of 30° or more.[2,5] Postoperative complications may include posterior subluxation of the tibia and inconsistent muscular response secondary to loss of muscle strength and possible scar tissue formation, both of which may lead to further joint stiffness and recurrence of contracture. A distal femoral osteotomy may be more successful in realigning the knee joint in such cases.[2] Knee extension contractures have a more favorable outcome and are addressed by quadricepsplasty (surgical repair of the quadriceps).[18]

Upper Extremity

If muscle strength and control are adequate, the upper extremities are placed in the optimum position for long-term function and ADLs: one elbow in extension (to reach the perineum), and the other in flexion (for feeding).[2,5,19] Shoulder range of motion (ROM) usually is adequate for self-care, and surgery is rarely required. The best surgical candidates for tendon transfers of the upper extremity are children over 4 years of age who have full passive ROM of the elbow in the dominant arm and at least grade 4 muscle strength of the muscle tendons to be transferred.[20] Usually the pectoralis major, triceps brachii, or latissimus dorsi[21] is used in tendon transfers to restore active elbow flexion. Wrist deformities are treated aggressively in infants and young children using passive stretching, serial casting, and custom wrist orthotics.[22] Using conservative management, Smith and Drennan[22] found that those with distal AMC had the greatest improvement in passive ROM, were functionally independent at follow-up, and had no recurrence of deformity. Those with classic AMC had rigid wrist flexion contractures and a 75% incidence of deformity recurrence. Surgical correction of the wrist involves anterior wrist capsulotomy and placement of the wrist in a neutral or slight dorsiflexion position. Long-term protective splinting is required.[5]

Spine

Approximately one fifth of children and adolescents with AMC have a long "C" thoracolumbar scoliosis (Figure 23-4).[2] When the curve is less than 30°, the scoliosis is managed conservatively with bracing in ambulators.[23] If the curve progresses, combined anterior and posterior spinal arthrodesis yields the best results.[23]

Rehabilitation Management: Evaluation, Intervention, and Clinical Implications

A multidisciplinary team is involved in the evaluation of a child with AMC. The aim of the initial evaluation is to establish a baseline from which to set realistic goals. Photographs and videos should be taken every 2 to 3 months for at least 2 years, detailing appropriate positioning and stretching of various joint contractures, to provide objective documentation.

Baseline goniometry is necessary, including passive ROM and the resting position of each joint, together with active ROM. Functional ROM (e.g., hand to mouth, hand to the top of the head, hand to forehead, hand to ear, and hand to the back of the neck) also should be assessed.[2] In infants and small children, muscle strength is evaluated

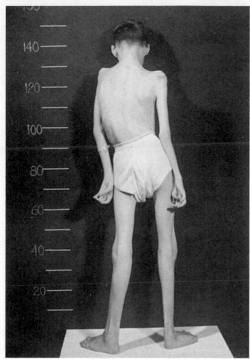

Figure 23-4

This patient, who has anterior cell arthrogryposis, has had a number of orthopedic procedures. Marked scoliosis and generalized muscle wasting, particularly of the shoulder girdle, are clearly demonstrated. (From Swaiman KF, Ashwal S, Ferriero DM: *Pediatric neurology: principles and practice,* ed 4, p 1872, Philadelphia, 2006, Elsevier.)

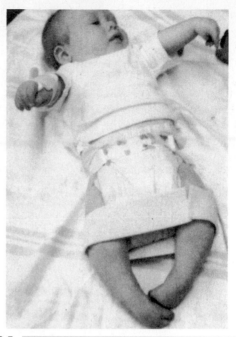

Figure 23-5

This child with arthrogryposis multiplex congenita is wearing a wide Velcro band strapped around the thighs to keep the legs in more neutral alignment. (From Donohoe M: Arthrogryposis multiplex congenita. In Campbell SK, Vander Linden DW, Palisano RJ, editors: *Physical therapy for children,* ed 3, p 388, Philadelphia, 2006, WB Saunders.)

by muscle palpation and observation of extremity movement against gravity. Gross motor function and developmental milestones should be evaluated.[2] Formal manual muscle testing (MMT) should begin when appropriate, because the strength of the extensor muscles of the lower extremity determines the appropriate level of bracing.

Current and potential gross motor skills and functional mobility, including the use of assistive devices and a manual or power wheelchair, should be evaluated. ADL skills, movement patterns, and muscle substitutions must be assessed to establish a treatment plan, with the family and the child as active team members. The ultimate goal is to maximize the child's independence in ADLs and mobility.

Family education, stretching, positioning, thermoplastic serial splinting, strengthening activities through play, facilitation of developmental activities, and teaching of compensatory strategies (especially in alternate modes of mobility) form the mainstay of physical therapy (PT) treatment in infancy and early childhood. Stretching needs to be incorporated into the daily care of infants. For example, stretching of the lower extremity can be done during diaper changes. During feeding, bathing, and dressing, both the lower and upper extremities can be stretched. The recommended regimen is 3 to 5 sets of stretches per day, with 3 to 5 repetitions in each set, and each repetition held for 20 to 30 seconds.[2] Low load, prolonged stretching is

preferred over maximum load stretching for prolonged periods because the latter may cause skin breakdown and intolerance to splints. For infants with the first clinical presentation of AMC described earlier, prone positioning for the first 3 months is essential to stretch the hip flexor muscles. Children with the second clinical presentation of AMC have more positioning options. These patients usually are frustrated with prone positioning because they are unable to prop themselves when placed on a wedge or roll. For these children, Velcro straps should be used to position the hips in a neutral position when the child is supine, and a towel roll should be used along the lateral borders of the thigh when the child is sitting (Figure 23-5).

Splints are adjusted for growth and improvement every 4 to 6 weeks. For the newborn, cock-up splints usually are provided 3 months after birth. AFOs to correct clubfeet should be worn 22 hours a day.[2] For the first 3 to 4 months, anterior thermoplastic knee flexion splints for extension contractures or posterior knee extension splints for flexion contractures should be worn 20 hours a day.[2] Knee flexion splints should not be worn at greater than 50° of flexion for sleeping, because this may encourage hip flexion. After 4 months of splinting, knee extension splints can be worn for standing activities and sleeping to help stretch the hip flexors; this encourages optimum lower extremity positioning during independent floor mobility.

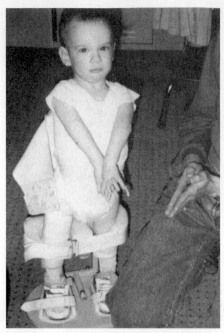

Figure 23-6

Child with arthrogryposis multiplex congenita using a standing frame. (From Donohoe M: Arthrogryposis multiplex congenita. In Campbell SK, Vander Linden DW, Palisano RJ, editors: *Physical therapy for children*, ed 3, p 389, Philadelphia, 2006, WB Saunders.)

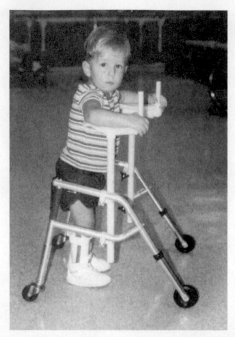

Figure 23-7

Thermoplastic forearm supports can be customized to the walker for a child with arthrogryposis multiplex congenita. (From Donohoe M: Arthrogryposis multiplex congenita. In Campbell SK, Vander Linden DW, Palisano RJ, editors: *Physical therapy for children*, ed 3, p 393, Philadelphia, 2006, WB Saunders.)

Reducing disability related to immobility is a major goal of treatment; therefore key functional motor skills should be addressed, such as rolling, hitching on the buttocks, and standing. Strengthening of muscles that help maintain an upright posture is important during the first 2 to 3 years and can be accomplished through developmental play. For example, dynamic trunk strengthening is achieved by having the child manipulate or reach for toys in various positions of sitting or static standing. Standing is an integral component and should begin by 6 to 9 months of age. Standing is initiated in standing frames with the lower extremities held in as optimally correct position as possible with the help of splints and high-top shoes (Figure 23-6). Advantages of standing include self-stretching of the feet and commencement of ambulation. Floor to stand and sit to stand activities begin once the child is ambulating. Limitations in strength and ROM in the lower extremities are addressed through splinting or bracing. If MMT results are less than fair in the hip extensors (3/5), bracing is required above the hip. If MMT results are less than fair in the knee extensors, bracing is required above the knee.[2]

In the preschool period, goals should emphasize ability versus disability, improving the child's function in basic ADLs, and enhancing independence in mobility and ambulation with minimal bracing and assistive devices. Gait assessment includes evaluating distance, use of assistive devices, speed, symmetry of step length and any gait deviations. Children with adequate strength and ROM generally require AFOs while walking to prevent recurring clubfeet deformities. Articulating AFOs may be more desirable and appropriate than static AFOs because they provide forefoot control, allow ankle dorsiflexion, and stretch the hindfoot during gait. Ideally, the least amount of bracing should be used; however, if less bracing causes the child to use assistive devices (i.e., walker, crutches, or canes) that previously were not required, then increased bracing is acceptable. Assistive devices can be customized with thermoplastic material to allow for less awkward handgrips. Forearm supports and other modifications can be added to walkers and other assistive devices when required (Figure 23-7). Shoes may need external wedges to compensate for hip and knee flexion contractures.[2] Children learning to walk may be limited in their independence if they do not have adequate strength and ROM to manipulate assistive devices. Walkers can be cumbersome and less energy efficient for such children, who typically have inadequate protective responses to falls. Power mobility may be the most energy-efficient means of ambulation for such children.

Families may need assistance in identifying and removing architectural and environmental barriers that impede their child's independence at home. The child should be encouraged to interact with nondisabled peers in school and to participate in extracurricular activities, such as swimming classes. Additional educational and therapy services are essential at this stage to maximize the child's potential.

moderate to severe
HKAFO without the l
helps lock the hips an
joints may be added
and strength increase
standing frames to or
foot-orthoses (KAFO
locked in full extensio
various walkers or cru
for children with m
mobility caster carts a
sidered for children
explore their enviro
should be encouraged
control and the cogni

Down Syndrom

Definition and Clas

First described by Le
or trisomy 21, is the
arising from faulty c
somes instead of the
are nondisjunction, t
junction occurs in 9
form, an extra sma
twenty-first pair of c
3% to 4% of affected
homologous chromc
subsequently reattacl
Mosaicism occurs in
type of DS in which
and others are nor

Table 23-1
Neuropathological a

Neuropathological a

Decreased weight (76
Microcephaly
Decreased anteropost
Microbrachycephaly
Changed convolution
Decreased number of
Lack of myelination c
  precentral areas and
Structural abnormalit
  pyramidal neurons c
Decreased synaptoge
Decreased number ol
  hippocampus
Increased neurofibrill
Increased senile plaqu

Osteogenesis Imperfecta

Definition and Classification

Osteogenesis imperfecta (OI) is an inherited disorder of connective tissue characterized by increased bone fragility.[24-29] The bone fragility is secondary to decreased bone mass, disturbed organization of bone tissue, and altered bone geometry. OI comprises several distinct syndromes and is genetically heterogeneous with a range of clinical presentations.[30] The classification system developed by Sillence is widely accepted and is based on clinical, genetic, and radiological findings.[30-32] Sillence divided OI into four types: types I and IV are autosomal dominant conditions that have a milder presentation; types II and III are autosomal recessive disorders that present with severe bone fragility and fractures at birth.[30-32]

Etiology, Epidemiology, and Pathophysiology

In most cases, OI is caused by mutations in one of the two genes encoding typeI collagen; the result is a qualitative and quantitative defect in collagen synthesis.[24,27-29] The incidence of OI is reported to be 1 in 20,000 to 30,000 live births,[25,28,31] and the prevalence is 16 per 1 million.[25] The defect in collagen synthesis results from an abnormality in the processing of procollagen to type I collagen, which leads to brittle bones. It affects the formation of both endochondral and intramembranous bone. The collagen fibers fail to mature beyond the reticular fiber stage.[25] Osteoblasts have normal or increased activity but fail to produce and organize collagen. Osteocytes are relatively abundant, but intracellular matrix is deficient.[25]

Diagnosis and Prognosis

The diagnosis is made primarily from clinical and radiographic findings. No definitive laboratory tests exist to identify OI. In severe OI, the child is born with multiple fractures sustained in utero or during the birth process; these cases have a high mortality rate. Infants and children with moderate OI are identified after they experience several fractures from light trauma or a fracture of unknown origin at a young age. In milder forms of OI, pathological fractures occur late in childhood. Joints are hypermobile, and the lower extremities are severely malaligned. Muscle strength is normal in type I OI except in the periarticular muscles of the hip joint; patients with type III OI have decreased muscle strength around the hip joint.[25] Developmental progress depends on the type and severity of OI.[31]

Milder presentations of OI need to be differentiated from multiple fractures sustained through child abuse.[26,33] Other differential diagnostic conditions include juvenile osteoporosis and rickets.[33]

It is important to note that Sillence's classification system does not predict functional outcome, particularly in patients with type III OI, because disuse, weakness, and osteoporosis secondary to immobilization may be prove to be more of a handicap to the child than the underlying disease.[34] Factors that affect independence and mobility include joint contractures, muscle weakness, and endurance capabilities, especially in the child with severe OI.[31]

Clinical Manifestations and Primary Impairments

The clinical features of OI are extremely variable and depend on the type and severity of the disorder. Primary impairments include bone fragility, short stature, scoliosis, defective dentinogenesis, blue sclerae and tympanic membrane, lax ligaments, weak muscles, failure of postnatal growth, and multiple, recurrent fractures sustained from minor or no trauma.[25,33] Bones are diffusely osteoporotic and have thin cortices and an altered trabecular pattern.

Long bones have narrow diaphyses; therefore bowing and resultant deformity are common. Lack of weight bearing in the long bones leads to a honeycomb pattern of ossification. The metaphyseal and epiphyseal areas of long bones show popcorn calcifications secondary to fragmentations of cartilaginous growth plates.[25] The pelvis has a trefoil shape, and protrusio acetabuli (protrusion of the femoral heads through a shallow acetabulum) is common secondary to repeated fractures.[25,33] Osteoporotic vertebrae fracture easily, resulting in a flattened, biconcave shape.[25]

Malformed ribs cause respiratory compromise, and ligamentous laxity results in an increased incidence of joint dislocation. Dentinogenesis imperfecta results in soft, translucent, brownish teeth. Umbilical, inguinal, and diaphragmatic hernias are common.[25,33] Metabolic abnormalities have also been reported in individuals with OI, including increased sweating, heat intolerance, elevated body temperature and resting tachycardia and tachypnea.[33]

Medical and Surgical Management

Improvements in medical care of respiratory tract infections and orthopedic management have led to better outcomes for children with OI.[25] No effective medications are available to strengthen skeletal structures and reduce or prevent fractures.[25] Investigators have studied various agents, including calcitonin, fluoride, growth hormones, and vitamins C and D, but none of these have proved efficacious in reducing bone fragility.[35,36]

Recently, the use of bisphosphonates (specifically pamidronate) has been associated with increased bone mineral density and ambulation, decreased bone pain and fracture incidence, improved vertebral shape and mass, greater cortical width, increased cancellous bone volume, and suppressed bone turnover.[24,37,38] Letocha et al.[37] conducted

developmental activiti
ting, should be encou
attempts to roll over,
the head. Supportec
inserts or corner chair
begins on a parent's l;
achieved, short-sit an
ster, or caregiver's le;
mote equilibrium res
for the lower extrem;
indicated; instead, tl
the shoulders when
on trunk control ov
the child through the
extremities.

Pool exercises ma
is to promote active
water. Alternatively,
objective. The child
neck and trunk flo
should wear long-sl
the absorbed water
limb and thus provi
movements in water

An important gc
age child is preven
tion and reduced ii
by the initial impai
opportunities for n
gait training in par
parent education. I:
ments include bor
muscle strength. S
atrophy and osteof
zation.[25] A major
be optimally mobil
with peers. If chilc
this stage, further
will occur, the mo
lateral bowing anc
be controlled wi
devices, such as
(Figure 23-10).

Rehabilitation i
adequate upright
mobility for enhar
ing, handling, anc
to the child's activ
pendence.[25] Activ
increase muscle s;
and abductors.[25,3]
play techniques, s
which the child at
porting the child'
by using a lower

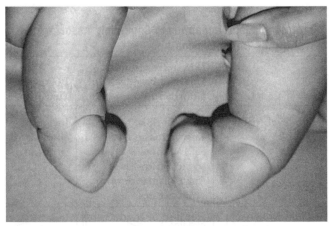

Figure 23-20
Infant with bilateral clubfeet demonstrates the deformities that are part of clubfeet. The infant is prone, a position that reveals the varus deformity of the hindfeet. The crease in the arch shows that these feet have a cavus deformity. The feet are internally rotated and in equinus. (From Grosfeld JL, O'Neill J, Coran A, Fonkalsrud E: *Pediatric surgery*, ed 6, vol 2, Philadelphia, 2006, Elsevier.)

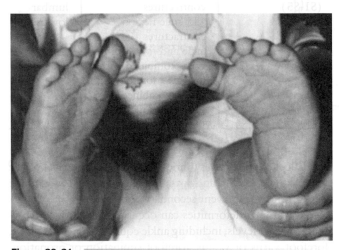

Figure 23-21
Metatarsus adductus. (From Grosfeld JL, O'Neill J, Coran A, Fonkalsrud E: *Pediatric surgery*, ed 6, vol 2, Philadelphia, 2006, Elsevier.)

contractures increase in frequency and severity in all lesion levels from early childhood into adolescence. Genu varus and valgus deformities are also found, along with lateral tibial torsion.

Hip deformities are common and include flexion and extension contractures, subluxation and dislocation, and torsional deformities of anteversion and retroversion. Many individuals with high lumbar lesions experience hip deformities as a result of the unopposed voluntary muscle activity of the hip flexors and adductors.[203] Hip flexion and adduction contractures increase the risk of hip subluxation or dislocation.[192,204] The frequency and severity of hip contractures reportedly is lower with low level lesions.[200]

Spinal deformities, such as scoliosis, kyphosis, and hyperlordosis, also are frequently associated with myelomeningocele. Scoliosis deformities may be congenital (secondary to vertebral anomalies) or acquired (secondary to muscle imbalances and positional deforming forces).[199] According to Trivedi et al.,[205] the prevalence of scoliosis is as high as 90% in patients with myelomeningocele, and approximately half of the spinal curves develop before 9 years of age. Scoliosis is more frequently observed with higher level lesion groups and becomes more prevalent and severe with increasing age in all groups.[199] Trivedi et al.[205] found that the most useful early predictor of the development of scoliosis is the level of the last posterior arch; thoracic level lesions lead to scoliosis in 89% of cases, high lumbar lesions (L1-L3) lead to scoliosis in 44% of cases, and low lumbar lesions (L4-L5) lead to scoliosis in 12% of cases. Kyphosis may be an isolated abnormality or may occur in conjunction with scoliosis; it may be limited to the lumbar spine or may involve the entire spinal column. Hyperlordosis is more prevalent in higher level lesions of myelomeningocele.

Two of the most obvious primary impairments are motor paralysis and abnormal or complete loss of sensation, especially of proprioception and kinesthetic awareness. The lower extremities are most affected; however, motor weakness in the upper extremities can occur and often is a sign of progressive neurological dysfunction. Osteopenia and the risk of fracture are increased in the lower extremities because of the decreased active muscle contraction forces through the long bones.[183] Sensory loss, which may not correlate with motor level involvement, also is common in the lower extremities, and lack of protective sensation often leads to skin breakdown. According to Shurtleff,[187] by young adulthood, 85% to 95% of patients will have suffered decubitus ulcers or other skin breakdown from tissue ischemia caused by excessive pressure, casts or orthoses, urine and stool soiling, friction and shear forces, and excessive weight bearing over bony prominences.

Many authors have confirmed the presence of abnormal sensory function related to proprioceptive and kinesthetic awareness deficits, which preferentially affect the upper extremity. Fine motor skills are impeded by slowness and inadequate adjustments of manipulative forces, and postural sway is affected by abnormal body position sense, possibly resulting from cerebellar ataxia, motor cortex or pyramidal tract damage, or motor learning deficits.[183,206-209] The motor level is defined as the lowest intact functional neuromuscular segment. Criteria for establishing motor levels were developed by the International Myelodysplasia Study Group using manual muscle testing.[183] Sensory levels do not consistently correlate with motor levels, therefore testing of dermatomes is imperative for light touch, pinprick, and vibration sense.[183,210]

Many other impairments or complications are associated with myelomeningocele. According to Barker et al.,[189]

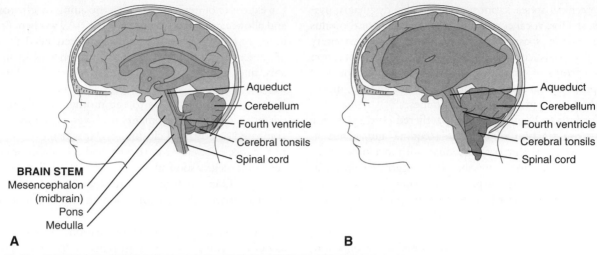

A, Normal brain with cerebrospinal fluid (CSF) circulation. **B,** Arnold-Chiari type II malformation with enlarged ventricles; this condition predisposes a child with myelomeningocele to hydrocephalus. The brain stem, the fourth ventricle, part of the cerebellum, and the cerebral tonsils are displaced downward through the foramen magnum, which leads to blockage of CSF flow. Also, pressure on the brain stem, which houses the cranial nerves, may result in nerve palsies. (From Goodman CC, Boissonnault WG, Fuller KS: *Pathology: implications for the physical therapist,* p 840, Philadelphia, 2003, WB Saunders.)

hydrocephalus occurs in 70% to 90% of individuals with myelomeningocele, and Bowmen et al.[190] reported that 80% to 90% of individuals with spina bifida require some form of central spinal fluid diversion (Figures 23-22 and 23-23). Shunt malfunction is a common complication caused by mechanical problems or infection, and as Caldarelli et al.[211] reported, almost half of patients with myelomeningocele require a shunt revision in the first year of life. Early symptoms of shunt complications related to increased intracranial pressure include alterations in the level of consciousness, restlessness, irritability, headache, respiratory changes, fever, and abdominal pain.[189]

Symptoms of Shunt Complications

- Altered level of consciousness
- Restlessness
- Irritability
- Headache
- Respiratory changes
- Fever
- Abdominal pain

Hydrocephalus frequently is associated with Arnold-Chiari type II malformation, characterized by a decent of the cerebellar vermis, fourth ventricle, and brain stem into the cervical spine.[189,212,213] Arnold-Chiari type II malformation is associated with multiple anomalies and may cause depressed respiratory drive (including apneic attacks), caudal cranial nerve palsies, or tetraparesis in the newborn. More often, symptoms arise in infants and children in the

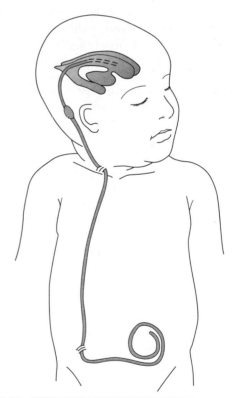

Figure 23-23

Ventriculoperitoneal shunt provides primary drainage of cerebrospinal fluid from the ventricles to an extracranial compartment, usually either the heart or the abdominal or peritoneal cavity, as shown. Extra tubing is left in the extracranial site to uncoil as the child grows. A unidirectional valve designed to open at a predetermined intraventricular pressure and to close when the pressure falls below that level prevents backflow of fluid. (From Goodman CC, Boissonnault WG, Fuller KS: *Pathology: implications for the physical therapist,* p 841, Philadelphia, 2003, WB Saunders.)

form of central apnea, cyanosis, bradycardia, dysphagia, nystagmus, stridor, vocal cord paralysis, torticollis, opisthotonus (severe muscle spasm), hypotonia, and upper extremity weakness or spasticity.[212-214] Hydromyelia is a complication with symptoms of rapidly progressive scoliosis, weakness of the upper extremities, spasticity, and ascending motor strength changes in the lower extremities.[189]

According to Wagner et al.,[213] tethered cord syndrome results from traction of the cauda equina and occurs in approximately one third of individuals with myelomeningocele. It most commonly presents with progressive scoliosis, gait changes, spasticity, or pain; less commonly, back pain, weakness, contractures of the lower extremities, or changes in bladder function may herald tethered cord syndrome.[190,215] Seizures secondary to brain malformation, cerebrospinal fluid (CSF) shunt malfunction or infection, and residual brain damage from a previous shunt infection or malfunction occur in 10% to 30% of children and adolescents with myelomeningocele.[183]

Other complications include bladder and bowel control difficulties caused by partial or complete denervation of S2-S4. These complications, which may result from spinal cord tethering, lead to neurogenic bladder.[183,189] According to Reigel,[216] fewer than 5% of children with myelomeningocele develop voluntary control of the urinary or anal sphincter.[183] Urinary tract infections are a common problem.[189]

In a study by Yeates et al.,[217] 50% of individuals with spina bifida had patterns of assets and deficits consistent with nonverbal learning disabilities. Dennis and Barnes[218] found that alterations in functional numeracy, which is predictive of higher social, personal, and community independence, were directly related to the number of shunt revisions. Latex allergies, which are thought to arise from repeated exposure and contact with latex products during both diagnostic and therapeutic interventions, occur in up to 73% of children and adolescents with spina bifida.[189,192,219] Finally, 50% or more of children with spina bifida age 6 years or older are overweight, and more than half of their adolescent and adult counterparts are obese.[189] Obesity leads to the recurrence of spinal deformities, hip and knee flexion contractures, and numerous health problems, including hypertension, skin infections, pressure sores, respiratory disease, heart disease, diabetes, impaired mobility, poor performance of ADLs, and decreased self-esteem.

Medical and Surgical Management

The primary neurosurgical intervention is repair of the open neural tube defect, usually within 48 to 72 hours after birth. The treatment goals are elimination of CSF leakage, preservation of neural function, and prevention of infection and secondary tethering of the spinal cord.[213] In utero repair aims to improve the functional outcome by reducing the exposure of nervous tissue to the amniotic environment and allowing nerve repair to proceed.[193] Two benefits of in utero repair have been found: a reduced need for shunt placement as a result of a reduced incidence of hydrocephalus, and reduced or even prenatal reversal of hindbrain herniation.[213,220] Fetal surgery remains controversial because of the high risks to the mother and fetus, and it has not yielded improvements in lower extremity function compared to postnatal closure.[193] Most babies with myelomeningocele are either born with hydrocephalus or develop ventriculomegaly soon after the neural tube defect is repaired. These children undergo ventriculoperitoneal shunting to manage excess CSF accumulation in the ventricles of the brain.[221]

Arnold-Chiari type II malformation, which usually is associated with hydrocephalus, remains an important cause of death and disability for individuals with myelomeningocele; therefore early detection and appropriate management are imperative. Before surgical intervention, the shunt must be evaluated for malfunction, because this may provoke or worsen a Arnold-Chiari malformation.[213] According to Griebel et al.,[222] surgical decompression of the Arnold-Chiari malformation has shown benefit in reducing upper and lower limb spasticity.

Although a goal of myelomeningocele repair is to prevent secondary tethering of the spinal cord, one third of individuals develop symptomatic spinal cord tethering.[213] Phuong et al.[223] reported that the progression of symptoms related to cord tethering was insidious; no effective method is available to prevent retethering, and 90% of individuals eventually undergo surgery to treat recurrent symptoms.[213,223] The surgical goal is to untether the spinal cord by dissecting the encasing arachnoidal adhesions.[213,224]

Most surgeons agree that no intervention is necessary for an individual with myelomeningocele with bilateral hip dislocations; however, whether to intervene with unilateral hip dislocation remains controversial.[193,199] In studying hip dislocation and its relation to functional gait, Gabrieli et al.[225] found that gait symmetry corresponded to the absence of hip contractures or bilateral symmetrical contractures but showed no relation to the presence of hip dislocation. These authors recommended addressing gait asymmetry by reducing soft tissue contractures rather than by surgically reducing unilateral hip dislocation.[193,225] In contrast, Lorente Moltó and Garrido[191] found that iliopsoas posterolateral transfer performed on subluxed or dislocated hips was effective in obtaining hip stability in properly selected patients with a lesion at level L3. Mayfield[199] states that a level pelvis and good range of motion are more important for function than hip reduction. Furthermore, surgery may be indicated for an individual with a lesion at level L3 or lower if quadriceps function is present and the potential exists for ambulation into adulthood.[183]

Surgical release of hip flexion contractures frequently is required in this patient group.[204] Complete posterior release and posterior knee capsulotomies often are recommended for individuals with knee flexion contractures of 20° or more. For both knee and hip procedures, upright standing in the early postoperative period and limited immobilization time are recommended for successful outcomes. Knee flexion contractures do recur, usually because of inadequate bracing, postoperative fractures, lack of postoperative physical therapy, obesity, or poor motivation to stand and walk.[226]

Derotational osteotomies for excessive lateral tibial torsion also have been studied. Vankoski et al.[227] found that children with lateral tibial torsion greater than 20° who failed to exhibit improved knee extension and extension moments in AFOs may benefit from derotational osteotomies.[227]

Numerous foot deformities can occur with all levels of myelomeningocele, leading to an array of surgical corrective procedures. Hindfoot valgus is commonly found in low level myelomeningocele. Medial displacement osteotomy of the calcaneus was studied by Torosian and Dias,[228] who found it to be a straightforward and successful procedure; the long-term benefit is preservation of subtalar motion. This procedure is indicated for patients with severe hindfoot valgus, associated pain, ulceration, and difficulty wearing a brace.

Surgical treatment for scoliosis is reserved for curves greater than 20°, because smaller curves often resolve without intervention.[205] The ideal minimum age for spinal fusion is 10 to 11 years old in girls and 12 to 13 years old in boys.[183,199] Several authors recommend combined anterior and posterior spinal fusion, each with instrumentation for individuals with thoracic level lesions.[192] Nutritional support, use of antibiotics, early mobilization, wearing a brace for 1 year, and family education are stressed.[192,229] The surgical procedure performed to reduce kyphosis is a kyphectomy. Although kyphectomy without instrumentation initially was reported to give excellent results, the recurrence of kyphosis was significant.[193,230] Therefore the use of instrumentation with transverse fixation is recommended to improve stability. A thorough assessment of the individual's status, including body weight and indications of osteopenia, should also be done.[231]

Rehabilitation Management: Evaluation, Intervention, and Clinical Implications

A child with myelomeningocele requires multidisciplinary care, and special consideration should be given to coordinating goals for the child and providing consistent information to the family. Evaluation and intervention should focus on enhancement of the child's development through management and reduction of impairments and maximization of the child's future functional potential through anticipation of secondary impairments.

After a complete history is obtained, the newborn should be evaluated for motor and sensory function before and after closure of the neural tube defect. This baseline information provides a foundation for planning and prioritizing interventions and family education, anticipating future functional potential and needs, and establishing the newborn's neurological status in order to monitor any changes. The newborn should be examined in the side lying position to prevent further injury to the lesion.[232] The infant should be in a quiet state when light touch and pinprick sensation are tested, and the testing should begin at the lowest level of sacral innervation and progress to higher levels until a response is elicited. Both deep tendon reflexes and primary reflexes should be examined.

Motor function testing should be done while the infant is in an alert state; these results can be documented as present or absent or as normal, weak, or absent. Techniques to elicit voluntary movement include placing the extremity in a gravity-dependent position to see whether the newborn holds the position; placing the extremity in an end range position to see whether the newborn moves out of the position; tickling; or using a variety of toys to prompt the newborn to move in response to auditory or visual stimuli. A knowledge of motor function can help the clinician predict habitual positioning and joint contractures that may not reduce spontaneously because of decreased active muscle contraction.

The newborn's bilateral upper and lower extremity ROM should be assessed, and the examiner should keep in mind that the observed degree of flexion may be greater than the expected physiological flexion secondary to intrauterine positioning and decreased voluntary movement in the womb. Paralyzed limbs should be moved delicately to prevent factures. Hip adduction should be assessed in the neutral position to prevent hip dislocation or subluxation of an unstable hip.

Baseline muscle tone should be assessed bilaterally in the upper and lower extremities of the newborn. Hypotonia throughout the body is common, especially in the neck and trunk; however, hypotonia or hypertonia can be found in the limbs as well. Early bilateral examination of the hips and feet should be performed, because hip and foot deformities are common.

Families should be educated in the handling and positioning of the newborn after closure of the neural tube. They also should be given verbal and written instructions on appropriate range of motion, stretching, and soft tissue mobilization techniques, as well as initial developmental activities to facilitate head and trunk control.

During the child's infancy, clinicians should continue to monitor joint alignment, muscle imbalance, and the development of joint contractures. Hip and knee flexion contractures are typical and can be combined with lateral rotation at the hips, especially when hip muscles are very weak or absent. It is imperative to monitor ROM and muscle extensibility closely and to initiate stretching exercises early, with the goal of achieving and maintaining full range

The goals of rehabilitation after fracture are to resolve impairments of mobility, strength, and function. Unlike adults, children often are not as restricted by the immobilization and have less deconditioning. They may be able to restore mobility and function independent of active physical therapy intervention, although this is somewhat site dependent.

Stress Fractures

Stress fractures are a type of overuse injury most often seen in the lower extremity. With normal use, microfractures occur and heal as part of the normal strengthening process of bone. As stresses to the bone increase, the extent of microfractures also increases. During periods of dramatically increased training, the number of microfractures increases faster than the body's ability to repair the fractures. These microfractures can coalesce into a stress fracture.

A stress fracture should be suspected in a child with a history of activity-related pain who reports a recent increase in activity level. Plain radiographic films frequently are negative, and a bone scan, computed tomography (CT), or magnetic resonance imaging (MRI) often is required to confirm the diagnosis (Figure 24-5). Other contributing factors, such as anorexia, menstrual irregularity, rheumatoid arthritis, neuropathy, and metabolic diseases, can increase the incidence of stress fractures, and the clinician must always consider these risk factors.[31]

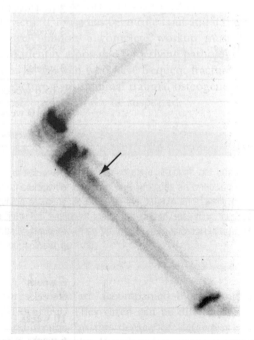

Figure 24-5
Bone scan of the tibia showing increased uptake of radioisotope consistent with a stress fracture.

Risk Factors for Stress Fractures
• Dramatic increase in activity
• Anorexia
• Menstrual irregularity
• Rheumatoid arthritis
• Neuropathy
• Metabolic diseases

Usually a period of relative rest is sufficient; this may be limited to restriction from athletics or may include limited weight bearing and immobilization for 4 to 8 weeks. It is important that the patient not return to activity until pain free; it is equally important that the return be gradual and that any underlying muscle weaknesses are corrected. If the patient had multiple stress fractures, a bone density radiograph (dual energy x-ray absorptiometry [DEXA]) should be obtained. Physical therapy can address specific impairments of mobility, strength, and muscle imbalances.

Shoulder Physeal Stress Fracture (Little Leaguer's Shoulder)

"Little leaguer's shoulder," or proximal humeral epiphysiolysis, is a stress fracture of the proximal humeral physis. Pitching, throwing, and certain racquet sports produce repeated torsional stresses across the physis, causing cartilaginous microfractures that result in widening of the physis from lateral to medial. The number of throws, not the technique, is the critical risk factor, therefore the number of throws the child is allowed to do each week should be controlled. No long-term problems after this injury have been reported.

Pain is the most commonly presenting symptom. It increases with the duration of pitching or throwing and usually is severe enough to prevent the child from participating. The pain localizes to the proximal lateral humerus and is worsened by medial or lateral rotation of the arm while the shoulder is in 90° abduction. Radiographic films of both shoulders (anteroposterior [AP] medial and lateral rotation views) usually are sufficient to demonstrate the lesion (Figure 24-6). Further imaging is rarely needed. On the radiographic films, the lateral aspect of the physis is widened compared to the rest of the physis or the opposite side.

Treatment includes stopping throwing or racquet sports until the pain resolves, usually a minimum of 6 to 12 weeks. A stretching and strengthening program to restore and improve throwing mechanics is then begun. A gradual return to the sport is instituted, with an emphasis on the pitch count. Fewer than 300 skilled throws per week is considered safe.[32] Coaches, the athlete, and the parents should be instructed to include pitches at practice, home,

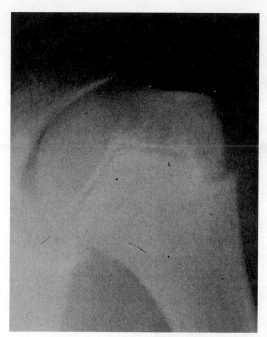

Figure 24-6
Anteroposterior (AP) image of the proximal humerus showing a widened lateral physis, indicative of a stress fracture of the physis.

and during games in the pitch count. Proper form and body mechanics are essential. General conditioning and pregame, postgame, and practice warm-up and cool-down activities are required, with emphasis on long-term results rather than quick return to play.

The clinician should identify movement impairments. The program should include restoring range of motion, with special attention to stretching the posterior capsule (e.g., sleeper stretch). A comprehensive rotator cuff and periscapular strengthening program is begun once the child is asymptomatic. Improving the performance of the dynamic stabilizers is essential. Return to throwing progresses in a very structured pattern, with emphasis on re-establishing proper throwing techniques. Rehabilitation professionals play an important role in educating parents, coaches, and athletes in the prevention of onset or further progression of dysfunction.

Prevention and Treatment of Overuse Injuries in Throwing Athletes

- Ensure proper conditioning, training practices, and warm-ups
- Keep sessions short
- Limit volume (i.e., innings, pitches)
- Ensure 3 to 4 days of rest between games
- Provide coaching in proper techniques
- Discourage pitching at home during and after the season
- Discourage curve balls, sliders, and breaking balls

Microinstability in the Shoulder

Most shoulder injuries in the young are minor and resolve with rest. Trauma can cause fractures and dislocations, which are similar to those injuries in the adult. Repetitive, strenuous use of the shoulder can stretch the shoulder capsule, leading to several problems. Most microinstability occurs as the anterior capsule is stretched, and the condition is most common in throwers and swimmers. Pain, clicking, and labral damage can ensue. Eventually, subacromial impingement and rotator cuff damage can occur. Improper technique, muscle group strength and endurance imbalance, and overuse are commonly implicated.

Pain with or after throwing or swimming is the typical complaint, and clicking occurs as the process advances. Over time, impingement can occur, leading to pain with overhead use and night pain. The physical examination shows minor anterior laxity, tenderness on anterior glenohumeral joint palpation, pain with apprehension testing, and a possible labral click with various labral testing techniques. Advanced cases produce a positive result on impingement testing, and rotator cuff weakness may be present. Radiographs are normal. In the early stages, MRI results are normal. However, labral changes (best detected when contrast is used in the joint) may become evident later, and in advanced cases, rotator cuff damage is evident.[33]

In the *Cochrane Database of Systematic Reviews*, Handoll et al.[34] compared surgical to conservative management of primary dislocation of the shoulder in five studies, some involving patients as young as 16 years of age. They concluded that surgery was successful for young adults, primarily males, who were active and engaged in demanding physical activities. Each of the studies used different rehabilitation programs, and none was specific to the adolescent population.[34]

The causative activity (throwing or swimming) must be halted. Inflammation is mitigated with anti-inflammatory medicines. As with adults, muscle strength throughout the shoulder girdle and endurance disparities must be corrected. Static and dynamic stabilization of the scapular muscles, neuromuscular re-education, and proprioception are essential for retraining normal patterns of muscle activity. Finally, skill development and technique must be corrected to prevent recurrence. When this is ineffective, surgical repair of the labrum and tightening of the anterior capsule may be needed. Rotator cuff surgery rarely is needed in the young (Figure 24-7).

Little Leaguer's Elbow

"Little leaguer's elbow" consists of one or more of four injuries to the young elbow. These are medial epicondyle physeal injury ("apophysitis"), radiocapitellar osteochondritis dissecans, anterior elbow strain and contracture, and posterior ulnohumeral shear injury. The normal mechanics

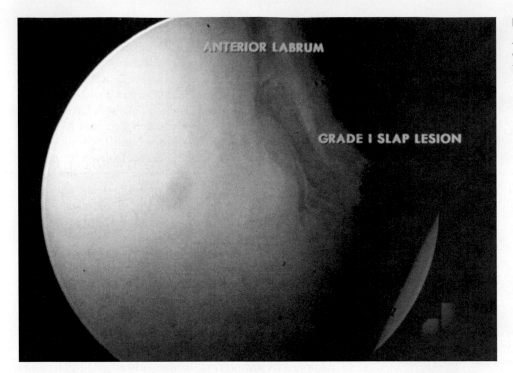

Figure 24-7
Arthroscopic view of early labral degeneration from excessive throwing.

of throwing (i.e., medial traction, lateral compression, anterior strain, and posterior shear) are the cause of this condition. Some evidence indicates that the number of throws is a more critical variable than the pitching style.[35] Typically, medial apophysitis occurs first, followed by a lateral osteochondral injury. Anterior strain and posterior ulnohumeral damage are late findings.

A young thrower with elbow pain should be questioned about the onset and the location or locations of pain, the number of pitches thrown per outing, rest between outings, and other positions played when not pitching. The typical case is a 12-year-old boy who does not count pitches, who pitches in multiple leagues, and who plays shortstop when not pitching.

The physical examination shows tenderness at the medial epicondyle, radiocapitellar joint, anterior soft tissues, and/or posterior ulnohumeral joint. In advanced cases, loss of terminal extension is seen. If an applied valgus stress causes pain and demonstrates laxity, a partial tear of the ulnar collateral ligament (UCL) should be suspected.

Plain radiographic films can show widening of the medial physis (Figure 24-8), radiocapitellar osteochondral damage, and loose bodies. An MRI scan commonly shows the extent of the osteochondral injury and the status of the UCL.

Early injury with minimal findings on imaging is treated with rest. In some cases, throwing must be halted for up to 1 full year. If the medial apophysis is displaced more than 5 mm, if the radiocapitellar osteochondritis dissecans (OCD) shows an unstable lesion, or if loose bodies are present, surgery is required. The medial apophysis can be

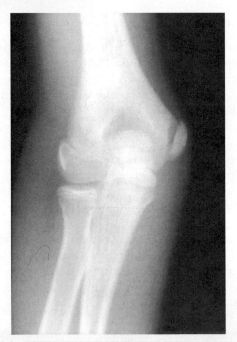

Figure 24-8
Anteroposterior (AP) radiograph showing widening of the medial apophysis. A comparison view of the opposite elbow can be obtained if necessary.

repaired with hardware, and the OCD lesion can be drilled, repaired, or debrided as needed. Loose bodies can be removed by open or arthroscopic techniques. A torn UCL in a child probably should be repaired or reconstructed if the child intends to return to pitching, but no studies exist that confirm this.

The goals of physical therapy are similar to those for little leaguer's shoulder: normalize ROM, strengthen the muscles that surround the joint, and improve muscle balance, proprioception, and throwing technique. For early symptoms, short periods of rest are necessary. This should be supported with strengthening and stretching of the elbow and forearm muscles. Longer rest and a progressive return to throwing are necessary for individuals with more persistent dysfunction.

Radial Head Dislocation (Nursemaid's Elbow)

"Nursemaid's elbow" is the distal dislocation of the radial head from the encircling annular ligament. It can be caused by a forceful traction on an extended, pronated forearm, such as occurs when an adult holding a child's hand pulls the child away from danger. The radial head becomes entrapped in the radiocapitellar joint. This dislocation occurs most often in children 1 to 4 years old; it is rare after 6 years of age, when the radial head is more fully formed.[36]

At the time of examination, the child presents with pain in the elbow, which is held in a slightly flexed position with the forearm pronated. If the history is appropriate, a reduction maneuver may be performed even before radiographs are obtained. Radiographic films are required for a first-time dislocation to ensure that no concomitant fracture is involved (e.g., Monteggia's fracture, which is a radial head dislocation with a fracture of the ulna); however, radiographic films of a radial head subluxation do not show a recognizable pattern. They may or may not show failure of the radial head to align with the capitellum. It also is important to differentiate nursemaid's elbow from congenital radial head dislocation, for which reduction is not successful.

Either of two reduction maneuvers may be used to treat radial head dislocation. One maneuver requires supination of the forearm with the elbow in slight flexion and the physician's thumb placed over the radial head. The other maneuver, which has been reported as being more successful, is hyperpronation followed by elbow flexion.[37] A successful reduction maneuver usually results in a pop, followed by resolution of the child's pain. The extremity can then be splinted for comfort, but no formal immobilization is required. If reduction is unsuccessful and radiographs are negative for fracture, a congenital dislocation should be considered, and surgical reduction may be warranted.

Gymnast's Wrist

Gymnasts, weight lifters, and cheerleaders often use their wrists as weight-bearing joints and in doing so place supraphysiological loads on the wrists. Repetitive loading of the wrists in this manner can lead to dorsal impaction and physeal damage. *Dorsal impaction* is the forceful loading of the wrist while it is in extension, leading to synovitis, edema,

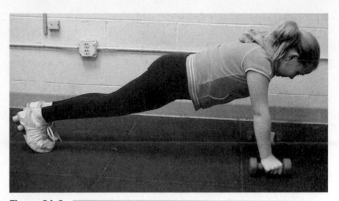

Figure 24-9

Dumbbells positioned correctly may help keep the wrists in neutral position to avoid hyperextension overuse injuries while exercises are performed.

and bone bruising at the radiocarpal joint. Chronic injury to the distal radial physis can lead to premature closure. Premature closure of the radial physis with continued growth of the distal ulna can lead to a shortened radius and positive ulnar variance. This, in turn, can lead to an ulnar impaction syndrome and pain.

Wrist pain in an individual at high risk should prompt a thorough examination. The pain may be localized to the distal radial physis, the dorsum of the wrist, or both. Initially, plain radiographs may be negative. As the process progresses, physeal bridging and positive ulnar variance may be seen. An MRI scan may reveal bone edema and synovitis before changes are seen on plain radiographs.

As with most overuse injuries, rest, using wrist splinting that limits dorsiflexion, can lead to healing and prevent further damage. Once physeal bridging occurs, surgical intervention is recommended, with resection of the physeal bar if it is less than 25% or an ulnar epiphysiodesis and/or shortening and radial osteotomy as needed.[38]

The clinician should assist coaches with proper training techniques. Taping, padding, or adapting exercise is helpful for reducing stress in hyperextension (Figure 24-9). Strengthening of the wrist flexors, as well as total arm strengthening, may reduce stress at the wrists. Ice is used to control pain after a workout.

Repetitive Strain Injuries from Computer and Video Game Use

Computers and video games are found in many schools and homes worldwide. Warning labels actually appear on the Web sites of video game manufacturers, warning against repetitive strain injuries and seizure activity related to extended use.[39] Rehabilitation professionals may be involved in educational programs to teach children and their parents appropriate sitting posture and to address specific injuries, such as carpal tunnel syndrome (CTS) or neck pain. Excessive use can lead to a sedentary lifestyle and result

Prevention of Computer and Video Game Overuse Injuries

1. Maintain a neutral sitting posture:
   - Back supported
   - No compression at popliteal angle
   - Feet on floor or footrest
   - Head on neck balance
   - Upper arm not abducted
   - Elbow angle at 90°
   - Neutral wrist
2. Follow a healthy lifestyle:
   - Nutrition
   - Stress management
3. Change tasks or take breaks.
4. Keep movements relaxed and use light force.
5. Prevent eyestrain:
   - Reduce glare
   - Adjust brightness, contrast

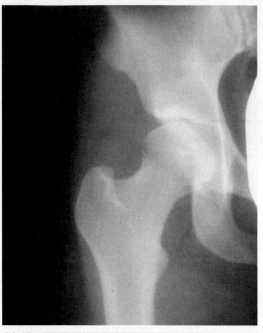

Figure 24-10
Adult with a shallow acetabulum from untreated hip dysplasia.

in poor fitness and obesity. Computer workstations or video game play stations should be ergonomically designed to fit children. Many of the principles that apply to adults also apply to children; only the size is different.

Hip Dysplasia

Developmental dysplasia of the hip (DDH) (originally called *congenital hip dysplasia* or *congenital dislocation of the hip*) occurs when the femoral head is subluxated or dislocated from the acetabulum (Figure 24-10) in the perinatal period. This disrupts the normal growth and development of the hip joint, leading to a shallow acetabulum with a flattened femoral head. The incidence is 1 to 5 per 1000 live births, although the rate has been reported as high as 35 per 1000 live births among Native Americans. Additional risk factors include first-born child, family history, female gender, and breech birth.[40-42] The prognosis is determined by the age at diagnosis and the degree of dislocation and deformity of the femoral head.

Risk Factors for Hip Dysplasia

- Race (white and Navajo Indian)
- First-born child
- Family history
- Female
- Breech birth

Perinatal screening focuses on two tests for detecting DDH: Barlow's test and Ortolani's test. Barlow's test is positive when the hip can be subluxated or dislocated from a reduced position; Ortolani's test is positive when the hip can be relocated from a dislocated position. These tests can be supplemented by ultrasound imaging in a perinatal child and radiographs once the child reaches 3 to 4 months of age. If the child is not screened, DDH often is not discovered until the child has difficulty walking or is noticed to walk with a waddling gait. A variant of the problem can present at several months of age after normal examinations earlier in life.[43]

If the dislocation is discovered in the perinatal period, treatment usually involves a Pavlik harness to hold the hip in a reduced position of abduction and lateral rotation. If the dislocation is discovered later or if closed reduction fails, a variety of surgical procedures can be performed, ranging from open reduction to femoral and acetabular osteotomies to reduce the hip and provide increased coverage for the femoral head. After any surgical treatment, the hip usually is protected by a hip spica cast for 6 to 18 weeks, and bracing then is used for up to an additional 6 to 12 months.

Physical therapists should instruct the family in activities of daily living (ADLs), how to put on and take off braces, and cast care. The Pavlik harness holds the hip in an abducted and flexed position, which looks like the letter M. It is worn full time for 6 to 8 weeks until the hip has stabilized. Children have a natural tendency to be unencumbered by the immobilization, which keeps the uninvolved extremities strong and flexible. However, exercise may be necessary, especially if treatment was delayed because of late diagnosis. After immobilization or surgery, the plan of care aims at improving resulting muscle weakness, ROM limitations, and gait deviations.

Snapping Hip

Snapping hip pain can be anterior or lateral. Anterior snapping hip usually refers to the movement of the iliopsoas tendon over the anterior hip. The iliopsoas tendon travels from the iliacus and psoas muscles on the interior pelvis over the anterior hip and attaches to the lesser trochanter. Snapping can be caused by an inflamed bursa, tightness in the tendon, or a prominent femoral head. Poor posture, with increased lumbar lordosis and more anterior pelvic rotation, allows greater lateral hip rotation but presents with a more prominent femoral head and shortens the psoas tendon. The tendon then snaps over the prominent femoral head or iliopectineal eminence, causing inflammatory changes and pain in the tendon. A snapping psoas causes anterior hip pain and a palpable snap. The snapping is best elicited by hip flexion followed by lateral rotation and extension. Although an MRI scan can show increased fluid in the psoas bursa, this is not diagnostic, and imaging studies rarely provide useful information.

Lateral hip snapping is caused by a tight iliotibial tract or band snapping over the greater trochanter; with lateral hip snapping, the iliotibial band (ITB) and tract are too tight and are overused. Overuse is thought to be the result of downhill running and weak core pelvic stabilizing muscles.

Oral anti-inflammatory drugs usually relieve the symptoms of both conditions. Resistant cases may require corticosteroid injections under fluoroscopic guidance, partial surgical release, or psoas or ITB lengthening. Treatment should include correction of lumbopelvic positional faults and correction of malalignment in the lower extremities. Identifying and resolving impairments of involved structures, muscle imbalances, and lack of flexibility are essential. Core stabilization and static postural training is followed by dynamic training with functional elements for the goal activities. Improper training techniques or biomechanics should be addressed and corrected.

Labral Tears of the Hip

Labral tears of the hip are recognized as a more common injury than once thought.[44] The tear is thought to be caused by a twisting injury, although underlying hip dysplasia can contribute to the labrum's susceptibility to damage. Labral damage frequently is accompanied by damage to the articular cartilage. A posterior hip subluxation due to trauma can cause a labral tear.

Hip pain and a palpable clunk with flexion, abduction, and external (lateral) rotation (i.e., the FABER test) are diagnostic for labral pathology. The pain usually can also be elicited by loaded hip rotation. An MRI arthrogram is useful for detecting labral lesions, and plain radiographs can be useful for detecting underlying acetabular dysplasia.

Arthroscopy is the treatment of choice for addressing labral lesions. As with meniscal lesions in the knee, treatment focuses on removing only the damaged portion of the lesion, leaving all intact labrum to help delay the appearance of osteoarthritis and further chondral injury. Recently, labral repairs have been attempted, but no data are available supporting the outcomes of labral repair. Preoperatively, physical therapy focuses on improving pain-free ROM through stretching and joint mobilization. Short axis distraction can be helpful for relieving pain and improving mobility. Postoperatively, impairments resulting from relative inactivity are resolved with progressive exercise.

Slipped Capital Femoral Epiphysis

Slipped capital femoral epiphysis (SCFE) is an acute or chronic fracture of the proximal femoral physis. Normally, in early adolescence the physis moves from a horizontal to an oblique orientation. This converts compressive stresses to shear stresses at the physis, putting the physis at risk for a Salter-Harris type I shear fracture. Other risk factors include male gender, high activity level, and obesity; 50% of patients have bilateral SCFE.[45] SCFE most commonly presents in boys in late childhood to early adolescence. Initially it may present as vague hip or knee pain that worsens with activity. An acute episode may occur, or the condition may be a chronic, low level, ongoing process. As the slip progresses, the patient has restricted range of motion, especially medial rotation. An overweight child with vague knee or hip pain may have SCFE. Radiographs, including an AP pelvis and frog lateral views, are useful for detecting the slip. Because slips may be subtle, careful radiograph analysis is necessary. The contralateral hip should always be evaluated. Further imaging rarely is required.

Risk Factors for Slipped Capitol Femoral Epiphysis

- Age (adolescence)
- Male
- High activity level
- Obesity

Surgical treatment is recommended for SCFE. If the slip is chronic, surgery may be delayed for several days. An acute slip is a relative emergency; it usually is stabilized with one or two screws across the physis within 24 hours. The screw acts to stimulate closure of the physis and prevent further migration. Non-weight-bearing is required until physeal closure is complete. Fifty percent of patients require pinning of the opposite side because of a slip there. A chronic slip typically is treated with a single in situ screw. An acute slip is treated with two screws. After surgery, the goals of rehabilitation are to normalize impairments of strength, flexibility, and gait. The clinician should assist the child and family in setting appropriate goals and plans for returning to activities and sports.

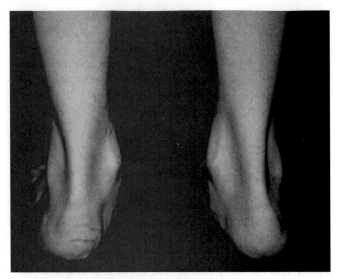

Figure 24-17
"Too many toes" laterally and a valgus heel are the hallmarks of hyperpronation and pes planus.

the individual has plantar fascial pain, or the cosmetic deformity is unacceptable. In these cases the first line of treatment is the use placement of functional orthotic inserts, which range from simple off-the-shelf arch supports to custom-molded devices. In rare cases a bony procedure, such as a calcaneal osteotomy, must be performed to correct the deformity.[84]

Plantar Fasciitis

Plantar fasciitis is manifested by patient complaints of pain at the proximal origin on the calcaneus. Pain in the sole of the foot is typical, especially in the morning on arising. Palpation demonstrates tenderness along the plantar fascia or at the medial calcaneal attachment. Imaging studies are not useful. Microtears occur in the fascial substance or attachment from repetitive traction. Achilles tendonitis and Sever's apophysitis frequently accompany plantar fasciitis in the child.

In all cases of plantar fasciitis, stretching of the calf and the plantar fascia is the primary treatment. Taping to support the plantar fascia can bring dramatic relief. Use of wooden rollers or tennis balls for direct massage is routinely successful. Use of functional orthotics has been advocated and can bring relief in many cases. On the other hand, orthotics can make plantar fasciitis more painful for some patients. No studies have clearly demonstrated which patients benefit from orthotics and which do not, and the podiatric literature has made the plea for more randomized, controlled studies.[85] Currently, there are strong advocates of orthotics only and as many or more for stretching only. Running and jumping must be reduced while treatment is undertaken. Night splints and surgical intervention are rarely used in the child.

Hallux Valgus

Hallux valgus in the immature or adolescent patient is a progressive valgus deformity of the hallux at the metatarsophalangeal joint. Hallux valgus is commonly called a "bunion" but the bunion, which consists of an exostosis, bursitis and a callus, is the result of a hallux valgus deformity. It usually is an inherited condition and frequently is accompanied by familial hyperlaxity and pes planus. The deformity results from altered foot mechanics caused by hyperpronation, a hypermobile first ray, and inherited bony malalignment. The deformity is apparent visually and progresses with time. It is rare in preadolescents. Radiographic films show increased intermetatarsal angles.

Observation is recommended for an asymptomatic adolescent hallux valgus. If pain develops or if the toes overlap, functional orthotics are helpful. Surgical correction is recommended only for the most severe, recalcitrant cases. A high recurrence rate is reported for surgically corrected hallux valgus in adolescents.[86]

Tarsal Coalition

Tarsal coalition is defined as a bony, cartilaginous, or fibrous connection between two or more of the bones in the midfoot or hindfoot. Approximately 90% are coalitions between the calcaneus and the navicular or between the middle facet of the talus and the calcaneus.[87] They are most commonly bilateral and occur in fewer that 1% of the general population. They are congenital and are thought to be caused by a failure of differentiation and segmentation. As the child matures, the coalition is thought to transform from a more cartilaginous union to a more rigid bony union that contributes to the pain.

The diagnosis usually is made in a child 11 to 15 years of age, with progressive flattening and increasing pain in one or both feet. The pain is worse with impact loading activities (which often coincide with an increase in athletic activities) and improves somewhat with rest. On physical examination, the child often has decreased subtalar motion and may have tight or spastic peroneal muscles. The child may also have a history of multiple ankle sprains. Although some of the coalitions may be seen on plain radiographs, a CT scan is the imaging study of choice.

Nonoperative therapies may be useful early in treatment; these include the use of orthotics, strengthening and stretching of the musculature, and possibly casting. When nonoperative therapy fails to provide sufficient relief, surgical procedures to excise the bony coalition with interposition of fat or muscle are suggested. When the coalition is unusually large or when degenerative changes in the subtalar joint have occurred, an arthrodesis may be required, although this is not the procedure of choice in an active young person. Patients may return to activities and sports after an appropriate rehabilitation program that involves restoring motion, strength, and function.

Spinal Injuries

Back pain is a common complaint in the general population; the lifetime prevalence is 60% to 90%. In the athletic population, it is a common reason for reporting injury and has a seasonal prevalence of 10% to 15%.[88] However, this is quite variable among different sports. In sports that emphasize the extremes of spinal motion, particularly when started at a young age (e.g., figure skating, ballet, and gymnastics), back injuries are seen in 30% of athletes or more.[89,90] For example, in one study of elite rhythmic gymnasts, back pain was reported in 85% of the athletes.[91] Prevention of these injuries is important for the young athlete with remaining spinal growth.

Multiple variables must be considered in the prevention and treatment of back injuries. The normal spinal development must be understood, as well as the ways repetitive forces may affect this development. Intrinsic biomechanics and sports-specific motion also are important co-factors of injury patterns. Finally, hormonal and nutritional factors may also be involved.

Spinal Anatomy, Development, and Biomechanics

The lumbar spine is a flexible structure that is positioned between two relatively inflexible entities, the sacrum and the thoracic spine. At the distal end of the lumbar spine, the lumbosacral juncture represents an abrupt lordotic transition to the pelvis. At the proximal thoracolumbar juncture, the transition is more gradual. The T1 to T10 segments are somewhat immobilized by the rib conjoined attachments, whereas T11 and T12 are free floating ribs with less immobilization. The distal lumbar spine is a common site of injury, possibly because of the more rigid fixation of the sacrum and pelvis and the acute lordotic angle of the lower lumbar spine.

The spine can be divided into anterior and posterior elements. The anterior elements include the intervertebral disc and the vertebral bodies. The posterior elements include the posterior arch with the pedicles, zygapophyseal joints (facets), lamina, spinous process, transverse processes, and attached ligaments (Figure 24-18). Essentially, each segment of the spine moves as a tripod (trijoint complex) with involvement of the intervertebral disc and two facet joints. Each joint is subject to force, depending on the position. In sitting and forward bending, the axis of rotation is at the intervertebral disc. With extension, such as a layback spin in figure skating, the axis of rotation changes to the facet joints, and pressure is applied to the pars interarticularis (pars), which is the thinnest part of the posterior arch between the facet joints (Figure 24-19). This is the location of a common stress fracture, or spondylolysis.

The intervertebral disc has two components. The outer ligamentous layers are well-organized sheaths of lamellae called the annulus. The outer third of the annulus is innervated. The inner gelatinous substance is the nucleus pulposus, which contains proteoglycans and type II collagen to maintain its osmotic gradient for a hydrated state.

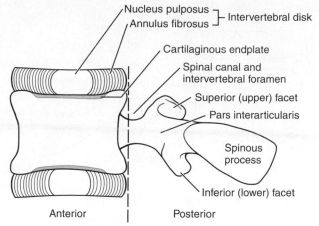

Figure 24-18
The anterior elements of the spine include the intervertebral disc and the vertebral bodies. The posterior elements include the posterior arch with the pedicles, zygapophyseal joints (facets), lamina, spinous process, transverse processes, and attached ligaments.

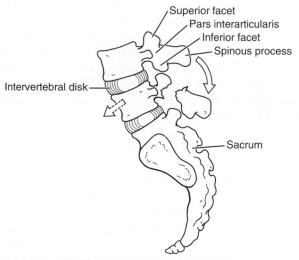

Figure 24-19
The pars interarticularis (pars) is the thinnest part of the posterior arch between the facet joints. This is the location of a common stress fracture, spondylolysis, which is caused by overloading with excessive extension.

The sacroiliac (SI) joint also is anatomically important in back injuries. The inferior one third of the SI joint is a true synovial joint with hyaline cartilage.[92] Forces such as landing from a jump, as is seen in skaters or gymnasts, are transmitted from the lower extremities to the trunk via the SI joint. Hip motion also affects the SI joint. For example, during hip flexion, a posterior pelvic tilt results in SI compression and lumbar flexion. Conversely, extension causes an anterior tilt, SI distraction, and lumbar extension.

Spinal development is a process that occurs from intrauterine development until the late teens. At birth each end of the vertebral body has an epiphyseal plate or ring epiphysis. On the intervertebral disc side, the epiphysis

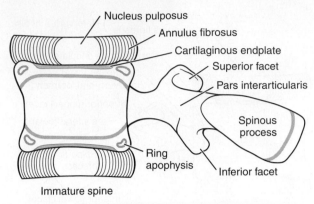

Figure 24-20
Around the circumference of the end plate is the apophyseal ring, which has inherent attachments to the annulus fibrosus.

functions as a cartilaginous end plate. Around the circumference of the end plate is the apophyseal ring, which has inherent attachments to the annulus fibrosus (Figure 24-20).[93] As the spine matures into adulthood, the end plate thickens with the development of subchondral bone. However, during adolescence, repetitive forces to the soft cartilaginous end plate and apophysis may cause growth abnormalities and disc herniation through these soft end plates (Schmorl's nodes). Furthermore, it has been shown that spondylolisthesis slippage occurs through the epiphysis during the growth spurt.[94]

Growth also affects the sagittal alignment of the spine. From the age of 6 through adolescence, thoracic kyphosis and lumbar lordosis increase progressively.[95] This is most notable in the prepubertal period.

Spinal motion relies on coordinated interaction of pelvic flexibility and trunk muscle activation. Hyperlordosis increases stress on the posterior elements. Factors that increase lordosis include iliopsoas inflexibility, thoracolumbar tightness, lower abdominal weakness, thoracic kyphosis, and genu recurvatum.[96] Trunk and lower extremity weakness are also risk factors for back injuries.[97,98] Core stabilization includes the intrinsic muscles of the multifidus, the transversus abdominis and internal obliques, that control segmental stability. It also includes the extrinsic group of muscles that connect the thorax and pelvis to the lower trunk (Figure 24-21). Proper coordination in the kinetic chain is important.

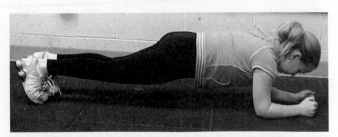

Figure 24-21
Planks are an excellent way to use body weight as resistance. Proper performance requires core strength and stabilization of the scapula.

Anterior Element Injury

Acute Disc Herniation. Acute lumbar disc herniations occur in about 2% of the general population.[99] They can occur in any patient as a result of repetitive loading in forward flexion. In the adolescent, they may present without radiating symptoms to the lower extremities and are most common at the L4-L5 and L5-S1 level. A variation of this is an acute annular tear without herniation of the nucleus pulposus. Apophyseal avulsion can occur, especially unique to the young athlete, in which the annulus pulls a piece of the ring apophysis from the vertebra. The presentation often is an inability to forward flex and a sciatic shift (lateral shift caused by pressure on the sciatic nerve) or scoliosis. Herniations usually are well demonstrated on an MRI scan.

These conditions usually are managed successfully in a conservative manner with relative rest and anti-inflammatory medication, which may include a fluoroscopically directed epidural corticosteroid injection. In the acute phase, a rigid brace in 15° extension often is useful for resolving the inflammation and mobilizing the patient into therapy. Gradually, an aggressive core stabilization program is started when the patient is able to do it. Surgical consideration is given to any progressive neurological deficit or refractory symptoms.

Clinical Point: Red Flag!

- Cauda equina symptoms with bowel or bladder dysfunction are a surgical emergency

Degenerative Disc Disease. In the adolescent, the predominant cause of low back pain is posterior element spondylolysis (47%). In the adult, the predominant cause is discogenic (48%).[100] Nonetheless, MRI changes in the disc have been noted in the young who perform repetitive flexion and extension, such as gymnasts. These changes include irregularities in the end plate and ring apophysis, as well as herniation of the disc through the end plate (Schmorl's node).[101] The risk of these changes is directly related to the amount of time spent in the activity; an excess of 15 hours per week increases the risk. When these end plate changes, such as Schmorl's nodes, occur at the thoracolumbar juncture, the condition is referred to as atypical Scheuermann's disease and often presents with a flat back. Pain caused by disc degeneration often is manifested by flexion-based activities. Peripheral symptoms usually do not occur except for some nonspecific referred pain.

Treatment involves a therapy program with cross training, core stabilization, and careful review of the biomechanics of the individual before return to competition. Extension bracing often is helpful in early mobilization and initial return to restricted activities. Well-defined periods of administration of anti-inflammatory medication are often useful. Epidural injections are more controversial with axial pain but may be considered in refractory cases. Adolescents with atypical Scheuermann's disc disease often benefit from extension bracing to help alleviate the flat back posture.

Posterior Element Injury

Spondylolysis and Spondylolisthesis. Spondylolysis is a stress fracture of the pars interarticularis. This injury most often occurs from repetitive hyperextension, in which the inferior articular facet impinges on the pars interarticularis and lamina below. In the nonathletic population, it has been demonstrated to occur in 5% of the population by the age of 6 and without symptoms or any long-term back pain.[102] However, in certain sports it has a higher frequency and is symptomatic; the incidence is as high as 33% in ballet and 32% in gymnastics. Furthermore, during the adolescent growth spurt, a small risk exists that spondylolysis will progress to spondylolisthesis. These adolescent patients present with activity-related pain that worsens on lumbar hyperextension, more specifically single leg hyperextension.[100]

Plain radiographs are not sufficiently sensitive to detect the stress fracture, which is diagnosed by single photon emission computed tomography (SPECT) bone scans. However, MRI techniques that focus on the posterior elements with 2 to 3 mm cuts are sensitive in the detection of spondylolysis without the adverse side effect of ionizing radiation.[103] A CT scan may be obtained to define the fracture's healing ability.

Treatment of spondylolysis involves antilordotic bracing and removal from activities that provoke symptoms for 6 weeks. During this time the patient may continue activities such as biking and aquatic exercise to maintain the level of conditioning. At the same time, a physical therapy program that addresses peripelvic flexibility and antilordotic strengthening should be initiated. After this period, once the adolescent is free of pain during hyperextension and at rest, a gradual return to preinjury activities is allowed, providing the patient remains pain free and continues to wear the brace. Using the brace during recreational or athletic activity inhibits extension and hyperextension activities, protecting the area. Ultimately, the rehabilitation program must stress full core stabilization with a flexion bias. Return to full recreational activities and athletics usually is not allowed for 4 months. Athletes with a minimal grade spondylolisthesis with a positive bone scan (a scan showing abnormal bone activity) are treated in a similar fashion. However, if the slippage is old, short-term bracing and similar therapy can be used. Uncommonly, these require a surgical fusion.

Lordotic Low Back Pain. During adolescence, lordosis normally increases. Cyclical loading of the posterior elements may cause excessive traction and compression of the spinous process and iliac crest apophyses, resulting in apophysitis. Furthermore, stress may be applied to the zygapophyseal joints resulting in chondromalacia and to transitional vertebrae pseudarthrosis (Bertolotti's syndrome). A transitional vertebra usually represents an incomplete segmentation of L5 with a bony extension to the ala of the sacrum. Bertolotti's syndrome usually is asymptomatic until repetitive extension is experienced. Collectively, these entities are referred to as lordotic low back pain. The adolescent often presents as in spondylolysis, with extension-based low back pain, except that the SPECT bone scan or MRI scan is normal.

Therapy emphasizes antilordotic strengthening but advances to full core and lower extremity strength. Bracing sometimes is useful in refractory situations.

Sacroiliac Inflammation. Sacroiliac (SI) inflammation may be caused by an acute traumatic fall on a unilateral ischium. Alternately, it may occur from repetitive asymmetrical forces applied to the pelvis from a limb length discrepancy or landing from jumps. This usually presents with unilateral back pain below the waistline. The clinician must always consider that stress fractures and SI infections may present in a similar fashion.

Treatment is directed at minimizing the asymmetrical force, possibly with a heel lift, and changing the offending activities. Stabilization is aimed at the muscle groups that stress the SI joint obliquely, such as oblique abdominals and the hip rotators, as well as hip abductors and extensors. Joint mobilization and SI corticosteroid injections may be helpful.

Spinal Curve Deformity

Adolescent Idiopathic Scoliosis. Adolescent idiopathic scoliosis is a common condition in young women and is seen in about 2% to 3% of the normal population.[104] Conditions known to cause spinal curve deformities are congenital spinal column abnormalities, neurological disorders, genetic conditions, and a multitude of other causes. Scoliosis caused by bony abnormalities of the spine present at birth is known as congenital scoliosis. In more than 80% of cases, a specific cause is not found, and such cases are defined as idiopathic or of undetermined cause. This is particularly so among the type of scoliosis seen in adolescent girls. School screening for scoliosis identifies asymmetries through the forward bending test. The student then is referred to a physician for further evaluation.

Some activities, such as ballet, produce asymmetrical forces across the immature spine; minor curves have been reported in 24% of dancers who started intense training at a prepubertal age.[105] Treatment for this condition follows standard guidelines for bracing of curves over 25° if sufficient growth remains. Also, cross training should be added to balance the spinal forces.

Common treatments for correction of the curvature are bracing, exercise, and electrical stimulation. A recent systematic review of clinical trials concluded that the effectiveness of bracing and exercise is not yet established.[106] Of the 436 studies found, only 13 were rated as randomized or controlled clinical trials. Additional effects of exercise with bracing or electrical stimulation with exercise also were not established. For subjects treated nonoperatively, the curve size was found to be significant for long-term results related to disability, quality of life, and psychological well-being. Pain was more significant in patients whose curves measured 45° or greater.[107]

Operative intervention is considered with curves that exceed 40°. Surgical goals include preventing or diminishing the progression of spinal deformity. The natural history of idiopathic scoliosis during adulthood tends to be progression if the curves are greater than 50° at the end of growth. The surgical procedure most often used to correct idiopathic adolescent scoliosis is a posterior spinal fusion with instrumentation and bone grafting. Postoperatively, patients are rapidly mobilized and resume daily activities, including return to school.[108]

Kyphosis. High levels of sporting activity during the growth spurt have been shown to increase both thoracic kyphosis and lumbar lordosis.[109] This has been demonstrated in a variety of athletes, most notably gymnasts participating in more than 400 hours of activity per year. Prevention of these spinal deformities may involve attention to upper back extension strengthening and abdominal strengthening. Kyphosis that exceeds 50° may require bracing.[105]

The role of physical therapy with all types of back pain and malalignments is to restore muscle balance and provide instruction in body mechanics and proper postures. If surgical intervention or bracing is needed, the patient requires instruction in mobility, ADLs, putting on and taking off the orthoses, and ambulation. The brace can be donned in bed or standing. Postoperatively, rotation should be minimized with logrolling. Breathing exercises may be necessary, because bracing can restrict chest expansion. Balance may need to be practiced initially. Light resistance exercise begins at 4 weeks and progresses slowly over the first 6 months. Return to full activities is allowed between 6 and 12 months, depending on the surgeon's protocol.

Compliance with exercise may be poor unless the child has experienced pain. Creative therapy provides interest for the child and provider. Regardless of the type of spinal pathology, exercise goals are trunk and pelvic strengthening and flexibility of the hip flexors, ITB, hamstrings, pectorals, and latissimus dorsi. For the patient with Scheuermann's kyphosis, extension of the thoracic segments is specifically addressed with manual therapy and the practice of extension exercises while maintaining a neutral lumbopelvic position. The patient progresses to static postural awareness and correction using the wall for proprioceptive feedback. Motor control in the new-found muscle balance in dynamic or functional movements is essential to returning to normal activity or sports while maintaining proper alignment.[110-113]

Backpack-Related Problems

The use of backpacks is no longer limited to hiking trails. Sports bags, particularly hockey bags, cause problems as well. Very young children bring their lunch and diapers to day care in backpacks. An association between the weight of a backpack and pain has been reported in adolescents.[114] Adolescents often are seen with a backpack slung over one shoulder or hanging very low on the back. Both the physiological and biomechanical effects of excessive weight in backpacks have been studied.[115] Compensatory measures are increases in trunk forward lean, cranovertebral angle, and lumbar lordosis.[115-117]

Prevention first is aimed at choosing a backpack that fits the child or adolescent properly. Shoulder straps should be padded and rest comfortably. The bottom of the pack should rest on the contour of the lower back rather than sagging onto the buttocks. The wearer should distribute the weight evenly by wearing both straps, and the contents of the backpack should be packed evenly, with compression straps adjusted to hold the contents stable. The heaviest items should be placed close to the spine. Students should be taught proper lifting techniques and to limit the weight of the contents. Suggestions for the weight of backpack contents range from 10% to 20% of the body weight.[115,117-119] It may be easier for the student to understand that the weight should be relatively easy to lift. For students already experiencing back pain, a second set of books for home or a wheeled pack is recommended (Figure 24-22).

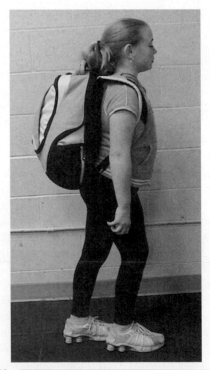

Figure 24-22

Proper backpack fit is essential to the prevention of back pain. Students should be instructed in proper packing of the backpack and should wear the pack using both straps and fit along the back, between the shoulders and the pelvis.

Postural Compensations When Wearing a Backpack

- Increased forward-leaning trunk
- Increased craniovertebral angle
- Increased lumbar lordosis

Some evidence indicates that back pain prevention programs in preadolescents have positive results.[120] Multidisciplinary approaches involving teachers, parents, physicians, physical therapists, and psychologists are encouraged to promote healthy habits in childhood. Working with injured students or students in school prevention programs provides more opportunities for encouraging overall physical fitness. More evidence is needed to confirm the long-term effects of these programs.

Summary

The clinician should fully evaluate the relationships of each element causing signs and symptoms, whether the impairments are in the spine or the extremities. Impairments at any joint can be compensated for by imbalances in muscle function or mobility at other joints. Both static (postural) and dynamic (functional movement) assessments should be performed. Alignment and muscle length throughout the kinetic chain should be assessed. Because of compensations and substitutions, the clinician must monitor and correct the performance of exercises throughout the rehabilitation process. Isolated training in open kinetic chain exercises is uniplanar; that is, it occurs in one plane only. For an individual to function in multiplanar activities, functional movement patterns, posture, balance, and proprioception must be included in the rehabilitation progression. All types of muscle contractions—isometric, concentric, and eccentric—must be used to achieve an effective and efficient return to activity-specific function.

Rehabilitation professionals also play a key role in the prevention of injuries. The work of coaches, teachers, and parents and education of the young are essential to preventing injury in children and adolescents. Training should include first aid, recognition of acute and overuse injuries, and return to play guidelines. Fundamental to this approach are protective equipment, proper training techniques, and skill development based on proper strengthening and conditioning programs. The participants' age and physical and sociological maturity need to be considered in program development, as well as their motivation to participate in the program for fitness, athletic training, or rehabilitation.

References

To enhance this text and add value for the reader, all references have been incorporated into a CD-ROM that is provided with this text. The reader can view the reference source and access it online whenever possible. There are a total of 120 references for this chapter.

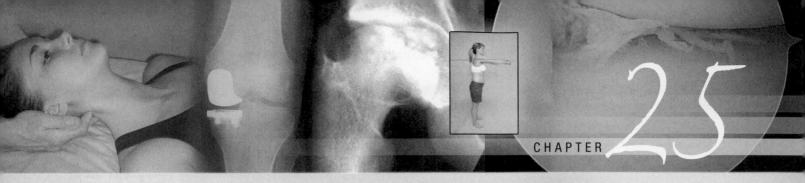

CHAPTER 25

SHOULDER ARTHROPLASTY

Timothy F. Tyler, Neil S. Roth, and Stephen J. Nicholas

Introduction

According to the American Academy of Orthopaedic Surgeons, about 4 million people in the United States seek medical care each year for shoulder problems. These conditions range from injuries such as dislocations and fractures to chronic debilitating diseases such as arthritis. Shoulder arthroplasty has been available to patients with severe, chronic, debilitating shoulder pathology since the early 1960s (Figure 25-1).[1-3] Like other joint replacement surgeries, it is designed to remove diseased portions of bone and joint and replace them with a prosthesis, thereby reducing the friction caused by disease and improving range of motion, eliminating the associated pain.

Prevalence of Shoulder Arthroplasty

The prevalence of total shoulder arthroplasty in the United States is less than that of total hip or knee arthroplasty but more than total elbow replacements. Shoulder arthroplasty has become the treatment of choice for many patients with a glenohumeral articular disease. The frequency of shoulder arthroplasties has increased substantially over the past decade, from approximately 10,000 in 1990 to 20,000 in 2000.[4] From 1990 to 1993, fewer than 5000 total shoulder arthroplasties were performed each year in this country; in comparison, combined hip and knee replacement operations exceeded 500,000 per year. According to an orthopedic news source, the prevalence of total shoulder arthroplasty in 1998 was 15,266, of which 8556 were hemiarthroplasties and 6710 were total shoulder athroplasties.[5] As the average age of the population increases and the outcome of shoulder arthroplasty continues to improve, the prevalence of this procedure will continue to rise.

Anatomy and Joint Design

Because of its anatomy and design, the glenohumeral joint does not lend itself to mechanical overload and cartilaginous breakdown. This non-weight-bearing joint is a ball and socket joint. The top of the humerus widens and forms the humeral head, which fits into a shallow socket of the scapula (glenoid fossa). During motion, the humeral head moves upon the glenoid fossa, providing a wide range of motion. Because of the fit of these two bones, very little surface area of the bones is actually in contact at any given moment, which may contribute to site-specific cartilage breakdown. The stability of the glenohumeral joint relies primarily on the joint capsule and the rotator cuff musculature. The tendons of the rotator cuff help create dynamic stability to the glenohumeral joint by connecting the humerus to the scapula. The primary force producer of the glenohumeral joint is the large deltoid muscle, which creates a force couple with the rotator cuff to allow normal kinematics to occur.

A layer of articular cartilage covers the head of the humerus and the surface of the glenoid fossa; in a healthy joint, this cartilaginous layer protects the bones against friction during movement. In addition, the glenoid labrum surrounds the periphery of the glenoid fossa and provides a slightly deeper socket for the humeral head to rest in. The joint capsule is lined with a synovial membrane, which provides synovial fluid to help reduce friction. In a normal glenohumeral joint, these parts work together to provide stability during a wide range of motion. When any of these joint surfaces become diseased, the normally smooth surface becomes rough, causing friction and pain (Figure 25-2). Arthritis leads to the breakdown of cartilage, allowing the bones to rub against each other. When this happens, scar tissue and bone spurs may also develop, leading to further pain and stiffness.

Indications for Shoulder Arthroplasty

Many different conditions can affect the glenohumeral joint and lead to a discussion about total shoulder replacement. (A hemiarthroplasty replaces the humeral head only, whereas a total shoulder arthroplasty involves replacing the glenoid

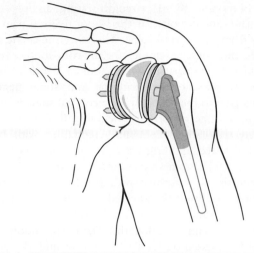

Figure 25-1
Components of a total shoulder arthroplasty.

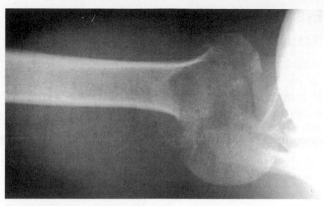

Figure 25-3
Proximal humeral fracture requiring shoulder arthroplasty.

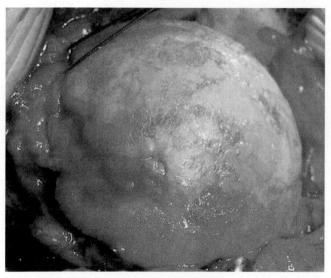

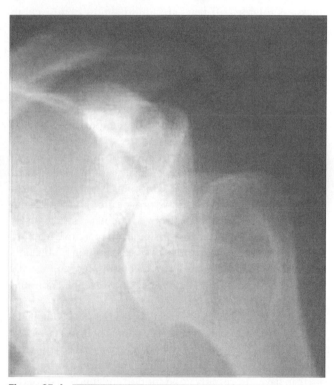

Figure 25-2
Humeral head with severe degenerative disease.

Figure 25-4
Inferior glenohumeral dislocation.

fossa as well.) Some of these conditions include rheumatoid arthritis, osteoarthritis, rotator cuff arthropathy, avascular necrosis, fractures of the shoulder region, and a failed shoulder prosthesis (from a previous joint replacement).[6-9] Some proximal humeral fractures (e.g., displaced anatomical neck fractures, four-part fractures, fracture-dislocations, and head-splitting fractures) are also indications for shoulder replacement (Figure 25-3).[10-13]

Deterioration of the glenohumeral joint after capsulorrhaphy for recurrent instability is more common in athletes; this condition arises more commonly after surgical procedures such as the Bristow procedure, the Magnuson-Stack procedure, and the Putti-Platt procedure and less commonly after the Bankart and capsular shift procedures.

Pain relief is the primary indication for total shoulder arthroplasty. Most surgeons are cautious about recommending shoulder replacement for improved range of motion and function. The most common reason for total shoulder arthroplasty, however, is arthritis. Because arthritis causes the cartilage to break down, it can cause a number of associated problems, such as scar formation and osteophytes. Post-traumatic arthritis is a form of osteoarthritis that develops after an injury, such as a fracture or dislocation of the shoulder (Figure 25-4). Arthritis also can develop after a rotator cuff tear. Rheumatoid arthritis is a systemic inflammatory condition of the joint lining that can affect people of any age and that usually affects multiple joints on both sides of the body.

Evaluation of the Arthritic Shoulder

History

Total shoulder arthroplasty has become the treatment of choice for most glenohumeral arthritides. A systematic, reproducible approach to each patient ensures comprehensive information gathering and therefore the proper diagnosis and choice of surgical procedure. Initially, the patient's age, hand dominance, occupation, athletic activities, medical history, and family history are recorded. Hand dominance is important to treatment recommendations, because the dominant arm of an active individual provides a different therapeutic challenge than the nondominant shoulder of a sedentary individual. Most arthritic shoulders and rotator cuff tears affect the dominant shoulder.[14] Although a patient's age is not necessarily diagnostic, full thickness rotator cuff tears are found almost exclusively in patients over 50 years of age. A complete general medical history should be obtained, with special attention given to any systemic or rheumatological disorders. In addition, a family history of generalized ligamentous laxity is important in the treatment of an arthritic patient with multidirectional shoulder instability. A previous incident of trauma can be the precursor of an arthritic shoulder; this can be an important piece of information in presurgical planning.

The patient' chief shoulder complaint usually consists of some element of pain, weakness, or loss of motion. Documenting the pattern of these symptoms is important, most notably the duration, severity, provocation, and location. Shoulder arthritis can arise from a traumatic event, but it often is atraumatic in origin, arising from repetitive loading. Severe night pain and pain at rest are common complaints in patients with mechanical shoulder pathology and usually are due to glenohumeral arthritis; however, infection and tumor must be ruled out.

Weakness of the affected shoulder is a frequent complaint, but splinting from pain commonly contributes to this lack of strength. Patients with concomitant large rotator cuff tears often report weakness or fatigue with overhead use, but they also can have surprisingly good motion and function once the arthritic shoulder has been replaced. Patients also may complain of "crackling" in their shoulders with motion; this can be due to a variety of disorders, including full thickness tears, which produce crepitus when the greater tuberosity comes into contact with the undersurface of the acromion; glenohumeral osteoarthritis; and acromioclavicular arthritis. However, when the "crackling" is accompanied by severe pain on movement, glenohumeral osteoarthritis needs to ruled out.

Physical Examination

Physical examination of the arthritic shoulder should proceed in an organized, reproducible manner. The examination consists of five basic parts: inspection, palpation, range of motion (ROM), strength testing, and provocative tests. The shoulder often is the site of referred pain, commonly from the cervical spine. Therefore the cervical spine must be thoroughly examined for any coexisting or referred pathology. Often a patient with shoulder arthritis has some degree of cervical spine arthritis and some degree of referred pain to the shoulder. The cervical spine is brought through a range of motion, including flexion, extension, and lateral rotation. Pain and crepitation with motion should be noted. Spurling's test, which is effective in distinguishing cervical spine radiculopathy from intrinsic shoulder arthritis, is performed with gentle cervical extension and rotation toward the affected shoulder with axial compression; a positive test result is indicated by posterior shoulder pain and radiculopathy. The deep tendon reflexes should be assessed bilaterally, and a thorough dermatomal sensory and motor evaluation should be performed.

Inspection

The patient should be examined with both shoulders exposed, which allows access anteriorly and posteriorly. A thorough inspection of the shoulder should note any muscular atrophy, hypertrophy, asymmetry, or deformity, as well as bony prominences. An arthritic shoulder sometimes presents as an extremely large mass on inspection. The examination may reveal a prominent scapular spine resulting from spinati atrophy; this often indicates a long-standing rotator cuff tear but may also be present with suprascapular nerve entrapment. The shoulder is evaluated for any deformity of the biceps muscle, because the long head of the biceps tendon often is ruptured in patients with rotator cuff disease and severe glenohumeral arthritis. Bony prominences and the contour of the shoulder also are noted, because a patient with glenohumeral arthritis loses normal contour and shows squaring and anterior fullness.

Palpation

Palpation around the shoulder joint should be done systematically so that each muscle, joint, and bony prominence is evaluated. The sternoclavicular joint; the clavicle; the acromioclavicular joint; the anterior, lateral, and posterior acromion; the anterior and posterior joint lines; and the biceps tendon each should be tested for discrete tenderness. Localized tenderness over the acromioclavicular (AC) joint often is overlooked as a source of symptoms and may be implicated in rotator cuff pathology or degenerative joint disease. Pain often is elicited by palpation of the greater tuberosity with rotator cuff pathology, but it also may be due to glenohumeral arthritis, and the finding should be correlated with rotational radiographs of the humerus (Figure 25-5). Tenderness in the bicipital groove may be present with involvement of the biceps tendon and can be implicated in both rotator cuff pathology and glenohumeral instability. Anterior and posterior joint line tenderness may be present with glenohumeral instability,

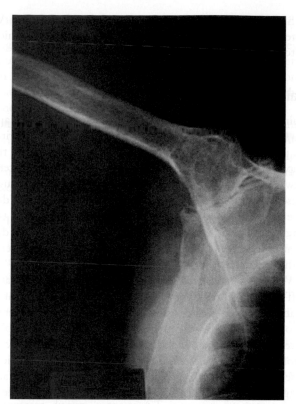

Figure 25-5
Radiograph confirming the diagnosis of severe glenohumeral arthritis.

whereas posterior joint line tenderness commonly is noted in patients with glenohumeral arthritis.

Range of Motion

The general motion of the shoulder complex is observed for glenohumeral rhythm, scapulothoracic motion, and overall synchrony of motion. The American Shoulder and Elbow Surgeons professional organization currently recommends that four functionally necessary arcs of motion be measured both actively and passively: total elevation, lateral rotation at neutral abduction, lateral rotation at 90° abduction, and medial rotation.[15,16] Patient's with limited motion in a single or multiple planes must be examined carefully to differentiate the possible etiologies, such as a rotator cuff tear, adhesive capsulitis, and glenohumeral arthritis.

In this patient population, total elevation, including both glenohumeral and scapulothoracic motion, may be more reproducibly measured than attempting to isolate glenohumeral motion and is more functionally relevant. However, both measurements are important for determining which joint is contributing to a functional loss. Passive elevation is more accurately measured in the supine position, whereas active elevation is measured erect. Lateral rotation is tested with the arm at the side and the patient supine, to eliminate trunk rotation, and also with the arm at 90° abduction.

Functional rotation ranges of motion are also documented. Functional medial rotation is measured according to the highest vertebral level an upright patient can reach with the thumb. Apley's scratch test evaluates the available functional lateral rotation ROM.

Strength Testing

The strength and integrity of joints, muscles, and tendons are important aspects of surgical planning. Manual strength testing may be difficult to assess quantitatively because of coexistent pain. Crepitation with motion from the glenohumeral joint, subacromial space, or scapulothoracic joint should be noted. Manual muscle testing of the supraspinatus is performed with the arm in 90° forward elevation and 20° medial rotation with the elbows extended (i.e., the empty can test). Manual muscle testing in lateral rotation is done with the elbow flexed and the arm at the side to prevent deltoid contribution; weakness in this position is a common finding with a tear involving the infraspinatus tendon. Weakness in lateral rotation at neutral may indicate a long-standing rotator cuff tear,[17] and with concomitant weakness in shoulder abduction, it shows a statistically significant correlation with the size of the tear.[18]

Manual muscle testing of the shoulder in lateral rotation above 45° abduction is done primarily to assess the teres minor. Patients with large or massive tears involving the infraspinatus often are unable to maintain the arm in lateral rotation at neutral and when the arm is abducted. The lateral rotation lag sign is designed to test the integrity of the supraspinatus and infraspinatus tendons; it is performed by passively flexing the elbow to 90° and the shoulder to 20° elevation and near maximum lateral rotation. The patient then is asked to maintain this position while the clinician releases the wrist; a positive result is a lag or angular drop.[19] The drop sign is designed to assess infraspinatus function; for this test, the patient is seated with her back to the clinician, who holds the affected arm at 90° elevation and maximum lateral rotation with the elbow at 90° flexion. The patient is asked to maintain this position while the physician supports the elbow and releases the wrist; the result is positive if a lag occurs.

Patients with subscapularis tears have an increased passive lateral rotation ROM and weakness of medial rotation. The competence of the subscapularis muscle can be assessed using the lift off test, which has been shown to be both sensitive and specific for a tear in the subscapularis tendon. Originally, the lift off test was determined to be positive (i.e., poor subscapularis function) when a patient could not lift the hand posteriorly off the lumbar region; however, recently the test was modified to achieve even greater sensitivity for subscapularis tears.[20] In the modified lift off test, the examiner places the arm in maximum medial rotation by passively lifting the patient's arm posteriorly off the lumbar region; the test result is positive (poor subscapularis function) if the patient is unable to maintain that position and the arm falls onto the back.

The internal rotation lag sign was recently described to assess subscapularis competency. It is similar to the modified

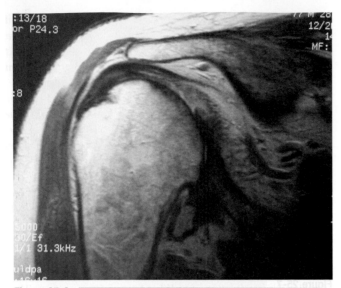

Figure 25-9
MRI demonstrating humeral head migration superiorly with rotator cuff arthropathy.

Other Modalities

When systemic disorders are suspected, routine blood tests to evaluate for rheumatological disorders, infection, and tumors should be considered. A complete blood count with differential, a sedimentation rate, a C-reactive protein level, chemistry profile, latex fixation test, serum protein electrophoresis, and an acid phosphatase level should be obtained as part of preoperative testing (Table 25-1). This panel allows the surgeon to rule out any other significant factors and pathology and provides a baseline for comparison after surgery if necessary.

Young Shoulder Arthroplasty Patients

Shoulder arthroplasty is becoming more common in young patients. Although trauma to the glenohumeral joint is associated with a dislocation episode, little is known about the incidence of shoulder arthroplasty in patients with shoulder instability. The long time span between dislocation and the development of arthritis makes determining any cause and effect relationship difficult.

Severe damage to the humeral head cartilage can occur after a dislocation. Taylor and Arciero[29] reported on 63 young patients under 24 years of age with first-time, traumatic anterior shoulder dislocations who were evaluated arthroscopically within 10 days of dislocation. Fifty-seven patients had Hill-Sachs lesions. However, osteochondral lesions of the humeral head were identified in 34 patients, and chondral lesions were noted in an additional 24, providing evidence that humeral head damage occurs. Hovelius et al.[30] followed 245 patients 10 years after primary anterior dislocations of the shoulder. The patients' ages at the time of dislocation ranged from 12 to 40 years. Radiographs taken on 185 shoulders at the time of primary dislocation demonstrated a Hill-Sachs lesion in 99 shoulders. This finding was associated with a significantly worse prognosis with regard to recurrent instability but had no effect on the development of arthritis. Radiographs

Table 25-1

Preoperative Tests with Normal Ranges

CBC W/Diff and PLT		Complete Metabolic Panel	
WBC	3.8-10.83/μL	Glucose	65-139 mg/dL
RBC	3.80-5.106/μL	Sodium	135-146 mmol/L
Hemoglobin	11.7-15.5 g/dL	Potassium	3.5-5.3 mmol/L
Hematocrit	35-45 %	Chloride	98-110 mmol/L
MCV	80-100 fL	Carbon dioxide	21-33 mmol/L
MCH	27-33 pg	Urea nitrogen	7-25 mg/dL
MCHC	32-36 g/dL	Creatinine	0.5-1.2 mg/dL
RDW	11%-15%	BUN/creatinine ratio	6-25
Platelet count	140-4003/μL	Calcium	8.5-10.4 mg/dL
MPV	7.5-11.5 fL	Protein, total	6.0-8.3 g/dL
Total Neutrophils, %	38%-80%	Albumin	3.5-4.9 g/dL
Total Lymphocytes, %	15%-49%	Globulin, calculated	2.2-4.2 g/dL
Monocytes, %	0%-13%	A/G ratio	0.8-2
Eosinophils, %	0-8%	Bilirubin, total	0.2-1.3 mg/dL
Basophils, %	0-2%	Alkaline phosphatase	20-125 U/L
Neutrophils, absolute	1500-7800 cells/μL	AST	2-35 U/L
Lymphocytes, absolute	850-3900/μL	ALT	2-40 U/L
Monocytes, absolute	200-950 cells/μL		
Eosinophils, absolute	15-550 cells/μL		
Basophils, absolute	0-200 cells/μL		

made for 208 shoulders at the 10-year follow-up examination were evaluated for post-traumatic dislocation arthritis. Twenty-three shoulders, or 11%, had mild arthritis, and 18, or 9%, had moderate or severe arthritis. No further instability was reported in some of the shoulders that had arthritis.

The most defining study to date was published by Marx et al.,[31] who used a case-control study to examine whether shoulder dislocation was associated with the development of arthrosis. Patients with osteoarthrosis who had undergone hemiarthroplasty or total shoulder arthroplasty were asked whether they had ever sustained a shoulder dislocation. Ninety-one patients who had undergone shoulder arthroplasty and 282 control subjects responded. The authors concluded that the risk of developing severe arthrosis of the shoulder is 10 to 20 times greater for individuals who have had a dislocation of the shoulder. It is evident that some degree of chondral injury and hemarthrosis may be associated with a shoulder dislocation and is not beneficial to the glenohumeral joint. Whether the hemarthrosis predisposes this patient population to arthritis and an eventual shoulder arthroplasty remains unclear.

One thing that is clear is the effect of overconstraining the glenohumeral joint during surgery for shoulder instability. Sperling et al.[32] reported on the intermediate to long-term results of shoulder arthroplasty performed to treat osteoarthritis after instability surgery in 33 patients with glenohumeral arthritis. The mean age at the time of the shoulder arthroplasty was 46 years. Twenty-one patients who had a total shoulder arthroplasty and 10 who had a hemiarthroplasty were followed for a minimum of 2 years. Shoulder arthroplasty was associated with significant pain relief and significant improvement in lateral rotation and active abduction. Interestingly, no significant difference was seen between the hemiarthroplasty group and the total shoulder arthroplasty group with regard to postoperative lateral rotation, active abduction, or pain. This study suggests that shoulder arthroplasty for the treatment of osteoarthritis of the glenohumeral joint after instability surgery in a group of young patients provides pain relief and improved motion. However, it may be associated with a higher incidence of revision surgery. Three patients in the hemiarthroplasty group and eight patients in the total shoulder arthroplasty group underwent revision surgery. In contrast, this was not the case in a series of 22 shoulder arthroplasties followed up over an average of 6 years. Burroughs et al.[33] reported no evidence of accelerated deterioration of shoulder function, and only two patients underwent revision surgery.

Given this conflict in the literature, little information is available to guide clinical decision making with regard to shoulder arthroplasty after instability surgery. The management of these patients requires a thorough preoperative evaluation and a careful review of diagnostic modalities. The severity of glenoid wear should be assessed using CT scans to determine the need for glenoid bone grafting. In addition, the surgeon should obtain the previous operative reports to determine the type of stabilization performed; this allows the surgeon to recognize frequently distorted anatomy and facilitates safe, effective soft tissue releases. The decision to proceed with a shoulder arthroplasty in a patient who has had a previous stabilization procedure should be made with caution. The surgeon should be prepared to address associated soft tissue contracture and potential bone deficiency.

Shoulder arthroplasty in the young patient for osteoarthritis of the glenohumeral joint after instability surgery provides satisfactory pain relief and improvement in motion but may be associated with a high rate of revision surgery and unsatisfactory results as a result of implant failure, instability, and painful glenoid arthritis.[33]

Preoperative Rehabilitation

Accepting differences in expectations, patient goals, physician goals, and physical therapist goals is essential. The physical therapist ideally should meet with the patient and the patient's caregiver before the surgery. At this time, the rehabilitation team can set reasonable goals for both early and eventual outcomes (Table 25-2). At this point, when the patients are not under the influence of pain medications, feeling ill, or experiencing pain, they can better comprehend the rehabilitation program, precautions, and expectations. This allows the patient and physical therapist to establish a relationship that will foster better cooperation during the sometimes painful and frustrating rehabilitation process. After the educational process, the preoperative assessment should include the available range of motion, strength, and the presence of visible atrophy, sensation, pain, and functional evaluation.

The educational process is essential for informing the patient of the risks and complications of surgery and anesthesia.[34] These risks for shoulder replacement surgery include injury to nerves and blood vessels; stiffness or instability of the shoulder joint; loosening of the prosthetic parts, requiring additional surgery; tearing of a rotator cuff tendon; and fracture of the humerus. In addition, total shoulder replacement carries with it the normal risks of any elective surgery, such as complications from anesthesia, excessive bleeding, infection, blood clots, and ultimately death.[35-37] The surgical procedure and the components of shoulder arthroplasty also are explained.

The educational process is essential for informing the patient of the restriction on the use of the shoulder and the impact on activities of daily living for at least the next 6 weeks. Because the subscapularis muscle is cut to expose the shoulder joint, no active medial rotation motion is permitted. For the patient, this means no violent squeezing, hugging, or slamming of car doors. However, the patient

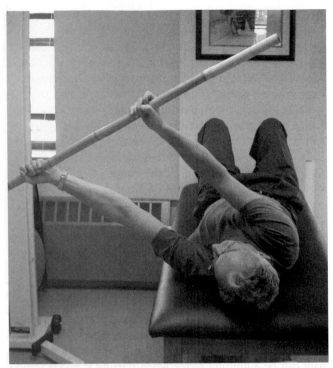

Figure 25-24
Horizontal abduction and adduction can be accomplished with the use of a cane.

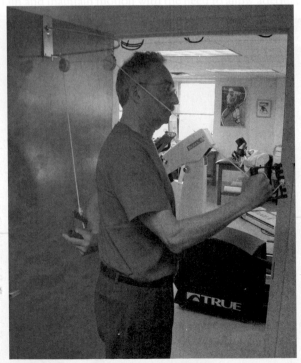

Figure 25-25
Use of the pulleys to regain functional internal rotation range of motion.

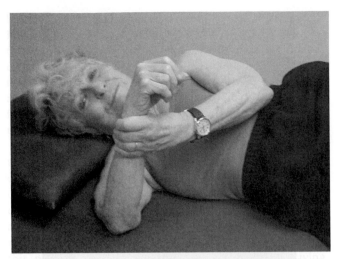

Figure 25-26
Sleeper stretch.

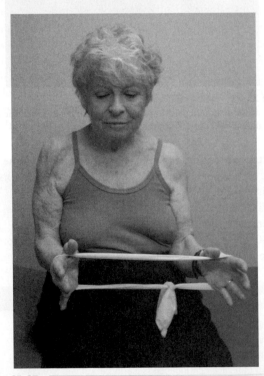

Figure 25-27
Early external rotation strengthening.

upper body ergometer (UBE) using light resistance can be beneficial at this time (4 weeks) to facilitate ROM and initiate active muscular control of the shoulder. The axis of rotation of the UBE should remain below the level of the shoulder joint so that forward flexion is not forced above 80°. The authors also stress the retro component of performing the UBE. By performing retro UBE (going backward), the authors hypothesize, the patient mobilizes the scapula and encourages proper posture.

Early strengthening of the serratus anterior muscle also is encouraged, provided the arm is maintained slightly below 90° of shoulder flexion and movement is pain free. Subsequent atrophy of the serratus anterior muscle, as a result of disuse, may allow the scapula to rest in a downwardly rotated position, causing inferior border prominence. Decker et al.[80] used electromyography (EMG) to determine which exercises consistently elicited the highest percentage of the maximum voluntary contraction (MVC) of the serratus anterior. They found that the serratus anterior punch out, scaption, dynamic hug, knee push-up plus, and push-up plus exercises consistently elicited over 20% MVC. Most important, they determined that the push-up plus and the dynamic hug exercises maintained the greatest percentage of the MVC and maintained the scapula in an upwardly rotated position. Although the early postoperative phase is too early in the rehabilitation process to perform these late exercises, Decker et al.[80] highlighted the serratus anterior punch out as a valuable exercise. Performed in a controlled, supervised setting, this is an excellent choice to initiate early serratus anterior neuromuscular re-education (Figure 25-28). Progression to the more challenging serratus anterior strengthening exercises can be considered during the intermediate phase of rehabilitation, keeping in mind that the patient is instructed to avoid heavy pushing, pulling, and lifting

for the first 6 weeks, and no upper extremity weight-bearing activities are allowed for 3 months.

A delicate balance exists between pushing patients too hard and progressing them as planned. Too often the patient may feel better rather than worse during this early protective phase; therefore the clinician must always respect the laws of tissue healing.

Milestones the authors look to achieve for progression to the next rehabilitation period are (1) toleration of submaximum isometrics of the rotator cuff muscles at 0° abduction; (2) attaining symmetrical mobility of the sternoclavicular, acromioclavicular, and scapulothoracic joints; and (3) protraction, retraction, elevation, and depression of the scapula against submaximum manual resistance. Adequate passive range of motion in flexion, abduction, adduction, and medial rotation at 45° abduction (50% to 75% of the uninvolved side) also should be attained before the patient is progressed.

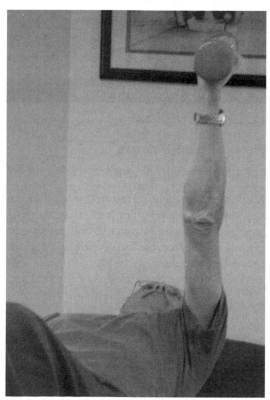

Figure 25-28
Serratus anterior strengthening in the supine position.

Early Postoperative Phase Milestones

- Ability to tolerate submaximum rotator cuff isometrics at 0°
- Symmetrical mobility of sternoclavicular, acromioclavicular, and scapulothoracic joints
- Ability to protract, retract, elevate, and depress scapula against submaximum manual resistance
- Adequate passive range of motion (50% to 75% of uninvolved side) at 45° abduction

Intermediate Postoperative Phase (Weeks 6 to 12)

During the intermediate postoperative phase of rehabilitation, the patient attempts to regain all available range of motion, including passive medial rotation. Initiation of passive lateral rotation range of motion at 0°, 45°, and 90° abduction and stretching beyond neutral rotation position are emphasized. Advancement to terminal ranges in all planes of motion is advocated unless otherwise specified by the referring surgeon. Medial rotation submaximum resistive exercise progressions also are initiated during this phase. A traditional rotator cuff isotonic exercise program is started, which includes side lying lateral rotation, prone extensions, and prone horizontal abduction (which may need to be limited between neutral to the scapular plane position initially, with progression to the coronal plane as ROM improves). Biceps and triceps curls in the standing position with glenohumeral joint rotation in a neutral resting position are begun. In addition, oscillation exercises with Flexbar or a Body Blade can begin. Rhythmic stabilization in open kinetic chain (Figure 25-29) and closed kinetic chain (Figure 25-30) environments can begin, with caution in shoulder arthroplasty patients who will be placing higher demands on the shoulder.

most patients work with a physical therapist only once or twice a day at most.

Aerobic Capacity and Endurance Training

Early focus on aerobic capacity training often is accomplished merely by the effort required of patients for basic functional mobility. For the more advanced patient, increasing the distance ambulated in the hospital and the frequency of ambulation taxes the cardiopulmonary system adequately for a training effect. For patients with underlying comorbidities in these areas, specific training parameters should be set, and the patient should use either heart rate or the rating of perceived exertion (RPE) scale as a guide to the amount of activity that is appropriate for aerobic capacity training.

Because the LOS after TKA has declined significantly over the past decade, patients routinely are discharged from the acute care setting in 3 to 4 days. Many patients return directly home, whereas others need additional care in a subacute care setting. The clinician is responsible for providing input on discharge planning and this begins on the initial day of intervention. Interdisciplinary collaboration among the patient's health care providers is important for determining the best discharge plan for the patient's unique needs. Factors that are important to consider include the presence and extent of any comorbidities that will influence the expected rate of recovery; the amount of support the patient will have at home from family or friends to assist in ADLs, basic household management, meal preparation, and food shopping; and the physical environment to which the patient is returning. Patients who live alone, have multiple comorbidities, or have an environmentally challenging home situation may need to be discharged to an inpatient facility for ongoing rehabilitation until the patient has achieved a level of function sufficient to return to the home setting.[45] On the other hand, patients with minimal medical issues, available social support, and a home environment that has minimal physical obstacles should be able to go directly home from the acute care facility and continue their rehabilitation either through home care services or in an outpatient setting.

Factors to Consider in Discharge Planning

- Presence and extent of comorbidities
- Social support for the patient at home
- Physical environment to which the patient is returning
- Patient's level of function (physical capacity)
- Patient's ability to use or need for assistive devices

Regardless of the discharge destination after the acute care stay, patients need some training and support with assistive devices for basic ADLs before they are discharged home. For

some, this training occurs in the acute care facility; patients transferred to a subacute facility receive their training and equipment there. The most common items issued for patients include long-handled implements, such as a bathing sponge, dressing aid, and reacher to assist the patient in gaining complete independence in bathing and dressing activities. Additional items may include elastic shoelaces, depending on the type of footwear the patient owns and wears. For a taller patient who may have difficulty with sit to stand transfers, a raised toilet seat may help the patient gain complete independence in toileting, and a tub bench is recommended to allow the patient to remain seated during showering for safety reasons. Additional modifications to the home may include grab bars in the bathroom for safety and ramps for home entrances if the patient has difficulty on stairs.

Subacute Care Rehabilitation

The subacute care level of rehabilitation may be provided in an inpatient facility such as a rehabilitation hospital, a transitional care unit, or skilled nursing facility. Regardless of the setting, the goal of rehabilitation is an extension of the care initiated in the acute care setting (Table 27-3). Patients typically remain at this level of care after discharge from the acute care setting, often on POD 3-5, and continue care for 10 to 14 days on average. Predictors of increased LOS for inpatient rehabilitation include age over 80 years, revision surgery, and multiple comorbidities or illnesses.[46]

The primary goal in the subacute setting is to progress the patient's mobility and safety to a level sufficient to allow the patient to return home. As with discharge from the

Table 27-3
Goals of Subacute Care/Home Rehabilitation and Types of Interventions

Goals	Types of Interventions
Maximize knee range of motion (ROM): 0° to 120° flexion	ROM exercises Prolonged stretching Continuous passive motion (CPM)
Improve strength and motor control	Therapeutic exercise focusing on strength
Achieve independent transfers	Transfer training
Achieve independent ambulation	Gait training with assistive device
Achieve independent basic self-care, activities of daily living (ADLs)	Assistive devices and training
Maximize aerobic capacity and endurance	Aerobic capacity training

acute care setting, social supports, environmental constraints, and the patient's overall physical capacity affect how quickly the individual returns home. Many patients discharged from a subacute care facility continue their rehabilitation through home care services until they are ready for an outpatient setting.

Interventions in the subacute care setting primarily continue with the treatments established in the acute care setting. Attention to maximizing ROM of the knee and quadriceps strength to allow independence in transfer and ambulation are the prime focus of treatment. Many of these patients have additional comorbidities that slow their progress in achieving independence in functional milestones. Frequently, pathology of the cardiovascular and/or pulmonary systems requires a slower pace in this rehabilitative setting. These patients tend to be more deconditioned going into surgery and require pacing strategies until their aerobic capacity increases. If they have significant limitations because of an underlying pathology that is not amenable to treatment, compensatory strategies need to be implemented, such as pacing strategies and modifications of home environmental constraints to allow the patient to achieve safe and effective functional mobility.

Strength training and aerobic conditioning are additional components of the rehabilitation program that can be implemented in the subacute care setting, because patients typically have less pain that limits their tolerance of treatment. Exercises such as upper body ergometry and progression to stationary biking can be initiated once the patient has sufficient ROM to allow full cycling with the pedals. Discharge from the subacute care setting to home occurs when the patient can demonstrate the ability to achieve independence in transfers, ambulation, ADLs, and instrumental activities of daily living (IADLs), including household management for patients returning to home alone (see volume 1 of this series, *Orthopedic Physical Assessment,* Chapter 1).

Home Care Rehabilitation

Once the patient has arrived home after discharge from either the acute care or subacute care setting, home care services can provide ongoing rehabilitation services if deemed necessary. Home care rehabilitation services often are provided to evaluate the patient's ability to negotiate the home environment safely and to provide ongoing interventions for functional training and therapeutic exercise. The primary reason patients continue with home care services after a subacute care inpatient stay is inadequate knee ROM (<90° flexion) for functional activities. Patients can follow independent exercise programs to maintain and gain ROM independently, but the shift in home exercise programs now focuses more on strength gains and endurance training (see Table 27-3). Patients can use walking, swimming, or stationary biking for endurance and aerobic

capacity training in addition to strengthening exercises that emphasize the quadriceps and hip musculature.

Outpatient Rehabilitation

When the patient is able to get out into the community and has transportation to an outpatient rehabilitation facility, care is transitioned from the home care setting to the outpatient setting. At this point the patient is not considered homebound and does not qualify for ongoing home care services under Medicare rules in the United States.[47] In addition, the outpatient clinic offers a variety of options in equipment to supplement the rehabilitation process.

The primary focus of treatment in the outpatient setting is strengthening, to facilitate the patient's return to full function. Residual deficits in ROM also are addressed through passive stretching and exercises that can be augmented with modalities as indicated (e.g., superficial heat, ultrasound, diathermy). For patients with residual strength deficits, electrical stimulation can be used to enhance strength training regimens.[48,49] The continuum of rehabilitation in the outpatient setting takes the patient to the end point in functional rehabilitation after TKA and should include return to sport-specific activities if the patient so desires. Additional exercise equipment, such as isokinetic devices, pulley systems, and stair climbers, can be used for strengthening purposes. Aerobic conditioning can be performed by walking and with stationary bicycles, upper body ergometers, elliptical and standard treadmills, and cross-country ski machines, depending on the patient's overall endurance, balance, agility, and preferred mode of exercise.

Rehabilitation programs continue to be supplemented by progressive home exercise programs that focus on the goals of the rehabilitation program (Table 27-4). These most often include resistive exercises with cuff weights,

Table 27-4
Goals of Outpatient Rehabilitation and Types of Interventions

Goals	Types of Interventions
Maximize knee range of motion (ROM)	ROM exercises Prolonged stretching Manual techniques
Maximize strength	Aggressive strength training
Achieve normal gait without assistive device	Gait training Balance training
Achieve independence in self-selected activities (sports, leisure)	ROM Strengthening exercises Balance exercises Endurance training as required for activity

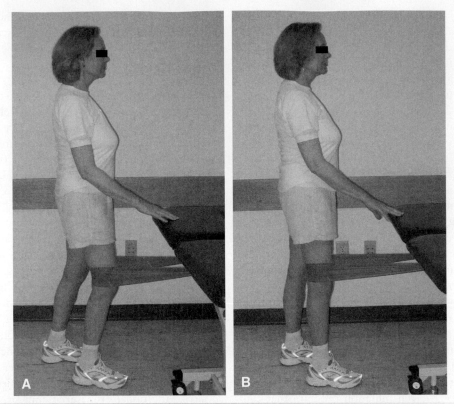

Figure 27-4
Quadriceps strengthening in closed chain using resistive elastic bands. **A,** Starting position (knee flexed).
B, Finishing position (knee extended).

resistance bands (Figure 27-4), or body weight in closed chain exercises, as well as ROM exercises with an emphasis on prolonged stretches to regain end range flexion or extension, depending on the patient's presentation. Gait training often continues in the outpatient setting; initially the patient is weaned off any assistive devices, and then the gait is fine-tuned as ROM and strength improve to restore a normal gait pattern and minimize any excessive loading on the joints from abnormal gait patterns. The frequency and duration of treatment are based on the patient's presentation and goals; however, a greater number of visits may be required if the patient needs manual techniques and stretching to improve ROM or if a treatment requires specific equipment (e.g., electrical stimulation). Outpatient rehabilitation often lasts at least 6 to 8 weeks because of the time needed to achieve true strength gains.

Regrettably, many patients stop participating in sports-related activities because of the pain associated with increased activity and advanced arthritis. For an increasing number of patients, TKA offers the hope of returning to meaningful activities, including a variety of sports and leisure activities. Sport-specific training often is included at the end of the rehabilitation process. A number of high loading, repetitive sports activities, such as running, basketball, soccer, high

impact aerobics, singles tennis, squash, racquetball, and Alpine skiing, are not recommended after TKA because these types of activities have been associated with early arthroplasty failure.[50] Lower load activities, such as walking, biking, golfing, swimming, tai chi, and bowling are encouraged, because these activities help maintain strength gained in rehabilitation and provide the overall health benefits derived from regular physical activity.

When patients have completed rehabilitation after TKA, they may choose to seek out additional assistance in returning to a specific leisure activity. Their sport of choice may have specific ROM, strength, or endurance requirements that call for additional training to allow the patient to participate fully at peak performance. Patients who want to return to cycling may need adjustments to their bicycles and additional work on ROM to maximize their tolerance of this activity. Golfers may need to address balance issues for the uneven terrain of the golf course to function confidently in this sport and may also need additional flexion to allow them to squat to view lines for putting. Often the patient can identify the obstacles that impede the ability to participate fully in a sports activity, and this information can help guide both the examination and treatment focus of sport-specific rehabilitation.

Caution: High Load Activities Not Recommended after Total Knee Arthroplasty

- Running
- Basketball
- Soccer
- High impact aerobics
- Singles tennis
- Squash
- Racquetball
- Alpine skiing

Additional Surgical Considerations for Knee Arthroplasty Patients

Unicompartmental knee arthroplasties increasingly are performed for patients with advanced arthritic changes in one compartment of the knee, most often the medial compartment. These patients undergo a similar surgical event except that the prosthesis implanted resurfaces only one compartment (medial or lateral) of the tibiofemoral joint (Figure 27-5). After surgery, these patients follow a rehabilitation protocol that parallels that of patients who have had a TKA. The primary difference in patients with a unicompartmental knee arthroplasty is that they undergo a less invasive surgical procedure that preserves more of the joint

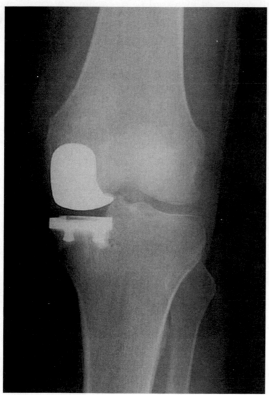

Figure 27-5
Anteroposterior radiograph of unicompartmental knee arthroplasty.

anatomy. Therefore they often have less blood loss at surgery, a shorter duration of anesthesia, and often less postoperative pain.[51,52] All these factors result in a faster recovery. Most of these patients are discharged directly home after the acute care stay, and they often are discharged home on POD 2 or 3. They may require some rehabilitation services in the home initially but are moved into the outpatient setting more quickly and follow an outpatient rehabilitation process similar to that for primary TKA.

The other surgical arthroplasty consideration involves patients with bilateral knee OA. Because of the pathophysiology of OA, more than 80% of patients presenting with debilitating knee pain for evaluation have bilateral symptoms. In fact, in a study by Mont et al.,[53] 43% of those presenting for unilateral TKA eventually had the other knee replaced as well; other researchers have had similar findings.[54,55] Patients who need bilateral knee replacements have a choice regarding the timing of the two procedures. A one-stage bilateral TKA may be done, in which one TKA is performed, the tourniquet is deflated, and the contralateral tourniquet is inflated and the second TKA is performed. As an alternative, the patient may opt for two separate procedures done days, weeks, or months apart (two-stage TKA).

The overall complication rates in patients undergoing bilateral rather than unilateral TKA are similar, which suggests that for the average patient, the larger bilateral surgery appears to pose no increased risk.[56,57] However, it is clearly evident that the operative insult of bilateral one-stage procedures is greater, involving increased blood loss, greater hemodynamic effects, an increased risk of anesthetic complications from longer operative times, and a greater risk of embolization of fat and marrow contents. For these reasons, patients older than 75 years and those with significant cardiovascular comorbidities are at increased risk of fatal complications and therefore should undergo a two-stage procedure.[57,58]

Patients who undergo a two-stage TKA follow the rehabilitation course outlined previously. Depending on the surgeon's and the patient's preferences, the second TKA may be performed as early as 10 days after the first, or the two stages may be done 3 or more months apart. For patients with a short interval between the two surgeries, the primary focus after the first procedure is to gain sufficient ROM and strength in the quadriceps muscle to allow this leg to act as the "strong" leg after the second procedure. These patients then follow a rehabilitation process similar to that outlined in the next paragraph for patients who undergo a one-stage bilateral TKA. Patients who have several months between procedures focus on fully rehabilitating the first knee before the second surgical procedure is performed.

One-stage bilateral TKAs present a unique challenge to the patient and rehabilitation professional. These patients need intensive rehabilitation services, because both knees

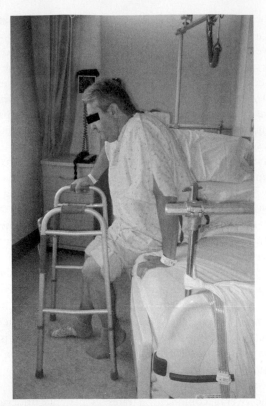

Figure 27-6
Assisted sit to stand transfers using elevation of the bed.

require treatment to address ROM and strength issues as outlined for single TKAs. Early postoperative functional training poses additional challenges, because the patient often does not have sufficient knee ROM or strength to succeed in sit to stand transfers. Compensatory strategies, such as elevating the bed (Figure 27-6) and using knee immobilizers, may help the patient succeed with transfers the first few days after surgery. CPM is alternated between the knees, because the size of the CPM machine makes it difficult to position the patient on two at one time. Despite the increased time on CPM, it is still important for patients to be out of bed and working on functional activities as well. Sufficient pain management is paramount in these patients, because pain often impairs motor control. These patients usually require discharge to an inpatient rehabilitation facility for ongoing rehabilitation, because most patients who have one-stage bilateral TKAs do not achieve independence in functional mobility until 10 to 14 days after surgery. These patients' condition also is influenced by longer anesthetic times and increased blood loss and their associated side effects, which hamper progress in rehabilitation. The advantage of this procedure is that once patients have progressed through the initial phases of rehabilitation, they do not have a knee with advanced OA impeding their progress in rehabilitation, as is often seen in patients with bilateral knee OA who opt for two procedures many months apart.

Complications after Total Knee Arthroplasty

Common complications immediately after surgery include pulmonary complications, such as postoperative atelectasis and pneumonia; vascular complications, including DVT and pulmonary embolus (PE); and local wound problems or infection. For clinician, a knowledge of the complications that may arise after TKA is important for early detection and referral to appropriate providers for management. Careful monitoring of the patient's heart rate, respiratory rate, oxygen (O_2) saturation levels, and body temperature can aid early detection of pulmonary complications. Interventions such as instruction in deep breathing exercises and manual techniques can help prevent and/or treat these pulmonary complications, which can be life threatening in older patients.

The frequency of thromboembolic disease in individuals who do not receive prophylactic therapy can be as high as 50%.[59] The risk of DVT is highest in the early postoperative period. Coumadin and low molecular weight heparins (blood thinning drugs) reduce the risk of postoperative DVT in patients with TKA. Physical methods, including compression stockings, pneumatic compression devices, CPM machines, and early mobilization, are useful adjuncts for preventing DVT but have not been proven to substitute for pharmacological prophylaxis. Although the overall incidence of DVT after TKA is low,[60] the seriousness of this complication warrants close observation and prophylactic anticoagulation. Patient reports of increased pain, swelling, warmth, and/or redness in the leg may accompany the development of DVT and warrant further examination by the surgeon.

Complications of Total Knee Arthroplasty

- Atelectasis (collapse of alveoli)
- Pneumonia
- Deep vein thrombosis
- Pulmonary embolism
- Wound problems
- Infection
- Medial collateral ligament injury
- Extensor mechanism failure (patellar tendon rupture)
- Arthrofibrosis (stiff knee)
- Periprosthetic fracture
- Unstable or loosened prosthesis
- Heterotopic ossification

Immunosuppression, diabetes, smoking, previous knee surgery, and obesity are known risk factors for postoperative knee infection, which can be a devastating complication requiring emergent irrigation and debridement and long-term intravenous (IV) antibiotics. Infection can be prevented by perioperative use of IV antibiotics (typically Ancef) and attention to careful surgical technique and soft tissue handling, which have been shown to minimize wound healing problems. In addition, laminar airflow and having a dedicated surgical team and reduced surgical time have been shown to reduce the risk of infection in patients with TKA.[61,62] Early signs and symptoms of infection, which present primarily in the area of the incision, include increased redness, warmth, edema, and possibly drainage from the surgical wound. Infection after wound closure can be either superficial (e.g., a cellulitis) or a deep infection in the joint or bone. Symptoms of progressively worsening pain accompanied by cardinal signs of systemic infection (e.g., fever, rigors [shivering]) should prompt the clinician to notify the surgeon, because early management of infection is critical for a successful outcome.

Additional mechanical complications in TKA can include medial collateral ligament (MCL) injury, extensor mechanism failure, arthrofibrosis, and/or periprosthetic fracture. Iatrogenic intraoperative disruption of the MCL during TKA typically has been treated with implantation of a more constrained prosthesis that provides varus/valgus restraint. Also, repair and/or reattachment of the ligament has proven successful, with postoperative knee scores and ROM equivalent to those in knees without this complication. Rehabilitation for these patients must be modified slightly, because they wear a brace for 6 weeks after surgery and follow an MCL injury protocol to allow healing of the ligament.

Rupture of the patellar tendon is the most common complication of knee arthroplasty. Nonsurgical treatment and primary repair have not proven successful. Reconstruction with fresh frozen extensor mechanism allograft is preferred because of the improved ability of both bone and tendon to incorporate. Nonabsorbable suture fixation of the allograft tendon onto a broad base of healthy quadriceps musculature allows reliable incorporation. Furthermore, fracture of the patella may also occur. Three aspects of the extensor mechanism must be assessed: whether the patellar component is loose, whether the extensor mechanism is partly or completely disrupted, and the extent of the remaining patellar bone. Nonsurgical treatment is successful if the extensor mechanism remains functional and the patellar component remains well fixed. Surgery is indicated in patients showing marked disruption of the extensor mechanism.[63,64]

Postoperative stiff knee is a sign of failure of TKA and remains an unsolved problem. The best predictor of postoperative ROM is preoperative motion. When arthrofibrosis is diagnosed early, it can be managed successfully with manipulation under anesthesia. Late treatment of stiffness is less likely to respond to manipulation.

Although the prevalence of postoperative periprosthetic fracture is fairly low (less than 2% of cases), treatment remains a challenge to all orthopedic surgeons, and the complication rates remain high. The main goal of treatment is to maintain alignment and fracture stability, and early ROM is essential to prevent stiffness. Surgery is indicated when the fracture is significantly displaced, the stability of

the prosthesis is compromised, and the quality of bone is suboptimal. Failed prosthesis, demonstrated by a loose implant, requires revision arthroplasty. Displaced fractures associated with well-fixed implants are best treated with reduction and rigid fixation to allow early range of motion.

Heterotopic ossification, another potential complication, results in calcium deposition within soft tissues around the joint. Although uncommon, this complication may directly impede progress with ROM and possibly strengthening exercises. Management may involve medication, radiation therapy, and possibly surgical excision, which will clearly alter the goals and rehabilitation treatment program.

The survival rate for TKA implants is 95% 10 to 15 years after the surgery. Late complications after TKA primarily include prosthetic loosening.[65] A new onset of pain in either the distal thigh or leg may indicate loosening of the prosthesis, and these symptoms typically worsen with weight-bearing activities and progressively worsen over time. Again, early referral to the surgeon is indicated, because appropriate surgical intervention is required. A painful TKA requires a broad systemic workup that includes both intrinsic (knee related) and extrinsic sources of pain. It is important to note that despite the widely taught precept that knee pain can originate outside the knee, patients continue to present to referral centers with pain in a replaced knee following an extensive and inconclusive work up of the knee joint when the origin of their pain is from an arthritic hip or lumbar spine.[6] Therefore protocols for evaluating a painful TKA begin with clinical and radiographic examination of extra-articular sites. Routine aspiration should be performed for a replaced knee suspicious for infection. White blood cell counts of 25,000/mm^3 or higher provide a strong suspicion for an infected TKA that needs to be surgically debrided.[61,62,66]

Failure of a replaced knee results in rapid acceleration of pain symptoms, functional decline, and the need for revision arthroplasty. Revision surgery is indicated for gross loosening of the implants, instability, infection, malalignment, wear, osteolysis, or disruption of the extensor mechanism. Gross loosening of the implants may occur secondary to wear and osteolysis, malalignment, or infection. Therefore routine knee aspiration is indicated.[67] A midline incision is made, but when multiple incisions are present, it is important to use the most lateral incision because of the soft tissue blood supply. It also is important to assess the bone integrity, remaining bone stock, and the extensor mechanism and collateral ligament integrity. Furthermore, it is important to restore the anatomical joint line, which generally is 1.5 cm (0.6 inch) proximal to the tip of the fibula. Elevation of the joint line results in patellar impingement and reduced quadriceps strength. The complication rate for revision TKA is much higher than for primary TKA, approaching 25%. Infection, dysfunction of the extensor mechanism, instability, fixation failure, and periprosthetic fracture all can compromise the outcome of revision surgery. Although most of these complications require intervention from providers other than the physical therapist, early recognition of complications and appropriate referral are important.

Outcomes of Total Knee Arthroplasty

Outcomes after TKA have been reported in the literature for decades, and the majority of studies have focused on the technical aspects of prosthetic implant survivability and design. More recent research has embraced the need also to address the impact of this procedure on quality of life issues important to the patient. More standardized outcome tools are being used to assess patient outcomes. However, a single ideal outcome tool to assess patients after TKA does not exist.

Overall, TKA for patients with end stage OA is considered a successful surgical intervention, with implant survivability reported to be 95% 10 to 15 years after surgery.[65] Factors that influence ROM outcomes include the design of the prosthesis, preoperative ROM, and obesity.[68] Controversy still exists as to whether a PCL-sparing or substitution prosthetic design provides greater flexion ROM by the end of rehabilitation.[60,65,68] This is partly influenced by the ongoing evolution of prosthetic design. However, it is important for the clinician to have an understanding of the type of implant used and the expected ROM that can be achieved to establish realistic ROM goals for the patient. Constrained and rotating hinge devices, which are inherently more stable by design, tend to limit flexion ROM and have the potential to transfer more shear and rotatory forces to the bone-prosthesis interface, potentially contributing to early loosening of the prosthesis.[65]

Unicompartmental arthroplasty has a reported 85% survival at 10 years. The most common reason for early failure is a lack of symptomatic improvement in patients who undergo conversion to a TKA. Appropriate patient selection is the key to preventing early conversion to TKA.[69,70]

Additional considerations on prosthetic design have focused on the effect of preserving the PCL as a soft tissue structure that can contribute proprioceptive and kinesthetic input to the knee. The rationale for leaving the PCL intact is to enhance joint position sense and provide important feedback for balance mechanisms. Studies have shown that proprioception and kinesthesia improve after TKA, most likely because of the reduction in pain and inflammation and postoperative changes to the capsuloligamentous structures, not necessarily because of preservation of the PCL.[71] Further studies that specifically address balance and proprioceptive training after TKA with both PCL-sparing and PCL-substituting devices may shed more light on this design feature.

Preoperative ROM and function are predictive of postoperative outcomes for patients with TKA.[8,9] The timing of measurement and the tools used to measure function vary in the literature. The Western Ontario and McMaster Universities Osteoarthritis Index (WOMAC) and the 6 Minute Walk Test (6MWT) have been reported to be most responsive when patients are examined 0 to 4 months after surgery.[72] Performance-based testing after TKA needs to consider the recovery time frame. Early postoperative assessments should include the 6MWT as the most responsive test. The timed stair ascent is not responsive early on, because many patients are unable to complete this task in the first 4 months after surgery.[72]

The Knee Society Clinical Rating Scale and the WOMAC are the most responsive outcome measures for TKA.[73] Both are disease-specific scales that rate function, pain, and stiffness; the primary symptoms associated with OA. Patient perception of functional recovery has multiple interactions, including psychological issues, which may influence the patient's report of function.[74-76] Comprehensive management, which includes psychological aspects, should be considered in the overall patient care plan.

A major focus in recent outcomes studies on patients who underwent TKA has been the correlation between strength and function. Many studies have reported residual weakness in patients who have completed rehabilitation,[74,77-79] which affects the patients' gait speed[80,81] and stair ascent strategy.[82] Experimental designs that focus specifically on additional interventions to address strength deficits have shown promise in improving strength and related functional activities.[80,83-85] Further research into interventions is important, to determine the optimum treatment for developing postoperative protocols that will rehabilitate patients to their fullest potential and restore their functional ability to that of age- and gender-matched controls. As patients' expectations for postoperative function change, rehabilitation programs must evolve to meet these needs fully.

Summary

Total knee arthroplasty is a successful intervention for patients with end stage arthritis of the knee. Rehabilitation is an essential component of the overall management of these patients. Coordinated, individualized care from all health care providers, from the preoperative phase through the continuum of postoperative rehabilitation, maximizes the patient's functional level and ability to resume meaningful activities. Ongoing advancements in surgical instrumentation and techniques, coupled with progressive rehabilitation programs, will continue to improve the long-term results and expectations for TKA.

References

To enhance this text and add value for the reader, all references have been incorporated into a CD-ROM that is provided with this text. The reader can view the reference source and access it online whenever possible. There are a total of 85 references for this chapter.

CHAPTER 28

MANAGEMENT OF OSTEOARTHRITIS AND RHEUMATOID ARTHRITIS

Maura Daly Iversen and Linda Steiner

Introduction

The term *arthritis* comprises a complex of diseases that affect more than 70 million people in the United States.[1] Arthritis can manifest in more than 100 forms. This chapter focuses on rheumatoid arthritis and osteoarthritis and provides an analysis and discussion of the rehabilitation management of these two conditions.

Osteoarthritis

Epidemiology and Pathophysiology

Osteoarthritis (OA) involves the entire joint but is primarily a disease of the cartilage (Figure 28-1). OA affects nearly 40 million people in the United States and is the second leading cause of disability. The exact pathogenesis is unknown. The most commonly affected and symptomatic joints are the apophyseal joints of the spine, the distal and proximal interphalangeal joints, the carpometacarpal joints, the first metatarsophalangeal joint, and the knee, hip, and patellofemoral joints.[2] The clinical features of OA are presented in Table 28-1.

Joints Commonly Affected by Osteoarthritis

- Spinal apophyseal joints
- Proximal interphalangeal (PIP) joints
- Distal interphalangeal (DIP) joint
- Carpometacarpal (CMC) joints
- First metatarsophalangeal (MTP) joint
- Hip
- Knee
- Patellofemoral joints

Risk factors for OA can be classified into two major categories: intrinsic risk factors and extrinsic risk factors. Intrinsic factors include knee alignment (a determinant of joint load), muscle strength, obesity, ligament laxity, and proprioception. Extrinsic factors include repetitive physical activity and injury.[2] Osteoarthritis is commonly referred to as *osteoarthrosis*. Although OA used to be considered a degenerative joint disease, this designation is no longer appropriate. Scientists now recognize that OA is a slowly progressing, dynamic disease that involves biomechanical, environmental, genetic, and biochemical factors (e.g., cytokines).[3]

Categories of Osteoarthritis

- Primary osteoarthritis: Results in articular changes, although the etiological basis for the disease is unknown
- Secondary osteoarthritis: Caused by underlying factors that accelerate age-related degeneration of cartilage
- These factors include inflammatory arthritis (e.g., rheumatoid arthritis or spondyloarthritis), hypermobility syndromes, metabolic diseases (e.g., diabetes), and congenital and acquired joint surface incongruities that accelerate damage to the cartilage, as well as trauma or sports-related injuries

Our understanding of OA has increased considerably over the past 10 years, partly as a result of advances in cartilage imaging techniques. Early OA is a focal disease that presents as a distinct lesion of the cartilage.[4,5] Patients with early OA have joint stiffness and progressive cartilage destruction with pain on loading of the affected joint. Over time, OA involves the entire joint, including the subchondral bone. Lesions progress with repeated biomechanical loading, synovial membrane inflammation, and release of

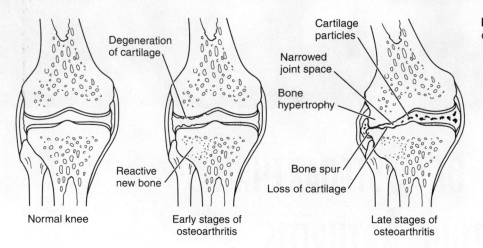

Figure 28-1
Osteoarthritis of the knee.

Table 28-1
Pathology and Clinical Features of Rheumatoid Arthritis and Osteoarthritis

Disease	Tissue Predominantly Involved	Clinical Features	Radiographic Features
Rheumatoid arthritis (RA)	Synovium (inflammation)	Symmetrical and bilateral joint involvement Joint pain, swelling, stiffness, and contracture Muscle weakness and fatigue *Acute*: Red, hot, swollen, painful joints; boggy feel, fatigue, with or without fever; ligamentous laxity; morning stiffness up to a few hours *Subacute*: Effusion, reduced redness and pain *Stable*: Generally no effusion, minimal stiffness	Periarticular swelling, joint effusion, regional osteoporosis, subchondral osteolytic erosions, joint subluxation
Osteoarthritis (OA)	Cartilage (degradation)	Affects hips, knees, spine, ankles, distal interphalangeal (DIP) joints, proximal interphalangeal (PIP) joints, and metacarpophalangeal (MCP) joints Joint pain, malalignment Decreased proprioception Muscle weakness *Early*: Focal cartilaginous lesions *End stage*: Loss of cartilage, bone on bone	Osteophytes at joint margins, joint space narrowing, subchondral sclerosis and cysts

Modified from Iversen MD, Liang MH, Bae SC: Exercise therapy in selected arthritides: rheumatoid arthritis, osteoarthritis, systemic lupus erythematosus, systemic sclerosis and polymyositis/dermatomyositis. In Frontera WR, Dawson DM, Slovik DM, editors: *Exercise in rehabilitation medicine*, Champaign, IL, 1999, Human Kinetics.

cytokines; this stimulates the production of matrix metalloproteinases, which cause cartilage degradation and loss. Eventually the joint surface is destroyed. The classic appearance of primary OA on radiographs is localized disease with evidence of unequal joint space narrowing, eburnation (a hard, white appearance) of the subchondral bone, osteophytes, and subchondral cysts (Figure 28-2). These findings increase in frequency after age 50. Only 40% of patients with severe radiographic features present with pain.[6,7]

The radiographic features of OA are graded according to specific criteria. The Kellgren scale is commonly used for this purpose (Table 28-2). On radiographs, secondary OA may appear as diffuse or localized disease, depending on the etiology (e.g., rheumatoid arthritis [RA], diabetes, or trauma). Secondary contractures occur around the involved joint and contiguous joints. These contractures alter joint alignment and can increase the biomechanical forces on the joint, accelerating cartilage loss and increasing energy requirements for activities.

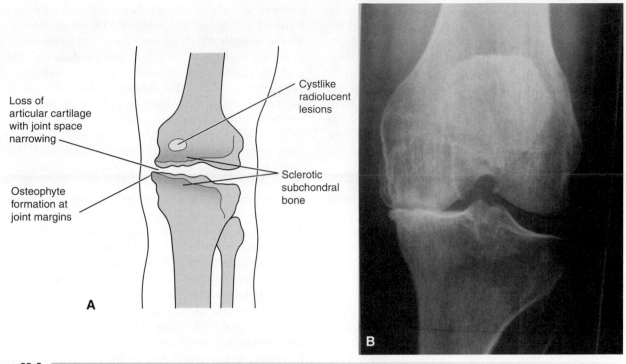

Loss of articular cartilage with joint space narrowing

Osteophyte formation at joint margins

Cystlike radiolucent lesions

Sclerotic subchondral bone

A

B

Figure 28-2

A, Radiographic hallmarks of osteoarthritis (Kellgren scale). **B,** Radiograph showing the main radiological signs of osteoarthritis. (**A** redrawn from McKinnis LN: *Fundamentals of orthopaedic radiology,* p 63, Philadelphia, 2005, FA Davis; **B** from Harris ED, Budd RC, Firestein GS et al: *Kelley's textbook of rheumatology,* ed 7, p 1514, Philadelphia, 2005, WB Saunders.)

Classic Radiographic Appearance of Primary Osteoarthritis

- Unequal joint space narrowing
- Eburnation (hard, white appearance) of subchondral bone
- Osteophyte formation
- Subchondral cysts

Table 28-2

Kellgren-Lawrence Classification of Radiological Joint Changes in Osteoarthritis

Classification	Description
Grade 0	No features
Grade 1	Doubtful: Minute osteophyte, doubtful significance
Grade 2	Minimal: Definite osteophyte, unimpaired joint space
Grade 3	Moderate: Moderate diminution of joint space
Grade 4	Severe: Greatly impaired joint space with sclerosis of subchondral bone

From Kellgren JH, Lawrence JS: Radiological assessment of osteoarthrosis, *Ann Rheum Dis* 16:494-501, 1957.

Signs, Symptoms, and Impairments

Joint Pain, Stiffness, Restricted Motion, and Alterations in Alignment

Osteoarthritis causes pain, aching, or stiffness and eventually altered joint alignment. Cartilage does not have nerve endings; therefore the pain of OA may be caused by stretching of the joint capsule as a result of inflammation, the release of inflammatory cytokines in the synovial fluid, muscle spasms, and pressure on the subchondral bone.[8] Patients frequently report that the pain increases with activity and is relieved by rest. Some patients have nighttime pain and report stiffness on waking. The stiffness often resolves in less than an hour and may be present after rest or with prolonged sitting.

Limitations in joint range of motion (ROM) are the result of osteophyte formation, soft tissue and tendon contractures surrounding a joint, periarticular muscle spasm, destruction of joint cartilage, persistent faulty posture, or muscular imbalance. Although a flexed position minimizes intra-articular pressure and reduces pain, it leads to flexion contracture. Crepitus may be felt when the joint is passively moved through the ROM; this results when irregular opposing cartilage surfaces rub together. Localized joint swelling is evident in patients with erosive OA and presents as warmth and soft tissue swelling.[9]

With hip OA, pain may be present in the hip, groin, anterior thigh, knee, or buttocks. ROM often is restricted, particularly internal rotation, and may be accompanied by crepitus. Patients may experience difficulties with mobility and personal hygiene, as well as increased energy expenditure with activities. Loss of hip range adversely affects the spine and other joints, including the knee and ankle. Preventive stretching is important and should be initiated early and often. Functionally based exercises, such as repetitive sit to stand, help maintain strength in hip and knee extensors. For patients unable to tolerate full gravity exercise, water (aquatic therapy) can be used to allow exercise with reduced load.[8]

Signs and Symptoms of Osteoarthritis

- Pain or aching with activity
- Morning stiffness
- Altered joint alignment
- Limited range of motion
- Joint contracture
- Crepitus
- Joint swelling

The knee is the most commonly affected weight-bearing joint. Malalignment of the knee, either varus or valgus, may be evident with severe disease (Figure 28-3). Knee varus is the more common presentation in knee osteoarthritis. The

presence of varus or valgus is associated with a threefold to fourfold increase in the odds of OA progression in the medial compartment of the knee.[2] Malalignment and abnormal tracking of the patella may produce retropatellar pain and chondromalacia patellae. Retropatellar pain often is experienced when the individual walks upstairs or on inclines or sits for prolonged periods. Knee pain can lead to disuse atrophy and deconditioning.[2,10] However, one research study suggested that muscle weakness may be a cause rather than a result of knee osteoarthritis.[11] Muscle weakness leads to changes in joint biomechanics and unequal forces across the joint surface. Joint laxity from muscle inhibition and joint space narrowing distributes the forces across the cartilage surface unequally and can accelerate the process of cartilage degeneration.[8]

Common features of hand OA are Heberden's and/or Bouchard's nodes, which are the result of bony overgrowths (Figure 28-4). Heberden's nodes appear at the medial and dorsolateral aspects of the distal interphalangeal (DIP) joints, and Bouchard's nodes appear at the proximal interphalangeal (PIP) joints. The finger joints appear bony and become less stable and less functional. Effusions may be present and over time lead to joint ankylosis. As a result of these deformities, patients lose their ability to grip small objects or to make a tight fist.

OA of the spine, also known as *spondylosis*, may affect the cervical, thoracic, and/or lumbar regions. Common changes evident on radiographs include osteophytes, which may form adjacent to the end plates and reduce blood supply to the vertebrae; stiffening and sclerosis (thickening or hardening) of the bone; facet joint degeneration; and degeneration of the disc. Severe OA of the facet joints can lead to spinal stenosis. Limited range of motion, especially

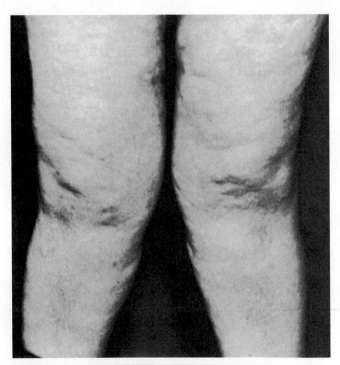

Figure 28-3

Valgus deformity of the knees. This is a common knee deformity that develops in patients with osteoarthritis of the lateral compartment. (From Polley HF, Hunder GG: *Rheumatologic interviewing and physical examination of the joints,* ed 2, p 214, Philadelphia, 1978, WB Saunders.)

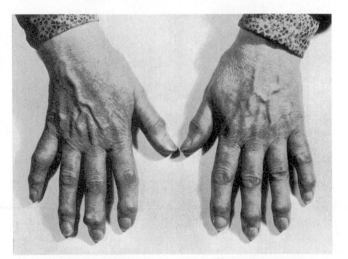

Figure 28-4

Osteoarthritic joint changes of the hand, including Heberden's nodes at the distal interphalangeal joints and Bouchard's nodes at the proximal interphalangeal joints. (From Polley HF, Hunder GG: *Rheumatologic interviewing and physical examination of the joints,* ed 2, p 120, Philadelphia, 1978, WB Saunders.)

rotation of the neck, is evident with cervical OA, along with pain and stiffness with movement.[3]

Muscle Weakness

Periarticular muscular weakness adds to the progression of disease through functional instability and diminished neuromuscular protective mechanisms.[9] Disuse atrophy probably results from ligament stretching, reflex inhibition from pain, capsular contraction, and joint irritation caused by pain and effusion.[8] Atrophy of the muscles because of reflex inhibition starts a vicious circle (Figure 28-5), increasing force across the damaged cartilage and altering the mechanics of the joint.

Proprioceptive Deficits

Proprioceptive changes occur with age,[12] with sedentary lifestyles, and with joint instability. These factors may contribute to or result from osteoarthritis. Proprioception is necessary for appropriate spatial and temporal coordination of the limb during movement. This increased coordination enhances stability and leads to more normal load distribution, reducing the risk of injury. Changes in proprioception may result from destructive alterations in the ligaments, cartilage, capsule, or muscle and tendon that alter joint alignment.[8] On examination, reduced joint proprioception may be present along with joint hypermobility. Barrett et al.[13] demonstrated that individuals with knee osteoarthritis have poorer knee proprioception than their healthy older counterparts. In another study, 28 adults with unilateral knee osteoarthritis (Kellgren scale grade 2 or higher) and 29 adults without knee osteoarthritis were recruited to allow examination of the impact of OA on joint proprioception.[14] A computer device and a stepper motor provided angular motion at 0.3°/sec and recorded angular displacement as patients reported the point at which they detected knee joint deflection. Patients with unilateral knee osteoarthritis demonstrated worse proprioception than their healthy counterparts.

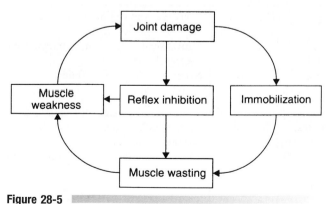

Figure 28-5
Vicious circle of injury. (Redrawn from Stokes M, Young A: The contribution of reflex inhibition to arthrogenous muscle weakness, *Clin Sci* 67:7-14, 1984.)

Basic Principles of Rehabilitation and Studies on the Effects of Exercise in Patients with Osteoarthritis

Goals of Rehabilitation and Studies on the Effects of Exercise

The goals of rehabilitation in OA are to maximize function and muscle force production and to reduce the deconditioning associated with OA of the weight-bearing joints. Evaluations of regimens to correct or prevent contractures are almost nonexistent. Heat, followed by passive ROM exercises and joint mobilization, is used clinically to reduce contractures. Proper posture and positioning during extended inactivity or sleep, along with active ROM exercises, are used to maximize functional range and strength. In difficult cases, serial casting or splinting can reduce contracture when followed by maintenance exercises.

Goals of Osteoarthritis Rehabilitation

- Maximize function
- Maximize strength
- Reduce deconditioning

In a systematic review of exercise therapy for knee and hip osteoarthritis, van Baar et al.[15] found that exercise interventions of varying modes yielded small reductions in disability, small to moderate effects on pain, and moderate effects of exercise on self-reported global assessments. Although studies have examined the impact of exercise on function, few investigators have examined the impact of strengthening programs on cartilage. Table 28-3 presents a summary of the various exercise studies designed for individuals with knee OA.

Few studies specifically measure changes in joint proprioception or the impact of exercise programs on joint proprioception. However, some studies emphasize the role of progressive balance activities (e.g., double-limb stance activities to single-limb stance) as methods of improving joint proprioception and strength, based on the assumption that proprioception does not spontaneously return when pain diminishes.[16,17] A variety of exercises, such as standing on unsteady surfaces, using biomechanical ankle platform system (BAPS) boards, and tilt/rocker boards, are used for balance and proprioception training. Although the way that exercise influences proprioception is unclear, clinicians agree that addressing proprioception is important in the rehabilitation program.

In one small trial, patients with hand OA were instructed in yoga and relaxation techniques for 10 weeks. At the end of the trial, patients reported decreased pain and tenderness and improved motion of finger joints.[18]

Most studies on the effects of exercise focus on strengthening exercises for patients with mild to moderate OA.

Table 28-3
Randomized, Controlled Trials of Exercise in Hip and Knee Osteoarthritis

Author	Sample	Intervention/Groups	Duration	Study Outcomes
Studies That Included Aerobic Exercise				
Minor et al.[24] (1989)	80 Patients with KOA 40 Patients with RA, mild to moderate disease	1. Stretching and isometric exercise 3 times/week for 1 hour plus aerobic walking, 30 minutes 2. Stretching and isometric exercise plus aerobic pool activities, 30 minutes 3. Stretching and isometric exercise 3 times/week for 1 hour	12 weeks	Pool and walking programs increased aerobic capacity 20% and 19% respectively; control group had no change No exacerbation of joint symptoms in the two aerobic groups On average, pain decreased by almost 10% and morning stiffness by 20 minutes in aerobic groups Physical activity, anxiety, and depression improved significantly in both aerobic groups more than for controls
Kovar et al.[25] (1992)	102 Patients with chronic, stable KOA	1. Supervised light stretching and strengthening plus education, followed by up to 30 minutes of walking 2. Control: Routine follow-up care, telephone follow-up calls 3 times/ week	8 weeks	Walking distance increased 18.4% in exercise group and decreased in control group Exercisers reported 39% improvement in activity (WOMAC), 27% decrease in pain, and decreased use of medications
Ettinger et al.[26] (1997)	439 Patients with radiographic evidence of KOA and disability	1. Aerobics for 60 minutes at 60% to 80% maximum HR 2. Resistive exercise 3. Education	18 months	83% of participants completed the study Adherence rate was 68% in aerobic group and 70% in strengthening group Aerobic exercisers showed 10% decrease in disability, 12% less knee pain, and improved walk time, stair climbing, and carrying ability compared to controls Strength group showed 8% decrease in disability and knee pain, improved walk time, stair climbing, and carrying ability compared to controls No radiographic changes seen in any group
Bautch et al.[29] (1997)	30 patients with KOA	1. Low resistance strengthening exercises, 3 times/week, 3 repetitions of each exercise, increased to 10 repetitions at 4 weeks plus low intensity treadmill walking plus education 1 time/week 2. Education only	12 weeks	Exercisers showed decreased pain levels Educational only group demonstrated better AIMS scores No change in synovial fluid composition
Messier et al.[28] (2000)	103 Patients with KOA	1. Aerobic exercise for 50 minutes, 5-minute warm-up and cool-down, with 40 minutes of walking at 50% to 85% maximum HR, 3 times/ week (3 months at center and 15 months at home)	18 months	Both exercise groups improved compared to controls Balance and postural sway improved in exercise groups

Table 28-3
Randomized, Controlled Trials of Exercise in Hip and Knee Osteoarthritis—Cont'd

Author	Sample	Intervention/Groups	Duration	Study Outcomes
		2. Weight-training exercises for upper and lower extremities, 2 sets of 10 repetitions of each exercise, 3 times/week (3 months at center and 15 months at home) 3. Monthly education group sessions plus scheduled contact from research team		
Penninx et al.[30] (2001)	250 Patients with KOA	1. Aerobic exercise, walking program 3 times/week for 60 minutes 2. Resistance exercises, 3 60-minute sessions per week using nine different exercises	3 months	Both exercise groups reduced their disability in ADLs as measured by a self-report questionnaire
Fransen et al.[107] (2001)	126 Patients with KOA; grades I, II	1. Individualized aerobic and strengthening led by the PT 2. Group aerobic and strengthening exercise, 2 times/week for 1 hour, supervised by a PT plus home exercise program 3. Wait list control	8 weeks	Both PT treatment groups showed significant improvements in pain, physical function, and health-related quality of life Improvements were maintained for 2 months No difference in outcomes was seen between the PT groups

Studies of Strengthening, Flexibility and Other Interventions

Author	Sample	Intervention/Groups	Duration	Study Outcomes
Callaghan et al.[31] (1985)	27 Patients with KOA	1. PT-led exercises, 3 sets of 10 exercises, 4 times/week for 20 minutes 2. Education plus repeated sit to stand exercises, no intensity specified 3. Sham electrical stimulation	2 weeks	No differences were seen between groups on any outcome measures
Borjesson et al.[32] (1996)	68 Patients with medial KOA (scheduled for surgery); grades I-III	1. PT-led exercises, 40-minute session, 3 times/week; included warm-up for 10 minutes, knee flexion/extension with 1-3 kg (2.2-6.6 pounds) weight, toe and heel standing, and hip dynamic exercises; 2 sets of 10 repetitions for each exercise and isometrics using 10-second hold and stretches 2. Control	5 weeks	No significant differences in gait, ROM, or isokinetic strength were seen between groups Patients in the PT group increased their ability to descend stairs and reported improved mood
Schilke et al.[108] (1996)	20 Patients with KOA	1. Isokinetic exercise, 6 sets of 5 MVCs of knee flexors and extensors 2. Control: No prescription	8 weeks	Significant decrease in pain, stiffness, and AIMS activity and OASI scores Increased mobility in the exercise group Control group increased right knee flexion and left knee extension

Table 28-3
Randomized, Controlled Trials of Exercise in Hip and Knee Osteoarthritis—Cont'd

Author	Sample	Intervention/Groups	Duration	Study Outcomes
Van Baar et al.[33] (1998)	201 Patients with HOA or KOA	1. Individual exercises 1-3 times/week for 30 minutes 2. Education	12 weeks	Exercisers showed 17-point decrease in pain and 19-point reduction in disability (effect sizes were medium to small, respectively)
Rogind et al.[22] 1998	25 Patients with KOA (Kellgren grade 3 on radiograph)	1. PT-led outpatient exercise, including general fitness, balance, coordination, flexibility, and strengthening exercises, 2 times/week 2. Control	12 weeks	78% Adherence Exercise group increased quadriceps strength by 20% At 1 year, walking speed improved by 13%, decreased 3.8 points, pain reduced by 2 points Increase in palpable effusions
O'Reilly et al.[109] (1999)	191 Patients with KOA symptomatic	1. Home exercises, including isometric knee exercise (5-second hold), dynamic knee and stepping exercises performed daily 2. Control	6 months	Decrease in WOMAC pain score by 22.5% and by 6.2% in controls Significant improvement in VAS pain and 17.4% change in function among exercisers
Deyle et al.[110] (2000)	83 Patients with KOA, grades I, III	1. Manual therapy to the knee, spine, hip, and ankle plus dynamic exercises for the hip and knee, as well as stretching exercise, 2 times/week for 30 minutes, plus a home exercise program 2. Subtherapeutic ultrasound	4 weeks	At 4 and 8 weeks, significant improvements in exercisers for 6MWT and WOMAC scores At 8 weeks, 6MWT improved 13.1% and WOMAC improved 55.8% compared to controls Gains still evident at 1 year
Hopman-Rock and Westhoff[21] (2000)	103 Patients with HOA or KOA	1. Peer-led educational program lasting 1 hour, plus 1 hour of PT-led dynamic and static exercises for the hip and knee, 1 time/week 2. Control	6 weeks	Significant improvements in pain, quadriceps strength, knowledge, and self-efficacy at postassessment Benefits still evident at 6 months in exercise group
Petrella and Bartha[19] (2000)	179 Patients with KOA, mild to moderate (medial compartment)	1. Progressive home-based exercise. Simple ROM and resistance exercises plus oxaprozin 2. Oxaprozin alone	8 weeks	Improvement seen in activity (self-paced walking, stepping) and activity-related pain in both exercise groups
Baker et al.[111] (2001)	46 Patients with KOA	1. Progressive strength training program (squats, step-ups, isotonic exercises of the lower limbs)	16 weeks	Improvements seen in strength, pain, physical function, and quality of life
Quilty et al.[112] (2001)	87 Patients	1. Nine 20-minute PT sessions, including quadriceps exercises, postural exercises and education, functional exercises, footwear recommendations, and patellar taping. Exercises performed at home, 10 times/day 2. Usual care	10 weeks	At 5 months, treatment group showed small decrease in pain and significant improvement in quadriceps strength No difference at 1 year

Table 28-3
Randomized, Controlled Trials of Exercise in Hip and Knee Osteoarthritis—Cont'd

Author	Sample	Intervention/Groups	Duration	Study Outcomes
Foley et al.[20] (2003)	105 Patients over age 50 with hip OA or KOA	1. Hydrotherapy, 3 times/week 2. Gym exercise, 3 times/week 3. Control	6 weeks	Both exercise programs produced functional gains and improved quadriceps strength compared with the control group Compliance was similar for the two exercise groups Compliance was similar for the two exercise groups Hydrotherapy group had increased their distance walked compared to control group Gym exercise group showed increased walking speed and self-efficacy compared to control group
Gur et al.[34] (2002)	23 Patients with bilateral KOA, grade II or III	1. 12 Concentric knee exercises performed 3 times/week 2. 6 Repetitions of concentric and 6 repetitions of eccentric knee exercises, at angular velocities of 30°-180%/sec 3. Control: Usual activity	8 weeks	Both exercise groups improved functional capacity, peak torque of knee, and pain relief Concentric-eccentric group performed better on the stair climbing/descending than the concentric group, and the concentric-eccentric group showed more reduction in pain Usual activity group did not show any improvements
Topp et al.[35] (2002)		1. Dynamic resistance Thera-Band exercises for 40 minutes (10-minute warm-up and cool-down), 3 times/week 2. Isometric exercises, 3 times/week	16 weeks	Isometric group decreased their time to perform functional tasks by 16% to 23% A 13% to 17% decrease in time to ascend/descend stairs was seen in the dynamic group Pain decreased in both groups No change was seen in controls
Hoeksma et al.[23] (2004)	109 Patients with hip OA	1. Manual therapy manipulations of the hip by manual therapist 2. Active exercises for the hip (nine sessions) plus home program with weights, endurance training, ROM, and stretching	5 weeks	An 81% improvement was seen in the manual therapy group compared to a 50% improvement in the exercisers

KOA, Knee osteoarthritis; *HOA*, hip osteoarthritis; *RA*, rheumatoid arthritis; *WOMAC*, Western Ontario and McMaster Universities Osteoarthritis Index; *AIMS*, Arthritis Impact Measurement Scale; *HR*, heart rate; *MVC*, maximum voluntary contraction; *ADLs*, activities of daily living; *PT*, physical therapist; *OASI*, Osteoarthritis Screening Index; ROM, range of motion; *VAS*, Visual Analogue Scale; *6MWT*, 6-Minute Walk Test.

In Table 28-3, randomized, controlled trials of exercise for hip and knee osteoarthritis are described. In an innovative study by Petrella and Bartha,[19] patients with knee OA were randomized to either a progressive resistive exercise program using common household items and nonsteroidal anti-inflammatory drugs (NSAIDs), or a progressive resistive exercise program using common household items combined with simple ROM exercises and NSAIDs, or NSAIDs alone. At the end of 8 weeks, patients in both exercise groups reported improvements in pain and functional performance compared to the group that received NSAIDs alone.

Foley et al.[20] randomly assigned 105 community dwelling patients with OA of the hip or knee to a gym-based or hydrotherapy exercise program or to a control group. The exercise groups attended exercise class 3 times a week for 6 weeks. Both the gym-based and hydrotherapy-based exercise groups showed increased quadriceps muscle strength and function compared to the control group. However, the hydrotherapy group tended to show greater gains in aerobic qualities of function, such as distance walked, whereas the gym-based group showed greater self-efficacy (i.e., confidence in self-management).

Hopman-Rock and Westhoff[21] randomized 103 patients with hip and knee OA to a program of health education and exercise. The program lasted 6 weeks and consisted of weekly sessions lasting 2 hours. The sessions included 1 hour of education and self-management led by a peer and 1 hour of exercise led by a physical therapist. The exercise program included a 15-minute discussion of the pros and cons of exercise and the importance of rest and alternating activities; this was followed by a warm-up, static and dynamic strengthening exercises for the hip and knee, and a cool-down. Patients not allocated to the education and exercise group received usual care. Significant improvements were found for pain, quality of life, quadriceps strength, knowledge, self-efficacy, and a physically active lifestyle in the intervention group. The effects were present, although to a lesser degree, at the 6-month assessment.

Rogind et al.[22] found positive outcomes in patients with severe knee OA who combined strengthening exercises and balance and coordination activities.[22] In this trial, 25 subjects were allocated to a 3-month training program that consisted of general fitness exercises, balance and coordination activities, stretching, and lower extremity strengthening plus a home program at an outpatient clinic, or control. Subjects exercised in groups twice a week. At the 3-month assessment, quadriceps strength had increased 20%, as measured by isokinetic testing. At 1 year, improvements were found in pain (a reduction of two points) and in functional index scores (a 3.8 reduction) compared to controls.

Few randomized, controlled studies have examined the impact of manual mobilization techniques combined with exercise in patients with OA. Hoeksma et al.[23] allocated 109 patients with hip OA to 5 weeks of either manual therapy and manipulations or active resistive hip exercises plus endurance training, ROM, and stretching. At the end of the trial, the manual therapy group demonstrated an 81% improvement compared with a 50% improvement in the exercise and stretching group.

Aerobic walking at moderate intensity appears to improve aerobic capacity by up to 20% without exacerbation of symptoms. In studies by Minor et al.[24] and Kovar et al.,[25] patients with mild to moderate osteoarthritis of the hips and knees not only improved aerobic capacity but demonstrated improvements in mood when aerobic walking was coupled with supervised stretching and strengthening exercises.

Ettinger et al.[26] studied the effects of exercise in a less controlled setting. In this study, 439 community dwelling subjects age 60 or older who had radiographic hallmarks of knee OA, pain, and physical disability were randomly allocated to an aerobic exercise program at 60% to 80% maximum heart rate, a resistance exercise program, or a health education program. At 18 months, patients in the aerobic and resistance exercise groups demonstrated modest improvements in pain (12%) and disability (10%), and better

scores on timed walk, stair climbing, and carrying ability than those in the health education group. The authors noted that education alone produced small improvements in outcomes, and this change may have led to the small differences between groups. Previous exercise behavior was the strongest predictor of exercise compliance in this sample.[27]

In a similarly designed study, Messier et al.[28] showed that aerobic exercise and strengthening programs improved balance and postural control. They enrolled 103 patients with knee osteoarthritis in an 18-month trial and allocated them to one of three groups: (1) supervised aerobic exercise at 50% to 85% of the maximum heart rate for 50 minutes, 3 times a week, for 3 months, followed by a home prescription; (2) supervised upper and lower extremity weight-training, 2 sets of 10 repetitions, 3 times a week, for 3 months, followed by a home exercise prescription; or (3) monthly educational sessions and scheduled contacts from the research team. At the end of the trial, patients in the exercise groups showed improved balance and postural stability.

Conclusions about Exercise and Osteoarthritis

The evidence from the preceding studies and others demonstrates that patients with mild to moderate knee and hip osteoarthritis can safely engage in effective aerobic and strengthening exercise without exacerbating joint symptoms. Improvements in mood, strength, and aerobic capacity are found, ranging from 15% to 40%, depending on the intensity of the prescribed exercise.[8] Gains in functional performance and reductions in limitations are greatest when the program lasts at least 8 weeks and exercises are performed at least 3 times a week.[20,24,25,28-35] As with other populations, compliance with an exercise program is critical to its effectiveness for the arthritic patient. Efficacy can be improved when home exercise is supplemented with a supervised program.

Clinical Point

Few studies have addressed the impact of resistance or aerobic exercise on patients with severe osteoarthritis, and the long-term effects of exercise on joint integrity and disability are unknown.

Aerobic exercise improves endurance, reduces fatigue, and has modest effects on muscle strength. With structured exercise (3 times a week over 4 months), individuals can improve strength and endurance, leading to decreased dependency and pain and increased functional activity. Some of these benefits continue for up to 8 months after an intense program.[36] The role of aerobic exercise in the management of patients with OA, particularly of the hips and knees, has received greater attention over the past 10 years. The concept that inactivity is a risk factor for osteoarthritis, rather than just an outcome of the disease, emphasizes the importance of aerobic exercise in disease management.

Achieving a Therapeutic Effect with Exercise. Some evidence indicates that exercises that focus on proprioception and balance may reduce disability and improve strength. However, more research is needed in this area. Despite the evidence that symptoms of OA of the hip and knee can be improved with exercise and that exercise is recommended in practice guidelines, most patients with OA have not had a prescription for exercise. Even when physicians prescribe exercise, only a small percentage of patients exercise in a manner that can achieve a therapeutic effect.[37] Certain patients with osteoarthritis of the hip can exercise at home as effectively as with outpatient hydrotherapy to improve joint mobility and increase muscle strength.[38] Including manual therapy with the exercise programs appears to provide added benefits. Caution needs to be applied in patients with lax or malaligned knees, especially with tibiofemoral OA, in which quadriceps strengthening may exacerbate symptoms. Table 28-4 summarizes the exercise recommendations for OA based on pain level and pathology.

Gait Problems and Use of Assistive Devices

A flexion contracture across the acetabulum toward the lateral margin[39] increases valgus forces at the knee and ankle and causes inefficient gait patterns and increased energy expenditure. Patients describe difficulty and pain when walking or climbing stairs and reduced functional independence. Decreased muscle strength and reduced joint proprioception also are associated with an increased incidence of falls.[17]

In one study, an exercise program consisting of individualized progressive training, including isometric and dynamic exercises for patients with knee osteoarthritis, significantly improved muscle function, functional capacity, and walking time (as much as 21%) and reduced self-reported difficulty with walking and pain.[36] Stationary cycling also has demonstrated improvements in walking speed, aerobic capacity, and pain.[40]

In a study by Leivseth et al.,[41] six patients with severe OA of the hip who were awaiting total hip arthroplasty (THA) increased hip adduction by 8.3°, increased the type I and II fiber cross-sectional area, and increased glycogen levels after passive muscle stretching perpendicular to the direction of

Table 28-4
Summary of Rehabilitation Interventions for Osteoarthritis

Type of Osteoarthritis (OA)	Recommendations
OA of the hip and knee Mild pain	AROM exercises (10 repetitions), 3 to 5 repetitions of flexibility and static exercises (8 to 10 repetitions of 6 seconds' duration) Dynamic exercises, especially of the quadriceps and hamstrings (8 to 10 repetitions) Low impact aerobic activities (pool, bicycling) 20 minutes, 3 times/week Balance activities (BAPS and tilt boards), single-limb stance
Moderate pain	Static and dynamic exercises—reduce to 5 repetitions. Flexibility exercises, 3 to 5 repetitions Low impact aerobic exercises (pool, bicycling) for 20 minutes, 3 times/week Balance and proprioception activities—bilateral Use of cane or lateral heel wedge foot orthosis, neoprene knee sleeve
Severe pain	Static and dynamic exercises (no resistance), 3 to 5 repetitions except with internal joint derangement Low to no impact aerobic exercises (pool) Note: Advise functional activities to keep moving
Bone on bone	Same as for severe form but few or no repetitions of dynamic exercises; patient education is very important Note: Caution should be used in prescribing quadriceps strengthening exercises for patients with ligamentous laxity and malalignment Orthosis: Varus unloader–type knee orthosis; may need crutches or walker
OA of the hand	Active movements, few repetitions, low resistance Teach home exercises, which the patient should repeat daily Aim to maintain full range of motion of MCP, PIP, and DIP joints

Modified from Iversen MD, Liang MH, Bae SC: Exercise therapy in selected arthritides: rheumatoid arthritis, osteoarthritis, systemic lupus erythematosus, systemic sclerosis and polymyositis/dermatomyositis. In Frontera WR, Dawson DM, Slovik DM, editors: *Exercise in rehabilitation medicine*, Champaign, IL, 1999, Human Kinetics.
AROM, Active range of motion; *BAPS*, biomechanical ankle platform system; *MCP*, metacarpophalangeal; *PIP*, proximal interphalangeal; *DIP*, distal interphalangeal.

the adductor muscle (without hip movement). The subjects stretched with a force of 20 to 30 kg (44.1 to 66.1 lbs) applied manually for 30 seconds, rested for 10 seconds, and repeated; the sessions lasted 25 minutes and were performed 5 days a week for 4 weeks.[41] Recent studies have also demonstrated improved rates of recovery in patients with end stage hip arthritis after preoperative and perioperative exercise programs for THA.[42,43]

Gait problems are common in patients with OA of any of the weight-bearing joints and are a clue to underlying pathology of the soft tissues or the joints themselves. Left untreated, they can cause problems. Clinicians should be attentive this diagnosis and design treatments that maximize joint function.

Orthoses for Osteoarthritis

Much of the research into bracing for OA has concentrated on devices to relieve knee pain and disability. In OA, the knee is subjected to increased medial compartment pressures secondary to varus loading during gait. Two main methods have been advanced to reduce these excessive forces: unloader-type knee orthoses (KO) or lateral wedge insoles at the foot. An unloader KO for varus gonarthrosis, or knee varus, can be either a thrust-type (Figure 28-6) or prestressed brace. The thrust-type, hinged KO has a single upright designed to create a valgus correcting force at the knee to unload the medial compartment.[44] Kirkley et al.[45] compared use of a varus unloader KO to a neoprene sleeve or to medical treatment alone in a group of 119 subjects with OA. After 6 months, the subjects who wore the unloader KO showed a significant difference in pain relief with functional tasks (e.g., a 6-minute walk and a 3-minute stair climb) compared to the group who

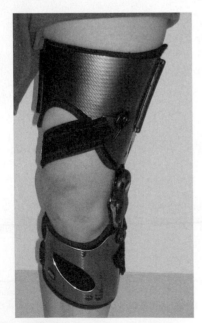

Figure 28-6
Varus unloader knee brace.

wore the neoprene sleeve. Both groups performed better than the nonbrace group.

Lindenfeld et al.[46] assessed the biomechanical properties of the brace to actually reduce the varus forces as well pain. They compared 11 subjects with OA before and after 4 weeks of brace wear and then compared them to 11 healthy controls. As measured on the Cincinnati Knee Rating System, pain, function, and biomechanical alignment all improved in the brace group. Alignment levels were reported to approach that of the normal control group.

Lateral wedge insoles or a variant, subtalar strapped insoles, are prescribed to make use of the closed chain properties of a foot orthosis (FO) on reducing compressive forces on the medial tibiofemoral joint compartment. Brouwer et al.[47] concluded that some limited evidence indicated that lateral wedges reduced the use of pain medication by OA patients when compared those who wore a neutral insole. However, function, as measured by the Western Ontario and McMaster Universities Osteoarthritis Index (WOMAC) functional scale, was not improved over the group that used neutral insoles after 6 months of wear. These researchers also reported that a lateral wedge insole with strapping for the subtalar joint demonstrated a biomechanical realignment effect, as measured by the femorotibial angle (FTA), but that those wearing these insoles reported more low back and foot pain with use. As yet, no studies have directly compared the use of an unloader KO with a lateral wedge insole or strapped subtalar lateral wedge insole. The clinical decision for use of these devices should be based on the patient's degree of disability and potential for compliance with an orthosis and the cost of the device.

Case Study in Osteoarthritis

John is a 77-year-old male who presents with a diagnosis of right hip OA. His radiographic findings suggest decreased joint space with small acetabular osteophytes off the anterior aspect of the joint. He has opted to delay surgical intervention and wants to use physical therapy to enhance his overall physical status. He reports minimal difficulty with activities of daily living (ADLs) and instrumental activities of daily living (IADLs) (see volume 1 of this series, *Orthopedic Physical Assessment*, Chapter 1). However, he has been increasingly sedentary since retiring from the post office 10 years ago. Currently, he reports late afternoon soreness on the anterior aspect of the leg and along the groin to his medial thigh, especially after doing a lot of walking.

On examination, John walks with a slow, deliberate gait pattern. He demonstrates decreased stance time on the right leg, and his right hip is maintained in flexion throughout the gait cycle. Decreased step length is noted on the left, and a positive Trendelenburg's sign on the right. Right hip ROM is 20° to 100° with a firm, unyielding end feel; internal rotation and abduction is 0° to 20° with a firm end feel; and external rotation is 0° to 35°. Left hip ROM is within normal limits. Right hip muscle strength is in the fair range. Lower abdominal strength is poor. Knee strength is good, and ankle strength is within normal limits (WNL). The patient has a positive Thomas test (20°) on the right. He demonstrates an inability to squat without visible muscle shaking and altered posture, a positive Trendelenburg's sign with unilateral squat, and increased trunk flexion with bilateral squat. Sensation is intact to light touch, but right hip kinesthesia and proprioception are reduced. He is able to maintain single-limb stance for approximately 5 seconds with eyes open. His past medical history is significant for coronary artery disease (no history of myocardial infarction), hypercholesteremia, gastroesophageal reflux disease, and a weight gain of 13.6 kg (30 lbs) over the past 10 years. His body mass index (BMI) is 27. He currently is taking the following medications: Zesteril, Lipitor, and Prilosec.

Questions: What rehabilitation program would you advise? What education about restrictions to his activities would you recommend? What type of exercise would you recommend? Do you think an assistive device would be useful?

Case Discussion

The patient's impairments of decreased hip muscle flexibility, poor muscle performance of the hip and trunk, poor motor control, pain, joint mobility, and diminished proprioception contribute to his altered gait and should be addressed in the rehabilitation program. Flexibility exercises and joint mobilization will help restore mobility and unload the hip joint while allowing a more normal gait pattern. Depending on the degree of pain, short-term use of a straight cane can further unload the joint for long distance walking. He will benefit from an exercise program that emphasizes strengthening of the proximal musculature of the hip, especially the weak gluteus medius. An exercise program should be started that incorporates stability exercises in weight bearing, such as rhythmic stabilization in standing, and progresses to unilateral static and dynamic control. The progression should take place as pain diminishes and proximal motor control improves. These activities not only improve motor coordination and strength, but also enhance proprioception. Aerobic exercise, such as aquatic classes and/or elliptical training, performed at 60% to 80% of his maximum heart rate, 3 times per week, should be incorporated into his program. The patient needs to learn how to modify his exercise regimen to adjust for his level of pain and to progress his exercises over time.

Rheumatoid Arthritis

Epidemiology and Pathophysiology

Classic rheumatoid arthritis is a chronic inflammatory disorder that not only affects joints, but also has multiple systemic manifestations. It affects approximately 1% to 2% of the U.S. population,[48] and it shortens life expectancy by about 10 years.[49] RA begins in early to middle life, affects women more often than men and the incidence increases with age.

The predominant pathology in rheumatoid disease is an inflammation of the synovium of diarthrodial joints, leading to a state of chronic synovitis. Synovitis that goes uncontrolled can lead to joint destruction (see Table 28-1). RA is characterized by periods of exacerbation and remission. The chronic fluctuating course of RA can follow various patterns. Patients may experience a continuous, low grade exacerbation or have periods of remission followed by exacerbations of various intensities. Although exacerbations are a feature of the disease, they can be triggered by infection or trauma or can occur after medications have been stopped. Fewer than 10% of patients with RA go into prolonged remissions.[50]

The pattern of joint involvement generally is symmetrical and polyarticular. Nearly 10% of those affected develop some joint deformities within 2 years of diagnosis. Radiological changes often are seen earliest in the feet and hands. The Sharp score, as modified by van der Heijde,[51] is a method of documenting the progression of the disease. Radiologists score the number of bony erosions and areas of joint space narrowing in 30 to 32 joints of the hand and 12 joints in the feet. The total score is recorded (maximum involvement equals 448 points) and monitored on successive radiographs to track progression.

Although RA can affect any area, the most commonly affected joints are the wrists, metacarpophalangeal (MCP) joints, and PIP joints in the upper extremity (Figure 28-7) and the ankle and foot (Figure 28-8) in the lower extremity. In the spine, RA is more common in the cervical area but can involve all segments. Because this is a systemic disease, extra-articular clinical symptoms may involve the cardiovascular system, pulmonary system, integument, and nervous system. Pleurisy, often presenting as shortness of breath or dyspnea on exertion, has been found in up to 70% of patients with RA. Pericarditis, myocarditis, and vasculitis, which may affect about 30% of patients, as well as renal effects secondary to vasculitis or to the toxic effects of long-term drugs used to control the disease, are all conditions that affect the physical functioning and exercise tolerance of patients with RA.[49,50,52]

Joints Commonly Affected by Rheumatoid Arthritis

- Wrist
- Metacarpophalangeal (MCP) joints
- Proximal interphalangeal (PIP) joints
- Foot
- Ankle
- Knee

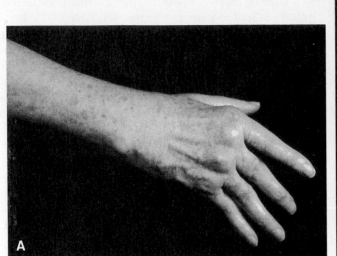
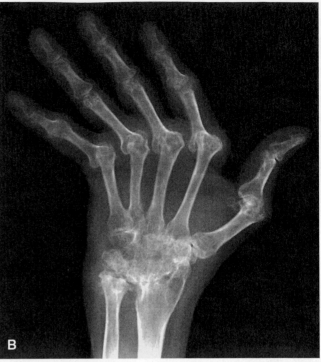
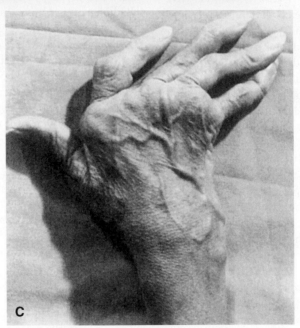

Figure 28-7

A, Ulnar deviation at the metacarpophalangeal (MCP) joints. This is a common deformity in patients with inflammatory arthritis, such as this patient with rheumatoid arthritis (RA). **B,** Ulnar deviation in rheumatoid arthritis. Severe ulnar deviation can be seen at the MCP joints with extensive erosions. Pancompartmental bony ankylosis and erosion are also seen at the wrist. **C,** Rheumatoid arthritis of the hand, showing advanced changes with ulnar drift and palmar subluxation at the MCP joints and swan neck and boutonniere deformities in the fingers. (**A** and **B** from Harris ED, Budd RC, Firestein GS et al: *Kelley's textbook of rheumatology,* ed 7, pp 491, 745, Philadelphia, 2005, WB Saunders; **C** from Swanson AB: Pathomechanics of deformities in the hand and wrist. In Hunter J, Schneider LH, Mackin EJ, Callahan AD, editors: *Rehabilitation of the hand: surgery and therapy,* p 895, St Louis, 1990, Mosby.)

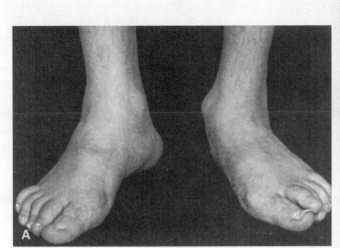
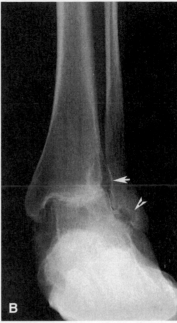

Figure 28-8

A, Valgus of the ankle, pes planus, and forefoot varus deformity of the left foot related to painful synovitis of the ankle, forefoot, and metatarsophalangeal joint in a 24-year-old man with severe rheumatoid arthritis. **B,** Rheumatoid arthritis of the ankle, showing diffuse loss of cartilage space with erosions of the fibula *(arrow and arrowhead)*. The scalloping along the medial border of the distal fibula *(arrow)* is called the fibular notch sign and is a characteristic finding in rheumatoid arthritis. The hindfoot is in valgus alignment. (From Harris ED, Budd RC, Firestein GS et al: *Kelley's textbook of rheumatology,* ed 7, pp 746, 1054, Philadelphia, 2005, WB Saunders.)

Bone loss leading to osteoporosis is greater than in age-matched cohorts[53,54] for both men and women with RA. In addition to the risk factors normally seen with primary osteoporosis, individuals with RA have factors such as periods of immobilization and long-term use of corticosteroids and disease-modifying antirheumatic drugs (DMARDS) (see volume 2 of this series, *Scientific Foundations and Principles of Practice in Musculoskeletal Rehabilitation,* Chapter 12). Studies have shown that patients with RA have a 1.5 to 3 times greater risk of osteoporotic fractures at the hip.[55,56] Vertebral deformities caused by osteoporotic fractures are 2 to 3 times more prevalent in those with RA.[57] However, a recent study by Haugeberg et al.[58] indicated that even with the use of DMARDS and corticosteroids, bone loss can be mitigated in a patient with RA if the individual is treated with antiresorptive drugs, calcium, and vitamin D.

Another common symptom of RA is fatigue, which may result from a combination of cytokine production, deconditioning from lack of exercise or activity, and altered biomechanics of involved joints. As with other chronic diseases, the patient has a higher risk of depression, which may contribute to the fatigue. In addition, the systemic nature of RA and the increased metabolic cost of normal living may significantly limit a person's function and restrict the level of independence as the disease progresses. The American College of Rheumatology has recommended a system to help clinicians classify the effect of the multiple impairments on the patient's global functional capacity (Table 28-5).[59]

Table 28-5

American College of Rheumatology's Classification of Global Functional Status in Rheumatoid Arthritis

Classification	Description
Class I	Completely able to perform usual activities of daily living (self-care, vocational, and avocational*)
Class II	Able to perform usual self-care and vocational activities but limited in avocational activities
Class III	Able to perform usual self-care activities but limited in vocational or avocational activities
Class IV	Limited in ability to perform usual self-care, vocational, and avocational activities

From Hochberg MC, Chang RW, Dwosh I et al: The American College of Rheumatology 1991 revised criteria for the classification of global functional status in rheumatoid arthritis, *Arthritis Rheum* 35:498, 1992.
*Self-care activities include dressing, feeding, bathing, grooming, and toileting; avocational activities (recreational and/or leisure activities) and vocational activities (work, school, homemaking) are patient desired and age and gender specific.

RA may also affect children. Juvenile rheumatoid arthritis (JRA) (referred to as *juvenile idiopathic arthritis* [JIA] by the European League Against Rheumatism) is diagnosed when the onset of symptoms occurs before age 16 and the symptoms persist for at least 6 consecutive weeks. No specific diagnostic tests can be used to confirm JRA; rather, several tests can be performed to support the clinical impression of the disease. The three primary subtypes of JRA established by the American College of Rheumatology are pauciarticular JRA, polyarticular JRA, and systemic JRA. These subtypes are based on the number of joints involved, the presence or absence of systemic features and, in some cases, the age of onset.[60] Because these classifications are based on the characteristics of the disease at onset, they may not indicate its course over time.[61]

Pauciarticular JRA is defined as synovitis in four or fewer joints, usually the elbows, knees, and ankles. The arthritis, which most often is asymmetrical, presents in the absence of systemic features. In pauciarticular JRA, the rheumatoid factor usually is negative. Pauciarticular JRA has two subtypes, based on the onset of disease and the clinical presentation. Early onset pauciarticular disease often occurs in girls before the age of 5. Late onset pauciarticular disease occurs around the ages of 10 to 12 years and most often affects the large weight-bearing joints (hips and knees) and entheses (muscle insertions). Stiffness and pain are the predominant complaints.[61]

Classification of Rheumatoid Arthritis in Children

- Pauciarticular (four or fewer joints)
  - Early onset
  - Late onset
- Polyarticular (five or more joints)
- Systemic

Polyarticular JRA affects girls more often than boys. It is characterized by synovitis in five or more joints, and patients may present with systemic features of the disease. The synovitis often is symmetrical. Although polyarticular JRA may involve any joint, the cervical spine frequently is affected. It is important to note that polyarticular JRA affects normal growth and development.[61]

Systemic JRA can occur at any age and is gender neutral. It is characterized by high, spiking fevers, a classic rash (pink to salmon colored) that often occurs on the trunk and proximal extremities, and synovitis in one or more joints. The fever generally is the first symptom and may precede other symptoms by up to months. Malaise, anemia, pericarditis, thrombocytopenia, lymphadenopathy, hepatomegaly, and other systemic features evident with adult RA may be present. These children are so ill that they often present with severe functional limitations and growth retardation (below the 5th percentile).[61]

Signs, Symptoms, and Impairments

Pain, Stiffness, and Swelling

RA can cause adaptive shortening of the soft tissues, tendons, and joint capsules. Bone erosion and cartilage loss reduce joint space and may contribute to subluxation-limiting joint motion. Swelling associated with joint effusion and extra-articular edema further reduces mobility. These changes result in significant mobility impairments and pain, especially during exacerbations. Analgesic and anti-inflammatory medications are the mainstays of medical management for these patients (see volume 2 of this series, *Scientific Foundations and Principles of Practice in Musculoskeletal Rehabilitation*, Chapter 12). However, physical modalities and exercise play an important role in reducing functional loss.

Signs and Symptoms of Rheumatoid Arthritis

- Chronic inflammation
- Exacerbations and remissions
- Symmetrical, polyarticular joint involvement
- Osteoporosis
- Fatigue
- Pain
- Deformity (subluxations)
- Mobility impairment
- Muscle weakness
- Depression

Studies that Address Pain, Stiffness, and Swelling. Cold helps reduce inflammation and pain when the joints are acutely inflamed. Heat should be avoided at this time, because it may exacerbate the inflammatory process.[62] When the inflammation resolves, either heat or cold can be used to relieve pain.[63] Local heat may be preferred before gentle exercise to reduce join stiffness. In general, few studies examine the effectiveness of modalities in the management of RA. A recent Ottawa Panel[64] concluded that some (but limited) evidence supports the use of ultrasound, paraffin, transcutaneous electrical nerve stimulation (TENS), and low level laser therapy in the management of pain and flexibility. The panel's guideline further stated that evidence for including or excluding electrotherapy modalities is inconclusive at this time.

Exercise may be used to reduce joint pain and stiffness through the stimulation of endogenous opiates. Ekdahl et al.[65] studied endorphin levels in patients with RA during exercise. They showed that a rise in serum levels of these internal opiates is directly related to the intensity and frequency of active exercise. Numerous research studies have found that ROM exercises safely and efficiently maximize joint motion in patients with RA even when performed for long periods.[66-70] Patients with early or stage I disease can safely perform daily exercise, including active flexibility and ROM, doing a few repetitions at each joint. Passive stretching should be deferred until the joints are not in an active exacerbation.[8]

Muscle Weakness

Muscle weakness is common with RA. Compared to age-matched healthy individuals, individuals with RA are as much as 33% to 55% weaker in knee flexion and extension.[62,71] The weakness is attributable to a number of causes, such as myositis or muscle fiber atrophy. Myositis, characterized by inflammation within the muscle itself, is not always apparent but can be assessed through muscle enzyme testing. If myositis is not present or is minimal, muscles can be exercised sufficiently so that training effects for muscle strengthening can be achieved.[72] Atrophy has been shown to occur in both type I and type II muscle

fibers and may stem either from disuse or from changes to the muscle tissue itself.[73]

Studies of Strength Training. Studies of strength training for patients with RA have focused on both effectiveness and safety.[74-76] Early studies of strength training focused on the impact of low intensity training, such as active ROM, isometric, or low load resistance exercise programs.[74] These studies incorporated exercise of varying intensity, frequency, and duration to avoid exacerbation of symptoms. More recent investigations studied moderate to high intensity strength training programs, defined as 50% or greater of maximum voluntary contraction (MVC). Considerable emphasis was placed on determining whether patients with RA could tolerate higher loads without sacrificing joint integrity. The randomized, controlled trials of exercise in patients with RA are reviewed in Table 28-6.[75-82]

Table 28-6
Randomized, Controlled Trials of Exercise in Rheumatoid Arthritis

Author	Sample	Intervention/Groups	Duration	Study Outcomes
Studies That Included Aerobic Exercise				
Ekblom et al.[113] (1975)	34 Patients with nonactive disease, class II, III	1. General rehabilitation (3 times/day) and ROM 2. Strength training and aerobic bicycle ergometry, 5 days/week, 20 to 40 minutes/day	6 Weeks	Trained group showed significant improvement in muscle strength and aerobic capacity measures, such as VO_2 max, decreased perceived exertion, and stair climbing. Control group showed no changes. Joint status was unchanged with exercise
Ekblom et al.[67] (1975)	30 Patients with nonactive disease, class II, III	1. 6-Month follow-up on patients enrolled in study by Ekblom et al. above	6 Weeks	6 Patients who exercised 4 times/week or more demonstrated sustained benefits
Harkcom et al.[84] (1985)	20 Patients with nonactive disease, class II	1. Low intensity biking, 3 times/week at 50 rpm for 15 minutes 2. Low intensity biking for 25 minutes 3. Low intensity biking for 35 minutes 4. Control	12 Weeks	All exercisers improved aerobic capacity (VO_2 max) and exercise duration. Only the group that exercised for 35 minutes showed differences in aerobic capacity. Exercise tolerated by subjects in all exercise groups
Minor et al.[24] (1989)	40 Patients with variable disease activity	1. Aerobic walking 2. Aqua aerobics 3. ROM exercise all groups; weekly aerobic exercise at 60% to 80% max HR, 3 times/week for 1 hour	12 Weeks	Significant improvement was seen in aerobic capacity, 15.2 m (50 feet) walk time, and daily physical activity in aerobic groups versus ROM group. No difference was seen between groups with regard to morning stiffness, flexibility, clinically active joints, or grip strength

Table 28-6
Randomized, Controlled Trials of Exercise in Rheumatoid Arthritis—Cont'd

Author	Sample	Intervention/Groups	Duration	Study Outcomes
Baslund et al.[114] (1993)	18 Patients with moderate disease activity	1. Progressive biking, 4 to 5 times/week at 80% VO_2 max for 35 minutes	8 Weeks	VO_2 max uptake increased 18% in the trained versus the control groups HR at stage 2 and BORG decreased No change seen in immune response
Hansen et al.[115] (1993)	75 Patients with mixed disease activity, class I, II	1. Individualized general exercise, 15 minutes, plus aerobic exercise, 2 to 3 times/week for 30 minutes 2. Group exercise SE plus weekly group 3. PT exercisers 4. No exercise	2 Years	No effect was seen on stiffness, pain scores, number of swollen joints, or functional scores; muscle strength improved in all groups, but no change was seen in aerobic fitness 50% Attendance in program was achieved by half of participants 25% Reported wanting to do more intense program
Van den Ende et al.[70] (1996)	100 Patients with stable disease	1. High intensity group: Walking/biking at 70% to 85% maximum HR plus strengthening exercise, 3 times/week for 1 hour 2. Low intensity group: ROM and isometrics, 2 times/week for 1 hour 3. Low intensity individual program: 2 times/week 4. Low intensity home program: 2 times/week	12 Weeks	High intensity group improved the most compared to other exercisers in aerobic capacity, muscle strength, and joint mobility significantly No differences were seen in deterioration of disease activity Follow-up at 12 weeks after program ended showed loss of aerobic capacity gains in high intensity group with no exercise
Hall et al.[86] (1996)		1. Hydrotherapy, 2 times/week for 30 minutes 2. Land exercises, 2 times/week for 30 minutes 3. Relaxation training	4 Weeks	All groups reported improved mood Hydrotherapy group had 27% less joint tenderness than other groups and increased knee ROM by 6.6° Changes in mood for hydrotherapy group remained at follow-up
van den Ende et al.[85] (2000)	64 Patients with active RA, no TKR, mean disease of 8 years, in hospital for care	1. Intensive exercise biking, 3 times/week, resistance exercise at 70% MVC 2. Conservative exercises, ROM and isometric exercise	1 Month	Significant increases seen in muscle strength, as well as improvement in disease activity (swollen joints decreased at 6-month follow-up for intensive exercise group) No differences seen in pain or joint mobility between groups
Westby et al.[116] (2000)	30 Women with class I, II disease; low dose steroids	1. Weight-bearing aerobic dance and strength exercise 3 times/week for 45 to 60 minutes 2. Usual activity with written information about exercise	12 Months	8% Decrease in active joints among the exercise group compared to a 2% decrease in control group

Table 28-6
Randomized, Controlled Trials of Exercise in Rheumatoid Arthritis—Cont'd

Author	Sample	Intervention/Groups	Duration	Study Outcomes
				Exercisers had a 21% reduction in ESR values versus a 13% increase in controls. Significant changes were seen in HAQ and fitness level No change was seen in bone density
Bilberg et al.[87] (2005)	46 Patients with class I, III disease; stable medications	1. Group pool exercise, moderate intensity aerobic and strength exercise 2. Home exercise	12 Weeks	Moderate pool exercise resulted in significant improvement in muscle endurance and vitality score on SF-36 No significant difference was seen in aerobic capacity measured by submaximum cycle ergometer

Studies of Strengthening Exercises, Flexibility, and Other Interventions

Author	Sample	Intervention/Groups	Duration	Study Outcomes
Wessel and Quinney[117] (1984)	32 Patients with stable disease, class II	1. Isometric knee exercise, 3 times/week 2. Isokinetic knee exercise, 3 times/week 3. Control	7 Weeks	Pain (both VAS and modified BORG scale) was significantly higher at all tests for isometric exercises than for isokinetic exercises at 180°/sec Swelling was not detected in any group
Ekdahl et al.[65] (1990)	67 Patients with low to moderate disease activity, class II	Home exercises supervised PT visits four groups: 1. Dynamic plus 12 PT visits 2. Dynamic plus 4 PT visits 3. Static exercise plus 12 PT 4. Static plus 4 PT visits; HEP for additional 3 months	6 Weeks	Dynamic exercisers had significantly greater increases in strength, aerobic capacity, endurance, and functional ability than static exercisers; effects persisted at 3 months No joint flares occurred in either group
Brighton et al.[66] (1993)	44 Patients with class I disease	1. Hand exercises daily 2. No exercise or active disease	48 Months	Significant increases were seen in strength and pinch grip in the exercisers Deterioration was noted in controls
Hoenig et al.[118] (1993)	57 Patients with class II, III disease	All patients performed exercises 2 times/daily for 10 to 20 minutes 1. Hand ROM exercises 2. Hand resistance exercise 3. Hand ROM plus resistive exercises 4. Control	3 Months	ROM improved hand joint count Resistance and dexterity improved
Hakkinen et al.[77] (1994)	43 Patients	1. Progressive dynamic strength training, 2 to 3 times/week at 40% to 60% max RM 2. Habitual physical activity	10 Months	Exercise group significantly improved bilateral dynamic strength (32%) and unilateral strength; ESR levels and function increased Only slight changes were seen in joints

Table 28-6
Randomized, Controlled Trials of Exercise in Rheumatoid Arthritis—Cont'd

Author	Sample	Intervention/Groups	Duration	Study Outcomes
Stenstrom et al.[119] (1975)	54 Patients with class I, II disease	Two groups: 1. Dynamic exercise, 3 times/week for 30 minutes 2. Relaxation training, 3 times/week for 30 minutes	3 Months	Dynamic group showed less perceived exertion with activity and improved scores on walking tasks Relaxation group improved in health-related perception, had less joint tenderness, and better LE muscle function
Rall et al.[78] (1996)	30 Patients with controlled disease	Four groups: 1. 8 Healthy elderly adults 2. 8 Patients with RA 3. 8 Young, healthy patients who performed resistance exercises 2 to 3 times/week at 80% IRM 4. 6 Elderly adults who did warm-up swimming exercise	12 Weeks	Exercisers increased muscle strength compared to controls: RA, 57%; young exercisers, 44%; elderly exercisers, 35%; no change was seen in joint symptoms No change was seen in joint symptoms RA patients reported improvements in pain and fatigue
Komatireddy[120] (1997)	49 Patients with class II, III disease	1. Progressive resistive circuit exercises at 30% to 40% of maximum load, more than 3 times/week for 20 to 30 minutes, plus video 2. No exercise	12 Weeks	Exercisers had significant improvements in self-reported joint counts and number of painful joints, knee extension HAW scores, and sit to stand time No significant changes were seen in VO$_2$ max or treadmill time
Stenstrom et al.[121] (1997)	54 Patients with class I, II disease	Two groups: 1. Dynamic training 2. Relaxation exercises for 30 minutes 5 times/week for 3 months then 2 to 3 times/week for 9 months (total time is 1 year)	12 Months	Improved physical and work impact was seen among dynamic exercisers, as measured by AIMS2 Relaxation group reported less pain, emotion reaction No significant differences were seen in health status or joint tenderness between the groups Compliance was about 65% for both groups over 1 year
Bostrom et al.[122] (1998)	45 Patients with mild RA	1. Progressive dynamic shoulder exercises at 30% maximum load, 3 times/week for 40 to 60 minutes 2. Static shoulder exercises	10 Weeks	Both groups reported fewer UE swollen joints and less shoulder-arm pain Dynamic exercisers showed improvements in physical and overall dimensions in the Sickness Impact Profile
McMeeken et al.[83] (1999)	36 Patients with nonacute RA	1. Knee extensor and flexor strengthening at 70% max RM, 2 to 3 times/week for 45 minutes 2. Attention control	6 Weeks	Exercisers reported significantly less pain and had improved knee extension/flexion strength and improved function as measured by HAQ and increased TUG time

Table 28-6
Randomized, Controlled Trials of Exercise in Rheumatoid Arthritis—Cont'd

Author	Sample	Intervention/Groups	Duration	Study Outcomes
Hakkinen et al.[123] (1999)	67 Patients with recent onset disease (<2 years)	1. Dynamic whole body exercises at 50% to 60% maximum load, 2 times/week for 45 minutes 2. ROM exercises 2 times/week and normal recreational activities	12 Months	Significant strength increases (22% to 35%) were seen in the dynamic group versus 3% to 24% in the ROM group No significant changes were seen in BMD
Hakkinen et al.[79] (2001)	70 Patients with recent onset disease (<2 years)	1. Dynamic whole body strengthening at 50% to 70% max RM, 2 times/week for 45 minutes 2. 2 times/week for 24 months; all patients were encouraged to participate in recreational activities 2 times/week	24 Months	62 Patients completed the study. Muscle strength disease activity (HAQ) and function improved in both groups, but greater improvements were seen in those who did dynamic exercises (19% to 59% increase in muscle strength) ROM group showed decreased BMD, whereas dynamic exercisers showed slight improvements in BMD femoral neck ($0.51 \pm 1.64\%$) and spine ($1.17 \pm 5.34\%$)
DeJong et al.[75] (2003)	309 Patients with class I-III disease	1. High intensity bicycle, circuit exercises, sports 2. Usual care	2 Years	Significant improvements were seen in aerobic fitness, muscle endurance, and self-reported improved function (MACTAR); no significant effect was seen on the small joints of the hands and feet No mean radiological changes were seen in the large joints except in those with baseline moderate changes
Hakkinen et al.[81] (2004)	70 Patients with recent onset disease (<2 years)	5-Year follow-up study of above groups	24 Months, monitored by researchers; 36 months, self-monitored	59/62 Subjects were re-evaluated at 5 years Gains in muscle strength in exercisers were maintained with self-monitored exercise BMD values remained unchanged from 2-year status Few joint changes were seen
DeJong et al.[88] (2004)	309 Patients with stable disease, class I-III	1. High intensity weight-bearing exercise 2. Usual care	2 Years	Exercise groups showed significant improvement in aerobic fitness and a decrease in radiological joint changes in the feet Increase in BMD of the hips was seen in the weight-bearing group

IRM, Illness Representation Model; *AIMS2,* Arthritis Impact Measurement Scale 2; *BMD,* bone mineral density; *BORG,* Borg scale of perceived exertion; *ESR,* erythrocyte sedimentation rate; *HAQ,* Health Assessment Questionnaire; *HEP,* home exercise program; *HR,* heart rate; *LE,* lower extremity; *MACTAR,* McMaster Toronto Arthritis Patient Preference Questionnaire; *max RM,* repetition maximum; *MVC,* maximum voluntary contraction; *PT,* physical therapist; *RA,* rheumatoid arthritis; *rpm,* revolutions/minute; *SE,* standard exercise; *SF-36,* McGill Pain Questionnaire and Short Form SF-36; *TKR,* total knee replacement; *TUG,* timed up and go test; *UE,* upper extremity; *VAS,* Visual Analogue Scale; *VO₂ max,* maximum amount of oxygen in milliliters.

In the aggregate, studies show that both static and dynamic strengthening programs improve strength and function in patients with RA in the range of 15% to 50%. Most of the studies included exercise at a frequency of 2 to 3 times a week. Studies of low to moderate intensity (25% to 50% MVC) demonstrated improvements in strength of approximately 15% to 30%; those of higher intensity showed greater gains. For example, McMeekan et al.[83] assigned 36 patients with nonactive RA either to a control group or to a group that performed knee flexor/extensor strengthening exercises at 70% MVC for 45 minutes, 2 to 3 times a week, for 6 weeks. At the 6-week follow-up, patients in the exercise group were able to generate significantly greater isokinetic torque than the control group. In addition, the exercise group reported less pain and greater function and mobility on a Health Assessment Questionnaire (HAQ).

Hakkinen et al.[80] compared the effect of a home strength training program performed at 50% to 70% maximal repetitions for upper extremity (UE) and lower extremity (LE) muscle groups with a home program of ROM exercises; both groups exercised twice weekly. Both groups also performed an aerobic exercise program 3 times a week. Variables studied included knee extension and hand grip strength, bone mineral density (BMD) of the femoral neck and lumbar spine, and radiographic joint changes. At the 2-year point, 62 patients completed the program. The exercise group showed a significant difference in maximum strength on a dynamometer and little joint damage. BMD showed little or no change. The subjects continued the exercise program on a self-monitored basis for 3 years. At the end of 3 years (5 years total of exercise), 59 of the original 62 patients were evaluated again. Strength gains were maintained for the resistance-trained groups through the subsequent 3-year self-monitored phase. BMD was unchanged, and radiographic evidence of joint damage continued to be low.

Fatigue and Endurance

Studies demonstrate that patients with RA have decreased aerobic capacity compared to healthy subjects. This is the result of deconditioning secondary to inactivity and pain, as well as the direct effects of the disease on the cardiovascular or pulmonary systems. However, with short-term conditioning programs, physical function can increase and cardiovascular fitness can be improved by 20%, as measured by VO_2 max.[67,70] The greatest improvements in aerobic capacity are gained with exercise regimens at 50% to 80% of VO_2 max.[8]

Aerobic exercise programs for patients with RA should be designed to accommodate the patient's functional limitations and degree of joint involvement. Non-impact-loading forms of land exercise, such as walking or cycling, should be considered to reduce stress to joints. Swimming and other aquatic exercise regimens have the advantage of using the buoyancy of water to reduce load. The recommended water temperature for patients with arthritis is 37° to 40°C (98.6° to 104°F), warm enough to help control pain and reduce muscle tension and joint stiffness.[72]

Studies of Aerobic Exercise. Initial studies of aerobic exercise enrolled patients with nonactive disease and used bicycle ergometry as the mode of exercise. In the earlier trials, exercise prescriptions were maintained at a relatively low intensity. Harkcom et al.[84] examined the impact of short burst (e.g., 15, 25, or 35 minutes), low intensity aerobic conditioning over 12 weeks. Only subjects assigned to the 35-minute low-intensity conditioning program demonstrated statistically significant improvements in aerobic capacity (6.9 mL/kg/minute, on average). Improvements among exercisers in the 25- and 15-minute programs were not statistically significant. All exercisers reported significant decreases in joint pain and swelling compared to nonexercising controls (p <0.01).

Van Ende et al.[85] studied 100 patients with RA in a 12-week program of high intensity exercise versus ROM and isometric exercises. The high intensity program included weight-bearing exercises and bicycling at 70% to 85% of the patient's age-predicted maximum heart rate. The low intensity groups did ROM and static strengthening exercises for the trunk and lower extremity; or an individual low intensity ROM and static exercise program, with instruction from a physical therapist; or a written home program of ROM and static exercises. At the end of 12 weeks, those exercising at the higher intensities showed significant improvement in aerobic capacity and knee muscle strength and mobility. An important find was that no exacerbation of joint symptoms was seen in any group, and joint symptoms actually decreased among the high intensity exercisers. Muscle strength gains were maintained, but aerobic gains were lost at a follow-up 12 weeks after the program ended.

Research on alternative forms of aerobic exercise, such as aquatic programs, has shown mixed results. Minor et al.[24] conducted a study of aerobic walking and aquatic programs that demonstrated improvements in both aerobic capacity and emotional satisfaction. Hall et al.[86] evaluated the effect of 4 weeks of seated immersion hydrotherapy versus land exercises or relaxation training. Each group met twice a week for 30 minutes. Subjects in the hydrotherapy group reported 27% less joint tenderness and an improvement in total combined knee motion.

In a more recent study, Bilberg et al.[87] assigned 46 subjects with class I to class III RA to either a treatment group, which participated in supervised aquatic therapy 2 times a week for 12 weeks, or to a control group, which continued with their regular activities. These authors found no significant aerobic effect from water exercise, as measured by cycle ergometry. However, they did report improved muscle endurance for both UE and LE muscle groups, as measured by isometric grip strength and a functional chair rise test.

Articular Changes

The effect of moderate to high intensity exercise on joint integrity has been a major focus of recent research. De Jong et al.[75,76,82,88] reported on a series of recent studies in which patients with stable class I to class III RA who participated in these higher levels of exercise were monitored over 2 years. In one study, 309 patients with stable RA who were enrolled in the Rheumatoid Arthritis Patients in Training (RAPIT) program were randomly assigned either to a usual care group or to an intensive supervised exercise group. The exercise group met for 75 minutes, 2 times a week, for 2 years. The exercise program was threefold: bicycle aerobic training for 20 minutes, a 20-minute exercise circuit consisting of 8 to 10 exercises, and a sport or game for 20 minutes. The exercise session also included warm-up and cool-down periods. Impact loading for joints included jumping during the warm-up and the selection of sports such as basketball, volleyball, indoor soccer, and badminton; 281 subjects finished the study.

The researchers assessed the effect of high intensity impact–generating exercise on the small joints of the feet and hands of 136 participants; 145 subjects had usual care. After 2 years, these researchers found that, not only did the rate of joint changes for the small joints not increase, but that the exercisers' feet showed less progression. In the larger weight-bearing joints (i.e., the knee and hip), the mean radiographic change was not significant for the whole group. However, participants who began the study with more radiological evidence of changes in the larger weight-bearing joints did show a progression of changes.[75,82] The researchers also reported improved aerobic capacity for the exercise group.

These studies suggest caution in prescribing exercise to patients who already have significant joint damage, especially in the large weight-bearing joints; however, they also support the use of such exercise in the small joints of the hands and feet.[76]

Basic Principles of Rehabilitation and Studies on the Effects of Exercise in Patients with Rheumatoid Arthritis

The goals of rehabilitation in the management of RA are to maximize strength, flexibility, endurance, and mobility and to promote independence while minimizing the potential for further joint destruction and deformity. A well-designed intervention program incorporates information about the extent of the joint impairments, as well as the patient's stage of disease, motivation, and adherence to therapy.[8] It is important to consider the patient's psychological state and motivation for rehabilitation. Depression and reduced self-efficacy are common in a chronic disease such as RA.[89,90] Interventions used in the management of RA include various forms of exercise, orthoses, adapted ambulatory aids, modalities, and patient education in energy conservation techniques.

Physical activity levels are low in patients with RA. A recent study on physical fitness and health perceptions of individuals with RA indicated that 47% of 298 participants reported low to fair levels of activity on a regular basis.[91] Patients with a chronic disease such as RA have to incorporate exercise and rehabilitation techniques into their daily lives; this makes adherence more difficult. In a recent trial by Munneke et al.[92] that examined exercise adherence in 146 patients with RA, 81% of the participants were still engaged in the supervised exercise program after 2 years. Patients with high disease activity and low functional ability at baseline were slightly more likely to drop out of the trial. However, strategies can be used to enhance adherence. Iversen et al.[93] found that a positive social support system can improve the adherence rate by 300%. It also is important to recognize the impact of the clinicians' own beliefs and expectations on the patient's adherence to therapy. Provider expectations and beliefs about various modes of exercise have been shown to affect patient adherence to exercise prescriptions.[94,95]

Rehabilitation Goals for Rheumatoid Arthritis

- Maximize strength
- Maximize flexibility and mobility
- Maximize endurance
- Promote independence
- Minimize deformity and joint destruction

Summary of Exercise Recommendations for the Patient with Rheumatoid Arthritis

Exercise should be considered an important, lifelong component of the management of rheumatoid arthritis. It has been shown to improve mobility, strength, endurance, function for daily tasks, and mood in patients with RA. Table 28-7 summarizes the exercise recommendations at various levels of disease presentation for RA. Daily ROM exercises should be performed on affected joints to maintain mobility and prevent contractures. During an exacerbation, 2 to 3 repetitions of active range of motion (AROM) exercises can be performed without unduly stressing the joints. Byers[96] recommends that patients exercise in the evening to help reduce the morning stiffness associated with RA. When the disease is in remission, ROM exercises can be increased to 8 to 10 repetitions a day for each involved joint.

Strengthening programs can incorporate isometric or active exercises with resistance when the patient is not experiencing an active flare-up (also called a *flare*), or exacerbation. Isometric exercise generally results in less inflammation, less of an increase in intra-articular pressure, and less shear.[62,97] The clinician must keep in mind, however, that sustained exercises of large muscle groups may put an increased load on the cardiovascular system and may be contraindicated in patients with RA who have cardiac problems.

Clearly, aerobic exercise programs, including those with weight-bearing components, appear to be better tolerated

Table 28-7

Summary of Rehabilitation Interventions for Rheumatoid Arthritis

Form of Rheumatoid Arthritis	Recommendations
Acute flare (hot joint)	AROM exercises for involved joints, 2 repetitions/joint/day Resting orthoses and assistive devices with built-up handles or platform attachments
Subacute	AROM exercises, 8 to 10 repetitions/joint/day Static exercises, 4 to 6 contractions lasting 6 seconds each Isotonic exercises with light resistance (avoid if joints are unstable or with tense popliteal cysts or internal joint derangement) Aerobic training, 15 to 20 minutes, 3 times/week. Cardiac evaluation is recommended for men over age 35 and women over age 45. Establish heart rate parameters and use perceived rating of exertion scale (e.g., Borg scale of perceived exertion)
Stable or inactive	AROM and flexibility exercises Static and dynamic strength training (avoid dynamic exercises if joints are unstable or with tense popliteal cysts) Aerobic training, 15 to 20 minutes, 3 times/week. Cardiac evaluation is recommended for men over age 35 and women over age 45. Establish heart rate parameters and use perceived rating of exertion scale Orthoses: Lower extremity—accommodative or custom foot orthoses in extra depth shoes or moldable shoes; upper extremity—consider working wrist/hand support

Modified from Iversen MD, Liang MH, Bae SC: Exercise therapy in selected arthritides: rheumatoid arthritis, osteoarthritis, systemic lupus erythematosus, systemic sclerosis and polymyositis/dermatomyositis. In Frontera WR, Dawson DM, Slovik DM, editors: *Exercise in rehabilitation medicine*, Champaign, IL, 1999, Human Kinetics.
AROM, Active range of motion.

than previously thought, at least in patients with stable disease (i.e., disease that is not in a period of active flare-up). The effect of more intensive exercise on patients with a more aggressive disease process is not yet clear, but the most recent studies recommend caution with high intensity or impact loading on the larger weight-bearing joints if the patient shows significant radiological joint changes. In addition to other signs of inflammation, pain should be a guide to determining the appropriate intensity of the program. Acute pain during exercise indicates a need to modify the program; vague, diffuse pain that resolves in less than 2 hours does not indicate a need for program modification.[63] Patients must recognize the signs of an acute flare (i.e., redness, inflammation, pain, and stiffness) and reduce the frequency and intensity of exercise. Exercise prescriptions should include the intensity, frequency, and duration at which each exercise should be performed and take into account the current stage of the disease.

Orthoses for Rheumatoid Arthritis

Orthoses, splints, and special shoes often are recommended, with the stated goals of relieving pain, reducing edema, providing increased joint stability, and thereby improving overall function. The most commonly prescribed devices are wrist and hand splints, extra depth shoes, and custom or prefabricated insole or foot orthoses.

Wrist and hand splints are categorized as resting splints and working splints (those designed to be worn for functional activities). Such splints can be custom-made for the individual or purchased over the counter. Janssen et al.[98]

evaluated the effect of using a resting splint on pain, grip strength, and swollen joints and found no difference between use and nonuse. Similarly, Kjeken et al.[99] found no differences in pain, stiffness, grip strength or self-reported quality of life between patients who used a working splint and those who did not. However, they did find evidence of some loss of motion while the splint was worn for work tasks. Stern et al.,[100] on the other hand, evaluated three common commercial elastic working splints and found no difference in dexterity with or without the splints in any of the ones used. Egan et al.,[101] in a recent Cochrane review, concluded that, since working wrist splints do not appear to be detrimental in terms of motion, they might be useful for a degree of pain relief in some patients. They further concluded that the evidence currently is insufficient to support the use of resting splints, although they acknowledged that some patients report a preference for wearing them for comfort reasons during acute exacerbations.

In the foot, a loss of plantar fat and muscle atrophy of interossei often are seen. Along with subluxation of tendons, these can led to deformities, especially of the forefoot, such as hammer toes and metatarsal subluxation.[102] Loss of support for the medial arch from overstretching of repetitively inflamed soft tissues may lead to significant overpronation. Extra depth shoes and shoes made of heat-moldable material are commonly prescribed footwear.[103] The extra depth shoe has an additional 0.64 to 0.95 cm (0.25 to 0.38 inch) of volume to accommodate any foot deformities and to allow use of an insert or foot orthosis (Figure 28-9). Inserts in the

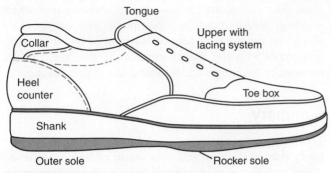

Figure 28-9
Extra depth foot segments and shoe design. (From the Association of Rheumatology Health Professionals: *Clinical care in the rheumatic diseases,* ed 3, p 268, Atlanta, 2007, The Association.)

form of both accommodative and custom posting often are prescribed. In one study, patients who wore extra depth shoes with a semirigid orthotic for 12 weeks reported less pain than when they wore just an extra depth shoe.[104] Soft inserts were not found to provide any further pain relief over just wearing the extra depth shoe alone. However, in another study, use of a functionally posted, semirigid foot orthosis alone did not appear to make a difference in pain or disability measures compared to a placebo insert.[105]

Ambulatory Aids and Adaptive Equipment

Many patients with RA have significant upper extremity joint dysfunction, especially of the hands and wrists, that makes use of a cane, crutch, or walker difficult or painful. An adaptation that can help is the use of platform attachments that distribute weight-bearing forces over the forearm. Devices with wider, flatter handgrips often are more comfortable than the standard grip. Cone-type handgrips are designed so that the ulnar side of the hand is on the wider part of the cone; this improves grip strength and resists the tendency for ulnar drift or deviation. A low cost alternative is to build up the handgrip of ambulatory aids or utensils and writing implements with moldable foam; this helps prevent compression on vulnerable joints while improving the ability to grip.

Energy Conservation Techniques

Because RA is a systemic disease, patients can easily become fatigued. Although all patients should be encouraged to participate in exercise programs as appropriate, educating patients in strategies for conserving energy while performing routine ADLs is equally important.[106] This becomes imperative during periods of exacerbation.

Energy Conservation Strategies[104]

- Schedule activities so that demanding physical tasks are alternated with less strenuous ones
- Sit to perform tasks when possible
- Gather all necessary supplies before a task
- Limit trips, especially up and down stairs
- Schedule adequate rest periods

In addition, patients should be taught to avoid positions and activities that perpetuate joint deformity. Squeezing a ball for hand exercise should be avoided, because it may contribute to subluxation at the MCP and interphalangeal (IP) joints as a result of excessive force on the ulnar side of the joints. Prolonged flexed positions of the hands and other extremity joints may shorten soft tissue and contribute to contractures.

Suggestions for Patient Education

- Provide simple, clear instructions
- Link the exercise or modality to a clear outcome and explain its use
- Provide patients with key symptoms they need to recognize that indicate a flare and the need for exercise modification
- Provide guidelines for modifying an exercise
- Encourage social support for exercise
- Ask patients to explain their expectations and attitudes toward exercise to help determine their willingness to exercise and perceived barriers to exercise

---

Case Study in Rheumatoid Arthritis

Holly is a 38-year-old female who presents with 5 months of bilateral knee, wrist, and hand pain. Upon examination, she exhibits pain (Visual Analogue Scale [VAS] score, 6/10) and 2+ swelling in the PIP joints, MCP joints, and wrist, with limited ROM. Several PIP joints exhibit 15° hypertension, and subcutaneous nodules are evident on the right fourth and fifth PIP joints. Slight ulnar deviation of the MCP joints is seen, left greater than right. Her knees are warm, painful, and swollen, and these symptoms are greater on the left than the right. The patella ballottement test is positive bilaterally. She has restricted ROM in her left knee of 10°. Both feet show hallux valgus and hammer toe deformities. The stiffness and swelling in her fingers, wrists, feet, and knees are worse in the morning, lasting up to 3 hours. By late afternoon, her hands, wrists, feet, and knees are aching, and she states that aspirin does not alleviate her pain. She is having difficulty performing her job as a university professor. Her typing is labored, and she has trouble demonstrating manual skills that require hand dexterity; she also has trouble with prolonged standing while conducting her laboratory courses. She saw her rheumatologist, who prescribed prednisone (10 mg), methotrexate, folic acid, and a multivitamin and referred her to physical therapy.

Case Discussion

This patient is in a flare. The prescribed medical therapy—a fast-acting pharmaceutical agent (prednisone) combined with a slow-acting disease-modifying drug (methotrexate)—hopefully will bring the disease under control. Her rehabilitation program should include gentle ROM exercises for the whole body, with special emphasis on her wrist, hands, fingers, knees, and feet. The synovitis evident in her hands and knees can lead to stretching of the joint capsule and ligaments. With synovitis, biomechanical forces across the joint are increased, and ligaments and tendons can become involved, leading to joint instability. Common changes evident in the hands (the joints commonly involved first) are radial deviation of the wrist, subluxation of the proximal carpal row, and radial rotation of the distal carpal bones. Therefore it is important to check for volar drop of the MCP joints by palpating the heads of these joints in relation to the extended first phalanx. Although flexed posturing generally is more comfortable, flexion can lead to intrinsic tightness. Resting splints for evening and dynamic splints may help maintain alignment during physical activities. Resistive dynamic exercises should be avoided with synovitis. In the hand, forceful squeezing results in joint deformities and may result in pathomechanical changes. ROM and isometric exercises are preferred, along with the use of ice to reduce swelling. A can of food or a cylinder can be used to perform isometric grasping and is preferred to ball squeezing, which can lead to ulnar drift.

Proper footwear that provides adequate support and allows accommodation of her foot deformities should be recommended. An extra depth shoe allows for use of a soft insole with enough room to accommodate the foot deformities. An ergonomic evaluation of her work space and home environment should be done so that recommendations can be made for individualized energy conserving techniques. She may benefit from an ergonomically designed computer keyboard and/or mouse that minimizes

ulnar drift and allows an easier grasp. Because prolonged standing is fatiguing, an appropriate supportive chair should be sought. Frequent monitoring of blood pressure is required with the use of steroids, because these drugs can lead to weight gain and subsequent hypertension.

Summary

This chapter discussed the roles of exercise therapy, ambulatory aids, modalities, and orthoses in addressing osteoarthritis and rheumatoid arthritis. The evidence supporting the use of various types of exercise, the strengths and limitations of these studies, and new recommendations were presented. The importance of prescribing the correct frequency, duration, intensity, and type of exercise for the various stages of disease was highlighted, as was the current data on the use of orthoses and appropriately adapted aids and assistive devices. Suggestions were presented for important patient educational material that can be included in the intervention plan.

References

To enhance this text and add value for the reader, all references have been incorporated into a CD-ROM that is provided with this text. The reader can view the reference source and access it online whenever possible. There are a total of 123 references for this chapter.

CHAPTER 29

SYSTEMIC BONE DISEASES: MEDICAL AND REHABILITATION INTERVENTION

PART A   MEDICAL INTERVENTION

James W. Edmondson and Emily Veeneman

PART B   REHABILITATION INTERVENTION

Jennifer L. Baird

PART A
Introduction

The human skeleton plays significant roles in ambulation, protection of vital soft tissues, and calcium ion and other mineral homeostasis. Disease may compromise one or more of these skeletal functions. *Systemic bone disease* is the term used to describe a heterogeneous group of skeletal disorders that involve global parts of the skeleton. It follows from this description that localized skeletal disease, such as osteomyelitis, is not considered systemic bone disease.

Among the systemic bone diseases, some disorders may compromise ambulatory and protective functions, whereas others may interfere with homeostatic function, producing either increments or decrements in mineral ion flux through tissues and blood.

This chapter addresses three common systemic bone diseases: osteoporosis, primary hyperparathyroidism, and Paget's disease of bone. Other, less prevalent diseases are described elsewhere.[1]

Common Systemic Bone Diseases

- Osteoporosis
- Primary hyperparathyroidism
- Paget's disease

Osteoporosis

The term *osteoporosis* literally means "soft bones." As the name implies, the most important sequela of osteoporosis is loss of structural integrity (i.e., fracture). Individual bodies vary in the amount of bone they have, a fact that has been recognized for at least 2500 years. In 440 BC, Herodotus noted:

> On the field where this battle was fought, I saw a very wonderful thing which the natives pointed out to me. The bones of the slain lie scattered upon the field in two lots, those of the Persians in one place by themselves, as the bodies lay at the first, those of the Egyptians in another place apart from them. If, then, you strike the Persian skulls, even with a pebble, they are so weak, that you break a hole in them; but the Egyptian skulls are so strong, that you may smite them with a stone and you will scarcely break them in. They gave me the following reason for this difference, which seemed to me likely enough: The Egyptians (they said) from early childhood have the head shaved, and so by the action of the sun the skull becomes thick and hard. The same cause prevents baldness in Egypt, where you see fewer bald men than in any other land. Such, then, is the reason why the skulls of the Egyptians are so strong. The Persians, on the other hand, have feeble skulls, because they keep themselves shaded from the first, wearing turbans upon their heads. What I have here mentioned I saw with my own eyes, and I observed also the like at Papremis, in the case of the Persians who were killed with Achaemenes, the son of Darius, by Inarus the Libyan.[2]

Although the causative speculations of Herodotus are not supported by contemporary understanding of the pathophysiology of osteoporosis, he did make noteworthy observations about skeletal frailty and racial variations in bone strength. Today, osteoporosis affects the lives of nearly 45 million in the United States; 10 million Americans already have osteoporosis and another

34 million have low bone mass or osteopenia.[3] It is important to understand that with osteoporosis, the quality or makeup of the bone is normal, but the amount is reduced. That is, the total bone mass per unit volume of bone is decreased, but no changes occur in chemical composition (i.e., the calcium/protein ratio is normal). Osteoporosis is a silent, progressive disease that has a long latency period before clinical symptoms develop. Cancellous or trabecular bone is primarily affected because it is the metabolically more active.

Osteoporosis can be categorized as primary osteoporosis (type I is postmenopausal osteoporosis, and type II is age related, or senile type, osteoporosis) and secondary osteoporosis, which occurs as a result of other conditions.

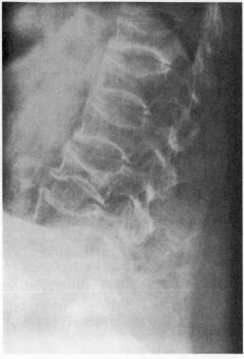

Figure 29-1
Lateral radiograph of the lumbar spine showing the biconcave appearance and compression of vertebral bodies seen in senile osteoporosis. (From Gartland JJ: *Fundamentals of orthopedics,* p 120, Philadelphia, 1979, WB Saunders.)

Common Causes of Secondary Osteoporosis

- Endocrine disorders
- Decreased physical activity
- Drugs (e.g., steroids, immunosuppressives, heparin)
- Reflex sympathetic dystrophy
- Inherited disorders (e.g., osteogenesis imperfecta)
- Malignancy
- Female athlete triad (eating disorder, amenorrhea, osteoporosis)

The most common morbid event in osteoporosis is fracture, and the most common sites of osteoporotic fractures are the spine, wrist, and hip (Figure 29-1).[4]

The two circumstances that are the immediate precursors of fracture are low bone density and increased frequency of falling.[5] Understandably, then, much of the clinical interest in osteoporosis has been directed toward understanding the determinants of bone density and falling. In boys and girls, bone mass steadily increases from birth and reaches its peak early in the 3rd decade of life.[6] When disease or malnutrition does not intervene, peak bone mass is set by gender, race, and heredity. Those fortunate enough to inherit a high peak bone mass are less likely to sustain fractures unless they take medications or are affected by other illnesses that rob the skeleton of minerals, leading to unanticipated fracture. Common diseases and conditions that result in osteoporosis include illnesses for which steroid therapy is part of the treatment (e.g., rheumatoid arthritis), premature menopause, hyperthyroidism, hyperparathyroidism, and organ transplantation.[7] Illnesses that lead to an increased frequency of falling, including Parkinson's disease, multiple sclerosis, and vitamin D deficiency, also raise fracture rates.[8-10]

Risk Factors in the Development of Osteoporosis

- Inactive lifestyle
- Early or surgically induced menopause
- Low dietary calcium intake
- Steroid medication
- Low weight, small build
- Caucasian
- Family history
- Scoliosis
- Northwestern European background
- Blonde or red hair
- Easily bruised
- Freckles
- Hypermobility
- Poor teeth

From Lane JM, Vigorita VJ: Osteoporosis, *Orthop Clin North Am* 15:716, 1984.

Bone Densitometry

Methodology

X-rays penetrate tissues with remarkable ease. This fundamental physical property underlies the utility of x-rays in both radiographic imaging and bone densitometry. The skeleton is a tissue

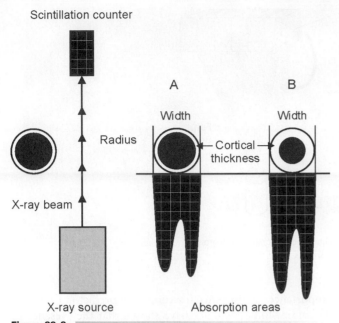

Figure 29-2

Bone densitometry: Photon absorptiometry of the radius.
In **A**, cortical thickness is smaller than in **B**; therefore,
the absorption area is smaller than that in **B**.

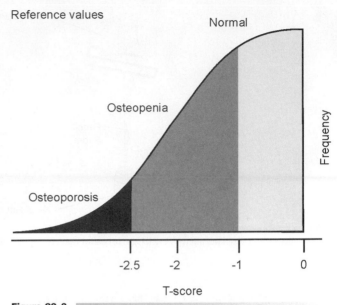

Figure 29-3

World Health Organization's definitions of bone density classification.

that partly prevents x-ray penetration, and the degree of absorption is directly related to the amount of mineral present.[11]

In Figure 29-2, the radius is seen to pass through a collimated x-ray beam. As the radius completes its passage through an x-ray beam, a characteristic w-shaped absorption curve is described. The width of the absorption curve is equal to the width of the radius, and the area of the absorption curve is directly related to the mineral content of the skeleton through which the beam passes. In Panel A, cortical thickness is smaller than in Panel B; therefore, the absorption area is smaller than that in Panel B. In single and dual energy absorptiometry scanning, cortical thickness is calculated as bone mineral content divided by area scanned; it is an area rather than a volumetric measurement.[12]

In 1994 the World Health Organization (WHO) expert panel refined the diagnostic criterion for osteoporosis. It now is based on bone density, and a previous fracture is no longer required (Figure 29-3).[13]

Although the WHO criterion has been the subject of considerable controversy, a quantifiable diagnostic criterion for osteoporosis has led to enhanced recognition of the importance of the disease, and as a result, many patients have received fracture-sparing therapy in cases in which previously no treatment would have been offered. The emergence of new, effective treatments for osteoporosis also has contributed greatly to awareness of the disease in the general population. Unfortunately, many still erroneously consider osteoporosis a disease of elderly women.[14]

Bone densitometry began as a research tool that was able to measure only the bone density of the forearm. Now, with a variety of radiological and ultrasound techniques, routine measurement of skeletal density is possible at multiple skeletal sites, including the spine, hip, total body, forearm, finger, and heel. Of the currently available methodologies, dual energy x-ray absorptiometry (DEXA) (Figure 29-4) of the central skeleton (spine and hip) has become the apparent gold standard because of its widespread availability in clinical practice, the prevalence of its use in osteoporotic fracture therapy trials, its relatively high precision, and the comparatively low radiation exposure needed to complete a scan.[15]

Kanis and Johnell[16] estimated that to undertake widespread screening of all at-risk individuals, approximately 11 densitometry units per 1 million population in Europe would be needed. The United States currently has almost 36 units per 1 million population, even though bone densitometry is performed on only about 25% of the at-risk population. Identifying patients with osteoporosis is now the most important goal for preserving and maintaining skeletal health in this country.[16]

Recognition of the importance of osteoporosis as a public health problem has been largely driven by national and international organizations, including WHO and the National Osteoporosis Foundation, and by the pharmaceutical industry, which has developed therapies that significantly reduce the risk of osteoporotic fractures in postmenopausal women, in men with osteoporosis, and in patients receiving glucocorticoid therapy.[17-20]

Determinants of a Fracture

Bone Density

Shortly after bone densitometry was developed, it became apparent that this technique was a powerful tool for fracture prediction, and that the relative fracture risk more

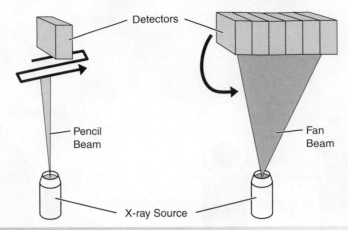

Figure 29-4

Dual energy x-ray absorptiometry (DEXA) source and detection systems. Pencil beam versus fan beam technology.

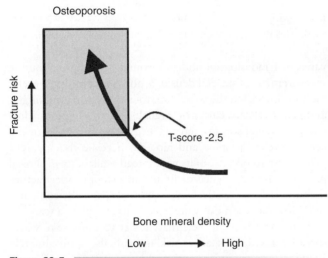

Figure 29-5

Relationship between bone density and risk of fracture.

than doubled with each standard deviation decline in bone density below the young adult mean bone density (Figure 29-5).[21]

Age

With the availability of bone density as a research tool, several researchers have shown the predictive importance of age for fractures.[22,23] De Laet et al.[22] studied the independent effects of age and bone density on the absolute risk of hip fracture (Figure 29-6). At all ages, the fracture risk rises as bone density falls. Between the ages of 50 and 80, the absolute fracture risk triples for the T score of −2.5.[22]

Previous Fracture

The important studies of Wasnich et al.[24] and Davis et al.,[25] as well as data from the placebo arms of clinical trials of osteoporotic pharmaceutical research, emphasized the

importance of previous fracture as a predictor of future fracture. Multiple studies have shown that the presence of a previous osteoporotic fracture increases the risk of a new osteoporotic fracture by at least fourfold. The work of Lindsay et al.[26] showed that the risk of a subsequent fracture is greatest for 1 year after fracture.

Smoking

The meta-analysis presented in Figure 29-7 shows the impact of smoking on the risk of hip fracture.[27] As anticipated, these data not only show the impact of age on the risk of hip fracture, but also the disproportional effect of smoking at advanced age.

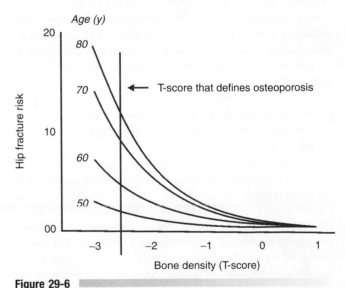

Figure 29-6

Age and bone density are independent predictors of the risk of hip fracture. (From De Laet C, Kanis JA, Oden A, Johanson H et al: Body mass index as a predictor of fracture risk: a meta-analysis, *Osteoporos Int* 16:1330-1338, 2005.)

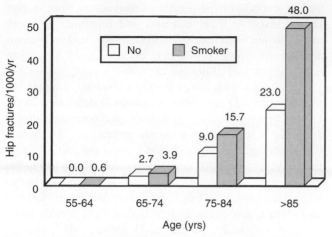

Figure 29-7

Effect of smoking on hip fractures in 11,861 subjects. (Redrawn from Law MR, Hackshaw AK: A meta-analysis of cigarette smoking, bone mineral density and risk of hip fracture: recognition of a major effect, *Br Med J* 315:841-846, 1997.)

Other Clinical Risk Factors

Cummings et al.[28] showed that among postmenopausal women, many risk attributes can be identified that raise the probability of hip fracture. Several properties, when present independently, increase the risk of a hip fracture among postmenopausal older women.

Clinical Factors that Independently Predict Hip Fractures

- Weight loss since age 25 years
- Inability to stand from seated position
- History of hyperthyroidism
- Age over 80 years
- Maternal hip fracture
- Anticonvulsant therapy
- Height at age 25 over 168 cm (5 feet, 6 inches)
- Poor depth perception
- Any prior fracture
- Caffeine (more than 2 cups a day)
- On feet less than 4 hours a day
- Fair, poor health
- Pulse over 80 beats per minute
- Long-acting benzodiazepine therapy

The value of these factors is that they can be quickly and easily assessed during a routine examination; their independent and additive nature is shown in Figure 29-8. The most useful clinical risk factors are an inability to stand without using the hands, age over 80 years, height, previous fractures, and a history of hyperthyroidism. On-line and personal data assistant (PDA) hip fracture risk calculators based on these clinical risk factors and on bone density T scores are now available.

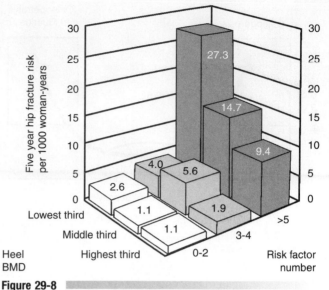

Figure 29-8

Independent and additive clinical risk factors predictive of hip fracture in older menopausal women. (Redrawn from Cummings SR, Nevitt MC, Browner WS et al: Risk factors for hip fracture in white women: Study of Osteoporotic Fractures Research Group, *N Engl J Med* 332:767, 1995.)

Bone Mineral Density and Fractures

The importance of bone mineral density (BMD) as a predictor of fracture has been well established. However, the experience gained from the use of pharmaceutical agents has identified inconsistencies in the notion that BMD is the only important skeletal property that controls fracture risk. In the initial months of treatment with most osteoporosis agents, the fracture risk declines significantly even though BMD changes minimally. Furthermore, the long-term increase in BMD attained with therapy does not account for the observed reductions in fracture risk.[29] Pharmaceutical agents are thought to modify skeletal strength by mechanisms other than their effect on bone mineral density. In some circumstances, bone mineral density increases and the fracture risk does not decline and may even increase. Examples include the genetic skeletal disorder osteopetrosis (an osteoclast-inactivating disorder and another metabolic bone disease) and during fluoride therapy.[30,31]

These observations have led to the belief that an optimum bone mineral density exists for preventing fracture. Many of the current therapy efforts have been directed toward individuals with low bone density (i.e., those with bone mineral density T scores in the osteoporotic range). However, data from the National Osteoporosis Risk Assessment (NORA) and other studies indicate that in approximately 50% of those with osteoporotic fractures (i.e., of the spine, hip, and radius), the BMD has not reached the osteoporotic range.[4] The importance of density-independent risk factors is not being widely addressed in the therapy of osteoporosis (Figure 29-9).

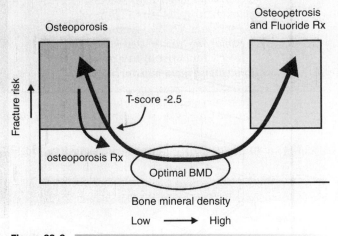

Figure 29-9
Optimum bone mineral density.

The optimum daily calcium intake for adolescents and adult women is thought to be approximately 1500 mg, plus 800 IU of vitamin D, which is needed to enhance intestinal calcium intake and skeletal mineralization. Recently, suboptimum blood levels of vitamin D have been found in many elderly patients with osteoporosis, particularly those living in northern latitudes of the United States.[32-34] The vitamin D metabolite 25-hydroxyvitamin D (25-OH D) is used as a marker of vitamin D adequacy. The optimum range is 30-50 ng/mL; vitamin D insufficiency is 10-30 ng/mL; and vitamin D deficiency is less than 10 ng/mL. The widespread prevalence of vitamin D insufficiency and deficiency has prompted one pharmaceutical company to combine vitamin D with its osteoporosis therapeutic agent.

Vitamin D Deficiency and Osteoporosis

An understanding of the importance of vitamin D in the pathophysiology of osteoporosis requires a review of the feedback loop involving parathyroid hormone (PTH), calcium, phosphorus, and vitamin D.[35] Vitamin D is obtained from two main sources, diet and the conversion of 7-dehydrocholesterol to cholecalciferol through ultraviolet sunlight through the skin. Next, the liver hydroxylates the cholecalciferol into 25-cholecalciferol, which represents the stores of vitamin D in the body. The 25-cholecalciferol is converted into the active form of vitamin D, or 1,25 vitamin D. Active vitamin D is vital to bone metabolism, calcium balance, and phosphorus homeostasis. Vitamin D increases both serum calcium and phosphorus levels through the mechanisms of principally increasing calcium absorption in the gastrointestinal tract and, to a lesser extent, enhancing intestinal phosphate reabsorption. Individuals deficient in vitamin D have hypocalcemia, hypophosphatemia, and a secondary hyperparathyroidism. A high alkaline phosphatase can be a clue to a high turnover state,

such as secondary hyperparathyroidism arising from vitamin D deficiency. As PTH increases and functions to resorb more calcium from the bone through increased osteoclastic activity, the hypocalcemia may be attenuated somewhat, resulting in a low to normal calcium.

Interference with any of the steps involved in the activation of vitamin D can result in vitamin D deficiency. In the United States and other well-developed countries, people are living longer than in previous generations. As a result, the percentage of the population comprising individuals in their 70s, 80s, and 90s is growing. This elderly group has its own subset of unique characteristics, including a higher incidence of vitamin D deficiency. For Americans, fortified milk, bread, and cereal, as well as fatty fish, provide much of the dietary source of vitamin D. Often, elderly patients ingest a diet poor in vitamin D or have malabsorption conditions, such as pancreatic insufficiency, small bowel disease (i.e., celiac sprue), or inflammatory bowel disease; or, vitamin D deficiency may be seen after gastrectomies that limit the amount of dietary vitamin D absorbed. Furthermore, a large percentage of older patients suffer from decreased mobility and spend most of their time indoors. Consequently, they have a reduced exposure to sunlight, an essential component of the ultraviolet (UV) light needed to activate vitamin D. Similar decreased sunlight intake is seen in cultures that promote the wearing of traditional clothing that covers any exposed skin. Even the location of inhabitance with relation to distance from the equator is important in the amount of exposure to UV light. Seasonal effects, such as lower levels of vitamin D in the winter months, have been described in various studies.

As people age, liver and kidney functions tend to decline, and if this effect is severe enough, problems with hydroxylation of vitamin D can occur. Medicines that increase P-450 enzymatic activity can result in the inactivation of vitamin D and reduce hepatic conversion of cholecalciferol to 25-cholecalciferol. Such drugs include the anticonvulsants carbamazepine, phenytoin, and phenobarbital; theophylline; and isoniazid. Finally, end organ resistance to vitamin D can thwart the final necessary step in the actions of vitamin D on bone and calcium homeostasis.

Vitamin D deficiency ultimately can result in myopathy, osteomalacia, and osteoporosis.[36] Studies such as the National Health and Nutrition Examination Survey (NHANES-III) have found that postmenopausal women with low levels of 25-vitamin D stores have lower DEXA scores.[34] Some controversy exists as to whether calcium supplementation independently, vitamin D supplementation independently, or supplementation of both is the ideal treatment for patients with osteoporosis. However, most clinicians agree that a daily intake of 800 IU of vitamin D and 1500 mg of elemental calcium is best. Many calcium tablets now are marketed as a combination tablet with both calcium and vitamin D. In addition, combination packages of bisphosphonate and calcium, as well as a pill containing bisphosphonate and vitamin D, are now clinically available. For patients with frank vitamin D deficiency (i.e., levels under 10 ng/mL), higher supplementation of vitamin D, on the order of 50,000 IU a week for several weeks, may be needed to replenish the vitamin D stores.

Osteoporosis Pharmacotherapy

Up until 5 years ago, all osteoporosis therapeutic agents were classified as inhibitors of bone resorption, because a primary mechanism of their efficacy was mediated through osteoclast inhibition. Anabolic agents target new bone formation by stimulating osteoblasts. Table 29-1 summarizes pertinent properties of these classes of osteoporotic agents.

Pharmacotherapy customarily is directed at men and women age 50 to 65 with an osteoporotic BMD (i.e., a T score of −2.5 or lower); older men and women (age 65 or older) with a T score below −2; and individuals receiving glucocorticoid therapy for 2 months or longer with a T score below −2 and with osteopenic densities and multiple clinical risk factors (Figure 29-10).

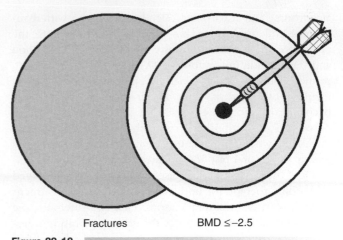

Fractures   BMD ≤−2.5

Figure 29-10
Therapy for osteoporosis.

Bone Resorption Inhibitors

- Bisphosphonates
- Selective estrogen receptor modulators (SERMs)
- Calcitonin

Bone Formation Stimulators (Anabolic Agents)

- Teriparatide
- Strontium ranelate

Bisphosphonates

Formulations and Mechanism of Action. Seven different bisphosphonates are available in the United States: alendronate, etidronate, ibandronate, pamidronate,

risedronate, tiludronate, and zolendronate. All are used routinely in the treatment of osteoporosis except etidronate and tiludronate. Alendronate, ibandronate, and risedronate are available as oral formulations. Pamidronate and zolendronate are intravenous (IV) options. All bisphosphonates inhibit osteoclastic bone reabsorption. This antiresorptive action is especially pronounced at sites of increased active absorption; therefore bisphosphonates have a potent ability to help counterbalance the increase in the resorption/formation ratio characteristically seen in osteoporotic bone.

In addition to inhibiting bone resorption, individual formulations of bisphosphonates also can inhibit bone mineralization to differing degrees. For example, etidronate, the first clinically available bisphosphonate, was shown to inhibit both bone resorption and bone mineralization in the same concentration (1:1), which raised concern about the side effect of osteomalacia. In contrast, the dose of alendronate that inhibits bone mineralization is 1000 times the dose that inhibits resorption; this makes alendronate a more attractive osteoporosis therapy agent. Consequently, alendronate has bypassed etidronate for long-term, chronic treatment of osteoporosis. Etidronate and tiludronate are much less potent in their bone resorption properties than

Table 29-1
Properties of Antiosteoporotic Agents

	Bisphosphonates	Raloxifene	Calcitonin	Teriparatide
Class of agent	Resorption inhibitor	Resorption inhibitor	Resorption inhibitor	Anabolic agent
Administration	Oral	Oral	Intranasal	Subcutaneous
Vertebral fractures	X	X	X	X
Hip fractures	X			
Peripheral fractures	X	X		X
Male osteoporosis	X			
Glucocorticoid-induced osteoporosis	X			
Cost (dollars/month)	65	70	40	500

alendronate and risedronate. Alendronate, along with ibandronate and risedronate, has been approved for both the prevention and treatment of osteoporosis by the U.S. Food and Drug Administration (FDA). The IV preparation, pamidronate, lacks the official FDA indication for the treatment of osteoporosis while zoledronic acid has recently been approved for the treatment of postmenopausal osteoporosis. However, both are routinely used for this purpose in patients who are unable to tolerate oral bisphosphonates and in whom oral bisphosphonates are not effective.

Over the past few years, bisphosphonates have emerged as first-line therapy for both the prevention and treatment of osteoporosis for several reasons. First and foremost, the clinical literature demonstrates the efficacy of bisphosphonates in the prevention of peripheral, vertebral, and hip fractures. Their efficacy has been shown in postmenopausal women, males with osteoporosis, and patients of both genders with glucocorticoid-induced osteoporosis. Furthermore, they are relatively easy to administer, are generally well tolerated, and have minimal side effects. In addition, these medicines are not as expensive as some of the newer agents, such as teriparatide.

Before the results of the Women's Health Initiative, a large clinical trial, were released, estrogen rivaled bisphosphonates for the role of first-line treatment of osteoporosis. Estrogen also had previously proved effective in preventing peripheral, vertebral, and hip fractures. However, the Women's Health Initiative raised concerns about the increased risk of thromboembolic and cardiovascular disease, breast cancer, and stroke with hormone replacement therapy. As a result, many women chose to discontinue estrogen therapy and turn to an alternative for osteoporosis treatment. Many health care workers shared this concern about the risk/benefit ratio of using estrogen as the sole primary therapy for osteoporosis. Many of these postmenopausal women with osteoporosis, who previously had taken estrogen, began taking bisphosphonates instead. Consequently, bisphosphonates became even more important as therapy for osteoporosis.

Dosages and Administration. The five bisphosphonate agents clinically used for osteoporosis and their doses are listed in Table 29-2.

Initially, alendronate and risedronate were administered as a once daily oral regimen. However, later studies showed that dosing once weekly had equivalent efficacy to the daily dosing. Advantages of dosing once weekly included improved compliance and fewer absolute days with a chance for gastrointestinal side effects. Ibandronate, which came on the market in 2003, is dosed orally once a month and intravenously at quarterly intervals

The absorption of bisphosphonates is 1% to 5% of the oral dose. Because of this poor absorption, proper administration is vital to successful, effective therapy. Oral bisphosphonates should be taken on an empty stomach with no other medicines. The patient should not eat any food or

Table 29-2
Bisphosphonates Used to Treat Osteoporosis

Drug	Prophylaxis and Treatment
Alendronate[37,38]	Prophylaxis: 5 mg given orally once a day, or 35 mg given orally once a week Treatment: 10 mg given orally once a day, or 70 mg given orally once a week
Ibandronate	Prophylaxis and treatment: 150 mg given orally once a month; 3 mg intravenous (IV) push given quarterly
Pamidronate	(Not approved by the U.S. Food and Drug Administration [FDA]): 90 mg IV infusion given at six month intervals
Risedronate[39,40]	Prophylaxis and treatment: 5 mg given orally once a day, or 35 mg given orally once a week
Zolendronate	(Not FDA approved): 4 mg IV infusion given yearly

take any medicines for 30 to 45 minutes after administration. A full 8-ounce glass of water should be taken with the pill, and other liquids should not be used as aids for swallowing the medication. Patients should be instructed to remain upright for at least 30 minutes after administration. Lying down or reclining within 30 minutes after taking the bisphosphonate can exacerbate the gastrointestinal side (see the next section). Approximately 20% of the medicine is expected to be taken up by the bone, and the remainder of the drug is excreted by the renal system. The serum half-life is approximately 1 hour, but bisphosphonates persist in the bone for a much longer time (estimated to be months to years).

Side Effects and Precautions. The main concerns with bisphosphonate therapy are the gastrointestinal (GI) effects. Pill-induced esophagitis, esophageal ulcers, exacerbation of gastroesophageal reflux disease (GERD) symptoms, and esophageal stricture have been reported. GI effects are more common in patients who do not properly follow the administration precautions previously discussed. Patients with impaired swallowing mechanisms (i.e., patients who have suffered a stroke, are struggling with multiple sclerosis, or have an esophageal pathology, such as achalasia) also are at higher risk for GI complications. Caution should be used with patients who have moderate to severe GERD and dyspepsia symptoms. Many health care providers choose to avoid oral bisphosphonates for these patients and consider IV forms as an alternative. However, transient, flulike, febrile illnesses, as well as transient lymphopenia, have been reported with IV administration of bisphosphonates.

Endocrine and metabolic side effects of hypocalcemia and hypophosphatemia have been reported, with hypocalcemia affecting approximately 18% of patients and hypophosphatemia about 10%. Both are usually mild and transient. In most cases the hypocalcemia is asymptomatic unless the patient has another predisposing risk factor, such as vitamin D deficiency. Patients taking oral bisphosphonates also should take at least 1000 to 1200 mg of elemental calcium and 400 IU of vitamin D a day.

Because of the high clearance of bisphosphonates by the kidneys, these drugs should be used with caution in patients with renal insufficiency. Worsening of renal function has been described after administration of bisphosphonates in these patients. Methods to avoid worsening renal function include giving a lower dose and infusing the IV dose over a longer period.

Recently, a concern has emerged about osteonecrosis of the jaw with prolonged use of bisphosphonates. Most of these cases have occurred in oncology patients receiving chronic, multiple IV doses of bisphosphonates. However, rare cases of similar avascular necrosis of the jaw have been reported with oral bisphosphonate use in postmenopausal women. The significance of this potential complication in patients with osteoporosis on oral bisphosphonate therapy warrants further investigation.

Raloxifene[40-42]

Formulation and Mechanism of Action. Raloxifene belongs to the class of antiresorptive agents used to treat osteoporosis. It functions as a selective estrogen receptor modulator (SERM). Two of the SERMs, raloxifene and tamoxifen, are often used clinically. Raloxifene is prescribed mostly for osteoporosis, whereas tamoxifen is prescribed as an anticancer agent. SERMs are unique in that they act in both an agonistic and an antagonistic manner at the site of estrogen receptors. The target organ determines whether the drug functions as an agonistic or an antagonist. For example, in bone, SERMs mimic the action of estrogen and prevent bone loss. SERMs also lower total cholesterol and low density lipoprotein (LDL) cholesterol, much as estrogen does. Their antiestrogenic effects on the uterus and breast diminish the risk of uterine and breast cancer.

Dosage and Indications. The customary dosage of raloxifene is a 60 mg tablet taken once a day. The drug is FDA approved for both the prevention and treatment of osteoporosis. Studies have shown raloxifene to be effective for fractures of the vertebral column as well as peripheral fractures. In comparison, the bisphosphonates protect against hip fractures, a site where raloxifene is not indicated.

Raloxifene can be taken with or without food at any time of day. Approximately 60% of the drug is absorbed, and it is highly protein bound in the serum. The onset of action is not typically observed until after it has been taken for 2 months.

Two commonly prescribed medicines, cholestyramine and ampicillin, reduce the absorption of raloxifene.

Side Effects and Precautions. One of the main concerns with raloxifene is the increased risk of superficial thrombophlebitis and deep vein thrombosis (DVT). Studies have found the risk of DVT to be comparable to that seen with the use of estrogen in hormone replacement therapy in postmenopausal women. Therefore, use of SERMs is not recommended in patients with other risk factors for DVT or pulmonary embolism, or a history of either of these conditions. Furthermore, women with a history of uterine or cervical cancer are not good candidates for SERMs. The cardiovascular effects of SERMs have not been well defined. However, the data from the Women's Health Initiative study that showed an increased risk of cardiovascular events in postmenopausal women with known coronary artery disease (CAD) who were in the hormone replacement group has led many clinicians to avoid the use of SERMs in patients with known CAD. Finally, raloxifene should not be used in pregnant women or women intending to conceive.

Some women experience significant hot flashes with raloxifene therapy. Frequently, these episodes are severe enough to prevent the further use of raloxifene as an antiosteoporotic agent. Other side effects that may limit its use include sinusitis and flulike symptoms. Arthralgias have been reported in approximately 10% of patients taking raloxifene. Hypertriglyceridemia occurs, especially in patients whose triglycerides increased during estrogen therapy.

Calcitonin[43,44]

Formulations and Mechanism of Action. Calcitonin is an antiresorptive agent. Its mechanism of action involves banding to osteoclasts to inhibit bone resorption. Both human and salmon calcitonin are prescribed clinically, and salmon calcitonin is the form of choice in most cases. Typically, the affinity of salmon calcitonin for the calcitonin receptor is approximately 40 times higher than that of human calcitonin. Also, salmon calcitonin has a longer half-life because of its slow clearance rate.

Calcitonin is available as intranasal, intramuscular, and subcutaneous preparations. Each form has advantages and disadvantages. Nasal calcitonin, the preferred mode of administration, has fewer side effects and more potent analgesia. However, nasal calcitonin has a delayed absorption time compared to the other forms and only about 25% of the bioavailability of the intramuscular version.

Dosage and Indications. With the nasal preparation, a dose of 200 units (1 spray) per day typically is used. Intramuscular and subcutaneous doses are 100 units a day. All preparations usually are stored in the refrigerator before initial use. After initial use, the injection remains stable at room temperature for 2 weeks, and the nasal pump should be stored at room temperature.

Studies have found calcitonin to be effective for fractures of the spine but not for peripheral or hip fractures. Therefore it is less potent for osteoporosis therapy overall than the antiresorptive bisphosphonates. Many clinicians consider calcitonin a second-line agent for the treatment of osteoporosis. In a head-to-head trial of alendronate versus calcitonin, DEXA scores improved at both the spine and hip to a greater degree with the bisphosphonate.

One feature that seems to be unique to calcitonin is its ability to reduce pain in patients with an acute fracture. The mechanism of action involved in this analgesic property is not clearly known. One hypothesis is that calcitonin increases the level of endorphins in the body. Therefore, in a patient with significant pain from an osteoporotic fracture, one choice of therapy is initially treating with calcitonin and then changing to another, more potent antiresorptive agent once the pain has subsided. From a cost perspective, calcitonin is the least expensive of the osteoporosis therapy agents.

Side Effects and Precautions. The most commonly reported side effects of calcitonin include flushing, nausea and vomiting, anorexia, and diarrhea. The incidence of these side effects is reduced when the drug is administered intranasally, but nasal irritation can result from use of the spray form. Flushing usually lasts less than 1 hour, and the unpleasantness of this side effect can be minimized if the medication is taken at bedtime just before sleep.

Calcitonin reduces renal tubular reabsorption and consequently results in an increase in the excretion of calcium, potassium, magnesium, phosphorus, and sodium by the kidneys. Monitoring of patients on calcitonin therapy involves following the serum calcium and electrolytes. Special caution and monitoring are recommended in patients taking other drugs that can lower the level of calcium in the blood, such as plicamycin. Sufficient dietary intake of calcium and vitamin D should be encouraged in patients with osteoporosis who take calcitonin.

Hypersensitivity to salmon calcitonin can be a significant problem. Some clinicians prefer to conduct a skin test in a supervised environment, with epinephrine readily available, before starting therapy with salmon calcitonin. Another concern with long-term use of calcitonin for osteoporosis is the possibility of resistance to therapy. The emergence of antibodies to calcitonin has been reported in patients with Paget's disease of bone who were chronically treated with salmon calcitonin. Once the antibodies had developed, active disease returned in many of these patients, signified by an increase in alkaline phosphatase. A similar reduction in efficacy as a result of the development of antibodies remains a potential limitation of the use of calcitonin in long-term treatment of osteoporosis.

Teriparatide[45,46]

Formulations and Mechanism of Action. Teriparatide became available in the United States for the treatment of osteoporosis in 2002. Teriparatide is recombinant human parathyroid hormone 1–34 (PTH) and is given as a subcutaneous injection. As an anabolic agent, it offers an important addition to the therapies already on the market. It may seem counterintuitive that a form of PTH would be beneficial to bone health, because the actions of endogenous PTH include resorption of calcium from the bone. However, when teriparatide is administered intermittently as a subcutaneous injection, it stimulates osteoblast function to promote bone formation. It also increases both renal tubular reabsorption and GI absorption of calcium. Consequently, bone mass, BMD, and bone strength are all increased.

Dosage and Indications. The dosage of teriparatide is 20 μg a day given as a subcutaneous injection. The drug is packaged in a prefilled syringe. Recommended sites for injection include the abdominal wall and the thigh area. Orthostasis has been described with the initial dose, therefore the first dose usually is given under supervision in a place where the patient can lie or sit down if necessary. The injector/pen should be stored in the refrigerator and should be discarded after approximately 28 days. Teriparatide usually is given for 18 to 24 months.

Teriparatide has been shown to be effective in reducing vertebral and peripheral fractures. It is indicated for both men and women at high risk for fractures. Such patients include those in whom other therapies have failed or who cannot tolerate other, more conventional osteoporosis therapies; those with a history of previous fractures; and those with several risk factors for fractures. For example, high risk patients with contraindications for bisphosphonate therapy constitute a large percentage of the individuals who are good candidates for teriparatide therapy.

The release of teriparatide drew an enthusiastic response from health care workers and researchers, who hoped that a combination therapy of teriparatide and bisphosphonates would provide an increased cumulative benefit for bone health. Theoretically this seemed logical, because one is an anabolic agent and the other is an antiresorptive agent. However, trials that tested this hypothesis did not show an additive benefit, and in fact some data suggested that concurrent use of a bisphosphonate and teriparatide reduces the overall anabolic effect of teriparatide. Therefore, in most patients treated with a bisphosphonate initially, this antiresorptive agent usually is stopped before teriparatide administration is started. After 18 to 24 months of teriparatide therapy, it is important to stop the teriparatide and restart the bisphosphonate to prevent the loss of the improvement in bone mass gained from PTH.

Side Effects and Precautions. As mentioned previously, orthostasis has been seen with the initiation of teriparatide therapy. Symptoms tend to improve after repeat administration of the drug. Headache is another significant central nervous system side effect. Nausea and dyspepsia also have been reported (approximately 9% and 5% of patients, respectively). Musculoskeletal side effects include leg cramps and arthralgias.

Transient hypercalcemia has been described and occurs most often 4 to 6 hours after administration of the dose. Monitoring of serum laboratory results involves calcium, phosphorus, and uric acid. The drug is not recommended for use in patients with a history of hypercalcemia, hyperparathyroidism, or skeletal cancer metastases.

A theoretical risk of osteosarcoma exists with the use of teriparatide. Studies with rats have found an association with osteosarcoma when the rats were exposed to high doses of teriparatide for most of their lifetime. No case reports of a similar occurrence of osteosarcoma in humans have been described. However, because osteosarcoma appears most often in children and young adults, careful consideration and caution should be exercised in the use of teriparatide in young adults. It is not approved for use in pediatric patients.

Teriparatide is costly (as much as $7,000 per year), which can put limitations on its use. Because it is not covered by insurance, the cost can be prohibitive. Teriparatide therefore usually is reserved for patients in whom other therapies have failed (e.g., patients who continue to have fractures despite bisphosphonate therapy).

Strontium Ranelate[47,48]

Formulations and Mechanism of Action. Strontium ranelate is a bone-stimulating agent. It is composed of an organic moiety, ranelic acid and two atoms of stable strontium. An advantage of strontium ranelate over teriparatide, the other major anabolic agent, is that strontium ranelate is available as an oral agent. Therefore many patients may prefer it over teriparatide, which requires a daily subcutaneous injection. Data from animal studies support the effectiveness of strontium ranelate's mechanism of action both in stimulating bone formation and inhibiting bone resorption.

Dosage and Indications. Several studies using human subjects have been performed with strontium ranelate, and its efficacy in treating women with osteoporosis appears to be dose dependent. Most studies have used a dosage of 2 g a day. Data show a significant increase in bone mineral density T scores in both the vertebral spine and the femoral neck. In addition, strontium ranelate appears to reduce the incidence of new vertebral fractures in women with known osteoporosis. Whether it is protective in the prevention of osteoporosis has not yet been determined.

Side Effects and Precautions. Although it has been shown to be effective in the treatment of osteoporosis in women with known osteoporosis, strontium ranelate currently is not clinically available. The main side effect of strontium ranelate is diarrhea. In most cases the diarrhea remits after the first 3 months of therapy. Strontium ranelate offers promise as a future bone-stimulating agent in the therapy of osteoporosis, but this agent is currently unavailable in the United States.

Primary Hyperparathyroidism

Primary hyperparathyroidism is the most common cause of hypercalcemia. Among ambulatory patients, primary hyperparathyroidism accounts for 75% of all causes of hypercalcemia. Figure 29-11 presents the typical causes of disorders of calcium homeostasis.

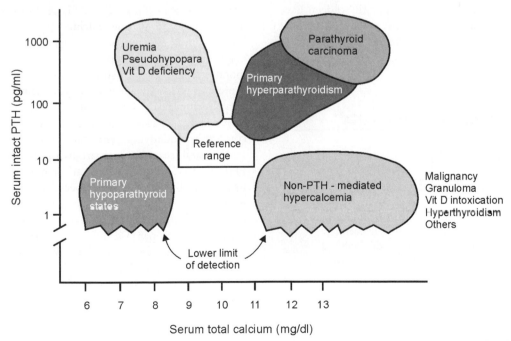

Figure 29-11
Calcium–intact parathyroid hormone (iPTH) relationships.

The parathyroid glands were first recognized in an Indian rhinoceros in 1880 by the anatomist Ivar Sandstrum, although their function was not discovered until a few decades later.[49] Hyperparathyroidism was first conjectured and later confirmed to be the problem of Albert J, a Viennese streetcar conductor who suffered from chronic skeletal pain and decalcification from 1919 to 1924.[50] From this uncertain beginning, primary hyperparathyroidism has emerged as a common and easily diagnosed endocrine disease now known largely to affect postmenopausal women.

Currently, about 80% of those with primary hyperparathyroidism have few or no symptoms directly attributable to parathyroid gland hyperactivity. The old adage that patients with hyperparathyroidism have "stones, bones, or abdominal groans" now is less applicable.[51]

In most patients with primary hyperparathyroidism, one or more mutations cause the parathyroid gland autonomy. However, in the most common forms of primary hyperparathyroidism, the molecular abnormality is still unknown.[52] The disorder is nonhereditary in 95% of patients. Yet the pathophysiology is best understood in the 5% with genetic diseases. Table 29-3 summarizes the current understanding of the forms of primary hyperparathyroidism.

The nearly invariant features of primary hyperparathyroidism are an elevated serum calcium level (hypercalcemia) and a frankly elevated or inappropriately high (for the level of serum calcium) intact parathyroid hormone (iPTH) level. For most clinical laboratories, the reference range for serum iPTH is 10-65 pg/mL. iPTH values over 40 pg/mL accompanied by hypercalcemia strongly point to a diagnosis of primary hyperparathyroidism.

Most patients with primary hyperparathyroidism have a sporadic disease, usually a chief cell adenoma involving one or more of the parathyroid glands.[53] Treatment with lithium and head or neck radiation therapy may induce

autonomous parathyroid function, although the exact mechanisms are not understood.[54,55] For most patients, the diagnosis rests on measurement of the calcium and iPTH levels.

Genetic primary hyperparathyroidism is the less often seen but, ironically, better understood form of primary hyperparathyroidism. In multiple endocrine neoplasia type 1 (MEN-1), inactivation of the tumor suppressor gene menin leads to neoplastic transformation of cells within the parathyroid glands, endocrine pancreas, and pituitary.[56] In this autosomal dominant inherited disease, primary hyperparathyroidism is present with a penetrance of 98% by age 40. Hyperparathyroidism commonly is identifiable by age 20. Pancreatic islet cell and pituitary tumors are less highly penetrant. Carcinoid tumors may also be present in patients with MEN-1.

MEN-2A and MEN-2B affect different families from those affected by MEN-1. In patients with MEN-2A, mutations within the RET oncogene lead to medullary carcinoma of the thyroid, pheochromocytoma, and occasionally to primary hyperparathyroidism.[57] Throughout the entire age spectrum, hyperparathyroidism has a penetrance of approximately 15%. MEN-2B is a considerably less common disease than MEN-2A and is characterized by a more aggressive form of medullary thyroid cancer, and mucosal neuromas of the lips and tongue, and a Marfan-like habitus.

Familial hypocalciuric hypercalcemia (FHH), also known as *benign familial hypercalcemia (BFH)*, produces hypercalcemia and inappropriate levels of iPTH by means of inactivating mutations in the calcium-sensing receptor genes in parathyroid and renal tubular cells.[58] Patients with FHH typically manifest mild hypercalcemia (serum calcium levels of 10.5-11.2 mg/dl), iPTH levels of 45-70 pg/mL, underexcretion of urine calcium (less than 150 mg/24 hours), and no symptoms of hyperparathyroidism. The diagnosis of FHH may be confirmed by detection of the mutation or mutations; suspicion is raised if hypercalcemia is present in close relatives or if the patient has minimal urinary calcium excretion. Parathyroidectomy is ill-advised treatment for patients with FHH, because it does not correct the underlying genetic abnormality.

Neonatal severe hyperparathyroidism is a variant of FHH that typically is present at birth and is characterized by marked, life-threatening hypercalcemia.[56] In most cases patients with neonatal severe hyperparathyroidism have a homozygous form of FHH, having acquired the mutated gene from both parents. Emergency parathyroidectomy is nearly always necessary. Patients with homozygous FHH mutations have now been identified with mild hypercalcemia and a clinical syndrome similar to that seen in typical heterozygous FHH.

Hyperparathyroidism–jaw tumor syndrome is a recently discovered and uncommon form of hyperparathyroidism that thus far has been described in only a limited number of families.[59] The noteworthy feature of

Table 29-3
Forms of Primary Hyperparathyroidism ($\uparrow$Ca^{2+} + $\uparrow$PTH)

Sporadic (95%)	Chief cell mutations Lithium induced Radiotherapy induced
Genetic (5%)	MEN-1 (98% penetrance by age 40) MEN-2A and MEN-2B (15% penetrance) Familial hypocalciuric hypercalcemia (heterozygous mutation of CaSR) Neonatal severe hyperparathyroidism (homozygous CaSR mutation) Hyperparathyroidism jaw tumor syndrome (low age-related penetrance) Familial isolated hyperparathyroidism

Ca^{2+}, calcium; *CaSR*, calcium-sensing receptor; *MEN-1*, multiple endocrine neoplasia type 1; *PTH*, parathyroid hormone.

hyperparathyroidism–jaw tumor syndrome is the unexpectedly high prevalence of parathyroid carcinoma, that approaches 15% of affected individuals.

Calcium-Sensing Receptor

Largely through the important work of Tfelt-Hansen and Brown, the calcium-sensing receptor (CaSR) has been shown to be the mechanism by which parathyroid and other cells recognize and respond to the calcium ion concentrations of the extracellular fluid.[58] Through this G-coupled transmembrane protein, parathyroid cells distinguish ambient levels of ionized calcium and regulate the synthesis and secretion of iPTH. The molecular mechanisms underlying activating and inactivating mutations of the CaSR are shown in Figure 29-12. On the vertical axis is the percentage of the maximum cellular response; this could be the percentage of the maximum generated amount of the intracellular signal IP_3, which is regulated by the calcium ion concentration and its interaction with CaSR. The EC50 is the ambient calcium ion concentration that produces 50% of the maximum response. Inactivating mutations of the CaSR (the dashed line), as seen in FHH, shift the EC50 to a higher calcium ion concentration. A higher calcium ion concentration is needed to suppress iPTH secretion. By contrast, activating mutations of the CaSR shift the EC50 to the left and lead to suppression of iPTH at lower ambient calcium ion concentrations. Clinically, this disorder is recognized as autosomal dominant hypoparathyroidism, which closely mimics idiopathic hypoparathyroidism.

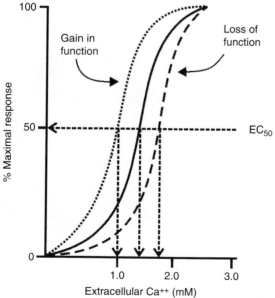

Figure 29-12

Functional changes arising from calcium-sensing receptor mutation.

Treatment of Primary Hyperparathyroidism

In October, 1990, the National Institutes of Health (NIH) convened a Consensus Development Conference on the Management of Asymptomatic Primary Hyperparathyroidism. Nearly 12 years later, a follow-up Workshop on Asymptomatic Primary Hyperparathyroidism: A Perspective for the 21st Century was convened to review and revise the recommendations made by the earlier conference.[60] According to the revised recommendations, surgical treatment of primary hyperparathyroidism can be considered if the patient has any of the following conditions:

- Kidney stones
- Fractures
- Peptic ulcer disease
- Serum calcium level more than 1 mg/dL above the reference range
- Urinary calcium excretion greater than 400 mg/24 hours
- Bone density T score of −2.5 or lower at any site
- Creatinine clearance reduced by 30%
- Age under 50 years
- Inability or unwillingness to be monitored

With these revisions, more patients with primary hyperparathyroidism meet the criteria for parathyroid surgery.

Parathyroid Surgery

As in most areas of medicine, technical advances have made elective parathyroid surgery both easier and safer for patients and surgeons, with no compromise in the success of surgery. One step forward that has simplified parathyroid surgery is the development of rapid iPTH measurements done intraoperatively. In less than 15 minutes after removal of the parathyroid adenoma, the surgeon can determine whether the intraoperative PTH level has declined by 50% compared to the preoperative value. This criterion has been used to confirm a successful parathyroidectomy.[61]

A second advantageous development has been the improvement in parathyroid scanning and ultrasonography. Sestamibi scanning has a positive predictive value of 95% for right and left inferior parathyroid adenomas, and ultrasonography has at least 65% positive predictive value for right and left inferior parathyroid adenomas.[62] The positive predictive value of sestamibi scanning for superior parathyroid adenomas exceeds 60%.

Some experienced parathyroid surgeons have used a handheld gamma probe to assist intraoperative localization of parathyroid adenomas. A potential limitation of this approach has been the accurate timing of preoperative sestamibi scanning.

Minimally Invasive Parathyroid Surgery[63,64]

Several centers in the United States and other countries have routinely and successfully undertaken parathyroidectomy using local anesthesia in patients in whom a single parathyroid adenoma can be successfully localized before surgery. This approach has allowed high risk surgical patients and others with primary hyperparathyroidism to undergo successful parathyroid surgery without hospitalization and general anesthesia. Minimally invasive parathyroid surgery (MIPS) currently is performed by only a few surgeons, but the number is growing. Obviously, not all patients with primary hyperparathyroidism are candidates for MIPS.

Exclusion Criteria for Minimally Invasive Parathyroid Surgery

- Multigland disease (e.g., familial hyperparathyroidism, multiple endocrine neoplasia)
- Previous neck radiotherapy
- Preoperative PTH measurement over 500 pg/mL (raises a question of parathyroid cancer)
- Goiter
- Substernal parathyroid adenoma
- Nonlocalization on preoperative testing
- Conflicting sestamibi and ultrasound localization

MIPS cannot be used for multiglandular primary hyperparathyroidism, because only one gland is approached in the procedure. Patients with MEN-1 and MEN-2 usually have a multiglandular disease. With previous radiotherapy to the neck, the tissue layers of the neck may not be cleanly dissectible, and a limited access procedure has a greater probability of failure. Also, the thyroid gland should be carefully evaluated to make sure that a thyroid carcinoma is not present in addition to primary hyperparathyroidism. Fortunately, parathyroid carcinoma is a rare disorder; however, hypercalcemia and iPTH levels over 400-500 pg/mL in the absence of impaired renal function raise diagnostic suspicion for parathyroid carcinoma. As noted earlier, patients with hyperparathyroidism–jaw tumor syndrome are more likely to have parathyroid carcinoma and are not good candidates for MIPS. A goiter may also complicate access to an abnormal parathyroid gland, thereby limiting the success of MIPS. A nearly absolute requirement for MIPS is the ability to localize the abnormal parathyroid gland before surgery. Failed or conflicting localization eliminates MIPS.

Medical Therapy for Primary Hyperparathyroidism

In 2004 the FDA approved the use of the CaSR agonist Cinacalcet to treat secondary hyperparathyroidism from chronic renal failure.[65] Subsequently, growing but off label use of cinacalcet has developed in the treatment of primary hyperparathyroidism.[66] Most patients with primary hyperparathyroidism require twice daily treatment with cinacalcet instead of the once daily therapy needed in secondary hyperparathyroidism. Potential limitations for the drug's use in primary hyperparathyroidism are the need for long-term therapy and its moderate expense ($300–$600 per month). Cinacalcet may not prevent the anticipated bone loss that occurs in untreated primary hyperparathyroidism

Paget's Disease of Bone (Osteitis Deformans)

Paget's disease of bone (PDB), described by Sir James Paget in 1877, is now thought to be a localized disorder of bone remodeling (Figure 29-13).[67] Although the etiology of PDB is incompletely understood, both genetic and viral mechanisms of the disease have gained strong research support.[68] Several pedigrees of families with multiple afflicted individuals have been described and provide a strong basis for a belief that in some patients, PDB is a genetic disease linked to chromosome 18q and other loci. In patients with nongenetic PDB, electron photomicrographs show paramyxoviral-like intranuclear inclusion bodies typical of the measles virus and the canine distemper virus in pagetic osteoclasts. To date no one has been able to recover infectious virus from pagetic bone.

Bone Remodeling

The mature skeleton uses a regenerative process called *bone remodeling* to repair damage that occurs during daily activities. Remodeling preserves skeletal strength using intrinsic bone cells called osteoclasts that remove and osteoblasts that subsequently replace localized areas of the skeleton.[69]

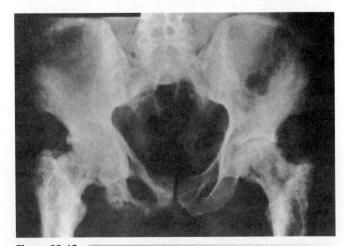

Figure 29-13
Radiograph of a pelvis affected by Paget's disease showing concentric-type Paget's arthritis of the right hip. (From Merkow RL, Lane JM: Current concepts of Paget's disease of bone, *Orthop Clin North Am* 15:761, 1984.)

The bone remodeling cycle is divided into four phases: activation, resorption, reversal, and formation.

Phases of the Bone Remodeling Cycle

- Activation
- Resorption
- Reversal
- Formation

With activation, osteoclasts are stimulated to remove localized packets of bone. Both the mineralized and the organic components of the skeleton are removed. Over several days, osteoclasts excavate a microtrench on the surface of the skeleton. With reversal, osteoclastic bone resorption abates and osteoblasts are stimulated to migrate onto the surface of the resorption cavity, where the organic components of the skeleton are laid down and subsequently mineralized (formation). In healthy individuals, the amount of resorbed skeleton is replaced by an equal amount of replaced bone, therefore no net loss of skeletal mass occurs. Temporally, the resorption phase of remodeling occurs more quickly than the formation phase; consequently, during periods of accelerated bone remodeling, a net loss of skeletal mass does occur. Virtually all circumstances in which remodeling is accelerated involve loss of bone mass. States of accelerated skeletal turnover include estrogen deprivation, primary hyperparathyroidism, and PDB. In Paget's disease, the localized nature of this disorder results in a minor reduction in total skeletal mass, but also localized disorganization of the skeletal architecture and a greater opportunity for fracture in the areas of pagetic bone.

Clinical Features[70-73]

PDB affects men and women with nearly equally frequency but is relatively uncommon before age 25. With advancing age, PDB is seen with increasing frequency, and it may affect 10% of the elderly population in areas of the world where PDB is noted frequently (e.g., the United States and southern Europe). PDB often is discovered as an incidental finding on radiographic evaluation for another problem. The most commonly affected parts of the skeleton are the skull, femur, pelvis, vertebra, and tibia. One skeletal site (mono-ostotic) or multiple sites (polyostotic) may be involved in Paget's disease. The diagnosis of PDB usually is made radiographically by the characteristic localized disruption of skeletal architecture, although pagetic bone can also be recognized on scintigraphic bone scans. Often the differential diagnosis includes PDB or osteoblastic malignancy (e.g., prostate cancer, thyroid cancer). Occasionally a bone biopsy is required to establish a specific diagnosis.

When Paget's disease is suspected, a careful history and physical examination should be performed to look for a hereditary link, a skeletal deformity of the tibia or skull, and a temperature change over the affected areas of bone. Pagetic bone may have an increased vasculature supply with increased warmth and occasionally a bruit. Patients with PDB of the basilar skull may have sensorineural hearing loss, and patients with polyostotic PDB may have congestive heart failure.

The most common symptom in PDB is pain, although the disease status commonly is inactive (asymptomatic PDB). The clinician often is confronted with the uncertainty of determining whether a patient's pain arises from pagetic bone or from the adjacent joint involved with degenerative arthritis.

The biochemical features of PDB are those of increased skeletal turnover; they include an elevated serum level of alkaline phosphatase or bone-specific alkaline phosphatase and increased urinary resorption makers, N-telo-peptide and CTX.[69] Disease activity often is directly related to the degree of elevation of the markers of bone turnover. With active PDB that involves an extensive proportion of the skeleton, the serum alkaline phosphatase may exceed the upper end of the reference range by tenfold. Occasionally, in patients with symptomatic but localized PDB, the serum alkaline phosphatase may not even be driven above the reference range. The biochemical markers of bone turnover typically are used to determine disease activity status and whether a patient should undergo therapy for PDB.

Treatment of Paget's Disease

The mainstays of treatment for PDB are the bone resorption inhibitors, which currently are dominated by bisphosphonates and may be administered orally or intravenously.[74,75]

For PDB, oral bisphosphonates are nearly always taken daily in doses similar to those used for weekly oral therapy of osteoporosis. In the United States, oral bisphosphonate therapy for PDB is dominated by alendronate and risedronate because of their effectiveness, availability, and ease of use. Oral bisphosphonate therapy is nearly always given for a finite period, which may be 2 to 3 months, depending on the agent selected. Intravenous bisphosphonates are most often used in patients with refractory PDB and those with severe PDB that requires more rapid resolution.

Subcutaneous and intramuscular calcitonin injections are also an effective therapy for PDB but are less frequently used because of the need for subcutaneous administration and because calcitonin therapy is less potent than bisphosphonate therapy. Concern also has been raised that calcitonin therapy may become ineffective with extended use. Little experience has been reported with the use of intranasal calcitonin for the treatment of PDB.

Part B   Rehabilitation Intervention

Osteoporosis

Clinicians do not usually see patients referred with a primary diagnosis of osteoporosis. They are much more likely to treat individuals who have sustained a fracture as a result of this underlying condition or who are referred for unrelated diagnoses. Osteoporosis accounts for more than 1.5 million fractures annually, of which 300,000 are hip fractures and 700,000 are vertebral fractures.[76] A knowledge of the impact and possible physical consequences of osteoporosis and of ways to develop a treatment plan for patients who have this condition, regardless of the referral diagnosis, is paramount.

Osteoporosis can be defined as a disease characterized by low bone mass and structural deterioration of bone tissue, leading to bone fragility and increased risk of fracture (Figure 29-14).[77] A BMD test can be done to clinically define osteoporosis or osteopenia (low bone mass) (Figure 29-15). The BMD refers to the relative fracture risk of a bone and the test used to classify bone health; the result is given as a T score of the hip BMD.

From an epidemiological perspective, approximately 10 million individuals in the United States have osteoporosis, and an additional 34 million have osteopenia. One in two women and one in four men over age 50 will have an osteoporosis-related fracture at some time in their life.[76] This means that clinicians working with those over age 50 are very likely to have patients with osteoporosis or osteopenia, and these patients therefore are at greater risk for injury or impairment related to these disease processes. For these reasons, consideration of the patient's bone status is vital, regardless of the referral diagnosis.

Although significantly more vertebral fractures occur than hip fractures, most rehabilitation clinicians think of a hip fracture when they think of osteoporosis. This is because these patients often are referred for rehabilitation after surgery. Individuals who have sustained vertebral fractures, on the other hand, often go undiagnosed;[77] the primary symptom of these fractures, back pain, often is attributed to "arthritis" or is thought to be a normal part of aging. Untreated vertebral fractures can result in increased kyphosis, which leads to changes in the postural position of the patient's cervical spine and head, bringing the center of mass further anterior to the spine (Figure 29-16). This postural alteration can result in a vicious cycle, causing a further increase in kyphosis. The kyphosis compresses the lungs and abdominal organs, making breathing and even eating difficult. These postural changes may also lead to a decrease in upper extremity function, especially with reaching, whereas increases in cervical lordosis lead to decreased

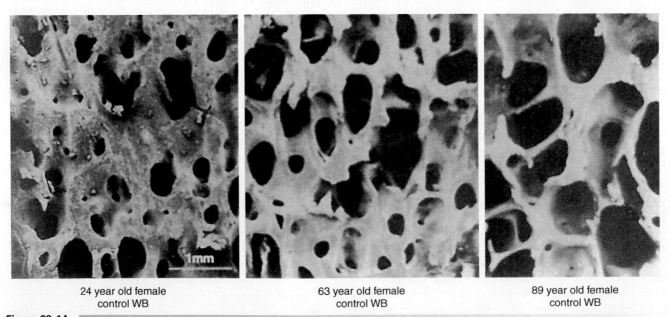

| 24 year old female | 63 year old female | 89 year old female |
| control WB | control WB | control WB |

Figure 29-14

Age-related changes in apparent density and architecture of human trabecular bone from the lumbar spine.
(Courtesy Marc D. Grynpas, PhD. In Buchwalter JA et al: *Orthopaedic basic science*, ed 2, American Academy of Orthopaedic Surgeons, 2000.)

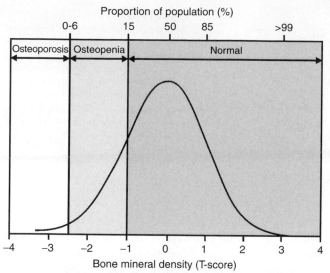

Figure 29-15

Normal distribution of bone mineral density (BMD) scores, represented as T scores. Note that a score of −1 to −2.5 represents osteopenia, and a score of −2.5 or lower indicates osteoporosis. (Redrawn from Kanis JA: Osteoporosis III: diagnosis of osteoporosis and assessment of fracture risk, *Lancet* 359:1929-1936, 2002.)

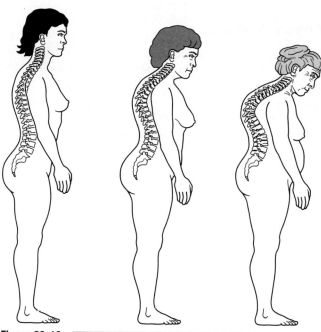

Figure 29-16

Increase in thoracic kyphosis commonly seen with advancing age and with vertebral compression fractures.

cervical flexibility and ultimately affect visual navigation of the environment.

The increased kyphosis must be counterbalanced by the back extensor muscles. However, if these muscles are too weak, they quickly fatigue while working to keep the spine extended. Clinicians responsible for the rehabilitative

management of patients with these types of problems must consider all these factors in designing a program to minimize kyphosis; the program must include education and counseling to make patients aware of the effects of inappropriate posture on their condition, bracing if appropriate, and improving the strength and endurance of the thoracic extensors and scapula retractors.

Clinicians must base their intervention not on the medical diagnosis, but on the resultant impairments and functional limitations found during the initial evaluation. Treatment of individuals with osteoporosis is no different. Therefore this section covers the past medical history, assessment, primary prevention, treatment of common impairments, effects of exercise on the skeleton, and kyphoplasty. The overriding objective for these patients is to improve functional ability and prevent fractures, which can lead to further significant declines in function. To this end, the goals of treatment include increasing strength, flexibility, and range of motion; improving balance (90% of hip fractures are the result of a fall);[78] correcting posture when possible; modulating pain; and educating the patient about lifestyle adaptations.

The Guide to Physical Therapist Practice[79] offers four classifications in the musculoskeletal preferred practice pattern, group 4, to guide decision making:

- 4A: Primary prevention/risk reduction for skeletal demineralization
- 4B: Impaired posture
- 4F: Spinal disorders
- 4G: Fracture

Group 4A is solely for use in primary prevention. Group 4B includes those who fall under the ICD-9-CM* codes for osteoporosis, kyphosis (acquired), abnormal posture, and pain in the thoracic spine. Group 4F also includes the ICD-9-CM code for osteoporosis. Group 4G includes the ICD-9-CM codes for osteoporosis, pathological fracture, fracture of the vertebral column without spinal cord injury, fracture of the pelvis, fracture of the neck of the femur, and fracture of other and unspecified parts of the femur.

Spinal Biomechanics

Any assessment or intervention for patients with or at risk for osteoporosis must take into consideration spinal biomechanics and safety. Spinal flexion requires a balance between flexor and extensor forces (Figure 29-17) (*force* is the capacity to do work; *work* is force exerted over a distance).

---

*ICD-9-CM is the International Classification of Diseases, 9th Edition, Clinical Modification. It is the official system of assigning codes to diagnoses and procedures associated with hospital utilization in the United States. The National Center for Health Statistics oversees diagnosis codes; the Centers for Medicare and Medicaid Services oversees procedure codes.

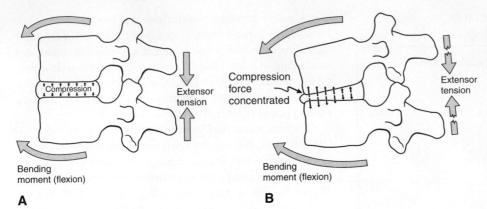

A, State of balance between flexors and extensors and the resulting biomechanics. **B,** State of increased flexor force and insufficient extensor force, resulting in compression on the anterior part of the vertebral body and the intervertebral disc. (Redrawn from Carlson JM: Clinical biomechanics of orthotic treatment of thoracic hyperkyphosis, *J Prosthet Orthot* 15: 31-35, 2003.)

Figure 29-17

Any force that falls anterior to the spine exerts a *flexion moment* (force acting at a distance perpendicular to a point) on the spine; any force that is posterior to the spine exerts an *extension moment* (Figure 29-18). Flexion moments include the *center of gravity* (the vertical displacement of the center of mass onto the ground). In older adults, this flexion moment often is increased because of the flexed posture they assume (see Figure 29-17, *B*). An increase in thoracic kyphosis (spinal flexion) increases the distance that the force acts on the spine.

The extensor muscles act to counteract the flexion moment. A patient with weak extensors has difficulty counteracting the flexion. Additional *stress* (a force exerted when one body or body part presses on, pulls on, pushes against, or tends to compress or twist another body or body part) or an increase in the flexor moment caused by asking these patients to participate in physical activities that increase flexion is contraindicated or requires a strong caution because these activities may increase the risk of anterior compression fractures and wedging of vertebral bodies. Flexion therefore is contraindicated in those with osteoporosis who have sustained a fracture and in those who have

not had a fracture but have a BMD T score of −2.5 or lower. Flexion is not recommended in those who show height loss and postural change but no current symptoms. Individuals who have not had a BMD test and who do not have signs or symptoms of osteoporosis can perform flexion, although clinicians should use discretion and appropriate judgment about which movements are safe. Spinal rotation and side bending are also cautioned against, although not as strongly as flexion, for the same groupings (Table 29-4).[80-82]

Primary Prevention

Bone density increases dramatically in the early years of childhood and adolescence. Once bone mass peaks, it is extremely difficult to increase bone mass further. However, the consequences of insufficient bone mass are not seen until old age, when levels become so low as to result in fractures. Consequently, osteoporosis is not a disease of old age, but a pediatric disease that does not manifest itself until old age.[83] Therefore the target population for prevention should be premenarcheal and young premenopausal women and young

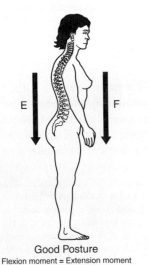
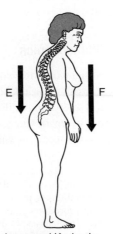
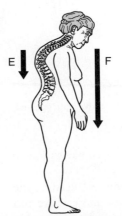
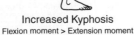

Good Posture
Flexion moment = Extension moment

Increased Kyphosis
Flexion moment > Extension moment

Significantly Increased Kyphosis
Flexion moment >> Extension moment

Figure 29-18

Changes in flexor and extensor moments of the thoracic spine with progressive increases in thoracic kyphosis. As the kyphosis increases, the flexor moment increases. The increase in flexor moment requires an equally large extensor moment to reduce force through the anterior part of the vertebral bodies. *E,* Extensor moment; *F,* flexor moment.

Table 29-4

Contraindications to Spinal Flexion Based on Bone Mineral Density Score

Bone Mineral Density Score	Spinal Flexion
T score of −2.5 or lower	Contraindicated
T score of −1 to −2.5	Not recommended; clinical judgment required
No bone mineral density (BMD) results available, but height loss, vertebral fracture, and kyphosis are present	Contraindicated

boys. Prevention is paramount. The goal of prevention is to maximize bone mass and bone mineral density. (Although density is "the mass of a substance per unit volume," [Merriam-Webster] and mass is "a measure of the amount of a material," the terms *bone mass* and *bone mineral density* often are used interchangeably.)

Exactly when bone mass peaks is the subject of debate; the suggested age ranges from middle to late teens[84-86] to the 20s.[87-89] However, according to Huijbregts et al.,[90] by the time girls are 12 years old, they have already achieved 80% of their adult BMD, and by the time boys have reached age 19 to 20, they have acquired 95% of their peak bone mass. Regardless of when peak bone mass is reached, it generally is agreed that the key ages for laying down bone mass are 11 to 16 in girls and a few years later in boys.[91] Genetics accounts for 70% of the variation seen in peak bone mass. However, strong support exists for the effect of three environmental factors on bone mass: habitual physical exercise, nutrition, and reproductive hormone status.[92]

Key Ages for Laying Down Bone Mass

- Girls: 11 to 16 years
- Boys: 13 to 18 years

Factors that Affect Bone Mass

- Physical activity
- Nutrition
- Reproductive hormone status

What are the roles of the various clinicians who focus on rehabilitation? A critical primary consideration is to educate patients and the public about the importance of exercise and appropriate nutrition for young children and adolescents. Research shows that in both children and adolescents, regular physical activity is directly related to increases in BMD[93-97] and to permanent increases in cross sectional areas of trained skeletal regions.[98,99] The only caveat is that the intensity of the exercise must not be so high as to cause the cessation of menses in females, which can lead to a decrease in BMD. This can be seen in the case of the female athlete triad, in which high level female athletes demonstrate disordered eating, amenorrhea, and osteoporosis. These three symptoms can lead to stress fractures caused by the premature bone loss. Appropriate nutrition also is vital; regular exercise combined with a sufficient intake of calcium can increase bone mass in adolescents.[93,100] A positive relationship exists between protein intake and bone mass gained during pubertal maturation.[84] Carbonated drinks are a significant risk factor for bone fractures, even after adjustments for age, weight, height, activity level, and total caloric intake in adults age 21 to 80.[101,102]

Female Athlete Triad

- Eating disorder
- Amenorrhea
- Osteoporosis

These factors can be discussed directly with children and adolescents and their parents, regardless of the reason the patient seeks therapy. Clinicians also should consider discussing the topic with any adult patient who has children or grandchildren. To be effective, education needs to be ongoing and aimed at various audiences. The settings and possibilities for education are many and varied.

Assessment of the Adult with Osteoporosis

Current and Past Medical History

Various factors that increase an individual's risk for osteoporosis were outlined in the previous section. Questions concerning these factors should be included in the past medical history form and discussed during the patient interview. Results of a BMD test are extremely helpful in guiding treatment. Clinicians also should keep in mind that a family history of a maternal hip fracture doubles the patient's risk for a hip fracture, regardless of current BMD levels.[28] Individuals with a vertebral compression fracture have a 15% higher mortality rate than those who do not experience fractures, and most compression fractures occur at T8–T12, L1, and L4.[77] Figure 29-19 presents a decision tree to help guide intervention.[103]

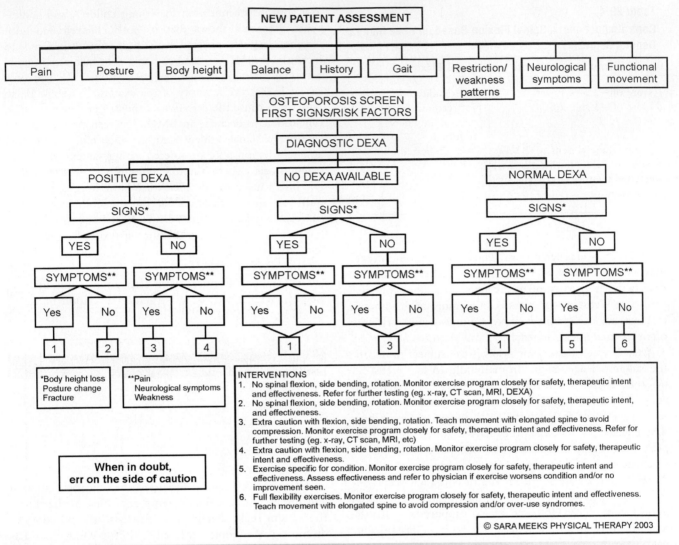

Figure 29-19
Decision tree for improved screening of patients for osteoporosis. (Modified from Meeks SM: The role of the physical therapist in the recognition, assessment, and exercise intervention in persons with, or at risk for, osteoporosis, *Topics Geriatr Rehab* 21:45, 2005.)

Examination. The objective examination can include tests and measures of height and weight, vision, cognition, posture, range of motion (ROM), strength, flexibility, balance, gait, and sensation, depending on the specific diagnosis. All these factors have the potential to contribute to falls; also, the findings provide a baseline measure before therapy is started and help guide the treatment plan. The following list is intended to guide the selection of specific tests and measures for patients with osteoporosis or to alert the clinician to factors to consider if these tests and measures are administered to individuals who may have osteoporosis or osteopenia but have been referred for an unrelated diagnosis. All measures should be as objective as possible.

Components of Examination for Osteoporosis

- Height and weight
- Vision
- Cognition
- Posture
- Range of motion
- Strength
- Flexibility
- Balance
- Gait
- Sensation

Height and Weight. Patients should be assessed standing without shoes. Regular measurement of height is important, because loss of height is one of the first signs of osteoporosis. A loss greater than 6 cm (2.4 inches) in those over age 60 and greater than 4 cm (1.6 inches) in those under age 60 suggests a vertebral fracture.[104] The current measurement is compared to the patient's recall of his or her tallest height.

Vision. Poor vision or visual field deficits can contribute to falls. Patients should be instructed to track the clinician's finger in all directions without moving the head to check for visual field deficits.

Cognition. The Beck Depression Inventory[105] can alert the clinician to possible depression, which may lead to decreased social interaction and physical activity, which can contribute to falls. Checking for orientation to time, place, and year can alert the clinician to overall cognitive status; if decreased, the patient may have difficulty following directions or in performing a home exercise program.

Posture. A photograph of the patient taken from the side and front (after receiving signed consent) allows the clinician to educate the patient about posture and demonstrate changes between specific follow-up evaluations and sessions. For repeatability, the patient should wear the same clothes each time a photograph is taken. A flexicurve can be used to measure the curves of the spine (http://www.umshp.org/pt/geritool). For cervical or thoracic deformity, the patient should be instructed to stand with the heels and buttocks against the wall, the head level, and the distance between the mastoid process and the wall should be measured in centimeters.[106]

Range of Motion. Regardless of which joints need to be measured, precautions for spinal motion should be followed, depending on the patient's BMD tests results and/or clinical presentation, as outlined under Spinal Biomechanics.

Strength. Key muscles include the trunk extensors, hip abductors (crucial to lateral balance control), and gastrosoleus (important for balance reactions). For very frail patients, the clinician must keep in mind that traditional manual muscle testing of the extremities requires stabilization at the trunk, which may be difficult or painful. For patients who can lie prone, trunk extensor endurance can be measured by placing a pillow under the pelvis and having the patient hold the sternum off a plinth for up to 20 seconds.[107] A 1 repetition maximum (1 RM) or 10 RM is another option for those who are not as frail. Trunk extensor endurance is more important than pure strength when these muscles are used for maintaining upright posture.

Balance/Gait. A standardized assessment, such as the Berg Balance Scale,[108,109] Tinetti Performance Oriented Mobility Assessment,[110] Activities-Specific Balance Scale,[111] or Dynamic Gait Index,[112,113] can be used to determine the fall risk and specific activities that are difficult for the patient.

Sensation. Tests of sensation, especially of the feet, may reveal changes in perception than can contribute to falls.

Functional Assessment. The Osteoporosis Functional Disability Questionnaire[114] can be used to establish the level of disability, which can aid goal setting. Pain can be assessed with the Visual Analog Scale. Repeating these tests and measures during reassessments provides solid, objective documentation of the patient's progress and response to the intervention program.

Intervention

Intervention for patients who have sustained a hip or Colles' fracture as a result of a fall will differ from those who have sustained vertebral fractures. Rehabilitation after a hip fracture or Colles' fractures should address impairments in lower or upper extremity strength and endurance, disturbances in balance, and gait impairments. Additional emphasis should be placed on education aimed at preventing further falls and establishing an appropriate exercise program for the patient to follow after discharge from physical therapy. (Additional detail about these diagnoses can be found in other sources.)

Based on the impairments uncovered, intervention for those who have sustained a vertebral fracture can be directed at reducing pain; improving posture, balance, strength, and flexibility/ROM; and patient education. Most of these interventions can be addressed by designing a comprehensive exercise program for the patient. A significant amount of research supports the use of a weight-bearing exercise program in older adults. Less research has been done on the value of such a program for adults with osteoporosis. In both cases, however, evidence exists of a carryover of benefits, including improved balance and a reduction in the number of falls.

General Principles of Exercise Intervention

Bone responds to force in a predictable manner, as described by Wolff's Law, which is the principle that every change in the form and function of a bone or in the function of the bone alone leads to changes in its internal architecture and in its external form. Bone is deposited and resorbed in accordance with the stresses placed upon it. Wolff's Law works not only through weight bearing through gravity (e.g., walking/running transmits forces through the limbs and results in increased BMD in the hip and lumbar spine) but also through the pull from tendons on bones that occurs when a muscle produces force. Hence, increases in strength through weight training or muscle contractions that are not directly in a weight-bearing position or are in a gravity-reduced or gravity-eliminated position (e.g., supine scapular retraction) cause increased force on the bone and result in increases in bone modeling. This law works both ways, however; in response to increased loads through weight training, for example, the bone responds by increasing its mass; however, once the exercise is stopped, the bone responds again by decreasing its mass, because the stress is no longer being applied.

Therefore an exercise intervention program must be continuous for the effects to be maintained.

The exercise also must follow other well-known principles of training, which many clinicians tend to forget when working with an older population. The exercise must be intense enough to challenge the system to adapt based on Wolff's Law, but not so intense as to cause a fracture. Unfortunately, there is no research to call upon regarding dose-response relationships to exercise; therefore no easy method is available to make this determination except clinical judgment. The fracture point of any bone is determined by its current BMD, the forces applied to the bone, and the moment caused by that force (the location of the application of the force; e.g., 2.3 kg [5 lbs] in the hand creates a greater moment at the shoulder than 2.3 kg [5 lbs] at the elbow). An adult with good posture who has a normal BMD can perform exercises that increase the flexion force on the spine, such as abdominal crunches, without risk of vertebral fracture. This is because the moment arm is small (see Figure 29-18), and the force is at a level the normal bone can tolerate. However, if a patient has osteoporosis and presents with a significant kyphosis (see Figure 29-18), the same exercise could result in an anterior vertebral fracture. In this case, the moment is much larger and the bones lack the BMD to withstand this amount of force.

The exercise intervention must also be specific to the anatomical site and varied so that the system continues to adapt and improve. If strengthening the back extensors is the goal, the clinician must ensure that the exercises prescribed specifically strengthen the extensors. In addition, the frequency and intensity of the exercise, as well as the manner in which the bone and muscle are used, must be varied so that they can adapt appropriately. For example, performing 10 repetitions of standing hip abduction against the resistance of light elastic bands or tubing 3 times a week for an entire month is not enough of a varied stimulus to achieve gains in bone or muscle. The intensity and/or frequency must be increased, and other exercises aimed at strengthening the same muscle must be incorporated into the treatment program.

Basic Principles of Osteoporosis Exercise Training

- Intensity must be sufficient to challenge the system
- Exercise must be specific to the anatomical site
- Exercise must be varied so that the system can continue to adapt

---

Effects of Exercise on the Skeleton

How do clinicians know that weight-bearing exercises are effective for adults with osteoporosis? This knowledge is based on the substantial evidence that elite athletes and long-term exercisers have greater bone mass and BMD at sites that undergo mechanical loading during exercise than age-matched sedentary individuals.[115-117] For example, runners age 50 to 72 have approximately 40% greater vertebral trabecular bone density than nonrunners.[116] Both male and female recreational and world-class weight lifters age 20 to 40 have 10% to 35% greater lumbar spine BMD[118-120] and vertebral trabecular bone density than controls.[121,122]

Effects of Exercise in Postmenopausal Women and Osteoporosis

Because women are much more likely to develop osteoporosis than men, most of the research on the effects of exercise in osteoporosis have included only women. In addition, much more research has been conducted on postmenopausal women than on postmenopausal women with osteoporosis. In postmenopausal women, Nelson et al.[123] found a reduced loss of trabecular bone density in the lumbar spine after a 1 year walking program. In their study, Chow et al.[124] used a control group, an aerobic exercise group, and an aerobic exercise plus weight training group. The two exercise groups were followed three times a week for 1 year. At the end of the study, both groups demonstrated a 4% to 8% increase in bone mass, whereas the control group had a 1.1% loss.

In a study involving postmenopausal women with osteoporosis, Krolner et al.[125] had women age 50 to 73 who had had a previous Colles' fracture participate in 8 months of aerobic exercise. The exercise group showed a 3.5% increase in lumbar BMD, whereas the control group showed a 2.5% decrease. Chow et al.[126] designed an exercise program to improve functional capacity and provide social interaction through 30 minutes of aerobic exercise, such as dance or walking, and 30 minutes of strength training performed at low loads with high (10 to 30) repetitions. After 2 years of three times weekly exercise, the exercise group demonstrated significantly fewer vertebral fractures than the control group: three of 53 women in the exercise group suffered fractures, compared to seven of 37 women in the control group.

Exercise has also been shown to be effective in the treatment of vertebral fractures and in increasing back extensor strength. Sinaki and Mikkelsen[81] studied women who had sustained a vertebral compression fracture. They found that resistance exercises to strengthen the back extensors led to a reduction in new fractures compared to controls, whereas exercises that strengthened the back flexors led to an increase in vertebral deformities.

Some of the most compelling research on the importance of back extensor strength was done by Sinaki et al.,[82] who performed a 10-year prospective study of the effects of back extensor strengthening on postmenopausal women. In their study, 65 women age 48 to 65 who were healthy, nonsmoking, and Caucasian and who did not participate in hormone replacement therapy (HRT) were randomized into a back exercise group or a control group. The exercise group wore a backpack containing weight equal to 30% of their maximum isometric back extensor strength and lifted the weight 10 times while prone. This was performed daily, 5 days a week. The weight was increased, but not to more than 22.7 kg (50 lbs). Every 4 weeks, muscle strength and physical activity were assessed, and proper lifting and good posture were reviewed with the subjects. After 2 years the exercise group discontinued the exercise, and the subjects were not monitored. Eight years later, the subjects were re-evaluated; 27 of the exercise group and 23 of the control group returned. Follow-up testing revealed more vertebral fractures in the control group than in the exercise group (30% versus 11% of subjects), a decrease in back extensor strength from baseline in both groups (16.5% in the exercise group and 27% in the controls), and significantly greater BMD of the spine in the exercise group.

Studies have shown that an increase in relative spinal extensor strength can lead to reduced thoracic kyphosis, fewer vertebral fractures, and less loss of height and anterior rib cage pain,[127-129] as well as to decreased pain, increased mobility, and overall improvement of quality of life.[130]

Key Points in the Treatment of Osteoporosis

- Exercise intervention in older adults with osteoporosis may not increase bone mineral density (BMD), but it can slow age-related loss of BMD
- Flexion is contraindicated in adults with osteoporosis and a low BMD score
- Strengthening of the back extensors is critical
- Osteoporosis is a childhood disease that does not manifest until old age; prevention is paramount

---

Even in light of the convincing evidence of the positive effects of increased trunk extensor strength, implementing extensor strengthening can be difficult in older adults. By the time they are seen for treatment, many of these patients have an increased thoracic kyphosis and a forward head that make even lying supine difficult. These postural deviations, along with decreased shoulder flexibility and decreased cervical rotation, can also make lying prone difficult, if not impossible. Starting in the supine position with pillows used as needed to support the flexed spine is a better idea. Initial treatments may be as basic as emphasizing attempts at lying supine with slowly decreasing support as the spine gently lengthens and extends so that the patient can eventually lie with one or no pillows under the head. This may not be a possibility for some patients because of long-standing bony deformities. Once a comfortable, lengthened, and extended supine position has been achieved, gentle cervical and thoracic extension can be initiated through isometrics, such as pushing the back of the head and the shoulders into a plinth. A comprehensive extension and postural re-education program designed specifically for this population is presented in *Walk Tall!* by Sara Meeks.[131] The book includes diagrams for each exercise and is spiral bound, making it easy to follow. Sitting is also a good option if the patient cannot tolerate the supine position. However,

the proprioceptive feedback from the plinth can help the patient maintain elongation in the spine, as opposed to tilting the head up, and also let the person know how far forward the head and/or shoulders are.

If the patient can tolerate lying prone, various extension exercises can be performed (Figure 29-20). These include arm and leg lifts, with the arms at the side, out to the side, or overhead. Combinations of arms only, legs only, or ipsilateral and contralateral arm and leg can all be used. Because these exercises can be difficult, the clinician should start with one extremity only and progress to alternating the same extremity. The last step in the progression should be extension of all four extremities together or alternating arm and leg extension, which can be difficult for patients to coordinate. For those who are familiar with yoga and have patients who practice it, poses such as the cobra and locust may be familiar (Figure 29-21). Patients are instructed to think of extending and lengthening through the extremities as they lift to promote elongation of the spine and to avoid compressing the back.

Older adults who tend toward a flexed posture likely have tight hip flexors, hamstrings, quadriceps, and calf muscles as well. These muscles all need to be stretched as the clinician works on gaining extension and length throughout the spine. The same difficulties in positioning need to be addressed to stretch the lower extremities as had to be addressed in working on spinal extension (e.g., supine with pillows under the head and progressing to fewer or no pillows). Positioning in side lying can be a good way for the clinician to stretch the quadriceps and hip flexors manually.

Compression Fractures

The primary goal of treatment for patients with vertebral fractures is the same for those without fractures: getting to a point where the patient can tolerate extension exercises. Initially, intervention is likely to focus on addressing pain, instructing the patient in proper body mechanics for transfers, and perhaps fitting the patient with a corset or lumbosacral orthosis.[132,133]

Fall Prevention

Because more than 90% of hip fractures occur as a direct result of a fall,[92] and two thirds of those who sustain a hip fracture do not return to their premorbid functional level,[134] a comprehensive treatment program for patients with osteopenia or osteoporosis must include interventions designed to prevent or reduce the likelihood of falling. Inactivity and low physical activity levels, reduced muscle strength, and hyperkyphosis all have been shown to be risk factors for falling and hip fracture.[128,132,133,135-138] Conversely, a large body of research has shown that higher physical activity levels and greater strength lower the risk of falling and subsequent fractures in both women and men.[78,135,139-144] Clinicians can best address the risk of falling by stressing the importance of increased physical

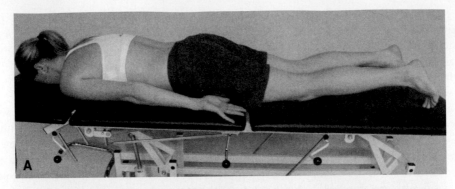

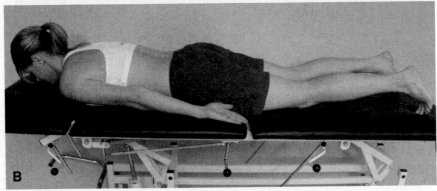

Figure 29-20

Upper back lift. This intermediate exercise strengthens the back muscles. **A,** The patient lies face down on the plinth with a pillow under the hips and lower part of the abdomen. A rolled towel may be used to cushion the forehead. Keeping the arms at the sides and the head in line with the neck and torso, the patient tightens the abdominal muscles. The individual must focus on keeping the shoulders down so that they do not shrug up toward the ears. **B,** The patient inhales and raises the head and chest a few inches off the plinth. Breathing normally, the patient holds this position for 5 seconds and then returns to the starting position. The patient rests for a few seconds and then repeats this exercise 5 to 10 times, as the person is able.

activity, even if the activity is not enough to increase strength in a very frail individual; they also can emphasize strengthening exercises for the muscle groups most likely to help improve balance, such as the hip abductors, hip extensors, and calf musculature, which are important in righting reactions. Clinicians should search for group or community programs in which patients can enroll if possible. This type of community and peer support may increase the likelihood of follow-through after discharge, as well as improve the patient's social interactions, which also makes carryover more probable. Clinicians must keep in mind that strengthening exercises need to be of sufficient intensity to achieve strength gains. Performing a 1 RM or a 10 RM test for lower extremity muscles can guide selection of the appropriate weight. Strength gains have been found in older adults with either increases in resistance or increases in repetitions;[145,146] gains in functional abilities have also been found with regimens that vary from 1 to 3 times a week.[146]

Other areas that must be addressed to reduce the risk of falls include vision; ROM limitations; the home setting (e.g., lighting, throw rugs, small pets underfoot); cognition;

a previous history of falling, which that may lead to fear of falls; co-morbidities; and medication use.

Surgical Management of Vertebral Fractures

Kyphoplasty

Kyphoplasty is a relatively new surgical procedure that can be performed on an outpatient basis to treat vertebral compression fractures (Figure 29-22). With the patient lying prone under local or general anesthesia, the surgeon inserts a tube into the collapsed vertebra. A balloon is passed through the tube and inflated to restore height to the spine and correct the kyphosis. The balloon is then removed, leaving space for the injection of cement. Vertebroplasty is a similar procedure in which the cement is injected but the balloon is not used to expand the vertebra.

Because kyphoplasty (and vertebroplasty) are such new procedures, no randomized, controlled trials are available on their efficacy. Because of the quick recovery and reduction in pain so often seen after the surgery, physicians have difficulty finding patients willing to be randomized

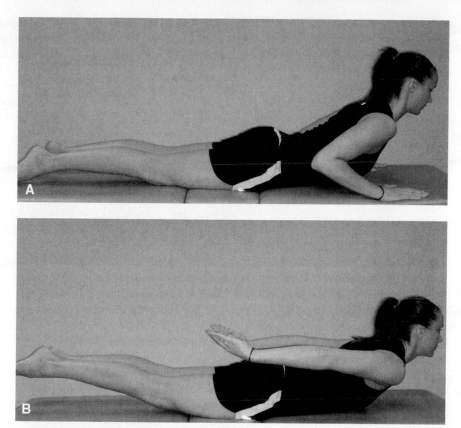

Figure 29-21

Yoga poses. **A,** Cobra pose. **B,** Locust pose.

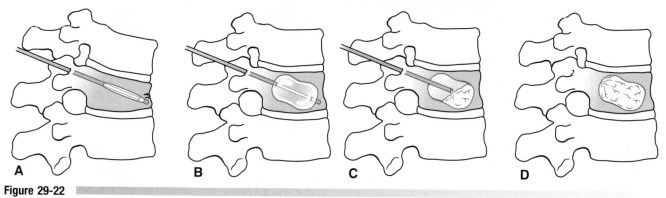

Figure 29-22

Kyphoplasty. **A,** Balloon tamp in place. **B,** Balloon tamp inflated and collapsed vertebral bone restored to near normal height. **C,** Cavity being filled with cement. **D,** Cavity completely filled with cement.

into a placebo group. However, the procedure is not without concerns. Because osteoporotic bone is a low density material, placement of a high density material, such as cement, adjacent to these vertebrae alters the biomechanical relationship between them and changes the transfer and absorption of forces. In a retrospective study of 38 patients, Fribourg et al.[147] found that 10 of these patients sustained an additional 17 fractures. Eight patients had a second fracture within 2 months of the procedure, and all had at least one fracture at an adjacent level. At this time, more research is needed on the

outcomes of this surgical procedure, especially with respect to long-term effects.

Although rehabilitation is not needed to help patients recover from kyphoplasty, these individuals would benefit from treatment to address other issues related to the fracture. They may need to be seen for the same issues that a person without a fracture would require rehabilitation: abnormal posture (increased kyphosis), weakness of the back extensors and lower extremity muscles required for balance, fall prevention and balance training, and education about lifestyle modifications.

Paget's Disease of Bone and Primary Hyperparathyroidism

Physical therapists are extremely unlikely to see patients referred with either PDB or primary hyperparathyroidism as a primary diagnosis. However, both conditions can result in osteopenia and osteoporosis and are therefore included to alert the clinician to other diagnoses that must be considered in the overall treatment of patients and to present some basic information about epidemiology, signs, and symptoms to facilitate proper diagnosis.

Paget's Disease of Bone

PDB is the most common bone disorder after osteoporosis. It affects approximately 3% of people in the United States over age 50 and 10% of those over age 80.[148] PDB is most common in the United Kingdom and in those of European descent; it is uncommon in Africans and Asians. This disease is often asymptomatic and is discovered incidentally through radiographs or an increase in serum alkaline phosphatase activity.[149] Bone pain is the most common symptom of the disease. Physical therapists may never see these patients, because medical intervention (e.g., a course of bisphosphonates) is very effective in reducing the bone pain, and this reduction can last for years after cessation of the medication.[148]

Because of the structural weakness of pagetic bone, the most common complications are pain, structural deformity, and fracture. If a diagnosis of PDB has not been made in an individual presenting for rehabilitation, specific physical symptoms can alert the clinician to this diagnosis.

Symptoms of Paget's Disease

- Bone pain from microfractures or osteoarthritis
- Bowing of a limb
- Thoracic kyphosis
- Loss of hearing
- Neurological symptoms from nerve compression caused by bone growth
- Spinal stenosis

The bone pain reported by patients with PDB can be distinguished from pain caused by osteoarthritis because the pain increases with rest, with weight bearing, when the limbs are warm, and at night. It is continuous and reported to be a dull, boring pain.[148] Rehabilitation is aimed primarily at reducing pain through the use of electrical stimulation or other physical agents, aquatic exercise, or land-based exercises that do not put stress on the affected bone or bones. In the case of fracture resulting from PDB, healing is slow because of the altered mechanical structure of the bone itself. Nonunion of fractures in PDB has been reported to be as high as 40%, especially when the fracture involves the proximal femur.[150,151] In addition, increased weight bearing through the bone, which stimulates bone growth and remodeling in healthy individuals, is a less effective process in individuals with PDB. Osteoarthritis secondary to Paget's disease eventually may require a total joint replacement or tibial osteotomy. Exercise intervention for those requiring joint replacement should take into consideration other lesions or areas affected by the disease that may require modification of traditional intervention so as to not cause fracture at another site. Also, as with fractures that are not treated surgically, rehabilitation will be extended because of the abnormalities of the bone structure. Other potential rehabilitation interventions include bracing for structural abnormalities (e.g., bowing of the lower limb) in attempts to realign the bones to provide for proper weight bearing; correction for leg length differences that may also result from bony deformities; and bracing for the spine in the case of spontaneous compression fractures resulting from unstable bone.

The key point that clinicians should remember with individuals with PDB, whether they are being treated for complications of the disease or for other diagnoses, is that the bone remodeling process in the affected areas is abnormal and produces a weak bone structure that is susceptible to fracture. Treatment of those who have undergone orthopedic surgery to repair fractures will likely be extended compared to those with normal bone status.

Primary Hyperparathyroidism

The function of the parathyroid glands is to maintain serum calcium concentrations and to regulate bone metabolism. In primary hyperparathyroidism, overproduction of PTH results in an increase in the release of calcium from the bones and into the blood. Hyperparathyroidism increases bone breakdown and replaces bone with fibrous tissue, resulting in generalized bone demineralization, resorption, and pathological fractures. Women are affected two to three times more often than men, and the average age at diagnosis is 55 years. Patients usually are asymptomatic, although they may have nonspecific back pain; those with symptomatic bone disease account for only 10% to 25% of patients.[152] BMD loss is greater in cortical bone (e.g., the forearm) than in trabecular bone (e.g., the spine) or in mixed cortical and trabecular bone (e.g., the hip).

Other than bone pain, symptoms can include thirst, generalized weakness, osteoporosis, kidney stones, polyuria, and constipation. In it severest form, pathological fractures occur as a result of advanced osteoporosis. However, it is extremely uncommon nowadays for the disease to progress to an advanced stage without being recognized during routine laboratory work.

For clinicians, the primary consideration in hyperparathyroidism is that osteoporosis at a relatively young age (around 55 years) should serve as a warning of the possibility of this condition.

References

To enhance this text and add value for the reader, all references have been incorporated into a CD-ROM that is provided with this text. The reader can view the reference source and access it online whenever possible. There are a total of 152 references for this chapter.

Other Resources

International Osteoporosis Foundation: http://www.osteofound.org/.

Medline Plus (search for osteoporosis): http://www.nlm.nih.gov/medlineplus/osteoporosis.html

National Osteoporosis Foundation: www.nof.org

National Institutes of Health, Milk Matters Campaign aimed at children: http://www.nichd.nih.gov/milk/milk.cfm

Osteoporosis Canada: http://www.osteoporosis.ca/english/home/default.asp?s=1

U.S. Bone and Joint Decade: http://www.usbjd.org/index.cfm

CHAPTER 30

MUSCLE DISEASE AND DYSFUNCTION

Ann-Marie Thomas and Walter R. Frontera

Muscular Dystrophies

The muscular dystrophies comprise a hereditary group of disorders arising from various genetic defects that alter the structure and function of a range of muscle proteins (Table 30-1).

Dystrophinopathies: Duchenne's Muscular Dystrophy and Becker's Muscular Dystrophy

Genetics/Epidemiology

Duchenne's muscular dystrophy (DMD) (also known as *pseudohypertrophic muscular dystrophy* or *pseudohypertrophic paralysis*) and Becker's muscular dystrophy (BMD) share a defect in the muscle protein dystrophin and an X-linked recessive mode of inheritance linked to a frame-shift mutation or a new mutation in the Xp21 gene locus.[1] DMD is characterized by severely reduced or absent dystrophin, whereas BMD involves a milder dystrophinopathy with decreased or altered dystrophin. Both conditions primarily affect young males. The incidence of DMD is 1 in 3300 male births worldwide, and the incidence of BMD is 1 in 14,000-31,000.[2]

Dystrophin is a key component of the sarcolemmal region of skeletal and cardiac muscle membranes. A deficiency of dystrophin leads to muscle membrane instability during contraction and relaxation (Figure 30-1).

Clinical Features: Duchenne's Muscular Dystrophy

At birth most male children with DMD appear normal. Subsequently, they show delayed milestones, especially with walking, running, jumping, and climbing stairs. The disorder has a characteristic pattern of progressive weakness and consequent functional decline. Proximal lower limb muscles, such as the hip extensors, usually are affected earlier than upper extremity and torso muscles; neck flexors are affected more than extensors, and progression is more rapid in the lower extremities than in the upper extremities.

Relative preservation is seen in the ankle plantar flexors and invertors, levator ani, external anal sphincter, and cranial nerve–innervated muscles except for the sternocleidomastoid.[2] By age 3 to 6, most boys have developed a wide-based, waddling gait and fall frequently. They also develop lumbar lordosis and use the characteristic Gower's maneuver (Figure 30-2) to rise from the floor.[2,3] By age 5 to 6, hypertrophy and sometimes pain develop in certain muscle groups, especially the calves, quadriceps, gluteals, and deltoids. Initially true hypertrophy of the calf muscle fibers occurs, but later pseudohypertrophy develops because muscle is largely replaced by fat and connective tissue (Figure 30-3).[3] By age 8, the child has difficulty with ambulation and climbing stairs, and by age 10, many patients depend on long leg braces to remain ambulatory; by age 12, most are wheelchair dependent. Bakker et al.[4] identified loss of hip extensor and ankle dorsiflexor strength as primary predictors of loss of ambulation.

Joint contractures and scoliosis occur frequently in DMD. By age 6 to 10, 70% of patients may have contractures of the iliotibial bands, hip flexors, and Achilles tendons. Ankle involvement can lead to toe walking. By age 8, most patients may also have contractures at the knee, elbow, and wrist extensors, which tend to worsen as the child spends more time in the wheelchair. Scoliosis may be seen in up to 90% of wheelchair-bound patients with DMD. As paraspinal muscles weaken, kyphoscoliosis worsens. This can complicate activities of daily living (ADLs) and positioning in bed or a wheelchair.

A more serious complication of kyphoscoliosis is respiratory impairment. Respiratory muscles usually are not significantly involved until the child becomes nonambulatory.[3] Respiratory muscle weakness, including the diaphragm and intercostals, is manifested by low maximum inspiratory and expiratory pressures and decreased vital capacity, forced vital capacity, and total lung capacity.[2] A restrictive defect results, with or without the previously mentioned scoliosis, and respiratory function becomes compromised.[5] Respiratory muscle

Table 30-1
Overview of the Muscular Dystrophies

Type	Mode of Inheritance/Gene Location/Gene Product	Clinical Presentation	Associated Features	Diagnosis	Treatment
Duchenne's muscular dystrophy (DMD)	XR Xp21 Dystrophin	Onset: Before age 5 Delayed milestones Progressive weakness of girdle muscles Calf hypertrophy Inability to walk after age 12 Joint contractures Scoliosis	Respiratory failure in 2nd to 3rd decade Cardiomyopathy Impaired intellectual function Acute gastric dilation	Clinical Increased CK EMG: Myopathic Muscle biopsy, dystrophin analysis DNA analysis	Pharmacological: Steroids Rehabilitative: PT/OT, ROM, contracture management, assistive devices, weight control, ambulation, seating, bracing Pulmonary: Assisted ventilation Surgical: Contracture release, spinal stabilization for scoliosis
Becker's muscular dystrophy	XR Xp21 Dystrophin	Onset: After age 5 Progressive weakness of girdle muscles Calf hypertrophy Inability to walk after age 15 Respiratory failure after 4th decade	Cardiomyopathy Impaired intellectual functioning	As in DMD	As in DMD
Facioscapulo-humeral muscular dystrophy	AD 4q35 Unknown	Onset: 1st to 5th decade Slowly progressive weakness of the face, shoulder girdle, scapular stabilizers, anterior leg	Pain in the neck, shoulders, Posterior chest, lower back Mild sensorineural hearing loss Retinal abnormalities Subclinical cardiomyopathy	Clinical CK: Normal/slightly elevated EMG: Myopathic Muscle bx: Necrotic fibers Variable inflammation DNA analysis	Pharmacological: None Rehabilitative: PT, OT, pain management Surgical: Scapular stabilization
Emery-Dreifuss muscular dystrophy	XR Xq28 Emerin AD 1q11 Lamin A/C	Triad 1. Early contractures 2. Slowly progressive muscle weakness in humeroperoneal distribution 3. Cardiac abnormalities	Increased resting energy expenditure	Clinical CK: Normal/slightly increased. ECG: Bradycardia, conduction block EDX: Myopathic Muscle bx: Immunochemistry shows absent emerin DNA analysis	Pharmacological: None Cardiac evaluations Rehabilitative: Contracture management Surgical: Contracture release Other: Increase caloric intake

(Continued)

Table 30-1
Overview of the Muscular Dystrophies—Cont'd

Type	Mode of Inheritance/Gene Location/Gene Product	Clinical Presentation	Associated Features	Diagnosis	Treatment
Limb-girdle muscular dystrophy	AD(6)/AR(10) Multiple Multiple	Onset: Childhood to adulthood Slowly progressive muscle weakness in pelvic girdle and lower limb Cardiac abnormalities (10%) Onset: Late childhood to adolescence	Respiratory insufficiency	Clinical, family history CK: Elevated EDX: Myopathic Muscle bx: Necrosis and regeneration, variable fiber size, increased connective tissue DNA analysis	Pharmacological: >Creatine monohydrate Cardiac monitoring Rehabilitative: PT, OT to maintain mobility, minimize contractures, provide assistive devices Ventilatory support
Myotonic muscular dystrophy	AD 19q13 Myotonic dystrophy Protein kinase	Onset: Any age Slowly progressive muscle weakness in face, distal limb Percussion myotonia	Cataracts, cardiac abnormalities, respiratory abnormalities, gastrointestinal abnormalities, CNS abnormalities, endocrine abnormalities	Clinical EDX: Myotonic discharges Muscle bx: Myopathic DNA analysis	Pharmacological: Medications for myotonia Rehabilitative: PT, OT for contracture management, assistive devices, modification of ADLs

AD, Autosomal dominant; *ADLs,* activities of daily living; *AR,* autosomal recessive; *bx,* biopsy; *CK,* creatine kinase; *CNS,* central nervous system; *DNA,* deoxyribonucleic acid; *ECG,* electrocardiography; *EDX,* electrodiagnostics; *EMG,* electromyography; *In↑,* increased; *OT,* occupational therapy; *PT,* physical therapy; *ROM,* range of motion; *XR,* X-linked recessive.

DMD: Etiology and Pathology

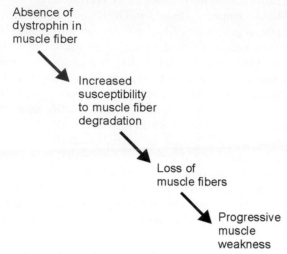

Figure 30-1
Dystrophin dysfunction.

weakness can also contribute to atelectasis and reduced thoracic compliance. Diaphragmatic weakness can contribute to nocturnal hypoxemia, hypoventilation, and hypercapnic respiratory failure.[5] Without aggressive pulmonary management,

respiratory insufficiency, with or without pneumonia, may result in death by age 20.[6] The age at which vital capacity falls below 1 L has been found to be a strong marker of mortality, with a 5-year survival rate of 8%.[7,8]

Dystrophin is also a component of cardiac muscle, smooth muscle, and brain. Therefore the heart, gastrointestinal (GI) tract, and central nervous system (CNS) may manifest abnormalities. Up to 90% of patients with DMD may show characteristic electrocardiographic abnormalities consisting of tall R waves and deep, narrow Q waves in leads I, aV_L, V_5, and V_6, attributable to fibrosis in the posterobasal left ventricle.[2,9] Other patients may show conduction defects, arrhythmias, sinus tachycardia, or cardiomyopathy.[2,9] Up to 40% of patients with DMD may succumb to cardiomyopathy if they also have ventilatory failure and pulmonary hypertension.[2] GI tract manifestations can include vomiting, abdominal pain, and distension caused by acute gastric dilation.[2,9] CNS involvement may include a lower intelligence quotient (IQ) (i.e., below 70-75) in approximately 20% to 30% of patients.[2,9] Bresolin et al.[10] found the mean IQ of patients with DMD to be 82.

DMD also can affect the skeletal system. Fractures occur in approximately 20% of these patients;[11] they can be caused by falls resulting from unsteady gait or can occur as a result of osteoporosis related to disuse in wheelchair-bound patients. The fractures usually heal normally.[3]

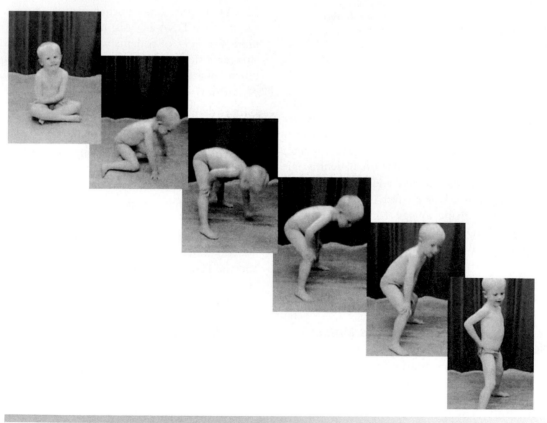

Figure 30-2
A 5-year-old with Duchenne's muscular dystrophy showing the typical Gower's maneuver while rising from the floor. (From Emery AEH, Muntoni F: *Duchenne muscular dystrophy,* ed 3, p 33, New York, 2003, Oxford University Press.)

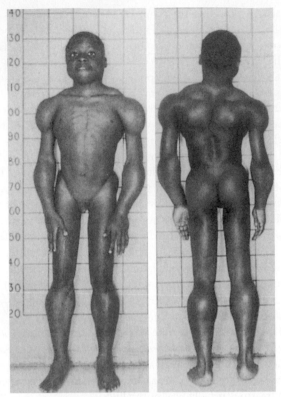

Figure 30-3
Pattern of muscle hypertrophy in Duchenne's muscular dystrophy. (From Emery AEH, Muntoni F: *Duchenne muscular dystrophy,* ed 3, p 31, New York, 2003, Oxford University Press.)

Clinical Features: Becker's Muscular Dystrophy

Patients with BMD show a pattern of muscle weakness and atrophy similar to that seen in DMD. Key differences include a later onset of clinical manifestations (usually after age 5) and the ability to ambulate past age 15.[2,3] Unlike with DMD, early in the course of BMD the patient is able to run, hop, lift the head off the bed, and get up from the floor without using Gower's maneuver.[3] Fifty percent of patients may be symptomatic by age 10 and 90% by age 20.[2] Patients with BMD usually are not wheelchair bound until late adulthood.[3] Respiratory failure usually does not occur until after the 4th decade.[2] Cardiac abnormalities are similar to those seen in DMD.[2,9] The mean age at death in a group of 51 patients with BMD was 42 years.[2]

Diagnosis of Duchenne's and Becker's Muscular Dystrophies

The presenting clinical features contribute to the diagnosis of DMD and BMD. These include a markedly elevated creatine kinase (CK), characteristic findings on muscle biopsy, electromyography (EMG) findings (Table 30-2),[12] and genetic tests. In DMD, CK may be elevated as much as 50 to 100 times normal very early in the course of the disease. It usually peaks by age 3 and falls by approximately 20% each year as a result of muscle loss.[2] In BMD, CK may by elevated 25 to 200 times normal during the first 10 years of life.

Muscle biopsy findings for DMD and BMD include necrosis, regeneration, fiber splitting, abnormal fiber size variation, endomysial and perimysial proliferation of connective tissue, internalized nuclei, and variable inflammatory response.[13] Eventually, muscle fibers are replaced by connective tissue and subsequently by adipose tissue, which results in pseudohypertrophy.[13] Less connective tissue proliferation may be seen in BMD than in DMD.

Motor and nerve conduction studies usually are normal except in extremely affected muscles, which may show a decrease in compound motor action potential.[14] Needle EMG findings show typical myopathic features (see Table 30-2).[12] Single fiber EMG may reveal increased fiber density as a result of fiber splitting, ephaptic (fiber to fiber) conduction, and remodeling of motor units.[14] As the percentage of fat and connective tissue increases, the number of motor units can be severely diminished and some areas of muscle may be electrically silent.

Dystrophin gene analysis can identify deletions and duplications in 60% to 65% of patients with DMD and in an even higher percentage of patients with BMD.[2] The deletions seen in BMD allow for production of some dystrophin.[2,9] Messenger ribonucleic acid (mRNA) analysis can identify mutations missed by deoxyribonucleic acid (DNA) analysis. Immunochemistry is more sensitive and specific than DNA analysis; it can confirm the diagnosis in more than 95% of patients with DMD. Immunochemistry also can differentiate between DMD and BMD.[2] All methods usually are not needed to make a diagnosis. If either disease was confirmed previously by gene or dystrophin protein analysis, a suspected case in the same family can be diagnosed based on clinical features alone.[2]

Treatment of Duchenne's and Becker's Muscular Dystrophies

The management of muscular dystrophies requires a multidisciplinary, multimodality approach to allow the patient and family the greatest quality of life (Figure 30-4).

Pharmacology. A report from the Quality Standards Subcommittee of the American Academy of Neurology and the Practice Committee of the Child Neurology Society reviewed multiple controlled trials that showed that prednisone at a dosage of either 0.75 mg/kg/day or 1.5 mg/kg/day was beneficial for boys with DMD; the lower dose was as effective as the higher dose.[15] Benefits included slowed progression of muscle weakness and increased muscle strength, performance, and pulmonary function.[15] Deflazacort, a prednisone derivative with similar effects, produces less weight gain at a dose of 0.9 mg a day or 2 mg every other day.[2,15,16] Additional controlled trials confirm the benefits of prednisone and deflazacort in prolonging ambulation and maintaining pulmonary function.[17]

Table 30-2

Electrodiagnostic Findings in Myopathies

Parameter	Muscular Dystrophy	Congenital	Metabolic	Inflammatory
DL	Normal	Normal	Normal	Normal
NCV	Normal	Normal	Normal	Normal
H reflex	Normal or absent	Normal or absent	Normal	Normal or absent
SNAP amplitude	Normal	Normal	Normal	Normal
CMAP amplitude	Normal or decreased	Normal or decreased	Decreased or normal	Normal or decreased
MUAP duration	Decreased and/or increased	Decreased or normal	Increased or normal	Increased
MUAP amplitude	Decreased and/or increased	Decreased or normal	Decreased or normal	Decreased and/or increased (IBM)
Polyphasics	Increased	Increased or normal	Increased or normal	Increased
Recruitment	Increased	Increased or normal	Increased or normal	Increased
Fibrillation and PSWs	Yes	Myotubular myopathy	Yes	Yes
CRDs	Yes	Myotubular myopathy	Yes	Yes
Myotonic potentials	Myotonic dystrophy	Myotubular myopathy	Acid maltase deficiency	No
Electrical silence	No	No	Contractures in McArdle's disease	

Modified from Krivickas L: Myopathies. In Tan FC, editor: *EMG secrets*, p 203, Philadelphia, 2004, Hanley & Belfus.
CMAP, Compound muscle action potential; *CRDs*, complex repetitive discharges; *DL*, distal latency; *IBM*, inclusion body myositis; *MUAP*, motor unit action potential; *NCV*, nerve conduction velocity; *PSWs*, positive sharp waves; *SNAP*, sensory nerve action potential.

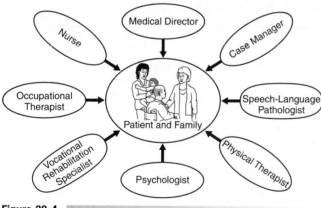

Figure 30-4

Multidisciplinary team.

An evidence-based review of all studies between 1989 and 2001 that used prednisone, deflazacort, or oxandrolone to treat DMD recommended that corticosteroids be started between ages 4 and 7 for the greatest benefit.[18] Common side effects, which may be improved with the lower dose, include irritability, hyperactivity, cushingoid appearance, GI complaints, skin rash, glucose intolerance, hypertension, and cataracts.[15] The patient should be monitored for these side effects, especially with long-term corticosteroid use.[15]

A pilot study suggested that the androgenic anabolic steroid oxandrolone may be beneficial in improving strength and function in DMD.[19] A 6-month randomized, double blind, placebo-controlled trial of oxandrolone to improve strength in DMD showed that this steroid may have some beneficial effect in slowing the progression of muscle weakness. It was suggested that this steroid be started before corticosteroids, because it has a better side effect profile.[20] Further studies are needed to establish the efficacy of oxandrolone in improving strength in neuromuscular disorders such as DMD and BMD. Oxandrolone has been approved by the U.S. Food and Drug Administration (FDA) for weight loss restitution in certain muscle wasting disorders, including DMD and BMD.[21] Additional studies are needed to further establish the effectiveness of this drug in improving strength and function in muscle wasting disorders.

Creatine monohydrate may play a small but significant role in improving muscle strength and performance of ADLs.[22,23] Possible side effects include elevation of transaminases and a decrease in high density lipoproteins (HDLs).[21]

A randomized, double blind, multicenter trial reported that early treatment with perindopril, an angiotensin-converting enzyme (ACE) inhibitor, delayed the onset and progression of prominent left ventricle dysfunction in children with DMD.[24]

Rehabilitation. Rehabilitation offers multiple approaches in the treatment of myopathies, as described by Hicks (Table 30-3).[25] Boys with DMD or BMD should be encouraged to lead active, normal lives during the early

Table 30-3
Rehabilitation Approaches to the Treatment of Myopathies

Approach	Comments
Patient evaluation	
Initial assessment	Needed to assess impairments, stage of illness, and overall disease activity and damage and to gauge responses to therapy
Function	Needed to assess ability to perform physical tasks, interact psychosocially, and communicate to establish level of disability and to follow outcomes of treatment strategies
Quality of life	Needed to assess overall satisfaction with life activities and make treatment recommendations to improve it
Exercise	
Range of motion and stretching	Needed to preserve, maintain, and increase joint motion
Isometric	Needed to increase muscle strength to perform tasks requiring isometric muscle contraction
Isotonic	Needed to increase muscle strength and endurance to perform tasks requiring isotonic muscle contraction
Aerobic	Needed to increase aerobic capacity and improve overall functional level
Recreational	Recommended to improve quality of life and provide socialization and informal exercise
Adaptive thinking	
Educational strategies	Instruction in energy conservation and compliance with exercise is essential
Assistive devices	Assistive devices can raise the individual's functional level from requiring the assistance of a person to independence with assistive devices
Heat and cold	Heat is used to increase collagen extensibility before tight joints are stretched. Cold is useful for reducing pain and muscle spasm
Orthotics	Short leg bracing is done in polymyositis and dermatomyositis and postpolio syndrome for quadriceps and ankle dorsiflexion weakness. Long leg braces are often needed in Duchenne's muscular dystrophy

From Hicks JE: Role of rehabilitation in the management of myopathies, *Curr Opin Rheumatol* 10:551, 1998.

stages of the disease, before the onset of difficulties with ambulation. Once ambulation is lost and the patient is wheelchair bound, contractures worsen, scoliosis develops or worsens, and pulmonary function deteriorates. Rehabilitation interventions in DMD focus on prolonging ambulation, preventing or slowing deformities such as joint contractures and scoliosis, and preserving respiratory function. In addition to psychological benefits,[26] the goal of rehabilitation is the highest quality of life for the patient and family. This is accomplished through weight control, passive and active exercises, use of orthotics and assistive devices, and selected surgical interventions.[3]

Preventing obesity is essential for optimum function in patients with DMD. Increased weight can result in greater difficulty with ambulation or elevation activities, such as rising from a chair. Weight control can be accomplished through diet regulation, monitoring weight at every medical visit, and patient and family education about the importance of weight control in maintaining function. Weight control becomes particularly difficult in wheelchair-bound patients.

Passive stretching exercises should be started early to prevent or reduce joint contractures; parents should be trained to carry out these daily stretching exercises.

Recommendations have been made regarding when to begin stretching various muscle groups (Table 30-4).[3] Night splints (ankle-foot orthosis [AFO]) can be effective in delaying heel cord tightness and should be prescribed when the ankles cannot be dorsiflexed beyond neutral.[3] Passive stretching combined with the use of night splints has been shown to be more effective than stretching alone.[27] Long leg splints also can be effective, but less patient compliance is seen because of the discomfort associated with wearing them. Once independent ambulation is lost, the patient may use a standing frame (Figure 30-5, A). The upright posture provides stretching in lower extremity joints and psychological benefits associated with standing. In a long-term retrospective study, Vignos et al.[28] described an effective contracture management regimen that included daily passive stretching of the hamstrings and Achilles tendons, prescribed standing and walking, Achilles tenotomy, posterior tibial tendon transfer, and knee-ankle-foot orthoses (KAFOs). This regimen allowed patients with DMD to continue ambulating to a mean age of 13.6 years. With bracing they were able to stand for an additional 2 years.

The ideal orthosis is a lightweight plastic or polypropylene KAFO with an ischial supporting lip (Figure 30-5, B).

Table 30-4

Prevention of Deformities in Duchenne's Muscular Dystrophy

Intervention	Timing	Comment
Achilles tendon stretching	As soon as contractures are present	Typically already at diagnosis
Night splints	If loss of ROM is 20° or more	Commonly a few years after diagnosis
Hip stretching	When contractures are detected	Common toward late phases of ambulation
Iliotibial band stretching	When contractures are detected	May occur during late phases of ambulation
Knee stretching	When contractures are detected	Rarely needed; may be found in children with asymmetrical ankle contractures

From Emery AEH, Muntoni F: *Duchenne muscular dystrophy,* ed 3, p 210, New York, 2003, Oxford University Press.

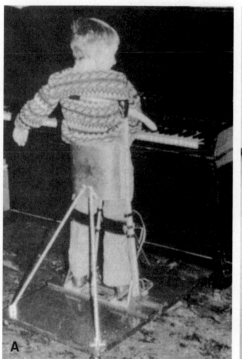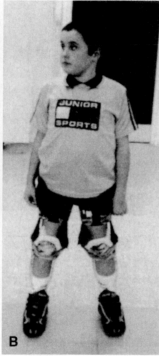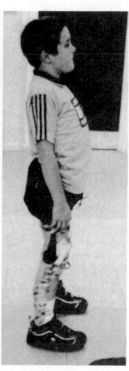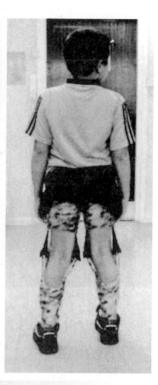

Figure 30-5

A, Simple standing frame. **B,** Standing child in knee-ankle-foot orthosis (KAFO). (From Emery AEH, Muntoni F: *Duchenne muscular dystrophy,* ed 3, pp 213-214, New York, 2003, Oxford University Press.)

An Achilles tenotomy, performed percutaneously, may be necessary to correct an equinovarus deformity and thus allow proper fitting of the orthosis. A program has been described involving fabrication of the orthosis 1 week before the tenotomy, fitting of the night splint in the operating room, and standing in the KAFOs by the next day.[3] The child is progressed over the next 1 to 1.5 weeks to independent ambulation. Important predictors of loss of ambulation in DMD include loss of hip extensor and ankle dorsiflexor strength.[4]

Scoliosis can be limited or delayed by prolongation of ambulation,[26] correct seating posture, and thoracic orthoses. The use of custom-molded, lightweight, thoracolumbar orthoses is recommended in patients with DMD who have a curvature greater than 30°.[3] The brace should be worn whenever the patient is seated. An orthopedic surgeon should evaluate patients with DMD who have scoliosis.

Ansved[29] completed a comprehensive review of exercise training in muscular dystrophies and reached the following conclusions:

1. Additional well-designed, controlled studies are needed to clarify the role of strength training in myopathic disorders.
2. High resistance strength training at submaximum or near-maximum levels is beneficial for slowly progressive myopathic disorders.

Table 30-5

Guidelines for Monitoring Pulmonary Function in Patients with Neuromuscular Disease

Baseline Evaluation	Basic Intervention/Training
History, physical examination/anthropometrics MIP/MEP PFT (if over age 5-6) Arterial blood gases Polysomnography Exercise (in selected cases)	Nutritional consultation and guidance Regular chest physiotherapy Use of percussive devices Respiratory muscle exercises Annual influenza vaccine
If VC is greater than 60% predicted and/or MIP/MEP is greater than 60 cm H_2O: Evaluate PFT every 6 months CXR, MIP/MEP, and polysomnography annually	If VC is less than 60% predicted and/or MIP/MEP is less than 60 cm H_2O: Evaluate PFT every 3 to 4 months CXR, MIP/MEP every 6 months Polysomnography every 6 months or annually

Modified from Gozal D: Pulmonary manifestations of neuromuscular disease with special reference to Duchenne muscular dystrophy and spinal muscular atrophy, *Pediatr Pulmonol* 29:148, 2000.

CXR, Chest x-ray; *MIP/MEP,* maximal inspiratory pressure/maximal expiratory pressure; *PFT,* pulmonary function test; *VC,* pulmonary capillary blood volume.

3. In rapidly progressive myopathies, such as DMD, high resistance training is controversial.

4. Regimens that may be beneficial in DMD include low resistance exercises started early in the disease, while a substantial amount of trainable muscle tissue remains.[29]

Normal physical activity is encouraged for as long as possible. Swimming makes exercises easier to perform. During periods of illness or injury, when bed rest may be required, the patient is at risk for disuse atrophy. As soon as the illness allows, a regimen of standing and dynamic exercises is recommended to minimize the effects of immobilization.[30]

Respiratory failure accounts for 90% of the morbidity and mortality in DMD. Respiratory function should be monitored frequently in patients with a neuromuscular disorder (NMD) (Table 30-5),[5] because these diseases produce well-recognized signs and symptoms of respiratory impairment (Table 30-6). Respiratory muscle exercises may be beneficial in patients with mild to moderate disease but do not prevent the eventual decline in pulmonary function. In a randomized, controlled trial,[31] respiratory muscle training (RMT) produced increased expiratory muscle strength and decreased respiratory load perception (modified Borg Visual Analog Scale, 0-10). After completion of the training regimen, muscle strength returned to baseline within 3 months, but respiratory load perception improvements persisted beyond 12 months. It was concluded that RMT could be associated with decreased respiratory symptoms. Koessler et al.[32] reported that inspiratory muscle training in patients with NMD and a vital capacity (VC) greater than 25% predicted resulted in increases in muscle strength and endurance.

Inspiratory muscle training in those with severely impaired lung function could be hazardous.[29] The American Thoracic Society issued a detailed Consensus Statement regarding the respiratory care of patients with DMD from

Table 30-6

Signs and Symptoms of Respiratory Impairment in Neuromuscular Disease

Signs	Symptoms

Vital signs
  Tachypnea
  Tachycardia
	Constitutional
	  Generalized fatigue
	  Weakness

Respiratory
  Use of accessory chest and abdominal muscles
  Paradoxical breathing pattern
  Diminished excursion
	Cardiopulmonary
	  Dyspnea
	  Lower extremity edema
	  Orthopnea
	  Secretion/retention

Cardiac
  Distended neck veins
  Edema
  Increased P2
  Cyanosis
	Central nervous system
	  Early morning headaches
	  Daytime hypersomnolence
	  Mood disturbances
	  Psychiatric disorders

	Sleep
	  Restless sleep
	  Nightmares
	  Enuresis
	  Frequent arousals

From Perrin C, Unterborn JN, Ambrosio CD, Hill NS: Pulmonary complications of chronic neuromuscular diseases and their management, *Muscle Nerve* 29:15, 2004.

baseline evaluation to end of life care.[33] The statement does not fully endorse recommendations regarding RMT and cites the need for further studies. Perrin et al.[34] suggest that a physical therapy program using deep breathing and forced expiratory maneuvers can improve symptoms and help preserve VC. Influenza and pneumococcal vaccination are recommended for wheelchair-bound patients.[3]

More agreement is seen regarding the use of mechanical noninvasive positive-pressure ventilation (and, when appropriate, continuous invasive ventilation) in chronic neuromuscular diseases, including DMD.[33-35] In patients with an impaired cough, a mechanical insufflator-exsufflator (MIE) can be beneficial for clearing secretions.[36]

Indications for Noninvasive Positive Pressure Ventilation in Chronic Neuromuscular Disease

- Symptoms such as fatigue, dyspnea, and morning headache plus one of the following physiological criteria:
  o Arterial carbon dioxide partial pressure (PaCO$_2$) over 45 mmHg (6kPa)
  o Oxygen saturation less than 88% for longer than 5 consecutive minutes on nocturnal oximetry
  o For progressive neuromuscular disease, a maximum inspiratory pressure less than 60 cm H$_2$O or a forced vital capacity less than 50% predicted

Modified from Perrin C, Unterborn JN, Ambrosio CD, Hill NS: Pulmonary complications of chronic neuromuscular diseases and their management, *Muscle Nerve* 29:20, 2004.

Surgical Care. Early release of contractures has not been found to be beneficial and is not recommended.[3] In addition to the Achilles tenotomy described previously for correcting an equinovarus deformity, a small percentage of patients with DMD may require release of hip flexion or iliotibial band contractures to allow proper fitting of KAFOs. Spinal surgery for scoliosis is recommended when the curvature is greater than 30° and has shown a tendency to deteriorate,[3] especially when the patient starts the pubertal growth spurt. The patient should have a forced VC greater than 25% to 35% of the predicted value before undergoing the procedure. The Luque operation, in which each vertebra is individually wired to two stainless steel rods, is the preferred procedure. After spinal stabilization and its consequent spinal rigidity, more frequent position changes overnight are advised.[3] Wheelchair-bound patients with DMD should be monitored every 4 to 6 months until they undergo spinal surgery or stop growing.[3] In contrast to some reports,[37-39] it now is not certain that spinal stabilization prolongs survival.[3,40,41] Most agree that it may improve quality of life.

Facioscapulohumeral Muscular Dystrophy

Genetics/Epidemiology

Facioscapulohumeral muscular dystrophy (FSHD) (also known as *Landouzy-Dejerine dystrophy*) is the third most common muscular dystrophy after DMD and myotonic dystrophy. The onset usually occurs in childhood or young adulthood (range, age 3 to 44).[42] By age 30, 98% of patients manifest symptoms.[42] The incidence of FSHD is approximately 1 in 20,000, and the prevalence is variable, ranging from 1 in 20,000 to 1 in 455,000, depending on the geographical region.[42,43] The disorder has an autosomal dominant pattern of inheritance linked to chromosome 4q35.[1,44]

Clinical Features

Patients with FSHD usually present in the 1st to 5th decades with a characteristic pattern of facial muscle weakness. This leads to the appearance of an expressionless face with a decreased ability to smile, whistle, or fully close the eyes because of weakness in the zygomaticus, orbicularis oris, and orbicularis oculi, respectively. The onset usually is insidious. The disorder is slowly progressive and can vary in the location and severity of the weakness.[1,45] Shoulder girdle weakness may also be noted at presentation.[45] Patients with an earlier onset of symptoms may be more severely affected,[45] although some researchers have found no difference in the clinical severity of the early and late onset forms.[46]

The patient complains of difficulty with activities that require arm elevation, such as combing the hair. The scapular stabilizers can be affected; therefore scapular winging may be noted with attempts to elevate the arm during the physical examination. The deltoids usually remain strong. The biceps may be involved more than the triceps, with sparing of the forearm muscles; this gives the arms a "Popeye" appearance.

Less commonly, the pelvic girdle and abdominal muscles are involved. The lower limb muscles usually are not affected, but weakness has been noted in the tibialis anterior.[45] Prolonged weakness in the ankles may lead to contractures. Gait usually is normal, and only 20% to 25% of those affected progress to being wheelchair bound.[1,45]

Symptoms usually progress in a descending, stepwise pattern. Life expectancy is normal. Respiratory muscle weakness that leads to respiratory failure has been reported, especially in those with severe weakness, wheelchair dependency, and kyphoscoliosis.[47] Associated features include pain in the neck, shoulder, posterior chest, and lower back and mild hearing loss. A recent report showed subclinical cardiac muscle involvement in patients with FSHD, which may put them at risk for ventricular arrhythmias and heart failure.[48]

Diagnosis

Creatine kinase usually is normal or only mildly elevated. EMG shows a typical myopathic pattern in affected muscles.[14] Muscle biopsy may show isolated, angular, necrotic fibers with a moth-eaten appearance. Many patients may have an inflammatory component on muscle biopsy.[42] Reliable DNA analysis that can identify the 4q35 deletion has become commercially available.

Diagnostic Criteria for Facioscapulohumeral Muscular Dystrophy[45]

- Muscle wasting and weakness that begins in the face or shoulders
- Facial weakness in at least 50% of affected family members
- No clinical cardiac involvement

Treatment

Pharmacology. No effective pharmacological treatments are available for FSHD. Albuterol combined with strength training was shown to have a limited positive outcome, but the effects of long-term use have not been evaluated.[49] A randomized, double blind, placebo-controlled trial of albuterol in FSHD showed a statistically significant increase in muscle mass and grip strength but no improvement in global strength (as measured by maximum voluntary isometric contraction testing) or in function.[43] Creatine monohydrate may produce mild improvements in muscle strength and ADLs.[22] Prednisone has not been shown to be beneficial.[50]

Rehabilitation. Features of FSHD amenable to rehabilitative interventions include footdrop, pain, and mobility deficits. A lightweight AFO may be beneficial for footdrop. Figure-of-eight bracing may help relieve shoulder pain, and assistive devices ranging from straight canes to motorized wheelchairs may be needed, depending on the severity of the mobility deficit. For many patients, pain may be the most debilitating feature of FSHD.[2,51] Nonsteroidal anti-inflammatory drugs (NSAIDs) may be beneficial, but if the pain is severe, long-acting narcotic analgesics may be necessary. An extensive Cochrane review of randomized trials addressing strength training and aerobic exercise in muscle diseases concluded that in FSHD, moderate intensity strength training appears not to cause harm; however, the evidence was insufficient to establish that it offers benefit.[52]

Surgical Care. Scapular winging may be amenable to surgical fixation of the scapula to the thorax for stabilization.[53] Scapulocostal fixation can afford over 20° to 30° additional movement, which may improve the patient's ability to lift or carry objects. Rare complications include brachial plexopathy and frozen shoulder.[54] Unfortunately, the effects tend to be temporary, and any benefit must be weighed against the risks of surgery and the necessary postoperative immobilization.[42] Fortunately, most patients learn to compensate for the limited arm elevation and do not opt for surgery.[42]

Emery-Dreifuss Muscular Dystrophy

Genetics/Epidemiology

Emery-Dreifuss muscular dystrophy (EDMD) (also known as *Emery muscular dystrophy type I* or *humeroperoneal dystrophy*) is an inherited disorder caused by mutations in the STA gene, which codes for the key nuclear protein emerin (X-linked EMD) and the LMNA gene, which codes for lamins A and C in autosomal dominant (AD) EMD.[55] The STA gene maps to chromosome Xq28 and the LMNA gene to chromosome 1q21.[56] The X-linked form primarily affects males, and the disease frequency is approximately 1 in 100,000.[57] The AD form affects males and females equally, and the disease frequency is unknown.[57] The underlying pathophysiology is not known.

Clinical Features

EDMD is characterized by a triad of clinical features: (1) early contractures in the elbows, Achilles tendon, and posterior cervical spinal muscles; (2) slowly progressive muscle weakness, which begins in a humeroperoneal distribution (X-linked form) or a scapulohumeroperoneal distribution (AD form); and (3) cardiac abnormalities.[58] The muscle weakness and contractures usually present before the cardiac abnormalities. Contractures usually precede muscle weakness in the X-linked form, and vice versa for the AD form. Contractures are especially common in the biceps and medial head of the gastrocnemius[59] and can worsen during the adolescent growth spurt. Late complications of the weakness can include lumbar lordosis and spinal rigidity.

The cardiac abnormalities include conduction defects, atrial and ventricular arrhythmias, and/or dilated cardiomyopathy.[57,58,60-65] In an extensive review, arrhythmias were noted in 92% of patients after age 30, and heart failure was seen in 64% after age 50.[66] The risk of sudden death can be as high as a 46% in EDMD, because many patients are symptom free.[58,61,63,66]

Diagnosis

The diagnosis is based mostly on clinical findings. Immunohistochemistry staining of a muscle biopsy sample showing the absence of emerin,[57] as well as DNA analysis,[62] can confirm the diagnosis.

Treatment

No specific pharmacological remedies are available for EDMD. All patients should have a comprehensive cardiac evaluation and regular follow-up to identify arrhythmias that may be amenable to pacemaker or defibrillator implantation; unfortunately, this is no guarantee that sudden death will be prevented.[66] Anticoagulation is recommended for individuals with atrial flutter or fibrillation or atrial standstill to prevent disabling embolic strokes.[62,63] Diuretics and angiotensin-converting enzyme (ACE) inhibitors may be beneficial in patients with significant ventricular dysfunction.

Rehabilitative interventions should seek to maintain function and mobility. The contractures usually are not preventable but may be minimized by stretching exercises. Achilles tenotomy may be required to correct an equinus deformity of the foot, and a rigid, hyperextended neck may be improved by orthopedic intervention. Patients with EDMD have been found to have an increased resting energy expenditure, which requires an increase in caloric intake to prevent further decline in muscle function.[67]

Limb-Girdle Muscular Dystrophies

Genetics/Epidemiology

The limb-girdle muscular dystrophies (LGMDs) (also known as *limb-girdle syndrome*) constitute a genetically heterogeneous group of disorders with an AD (6) or AR (10) mode of inheritance.[1,68] The prevalence is approximately 8.1 in 1 million.[69] The affected genes code for various muscle proteins associated with sarcolemma, nuclear membrane, contractile apparatus, and enzymatic functions.[70] The 6 AD forms of LGMD have been classified as LGMD 1A-1F and the AR forms as LGMD 2A-2J.[70] LGMDs 2C-2F have been classified as the sarcoglycanopathies, because the proteins affected are subtypes of the transmembrane protein sarcoglycan.[70] The exact underlying pathophysiology is as yet unknown.

Clinical Features

Patients with LGMD can present at any age from childhood to adulthood. Common features include preferential proximal lower limb and pelvic girdle weakness, with upper limb weakness and scapular winging occurring later.[70] The weakness is slowly progressive, and some patients become wheelchair dependent. Facial and extraocular muscles usually are spared. Severe diaphragmatic weakness can result in chronic alveolar hypoventilation and respiratory failure. Elbow, Achilles tendon, and hip flexion contractures may occur in certain subtypes.[68] Each LGMD has a characteristic phenotype, and varying patterns of muscle involvement are seen.[68] Cardiac abnormalities have been noted to occur in LGMD.[71] In one review of 97 patients with LGMD, 10% were found to have clinically relevant cardiac abnormalities, including conduction defects and dilated cardiomyopathy.[72,73] The wide variability in the clinical findings among the subtypes was extensively described by an international workshop on the LGMDs.[68]

Diagnosis

Diagnosis of LGMD requires a complete physical examination and history, including as complete a family history as possible to identify clinical patterns attributable to a particular subtype of LGMD. Creatine kinase can be markedly elevated. Genetic analysis and muscle biopsy are important to make the diagnosis and to rule out other myopathies that may present with a limb-girdle distribution of weakness. Muscle biopsy can be nonspecific and usually reveals necrosis and regeneration, increased internalized nuclei, marked variability of fiber size, increased fibrous and adipose tissue, and fiber hypertrophy.[74] Biopsy may also show many lobulated and moth-eaten fibers.[75]

Treatment

No pharmacological treatment is available for LGMD. Creatine monohydrate was shown to have a small but significant effect in improving muscle strength and performance of ADLs.[22] Cardiac monitoring throughout the disease is recommended.[70] In the more severe cases, especially when the patient is wheelchair bound, respiratory failure may need to be addressed with ventilatory devices.[35] Rehabilitative efforts should focus on maintaining mobility and minimizing contractures. Stretching exercises are important for maintaining joint range of motion, and AFOs may help compensate for distal lower extremity weakness. The patient's functional status should be monitored closely and can be a more sensitive indicator of disease progression than manual muscle testing.[76]

Myotonic Dystrophy

Genetics/Epidemiology

Myotonic dystrophy (MD) (also known as *myotonic muscular dystrophy* or *myotonic muscular dystrophy type 1*) is the most common of a heterogeneous group of myotonic disorders. It has an AD mode of inheritance mapped to chromosome 19q13,[56] which codes for myotonic dystrophy protein kinase (DMPK).[77] The incidence of MD is approximately 13.5 in 100,000 live births, and the prevalence is 3-5 per 100,000.[14]

Clinical Features

The muscle weakness of MD can begin at any age, including the neonatal period. It is slowly progressive, symmetrical, and manifested predominately in the muscles of the face, jaw, anterior neck, and distal (more than proximal) limbs.[77] Frontal baldness, ptosis, and atrophy in the temporalis and masseter muscles result in a characteristic "hatchet-faced" appearance. Dysarthria and dysphagia can result from pharyngeal and lingual muscle weakness. Myotonia is a delayed relaxation of a contracted muscle that the patient may describe as stiffness. This myotonia is most prominent in the hands and can be reproduced by percussion of muscle groups such as the thenar eminence. Patients with MD often do not notice or may deny their weakness and myotonia.

Many other systems are involved in MD (Table 30-7).[77] A relatively recently recognized related disorder is type 2 myotonic dystrophy, or proximal myotonic myopathy. It is also autosomal dominant and shows multisystem involvement. Important differences include gene mapping to chromosome 3q, later onset of symptoms, more proximal weakness, and minimal or clinically absent myotonia.[77]

Diagnosis

The diagnosis is based on a careful history, including a family history, physical examination, and commercially available DNA analysis. Creatine kinase may be normal or slightly elevated. EMG and muscle biopsy usually are not needed to make the diagnosis.[77] When used, needle EMG shows myotonic discharges with a characteristic pattern of waxing and waning of the frequency and amplitude.[14] Muscle biopsy is rarely needed.

Treatment

Myotonia can be controlled with medications such as mexiletine, phenytoin, quinine, and procainamide. Quinine and procainamide should be avoided if the patient has cardiac

Table 30-7

Systemic Involvement in Myotonic Dystrophy

System	Principal Involvement
Smooth muscle	Esophagus, colon, anal sphincter, uterus (other sites may also be affected)
Heart	Conduction defects, in particular heart block, atrial arrhythmias; less commonly, cardiomyopathy
Lungs	Aspiration pneumonia from esophageal and diaphragmatic involvement, hypoventilation
Peripheral nerve	Variable and rarely clinically significant; minor sensory loss possible
Brain	Severe involvement in congenital form; mild cognitive and psychological changes frequent in adults; hypersomnia
Endocrine system	Testicular tubular atrophy; diabetes (rarely clinically significant); sometimes abnormalities of growth hormone and other pituitary functions
Eye	Cataract, retinal degeneration, ocular hypotonia, ptosis, extraocular weakness
Skeletal system	Cranial hyperostosis, air sinus enlargement; jaw and palate involvement; talipes (childhood cases); scoliosis (uncommon)
Skin	Premature balding; calcifying epithelioma

From Engel AG, Franzini-Armstrong C, editors: *Myology*, ed 3, vol 2, p 1044, New York, 2004, McGraw-Hill.

conduction abnormalities. All of these medications should be used only in severe cases.

Rehabilitation interventions can be important for managing the musculoskeletal complaints. Distal lower limb weakness or footdrop can be treated with lightweight orthoses, and neck muscle weakness may require a cervical collar or head support. Assistive devices such as canes and walkers may prolong mobility. In severe cases, wheelchairs may be prescribed, especially for long distances or outdoor use. Most patients with MD remain ambulatory.[77] Dysphagia may be amenable to speech and language pathology interventions, which may help minimize the risk of aspiration. Feeding tubes may be necessary with severe dysphagia. The multiple systemic problems require additional management (Table 30-8).

Congenital Myopathies

The congenital myopathies constitute a heterogeneous group of nonprogressive or slowly progressive muscle disorders that present in the neonatal period. They were deemed myopathies instead of dystrophies because they originally were all thought to be nonprogressive. They show distinctive morphological abnormalities on muscle biopsy and share certain clinical features, such as generalized weakness, hypotonia (floppy infant), hyporeflexia, delayed motor milestones, decreased muscle bulk, and various dysmorphic features attributable to the myopathy.[78]

Laboratory findings usually include a normal or minimally elevated CK, which can help distinguish these disorders from the muscular dystrophies. Motor and sensory nerve conduction studies are normal, and needle EMG findings usually are normal or show small, polyphasic motor unit potentials.[14]

The congenital myopathies have common management options that use a multidisciplinary approach to maximize the patient's quality of life (Table 30-9). North[78] suggests the following general approach to management:

1. Prevention
2. Monitoring
3. Risk management during procedures
4. Symptomatic therapy and rehabilitation

Prevention can be accomplished through genetic counseling and prenatal diagnosis. Monitoring allows early detection of disease manifestations and complications with early referral to a multidisciplinary team under the direction of a coordinating physician who can do regular checkups and make appropriate referrals. Decreased respiratory capacity is one of the primary sources of disability and eventual mortality; respiratory capacity should be monitored through pulmonary function testing, oximetry, and evaluation of carbon dioxide (CO_2) during sleep and while awake.[14]

Screening for scoliosis is an integral part of monitoring of respiratory capacity. The possible need and options for assisted ventilation should be discussed with the family. Chest physical therapy and postural drainage are important therapies for managing secretions. Feeding difficulties may require input from a speech pathologist, and gastrostomy tube placement may be necessary in severe cases.

Mobility and ADL deficits require ongoing input from a physical therapist and an occupational therapist.

Some of the better-defined congenital myopathies are discussed in more detail in the following sections; these include central core disease, nemaline disease, and myotubular/centronuclear myopathy.

Central Core Disease

Central core disease (CCD) is a genetic disorder with an autosomal dominant mode of inheritance mapped to chromosome 19q12-q13.2, which codes for the ryanodine receptor gene.[79] The resultant defect in skeletal muscle is thought to be related to abnormalities in calcium ion (Ca^{2+}) regulation.[80] In addition to the common features mentioned previously, most patients show decreased muscle bulk, slender frame, and only mild, symmetrical weakness. The weakness is predominantly in the proximal lower limbs, but the face and neck can also be involved.[78] Overall, little disability is seen, and most patients are able to walk by age 3 to 4.[78] Other frequent features include kyphoscoliosis,

Table 30-8
Management of Myotonic Dystrophy

Problem	Management
Cardiorespiratory	
Arrhythmias and other heart conduction defects	Regular electrocardiograms, full cardiac investigation if defects significant; drug management of acute episodes as appropriate for particular arrhythmia; pacemaker if conduction defect severe or episodes of significant heart block; avoid aggravation by antimyotonic drugs
Bronchial aspiration	Avoid by adjusting diet, sleeping propped up; investigate esophageal function if suspected
Hypoventilation	Consider assisted nocturnal ventilation
Central Nervous System	
Somnolence	Exclude hypoventilation as cause; consider use of modapinil if severe
Depression	Treat on its own merits
Gastrointestinal	
Swallowing difficulty	Investigate fully to identify site of problem
Gastroparesis	Metoclopramide may be helpful
Constipation	Avoid liquid paraffin; treat as for irritable bowel syndrome
Gallbladder problems	Surgery is particularly hazardous; avoid if possible or use minimally invasive techniques
Endocrine	
Diabetes	Detect by urine and blood glucose monitoring
Other endocrine problems	Rarely clinically significant
Ophthalmic	
Cataract	Good results from extraction; look for retinopathy if vision remains poor
Strabismus	Good results from correction (usually in childhood)
Surgery and Anesthesia	Awareness of hazards avoids most risks; preoperative and postoperative measures; abdominal surgery is particularly hazardous

From Engel AG, Franzini-Armstrong C, editors: *Myology,* ed 3, vol 2, p 1070, New York, 2004, McGraw-Hill.

Table 30-9
Management of Patients with Congenital Myopathies

Problem	Referral	Possible Interventions
Skeletal muscle involvement Hypotonia Weakness Contractures	Physical therapy Occupational therapy	Objective testing of muscle strength Regular exercise program Active and passive stretching Standing frame Orthotics/splinting (upper and lower limb) Serial plaster casting Enhance mobility (walking frames or wheelchair) Liaise with local services
Respiratory muscle involvement Reduced respiratory capacity Recurrent chest infection Aspiration Nocturnal hypoxia Respiratory failure	Physical therapy Lung function tests Sleep study Respiratory physician Occupational therapy	Breathing exercises Chest physiotherapy to clear secretions Seating assessment Influenza vaccination Aggressive management of acute infections, including antibiotic therapy Nocturnal ventilation Assisted ventilation Liaise with local services
Bulbar involvement Feeding and swallowing difficulties Failure to thrive	Speech pathologist Dietitian Gastroenterologist	Speech therapy Modified barium swallow Caloric supplementation/thickened feed Gavage feeding or gastrostomy feeding

(Continued)

Table 30-9
Management of Patients with Congenital Myopathies—Cont'd

Problem	Referral	Possible Interventions
Bulbar involvement Dysarthria Excessive drooling	Speech pathologist Surgeon	Speech therapy Anticholinergic medications Pharyngoplasty Salivary duct surgery
Developmental or psychosocial delay	Occupational therapy Physical therapy Speech pathology Psychologist Developmental physician	Assessment Advice about appropriate intervention/liaise with local services Developmental stimulation Home programs Reassessment if deterioration occurs
Scoliosis	Physiotherapy Orthopedic surgeon	Baseline assessment, including spinal radiographs Monitoring of degree of curve Bracing Corrective surgery
Foot deformities	Physical therapy Orthopedic surgeon	Splinting/serial casting Corrective surgery
Cardiac involvement Conduction defects Cardiomyopathy Cor pulmonale	Cardiologist	Electrocardiogram, Holter monitor, cardiac echocardiogram Medication if indicated

Inability to perform activities of daily
   living (ADLs)
Inability to achieve independence with
   bathing, toileting, dressing, feeding
Difficulties with access
Handwriting difficulties
	Occupational therapy
	Community nurse
		Aids for individual ADLs
		Wheelchair assessment
		Home nursing assistance
		Home visit and modifications
		School visit and modifications
		Typing and computer programs
		Car modifications
		Liaise with local services

Excessive weight gain Limits mobility and exacerbates weakness	Dietitian Physical therapy	Calorie-controlled diet Exercise program

Inability to participate in sport/leisure
   activities
	Physical therapy
	Occupational therapy
		Liaise with/visit schools
		Contact with sporting organizations for people
		   with disabilities
		Hydrotherapy

Constipation	Dietitian Physician Gastroenterologist	High fiber diet Laxatives/enemas
Depression or behavioral problems	Psychologist	Individual or family therapy Medication
Family financial and social difficulties	Social work Muscular Dystrophy Association Government assistance agencies	Disability allowance/pension Caregivers' allowance Support groups Financial assistance with equipment and home modifications Transport and travel assistance
Planning future pregnancies	Geneticist Genetic counselor	Genetic counseling Planning prenatal diagnosis
Planning surgery	Consult with anesthetist Respiratory physician	Malignant hyperthermia precautions Lung function tests and physiotherapy before surgery

(Continued)

Table 30-9
Management of Patients with Congenital Myopathies—Cont'd

Problem	Referral	Possible Interventions
Planning future employment	Vocational counseling service Occupational therapy	Planning school studies Vocational planning Work experience Training, work placement and support
Coordination of care	Pediatrician or subspecialist with an interest Neurologist, geneticist, or rehabilitation specialist	Contact with general practitioner by telephone Liaise with local services Copy of all correspondence to key personnel Arrange case conferences when necessary Determine timing of respiratory, orthopedic, and palliative interventions

From Engel AG, Franzini-Armstrong C, editors: *Myology,* ed 3, vol 2, pp 1521-1522, New York, 2004, McGraw-Hill.

pes cavus, pes planus, and congenital dislocation of the hip.[78] Patients with CCD usually have normal intelligence,[78] although they also have an increased risk of malignant hyperthermia.[81]

Laboratory tests reveal the common features mentioned previously. Muscle biopsy shows characteristic cores that run the length of most of the type I fibers. These cores are single, centrally located, and circular, and electron microscopy shows that they lack mitochondria or sarcoplasmic reticulum.[78]

A pilot study has suggested that the β_2-agonist salbutamol may be beneficial for improving muscle strength and functional abilities in patients whose CCD is severe enough to require treatment.[82] Larger prospective, randomized, double blind, placebo-controlled trials are needed to confirm these findings. Lower limb weakness can be treated with bracing (see Table 30-9).

Nemaline (Rod) Disease

Nemaline (rod) disease (ND) or myopathy is a congenital disorder with an autosomal dominant, recessive, or sporadic mode of inheritance mapping to multiple genes that code for components of the sarcomeric thin filaments.[83-89] The two most commonly affected genes are the nebulin and actin genes.[90] Patients with ND are classified according to age of onset and clinical severity into one of five forms: severe congenital, intermediate congenital, typical congenital, childhood, or adult onset, although the forms can overlap.[78,91,92]

In addition to the common features of congenital myopathies mentioned previously, the clinical findings in ND include more prominent weakness in the face, neck, and trunk flexors, dorsiflexors, and toe extensors.[93] In the late onset form, the weakness does not present until age 20 to 50 and may progress rapidly; it may be accompanied by myalgia.[78] Infants often have difficulty with sucking and swallowing and consequent feeding problems. Infants and young children may have hypermobility in joints and later

develop contractures and deformities.[78] Kyphoscoliosis and the subsequent restricted respiratory capacity appear to affect the prognosis. The CNS usually is spared, and these patients have a normal IQ.[93]

The laboratory findings for ND are those common for congenital myopathies mentioned previously. In addition, muscle biopsy reveals characteristic threadlike structures (rods) in the Z-line plane of muscle fibers; the rods consists of Z-line protein material.[78,90,94] It should be noted that these rods have been associated with other disorders.[95,96] The muscle biopsy also shows a predominance of type I fibers.

Pilot studies have suggested that L-tyrosine may be beneficial in improving muscle strength, appetite, and weight gain and for reducing oral secretions.[90] Wallgren-Pettersson[97] suggested that rehabilitation should focus on maintaining cardiorespiratory capacity through exercise and the prevention and treatment of scoliosis. Long periods of immobilization can lead to disuse atrophy with worsening weakness and therefore should be avoided. Respiratory infections require rapid, aggressive treatment, and respiratory function should be monitored regularly for hypoventilation.[98] Respiratory insufficiency may require consultation with an otolaryngologist and eventually assisted ventilation (see Table 30-9).[99]

Myotubular/Centronuclear Myopathy

Myotubular/centronuclear myopathy (MTM) is a congenital disorder with two forms. The first (myotubular) has an X-linked mode of inheritance mapped to chromosome Xq28. The other, rare form (centronuclear) has an autosomal recessive mode of inheritance with an unknown gene location.

In the X-linked (myotubular) form, affected males present at birth with severe hypotonia, weakness, feeding difficulties, respiratory distress, bilateral ptosis, limited eye movements, and absent tendon reflexes.[78] Associated features include pectus carinatum and hip and knee contractures.[78] Death from respiratory failure used to occur in the first year, but this has been improving with the use of assisted ventilation. More than 50% of patients can now be expected to live beyond the first year.[78] Cognitive function usually is normal unless the patient experienced hypoxia.

The autosomal recessive (centronuclear) form mostly presents in infancy, early childhood, or occasionally early adulthood; in general, later than the X-linked form.[78] In addition to the clinical features common to congenital myopathies mentioned previously, associated findings include bulbar weakness, respiratory distress, ophthalmoplegia, high-arched palate, pectus excavatum, talipes equinovarus, and depressed or absent reflexes.[78] The weakness usually is more proximal and precludes the ability to run. Although the course is slowly progressive, the patient may develop scoliosis and loss of ambulation by adolescence.[78]

In addition to the laboratory and EMG findings common to the congenital myopathies mentioned previously, the two forms share characteristic findings on muscle biopsy, including a predominance of type I muscle fibers with centrally placed nuclei. Pulmonary function tests may show a restricted pattern.

Treatment for most congenital myopathies requires a multidisciplinary approach that includes various specialties (see Table 30-9).

Inflammatory Myopathies

Polymyositis and Dermatomyositis

Polymyositis (PM) and dermatomyositis (DM) are idiopathic inflammatory disorders with an incidence of approximately 1 in 100,000.[100] PM usually presents in those over age 20, whereas DM has a bimodal age distribution, occurring more commonly in childhood to early adulthood and in the 40s-50s. The female to male ratio is approximately 2:1.[101] The underlying etiology remains unknown. Current knowledge favors a combination of environmental risk factors and genetic susceptibility.[102,103]

Clinical Presentation

Both PM and DM present with a progressive, symmetrical, proximal (more than distal) pattern of muscle weakness. Patients may complain of difficulty rising from a seated position or with overhead activities such as brushing the hair. Muscle pain and tenderness affect approximately one third of these patients and affects the upper extremity more commonly than the lower extremity. Later in the course of the disease, neck, swallowing, and respiratory muscles may become affected, resulting in aspiration pneumonia and respiratory failure.[104] Arthralgia may occur in as many as 50% of patients with PM.[100]

The adult and childhood forms of DM show characteristic erythematous skin lesions, predominantly in the periorbital,

perioral, malar, anterior neck, chest, and extensor surfaces of joints.[100] The periorbital rash usually is violaceous or heliotrope in color. Gottron's rash is a violaceous, raised, scaly rash over the knuckles. As the disease progresses, scaling, pigmentation, and depigmentation can occur in the area of the rash. The rash sometimes appears before the muscle weakness.[100]

PM and DM are associated with abnormalities in the cardiac and pulmonary systems and with certain malignancies.[100,105] Cardiomyopathy, pericarditis, left ventricular diastolic dysfunction, atrial arrhythmias and conduction defects are the most common cardiac abnormalities.[104,106-109] Interstitial lung disease (ILD) occurs in approximately 30% of patients with PM or DM.[104,110,111] It tends to be more severe and more refractory to corticosteroid treatment in DM.[112] Signs and symptoms suggesting ILD include fever, nonproductive cough, dyspnea, hypoxemia, and lung infiltrates. These signs and symptoms may even precede the skin or muscle abnormalities.[104,113] Patients with PM or DM may have a connective tissue disease, such as rheumatoid arthritis, systemic lupus erythematous, scleroderma, or Sjögren's syndrome.

Population-based cohort studies strongly suggest an association with malignancy.[114] Ovarian cancer and lung cancer appear to be more closely associated with DM, and lung cancer and non-Hodgkin's lymphoma are associated with PM.[114] Vasculitis that affects the GI tract may also be seen, especially in children.

Diagnosis

A comprehensive history, including a family history, physical examination, CK level, EMG, and muscle biopsy findings, forms the basis of diagnosis of PM and DM.[115] CK, aldolase, lactate dehydrogenase (LDH) and aspartate aminotransferase (AST) all can be elevated with muscle parenchymal damage. An elevated CK is the most specific of these muscle enzymes results for detecting active muscle disease, because the others also can be elevated with liver disease; CK can be elevated five- to 50-fold in PM. It is important to note that CK may be normal in some patients with PM or DM, especially juvenile DM.[100] The erythrocyte sedimentation rate (ESR) usually is normal or mildly elevated and does not accurately reflect disease activity or correlate with the severity of weakness.[100] Antinuclear antibodies may be found in approximately 50% of patients with myositis. Anti-Jo-1 antibodies may be seen in PM more often than in DM and may be associated with ILD.[116] The usefulness of the antinuclear antibody (ANA) test is limited, because a negative or low titer does not exclude the diagnosis.[100]

On electrodiagnostic testing, sensory and motor nerve conduction studies usually are normal. Needle EMG findings can include positive sharp waves (PSWs) and fibrillation potentials on needle insertion, which suggests membrane instability. This abnormal insertional activity is a good indicator of active disease and may be seen in more than 80% of patients with PM or DM.[117] In chronic disease with significant tissue loss, the PSWs and fibrillation potentials may be decreased; this also may occur after treatment, with resultant stabilization of the muscle membrane.[117] EMG may also reveal a decrease in the duration and amplitude of motor unit potentials, reflecting the diminished number of muscle fibers in the motor unit. Increased polyphasia may also be seen, reflecting asynchrony in the electrical activity of the remaining fibers. It should be noted that active disease can be present in scattered areas; therefore sufficient time is needed to assess multiple areas of multiple muscles to collect adequate information. Proximal, distal, and paraspinal muscles should be examined. Muscle biopsy findings include necrosis, regeneration, variation in fiber diameter, proliferation of connective tissue and collections of inflammatory cells.[100]

Treatment

Corticosteroids are an effective first-line treatment in most patients with DM or PM.[100,118] Adults usually require 30 to 40 mg a day initially. In more severe disease, adults may require 1 to 1.5 mg/kg/day, and children may need 1 to 2 mg/kg/day in divided doses. The steroid is given until the serum CK normalizes, which usually takes 6 to 12 weeks. It is then given in a single dose and gradually tapered over several months until a maintenance dose is reached in 4 to 6 months.[100] A gradual decline in serum CK usually indicates a favorable response. Improvement in strength can lag behind the CK improvement. Steroid myopathy (discussed later) is a possible complication. Other side effects of steroids include hypertension, glucose intolerance, weight gain, a cushingoid appearance, cataracts, glaucoma, and osteoporosis. Strategies to minimize these side effects include alternate-day dosing, vitamin D and calcium supplementation, control of food intake, and antacids.

Second-line treatments include azathioprine and methotrexate, which should be reserved for use when steroids are ineffective or the disease is severe.[100] Third-line therapies may include cyclosporin, mycophenolate mofetil, cyclophosphamide, intravenous immunoglobulins, or plasma exchange.[100] These are indicated when patients do not respond to first- and second-line treatments. Refractory ILD may respond to cyclospine[112] or to cyclophosphamide alone or in combination with corticosteroids.[111]

Rehabilitative interventions should focus on maintaining function and maximizing quality of life.[25] A recent review of studies on exercise in PM and DM reported a reduction in disability, an increase in muscle strength and aerobic capacity, and no change in disease activity from a variety of exercise regimens; larger multicenter, randomized, controlled trials are needed to establish the efficacy of various exercise regimens.[119] Range of motion and stretching exercises are essential for preventing contractures and should be initiated early in the course of PM or DM. As with other myopathic disorders, assistive devices and mobility aides may become necessary as function declines.

Outcome of Polymyositis and Dermatomyositis

The outcome in PM and DM is determined by multiple factors. A poor outcome is more likely with older age at presentation; severe disease; delay in diagnosis and treatment; significant cardiac, pulmonary, or GI symptoms; malignancy; and antisynthetase or anti-SRP autoantibodies levels.[105] In one study, 105 patients with DM or PM were found to have a significantly poorer quality of life than the normal population as measured by the Short-Form 36-Item Health Status Survey (SF-36); the mortality rate was approximately 14%.[120] In another study, the 10-year survival rates were 89.4% for PM and 86.4% for DM, and cardiac muscle involvement was the main predictor of death (p <0.01) (Table 30 10).[121]

Metabolic Myopathies

The metabolic myopathies constitute a heterogeneous group of disorders caused by genetic defects that compromise muscle energy production. The hydrolysis of adenosine triphosphate (ATP) to adenosine diphosphate (ADP)

Table 30-10
Overview of Polymyositis and Dermatomyositis

Disorder	Clinical Presentation	Associated Features	Diagnosis	Treatment
Polymyositis	Arthritis Symmetrical proximal muscle weakness Muscle pain, tenderness	Interstitial lung disease Cardiac abnormalities Gastrointestinal abnormalities Collagen vascular disease	Increased creatine kinase	Corticosteroids Range of motion, stretching
Dermatomyositis	As for polymyositis plus rash	Interstitial lung disease Cardiac abnormalities Gastrointestinal abnormalities Collagen vascular disease	Increased creatine kinase	As for polymyositis

generates the energy needed for muscle contractions. ATP is used and replenished by key metabolic processes, which require proper functioning of the multiple enzymes involved in this cascade of reactions. Enzyme dysfunction can result in an inadequate supply of ATP needed for muscle contraction. Glycogen is an important substrate in these metabolic processes. Eleven enzyme defects that affect glycogen synthesis (1), glycogenolysis (3), and glycolysis (7) have been well described (Figure 30-6).[122] The following sections discuss some of the more common metabolic disorders that result in myopathies, including myophosphorylase deficiency, phosphofructokinase deficiency, debrancher enzyme deficiency and acid maltase deficiency (Table 30-11).

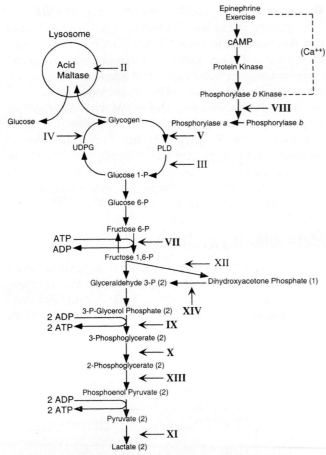

Figure 30-6

Schematic of glycogen metabolism and glycolysis. Roman numerals denote muscle glycogenoses caused by defects in the following enzymes: *II,* acid maltase; *III,* debrancher; *IV,* brancher; *V,* phosphorylase; *VII,* phosphofructokinase; *VIII,* phosphorylase *b* kinase; *IX,* phosphoglycerate kinase; *X,* phosphoglycerate mutase; *XI,* lactate dehydrogenase; *XII,* aldolase; *XIII,* enolase; *XIV,* triosephosphate isomerase. (From Dimauro S, Hays AP, Tsujino S: Nonlysosomal glycogenoses. In Engel AG, Franzini-Armstrong C, editors: *Myology,* ed 3, vol 2, New York, 2004, McGraw-Hill.)

Myophosphorylase Deficiency

During early exercise (within seconds) and with high intensity activity, energy metabolism in muscles predominantly depends on the breakdown of glycogen. Myophosphorylase is the enzyme that initiates the metabolism of glycogen. Myophosphorylase deficiency (also known as *glycogenosis type V* or *McArdle's disease*) leads to blocked glycogenolysis, resulting in low exercise tolerance. This deficiency is one of the more common glycogenoses, with a prevalence of approximately 1 in 100,000.[122] It has an autosomal recessive mode of inheritance mapped to chromosome 11 and a male to female ration of 3:1.

The onset usually occurs in childhood, and the child may complain of muscle aches and inability to keep up with peers during play. Most patients are diagnosed by early adulthood. Exercise intolerance is most evident during short bursts of high intensity activity, such as weight lifting, or during sustained moderate intensity activity, such as walking. This intolerance can present as myalgia, muscle stiffness, weakness, or early fatigue; rest usually relieves it. Patients can experience a "second wind," which consists of renewed endurance, if they rest at the onset of myalgia. Without rest, the patient may experience painful muscle cramps that may last for hours. Patients usually are asymptomatic between attacks, and most adapt well and do not lead sedentary lives.[124] Fixed, proximal (greater than distal) weakness can occur in approximately one third of patients, especially older patients.[122,125] A serious complication is muscle necrosis with myoglobinuria and acute renal failure. This can occur in as many as 15% of patients with McArdle's disease.[126-128] Tea-colored urine usually is one of the first clues to myoglobinuria and should spark an aggressive workup.

Diagnosis

Diagnosis of McArdle's disease includes a careful history, including a family history, CK level determination, electro-diagnostics, muscle biopsy, and genetic analysis. Physical examination findings usually are normal between episodes of muscle cramping or weakness. The serum CK is elevated in most patients with McArdle's disease even between episodes of muscle cramping. Motor and sensory nerve conduction studies usually are normal. Needle EMG findings can be normal between episodes of myoglobinuria, but as many as 50% of patients may still show evidence of membrane irritability with fibrillation potentials, PSWs, and myotonic discharges.[14] Electrical silence may be noted during times of maximum muscle contraction. In the forearm ischemic test, serial lactate and ammonia serum levels are measured after 1 minute of forearm exercise; both should increase threefold to fourfold. This test usually does not yield a significant increase in the venous lactate level in conditions such as the glycogen storage disorders, in which glycogen cannot be properly used. Muscle biopsy may reveal subsarcolemmal deposits of glycogen that appear as bulges. Similar deposits between myofibrils may result in a vacuolar appearance.[122]

Table 30-11
Metabolic Myopathies

Glycogenosis/Pattern of Inheritance	Abnormal Enzyme	Clinical Presentation	Diagnosis	Venous Lactate Response in Forearm Exercise Test	Treatment
Type V McArdle's disease (autosomal recessive)	Phosphorylase	Childhood onset Exercise intolerance Myalgias Myoglobinuria (15%)	Increased CK Muscle biopsy DNA analysis	No increase	Rest periods at onset of myalgia Supplemental sucrose ? Creatine High protein diet PT/OT exercises, orthotics
Type VII Tarui's disease (autosomal recessive)	Phosphofructokinase	Exercise intolerance Myalgias Nausea, vomiting Hemolytic anemia Gout	Increased CK	No increase	Rest periods PT/OT exercises, orthotics
Type III Cori-Forbes disease (autosomal recessive)	Debranching enzyme	Short stature Exercise intolerance Muscle weakness Cardiomyopathy Hepatomegaly	Increased CK	No increase	High protein diet PT/OT exercises, orthotics
Type II Acid maltase deficiency Pompe's disease (infantile form) (autosomal recessive)	Acid maltase (α-glucosidase)	Muscle weakness Infantile, childhood, adult forms	Increased CK, AST, LDH Muscle biopsy	No increase	?High protein diet PT/OT exercises, orthotics

AST, Aspartate aminotransferase; *CK,* creatine kinase; *DNA,* deoxyribonucleic acid; *LDH,* lactate dehydrogenase; *OT,* occupational therapy; *PT,* physical therapy.

Molecular analysis of blood can now be used to make the diagnosis, obviating the need for muscle biopsy.[129]

Treatment

Appropriate timing of rest periods at the onset of myalgia allows use of the second wind phenomenon and thus prolonged activity tolerance. Low dose creatine supplementation has shown modest benefits in a small number of patients.[130] A small, randomized, controlled study suggested that sucrose ingestion before exercise could improve exercise tolerance in patients with McArdle's disease.[131] Supplemental sucrose increased the mean plasma glucose level and resulted in marked improvement in exercise tolerance with a significant drop in heart rate (p <0.001) and a marked drop in the level of perceived exertion in patients compared to when they received the placebo. However, this supplementation has the potential to cause significant weight gain. Further multicenter collaboration and standardized treatment and assessment protocols are needed for future treatment trials. A recent Cochrane review of pharmacological and nutritional treatments in improving exercise performance and quality of life in McArdle's disease concluded that as yet, no specific treatment can be recommended for McArdle's disease.[130]

In any of the metabolic disorders, rehabilitation exercises may slow the onset of weakness and associated contractures. Lightweight orthotics may be beneficial for distal lower limb weakness to allow safe ambulation. In the rare cases of severe generalized weakness, the patient may require a wheelchair. In cases involving respiratory muscle weakness, chest physical therapy is important for clearing secretions.

Phosphofructokinase Deficiency

Phosphofructokinase (PFK) deficiency (also known as *glycogenosis type VII* or *Tarui's disease*) has an autosomal recessive mode of inheritance and is most common in the Ashkenazi Jewish population. Clinically, PFK deficiency is similar to McArdle's disease but is less common and less likely to cause myoglobinuria. Some differences include fewer occurrences of the "second wind" phenomenon and more frequent nausea and vomiting during the exercise-induced episodes of myalgia and weakness.[123] Jaundice, reflecting hemolytic anemia, and gouty arthritis can further distinguish PFK deficiency from McArdle's disease.[132,133]

Diagnosis

CK elevation and EMG and muscle biopsy findings are similar to those in McArdle's disease. Specific staining for PFK can aid the diagnosis.[134] In PFK deficiency, glycolytic intermediates can accumulate and can be detected as a distinct peak on phosphorus magnetic resonance spectroscopy testing after mild exercise; this does not occur in McArdle's disease. Molecular genetic analysis can provide a definitive diagnosis of PFK deficiency.

Treatment

No specific treatment is available for PFK deficiency. A high protein diet has been suggested, but its efficacy has not been proven. Unlike in McArdle's disease, glucose supplementation usually is not effective because it does not bypass the metabolic defect. Rest periods can prolong exercise tolerance. Rehabilitation involvement is the same as for McArdle's disease.

Debrancher Deficiency

Debrancher deficiency (DD) (also known as *glycogenosis type III*, *Cori-Forbes disease*, or *amylo-1,6-glucosidase deficiency*) usually is a benign genetic disorder of glycogen metabolism that mostly affects the liver and muscle. It has an autosomal recessive mode of inheritance mapped to chromosome 1p21.[135] Males are more frequently affected. During glycogenolysis, the peripheral chains of glycogen are shortened to a length of four glucosyl units. Further metabolism of glycogen requires the debrancher enzyme to remove these chain remnants. Debrancher enzyme deficiency results in a buildup of glycogen remnant in muscle and liver, leading to myopathy and hepatomegaly.[136]

DD usually presents in childhood with hypotonia, a decreased growth rate, and fasting hypoglycemia. The progression can be very slow and may improve in adolescence; most survive into adulthood. As in McArdle's disease and PFK deficiency, many patients with DD complain of exercise intolerance, but some do not.[137] The distal portions of the upper and lower limbs are more commonly affected than the proximal muscles, and myoglobinuria and cramps are much less frequent. A more generalized weakness can include the respiratory muscles and can manifest as respiratory failure.[137,138] Other clinical manifestations usually include hepatomegaly, hypoglycemia, hyperlipidemia, growth retardation, and cardiomyopathy.[139]

Diagnosis

The serum CK usually is elevated in patients with DD. EMG reveals myopathic features with fibrillations and positive sharp wave and complex repetitive discharges; fasciculations are rare.[14] Nerve conduction velocities usually are normal. Cardiac testing may show left ventricular or biventricular hypertrophy. Under normal circumstances, glucagon or epinephrine administered to a fasting patient would result in an increase in the blood glucose level; this does not occur in patients with DD. Muscle biopsy reveals glycogen-containing vacuoles in the subsarcolemmal and intermyofibrillar areas. The skin, liver, myocardium, and intramuscular nerves may also show glycogen deposits.[123] No rise in lactate is seen with the forearm ischemic test.

Treatment

A high protein diet during the day, with a high protein snack at night, has been reported to be beneficial.[137,140,141] The recommended distribution on nutrients is 45% carbohydrates, 25% protein, and 30% fat.[140] In severe cases, liver transplantation may be necessary. Cardiac status should be monitored regularly. Rehabilitation involvement is as in McArdle's disease.

Acid Maltase Deficiency

Acid maltase deficiency (AMD) (also known as *glycogenosis type II* or *Pompe's disease [infantile variant]*) is a genetic disorder with an autosomal recessive mode of inheritance mapped to chromosome 17q21-23. It results from a deficiency of the enzyme acid maltase, which is required to release glucose from maltose (a disaccharide), oligosaccharides, and glycogen. The acid maltase deficiency results in a buildup of glycogen in cardiac and skeletal muscle and the liver. Infantile, childhood, and adult forms have been described.

The infantile form is characterized by hypotonia, cardiomyopathy, and rapidly progressive skeletal muscle weakness that starts within months of birth.[142] This is further complicated by feeding and respiratory problems. Death usually occurs within 2 years as a result of cardiac or pulmonary failure. The heart, liver, and tongue often are enlarged because of glycogen deposits.

The childhood onset variant is characterized by slowly progressive muscle weakness and delayed motor milestones. The weakness occurs mostly in the proximal muscles and respiratory muscles; cardiac muscle usually is spared. Death from respiratory failure usually occurs in the 2nd decade.

The adult variant is characterized by the onset of myopathy after age 20. It is slowly progressive and mostly affects the proximal limb and trunk musculature. Respiratory failure may be the presentation in approximately one third of cases.[142,143] Obstructive sleep apnea also has been reported in association with macroglossia and tongue weakness.[144] Liver and cardiac enlargement usually is absent in the adult variant.

Diagnosis

AMD can be assayed in muscle fibers, leukocytes, fibroblasts, and urine.[142] Serum CK, AST, and LDH usually are elevated in all variants, and infants show the highest levels of CK and AST. CK usually is less than 10 times the upper limit of normal. On electrodiagnostic testing, all three forms reveal normal motor and sensory nerve conduction; EMG reveals a myopathic pattern, including myotonic discharges without clinical myotonia.[14] Muscle biopsy reveals a vacuolar myopathy in all variants.[142] Cardiac workup may reveal left ventricular hypertrophy and electrocardiographic abnormalities such as left axis deviation, short PR interval, inverted T waves and large amplitude QRS complexes.[145] Pulmonary function testing usually reveals a restrictive pattern as a result of diaphragmatic muscle weakness. No rise in lactate is seen with the forearm ischemic test.

Treatment

Phase II clinical trials are beginning to show promising results with recombinant acid α-glucosidase (rhGAA) in patients with the infantile variant.[146] Earlier studies using mouse models demonstrated up to a 75% clearance of glycogen with rhGAA therapy.[147] In one report, reversible nephrotic syndrome resulted from treatment with rhGAA.[148] Gene therapy trials are underway using mouse models.[149-152] Respiratory failure can be addressed with bilevel positive airway pressure ventilation.[153] A high protein diet has not been consistently shown to be beneficial.[142] Rehabilitation involvement is as in McArdle's disease.

Endocrine Myopathies

Endocrine disorders frequently manifest with muscular impairment. The features of endocrine myopathies most amenable to rehabilitation intervention include muscle weakness and atrophy. Exercises, orthotics, or assistive devices may be necessary, depending on the severity of the deficits.

The following sections discuss corticosteroid myopathy and the myopathies associated with parathyroid and thyroid abnormalities.

Corticosteroid Myopathy

Corticosteroid myopathy (CSM) is the most common endocrine myopathy. It may result from excessive endogenous (Cushing's syndrome) or exogenous steroids. Exogenous sources are more common; the incidence is approximately 2.4% to 21% of patients treated with chronic steroids. Women may be as much as twice as vulnerable as men, and fluorinated corticosteroids (e.g., dexamethasone, beclomethasone, and triamcinolone) are more commonly implicated than nonfluorinated corticosteroids.[154] The severity of CSM may also depend on the treatment duration, dosage,[155] and treatment regimen. Repetitive burst treatments are thought to be worse than continuous treatment, even with the same dose.[156] Short-term treatment with massive doses, such as in the intravenous (IV) treatment of status asthmaticus or severe chronic obstructive pulmonary disease, may result in CSM.[155-157] Adrenal gland dysfunction, such as in Cushing's disease (cortisol excess) and ectopic adrenocorticotrophic hormone (ACTH) production, contributes to endogenous steroid excess.

Clinical Presentation

Patients with CSM usually describe an insidious onset of proximal muscle weakness and atrophy, with greater involvement of the lower limbs than the upper limbs. Distal limb involvement may be seen later in the course of CSM. The weakness can develop over weeks to years. A more acute form of CSM shows a more rapid onset of weakness over several days with greater involvement of respiratory muscles.[155,157,158] This acute form has been called *acute quadriplegic myopathy, critical illness myopathy (CIM)*, and *myopathy associated with loss of thick filaments*. Other clinical findings in CSM include fragile, pigmented skin; moon facies; osteoporosis; and truncal adipose tissue. Sensation and deep tendon reflexes usually are normal.

Diagnosis

Laboratory findings usually include normal CK, LDH, AST, and aldolase levels, except in the acute form of CSM, in which CK may be markedly elevated. Muscle biopsy usually shows preferential atrophy of type II fast twitch glycolytic fibers except in CIM, in which there is a more generalized muscle atrophy involving type I and type II fibers. Motor and sensory nerve conduction studies are expected to be normal, because the peripheral nerves are not affected. Needle EMG usually reveals normal insertional activity and low amplitude, short duration motor unit potentials, especially later in the course.[117] Diagnostic criteria have been described for CIM (Table 30-12).

Treatment

Treatment options for CSM include stopping the steroid, switching to alternate-day dosing, reducing the dose, or switching from a fluorinated steroid to an equivalent dose of a nonfluorinated steroid.[154] Endogenous steroid excess is best treated with removal of any glucocorticoid-excreting tumors.[154] The patient may not experience full recovery for several months.

Physical therapy, including strength training exercises, is important for helping the patient overcome the weakness and prevent further muscle wasting that may result from inactivity. Increased activity has been found to partly prevent glucocorticoid-induced atrophy.[159,160]

Hyperthyroidism

Varying degrees of weakness may occur in as many as 82% of thyrotoxic patients, and females are affected more

Table 30-12
Diagnostic Criteria for Critical Illness Myopathy*

Major Diagnostic Features	Supportive Features
1. Sensory nerve action potential amplitudes over 80% of lower limit of normal in two or more nerves	1. Compound muscle action potential amplitudes less than 80% of the lower limit of normal in two or more nerves without conduction block
2. Needle electromyogram with short duration, low amplitude motor unit potentials with early or normal full recruitment, with or without fibrillation potentials	2. Elevated serum cardiac enzymes, assessed in the first week of illness
3. Absence of a decremental response on repetitive nerve stimulation	3. Demonstration of muscle inexcitability
4. Muscle histopathological findings of myopathy with myosin loss	

From Engel AG, Franzini-Armstrong C, editors: *Myology,* ed 3, vol 2, p 1719, New York, 2004, McGraw-Hill.
*Definitive diagnosis is made when all four major diagnostic features are present; probable diagnosis is based on three major features and at least one supportive feature; possible diagnosis is based on major features 1 and 3 or 2 and 3 and at least one supportive feature.

frequently. The weakness usually is present by the end of the 5th decade, and the incidence appears to correlate with the duration of hyperthyroidism.[154] The pathogenesis is thought to be related to enhanced muscle protein catabolism with increased muscle amino acid release in response to stimulation by the elevated thyroxine.[161]

Clinical Presentation

The weakness seen in hyperthyroidism is mostly proximal, resulting in difficulty rising from a sitting position or performing overhead activities. It can be associated with muscle atrophy and may be much more severe than the atrophy would suggest. The patient may complain of fatigue, myalgia, and exercise intolerance. Respiratory muscle involvement can result in respiratory insufficiency, requiring mechanical ventilation.[154] Bulbar involvement can result in dysphagia and dysphonia.[117] Tendon reflexes usually are normal or brisk. A prospective cohort study in adults newly diagnosed with thyroid disease revealed that neuromuscular complaints were present in 67% of patients with hyperthyroidism, and 62% showed clinical weakness in at least one muscle group.[162] This weakness evolved rapidly and at an early stage of the disease compared to hypothyroidism.

Diagnosis

Laboratory testing in primary hyperthyroidism reveals elevated T_3 and T_4 and a low thyroid-stimulating hormone (TSH). CK, LDH, and myoglobin levels usually are normal. A recent study suggested that serum and urine levels of carnitine may be significantly reduced in hyperthyroidism and that normalization occurs after resumption of a euthyroid state.[163] EMG may reveal short duration motor unit potentials with increased polyphasic potentials. These EMG findings may be proportional to the severity of the atrophy and weakness but not to the amount of

thyrotoxicosis.[117] Motor and sensory nerve conduction studies are normal.[117] Abnormalities usually resolve with treatment of the hyperthyroidism and resumption of a euthyroid state.

Treatment

The myopathy usually improves with treatment of the underlying hyperthyroidism and return to a euthyroid state. It may take several months for strength to improve and even longer for normal muscle bulk to return. In the study mentioned previously, weakness resolved completely over an average of 3.6 months.[162] Active exercises with physical and occupational therapists can delay or even prevent the development of disuse atrophy. In more severe cases, assistive devices may be required.

Hypothyroidism

The primary myopathic clinical features associated with hypothyroidism are proximal muscle weakness, stiffness, fatigue, and slowed movements. A delay in the relaxation of deep tendon reflexes may also be seen and less commonly, the patient may complain of muscle cramps.[154] Muscle hypertrophy may be observed. Hoffman's syndrome is the name given to the combination of muscle hypertrophy, slow movements, weakness, and cramps in adults. Kocher-Debre-Semelaignet syndrome is the name given to the same findings, minus myalgia, in children. Myoedema is present when a localized contracture occurs in response to tapping or pinching of the muscle; it can occur in as many as one third of patients with hypothyroidism but is not specific for this disorder.[154] A prospective cohort study in adults newly diagnosed with thyroid disease revealed that neuromuscular complaints were present in 79% of those with hypothyroidism; 38% had clinical weakness in one or more muscle groups on manual muscle testing, 42% had signs of sensorimotor axonal neuropathy, and 29% had carpal tunnel syndrome (CTS).[162]

The serum CK usually is elevated, up to 100 times normal, but does not correlate with weakness; it usually normalizes after treatment of symptomatic patients. With primary hypothyroidism, T_3 and T_4 are depressed, whereas TSH is elevated. A recent study suggested that serum and urine levels of carnitine may be lower than normal in hypothyroidism and that normalization occurs after resumption of a euthyroid state.[163] Needle EMG can reveal PSWs and fibrillation potentials in a few cases; motor and sensory nerve conduction studies usually are normal unless the patient also has an entrapment neuropathy, such a CTS.[117] Complex repetitive discharges (CRDs) are uncommon. Myoedema usually is electrically silent. As in hyperthyroidism, treatment of the underlying thyroid dysfunction significantly improves the clinical findings, and active exercise prevents further weakness from disuse.

Hyperparathyroidism

Parathyroid hormone (PTH) is important for calcium and phosphorus homeostasis. In primary hyperparathyroidism, PTH may be elevated as a result of an adenoma or hyperplasia.[164] Renal disease usually contributes to secondary hyperparathyroidism. The effects of hyperparathyroidism or hypoparathyroidism on bone are well understood; the mechanism of weakness is not as well understood. One possible explanation cites an increase in protein degradation mediated by the increased calcium in hyperparathyroidism.[154]

Clinical Presentation

Patients with symptomatic hyperparathyroidism may present with proximal (greater than distal) symmetrical weakness and muscle stiffness. The lower limbs usually are more severely affected. The degree of weakness does not correlate well with the calcium or phosphate levels.[154] The patient may also have muscle atrophy and myalgia. Deep tendon reflexes may be hyperactive, and the patient may have a positive Babinski's sign. The patient may also complain of fatigue, polydipsia, dry skin, pruritus, memory loss, and anxiety.[165] Bulbar involvement may result in dysphagia and hoarseness.[166,167]

Diagnosis

In primary hyperparathyroidism, the serum CK and aldolase usually are normal; serum phosphate is low; and PTH, serum alkaline phosphatase, and calcium are elevated.[154] In secondary hyperparathyroidism caused by renal disease, serum calcium and active vitamin D levels are low. Motor and sensory nerve conduction studies are expected to be normal in primary hyperparathyroidism, whereas in secondary hyperparathyroidism, peripheral neuropathy associated with renal failure can result in decreased conduction velocities.[117] Needle EMG may show short duration, polyphasic

motor unit action potential (MUAP), especially in severe disease. Muscle biopsy may show selective atrophy of type II fibers.

Treatment

Patients with primary hyperparathyroidism usually respond well to parathyroidectomy.[154,165] In a prospective cohort study of 23 consecutive patients presenting for parathyroidectomy for the treatment of primary hyperparathyroidism, all 23 were noted to achieve normocalcemia, as well as a significant decline in disease-specific complaints, including muscle weakness.[165] In another series of 866 patients undergoing parathyroidectomy, 98.2% achieved normocalcemia.[164] Patients with secondary hyperparathyroidism require vitamin D and calcium supplementation or renal transplantation.

Hypoparathyroidism

Tetany resulting from hypocalcemia is the most common muscle disorder associated with hypoparathyroidism.[154] The patient may complain of perioral and distal numbness and paresthesias. Chvostek's sign is present when tapping the facial nerve at the external auditory meatus produces contractions in the ipsilateral facial muscles. Trousseau's sign (thumb adduction, metacarpophalangeal joint flexion, and interphalangeal joint extension) is also associated with the hypocalcemia. Overall, myopathy is unusual in hypoparathyroidism.

Laboratory tests may reveal a normal or slightly elevated serum CK, low PTH, low calcium, and high phosphate. Motor and sensory nerve conduction studies are normal, and the most significant findings on needle EMG are the spontaneous MUAPs that fire in rapid succession, producing the so-called doublets and triplets.[117]

Treatment includes correcting the hypocalcemia and hyperphosphatemia with vitamin D and calcium. Severe tetany may require IV administration of calcium. Long-term treatment of hypocalcemia requires daily doses of 2-5 g of elemental calcium daily plus 50,000-100,000 IU vitamin D.[154]

Toxic Myopathies

Table 30-13 summarizes some of the more common toxins that cause myopathy. Alcoholic myopathy is discussed in more detail.

Alcoholic Myopathy

Alcohol is one of the most common toxins that can cause myopathy. In addition to causing muscle weakness through peripheral neuropathy, alcohol can directly damage muscle. The recognized forms of alcoholic myopathy are acute necrotizing myopathy, hypokalemic myopathy, chronic alcoholic myopathy, and cardiomyopathy.

Table 30-13
Toxic Myopathies Secondary to Medications or Toxins

Myopathy	Medication/Toxin	Clinical Features	Laboratory Findings
Necrotizing	Statins, clofibrate, gemfibrozil Alcohol abuse	Painful proximal myopathy	Increased creatine kinase Possible myoglobinuria
Hypokalemic	Diuretics Laxatives Alcohol abuse Amphotericin B	Periodic weakness Absent/depressed reflexes	Increased creatine kinase Possible myoglobinuria Hypokalemia
Inflammatory	D-penicillamine Interferon-α Procainamide	Proximal muscle pain and weakness	Increased creatine kinase Possible myoglobinuria
Mitochondrial	Zidovudine	Proximal muscle pain and weakness	Normal or increased creatine kinase
Focal	Heroin Diazepam Lidocaine	Local pain, swelling Contracture of affected muscle	Normal or increased creatine kinase
Antimicrotubular	Colchicine Vincristine	Proximal muscle weakness Mild peripheral neuropathy	Increased creatine kinase

Acute necrotizing myopathy usually occurs in chronic alcoholics or after particularly heavy bouts of drinking. The patient can present with a weak, swollen, painful, tender limb, which frequently is mistaken for thrombophlebitis.[2] In most cases cessation of alcohol intake results in a full recovery within 2 weeks; severe cases may result in myoglobinuria and acute renal failure.[168] Acute hypokalemic myopathy manifests as isolated acute muscle weakness that evolves over days and is reversible with potassium repletion.[2,169] Chronic alcoholic myopathy may occur in up to two thirds of chronic alcoholics and typically evolves over weeks to months to affect the shoulders and hips equally.[168] CK may be elevated in only 10% to 50% of patients.[170] Treatment must include alcohol cessation, and even then residual weakness may be present. In severe cases the patient may require strengthening exercises, orthotics, or assistive devices.

Summary

Myopathies constitute a broad range of disorders with a heterogeneous range of etiologies and features. These muscle disorders can be hereditary or acquired. Myopathies can be categorized as muscular dystrophies or as congenital, inflammatory, metabolic, endocrine, or toxic myopathies. A common presenting feature is proximal (greater than distal) weakness. The rate of progression of the weakness, associated findings involving other organ systems, genetic testing where available, laboratory abnormalities, electrodiagnostic findings, and muscle biopsy features contribute to identification of a particular disorder. In many cases treatment does not cure the disorder, but rather provides support for the myriad of resulting physiological and functional deficits. Surgical intervention may be necessary in some cases to correct structural deficits to improve function. Rehabilitation, with its multidisciplinary approach, is vital for providing the bridge between disease-related dysfunction and an existence that includes functioning with a reasonable quality of life.

References

To enhance this text and add value for the reader, all references have been incorporated into a CD-ROM that is provided with this text. The reader can view the reference source and access it online whenever possible. There are a total of 170 references for this chapter.

CHAPTER 31

FIBROMYALGIA AND RELATED DISORDERS

Joanne Borg-Stein

Introduction

Clinicians all too often encounter patients with multiple complaints of widespread, somewhat diffuse pain and stiffness. Correctly or incorrectly, these patients often are given a diagnosis of fibromyalgia, myofascial pain syndrome, or some other label. The purpose of this chapter is to delineate what constitutes these conditions and how they are most appropriately managed.

Fibromyalgia syndrome (FMS) is a disorder of chronic, widespread pain of at least 6 months' duration marked by widespread musculoskeletal aching and accompanied by multiple, widespread tender points. Most patients (80%) are women.[1] In 1990 the American College of Rheumatology identified three distinct criteria that must be met before a patient can be diagnosed with fibromyalgia.

Fibromyalgia Criteria[1]

- Pain in the axial skeleton
- Pain above and below the waist
- Pain on palpation in at least 11 of 18 paired tender points throughout the body

Myofascial pain syndrome (MPS) is a condition in which pain originates from myofascial trigger points in skeletal muscle, either alone or in combination with other pain generators. Myofascial trigger points are discrete areas of focal tenderness in a muscle that are characterized by hypersensitive, palpable, taut bands of muscle that are painful to palpation. Manual pressure over these points reproduces the patient's pain and refers pain in a variety of characteristic patterns. Some clinicians prefer the designation *regional soft tissue pain* as a clinically useful term that encompasses pain and localized tenderness not only in muscle but also in other contiguous soft tissues, such as ligaments and tendons.[2]

Epidemiology

Fibromyalgia is present in 6 to 10 million Americans.[3] Of the general population, 10% report such complaints, which clearly indicates that chronic, widespread musculoskeletal pain is a major health problem in the Western world. The prevalence of fibromyalgia is reportedly 3% to 5%, with a significant female predominance.[4] Recent evidence suggests that fibromyalgia and related syndromes may share inheritable pathophysiological features, such as serotonin- and dopamine-related genes.[5]

Myofascial pain has a high prevalence among individuals with regional pain complaints. The prevalence varies, from 21% of patients seen in a general orthopedic clinic, to 30% of patients with regional pain in a general medical clinic, to as high as 85% to 90% of patients presenting to specialty pain management centers. Women and men are affected equally.[6-8]

Clinical Presentation

The symptoms of fibromyalgia consist of musculoskeletal pain and stiffness in a widespread distribution, usually involving the neck, shoulder, and pelvic girdle and all the extremities. Patients may present with pain predominantly in one or two regions (the low back and neck are the most common areas), but direct questioning often reveals pain in many other areas. Other common symptoms are general fatigue, poor sleep, and morning fatigue. Paresthesia is present in about 50% of cases, usually in the extremities, and may mimic nerve root compression. Associated conditions such as migraine, irritable bowel syndrome, and restless leg syndrome are common.[9]

The physical examination of a patient with fibromyalgia reveals pain on palpation over 11 of 18 characteristic tender points (Figure 31-1). The pressure applied should just blanch the fingernail bed of the examiner. Examination findings for the joints and nervous system are normal,

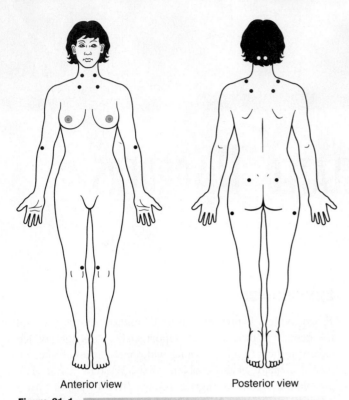

Anterior view   Posterior view

Figure 31-1
Fibromyalgia trigger points.

despite the reported symptoms of a swollen feeling in the joints and numbness. Range of motion of the cervical and lumbar spines may be slightly restricted because of pain. Diffuse soft tissue tenderness may be seen on palpation of the cervical, thoracic, and lumbar areas of the spine, including ligaments and paraspinal muscles.[10]

The characteristic symptoms of myofascial pain may begin after a discrete trauma or injury or may have an insidious onset. Patients note localized or regional deep aching sensations, which can vary from mild to severe.[11] The **myofascial trigger points (MTrPs)** of each muscle have their own characteristic pain pattern; therefore the distribution of pain can help identify which muscles may have the responsible MTrP.[12] Frequently, associated autonomic dysfunction may occur, including abnormal sweating, lacrimation, dermal flushing, and vasomotor and temperature changes.[13] Cervical myofascial pain may be associated with neuro-otological symptoms, including imbalance, dizziness, and tinnitus.[14] Functional complaints include decreased work tolerance, impaired muscle coordination, stiff joints, fatigue, and weakness. Other associated neurological symptoms include paresthesias, numbness, blurred vision, twitches, and trembling. Later stages can be compounded by sleep disturbance, mood changes, and stress.[15-17]

The physical examination of a patient with myofascial pain begins with a careful medical, neurological, and musculoskeletal examination. Posture, biomechanics, and joint function should be analyzed to identify any underlying factors that may have contributed to the development of the local or regional pain. An active MTrP usually is associated with a painful, restricted range of motion. The trigger point should be identified by gentle palpation across the direction of the muscle fibers. The examiner should detect a ropelike nodularity to the taut band of muscle. Palpation of this area is exquisitely painful and reproduces the patient's local and referred pain pattern.[18]

Laboratory Tests

The results of routine laboratory tests, such as a complete blood count (CBC), erythrocyte sedimentation rate (ESR), and chemistry profile, are normal in FMS and MPS. Thyroid function test results are normal, but these tests may be helpful for excluding hypothyroidism or hyperthyroidism in patients with muscle pain. Diagnostic imaging examinations (radiographs, computed tomography [CT] scans, magnetic resonance imaging [MRI]) are normal; however, coincidental osteoarthrosis or discogenic changes are common findings. The treating clinician must determine the relevance of these findings to the patient based on the clinical scenario.[19]

Well-controlled studies in patients with fibromyalgia and chronic muscle pain demonstrate normal muscle biopsy, electromyography (EMG), and nerve conduction studies.[20] Sleep electroencephalogram (EEG) studies may be requested to confirm clinical suspicion of sleep disorders, such as periodic limb movement disorder, rapid eye movement (REM) behavior disorder, and sleep apnea. Alpha intrusion into stage 4 delta wave is seen in about 40% of patients, but these studies should be ordered only if there is clinical suspicion of the previously mentioned sleep disorders.[21]

Differential Diagnosis

In clinical practice, the presentations of muscle pain disorders often overlap. The differences among myofascial pain, regional soft tissue pain, and widespread muscle pain often are indistinct. The differential diagnosis of muscle pain is broad. Specific critical questions may be useful for distinguishing the contributions of different factors and can help the clinician develop an appropriate and specific treatment plan.

Critical Questions for Development of a Treatment Plan for Myofascial Pain

- Is there regional myofascial pain with trigger points present?
- Is the myofascial pain the primary pain generator or are there other coexisting or underlying structural diagnoses?
- Is there a nutritional, metabolic, psychological, visceral, or inflammatory disorder that may contribute to or cause the myofascial pain or regional muscle pain?
- Is there widespread pain and other associated symptoms?

Differential Diagnosis Should Include but Should Not Be Limited to Elimination of the Following Conditions:

- Joint disorders: zygapophyseal joint disorder, osteoarthritis, loss of normal joint motion
- Inflammatory disorders: polymyositis, polymyalgia rheumatica, rheumatoid arthritis
- Neurological disorders: radiculopathy, entrapment neuropathy, metabolic myopathy
- Regional soft tissue disorders: bursitis, epicondylitis, tendonitis, cumulative trauma
- Discogenic disorders: degenerative disc disease, annular tears, protrusion, herniation
- Visceral referred pain: gastrointestinal, cardiac, pulmonary, renal
- Mechanical stresses: postural dysfunction, scoliosis, leg length discrepancy
- Nutritional, metabolic, and endocrine conditions: deficiency in vitamins B_1, B_{12}, and/or folic acid; alcoholic and toxic myopathy; iron, calcium, or magnesium deficiency; hypothyroidism
- Psychological disorders: depression, anxiety, disordered sleep
- Infectious diseases: viral illness, chronic hepatitis, bacterial or viral myositis
- Fibromyalgia or widespread chronic pain[2]

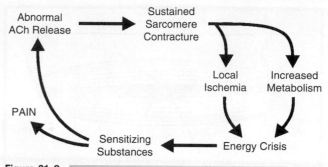

Figure 31-2

Simon's positive feedback loop. (Modified from Simons DG, Travell JG, Simons LS: *Myofascial pain and dysfunction: the trigger point manual, vol 1, Upper Half of Body,* ed 2, p 71, Baltimore, 1999, Williams & Wilkins.)

Pathophysiology of Fibromyalgia and Myofascial Pain Syndrome

Chronic muscle pain, regional myofascial pain, and fibromyalgia can be considered a spectrum of clinical disorders. They share pathophysiological mechanisms and often coexist in a patient. Although the following discussion is organized by neuroanatomical location, these processes are interrelated and should be considered in an integrated fashion.

Motor End Plate

An important finding in the pathophysiology of myofascial pain is a pathological increase in the release of acetylcholine (Ach) by the nerve terminal of an abnormal motor end plate under resting conditions, an event supported by electrodiagnostic evidence.[22,23] This abnormality is considered the primary dysfunction in the integrated hypothesis proposed by Simons et al.[12] and Mense et al.,[18] which postulates a positive feedback loop (Figure 31-2).

The concept of the abnormal motor end plate has been supported by electrodiagnostic studies, which have demonstrated end plate noise (EPN) significantly more frequently in MTrPs than in the same end plate zone outside the MTrP.[23,24] Because EPN is characteristic, but not diagnostic, of MTrPs, the significance of these findings is still a matter of debate. Increased EPN has been seen in response to many types of mechanical and chemical stimulation of

the end plate structure and does not appear to be specific to myofascial pain.[25,26]

Muscle Fiber

Some researchers hypothesize that increased release of acetylcholine may result in sustained depolarization of the postjunctional membrane of the muscle fiber and produce sustained sarcomere shortening and contracture. Simons referred to this maximally contracted sarcomere in the region of the motor end plate as a *contraction knot* (Figure 31-3).[12] Compelling histological support for this phenomenon is found in canine models of MTrPs: longitudinal sections of dog trigger points demonstrate this sarcomere shortening, and cross sections of dog and human MTrPs strongly suggest it as well.[27,28]

One consequence of chronically sustained sarcomere shortening may be greatly increased local energy consumption and reduction of local circulation, a combination that produces local ischemia and hypoxia. The sustained tension of muscle fibers in the taut band produces an enthesopathy at the myotendinous junction that can be identified as an attachment MTrP. Muscle stretching techniques are effective because they equalize sarcomere length throughout the affected muscle fibers and break the feedback cycle.

The localized muscle ischemias stimulate the release of neurovasoreactive substances such as prostaglandins, bradykinin, serotonin, and histamine, which sensitize afferent nerve fibers in muscle. These sensitized fibers may account for local muscle tenderness.[18]

Central Mechanisms: Spinal and Supraspinal

The referred pain that results from trigger points arises from central convergence and facilitation. Experimental data have shown that under pathological conditions, convergent connections from deep afferent nociceptors to dorsal horn neurons are facilitated and amplified in the spinal cord.[18,29] Referral to adjacent myotomes occurs as a result of the spread

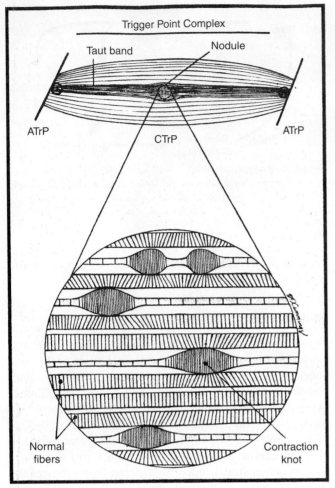

Figure 31-3

Simon's contraction knot. (Modified from Simons DG, Travell JG, Simons LS: *Myofascial pain and dysfunction: the trigger point manual, vol 1, Upper Half of Body*, ed 2, p 70, Baltimore, 1999, Williams & Wilkins.)

of central sensitization to adjacent spinal segments.[30,31] This pattern results in both referred pain and expansion of the region of pain beyond the initial nociceptive region.

At the level of the central nervous system (CNS), spinal neuroplastic changes occur in the second order neuron pool of the dorsal horn as a result of persistent pain. These changes produce a long-lasting increase in the excitability of nociceptor pathways. Central sensitization results, characterized by increased excitability of the neurons and expansion of the receptive pool of neurons. Neurotransmitters involved in the process of central sensitization include substance P, N-methyl-D-aspartate, glutamate, and nitric oxide.[22] In addition, impairments may occur in supraspinal inhibitory descending pain control pathways that release inhibitory neurotransmitters such as γ-aminobutyric acid (GABA), serotonin, and norepinephrine.[32] A recent study of opioid peptide levels in the cerebrospinal fluid (CSF) of patients with fibromyalgia demonstrated that opioid dysfunction may contribute to pain in fibromyalgia.[33]

In FMS, significant peripheral pathology is absent, and recent studies suggested central sensitization as the most important CNS aberration. Controlled studies have shown an increase in CSF substance P (which mediates pain transmission) and a decrease in serum serotonin (which mediates pain inhibition) and CSF 5HIAA (a metabolite of serotonin). These findings may explain amplified pain and a decreased pain threshold in FMS.[34,35] Sleep abnormality has been objectively documented by EEG studies. Disturbed stage 4 sleep may explain the reported decrease in serum insulin-like growth factor-1 (IGF-1), which reflects the integrated secretion of growth hormone.[36,37]

FMS is not a psychiatric condition; however, a psychological disturbance (e.g., anxiety, mental stress, depression) is present in 30% to 40% of patients with fibromyalgia (generally similar to the proportion seen in rheumatoid arthritis). Psychological factors seem to aggravate, but not cause, the pain. No correlation exists between psychological status and symptoms of FMS other than pain (e.g., a swollen feeling, paresthesia, and number of tender points).[38]

Most recent functional magnetic resonance imaging (fMRI) studies of the brain demonstrate that fibromyalgia is characterized by cortical or subcortical augmentation of pain processing. These studies provide further evidence of a physiological explanation for fibromyalgia pain.[39,40]

Treatment of Fibromyalgia and Myofascial Pain Syndrome

The following discussion refers to the management of muscle pain syndromes, including FMS and MPS. Much of the research has been done on one or both of these overlapping patient populations. Where clinically relevant, techniques specific to either MPS or FMS are noted.

Diagnosis and Education

The treatment of a patient with chronic muscle pain should proceed as follows:

1. Make a firm diagnosis of FMS or MPS based on its own characteristics; avoid unnecessary investigations but eliminate as much as possible the conditions listed previously as differential diagnoses.
2. Educate the patient about FMS and MPS. Explain the role of the CNS in chronic pain and reassure the patient that the muscles work normally. Provide an overview of treatment strategies and encourage the patient to read information from the Arthritis Foundation.
3. Reassure the patient that the muscle pain does not cause tissue damage.
4. Demonstrate an attitude of understanding and empathy; this is crucial for success in management. Never imply that symptoms are "all in your head."

5. Explain the probable mechanisms of pain to the patient in simple language (neuroendocrine dysfunction causes a chemical imbalance). Explain how a serotonin deficiency causes pain. If significant psychological factors are present, explain how they act as aggravating factors.

6. Recognize and address significant psychological factors such as depression, anxiety, mental stress (at home or work), and poor coping skills. The physician can use a written questionnaire or interview skills to help identify psychological factors. A minority of patients require referral to a psychiatrist for management of more severe psychiatric disease and psychopharmacological consultation and management.

7. Inquire about all aggravating factors that vary from patient to patient and provide individualized management. Some of these aggravating factors may include poor nutrition, poor ergonomics at home or work, and poor postural habits.

8. Help patients achieve restful sleep.

9. Encourage cardiovascular fitness by encouraging the patient to be more active (e.g., taking walks, swimming, jogging).

10. When appropriate, recommend physical therapy for management of regional musculoskeletal disorders. This may include manual therapy to promote optimum joint alignment and muscle flexibility and education in a proper exercise program.

11. Promote behavioral modification through education, including cognitive behavioral concepts.[9]

Pharmacological Management

Because of the considerable clinical overlap among myofascial pain, fibromyalgia, regional soft tissue pain, and tension headache, agents that are beneficial in one syndrome may be useful in another. In the absence of controlled data specifically examining drug efficacy in each disorder, clinicians often generalize from these associated disorders.

Nonsteroidal Anti-inflammatory Drugs

Minimal literature is available that evaluates the use of nonsteroidal anti-inflammatory drugs (NSAIDs) for chronic muscle pain. Several studies have found that NSAIDs have a small benefit in the management of pain in fibromyalgia if they are used in combination with alprazolam, amitriptyline, or cyclobenzaprine.[41-43] Interestingly, NSAIDs continue to be popular among patients; a recent study by Wolfe et al.[44] found that patients with fibromyalgia considered NSAIDs more effective than acetaminophen for pain management.

Tramadol

Tramadol is a combination of a weak opioid agonist and an inhibitor of the reuptake of serotonin and norepinephrine in the dorsal horn. No published, controlled trials are available on the use of tramadol for the treatment of myofascial pain; however, several studies support its efficacy in fibromyalgia, chronic low back pain, and osteoarthritis, all of which are commonly seen in association.[45-49]

Antidepressants

Tricyclic antidepressants (e.g., amitriptyline) have been shown to be effective for chronic tension-type headache, fibromyalgia, and intractable pain syndromes associated with muscle spasm.[50-53] Selective serotonin reuptake inhibitors (SSRIs) have not been specifically studied for myofascial pain, although their efficacy has been documented in fibromyalgia for improving pain, sleep, and a global sense of well-being.[49,54] More recent studies supported the use of dual reuptake inhibitors, (serotonin and norepinephrine) for the treatment of fibromyalgia. Evidence supports the use of venlafaxine, milnacipram, and duloxetine.[55-57]

α_2-Adrenergic Agonists

The two major α_2-adrenergic agonists available for clinical use are clonidine and tizanidine. Tizanidine acts centrally at the level of the spinal cord to inhibit spinal polysynaptic pathways and to reduce the release of aspartate, glutamate, and substance P.[58,59]

Anticonvulsants

To date, there has been one controlled trial of pregabalin in the treatment of fibromyalgia. The drug demonstrated reduction of pain, disturbed sleep, and fatigue compared with placebo.[60] An open label study of gabapentin in the treatment of chronic daily headache found possible efficacy.[61]

Botulinum Toxin

Botulinum toxin type A (Botox) appears to be emerging as a promising but expensive agent with efficacy in chronic myofascial pain syndromes and chronic daily headache.[62-64] Cheshire et al.[65] conducted a small, randomized, double blind, placebo-controlled trial of botulinum toxin type A and demonstrated a reduction of at least 30% in visual analogue pain scales, verbal pain descriptors, palpable muscle firmness, and pressure pain thresholds in the botulinum toxin group compared with a placebo (saline) group. Fishman et al.[66,67] demonstrated improvement in patients with piriformis syndrome with injection of botulinum toxins (type A and type B). Porta[68] compared botulinum toxin type A with steroid injection for the treatment of chronic myofascial pain and found greater improvement at 30 and 60 days after treatment in the group treated with botulinum toxin. By comparison, Wheeler et al.[69] were unable to demonstrate a statistically significant difference between botulinum toxin and placebo for the treatment of refractory unilateral cervicothoracic myofascial pain.

Both peripheral and central mechanisms may explain the apparent efficacy of botulinum toxin in the treatment of chronic muscle pain. First, blockade of Ach release at the neuromuscular junction reduces muscle hyperactivity, which in turn may reduce local ischemia. Second, if, as theorized, trigger points are sustained by excessive release of Ach and sarcomere shortening, botulinum toxin may disrupt the abnormal neurophysiology of the trigger point. Evidence also has been found of retrograde uptake of botulinum toxin into the spinal cord and nucleus raphe, structures that modulate expression of neurotransmitters important in pain perception (e.g., substance P, enkephalins).[70] In addition, botulinum toxin type A inhibits neurotransmitter release from primary sensory neurons in the rat formalin model. Through this mechanism, Botox inhibits peripheral sensitization in these models, which leads to an indirect reduction in central sensitization.[71]

Nonpharmacological Treatment of Muscle Pain

Postural, Mechanical, and Ergonomic Modifications

Although standard clinical practice and conventional wisdom include efforts to correct postural and ergonomic abnormalities, little direct data are available that support this approach in treating muscle pain. A study by Komiyama et al.[72] combined postural training and behavioral therapy in the treatment of myofascial oral pain and found that the subjects receiving the combination therapy were able to regain free, unassisted mouth opening earlier than those treated with behavioral therapy alone; however, the differences in outcome were clinically minor.

The occupational medicine literature provides evidence that injuries are more common when workers are subjected to greater loads and have undesirable postures during work.[73] Occupational muscle pain syndromes are theorized to occur as the result of repetitive microtrauma and myofascial shortening. Correction of awkward postures is a standard part of treatment of these disorders, although long-term efficacy studies are lacking.[74]

Stress Reduction

Stress reduction techniques, including cognitive-behavioral programs such as meditation, progressive relaxation training, and biofeedback, are often incorporated into chronic pain rehabilitation programs. However, few studies have specifically addressed the efficacy of these techniques for myofascial pain. Crockett et al.[75] compared a multifaceted relaxation program with (1) physical therapy, (2) dental splinting, or (3) transcutaneous electrical nerve stimulation (TENS) for management of chronic facial and masticatory myofascial pain. They found equivalent results and a good response among all the treatment groups. Interestingly, EMG biofeedback, as well as meditation-based stress reduction programs, are established as beneficial in fibromyalgia.[76,77]

Acupuncture

A growing body of evidence supports the efficacy of acupuncture in myofascial pain and fibromyalgia. The limited amount of high quality data suggests that real acupuncture is better than sham for relieving pain, improving global ratings, and reducing morning stiffness in fibromyalgia.[78] An exception to this is a recent randomized clinical trial of acupuncture compared with sham acupuncture in fibromyalgia, which did not demonstrate any difference between the patients in the sham groups and those in the treatment group.[79] The 1997 National Institutes of Health consensus statement on acupuncture concluded that "acupuncture may be useful as an adjunct treatment or an acceptable alternative to be included in a comprehensive management program" in the treatment of fibromyalgia, myofascial pain, low back pain, osteoarthritis, and lateral epicondylitis.[80] Birch and Jamison[81] found relevant acupuncture (over points relevant to myofascial neck pain) to be superior to both NSAID treatment and irrelevant acupuncture (superficial needling not related to neck pain) in a group of 46 patients with chronic myofascial pain. Interestingly, a remarkably close relationship has been described between acupuncture points and trigger points.[82] Questions that need to be answered in future randomized, controlled trials include the true benefit of acupuncture in chronic muscle pain, the duration of the benefit of acupuncture, the optimum acupuncture techniques, and the value of booster treatments for the treatment of muscle pain.

Massage, Transcutaneous Electrical Nerve Stimulation, and Ultrasound

Studies suggesting efficacy of massage as part of the treatment of muscle pain are scant. In a study by Gam et al.,[83] massage combined with stretching exercises was better than the control group in reducing the number and intensity of myofascial trigger points. Only a mild reduction was seen in neck and shoulder pain. Hernandez-Reif et al.[84] found that massage therapy was effective in reducing pain, increasing serotonin and dopamine levels, and reducing symptoms associated with chronic low back pain. However, this study did not specify the etiology of the pain.

TENS therapy has shown mixed results in the treatment of myofascial pain. One single blind study compared TENS with sham TENS in 10 patients for treatment of myofascial pain and found no benefit for pain reduction; however, the study used subthreshold TENS parameters.[85] Graff-Radford et al.[87] compared four different TENS settings to no-stimulation control in a double blind study and found that high frequency, high intensity TENS reduced myofascial pain.

Ultrasound in combination with massage and exercise has been tested in one randomized, controlled trial.[83] In this study, ultrasound, massage, and exercise had no additional benefit over sham ultrasound with massage and acupuncture for the treatment of myofascial trigger points.

Exercise for Fibromyalgia and Myofascial Pain

Stretching exercises form the basis of treatment for myofascial pain. This treatment addresses the muscle tightness and shortening that are closely associated with pain in these disorders and permits gradual restoration of normal activity. Slow, sustained stretching throughout the available range of motion is the most effective approach. Once muscle pain has decreased and range of motion has been restored, exercise to improve muscle strength and endurance should be instituted to maximize functional outcome. Aerobic exercise should also be included as part of an overall musculoskeletal and cardiovascular fitness program to prevent recurrence.[87]

Importance of Exercise for Myofascial Pain

Exercise is one of the most important aspects of the rehabilitation and management of chronic muscle pain syndromes.[88] The benefits of exercise include:

- Optimization of joint and soft tissue flexibility
- Improved functional status
- Improved mood
- Improved self-efficacy
- Reduction of pain

Patients should be encouraged to remain active but to perform daily activities in a gentle, lightly loaded manner. When a movement leads to pain, the patient should stop the movement at the point of beginning pain and slowly, gently explore extending the movement just a little farther to help release the muscle tightness. Clinical experience suggests that leaving a muscle in the shortened position aggravates myofascial trigger points.[2]

Trigger Point Injection for Fibromyalgia and Myofascial Pain

In general, trigger points are the hallmark of myofascial pain syndrome. Patients with generalized muscle pain, such as FMS, frequently have trigger points and painful, shortened areas of muscle. These local areas can be treated with trigger point injections.

As mentioned, stretching exercises are the mainstay of myofascial pain management, and injection therapy should be reserved to supplement or augment these exercises.[87] When MTrP injection is used as the primary therapy, patients are at risk of becoming dependent on this treatment for pain relief. Educating patients about the effectiveness of manual stretching techniques and instructing them in these techniques empower patients to self-manage their symptoms effectively. As pain relief and function increase, the patient resumes normal activity, which further helps to inactivate MTrPs. Optimum results are obtained when injections are preceded and immediately followed by manual MTrP release techniques, with the patient learning how to follow a continuing home program.[89]

When injection proves necessary for initiating therapy or for dealing with a recalcitrant area of myofascial pain, a series of injections should be started and the patient should be informed that this treatment has a limited role in the long-term management of myofascial pain. Often three consecutive visits for injection are recommended for chronic myofascial pain; the patient is reassessed after the third visit to evaluate the efficacy of the injections and to determine whether further injections are necessary.

MTrP injections may involve the use of no medication (dry needling) or the use of short- or long-acting anesthetics, steroids, or botulinum toxin. A number of techniques may be used, such as slow search,[90] fast in–fast out, superficial dry needling, intramuscular stimulation, twitch-obtaining intramuscular stimulation, and needling and infiltration with preinjection blocks. Several theories have been proposed regarding the mechanism of action of injections for myofascial pain.

Dry needling of trigger points with acupuncture needles provides as much pain relief as injection of lidocaine but causes more postinjection soreness.[91] The effectiveness of dry needling depends on the needle eliciting local twitch responses.[91] Presumably, the needle mechanically disrupts and terminates the dysfunctional activity of involved motor end plates, with or without injection. Longer acting anesthetics are more myotoxic and do not show a proven increase in MTrP pain relief. The effectiveness of injection steroids in MTrPs is controversial and without a clear rationale because little evidence exists to support an inflammatory pathophysiology for MTrPs. Injection of botulinum toxin is emerging as a good option for treatment of chronic muscle pain.[92]

In a recent systematic review article on needling therapies for MTrPs, Cummings and White[93] concluded that based on current medical evidence, the "nature of the injected substance makes no difference to the outcome and that wet needling is not therapeutically superior to dry needling." This is clearly an area in which more research is needed.

Hong's fast in–fast out technique[91] elicits local twitch responses more quickly than other techniques and presumably reduces needle trauma to muscle fibers from the twitch movement. Baldry et al.[94] recommend superficial dry needling, which they speculate may inactivate MTrPs through stimulation of cutaneous A delta fibers. A study by Chu,[95] based on the work of Gunn,[96] reported a technique in which neurogenically evoked muscle twitches relieved myofascial-type pain. The needling and infiltration technique described by Fischer and Imamura,[97] who used a preinjection block, permits more thorough injection of the trigger point and taut band region with reportedly less patient discomfort.

All of these techniques rely on accurate identification of MTrPs by means of palpation. No definitive evidence indicates that one technique is superior to another in long-term outcome. As Cummings and White[93] remarked, "Because no technique is better than any other, we recommend that the method safest and most comfortable for the patient should be used." Very slim acupuncture needles may have the advantage of minimizing tissue trauma and allowing the practitioner to needle four to six trigger points at one session.

Functional Outcomes in Chronic Muscle Pain

Outcome studies of myofascial pain and its treatment are few. In one study of pain, disability, and psychological functioning in chronic low back pain subgroups, patients with low back pain of myofascial origin had outcomes similar to or slightly worse than those with disc herniation, as measured by several standardized questionnaires on pain and disability.[98] Patients with myofascial pain have less accurate beliefs about their pain symptoms, express more dissatisfaction with physician efforts to treat their pain, and report receiving little information from their physicians.[99] A 1998 study by Heikkila et al.[100] investigated the outcome from a multidisciplinary rehabilitation program for patients with whiplash and myofascial pain. After the rehabilitation period, 49% of patients had improved their coping skills for managing chronic pain, and this figure rose to 63% after 2 years. In addition, 46% of patients had increased their life satisfaction. The myofascial pain group also reduced their sick leave time.[100]

In a national six-center longitudinal study, Wolfe et al.[101] determined the intermediate and long-term outcomes of fibromyalgia in patients seen in rheumatology centers that have a special interest in the syndrome. Although functional disability worsened slightly and health satisfaction improved slightly, measures of pain, global severity, fatigue, sleep disturbance, anxiety, depression, and health status were markedly abnormal at the initiation of the study and were essentially unchanged over the study period.

Summary

Chronic muscle pain is a common clinical complaint among patients who seek care for musculoskeletal disorders. The clinical presentation covers a spectrum ranging from focal or regional complaints to more widespread pain. Nevertheless, treatment paradigms overlap and are guided by the following major principles:

1. Be a sympathetic provider.
2. Make an accurate diagnosis of myofascial pain or fibromyalgia.
3. Identify and treat any peripheral pain generators (e.g., tendonitis, bursitis, radiculopathy) to reduce the peripheral nociceptive input to the CNS.
4. Treat the CNS dysfunction with a balanced, modern pharmacological approach.
5. Treat the associated symptoms (e.g. sleep, mood, headache, bowel, fatigue) or refer the patient to the appropriate provider.
6. Engage all patients in a comprehensive exercise and functional rehabilitation program.
7. Judiciously offer injection techniques for local trigger points or other peripheral pain generators to reduce pain and facilitate rehabilitation.
8. Educate all patients about the diagnosis and encourage self-management.
9. Incorporate mind-body techniques (e.g., meditation, relaxation training) to manage chronic pain.

References

To enhance this text and add value for the reader, all references have been incorporated into a CD-ROM that is provided with this text. The reader can view the reference source and access it online whenever possible. There are a total of 101 references for this chapter.

Index

Note: Page numbers followed by 'f', 't', 'b' indicate figures, tables, boxes respectively.